Y0-BYK-917

HEALTH CARE STATE RANKINGS
1999

Health Care in the 50 United States

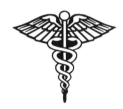

Kathleen O'Leary Morgan and Scott Morgan, Editors

Associate Editor: Kim Tiffany
Editorial Assistants: Pat Moffet and Emily Davis

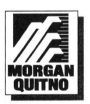

Morgan Quitno Press
© Copyright 1999, All Rights Reserved

512 East 9th Street, P.O. Box 1656
Lawrence, KS 66044-8656
USA
800-457-0742 or 785-841-3534
www.morganquitno.com
Seventh Edition

RA407.3
H423
1999

© Copyright 1999 by
Morgan Quitno Corporation
512 East 9th Street, P.O. Box 1656
Lawrence, Kansas   66044-8656

800-457-0742 or 785-841-3534
www.morganquitno.com

All Rights Reserved

No part of this book may be reproduced in any form, by photostat, microfilm, xerography, or any other means, or incorporated into any information retrieval system, electronic or mechanical, without the written permission of the copyright owner.   Copyright is not claimed in any material from U.S. Government sources. However, its arrangement and compilation along with all other material are subject to the copyright. If you are interested in reprinting our material, please call or write.   We would be happy to discuss it with you and are usually willing to allow reprinting with the following citation: "*Health Care State Rankings 1999*, Morgan Quitno Press, Lawrence, KS."

ISBN: 1-56692-333-6
ISSN: 1065-1403

Health Care State Rankings 1999 sells for $49.95 ($5.00 shipping) and is only available in paper binding. For those who prefer ranking information tailored to a particular state, we also offer *Health Care State Perspectives*, state-specific reports for each of the 50 states. These individual guides provide information on a state's data and rank for each of the categories featured in the national *Health Care State Rankings* volume. Perspectives sell for $19.00 or $9.50 if ordered with *Health Care State Rankings*. If crime statistics are your interest, please ask about our annual *Crime State Rankings* ($49.95 paper). If you are interested in city and metropolitan crime data, we offer *City Crime Rankings* ($37.95 paper). For a general view of the states, please ask about our annual *State Rankings* reference book ($49.95 paper). All of our data sets are also available in machine readable format. Shipping and handling is $5.00 per order.

Seventh Edition
Printed in the United States of America
April 1999

PREFACE

How many citizens in your state have no health insurance? How good is access to primary care physicians? Which states have the highest cancer death rates? You'll find the answers to these and hundreds of other health-related questions in *Health Care State Rankings 1999*. This seventh edition compares states in births and reproductive health, deaths, disease, insurance and finance, health care providers, facilities and physical fitness. In all, more than 500 tables of state comparisons give you all the information you need on virtually every aspect of health care in the 50 United States.

Important Notes About *Health Care State Rankings 1999*

Health Care State Rankings 1999 is the product of our year-long search for state health care data. We have contacted both government and private sector health care sources in an effort to bring you the best and most up-to-date collection of state health care information possible. Most tables were updated from last year, a few are new and a few others were deleted. However, in some cases updated information is not available and tables are repeated. Our regular readers will note that once again the finance chapter has a number of repeat tables. Unfortunately, the Health Care Financing Administration has not yet issued updates of its state estimates of health care expenditures (1993 are the latest). While we await the revised state numbers, we have included this year a table showing national health care expenditures for 1997 (see page 246).

Our annual review process may bring about a number of changes in our books, but there are many popular features that are retained. These include source information and other pertinent footnotes clearly shown at the bottom of each page and national totals, rates and percentages prominently displayed at the top of each table. In addition, every other line is shaded in gray for easier reading. We also provide numerous information finding tools: a thorough table of contents, table listings at the beginning of each chapter, a roster of sources with addresses and phone numbers, a detailed index and a chapter thumb index.

As in all of our reference books, the numbers shown in *Health Care State Rankings* require no additional calculations to convert them from millions, thousands, etc. All states are ranked on a high to low basis, with any ties among the states listed alphabetically for a given ranking. Negative numbers are shown in parentheses "( )." For tables with national totals (as opposed to rates, per capita's, etc.) a separate column is included showing what percent of the national total each individual state's total represents. This column is headed by "% of USA." This percentage figure is particularly interesting when compared with a state's share of the nation's population for a particular year (provided in an appendix).

If you need information for just one state, check out our *Health Care State Perspective* series of publications.

These 21-page comb bound reports feature data and ranking information for an individual state, as reported in *Health Care State Rankings 1999*. (For example *California Health Care in Perspective* features information about the state of California only.) They serve as handy, quick reference guides for those who do not want to page through the entire *Health Care State Rankings* volume searching for information for their particular state. When purchased by themselves, *Health Care State Perspectives* sell for $19. When purchased with a copy of *Health Care State Rankings*, these handy quick reference guides are just $9.50. For additional information, please call us toll-free at 1-800-457-0742.

Other Books From Morgan Quitno Press

In addition to *Health Care State Rankings*, our company offers three other rankings reference books. The first of these, *State Rankings*, provides a general view of the states. Statistics are featured in a wide variety of categories including agriculture, transportation, government finance, health, population, crime, education, social welfare, energy and environment. Our annual compilation of state crime data is featured in *Crime State Rankings*. This reference volume contains a huge collection of user friendly statistics on law enforcement personnel and expenditures, corrections, arrests and offenses. If city and metro area crime are your interest, *City Crime Rankings* compares crime in all metropolitan areas and cities of 75,000 or more population (approx. 300 cities). Numbers of crimes, crime rates, changes in crime rates over one and five years are presented for all major crime categories reported by the FBI. Final 1997 crime data are featured.

City Crime Rankings sells for $37.95. The *State Rankings* and *Crime State Rankings* books each are available for $49.95. (S/H $5 per order) All books are paperback. For true data aficionados, the information in our books also is available on diskette (PC format dbf, ASCII or Excel). This electronic format allows you to import our data into your computer program for tailor-made analysis.

New to the Morgan Quitno family of publications is *State Statistical Trends,* a monthly journal that examines changes in life and government for the 50 United States. Each 100-page monthly issue focuses on a different subject and provides a collection of tables, graphics and commentary showing state multi-year trends. For further information about *Trends* or any of our other publications, please call us toll-free at 1-800-457-0742.

Finally, thank you to the librarians, government and health care industry officials who help us each year with the development, design and production of this book. Your guidance is invaluable to this project. We also enjoy input from our readers, so please don't hesitate to keep those comments and suggestions coming our way.

THE EDITORS

WHICH STATE IS HEALTHIEST?

After years of second place finishes, Minnesota finally is in the spotlight as 1999's Healthiest State. Beating out Hawaii (the seemingly perennial winner) Minnesota shines as the state with the healthiest population and the best access to heath care providers. At the opposite end of the scale, Louisiana comes in as the least healthy state, bumping off Arkansas which had held the #50 spot for five years in a row.

Each year we take a step back from our objective reporting of health statistics, throw some basic figures into our computer and determine which is the Healthiest State. For this year, Minnesota comes out on top, followed by Hawaii, Vermont, New Hampshire and Nebraska. Joining Louisiana at the end of the scale were Mississippi, Alabama, Nevada and South Carolina.

A New Methodology

Twenty-one factors were chosen from our 1999 *Health Care State Rankings* book that reflect basic health care and access to health care (see box below.) Two factors, percent change in uninsured and hospitals per 1,000 square miles, were removed from this year's rankings. In addition, the cancer death rate factor was replaced with the age-adjusted death rate by malignant neoplasms. The 21 factors were divided into two groups: those that are "negative" where a high ranking would be considered bad for a state and those that are "positive" for which a high ranking would be considered good for a state. In previous years, rankings were determined based on a simple average of the state's rankings for these factors. This year, following the methodology used for our Dangerous State and Safest/Dangerous City Awards, a new approach was taken. Rates for each of the 21 factors were processed through a formula that measures how a state compares to the national average for a given category. The positive and negative nature of each factor was taken into account as part of the formula. Once these computations were made, the factors then were weighted (factors were weighted equally.) These weighted scores were then added together to get a state's final score ("SUM" on the table above.) This way, states are assessed based on how they stack up against the national average. The end result is that the farther below the national average a state's health ranking is, the lower (and less healthy) it ranks. The farther above the national average, the higher (and healthier) a state ranks.

The table above shows how each state fared in the 1999 Healthiest State Award as well as its placement in 1998. Caution is advised in comparing the two years' rankings because of the change in methodology. Congratulations to the very healthy citizens of Minnesota!   THE EDITORS

1999 HEALTHIEST STATE AWARD

RANK	STATE	SUM	'98	RANK	STATE	SUM	'98
1	Minnesota	18.49	2	26	Indiana	3.56	35
2	Hawaii	17.63	1	27	South Dakota	3.44	8
3	Vermont	16.76	4	28	Alaska	3.42	20
4	New Hampshire	15.96	3	29	Idaho	2.06	15
5	Nebraska	14.18	10	30	Illinois	1.44	26
6	Iowa	12.32	7	31	Oklahoma	1.13	38
7	Maine	11.77	14	32	North Carolina	(0.32)	27
8	Kansas	10.90	6	33	Michigan	(0.84)	31
8	Massachusetts	10.90	16	34	Georgia	(1.45)	21
10	Utah	10.72	5	35	Arizona	(1.78)	39
10	Washington	10.72	13	36	West Virginia	(1.94)	41
12	Montana	9.24	11	37	Kentucky	(2.71)	44
13	North Dakota	8.55	29	38	Missouri	(3.47)	48
14	Wyoming	7.57	18	39	Tennessee	(3.85)	47
15	Wisconsin	7.36	23	40	Delaware	(5.71)	32
16	Virginia	7.09	16	41	Texas	(7.33)	36
17	Oregon	6.64	24	42	Florida	(8.54)	42
18	Ohio	6.60	33	43	New York	(8.59)	28
19	California	6.44	12	44	New Mexico	(9.00)	34
20	Connecticut	6.38	9	45	Arkansas	(9.34)	50
21	Rhode Island	5.82	22	46	South Carolina	(10.96)	43
22	Pennsylvania	4.72	37	47	Nevada	(12.23)	39
23	New Jersey	4.39	25	48	Alabama	(12.57)	46
24	Colorado	4.10	30	49	Mississippi	(15.85)	45
25	Maryland	3.65	18	50	Louisiana	(17.92)	49

POSITIVE (+) AND NEGATIVE (-) FACTORS CONSIDERED:

1. Births of Low Birthweight as a Percent of All Births (Table 15) -
2. Births to Teenage Mothers as a Percent of Live Births (Table 30) -
3. Percent of Mothers Receiving Late or No Prenatal Care (Table 54) -
4. Age-Adjusted Death Rate (Table 78) -
5. Infant Mortality Rate (Table 85) -
6. Age-Adjusted Death Rate by Neoplasms (Table 153) -
7. Death Rate by Suicide (Table 176) -
8. Health Care Expenditures as a Percent of Gross State Product (Table 248) -
9. Per Capita Personal Health Expenditures (Table 249) -
10. Percent of Population Not Covered by Health Insurance (Table 294) -
11. Estimated Rate of New Cancer Cases (Table 355) -
12. AIDS Rate (Table 377) -
13. Sexually Transmitted Disease Rate (Table 410) -
14. Percent of Population Lacking Access to Primary Care (Table 439) -
15. Percent of Adults Who Are Binge Drinkers (Table 502) -
16. Percent of Adults Who Smoke (Table 503) -
17. Percent of Adults Overweight (Table 506) -
18. Number of Days in Past Month When Physical Health was "Not Good" (Table 507) -
19. Beds in Community Hospitals per 100,000 Population (Table 206) +
20. Percent of Children Aged 19-35 Months Fully Immunized (Table 408) +
21. Safety Belt Usage Rate (Table 511) +

TABLE OF CONTENTS

I. Births and Reproductive Health

TABLE OF CONTENTS (continued)

II. Deaths

TABLE OF CONTENTS (continued)

TABLE OF CONTENTS (continued)

III. Facilities

TABLE OF CONTENTS (continued)

TABLE OF CONTENTS (continued)

TABLE OF CONTENTS (continued)

V. Incidence of Disease

TABLE OF CONTENTS (continued)

VI. Providers

TABLE OF CONTENTS (continued)

VII. Physical Fitness

VIII. Appendix

IX. Sources

X. Index

I. BIRTHS AND REPRODUCTIVE HEALTH

1   Births in 1997
2   Birth Rate in 1997
3   Births in 1996
4   Birth Rate in 1996
5   Births in 1990
6   Birth Rate in 1990
7   Births in 1980
8   Birth Rate in 1980
9   Fertility Rate in 1997
10   Births to White Women in 1997
11   White Births as a Percent of All Births in 1997
12   Births to Black Women in 1997
13   Black Births as a Percent of All Births in 1997
14   Births of Low Birthweight in 1997
15   Births of Low Birthweight as a Percent of All Births in 1997
16   Births of Low Birthweight to White Women in 1997
17   Births of Low Birthweight to White Women as a Percent of All Births to White Women in 1997
18   Births of Low Birthweight to Black Women in 1997
19   Births of Low Birthweight to Black Women as a Percent of All Births to Black Women in 1997
20   Births to Unmarried Women in 1997
21   Births to Unmarried Women as a Percent of All Births in 1997
22   Births to Unmarried White Women in 1997
23   Births to Unmarried White Women as a Percent of All Births to White Women in 1997
24   Births to Unmarried Black Women in 1997
25   Births to Unmarried Black Women as a Percent of All Births to Black Women in 1997
26   Births to Teenage Mothers in 1997
27   Percent of Births to Teenage Mothers in 1997
28   Births to Teenage Mothers in 1996
29   Teenage Birth Rate in 1996
30   Births to Teenage Mothers as a Percent of Live Births in 1996
31   Births to White Teenage Mothers in 1996
32   Births to White Teenage Mothers as a Percent of White Births in 1996
33   Births to Black Teenage Mothers in 1996
34   Births to Black Teenage Mothers as a Percent of Black Births in 1996
35   Pregnancy Rate for 15 to 19 Year Old Women in 1995
36   Percent Change in Pregnancy Rate for 15 to 19 Year Old Women: 1992 to 1995
37   Births to Teenage Mothers in 1990
38   Teenage Birth Rate in 1990
39   Percent Change in Teenage Birth Rate: 1990 to 1996
40   Births to Teenage Mothers in 1980
41   Teenage Birth Rate in 1980
42   Births to Women 35 to 49 Years Old in 1996
43   Births to Women 35 to 49 Years Old as a Percent of All Births in 1996
44   Births by Vaginal Delivery in 1996
45   Percent of Births by Vaginal Delivery in 1996
46   Births by Cesarean Delivery in 1996
47   Percent of Births by Cesarean Delivery in 1996
48   Percent Change in Rate of Cesarean Births: 1989 to 1996
49   Births by Vaginal Delivery After a Previous Cesarean Delivery (VBAC) in 1996
50   Percent of Vaginal Births After a Cesarean (VBAC) in 1996
51   Percent of Mothers Beginning Prenatal Care in First Trimester in 1997
52   Percent of White Mothers Beginning Prenatal Care in First Trimester in 1997
53   Percent of Black Mothers Beginning Prenatal Care in First Trimester in 1997
54   Percent of Mothers Receiving Late or No Prenatal Care in 1996
55   Percent of White Mothers Receiving Late or No Prenatal Care in 1996
56   Percent of Black Mothers Receiving Late or No Prenatal Care in 1996
57   Percent of Births to Women Who Smoked During Pregnancy in 1996
58   Percent of Births Attended by Midwives in 1996

I. BIRTHS AND REPRODUCTIVE HEALTH
(CONTINUED)

Abortions

Births in 1997

National Total = 3,894,970 Live Births*

ALPHA ORDER

RANK	STATE	BIRTHS	% of USA
23	Alabama	61,038	1.6%
47	Alaska	9,705	0.2%
16	Arizona	75,753	1.9%
34	Arkansas	36,720	0.9%
1	California	526,033	13.5%
24	Colorado	56,539	1.5%
30	Connecticut	42,977	1.1%
45	Delaware	10,243	0.3%
4	Florida	192,556	4.9%
9	Georgia	118,347	3.0%
40	Hawaii	17,381	0.4%
39	Idaho	18,594	0.5%
5	Illinois	180,898	4.6%
13	Indiana	83,447	2.1%
33	Iowa	36,933	0.9%
32	Kansas	37,446	1.0%
25	Kentucky	53,228	1.4%
21	Louisiana	66,012	1.7%
42	Maine	13,670	0.4%
19	Maryland	70,267	1.8%
14	Massachusetts	82,448	2.1%
8	Michigan	133,621	3.4%
22	Minnesota	64,525	1.7%
31	Mississippi	42,747	1.1%
17	Missouri	74,747	1.9%
44	Montana	10,851	0.3%
37	Nebraska	23,327	0.6%
35	Nevada	27,039	0.7%
41	New Hampshire	14,433	0.4%
10	New Jersey	113,141	2.9%
36	New Mexico	26,874	0.7%
3	New York	263,339	6.8%
11	North Carolina	107,013	2.7%
48	North Dakota	8,356	0.2%
6	Ohio	152,265	3.9%
27	Oklahoma	48,110	1.2%
28	Oregon	43,895	1.1%
7	Pennsylvania	144,235	3.7%
43	Rhode Island	12,388	0.3%
26	South Carolina	51,904	1.3%
46	South Dakota	10,208	0.3%
18	Tennessee	74,577	1.9%
2	Texas	333,889	8.6%
29	Utah	43,885	1.1%
49	Vermont	6,667	0.2%
12	Virginia	91,990	2.4%
15	Washington	79,024	2.0%
38	West Virginia	20,752	0.5%
20	Wisconsin	66,602	1.7%
50	Wyoming	6,424	0.2%

RANK ORDER

RANK	STATE	BIRTHS	% of USA
1	California	526,033	13.5%
2	Texas	333,889	8.6%
3	New York	263,339	6.8%
4	Florida	192,556	4.9%
5	Illinois	180,898	4.6%
6	Ohio	152,265	3.9%
7	Pennsylvania	144,235	3.7%
8	Michigan	133,621	3.4%
9	Georgia	118,347	3.0%
10	New Jersey	113,141	2.9%
11	North Carolina	107,013	2.7%
12	Virginia	91,990	2.4%
13	Indiana	83,447	2.1%
14	Massachusetts	82,448	2.1%
15	Washington	79,024	2.0%
16	Arizona	75,753	1.9%
17	Missouri	74,747	1.9%
18	Tennessee	74,577	1.9%
19	Maryland	70,267	1.8%
20	Wisconsin	66,602	1.7%
21	Louisiana	66,012	1.7%
22	Minnesota	64,525	1.7%
23	Alabama	61,038	1.6%
24	Colorado	56,539	1.5%
25	Kentucky	53,228	1.4%
26	South Carolina	51,904	1.3%
27	Oklahoma	48,110	1.2%
28	Oregon	43,895	1.1%
29	Utah	43,885	1.1%
30	Connecticut	42,977	1.1%
31	Mississippi	42,747	1.1%
32	Kansas	37,446	1.0%
33	Iowa	36,933	0.9%
34	Arkansas	36,720	0.9%
35	Nevada	27,039	0.7%
36	New Mexico	26,874	0.7%
37	Nebraska	23,327	0.6%
38	West Virginia	20,752	0.5%
39	Idaho	18,594	0.5%
40	Hawaii	17,381	0.4%
41	New Hampshire	14,433	0.4%
42	Maine	13,670	0.4%
43	Rhode Island	12,388	0.3%
44	Montana	10,851	0.3%
45	Delaware	10,243	0.3%
46	South Dakota	10,208	0.3%
47	Alaska	9,705	0.2%
48	North Dakota	8,356	0.2%
49	Vermont	6,667	0.2%
50	Wyoming	6,424	0.2%
	District of Columbia	7,905	0.2%

Source: U.S. Department of Health and Human Services, National Center for Health Statistics
"National Vital Statistics Report" (Vol. 47, No. 4, October 7, 1998)
Data are preliminary estimates by state of residence.

Birth Rate in 1997

National Rate = 14.6 Live Births per 1,000 Population*

ALPHA ORDER

RANK	STATE	RATE
21	Alabama	14.1
6	Alaska	15.9
3	Arizona	16.6
13	Arkansas	14.6
4	California	16.3
15	Colorado	14.5
39	Connecticut	13.1
24	Delaware	14.0
39	Florida	13.1
7	Georgia	15.8
13	Hawaii	14.6
10	Idaho	15.4
11	Illinois	15.2
20	Indiana	14.2
42	Iowa	12.9
18	Kansas	14.4
34	Kentucky	13.6
11	Louisiana	15.2
50	Maine	11.0
27	Maryland	13.8
36	Massachusetts	13.5
32	Michigan	13.7
27	Minnesota	13.8
8	Mississippi	15.7
27	Missouri	13.8
45	Montana	12.3
21	Nebraska	14.1
5	Nevada	16.1
45	New Hampshire	12.3
24	New Jersey	14.0
9	New Mexico	15.5
15	New York	14.5
18	North Carolina	14.4
41	North Dakota	13.0
34	Ohio	13.6
15	Oklahoma	14.5
36	Oregon	13.5
47	Pennsylvania	12.0
44	Rhode Island	12.5
27	South Carolina	13.8
27	South Dakota	13.8
26	Tennessee	13.9
2	Texas	17.2
1	Utah	21.3
49	Vermont	11.3
32	Virginia	13.7
21	Washington	14.1
48	West Virginia	11.4
42	Wisconsin	12.9
38	Wyoming	13.4

RANK ORDER

RANK	STATE	RATE
1	Utah	21.3
2	Texas	17.2
3	Arizona	16.6
4	California	16.3
5	Nevada	16.1
6	Alaska	15.9
7	Georgia	15.8
8	Mississippi	15.7
9	New Mexico	15.5
10	Idaho	15.4
11	Illinois	15.2
11	Louisiana	15.2
13	Arkansas	14.6
13	Hawaii	14.6
15	Colorado	14.5
15	New York	14.5
15	Oklahoma	14.5
18	Kansas	14.4
18	North Carolina	14.4
20	Indiana	14.2
21	Alabama	14.1
21	Nebraska	14.1
21	Washington	14.1
24	Delaware	14.0
24	New Jersey	14.0
26	Tennessee	13.9
27	Maryland	13.8
27	Minnesota	13.8
27	Missouri	13.8
27	South Carolina	13.8
27	South Dakota	13.8
32	Michigan	13.7
32	Virginia	13.7
34	Kentucky	13.6
34	Ohio	13.6
36	Massachusetts	13.5
36	Oregon	13.5
38	Wyoming	13.4
39	Connecticut	13.1
39	Florida	13.1
41	North Dakota	13.0
42	Iowa	12.9
42	Wisconsin	12.9
44	Rhode Island	12.5
45	Montana	12.3
45	New Hampshire	12.3
47	Pennsylvania	12.0
48	West Virginia	11.4
49	Vermont	11.3
50	Maine	11.0

	District of Columbia	14.9

Source: U.S. Department of Health and Human Services, National Center for Health Statistics
   "National Vital Statistics Report" (Vol. 47, No. 4, October 7, 1998)
*Data are preliminary estimates by state of residence.

Births in 1996

National Total = 3,891,494 Live Births*

ALPHA ORDER

RANK	STATE	BIRTHS	% of USA	RANK	STATE	BIRTHS	% of USA
23	Alabama	60,488	1.6%	1	California	539,433	13.9%
47	Alaska	10,037	0.3%	2	Texas	330,406	8.5%
16	Arizona	75,322	1.9%	3	New York	263,963	6.8%
34	Arkansas	36,371	0.9%	4	Florida	189,392	4.9%
1	California	539,433	13.9%	5	Illinois	183,180	4.7%
24	Colorado	55,807	1.4%	6	Ohio	151,692	3.9%
28	Connecticut	44,469	1.1%	7	Pennsylvania	148,338	3.8%
46	Delaware	10,155	0.3%	8	Michigan	133,387	3.4%
4	Florida	189,392	4.9%	9	New Jersey	114,306	2.9%
10	Georgia	114,043	2.9%	10	Georgia	114,043	2.9%
40	Hawaii	18,401	0.5%	11	North Carolina	104,470	2.7%
39	Idaho	18,625	0.5%	12	Virginia	92,354	2.4%
5	Illinois	183,180	4.7%	13	Indiana	83,513	2.1%
13	Indiana	83,513	2.1%	14	Massachusetts	80,276	2.1%
32	Iowa	37,139	1.0%	15	Washington	77,945	2.0%
33	Kansas	36,651	0.9%	16	Arizona	75,322	1.9%
25	Kentucky	52,706	1.4%	17	Missouri	73,832	1.9%
21	Louisiana	65,204	1.7%	18	Tennessee	73,754	1.9%
42	Maine	13,774	0.4%	19	Maryland	71,533	1.8%
19	Maryland	71,533	1.8%	20	Wisconsin	67,106	1.7%
14	Massachusetts	80,276	2.1%	21	Louisiana	65,204	1.7%
8	Michigan	133,387	3.4%	22	Minnesota	63,700	1.6%
22	Minnesota	63,700	1.6%	23	Alabama	60,488	1.6%
31	Mississippi	40,987	1.1%	24	Colorado	55,807	1.4%
17	Missouri	73,832	1.9%	25	Kentucky	52,706	1.4%
44	Montana	10,856	0.3%	26	South Carolina	51,117	1.3%
37	Nebraska	23,286	0.6%	27	Oklahoma	46,193	1.2%
36	Nevada	26,125	0.7%	28	Connecticut	44,469	1.1%
41	New Hampshire	14,520	0.4%	29	Oregon	43,658	1.1%
9	New Jersey	114,306	2.9%	30	Utah	42,087	1.1%
35	New Mexico	27,228	0.7%	31	Mississippi	40,987	1.1%
3	New York	263,963	6.8%	32	Iowa	37,139	1.0%
11	North Carolina	104,470	2.7%	33	Kansas	36,651	0.9%
48	North Dakota	8,347	0.2%	34	Arkansas	36,371	0.9%
6	Ohio	151,692	3.9%	35	New Mexico	27,228	0.7%
27	Oklahoma	46,193	1.2%	36	Nevada	26,125	0.7%
29	Oregon	43,658	1.1%	37	Nebraska	23,286	0.6%
7	Pennsylvania	148,338	3.8%	38	West Virginia	20,750	0.5%
43	Rhode Island	12,652	0.3%	39	Idaho	18,625	0.5%
26	South Carolina	51,117	1.3%	40	Hawaii	18,401	0.5%
45	South Dakota	10,473	0.3%	41	New Hampshire	14,520	0.4%
18	Tennessee	73,754	1.9%	42	Maine	13,774	0.4%
2	Texas	330,406	8.5%	43	Rhode Island	12,652	0.3%
30	Utah	42,087	1.1%	44	Montana	10,856	0.3%
49	Vermont	6,767	0.2%	45	South Dakota	10,473	0.3%
12	Virginia	92,354	2.4%	46	Delaware	10,155	0.3%
15	Washington	77,945	2.0%	47	Alaska	10,037	0.3%
38	West Virginia	20,750	0.5%	48	North Dakota	8,347	0.2%
20	Wisconsin	67,106	1.7%	49	Vermont	6,767	0.2%
50	Wyoming	6,286	0.2%	50	Wyoming	6,286	0.2%
					District of Columbia	8,390	0.2%

Source: U.S. Department of Health and Human Services, National Center for Health Statistics
"Monthly Vital Statistics Report" (Vol. 46, No. 11, Supplement, June 30, 1998)
*Final data by state of residence.

Birth Rate in 1996

National Rate = 14.7 Live Births per 1,000 Population*

ALPHA ORDER			RANK ORDER		
RANK	**STATE**	**RATE**	**RANK**	**STATE**	**RATE**
21	Alabama	14.2	1	Utah	21.0
5	Alaska	16.5	2	Texas	17.3
3	Arizona	17.0	3	Arizona	17.0
15	Arkansas	14.5	4	California	16.9
4	California	16.9	5	Alaska	16.5
14	Colorado	14.6	6	Nevada	16.3
34	Connecticut	13.6	7	New Mexico	15.9
26	Delaware	14.0	8	Idaho	15.7
38	Florida	13.2	9	Georgia	15.5
9	Georgia	15.5	9	Hawaii	15.5
9	Hawaii	15.5	9	Illinois	15.5
8	Idaho	15.7	12	Mississippi	15.1
9	Illinois	15.5	13	Louisiana	15.0
17	Indiana	14.3	14	Colorado	14.6
41	Iowa	13.0	15	Arkansas	14.5
21	Kansas	14.2	15	New York	14.5
34	Kentucky	13.6	17	Indiana	14.3
13	Louisiana	15.0	17	New Jersey	14.3
50	Maine	11.1	17	North Carolina	14.3
23	Maryland	14.1	17	South Dakota	14.3
38	Massachusetts	13.2	21	Alabama	14.2
28	Michigan	13.9	21	Kansas	14.2
33	Minnesota	13.7	23	Maryland	14.1
12	Mississippi	15.1	23	Nebraska	14.1
30	Missouri	13.8	23	Washington	14.1
46	Montana	12.3	26	Delaware	14.0
23	Nebraska	14.1	26	Oklahoma	14.0
6	Nevada	16.3	28	Michigan	13.9
45	New Hampshire	12.5	28	Tennessee	13.9
17	New Jersey	14.3	30	Missouri	13.8
7	New Mexico	15.9	30	South Carolina	13.8
15	New York	14.5	30	Virginia	13.8
17	North Carolina	14.3	33	Minnesota	13.7
41	North Dakota	13.0	34	Connecticut	13.6
34	Ohio	13.6	34	Kentucky	13.6
26	Oklahoma	14.0	34	Ohio	13.6
34	Oregon	13.6	34	Oregon	13.6
46	Pennsylvania	12.3	38	Florida	13.2
44	Rhode Island	12.8	38	Massachusetts	13.2
30	South Carolina	13.8	40	Wyoming	13.1
17	South Dakota	14.3	41	Iowa	13.0
28	Tennessee	13.9	41	North Dakota	13.0
2	Texas	17.3	41	Wisconsin	13.0
1	Utah	21.0	44	Rhode Island	12.8
48	Vermont	11.5	45	New Hampshire	12.5
30	Virginia	13.8	46	Montana	12.3
23	Washington	14.1	46	Pennsylvania	12.3
49	West Virginia	11.4	48	Vermont	11.5
41	Wisconsin	13.0	49	West Virginia	11.4
40	Wyoming	13.1	50	Maine	11.1
				District of Columbia	15.4

Source: U.S. Department of Health and Human Services, National Center for Health Statistics
   "National Vital Statistics Report" (Vol. 47, No. 4, October 7, 1998)
Final data by state of residence.

Births in 1990

National Total = 4,158,212 Live Births*

ALPHA ORDER

RANK	STATE	BIRTHS	% of USA
23	Alabama	63,487	1.53%
44	Alaska	11,902	0.29%
21	Arizona	68,995	1.66%
33	Arkansas	36,457	0.88%
1	California	612,628	14.73%
26	Colorado	53,525	1.29%
27	Connecticut	50,123	1.21%
46	Delaware	11,113	0.27%
4	Florida	199,339	4.79%
10	Georgia	112,666	2.71%
39	Hawaii	20,489	0.49%
42	Idaho	16,433	0.40%
5	Illinois	195,790	4.71%
14	Indiana	86,214	2.07%
31	Iowa	39,409	0.95%
32	Kansas	39,020	0.94%
25	Kentucky	54,362	1.31%
20	Louisiana	72,192	1.74%
41	Maine	17,359	0.42%
15	Maryland	80,245	1.93%
13	Massachusetts	92,654	2.23%
8	Michigan	153,700	3.70%
22	Minnesota	68,013	1.64%
29	Mississippi	43,563	1.05%
16	Missouri	79,260	1.91%
45	Montana	11,613	0.28%
36	Nebraska	24,380	0.59%
38	Nevada	21,599	0.52%
40	New Hampshire	17,569	0.42%
9	New Jersey	122,289	2.94%
35	New Mexico	27,402	0.66%
3	New York	297,576	7.16%
11	North Carolina	104,525	2.51%
48	North Dakota	9,250	0.22%
7	Ohio	166,913	4.01%
28	Oklahoma	47,649	1.15%
30	Oregon	42,891	1.03%
6	Pennsylvania	171,961	4.14%
43	Rhode Island	15,195	0.37%
24	South Carolina	58,610	1.41%
47	South Dakota	10,999	0.26%
18	Tennessee	74,962	1.80%
2	Texas	316,423	7.61%
34	Utah	36,277	0.87%
49	Vermont	8,273	0.20%
12	Virginia	99,352	2.39%
17	Washington	79,251	1.91%
37	West Virginia	22,585	0.54%
19	Wisconsin	72,895	1.75%
50	Wyoming	6,985	0.17%

RANK ORDER

RANK	STATE	BIRTHS	% of USA
1	California	612,628	14.73%
2	Texas	316,423	7.61%
3	New York	297,576	7.16%
4	Florida	199,339	4.79%
5	Illinois	195,790	4.71%
6	Pennsylvania	171,961	4.14%
7	Ohio	166,913	4.01%
8	Michigan	153,700	3.70%
9	New Jersey	122,289	2.94%
10	Georgia	112,666	2.71%
11	North Carolina	104,525	2.51%
12	Virginia	99,352	2.39%
13	Massachusetts	92,654	2.23%
14	Indiana	86,214	2.07%
15	Maryland	80,245	1.93%
16	Missouri	79,260	1.91%
17	Washington	79,251	1.91%
18	Tennessee	74,962	1.80%
19	Wisconsin	72,895	1.75%
20	Louisiana	72,192	1.74%
21	Arizona	68,995	1.66%
22	Minnesota	68,013	1.64%
23	Alabama	63,487	1.53%
24	South Carolina	58,610	1.41%
25	Kentucky	54,362	1.31%
26	Colorado	53,525	1.29%
27	Connecticut	50,123	1.21%
28	Oklahoma	47,649	1.15%
29	Mississippi	43,563	1.05%
30	Oregon	42,891	1.03%
31	Iowa	39,409	0.95%
32	Kansas	39,020	0.94%
33	Arkansas	36,457	0.88%
34	Utah	36,277	0.87%
35	New Mexico	27,402	0.66%
36	Nebraska	24,380	0.59%
37	West Virginia	22,585	0.54%
38	Nevada	21,599	0.52%
39	Hawaii	20,489	0.49%
40	New Hampshire	17,569	0.42%
41	Maine	17,359	0.42%
42	Idaho	16,433	0.40%
43	Rhode Island	15,195	0.37%
44	Alaska	11,902	0.29%
45	Montana	11,613	0.28%
46	Delaware	11,113	0.27%
47	South Dakota	10,999	0.26%
48	North Dakota	9,250	0.22%
49	Vermont	8,273	0.20%
50	Wyoming	6,985	0.17%
	District of Columbia	11,850	0.28%

Source: U.S. Department of Health and Human Services, National Center for Health Statistics
    "Monthly Vital Statistics Report" (Vol. 41, No. 9, Supplement, February 25, 1993)
*Final data by state of residence.

Birth Rate in 1990

National Rate = 16.7 Births per 1,000 Population*

ALPHA ORDER

RANK	STATE	RATE
26	Alabama	15.7
1	Alaska	21.6
4	Arizona	18.8
29	Arkansas	15.5
3	California	20.6
20	Colorado	16.2
38	Connecticut	15.2
15	Delaware	16.7
32	Florida	15.4
9	Georgia	17.4
6	Hawaii	18.5
18	Idaho	16.3
10	Illinois	17.1
28	Indiana	15.6
48	Iowa	14.2
26	Kansas	15.7
43	Kentucky	14.8
10	Louisiana	17.1
49	Maine	14.1
13	Maryland	16.8
32	Massachusetts	15.4
16	Michigan	16.5
29	Minnesota	15.5
12	Mississippi	16.9
29	Missouri	15.5
45	Montana	14.5
32	Nebraska	15.4
8	Nevada	18.0
22	New Hampshire	15.8
22	New Jersey	15.8
7	New Mexico	18.1
16	New York	16.5
22	North Carolina	15.8
45	North Dakota	14.5
32	Ohio	15.4
39	Oklahoma	15.1
39	Oregon	15.1
45	Pennsylvania	14.5
39	Rhode Island	15.1
13	South Carolina	16.8
22	South Dakota	15.8
32	Tennessee	15.4
5	Texas	18.6
2	Utah	21.1
44	Vermont	14.7
21	Virginia	16.1
18	Washington	16.3
50	West Virginia	12.6
42	Wisconsin	14.9
32	Wyoming	15.4

RANK ORDER

RANK	STATE	RATE
1	Alaska	21.6
2	Utah	21.1
3	California	20.6
4	Arizona	18.8
5	Texas	18.6
6	Hawaii	18.5
7	New Mexico	18.1
8	Nevada	18.0
9	Georgia	17.4
10	Illinois	17.1
10	Louisiana	17.1
12	Mississippi	16.9
13	Maryland	16.8
13	South Carolina	16.8
15	Delaware	16.7
16	Michigan	16.5
16	New York	16.5
18	Idaho	16.3
18	Washington	16.3
20	Colorado	16.2
21	Virginia	16.1
22	New Hampshire	15.8
22	New Jersey	15.8
22	North Carolina	15.8
22	South Dakota	15.8
26	Alabama	15.7
26	Kansas	15.7
28	Indiana	15.6
29	Arkansas	15.5
29	Minnesota	15.5
29	Missouri	15.5
32	Florida	15.4
32	Massachusetts	15.4
32	Nebraska	15.4
32	Ohio	15.4
32	Tennessee	15.4
32	Wyoming	15.4
38	Connecticut	15.2
39	Oklahoma	15.1
39	Oregon	15.1
39	Rhode Island	15.1
42	Wisconsin	14.9
43	Kentucky	14.8
44	Vermont	14.7
45	Montana	14.5
45	North Dakota	14.5
45	Pennsylvania	14.5
48	Iowa	14.2
49	Maine	14.1
50	West Virginia	12.6
	District of Columbia	19.5

Source: U.S. Department of Health and Human Services, National Center for Health Statistics
   "Monthly Vital Statistics Report" (Vol. 41, No. 9, Supplement, February 25, 1993)
*Final data by state of residence.

Births in 1980

National Total = 3,612,000 Births*

ALPHA ORDER

RANK	STATE	BIRTHS	% of USA
21	Alabama	64,000	1.77%
48	Alaska	10,000	0.28%
26	Arizona	50,000	1.38%
34	Arkansas	37,000	1.02%
1	California	403,000	11.16%
26	Colorado	50,000	1.38%
33	Connecticut	39,000	1.08%
49	Delaware	9,000	0.25%
8	Florida	132,000	3.65%
10	Georgia	92,000	2.55%
39	Hawaii	18,000	0.50%
38	Idaho	20,000	0.55%
4	Illinois	190,000	5.26%
11	Indiana	88,000	2.44%
28	Iowa	48,000	1.33%
32	Kansas	41,000	1.14%
22	Kentucky	60,000	1.66%
13	Louisiana	82,000	2.27%
40	Maine	16,000	0.44%
22	Maryland	60,000	1.66%
17	Massachusetts	73,000	2.02%
7	Michigan	146,000	4.04%
19	Minnesota	68,000	1.88%
28	Mississippi	48,000	1.33%
14	Missouri	79,000	2.19%
41	Montana	14,000	0.39%
36	Nebraska	27,000	0.75%
43	Nevada	13,000	0.36%
41	New Hampshire	14,000	0.39%
9	New Jersey	97,000	2.69%
37	New Mexico	26,000	0.72%
3	New York	239,000	6.62%
12	North Carolina	84,000	2.33%
45	North Dakota	12,000	0.33%
5	Ohio	169,000	4.68%
24	Oklahoma	52,000	1.44%
30	Oregon	43,000	1.19%
6	Pennsylvania	159,000	4.40%
45	Rhode Island	12,000	0.33%
24	South Carolina	52,000	1.44%
43	South Dakota	13,000	0.36%
18	Tennessee	69,000	1.91%
2	Texas	274,000	7.59%
31	Utah	42,000	1.16%
50	Vermont	8,000	0.22%
15	Virginia	78,000	2.16%
19	Washington	68,000	1.88%
35	West Virginia	29,000	0.80%
16	Wisconsin	75,000	2.08%
47	Wyoming	11,000	0.30%

RANK ORDER

RANK	STATE	BIRTHS	% of USA
1	California	403,000	11.16%
2	Texas	274,000	7.59%
3	New York	239,000	6.62%
4	Illinois	190,000	5.26%
5	Ohio	169,000	4.68%
6	Pennsylvania	159,000	4.40%
7	Michigan	146,000	4.04%
8	Florida	132,000	3.65%
9	New Jersey	97,000	2.69%
10	Georgia	92,000	2.55%
11	Indiana	88,000	2.44%
12	North Carolina	84,000	2.33%
13	Louisiana	82,000	2.27%
14	Missouri	79,000	2.19%
15	Virginia	78,000	2.16%
16	Wisconsin	75,000	2.08%
17	Massachusetts	73,000	2.02%
18	Tennessee	69,000	1.91%
19	Minnesota	68,000	1.88%
19	Washington	68,000	1.88%
21	Alabama	64,000	1.77%
22	Kentucky	60,000	1.66%
22	Maryland	60,000	1.66%
24	Oklahoma	52,000	1.44%
24	South Carolina	52,000	1.44%
26	Arizona	50,000	1.38%
26	Colorado	50,000	1.38%
28	Iowa	48,000	1.33%
28	Mississippi	48,000	1.33%
30	Oregon	43,000	1.19%
31	Utah	42,000	1.16%
32	Kansas	41,000	1.14%
33	Connecticut	39,000	1.08%
34	Arkansas	37,000	1.02%
35	West Virginia	29,000	0.80%
36	Nebraska	27,000	0.75%
37	New Mexico	26,000	0.72%
38	Idaho	20,000	0.55%
39	Hawaii	18,000	0.50%
40	Maine	16,000	0.44%
41	Montana	14,000	0.39%
41	New Hampshire	14,000	0.39%
43	Nevada	13,000	0.36%
43	South Dakota	13,000	0.36%
45	North Dakota	12,000	0.33%
45	Rhode Island	12,000	0.33%
47	Wyoming	11,000	0.30%
48	Alaska	10,000	0.28%
49	Delaware	9,000	0.25%
50	Vermont	8,000	0.22%
	District of Columbia	9,000	0.25%

Source: U.S. Department of Health and Human Services, National Center for Health Statistics
    "Vital Statistics of the United States, 1980" and "Monthly Vital Statistics Report"
*Live births by state of residence.

Birth Rate in 1980

National Rate = 15.9 Births per 1,000 Population*

ALPHA ORDER				RANK ORDER		
RANK	**STATE**	**RATE**		**RANK**	**STATE**	**RATE**
27	Alabama	16.3		1	Utah	28.6
2	Alaska	23.7		2	Alaska	23.7
11	Arizona	18.4		3	Wyoming	22.5
27	Arkansas	16.3		4	Idaho	21.4
18	California	17.0		5	New Mexico	20.0
15	Colorado	17.2		6	Louisiana	19.5
50	Connecticut	12.5		7	South Dakota	19.2
33	Delaware	15.8		7	Texas	19.2
45	Florida	13.5		9	Mississippi	19.0
19	Georgia	16.9		10	Hawaii	18.8
10	Hawaii	18.8		11	Arizona	18.4
4	Idaho	21.4		11	North Dakota	18.4
20	Illinois	16.6		13	Montana	18.1
30	Indiana	16.1		14	Nebraska	17.4
24	Iowa	16.4		15	Colorado	17.2
15	Kansas	17.2		15	Kansas	17.2
27	Kentucky	16.3		15	Oklahoma	17.2
6	Louisiana	19.5		18	California	17.0
41	Maine	14.6		19	Georgia	16.9
43	Maryland	14.2		20	Illinois	16.6
49	Massachusetts	12.7		20	Minnesota	16.6
34	Michigan	15.7		20	Nevada	16.6
20	Minnesota	16.6		20	South Carolina	16.6
9	Mississippi	19.0		24	Iowa	16.4
30	Missouri	16.1		24	Oregon	16.4
13	Montana	18.1		24	Washington	16.4
14	Nebraska	17.4		27	Alabama	16.3
20	Nevada	16.6		27	Arkansas	16.3
39	New Hampshire	14.9		27	Kentucky	16.3
47	New Jersey	13.2		30	Indiana	16.1
5	New Mexico	20.0		30	Missouri	16.1
44	New York	13.6		32	Wisconsin	15.9
42	North Carolina	14.4		33	Delaware	15.8
11	North Dakota	18.4		34	Michigan	15.7
34	Ohio	15.7		34	Ohio	15.7
15	Oklahoma	17.2		36	Vermont	15.4
24	Oregon	16.4		37	Tennessee	15.1
46	Pennsylvania	13.4		37	West Virginia	15.1
48	Rhode Island	12.9		39	New Hampshire	14.9
20	South Carolina	16.6		40	Virginia	14.7
7	South Dakota	19.2		41	Maine	14.6
37	Tennessee	15.1		42	North Carolina	14.4
7	Texas	19.2		43	Maryland	14.2
1	Utah	28.6		44	New York	13.6
36	Vermont	15.4		45	Florida	13.5
40	Virginia	14.7		46	Pennsylvania	13.4
24	Washington	16.4		47	New Jersey	13.2
37	West Virginia	15.1		48	Rhode Island	12.9
32	Wisconsin	15.9		49	Massachusetts	12.7
3	Wyoming	22.5		50	Connecticut	12.5
					District of Columbia	14.7

Source: U.S. Department of Health and Human Services, National Center for Health Statistics
"Vital Statistics of the United States, 1980" and "Monthly Vital Statistics Report"
Live births by state of residence.

Fertility Rate in 1997

National Rate = 65.3 Live Births per 1,000 Women 15 to 44 Years Old*

ALPHA ORDER

RANK ORDER

RANK	STATE	RATE	RANK	STATE	RATE
28	Alabama	62.2	1	Utah	90.2
6	Alaska	70.6	2	Arizona	78.1
2	Arizona	78.1	3	Nevada	75.8
12	Arkansas	67.8	4	Texas	75.3
5	California	72.5	5	California	72.5
21	Colorado	64.2	6	Alaska	70.6
36	Connecticut	60.1	7	New Mexico	70.5
35	Delaware	60.2	8	Idaho	70.3
18	Florida	65.0	9	Hawaii	69.0
14	Georgia	66.2	10	Illinois	68.4
9	Hawaii	69.0	11	Mississippi	68.2
8	Idaho	70.3	12	Arkansas	67.8
10	Illinois	68.4	13	Oklahoma	67.6
24	Indiana	62.9	14	Georgia	66.2
33	Iowa	60.8	15	Kansas	66.0
15	Kansas	66.0	16	Louisiana	65.7
37	Kentucky	60.0	17	New York	65.4
16	Louisiana	65.7	18	Florida	65.0
50	Maine	49.5	19	Nebraska	64.6
42	Maryland	58.9	20	North Carolina	64.3
40	Massachusetts	59.3	21	Colorado	64.2
37	Michigan	60.0	22	New Jersey	64.0
30	Minnesota	61.4	23	South Dakota	63.8
11	Mississippi	68.2	24	Indiana	62.9
25	Missouri	62.8	25	Missouri	62.8
41	Montana	59.1	25	Oregon	62.8
19	Nebraska	64.6	27	Washington	62.5
3	Nevada	75.8	28	Alabama	62.2
48	New Hampshire	52.8	29	Wyoming	62.1
22	New Jersey	64.0	30	Minnesota	61.4
7	New Mexico	70.5	31	Tennessee	61.3
17	New York	65.4	32	North Dakota	61.0
20	North Carolina	64.3	33	Iowa	60.8
32	North Dakota	61.0	33	Ohio	60.8
33	Ohio	60.8	35	Delaware	60.2
13	Oklahoma	67.6	36	Connecticut	60.1
25	Oregon	62.8	37	Kentucky	60.0
46	Pennsylvania	55.9	37	Michigan	60.0
45	Rhode Island	56.3	37	South Carolina	60.0
37	South Carolina	60.0	40	Massachusetts	59.3
23	South Dakota	63.8	41	Montana	59.1
31	Tennessee	61.3	42	Maryland	58.9
4	Texas	75.3	43	Wisconsin	58.2
1	Utah	90.2	44	Virginia	58.1
49	Vermont	50.0	45	Rhode Island	56.3
44	Virginia	58.1	46	Pennsylvania	55.9
27	Washington	62.5	47	West Virginia	53.2
47	West Virginia	53.2	48	New Hampshire	52.8
43	Wisconsin	58.2	49	Vermont	50.0
29	Wyoming	62.1	50	Maine	49.5
				District of Columbia	61.5

Source: U.S. Department of Health and Human Services, National Center for Health Statistics
   "National Vital Statistics Report" (Vol. 47, No. 4, October 7, 1998)
*Data are preliminary estimates by state of residence.

Births to White Women in 1997

National Total = 3,085,477 Live Births to White Women*

ALPHA ORDER

RANK	STATE	BIRTHS	% of USA
25	Alabama	40,529	1.3%
48	Alaska	6,473	0.2%
16	Arizona	66,319	2.1%
33	Arkansas	28,227	0.9%
1	California	427,102	13.8%
21	Colorado	51,717	1.7%
29	Connecticut	36,213	1.2%
45	Delaware	7,496	0.2%
4	Florida	144,174	4.7%
11	Georgia	75,663	2.5%
50	Hawaii	4,479	0.1%
39	Idaho	18,012	0.6%
5	Illinois	138,912	4.5%
12	Indiana	74,764	2.4%
30	Iowa	34,830	1.1%
31	Kansas	33,403	1.1%
22	Kentucky	47,950	1.6%
28	Louisiana	37,643	1.2%
41	Maine	13,324	0.4%
23	Maryland	44,488	1.4%
13	Massachusetts	70,389	2.3%
8	Michigan	105,723	3.4%
19	Minnesota	57,349	1.9%
36	Mississippi	22,646	0.7%
17	Missouri	62,149	2.0%
43	Montana	9,431	0.3%
37	Nebraska	21,315	0.7%
34	Nevada	22,962	0.7%
40	New Hampshire	14,117	0.5%
9	New Jersey	84,620	2.7%
35	New Mexico	22,733	0.7%
3	New York	189,054	6.1%
10	North Carolina	75,882	2.5%
46	North Dakota	7,399	0.2%
6	Ohio	127,230	4.1%
27	Oklahoma	37,891	1.2%
26	Oregon	40,314	1.3%
7	Pennsylvania	120,222	3.9%
42	Rhode Island	10,862	0.4%
32	South Carolina	32,910	1.1%
44	South Dakota	8,455	0.3%
20	Tennessee	57,080	1.8%
2	Texas	284,245	9.2%
24	Utah	41,666	1.4%
47	Vermont	6,581	0.2%
15	Virginia	66,806	2.2%
14	Washington	68,340	2.2%
38	West Virginia	19,875	0.6%
18	Wisconsin	57,439	1.9%
49	Wyoming	6,099	0.2%

RANK ORDER

RANK	STATE	BIRTHS	% of USA
1	California	427,102	13.8%
2	Texas	284,245	9.2%
3	New York	189,054	6.1%
4	Florida	144,174	4.7%
5	Illinois	138,912	4.5%
6	Ohio	127,230	4.1%
7	Pennsylvania	120,222	3.9%
8	Michigan	105,723	3.4%
9	New Jersey	84,620	2.7%
10	North Carolina	75,882	2.5%
11	Georgia	75,663	2.5%
12	Indiana	74,764	2.4%
13	Massachusetts	70,389	2.3%
14	Washington	68,340	2.2%
15	Virginia	66,806	2.2%
16	Arizona	66,319	2.1%
17	Missouri	62,149	2.0%
18	Wisconsin	57,439	1.9%
19	Minnesota	57,349	1.9%
20	Tennessee	57,080	1.8%
21	Colorado	51,717	1.7%
22	Kentucky	47,950	1.6%
23	Maryland	44,488	1.4%
24	Utah	41,666	1.4%
25	Alabama	40,529	1.3%
26	Oregon	40,314	1.3%
27	Oklahoma	37,891	1.2%
28	Louisiana	37,643	1.2%
29	Connecticut	36,213	1.2%
30	Iowa	34,830	1.1%
31	Kansas	33,403	1.1%
32	South Carolina	32,910	1.1%
33	Arkansas	28,227	0.9%
34	Nevada	22,962	0.7%
35	New Mexico	22,733	0.7%
36	Mississippi	22,646	0.7%
37	Nebraska	21,315	0.7%
38	West Virginia	19,875	0.6%
39	Idaho	18,012	0.6%
40	New Hampshire	14,117	0.5%
41	Maine	13,324	0.4%
42	Rhode Island	10,862	0.4%
43	Montana	9,431	0.3%
44	South Dakota	8,455	0.3%
45	Delaware	7,496	0.2%
46	North Dakota	7,399	0.2%
47	Vermont	6,581	0.2%
48	Alaska	6,473	0.2%
49	Wyoming	6,099	0.2%
50	Hawaii	4,479	0.1%
	District of Columbia	1,973	0.1%

Source: U.S. Department of Health and Human Services, National Center for Health Statistics
    "National Vital Statistics Report" (Vol. 47, No. 4, October 7, 1998)
*Preliminary data by state of residence. By race of mother.

White Births as a Percent of All Births in 1997

National Percent = 79.2% of Live Births*

ALPHA ORDER

RANK ORDER

RANK	STATE	PERCENT		RANK	STATE	PERCENT
44	Alabama	66.4		1	Vermont	98.7
43	Alaska	66.7		2	New Hampshire	97.8
18	Arizona	87.5		3	Maine	97.5
34	Arkansas	76.9		4	Idaho	96.9
31	California	81.2		5	West Virginia	95.8
10	Colorado	91.5		6	Utah	94.9
26	Connecticut	84.3		6	Wyoming	94.9
39	Delaware	73.2		8	Iowa	94.3
37	Florida	74.9		9	Oregon	91.8
45	Georgia	63.9		10	Colorado	91.5
50	Hawaii	25.8		11	Nebraska	91.4
4	Idaho	96.9		12	Kentucky	90.1
35	Illinois	76.8		13	Indiana	89.6
13	Indiana	89.6		14	Kansas	89.2
8	Iowa	94.3		15	Minnesota	88.9
14	Kansas	89.2		16	North Dakota	88.5
12	Kentucky	90.1		17	Rhode Island	87.7
48	Louisiana	57.0		18	Arizona	87.5
3	Maine	97.5		19	Montana	86.9
47	Maryland	63.3		20	Washington	86.5
22	Massachusetts	85.4		21	Wisconsin	86.2
32	Michigan	79.1		22	Massachusetts	85.4
15	Minnesota	88.9		23	Texas	85.1
49	Mississippi	53.0		24	Nevada	84.9
29	Missouri	83.1		25	New Mexico	84.6
19	Montana	86.9		26	Connecticut	84.3
11	Nebraska	91.4		27	Ohio	83.6
24	Nevada	84.9		28	Pennsylvania	83.4
2	New Hampshire	97.8		29	Missouri	83.1
38	New Jersey	74.8		30	South Dakota	82.8
25	New Mexico	84.6		31	California	81.2
41	New York	71.8		32	Michigan	79.1
42	North Carolina	70.9		33	Oklahoma	78.8
16	North Dakota	88.5		34	Arkansas	76.9
27	Ohio	83.6		35	Illinois	76.8
33	Oklahoma	78.8		36	Tennessee	76.5
9	Oregon	91.8		37	Florida	74.9
28	Pennsylvania	83.4		38	New Jersey	74.8
17	Rhode Island	87.7		39	Delaware	73.2
46	South Carolina	63.4		40	Virginia	72.6
30	South Dakota	82.8		41	New York	71.8
36	Tennessee	76.5		42	North Carolina	70.9
23	Texas	85.1		43	Alaska	66.7
6	Utah	94.9		44	Alabama	66.4
1	Vermont	98.7		45	Georgia	63.9
40	Virginia	72.6		46	South Carolina	63.4
20	Washington	86.5		47	Maryland	63.3
5	West Virginia	95.8		48	Louisiana	57.0
21	Wisconsin	86.2		49	Mississippi	53.0
6	Wyoming	94.9		50	Hawaii	25.8

District of Columbia   25.0

Source: Morgan Quitno Press using data from U.S. Dept. of Health and Human Services, Nat'l Center for Health Statistics "National Vital Statistics Report" (Vol. 47, No. 4, October 7, 1998)
Preliminary data by state of residence. By race of mother.

Births to Black Women in 1997

National Total = 600,898 Live Births to Black Women*

RANK	STATE	BIRTHS	% of USA
15	Alabama	19,859	3.3%
41	Alaska	453	0.1%
32	Arizona	2,503	0.4%
21	Arkansas	7,905	1.3%
5	California	37,477	6.2%
30	Colorado	2,585	0.4%
24	Connecticut	5,238	0.9%
31	Delaware	2,512	0.4%
2	Florida	43,579	7.3%
3	Georgia	39,774	6.6%
39	Hawaii	578	0.1%
47	Idaho	68	0.0%
6	Illinois	35,453	5.9%
22	Indiana	7,633	1.3%
35	Iowa	1,109	0.2%
29	Kansas	2,817	0.5%
26	Kentucky	4,652	0.8%
8	Louisiana	27,126	4.5%
46	Maine	81	0.0%
10	Maryland	22,966	3.8%
20	Massachusetts	7,922	1.3%
9	Michigan	24,277	4.0%
27	Minnesota	3,252	0.5%
16	Mississippi	19,541	3.3%
19	Missouri	11,144	1.9%
49	Montana	31	0.0%
34	Nebraska	1,253	0.2%
33	Nevada	2,143	0.4%
43	New Hampshire	105	0.0%
13	New Jersey	20,846	3.5%
40	New Mexico	506	0.1%
1	New York	56,460	9.4%
7	North Carolina	27,476	4.6%
45	North Dakota	84	0.0%
11	Ohio	22,659	3.8%
25	Oklahoma	4,725	0.8%
36	Oregon	939	0.2%
14	Pennsylvania	20,408	3.4%
37	Rhode Island	931	0.2%
17	South Carolina	18,271	3.0%
44	South Dakota	91	0.0%
18	Tennessee	16,345	2.7%
4	Texas	39,476	6.6%
42	Utah	269	0.0%
50	Vermont	24	0.0%
12	Virginia	21,111	3.5%
28	Washington	3,214	0.5%
38	West Virginia	746	0.1%
23	Wisconsin	6,421	1.1%
48	Wyoming	63	0.0%

RANK	STATE	BIRTHS	% of USA
1	New York	56,460	9.4%
2	Florida	43,579	7.3%
3	Georgia	39,774	6.6%
4	Texas	39,476	6.6%
5	California	37,477	6.2%
6	Illinois	35,453	5.9%
7	North Carolina	27,476	4.6%
8	Louisiana	27,126	4.5%
9	Michigan	24,277	4.0%
10	Maryland	22,966	3.8%
11	Ohio	22,659	3.8%
12	Virginia	21,111	3.5%
13	New Jersey	20,846	3.5%
14	Pennsylvania	20,408	3.4%
15	Alabama	19,859	3.3%
16	Mississippi	19,541	3.3%
17	South Carolina	18,271	3.0%
18	Tennessee	16,345	2.7%
19	Missouri	11,144	1.9%
20	Massachusetts	7,922	1.3%
21	Arkansas	7,905	1.3%
22	Indiana	7,633	1.3%
23	Wisconsin	6,421	1.1%
24	Connecticut	5,238	0.9%
25	Oklahoma	4,725	0.8%
26	Kentucky	4,652	0.8%
27	Minnesota	3,252	0.5%
28	Washington	3,214	0.5%
29	Kansas	2,817	0.5%
30	Colorado	2,585	0.4%
31	Delaware	2,512	0.4%
32	Arizona	2,503	0.4%
33	Nevada	2,143	0.4%
34	Nebraska	1,253	0.2%
35	Iowa	1,109	0.2%
36	Oregon	939	0.2%
37	Rhode Island	931	0.2%
38	West Virginia	746	0.1%
39	Hawaii	578	0.1%
40	New Mexico	506	0.1%
41	Alaska	453	0.1%
42	Utah	269	0.0%
43	New Hampshire	105	0.0%
44	South Dakota	91	0.0%
45	North Dakota	84	0.0%
46	Maine	81	0.0%
47	Idaho	68	0.0%
48	Wyoming	63	0.0%
49	Montana	31	0.0%
50	Vermont	24	0.0%
	District of Columbia	5,795	1.0%

Source: U.S. Department of Health and Human Services, National Center for Health Statistics
"National Vital Statistics Report" (Vol. 47, No. 4, October 7, 1998)
*Preliminary data by state of residence. By race of mother.

Black Births as a Percent of All Births in 1997

National Percent = 15.4% of Live Births*

ALPHA ORDER				RANK ORDER		
RANK	**STATE**	**PERCENT**		**RANK**	**STATE**	**PERCENT**
6	Alabama	32.5		1	Mississippi	45.7
33	Alaska	4.7		2	Louisiana	41.1
37	Arizona	3.3		3	South Carolina	35.2
12	Arkansas	21.5		4	Georgia	33.6
30	California	7.1		5	Maryland	32.7
34	Colorado	4.6		6	Alabama	32.5
20	Connecticut	12.2		7	North Carolina	25.7
8	Delaware	24.5		8	Delaware	24.5
10	Florida	22.6		9	Virginia	22.9
4	Georgia	33.6		10	Florida	22.6
37	Hawaii	3.3		11	Tennessee	21.9
48	Idaho	0.4		12	Arkansas	21.5
14	Illinois	19.6		13	New York	21.4
25	Indiana	9.1		14	Illinois	19.6
39	Iowa	3.0		15	New Jersey	18.4
28	Kansas	7.5		16	Michigan	18.2
26	Kentucky	8.7		17	Missouri	14.9
2	Louisiana	41.1		17	Ohio	14.9
46	Maine	0.6		19	Pennsylvania	14.1
5	Maryland	32.7		20	Connecticut	12.2
23	Massachusetts	9.6		21	Texas	11.8
16	Michigan	18.2		22	Oklahoma	9.8
32	Minnesota	5.0		23	Massachusetts	9.6
1	Mississippi	45.7		23	Wisconsin	9.6
17	Missouri	14.9		25	Indiana	9.1
50	Montana	0.3		26	Kentucky	8.7
31	Nebraska	5.4		27	Nevada	7.9
27	Nevada	7.9		28	Kansas	7.5
45	New Hampshire	0.7		28	Rhode Island	7.5
15	New Jersey	18.4		30	California	7.1
41	New Mexico	1.9		31	Nebraska	5.4
13	New York	21.4		32	Minnesota	5.0
7	North Carolina	25.7		33	Alaska	4.7
42	North Dakota	1.0		34	Colorado	4.6
17	Ohio	14.9		35	Washington	4.1
22	Oklahoma	9.8		36	West Virginia	3.6
40	Oregon	2.1		37	Arizona	3.3
19	Pennsylvania	14.1		37	Hawaii	3.3
28	Rhode Island	7.5		39	Iowa	3.0
3	South Carolina	35.2		40	Oregon	2.1
44	South Dakota	0.9		41	New Mexico	1.9
11	Tennessee	21.9		42	North Dakota	1.0
21	Texas	11.8		42	Wyoming	1.0
46	Utah	0.6		44	South Dakota	0.9
48	Vermont	0.4		45	New Hampshire	0.7
9	Virginia	22.9		46	Maine	0.6
35	Washington	4.1		46	Utah	0.6
36	West Virginia	3.6		48	Idaho	0.4
23	Wisconsin	9.6		48	Vermont	0.4
42	Wyoming	1.0		50	Montana	0.3
					District of Columbia	73.3

*Source: Morgan Quitno Press using data from U.S. Dept. of Health and Human Services, Nat'l Center for Health Statistics
"National Vital Statistics Report" (Vol. 47, No. 4, October 7, 1998)*
Preliminary data by state of residence. By race of mother.

Births of Low Birthweight in 1997

National Total = 292,123 Live Births*

ALPHA ORDER

RANK	STATE	BIRTHS	% of USA
19	Alabama	5,677	1.9%
47	Alaska	573	0.2%
20	Arizona	5,227	1.8%
30	Arkansas	3,048	1.0%
1	California	32,614	11.2%
21	Colorado	4,975	1.7%
29	Connecticut	3,051	1.0%
42	Delaware	901	0.3%
4	Florida	15,404	5.3%
8	Georgia	10,415	3.6%
39	Hawaii	1,217	0.4%
40	Idaho	1,171	0.4%
5	Illinois	14,291	4.9%
16	Indiana	6,092	2.1%
34	Iowa	2,364	0.8%
32	Kansas	2,584	0.9%
26	Kentucky	4,152	1.4%
13	Louisiana	6,667	2.3%
44	Maine	807	0.3%
15	Maryland	6,183	2.1%
17	Massachusetts	5,771	2.0%
9	Michigan	10,289	3.5%
27	Minnesota	3,742	1.3%
24	Mississippi	4,317	1.5%
18	Missouri	5,756	2.0%
45	Montana	684	0.2%
38	Nebraska	1,633	0.6%
36	Nevada	2,082	0.7%
43	New Hampshire	837	0.3%
11	New Jersey	8,825	3.0%
35	New Mexico	2,096	0.7%
3	New York	20,540	7.0%
10	North Carolina	9,417	3.2%
49	North Dakota	518	0.2%
6	Ohio	11,724	4.0%
28	Oklahoma	3,512	1.2%
33	Oregon	2,414	0.8%
7	Pennsylvania	10,962	3.8%
41	Rhode Island	917	0.3%
22	South Carolina	4,723	1.6%
48	South Dakota	561	0.2%
14	Tennessee	6,563	2.2%
2	Texas	24,374	8.3%
31	Utah	2,896	1.0%
50	Vermont	420	0.1%
12	Virginia	7,083	2.4%
23	Washington	4,425	1.5%
37	West Virginia	1,722	0.6%
25	Wisconsin	4,263	1.5%
46	Wyoming	578	0.2%

RANK ORDER

RANK	STATE	BIRTHS	% of USA
1	California	32,614	11.2%
2	Texas	24,374	8.3%
3	New York	20,540	7.0%
4	Florida	15,404	5.3%
5	Illinois	14,291	4.9%
6	Ohio	11,724	4.0%
7	Pennsylvania	10,962	3.8%
8	Georgia	10,415	3.6%
9	Michigan	10,289	3.5%
10	North Carolina	9,417	3.2%
11	New Jersey	8,825	3.0%
12	Virginia	7,083	2.4%
13	Louisiana	6,667	2.3%
14	Tennessee	6,563	2.2%
15	Maryland	6,183	2.1%
16	Indiana	6,092	2.1%
17	Massachusetts	5,771	2.0%
18	Missouri	5,756	2.0%
19	Alabama	5,677	1.9%
20	Arizona	5,227	1.8%
21	Colorado	4,975	1.7%
22	South Carolina	4,723	1.6%
23	Washington	4,425	1.5%
24	Mississippi	4,317	1.5%
25	Wisconsin	4,263	1.5%
26	Kentucky	4,152	1.4%
27	Minnesota	3,742	1.3%
28	Oklahoma	3,512	1.2%
29	Connecticut	3,051	1.0%
30	Arkansas	3,048	1.0%
31	Utah	2,896	1.0%
32	Kansas	2,584	0.9%
33	Oregon	2,414	0.8%
34	Iowa	2,364	0.8%
35	New Mexico	2,096	0.7%
36	Nevada	2,082	0.7%
37	West Virginia	1,722	0.6%
38	Nebraska	1,633	0.6%
39	Hawaii	1,217	0.4%
40	Idaho	1,171	0.4%
41	Rhode Island	917	0.3%
42	Delaware	901	0.3%
43	New Hampshire	837	0.3%
44	Maine	807	0.3%
45	Montana	684	0.2%
46	Wyoming	578	0.2%
47	Alaska	573	0.2%
48	South Dakota	561	0.2%
49	North Dakota	518	0.2%
50	Vermont	420	0.1%
	District of Columbia	1,051	0.4%

Source: Morgan Quitno Press using data from U.S. Dept. of Health and Human Services, Nat'l Center for Health Statistics "National Vital Statistics Report" (Vol. 47, No. 4, October 7, 1998)

Estimates based on preliminary data by state of residence. Births of less than 2,500 grams (5 pounds 8 ounces).

Births of Low Birthweight as a Percent of All Births in 1997

National Percent = 7.5% of Live Births*

ALPHA ORDER			RANK ORDER		
RANK	STATE	PERCENT	RANK	STATE	PERCENT
3	Alabama	9.3	1	Louisiana	10.1
44	Alaska	5.9	1	Mississippi	10.1
34	Arizona	6.9	3	Alabama	9.3
12	Arkansas	8.3	4	South Carolina	9.1
42	California	6.2	5	Wyoming	9.0
6	Colorado	8.8	6	Colorado	8.8
30	Connecticut	7.1	6	Delaware	8.8
6	Delaware	8.8	6	Georgia	8.8
14	Florida	8.0	6	Maryland	8.8
6	Georgia	8.8	6	North Carolina	8.8
31	Hawaii	7.0	6	Tennessee	8.8
39	Idaho	6.3	12	Arkansas	8.3
15	Illinois	7.9	12	West Virginia	8.3
27	Indiana	7.3	14	Florida	8.0
37	Iowa	6.4	15	Illinois	7.9
34	Kansas	6.9	16	Kentucky	7.8
16	Kentucky	7.8	16	New Jersey	7.8
1	Louisiana	10.1	16	New Mexico	7.8
44	Maine	5.9	16	New York	7.8
6	Maryland	8.8	20	Michigan	7.7
31	Massachusetts	7.0	20	Missouri	7.7
20	Michigan	7.7	20	Nevada	7.7
46	Minnesota	5.8	20	Ohio	7.7
1	Mississippi	10.1	20	Virginia	7.7
20	Missouri	7.7	25	Pennsylvania	7.6
39	Montana	6.3	26	Rhode Island	7.4
31	Nebraska	7.0	27	Indiana	7.3
20	Nevada	7.7	27	Oklahoma	7.3
46	New Hampshire	5.8	27	Texas	7.3
16	New Jersey	7.8	30	Connecticut	7.1
16	New Mexico	7.8	31	Hawaii	7.0
16	New York	7.8	31	Massachusetts	7.0
6	North Carolina	8.8	31	Nebraska	7.0
42	North Dakota	6.2	34	Arizona	6.9
20	Ohio	7.7	34	Kansas	6.9
27	Oklahoma	7.3	36	Utah	6.6
49	Oregon	5.5	37	Iowa	6.4
25	Pennsylvania	7.6	37	Wisconsin	6.4
26	Rhode Island	7.4	39	Idaho	6.3
4	South Carolina	9.1	39	Montana	6.3
49	South Dakota	5.5	39	Vermont	6.3
6	Tennessee	8.8	42	California	6.2
27	Texas	7.3	42	North Dakota	6.2
36	Utah	6.6	44	Alaska	5.9
39	Vermont	6.3	44	Maine	5.9
20	Virginia	7.7	46	Minnesota	5.8
48	Washington	5.6	46	New Hampshire	5.8
12	West Virginia	8.3	48	Washington	5.6
37	Wisconsin	6.4	49	Oregon	5.5
5	Wyoming	9.0	49	South Dakota	5.5
				District of Columbia	13.3

Source: U.S. Department of Health and Human Services, National Center for Health Statistics
   "National Vital Statistics Report" (Vol. 47, No. 4, October 7, 1998)
*Estimates based on preliminary data by state of residence. Births of less than 2,500 grams (5 pounds 8 ounces).

Births of Low Birthweight to White Women in 1997

National Total = 200,556 Live Births*

ALPHA ORDER

RANK	STATE	BIRTHS	% of USA
23	Alabama	2,999	1.5%
49	Alaska	356	0.2%
15	Arizona	4,377	2.2%
33	Arkansas	2,032	1.0%
1	California	23,918	11.9%
14	Colorado	4,396	2.2%
28	Connecticut	2,318	1.2%
45	Delaware	517	0.3%
4	Florida	9,804	4.9%
12	Georgia	4,994	2.5%
50	Hawaii	219	0.1%
39	Idaho	1,135	0.6%
5	Illinois	8,890	4.4%
11	Indiana	5,009	2.5%
30	Iowa	2,159	1.1%
31	Kansas	2,138	1.1%
20	Kentucky	3,548	1.8%
26	Louisiana	2,635	1.3%
41	Maine	786	0.4%
24	Maryland	2,847	1.4%
13	Massachusetts	4,646	2.3%
8	Michigan	6,872	3.4%
22	Minnesota	3,154	1.6%
35	Mississippi	1,653	0.8%
17	Missouri	4,164	2.1%
43	Montana	575	0.3%
38	Nebraska	1,428	0.7%
36	Nevada	1,630	0.8%
40	New Hampshire	833	0.4%
9	New Jersey	5,416	2.7%
34	New Mexico	1,773	0.9%
3	New York	12,667	6.3%
10	North Carolina	5,388	2.7%
47	North Dakota	459	0.2%
6	Ohio	8,524	4.3%
27	Oklahoma	2,577	1.3%
32	Oregon	2,137	1.1%
7	Pennsylvania	7,814	3.9%
42	Rhode Island	749	0.4%
29	South Carolina	2,205	1.1%
46	South Dakota	473	0.2%
16	Tennessee	4,224	2.1%
2	Texas	18,476	9.2%
25	Utah	2,708	1.4%
48	Vermont	415	0.2%
18	Virginia	4,142	2.1%
19	Washington	3,622	1.8%
37	West Virginia	1,610	0.8%
21	Wisconsin	3,274	1.6%
44	Wyoming	555	0.3%

RANK ORDER

RANK	STATE	BIRTHS	% of USA
1	California	23,918	11.9%
2	Texas	18,476	9.2%
3	New York	12,667	6.3%
4	Florida	9,804	4.9%
5	Illinois	8,890	4.4%
6	Ohio	8,524	4.3%
7	Pennsylvania	7,814	3.9%
8	Michigan	6,872	3.4%
9	New Jersey	5,416	2.7%
10	North Carolina	5,388	2.7%
11	Indiana	5,009	2.5%
12	Georgia	4,994	2.5%
13	Massachusetts	4,646	2.3%
14	Colorado	4,396	2.2%
15	Arizona	4,377	2.2%
16	Tennessee	4,224	2.1%
17	Missouri	4,164	2.1%
18	Virginia	4,142	2.1%
19	Washington	3,622	1.8%
20	Kentucky	3,548	1.8%
21	Wisconsin	3,274	1.6%
22	Minnesota	3,154	1.6%
23	Alabama	2,999	1.5%
24	Maryland	2,847	1.4%
25	Utah	2,708	1.4%
26	Louisiana	2,635	1.3%
27	Oklahoma	2,577	1.3%
28	Connecticut	2,318	1.2%
29	South Carolina	2,205	1.1%
30	Iowa	2,159	1.1%
31	Kansas	2,138	1.1%
32	Oregon	2,137	1.1%
33	Arkansas	2,032	1.0%
34	New Mexico	1,773	0.9%
35	Mississippi	1,653	0.8%
36	Nevada	1,630	0.8%
37	West Virginia	1,610	0.8%
38	Nebraska	1,428	0.7%
39	Idaho	1,135	0.6%
40	New Hampshire	833	0.4%
41	Maine	786	0.4%
42	Rhode Island	749	0.4%
43	Montana	575	0.3%
44	Wyoming	555	0.3%
45	Delaware	517	0.3%
46	South Dakota	473	0.2%
47	North Dakota	459	0.2%
48	Vermont	415	0.2%
49	Alaska	356	0.2%
50	Hawaii	219	0.1%
	District of Columbia	116	0.1%

Source: Morgan Quitno Press using data from U.S. Dept. of Health and Human Services, Nat'l Center for Health Statistics "National Vital Statistics Report" (Vol. 47, No. 4, October 7, 1998)

Preliminary data by state of residence. Births of less than 2,500 grams (5 pounds 8 ounces). Calculated by the editors by multiplying total number of births to white women by percent of such births reported as being of low birthweight.

Births of Low Birthweight to White Women
As a Percent of All Births to White Women in 1997
National Percent = 6.5% of Live Births to White Women*

ALPHA ORDER

RANK	STATE	PERCENT
5	Alabama	7.4
46	Alaska	5.5
23	Arizona	6.6
9	Arkansas	7.2
44	California	5.6
2	Colorado	8.5
30	Connecticut	6.4
13	Delaware	6.9
15	Florida	6.8
23	Georgia	6.6
50	Hawaii	4.9
35	Idaho	6.3
30	Illinois	6.4
17	Indiana	6.7
37	Iowa	6.2
30	Kansas	6.4
5	Kentucky	7.4
12	Louisiana	7.0
41	Maine	5.9
30	Maryland	6.4
23	Massachusetts	6.6
26	Michigan	6.5
46	Minnesota	5.5
8	Mississippi	7.3
17	Missouri	6.7
40	Montana	6.1
17	Nebraska	6.7
10	Nevada	7.1
41	New Hampshire	5.9
30	New Jersey	6.4
4	New Mexico	7.8
17	New York	6.7
10	North Carolina	7.1
37	North Dakota	6.2
17	Ohio	6.7
15	Oklahoma	6.8
48	Oregon	5.3
26	Pennsylvania	6.5
13	Rhode Island	6.9
17	South Carolina	6.7
44	South Dakota	5.6
5	Tennessee	7.4
26	Texas	6.5
26	Utah	6.5
35	Vermont	6.3
37	Virginia	6.2
48	Washington	5.3
3	West Virginia	8.1
43	Wisconsin	5.7
1	Wyoming	9.1

RANK ORDER

RANK	STATE	PERCENT
1	Wyoming	9.1
2	Colorado	8.5
3	West Virginia	8.1
4	New Mexico	7.8
5	Alabama	7.4
5	Kentucky	7.4
5	Tennessee	7.4
8	Mississippi	7.3
9	Arkansas	7.2
10	Nevada	7.1
10	North Carolina	7.1
12	Louisiana	7.0
13	Delaware	6.9
13	Rhode Island	6.9
15	Florida	6.8
15	Oklahoma	6.8
17	Indiana	6.7
17	Missouri	6.7
17	Nebraska	6.7
17	New York	6.7
17	Ohio	6.7
17	South Carolina	6.7
23	Arizona	6.6
23	Georgia	6.6
23	Massachusetts	6.6
26	Michigan	6.5
26	Pennsylvania	6.5
26	Texas	6.5
26	Utah	6.5
30	Connecticut	6.4
30	Illinois	6.4
30	Kansas	6.4
30	Maryland	6.4
30	New Jersey	6.4
35	Idaho	6.3
35	Vermont	6.3
37	Iowa	6.2
37	North Dakota	6.2
37	Virginia	6.2
40	Montana	6.1
41	Maine	5.9
41	New Hampshire	5.9
43	Wisconsin	5.7
44	California	5.6
44	South Dakota	5.6
46	Alaska	5.5
46	Minnesota	5.5
48	Oregon	5.3
48	Washington	5.3
50	Hawaii	4.9
	District of Columbia	5.9

Source: U.S. Department of Health and Human Services, National Center for Health Statistics
"National Vital Statistics Report" (Vol. 47, No. 4, October 7, 1998)
*Preliminary data by state of residence. Births of less than 2,500 grams (5 pounds 8 ounces).

Births of Low Birthweight to Black Women in 1997

National Total = 78,117 Live Births*

<u>ALPHA ORDER</u>

RANK	STATE	BIRTHS	% of USA
16	Alabama	2,602	3.3%
41	Alaska	54	0.1%
31	Arizona	340	0.4%
21	Arkansas	996	1.3%
6	California	4,535	5.8%
27	Colorado	390	0.5%
24	Connecticut	634	0.8%
29	Delaware	354	0.5%
2	Florida	5,317	6.8%
3	Georgia	5,171	6.6%
40	Hawaii	57	0.1%
NA	Idaho**	NA	NA
4	Illinois	4,928	6.3%
20	Indiana	1,008	1.3%
35	Iowa	115	0.1%
28	Kansas	363	0.5%
26	Kentucky	558	0.7%
7	Louisiana	3,960	5.1%
NA	Maine**	NA	NA
10	Maryland	3,123	4.0%
23	Massachusetts	840	1.1%
9	Michigan	3,205	4.1%
29	Minnesota	354	0.5%
15	Mississippi	2,618	3.4%
19	Missouri	1,504	1.9%
NA	Montana**	NA	NA
34	Nebraska	147	0.2%
33	Nevada	294	0.4%
NA	New Hampshire**	NA	NA
12	New Jersey	2,856	3.7%
39	New Mexico	79	0.1%
1	New York	6,662	8.5%
8	North Carolina	3,737	4.8%
NA	North Dakota**	NA	NA
11	Ohio	3,082	3.9%
25	Oklahoma	581	0.7%
37	Oregon	104	0.1%
13	Pennsylvania	2,837	3.6%
36	Rhode Island	111	0.1%
17	South Carolina	2,467	3.2%
NA	South Dakota**	NA	NA
18	Tennessee	2,239	2.9%
5	Texas	4,895	6.3%
42	Utah	37	0.0%
NA	Vermont**	NA	NA
14	Virginia	2,660	3.4%
32	Washington	328	0.4%
38	West Virginia	95	0.1%
22	Wisconsin	854	1.1%
NA	Wyoming**	NA	NA

<u>RANK ORDER</u>

RANK	STATE	BIRTHS	% of USA
1	New York	6,662	8.5%
2	Florida	5,317	6.8%
3	Georgia	5,171	6.6%
4	Illinois	4,928	6.3%
5	Texas	4,895	6.3%
6	California	4,535	5.8%
7	Louisiana	3,960	5.1%
8	North Carolina	3,737	4.8%
9	Michigan	3,205	4.1%
10	Maryland	3,123	4.0%
11	Ohio	3,082	3.9%
12	New Jersey	2,856	3.7%
13	Pennsylvania	2,837	3.6%
14	Virginia	2,660	3.4%
15	Mississippi	2,618	3.4%
16	Alabama	2,602	3.3%
17	South Carolina	2,467	3.2%
18	Tennessee	2,239	2.9%
19	Missouri	1,504	1.9%
20	Indiana	1,008	1.3%
21	Arkansas	996	1.3%
22	Wisconsin	854	1.1%
23	Massachusetts	840	1.1%
24	Connecticut	634	0.8%
25	Oklahoma	581	0.7%
26	Kentucky	558	0.7%
27	Colorado	390	0.5%
28	Kansas	363	0.5%
29	Delaware	354	0.5%
29	Minnesota	354	0.5%
31	Arizona	340	0.4%
32	Washington	328	0.4%
33	Nevada	294	0.4%
34	Nebraska	147	0.2%
35	Iowa	115	0.1%
36	Rhode Island	111	0.1%
37	Oregon	104	0.1%
38	West Virginia	95	0.1%
39	New Mexico	79	0.1%
40	Hawaii	57	0.1%
41	Alaska	54	0.1%
42	Utah	37	0.0%
NA	Idaho**	NA	NA
NA	Maine**	NA	NA
NA	Montana**	NA	NA
NA	New Hampshire**	NA	NA
NA	North Dakota**	NA	NA
NA	South Dakota**	NA	NA
NA	Vermont**	NA	NA
NA	Wyoming**	NA	NA

District of Columbia 927 1.2%

Source: Morgan Quitno Press using data from U.S. Dept. of Health and Human Services, Nat'l Center for Health Statistics
"National Vital Statistics Report" (Vol. 47, No. 4, October 7, 1998)
*Preliminary data by state of residence. Births of less than 2,500 grams (5 pounds 8 ounces). Calculated by the editors by multiplying total number of births to black women by percent of such births reported as being of low birthweight.
**Not available.

Births of Low Birthweight to Black Women
As a Percent of All Births to Black Women in 1997
National Percent = 13.0% of Live Births to Black Women*

ALPHA ORDER				RANK ORDER		
RANK	STATE	PERCENT		RANK	STATE	PERCENT
21	Alabama	13.1		1	New Mexico	15.6
33	Alaska	11.9		2	Colorado	15.1
11	Arizona	13.6		3	Louisiana	14.6
25	Arkansas	12.6		4	Delaware	14.1
30	California	12.1		5	Illinois	13.9
2	Colorado	15.1		5	Pennsylvania	13.9
30	Connecticut	12.1		7	Nevada	13.7
4	Delaware	14.1		7	New Jersey	13.7
29	Florida	12.2		7	Tennessee	13.7
22	Georgia	13.0		7	Utah	13.7
42	Hawaii	9.8		11	Arizona	13.6
NA	Idaho**	NA		11	Maryland	13.6
5	Illinois	13.9		11	North Carolina	13.6
19	Indiana	13.2		11	Ohio	13.6
40	Iowa	10.4		15	Missouri	13.5
23	Kansas	12.9		15	South Carolina	13.5
32	Kentucky	12.0		17	Mississippi	13.4
3	Louisiana	14.6		18	Wisconsin	13.3
NA	Maine**	NA		19	Indiana	13.2
11	Maryland	13.6		19	Michigan	13.2
39	Massachusetts	10.6		21	Alabama	13.1
19	Michigan	13.2		22	Georgia	13.0
38	Minnesota	10.9		23	Kansas	12.9
17	Mississippi	13.4		24	West Virginia	12.8
15	Missouri	13.5		25	Arkansas	12.6
NA	Montana**	NA		25	Virginia	12.6
36	Nebraska	11.7		27	Texas	12.4
7	Nevada	13.7		28	Oklahoma	12.3
NA	New Hampshire**	NA		29	Florida	12.2
7	New Jersey	13.7		30	California	12.1
1	New Mexico	15.6		30	Connecticut	12.1
35	New York	11.8		32	Kentucky	12.0
11	North Carolina	13.6		33	Alaska	11.9
NA	North Dakota**	NA		33	Rhode Island	11.9
11	Ohio	13.6		35	New York	11.8
28	Oklahoma	12.3		36	Nebraska	11.7
37	Oregon	11.1		37	Oregon	11.1
5	Pennsylvania	13.9		38	Minnesota	10.9
33	Rhode Island	11.9		39	Massachusetts	10.6
15	South Carolina	13.5		40	Iowa	10.4
NA	South Dakota**	NA		41	Washington	10.2
7	Tennessee	13.7		42	Hawaii	9.8
27	Texas	12.4		NA	Idaho**	NA
7	Utah	13.7		NA	Maine**	NA
NA	Vermont**	NA		NA	Montana**	NA
25	Virginia	12.6		NA	New Hampshire**	NA
41	Washington	10.2		NA	North Dakota**	NA
24	West Virginia	12.8		NA	South Dakota**	NA
18	Wisconsin	13.3		NA	Vermont**	NA
NA	Wyoming**	NA		NA	Wyoming**	NA
					District of Columbia	16.0

Source: U.S. Department of Health and Human Services, National Center for Health Statistics
  "National Vital Statistics Report" (Vol. 47, No. 4, October 7, 1998)
*Preliminary data by state of residence. Births of less than 2,500 grams (5 pounds 8 ounces).
**Insufficient data.

Births to Unmarried Women in 1997

National Total = 1,261,970 Live Births*

ALPHA ORDER

RANK	STATE	BIRTHS	% of USA
21	Alabama	20,692	1.6%
47	Alaska	2,941	0.2%
13	Arizona	28,559	2.3%
31	Arkansas	12,558	1.0%
1	California	172,539	13.7%
28	Colorado	14,248	1.1%
29	Connecticut	13,925	1.1%
43	Delaware	3,687	0.3%
4	Florida	69,320	5.5%
9	Georgia	41,895	3.3%
39	Hawaii	5,180	0.4%
42	Idaho	3,849	0.3%
5	Illinois	60,420	4.8%
15	Indiana	26,870	2.1%
34	Iowa	9,676	0.8%
33	Kansas	10,335	0.8%
26	Kentucky	15,702	1.2%
12	Louisiana	28,979	2.3%
41	Maine	4,060	0.3%
18	Maryland	23,539	1.9%
19	Massachusetts	21,436	1.7%
8	Michigan	44,496	3.5%
25	Minnesota	15,938	1.3%
23	Mississippi	19,450	1.5%
17	Missouri	24,741	2.0%
46	Montana	3,125	0.2%
38	Nebraska	6,018	0.5%
35	Nevada	9,599	0.8%
44	New Hampshire	3,435	0.3%
11	New Jersey	31,453	2.5%
32	New Mexico	11,690	0.9%
3	New York	92,169	7.3%
10	North Carolina	34,458	2.7%
48	North Dakota	2,173	0.2%
6	Ohio	51,618	4.1%
27	Oklahoma	15,540	1.2%
30	Oregon	12,642	1.0%
7	Pennsylvania	47,309	3.7%
40	Rhode Island	4,088	0.3%
22	South Carolina	19,724	1.6%
45	South Dakota	3,175	0.3%
16	Tennessee	25,431	2.0%
2	Texas	102,504	8.1%
36	Utah	7,241	0.6%
50	Vermont	1,740	0.1%
14	Virginia	26,953	2.1%
20	Washington	21,416	1.7%
37	West Virginia	6,495	0.5%
24	Wisconsin	18,715	1.5%
49	Wyoming	1,754	0.1%

RANK ORDER

RANK	STATE	BIRTHS	% of USA
1	California	172,539	13.7%
2	Texas	102,504	8.1%
3	New York	92,169	7.3%
4	Florida	69,320	5.5%
5	Illinois	60,420	4.8%
6	Ohio	51,618	4.1%
7	Pennsylvania	47,309	3.7%
8	Michigan	44,496	3.5%
9	Georgia	41,895	3.3%
10	North Carolina	34,458	2.7%
11	New Jersey	31,453	2.5%
12	Louisiana	28,979	2.3%
13	Arizona	28,559	2.3%
14	Virginia	26,953	2.1%
15	Indiana	26,870	2.1%
16	Tennessee	25,431	2.0%
17	Missouri	24,741	2.0%
18	Maryland	23,539	1.9%
19	Massachusetts	21,436	1.7%
20	Washington	21,416	1.7%
21	Alabama	20,692	1.6%
22	South Carolina	19,724	1.6%
23	Mississippi	19,450	1.5%
24	Wisconsin	18,715	1.5%
25	Minnesota	15,938	1.3%
26	Kentucky	15,702	1.2%
27	Oklahoma	15,540	1.2%
28	Colorado	14,248	1.1%
29	Connecticut	13,925	1.1%
30	Oregon	12,642	1.0%
31	Arkansas	12,558	1.0%
32	New Mexico	11,690	0.9%
33	Kansas	10,335	0.8%
34	Iowa	9,676	0.8%
35	Nevada	9,599	0.8%
36	Utah	7,241	0.6%
37	West Virginia	6,495	0.5%
38	Nebraska	6,018	0.5%
39	Hawaii	5,180	0.4%
40	Rhode Island	4,088	0.3%
41	Maine	4,060	0.3%
42	Idaho	3,849	0.3%
43	Delaware	3,687	0.3%
44	New Hampshire	3,435	0.3%
45	South Dakota	3,175	0.3%
46	Montana	3,125	0.2%
47	Alaska	2,941	0.2%
48	North Dakota	2,173	0.2%
49	Wyoming	1,754	0.1%
50	Vermont	1,740	0.1%
	District of Columbia	5,028	0.4%

Source: Morgan Quitno Press using data from U.S. Dept. of Health and Human Services, Nat'l Center for Health Statistics "National Vital Statistics Report" (Vol. 47, No. 4, October 7, 1998)

Preliminary data by state of residence. Calculated by the editors by multiplying total number of births by reported percent of births to unmarried women.

Births to Unmarried Women as a Percent of All Births in 1997

National Percent = 32.4% of Live Births*

ALPHA ORDER

RANK	STATE	PERCENT
13	Alabama	33.9
29	Alaska	30.3
5	Arizona	37.7
11	Arkansas	34.2
20	California	32.8
46	Colorado	25.2
22	Connecticut	32.4
6	Delaware	36.0
6	Florida	36.0
9	Georgia	35.4
30	Hawaii	29.8
49	Idaho	20.7
16	Illinois	33.4
24	Indiana	32.2
41	Iowa	26.2
38	Kansas	27.6
32	Kentucky	29.5
2	Louisiana	43.9
31	Maine	29.7
15	Maryland	33.5
43	Massachusetts	26.0
17	Michigan	33.3
47	Minnesota	24.7
1	Mississippi	45.5
18	Missouri	33.1
34	Montana	28.8
45	Nebraska	25.8
8	Nevada	35.5
48	New Hampshire	23.8
37	New Jersey	27.8
3	New Mexico	43.5
10	New York	35.0
24	North Carolina	32.2
43	North Dakota	26.0
13	Ohio	33.9
23	Oklahoma	32.3
34	Oregon	28.8
20	Pennsylvania	32.8
19	Rhode Island	33.0
4	South Carolina	38.0
27	South Dakota	31.1
12	Tennessee	34.1
28	Texas	30.7
50	Utah	16.5
42	Vermont	26.1
33	Virginia	29.3
40	Washington	27.1
26	West Virginia	31.3
36	Wisconsin	28.1
39	Wyoming	27.3

RANK ORDER

RANK	STATE	PERCENT
1	Mississippi	45.5
2	Louisiana	43.9
3	New Mexico	43.5
4	South Carolina	38.0
5	Arizona	37.7
6	Delaware	36.0
6	Florida	36.0
8	Nevada	35.5
9	Georgia	35.4
10	New York	35.0
11	Arkansas	34.2
12	Tennessee	34.1
13	Alabama	33.9
13	Ohio	33.9
15	Maryland	33.5
16	Illinois	33.4
17	Michigan	33.3
18	Missouri	33.1
19	Rhode Island	33.0
20	California	32.8
20	Pennsylvania	32.8
22	Connecticut	32.4
23	Oklahoma	32.3
24	Indiana	32.2
24	North Carolina	32.2
26	West Virginia	31.3
27	South Dakota	31.1
28	Texas	30.7
29	Alaska	30.3
30	Hawaii	29.8
31	Maine	29.7
32	Kentucky	29.5
33	Virginia	29.3
34	Montana	28.8
34	Oregon	28.8
36	Wisconsin	28.1
37	New Jersey	27.8
38	Kansas	27.6
39	Wyoming	27.3
40	Washington	27.1
41	Iowa	26.2
42	Vermont	26.1
43	Massachusetts	26.0
43	North Dakota	26.0
45	Nebraska	25.8
46	Colorado	25.2
47	Minnesota	24.7
48	New Hampshire	23.8
49	Idaho	20.7
50	Utah	16.5
	District of Columbia	63.6

Source: U.S. Department of Health and Human Services, National Center for Health Statistics
    "National Vital Statistics Report" (Vol. 47, No. 4, October 7, 1998)
Data are preliminary estimates by state of residence.

Births to Unmarried White Women in 1997

National Total = 796,053 Live Births*

ALPHA ORDER

RANK	STATE	BIRTHS	% of USA
32	Alabama	6,849	0.9%
49	Alaska	1,385	0.2%
9	Arizona	23,013	2.9%
35	Arkansas	6,520	0.8%
1	California	138,808	17.4%
20	Colorado	12,360	1.6%
25	Connecticut	9,669	1.2%
45	Delaware	1,881	0.2%
4	Florida	39,071	4.9%
16	Georgia	14,830	1.9%
50	Hawaii	766	0.1%
40	Idaho	3,638	0.5%
6	Illinois	32,644	4.1%
10	Indiana	20,859	2.6%
29	Iowa	8,568	1.1%
30	Kansas	8,050	1.0%
21	Kentucky	12,227	1.5%
28	Louisiana	8,846	1.1%
39	Maine	3,931	0.5%
26	Maryland	9,120	1.1%
13	Massachusetts	15,908	2.0%
8	Michigan	25,479	3.2%
22	Minnesota	12,158	1.5%
38	Mississippi	4,461	0.6%
14	Missouri	15,786	2.0%
43	Montana	2,188	0.3%
37	Nebraska	4,796	0.6%
31	Nevada	7,509	0.9%
41	New Hampshire	3,346	0.4%
12	New Jersey	17,178	2.2%
27	New Mexico	9,002	1.1%
3	New York	51,990	6.5%
15	North Carolina	15,101	1.9%
48	North Dakota	1,576	0.2%
5	Ohio	33,843	4.3%
24	Oklahoma	9,890	1.2%
23	Oregon	11,248	1.4%
7	Pennsylvania	30,777	3.9%
42	Rhode Island	3,237	0.4%
33	South Carolina	6,845	0.9%
44	South Dakota	1,928	0.2%
17	Tennessee	13,185	1.7%
2	Texas	76,462	9.6%
34	Utah	6,542	0.8%
46	Vermont	1,724	0.2%
18	Virginia	13,094	1.6%
11	Washington	17,495	2.2%
36	West Virginia	5,923	0.7%
19	Wisconsin	12,637	1.6%
47	Wyoming	1,598	0.2%

RANK ORDER

RANK	STATE	BIRTHS	% of USA
1	California	138,808	17.4%
2	Texas	76,462	9.6%
3	New York	51,990	6.5%
4	Florida	39,071	4.9%
5	Ohio	33,843	4.3%
6	Illinois	32,644	4.1%
7	Pennsylvania	30,777	3.9%
8	Michigan	25,479	3.2%
9	Arizona	23,013	2.9%
10	Indiana	20,859	2.6%
11	Washington	17,495	2.2%
12	New Jersey	17,178	2.2%
13	Massachusetts	15,908	2.0%
14	Missouri	15,786	2.0%
15	North Carolina	15,101	1.9%
16	Georgia	14,830	1.9%
17	Tennessee	13,185	1.7%
18	Virginia	13,094	1.6%
19	Wisconsin	12,637	1.6%
20	Colorado	12,360	1.6%
21	Kentucky	12,227	1.5%
22	Minnesota	12,158	1.5%
23	Oregon	11,248	1.4%
24	Oklahoma	9,890	1.2%
25	Connecticut	9,669	1.2%
26	Maryland	9,120	1.1%
27	New Mexico	9,002	1.1%
28	Louisiana	8,846	1.1%
29	Iowa	8,568	1.1%
30	Kansas	8,050	1.0%
31	Nevada	7,509	0.9%
32	Alabama	6,849	0.9%
33	South Carolina	6,845	0.9%
34	Utah	6,542	0.8%
35	Arkansas	6,520	0.8%
36	West Virginia	5,923	0.7%
37	Nebraska	4,796	0.6%
38	Mississippi	4,461	0.6%
39	Maine	3,931	0.5%
40	Idaho	3,638	0.5%
41	New Hampshire	3,346	0.4%
42	Rhode Island	3,237	0.4%
43	Montana	2,188	0.3%
44	South Dakota	1,928	0.2%
45	Delaware	1,881	0.2%
46	Vermont	1,724	0.2%
47	Wyoming	1,598	0.2%
48	North Dakota	1,576	0.2%
49	Alaska	1,385	0.2%
50	Hawaii	766	0.1%
	District of Columbia	475	0.1%

Source: Morgan Quitno Press using data from U.S. Dept. of Health and Human Services, Nat'l Center for Health Statistics "National Vital Statistics Report" (Vol. 47, No. 4, October 7, 1998)
*Preliminary data by state of residence. Calculated by the editors by multiplying total number of births to white women by percent of such births reported as being to unmarried white women.

Births to Unmarried White Women
As a Percent of All Births to White Women in 1997
National Percent = 25.8% of Live Births*

ALPHA ORDER

RANK ORDER

RANK	STATE	PERCENT
49	Alabama	16.9
37	Alaska	21.4
2	Arizona	34.7
31	Arkansas	23.1
4	California	32.5
26	Colorado	23.9
13	Connecticut	26.7
22	Delaware	25.1
11	Florida	27.1
46	Georgia	19.6
48	Hawaii	17.1
43	Idaho	20.2
28	Illinois	23.5
8	Indiana	27.9
23	Iowa	24.6
24	Kansas	24.1
20	Kentucky	25.5
28	Louisiana	23.5
7	Maine	29.5
41	Maryland	20.5
34	Massachusetts	22.6
24	Michigan	24.1
39	Minnesota	21.2
45	Mississippi	19.7
21	Missouri	25.4
30	Montana	23.2
35	Nebraska	22.5
3	Nevada	32.7
27	New Hampshire	23.7
42	New Jersey	20.3
1	New Mexico	39.6
10	New York	27.5
44	North Carolina	19.9
38	North Dakota	21.3
14	Ohio	26.6
17	Oklahoma	26.1
8	Oregon	27.9
18	Pennsylvania	25.6
5	Rhode Island	29.8
40	South Carolina	20.8
33	South Dakota	22.8
31	Tennessee	23.1
12	Texas	26.9
50	Utah	15.7
15	Vermont	26.2
46	Virginia	19.6
18	Washington	25.6
5	West Virginia	29.8
36	Wisconsin	22.0
15	Wyoming	26.2

RANK	STATE	PERCENT
1	New Mexico	39.6
2	Arizona	34.7
3	Nevada	32.7
4	California	32.5
5	Rhode Island	29.8
5	West Virginia	29.8
7	Maine	29.5
8	Indiana	27.9
8	Oregon	27.9
10	New York	27.5
11	Florida	27.1
12	Texas	26.9
13	Connecticut	26.7
14	Ohio	26.6
15	Vermont	26.2
15	Wyoming	26.2
17	Oklahoma	26.1
18	Pennsylvania	25.6
18	Washington	25.6
20	Kentucky	25.5
21	Missouri	25.4
22	Delaware	25.1
23	Iowa	24.6
24	Kansas	24.1
24	Michigan	24.1
26	Colorado	23.9
27	New Hampshire	23.7
28	Illinois	23.5
28	Louisiana	23.5
30	Montana	23.2
31	Arkansas	23.1
31	Tennessee	23.1
33	South Dakota	22.8
34	Massachusetts	22.6
35	Nebraska	22.5
36	Wisconsin	22.0
37	Alaska	21.4
38	North Dakota	21.3
39	Minnesota	21.2
40	South Carolina	20.8
41	Maryland	20.5
42	New Jersey	20.3
43	Idaho	20.2
44	North Carolina	19.9
45	Mississippi	19.7
46	Georgia	19.6
46	Virginia	19.6
48	Hawaii	17.1
49	Alabama	16.9
50	Utah	15.7
	District of Columbia	24.1

Source: U.S. Department of Health and Human Services, National Center for Health Statistics
"National Vital Statistics Report" (Vol. 47, No. 4, October 7, 1998)
Preliminary data by state of residence. Calculated by the editors by multiplying total number of births to white women by percent of such births reported as being to unmarried white women.

Births to Unmarried Black Women in 1997

National Total = 415,221 Live Births*

<table>
<tr><td colspan="4"><u>ALPHA ORDER</u></td><td colspan="4"><u>RANK ORDER</u></td></tr>
<tr><td>RANK</td><td>STATE</td><td>BIRTHS</td><td>% of USA</td><td>RANK</td><td>STATE</td><td>BIRTHS</td><td>% of USA</td></tr>
<tr><td>15</td><td>Alabama</td><td>13,703</td><td>3.3%</td><td>1</td><td>New York</td><td>37,320</td><td>9.0%</td></tr>
<tr><td>40</td><td>Alaska</td><td>193</td><td>0.0%</td><td>2</td><td>Florida</td><td>29,329</td><td>7.1%</td></tr>
<tr><td>31</td><td>Arizona</td><td>1,619</td><td>0.4%</td><td>3</td><td>Illinois</td><td>27,299</td><td>6.6%</td></tr>
<tr><td>20</td><td>Arkansas</td><td>5,897</td><td>1.4%</td><td>4</td><td>Georgia</td><td>26,728</td><td>6.4%</td></tr>
<tr><td>6</td><td>California</td><td>23,348</td><td>5.6%</td><td>5</td><td>Texas</td><td>24,909</td><td>6.0%</td></tr>
<tr><td>33</td><td>Colorado</td><td>1,424</td><td>0.3%</td><td>6</td><td>California</td><td>23,348</td><td>5.6%</td></tr>
<tr><td>24</td><td>Connecticut</td><td>3,682</td><td>0.9%</td><td>7</td><td>Louisiana</td><td>19,856</td><td>4.8%</td></tr>
<tr><td>29</td><td>Delaware</td><td>1,789</td><td>0.4%</td><td>8</td><td>North Carolina</td><td>18,299</td><td>4.4%</td></tr>
<tr><td>2</td><td>Florida</td><td>29,329</td><td>7.1%</td><td>9</td><td>Michigan</td><td>18,281</td><td>4.4%</td></tr>
<tr><td>4</td><td>Georgia</td><td>26,728</td><td>6.4%</td><td>10</td><td>Ohio</td><td>17,493</td><td>4.2%</td></tr>
<tr><td>42</td><td>Hawaii</td><td>122</td><td>0.0%</td><td>11</td><td>Pennsylvania</td><td>15,877</td><td>3.8%</td></tr>
<tr><td>46</td><td>Idaho</td><td>31</td><td>0.0%</td><td>12</td><td>Mississippi</td><td>14,812</td><td>3.6%</td></tr>
<tr><td>3</td><td>Illinois</td><td>27,299</td><td>6.6%</td><td>13</td><td>Maryland</td><td>14,078</td><td>3.4%</td></tr>
<tr><td>21</td><td>Indiana</td><td>5,824</td><td>1.4%</td><td>14</td><td>New Jersey</td><td>13,800</td><td>3.3%</td></tr>
<tr><td>35</td><td>Iowa</td><td>835</td><td>0.2%</td><td>15</td><td>Alabama</td><td>13,703</td><td>3.3%</td></tr>
<tr><td>28</td><td>Kansas</td><td>1,958</td><td>0.5%</td><td>16</td><td>Virginia</td><td>13,405</td><td>3.2%</td></tr>
<tr><td>26</td><td>Kentucky</td><td>3,345</td><td>0.8%</td><td>17</td><td>South Carolina</td><td>12,771</td><td>3.1%</td></tr>
<tr><td>7</td><td>Louisiana</td><td>19,856</td><td>4.8%</td><td>18</td><td>Tennessee</td><td>12,014</td><td>2.9%</td></tr>
<tr><td>45</td><td>Maine</td><td>34</td><td>0.0%</td><td>19</td><td>Missouri</td><td>8,659</td><td>2.1%</td></tr>
<tr><td>13</td><td>Maryland</td><td>14,078</td><td>3.4%</td><td>20</td><td>Arkansas</td><td>5,897</td><td>1.4%</td></tr>
<tr><td>23</td><td>Massachusetts</td><td>4,698</td><td>1.1%</td><td>21</td><td>Indiana</td><td>5,824</td><td>1.4%</td></tr>
<tr><td>9</td><td>Michigan</td><td>18,281</td><td>4.4%</td><td>22</td><td>Wisconsin</td><td>5,291</td><td>1.3%</td></tr>
<tr><td>27</td><td>Minnesota</td><td>2,140</td><td>0.5%</td><td>23</td><td>Massachusetts</td><td>4,698</td><td>1.1%</td></tr>
<tr><td>12</td><td>Mississippi</td><td>14,812</td><td>3.6%</td><td>24</td><td>Connecticut</td><td>3,682</td><td>0.9%</td></tr>
<tr><td>19</td><td>Missouri</td><td>8,659</td><td>2.1%</td><td>25</td><td>Oklahoma</td><td>3,369</td><td>0.8%</td></tr>
<tr><td>NA</td><td>Montana***</td><td>NA</td><td>NA</td><td>26</td><td>Kentucky</td><td>3,345</td><td>0.8%</td></tr>
<tr><td>34</td><td>Nebraska</td><td>907</td><td>0.2%</td><td>27</td><td>Minnesota</td><td>2,140</td><td>0.5%</td></tr>
<tr><td>32</td><td>Nevada</td><td>1,470</td><td>0.4%</td><td>28</td><td>Kansas</td><td>1,958</td><td>0.5%</td></tr>
<tr><td>43</td><td>New Hampshire</td><td>54</td><td>0.0%</td><td>29</td><td>Delaware</td><td>1,789</td><td>0.4%</td></tr>
<tr><td>14</td><td>New Jersey</td><td>13,800</td><td>3.3%</td><td>30</td><td>Washington</td><td>1,748</td><td>0.4%</td></tr>
<tr><td>39</td><td>New Mexico</td><td>287</td><td>0.1%</td><td>31</td><td>Arizona</td><td>1,619</td><td>0.4%</td></tr>
<tr><td>1</td><td>New York</td><td>37,320</td><td>9.0%</td><td>32</td><td>Nevada</td><td>1,470</td><td>0.4%</td></tr>
<tr><td>8</td><td>North Carolina</td><td>18,299</td><td>4.4%</td><td>33</td><td>Colorado</td><td>1,424</td><td>0.3%</td></tr>
<tr><td>48</td><td>North Dakota</td><td>24</td><td>0.0%</td><td>34</td><td>Nebraska</td><td>907</td><td>0.2%</td></tr>
<tr><td>10</td><td>Ohio</td><td>17,493</td><td>4.2%</td><td>35</td><td>Iowa</td><td>835</td><td>0.2%</td></tr>
<tr><td>25</td><td>Oklahoma</td><td>3,369</td><td>0.8%</td><td>36</td><td>Oregon</td><td>626</td><td>0.2%</td></tr>
<tr><td>36</td><td>Oregon</td><td>626</td><td>0.2%</td><td>37</td><td>Rhode Island</td><td>600</td><td>0.1%</td></tr>
<tr><td>11</td><td>Pennsylvania</td><td>15,877</td><td>3.8%</td><td>38</td><td>West Virginia</td><td>568</td><td>0.1%</td></tr>
<tr><td>37</td><td>Rhode Island</td><td>600</td><td>0.1%</td><td>39</td><td>New Mexico</td><td>287</td><td>0.1%</td></tr>
<tr><td>17</td><td>South Carolina</td><td>12,771</td><td>3.1%</td><td>40</td><td>Alaska</td><td>193</td><td>0.0%</td></tr>
<tr><td>44</td><td>South Dakota</td><td>36</td><td>0.0%</td><td>41</td><td>Utah</td><td>149</td><td>0.0%</td></tr>
<tr><td>18</td><td>Tennessee</td><td>12,014</td><td>2.9%</td><td>42</td><td>Hawaii</td><td>122</td><td>0.0%</td></tr>
<tr><td>5</td><td>Texas</td><td>24,909</td><td>6.0%</td><td>43</td><td>New Hampshire</td><td>54</td><td>0.0%</td></tr>
<tr><td>41</td><td>Utah</td><td>149</td><td>0.0%</td><td>44</td><td>South Dakota</td><td>36</td><td>0.0%</td></tr>
<tr><td>NA</td><td>Vermont***</td><td>NA</td><td>NA</td><td>45</td><td>Maine</td><td>34</td><td>0.0%</td></tr>
<tr><td>16</td><td>Virginia</td><td>13,405</td><td>3.2%</td><td>46</td><td>Idaho</td><td>31</td><td>0.0%</td></tr>
<tr><td>30</td><td>Washington</td><td>1,748</td><td>0.4%</td><td>47</td><td>Wyoming</td><td>26</td><td>0.0%</td></tr>
<tr><td>38</td><td>West Virginia</td><td>568</td><td>0.1%</td><td>48</td><td>North Dakota</td><td>24</td><td>0.0%</td></tr>
<tr><td>22</td><td>Wisconsin</td><td>5,291</td><td>1.3%</td><td>NA</td><td>Montana***</td><td>NA</td><td>NA</td></tr>
<tr><td>47</td><td>Wyoming</td><td>26</td><td>0.0%</td><td>NA</td><td>Vermont***</td><td>NA</td><td>NA</td></tr>
<tr><td></td><td></td><td></td><td></td><td></td><td>District of Columbia</td><td>4,514</td><td>1.1%</td></tr>
</table>

Source: Morgan Quitno Press using data from U.S. Dept. of Health and Human Services, Nat'l Center for Health Statistics "National Vital Statistics Report" (Vol. 47, No. 4, October 7, 1998)
*Preliminary data by state of residence. Calculated by the editors by multiplying total number of births to black women by percent of such births reported as being to unmarried black women.

Births to Unmarried Black Women
As a Percent of All Births to Black Women in 1997
National Percent = 69.1% of Live Births*

ALPHA ORDER

RANK	STATE	PERCENT
21	Alabama	69.0
43	Alaska	42.5
30	Arizona	64.7
11	Arkansas	74.6
34	California	62.3
39	Colorado	55.1
18	Connecticut	70.3
17	Delaware	71.2
23	Florida	67.3
24	Georgia	67.2
48	Hawaii	21.1
42	Idaho	45.6
5	Illinois	77.0
6	Indiana	76.3
9	Iowa	75.3
20	Kansas	69.5
15	Kentucky	71.9
13	Louisiana	73.2
44	Maine	42.0
35	Maryland	61.3
36	Massachusetts	59.3
9	Michigan	75.3
29	Minnesota	65.8
8	Mississippi	75.8
3	Missouri	77.7
NA	Montana**	NA
14	Nebraska	72.4
22	Nevada	68.6
41	New Hampshire	51.0
27	New Jersey	66.2
37	New Mexico	56.7
28	New York	66.1
26	North Carolina	66.6
47	North Dakota	28.6
4	Ohio	77.2
16	Oklahoma	71.3
25	Oregon	66.7
2	Pennsylvania	77.8
31	Rhode Island	64.5
19	South Carolina	69.9
46	South Dakota	39.6
12	Tennessee	73.5
33	Texas	63.1
38	Utah	55.3
NA	Vermont**	NA
32	Virginia	63.5
40	Washington	54.4
7	West Virginia	76.1
1	Wisconsin	82.4
45	Wyoming	41.9

RANK ORDER

RANK	STATE	PERCENT
1	Wisconsin	82.4
2	Pennsylvania	77.8
3	Missouri	77.7
4	Ohio	77.2
5	Illinois	77.0
6	Indiana	76.3
7	West Virginia	76.1
8	Mississippi	75.8
9	Iowa	75.3
9	Michigan	75.3
11	Arkansas	74.6
12	Tennessee	73.5
13	Louisiana	73.2
14	Nebraska	72.4
15	Kentucky	71.9
16	Oklahoma	71.3
17	Delaware	71.2
18	Connecticut	70.3
19	South Carolina	69.9
20	Kansas	69.5
21	Alabama	69.0
22	Nevada	68.6
23	Florida	67.3
24	Georgia	67.2
25	Oregon	66.7
26	North Carolina	66.6
27	New Jersey	66.2
28	New York	66.1
29	Minnesota	65.8
30	Arizona	64.7
31	Rhode Island	64.5
32	Virginia	63.5
33	Texas	63.1
34	California	62.3
35	Maryland	61.3
36	Massachusetts	59.3
37	New Mexico	56.7
38	Utah	55.3
39	Colorado	55.1
40	Washington	54.4
41	New Hampshire	51.0
42	Idaho	45.6
43	Alaska	42.5
44	Maine	42.0
45	Wyoming	41.9
46	South Dakota	39.6
47	North Dakota	28.6
48	Hawaii	21.1
NA	Montana**	NA
NA	Vermont**	NA
	District of Columbia	77.9

Source: U.S. Department of Health and Human Services, National Center for Health Statistics
"National Vital Statistics Report" (Vol. 47, No. 4, October 7, 1998)
*Data are preliminary estimates by state of residence. By race of mother.
**Too few births for a reliable figure.

Births to Teenage Mothers in 1997

National Total = 498,556 Live Births*

ALPHA ORDER

RANK	STATE	BIRTHS	% of USA
15	Alabama	10,743	2.2%
47	Alaska	1,077	0.2%
14	Arizona	11,287	2.3%
26	Arkansas	7,050	1.4%
1	California	61,546	12.3%
27	Colorado	6,728	1.3%
36	Connecticut	3,524	0.7%
42	Delaware	1,373	0.3%
4	Florida	25,803	5.2%
7	Georgia	18,344	3.7%
40	Hawaii	1,912	0.4%
39	Idaho	2,361	0.5%
5	Illinois	22,612	4.5%
13	Indiana	11,849	2.4%
34	Iowa	3,952	0.8%
31	Kansas	4,868	1.0%
21	Kentucky	8,676	1.7%
11	Louisiana	12,278	2.5%
41	Maine	1,381	0.3%
24	Maryland	7,238	1.5%
28	Massachusetts	6,101	1.2%
8	Michigan	15,634	3.1%
29	Minnesota	5,614	1.1%
18	Mississippi	8,849	1.8%
16	Missouri	10,390	2.1%
44	Montana	1,324	0.3%
38	Nebraska	2,449	0.5%
35	Nevada	3,650	0.7%
46	New Hampshire	1,126	0.2%
19	New Jersey	8,825	1.8%
32	New Mexico	4,810	1.0%
3	New York	28,177	5.7%
9	North Carolina	15,303	3.1%
49	North Dakota	760	0.2%
6	Ohio	20,251	4.1%
23	Oklahoma	8,131	1.6%
30	Oregon	5,487	1.1%
10	Pennsylvania	15,000	3.0%
43	Rhode Island	1,326	0.3%
22	South Carolina	8,512	1.7%
45	South Dakota	1,245	0.2%
12	Tennessee	12,156	2.4%
2	Texas	53,756	10.8%
33	Utah	4,608	0.9%
50	Vermont	560	0.1%
17	Virginia	10,119	2.0%
20	Washington	8,693	1.7%
37	West Virginia	3,300	0.7%
25	Wisconsin	7,126	1.4%
48	Wyoming	906	0.2%

RANK ORDER

RANK	STATE	BIRTHS	% of USA
1	California	61,546	12.3%
2	Texas	53,756	10.8%
3	New York	28,177	5.7%
4	Florida	25,803	5.2%
5	Illinois	22,612	4.5%
6	Ohio	20,251	4.1%
7	Georgia	18,344	3.7%
8	Michigan	15,634	3.1%
9	North Carolina	15,303	3.1%
10	Pennsylvania	15,000	3.0%
11	Louisiana	12,278	2.5%
12	Tennessee	12,156	2.4%
13	Indiana	11,849	2.4%
14	Arizona	11,287	2.3%
15	Alabama	10,743	2.2%
16	Missouri	10,390	2.1%
17	Virginia	10,119	2.0%
18	Mississippi	8,849	1.8%
19	New Jersey	8,825	1.8%
20	Washington	8,693	1.7%
21	Kentucky	8,676	1.7%
22	South Carolina	8,512	1.7%
23	Oklahoma	8,131	1.6%
24	Maryland	7,238	1.5%
25	Wisconsin	7,126	1.4%
26	Arkansas	7,050	1.4%
27	Colorado	6,728	1.3%
28	Massachusetts	6,101	1.2%
29	Minnesota	5,614	1.1%
30	Oregon	5,487	1.1%
31	Kansas	4,868	1.0%
32	New Mexico	4,810	1.0%
33	Utah	4,608	0.9%
34	Iowa	3,952	0.8%
35	Nevada	3,650	0.7%
36	Connecticut	3,524	0.7%
37	West Virginia	3,300	0.7%
38	Nebraska	2,449	0.5%
39	Idaho	2,361	0.5%
40	Hawaii	1,912	0.4%
41	Maine	1,381	0.3%
42	Delaware	1,373	0.3%
43	Rhode Island	1,326	0.3%
44	Montana	1,324	0.3%
45	South Dakota	1,245	0.2%
46	New Hampshire	1,126	0.2%
47	Alaska	1,077	0.2%
48	Wyoming	906	0.2%
49	North Dakota	760	0.2%
50	Vermont	560	0.1%
	District of Columbia	1,233	0.2%

Source: Morgan Quitno Press using data from U.S. Dept. of Health and Human Services, Nat'l Center for Health Statistics "National Vital Statistics Report" (Vol. 47, No. 4, October 7, 1998)

*Preliminary data. Live births to women under the age of 20 years old. These numbers were calculated by the editors by multiplying the percent of live births to teenage women times total births. These are rough estimates and differ from other teenage birth numbers in this book in that they include births to women under the age of 15.

Percent of Births to Teenage Mothers in 1997

National Percent = 12.8% of Live Births*

ALPHA ORDER			RANK ORDER		
RANK	STATE	PERCENT	RANK	STATE	PERCENT
5	Alabama	17.6	1	Mississippi	20.7
31	Alaska	11.1	2	Arkansas	19.2
13	Arizona	14.9	3	Louisiana	18.6
2	Arkansas	19.2	4	New Mexico	17.9
29	California	11.7	5	Alabama	17.6
28	Colorado	11.9	6	Oklahoma	16.9
47	Connecticut	8.2	7	South Carolina	16.4
19	Delaware	13.4	8	Kentucky	16.3
19	Florida	13.4	8	Tennessee	16.3
12	Georgia	15.5	10	Texas	16.1
32	Hawaii	11.0	11	West Virginia	15.9
23	Idaho	12.7	12	Georgia	15.5
24	Illinois	12.5	13	Arizona	14.9
15	Indiana	14.2	14	North Carolina	14.3
35	Iowa	10.7	15	Indiana	14.2
22	Kansas	13.0	16	Wyoming	14.1
8	Kentucky	16.3	17	Missouri	13.9
3	Louisiana	18.6	18	Nevada	13.5
43	Maine	10.1	19	Delaware	13.4
42	Maryland	10.3	19	Florida	13.4
50	Massachusetts	7.4	21	Ohio	13.3
29	Michigan	11.7	22	Kansas	13.0
45	Minnesota	8.7	23	Idaho	12.7
1	Mississippi	20.7	24	Illinois	12.5
17	Missouri	13.9	24	Oregon	12.5
26	Montana	12.2	26	Montana	12.2
39	Nebraska	10.5	26	South Dakota	12.2
18	Nevada	13.5	28	Colorado	11.9
48	New Hampshire	7.8	29	California	11.7
48	New Jersey	7.8	29	Michigan	11.7
4	New Mexico	17.9	31	Alaska	11.1
35	New York	10.7	32	Hawaii	11.0
14	North Carolina	14.3	32	Virginia	11.0
44	North Dakota	9.1	32	Washington	11.0
21	Ohio	13.3	35	Iowa	10.7
6	Oklahoma	16.9	35	New York	10.7
24	Oregon	12.5	35	Rhode Island	10.7
41	Pennsylvania	10.4	35	Wisconsin	10.7
35	Rhode Island	10.7	39	Nebraska	10.5
7	South Carolina	16.4	39	Utah	10.5
26	South Dakota	12.2	41	Pennsylvania	10.4
8	Tennessee	16.3	42	Maryland	10.3
10	Texas	16.1	43	Maine	10.1
39	Utah	10.5	44	North Dakota	9.1
46	Vermont	8.4	45	Minnesota	8.7
32	Virginia	11.0	46	Vermont	8.4
32	Washington	11.0	47	Connecticut	8.2
11	West Virginia	15.9	48	New Hampshire	7.8
35	Wisconsin	10.7	48	New Jersey	7.8
16	Wyoming	14.1	50	Massachusetts	7.4
				District of Columbia	15.6

Source: U.S. Department of Health and Human Services, National Center for Health Statistics
   "National Vital Statistics Report" (Vol. 47, No. 4, October 7, 1998)
*Births to women 19 years old and younger.

Births to Teenage Mothers in 1996

National Total = 491,577 Live Births*

ALPHA ORDER				RANK ORDER			
RANK	STATE	BIRTHS	% of USA	RANK	STATE	BIRTHS	% of USA
15	Alabama	10,807	2.2%	1	California	63,222	12.9%
46	Alaska	1,096	0.2%	2	Texas	52,273	10.6%
14	Arizona	11,009	2.2%	3	Florida	24,806	5.0%
25	Arkansas	7,026	1.4%	4	New York	23,876	4.9%
1	California	63,222	12.9%	5	Illinois	22,831	4.6%
27	Colorado	6,541	1.3%	6	Ohio	19,851	4.0%
35	Connecticut	3,578	0.7%	7	Georgia	17,648	3.6%
41	Delaware	1,334	0.3%	8	Michigan	15,909	3.2%
3	Florida	24,806	5.0%	9	Pennsylvania	15,330	3.1%
7	Georgia	17,648	3.6%	10	North Carolina	15,296	3.1%
40	Hawaii	1,884	0.4%	11	Tennessee	12,061	2.5%
38	Idaho	2,486	0.5%	12	Louisiana	11,945	2.4%
5	Illinois	22,831	4.6%	13	Indiana	11,875	2.4%
13	Indiana	11,875	2.4%	14	Arizona	11,009	2.2%
34	Iowa	4,047	0.8%	15	Alabama	10,807	2.2%
32	Kansas	4,714	1.0%	16	Missouri	10,262	2.1%
18	Kentucky	8,786	1.8%	17	Virginia	9,912	2.0%
12	Louisiana	11,945	2.4%	18	Kentucky	8,786	1.8%
42	Maine	1,333	0.3%	19	New Jersey	8,639	1.8%
24	Maryland	7,186	1.5%	20	Washington	8,609	1.8%
28	Massachusetts	5,761	1.2%	21	Mississippi	8,451	1.7%
8	Michigan	15,909	3.2%	22	South Carolina	8,362	1.7%
30	Minnesota	5,417	1.1%	23	Oklahoma	7,780	1.6%
21	Mississippi	8,451	1.7%	24	Maryland	7,186	1.5%
16	Missouri	10,262	2.1%	25	Arkansas	7,026	1.4%
43	Montana	1,326	0.3%	26	Wisconsin	6,965	1.4%
39	Nebraska	2,434	0.5%	27	Colorado	6,541	1.3%
37	Nevada	3,402	0.7%	28	Massachusetts	5,761	1.2%
47	New Hampshire	1,072	0.2%	29	Oregon	5,681	1.2%
19	New Jersey	8,639	1.8%	30	Minnesota	5,417	1.1%
31	New Mexico	4,775	1.0%	31	New Mexico	4,775	1.0%
4	New York	23,876	4.9%	32	Kansas	4,714	1.0%
10	North Carolina	15,296	3.1%	33	Utah	4,438	0.9%
49	North Dakota	793	0.2%	34	Iowa	4,047	0.8%
6	Ohio	19,851	4.0%	35	Connecticut	3,578	0.7%
23	Oklahoma	7,780	1.6%	36	West Virginia	3,420	0.7%
29	Oregon	5,681	1.2%	37	Nevada	3,402	0.7%
9	Pennsylvania	15,330	3.1%	38	Idaho	2,486	0.5%
44	Rhode Island	1,285	0.3%	39	Nebraska	2,434	0.5%
22	South Carolina	8,362	1.7%	40	Hawaii	1,884	0.4%
45	South Dakota	1,189	0.2%	41	Delaware	1,334	0.3%
11	Tennessee	12,061	2.5%	42	Maine	1,333	0.3%
2	Texas	52,273	10.6%	43	Montana	1,326	0.3%
33	Utah	4,438	0.9%	44	Rhode Island	1,285	0.3%
50	Vermont	601	0.1%	45	South Dakota	1,189	0.2%
17	Virginia	9,912	2.0%	46	Alaska	1,096	0.2%
20	Washington	8,609	1.8%	47	New Hampshire	1,072	0.2%
36	West Virginia	3,420	0.7%	48	Wyoming	899	0.2%
26	Wisconsin	6,965	1.4%	49	North Dakota	793	0.2%
48	Wyoming	899	0.2%	50	Vermont	601	0.1%
					District of Columbia	1,354	0.3%

Source: U.S. Dept of Health & Human Services, National Center for Health Statistics (unpublished data)

*Live births to women age 15 to 19 years old by state of residence.

Teenage Birth Rate in 1996

National Rate = 54.4 Births per 1,000 Teenage Women*

ALPHA ORDER

RANK ORDER

RANK	STATE	RATE	RANK	STATE	RATE
7	Alabama	69.2	1	Mississippi	75.5
29	Alaska	46.4	2	Arkansas	75.4
3	Arizona	73.9	3	Arizona	73.9
2	Arkansas	75.4	4	Texas	73.5
14	California	62.6	5	New Mexico	70.9
25	Colorado	49.5	6	Nevada	69.6
42	Connecticut	37.4	7	Alabama	69.2
18	Delaware	56.9	8	Georgia	68.2
16	Florida	58.9	9	Louisiana	66.7
8	Georgia	68.2	10	Tennessee	66.1
26	Hawaii	48.1	11	North Carolina	63.5
27	Idaho	47.2	12	Oklahoma	63.4
17	Illinois	57.1	13	South Carolina	62.9
19	Indiana	56.1	14	California	62.6
41	Iowa	37.8	15	Kentucky	61.5
24	Kansas	49.6	16	Florida	58.9
15	Kentucky	61.5	17	Illinois	57.1
9	Louisiana	66.7	18	Delaware	56.9
48	Maine	31.4	19	Indiana	56.1
30	Maryland	46.1	20	Missouri	53.7
46	Massachusetts	32.2	21	Oregon	50.8
28	Michigan	46.5	22	Ohio	50.4
47	Minnesota	32.1	23	West Virginia	50.3
1	Mississippi	75.5	24	Kansas	49.6
20	Missouri	53.7	25	Colorado	49.5
40	Montana	38.6	26	Hawaii	48.1
39	Nebraska	38.7	27	Idaho	47.2
6	Nevada	69.6	28	Michigan	46.5
50	New Hampshire	28.6	29	Alaska	46.4
44	New Jersey	35.4	30	Maryland	46.1
5	New Mexico	70.9	31	Virginia	45.5
36	New York	41.8	32	Washington	45.0
11	North Carolina	63.5	33	Wyoming	44.0
45	North Dakota	32.3	34	Utah	42.8
22	Ohio	50.4	35	Rhode Island	42.5
12	Oklahoma	63.4	36	New York	41.8
21	Oregon	50.8	37	South Dakota	39.5
38	Pennsylvania	39.3	38	Pennsylvania	39.3
35	Rhode Island	42.5	39	Nebraska	38.7
13	South Carolina	62.9	40	Montana	38.6
37	South Dakota	39.5	41	Iowa	37.8
10	Tennessee	66.1	42	Connecticut	37.4
4	Texas	73.5	43	Wisconsin	36.8
34	Utah	42.8	44	New Jersey	35.4
49	Vermont	30.1	45	North Dakota	32.3
31	Virginia	45.5	46	Massachusetts	32.2
32	Washington	45.0	47	Minnesota	32.1
23	West Virginia	50.3	48	Maine	31.4
43	Wisconsin	36.8	49	Vermont	30.1
33	Wyoming	44.0	50	New Hampshire	28.6
				District of Columbia	102.1

Source: U.S. Department of Health and Human Services, National Center for Health Statistics
"Monthly Vital Statistics Report" (Vol. 46, No. 11, Supplement, June 30, 1998)
Women aged 15 to 19 years old.

Births to Teenage Mothers as a Percent of Live Births in 1996

National Percent = 12.6% of Live Births*

ALPHA ORDER

RANK	STATE	PERCENT
4	Alabama	17.9
32	Alaska	10.9
13	Arizona	14.6
2	Arkansas	19.3
28	California	11.7
28	Colorado	11.7
47	Connecticut	8.0
19	Delaware	13.1
19	Florida	13.1
12	Georgia	15.5
39	Hawaii	10.2
18	Idaho	13.3
25	Illinois	12.5
16	Indiana	14.2
32	Iowa	10.9
24	Kansas	12.9
7	Kentucky	16.7
3	Louisiana	18.3
42	Maine	9.7
41	Maryland	10.0
50	Massachusetts	7.2
27	Michigan	11.9
46	Minnesota	8.5
1	Mississippi	20.6
17	Missouri	13.9
26	Montana	12.2
35	Nebraska	10.5
22	Nevada	13.0
49	New Hampshire	7.4
48	New Jersey	7.6
5	New Mexico	17.5
44	New York	9.0
13	North Carolina	14.6
43	North Dakota	9.5
19	Ohio	13.1
6	Oklahoma	16.8
22	Oregon	13.0
38	Pennsylvania	10.3
39	Rhode Island	10.2
9	South Carolina	16.4
30	South Dakota	11.4
9	Tennessee	16.4
11	Texas	15.8
35	Utah	10.5
45	Vermont	8.9
34	Virginia	10.7
31	Washington	11.0
8	West Virginia	16.5
37	Wisconsin	10.4
15	Wyoming	14.3

RANK ORDER

RANK	STATE	PERCENT
1	Mississippi	20.6
2	Arkansas	19.3
3	Louisiana	18.3
4	Alabama	17.9
5	New Mexico	17.5
6	Oklahoma	16.8
7	Kentucky	16.7
8	West Virginia	16.5
9	South Carolina	16.4
9	Tennessee	16.4
11	Texas	15.8
12	Georgia	15.5
13	Arizona	14.6
13	North Carolina	14.6
15	Wyoming	14.3
16	Indiana	14.2
17	Missouri	13.9
18	Idaho	13.3
19	Delaware	13.1
19	Florida	13.1
19	Ohio	13.1
22	Nevada	13.0
22	Oregon	13.0
24	Kansas	12.9
25	Illinois	12.5
26	Montana	12.2
27	Michigan	11.9
28	California	11.7
28	Colorado	11.7
30	South Dakota	11.4
31	Washington	11.0
32	Alaska	10.9
32	Iowa	10.9
34	Virginia	10.7
35	Nebraska	10.5
35	Utah	10.5
37	Wisconsin	10.4
38	Pennsylvania	10.3
39	Hawaii	10.2
39	Rhode Island	10.2
41	Maryland	10.0
42	Maine	9.7
43	North Dakota	9.5
44	New York	9.0
45	Vermont	8.9
46	Minnesota	8.5
47	Connecticut	8.0
48	New Jersey	7.6
49	New Hampshire	7.4
50	Massachusetts	7.2
	District of Columbia	16.1

Source: U.S. Department of Health and Human Services, National Center for Health Statistics
(unpublished data)

*Live births to women age 15 to 19 years old by state of residence.

Births to White Teenage Mothers in 1996

National Total = 344,685 Live Births*

ALPHA ORDER

RANK	STATE	BIRTHS	% of USA
20	Alabama	5,565	1.6%
47	Alaska	620	0.2%
10	Arizona	9,471	2.7%
25	Arkansas	4,677	1.4%
1	California	52,805	15.3%
17	Colorado	5,803	1.7%
37	Connecticut	2,571	0.7%
46	Delaware	684	0.2%
3	Florida	15,337	4.4%
11	Georgia	8,920	2.6%
50	Hawaii	285	0.1%
38	Idaho	2,387	0.7%
6	Illinois	13,653	4.0%
9	Indiana	9,506	2.8%
32	Iowa	3,648	1.1%
30	Kansas	3,901	1.1%
14	Kentucky	7,485	2.2%
22	Louisiana	4,961	1.4%
40	Maine	1,299	0.4%
34	Maryland	3,116	0.9%
26	Massachusetts	4,506	1.3%
8	Michigan	10,226	3.0%
28	Minnesota	4,103	1.2%
35	Mississippi	3,062	0.9%
15	Missouri	7,368	2.1%
42	Montana	1,023	0.3%
39	Nebraska	2,020	0.6%
36	Nevada	2,749	0.8%
41	New Hampshire	1,043	0.3%
23	New Jersey	4,841	1.4%
29	New Mexico	4,049	1.2%
4	New York	14,887	4.3%
12	North Carolina	8,468	2.5%
48	North Dakota	615	0.2%
5	Ohio	14,394	4.2%
19	Oklahoma	5,581	1.6%
21	Oregon	5,185	1.5%
7	Pennsylvania	10,570	3.1%
43	Rhode Island	1,014	0.3%
31	South Carolina	3,893	1.1%
45	South Dakota	802	0.2%
13	Tennessee	7,999	2.3%
2	Texas	42,943	12.5%
27	Utah	4,185	1.2%
49	Vermont	593	0.2%
18	Virginia	5,704	1.7%
16	Washington	7,284	2.1%
33	West Virginia	3,215	0.9%
24	Wisconsin	4,704	1.4%
44	Wyoming	829	0.2%

RANK ORDER

RANK	STATE	BIRTHS	% of USA
1	California	52,805	15.3%
2	Texas	42,943	12.5%
3	Florida	15,337	4.4%
4	New York	14,887	4.3%
5	Ohio	14,394	4.2%
6	Illinois	13,653	4.0%
7	Pennsylvania	10,570	3.1%
8	Michigan	10,226	3.0%
9	Indiana	9,506	2.8%
10	Arizona	9,471	2.7%
11	Georgia	8,920	2.6%
12	North Carolina	8,468	2.5%
13	Tennessee	7,999	2.3%
14	Kentucky	7,485	2.2%
15	Missouri	7,368	2.1%
16	Washington	7,284	2.1%
17	Colorado	5,803	1.7%
18	Virginia	5,704	1.7%
19	Oklahoma	5,581	1.6%
20	Alabama	5,565	1.6%
21	Oregon	5,185	1.5%
22	Louisiana	4,961	1.4%
23	New Jersey	4,841	1.4%
24	Wisconsin	4,704	1.4%
25	Arkansas	4,677	1.4%
26	Massachusetts	4,506	1.3%
27	Utah	4,185	1.2%
28	Minnesota	4,103	1.2%
29	New Mexico	4,049	1.2%
30	Kansas	3,901	1.1%
31	South Carolina	3,893	1.1%
32	Iowa	3,648	1.1%
33	West Virginia	3,215	0.9%
34	Maryland	3,116	0.9%
35	Mississippi	3,062	0.9%
36	Nevada	2,749	0.8%
37	Connecticut	2,571	0.7%
38	Idaho	2,387	0.7%
39	Nebraska	2,020	0.6%
40	Maine	1,299	0.4%
41	New Hampshire	1,043	0.3%
42	Montana	1,023	0.3%
43	Rhode Island	1,014	0.3%
44	Wyoming	829	0.2%
45	South Dakota	802	0.2%
46	Delaware	684	0.2%
47	Alaska	620	0.2%
48	North Dakota	615	0.2%
49	Vermont	593	0.2%
50	Hawaii	285	0.1%
	District of Columbia	136	0.0%

Source: U.S. Dept of Health & Human Services, National Center for Health Statistics
(unpublished data)
*Live births to women age 15 to 19 years old by state of residence.

Births to White Teenage Mothers as a Percent of White Births in 1996

National Percent = 11.1% of White Live Births*

ALPHA ORDER			RANK ORDER		
RANK	STATE	PERCENT	RANK	STATE	PERCENT
11	Alabama	13.8	1	New Mexico	17.5
35	Alaska	9.1	2	Arkansas	16.8
7	Arizona	14.3	3	West Virginia	16.2
2	Arkansas	16.8	4	Kentucky	15.8
18	California	12.0	5	Oklahoma	15.2
23	Colorado	11.4	5	Texas	15.2
46	Connecticut	6.8	7	Arizona	14.3
35	Delaware	9.1	7	Mississippi	14.3
25	Florida	10.8	9	Tennessee	14.2
17	Georgia	12.2	10	Wyoming	13.9
49	Hawaii	5.9	11	Alabama	13.8
13	Idaho	13.2	12	Louisiana	13.3
30	Illinois	9.7	13	Idaho	13.2
14	Indiana	12.9	14	Indiana	12.9
29	Iowa	10.4	15	Oregon	12.8
21	Kansas	11.9	16	Nevada	12.3
4	Kentucky	15.8	17	Georgia	12.2
12	Louisiana	13.3	18	California	12.0
30	Maine	9.7	18	Missouri	12.0
46	Maryland	6.8	18	South Carolina	12.0
48	Massachusetts	6.5	21	Kansas	11.9
30	Michigan	9.7	22	North Carolina	11.5
45	Minnesota	7.2	23	Colorado	11.4
7	Mississippi	14.3	24	Ohio	11.3
18	Missouri	12.0	25	Florida	10.8
25	Montana	10.8	25	Montana	10.8
33	Nebraska	9.5	25	Washington	10.8
16	Nevada	12.3	28	Utah	10.5
44	New Hampshire	7.3	29	Iowa	10.4
50	New Jersey	5.6	30	Illinois	9.7
1	New Mexico	17.5	30	Maine	9.7
43	New York	7.8	30	Michigan	9.7
22	North Carolina	11.5	33	Nebraska	9.5
41	North Dakota	8.3	34	South Dakota	9.3
24	Ohio	11.3	35	Alaska	9.1
5	Oklahoma	15.2	35	Delaware	9.1
15	Oregon	12.8	35	Rhode Island	9.1
39	Pennsylvania	8.5	38	Vermont	8.9
35	Rhode Island	9.1	39	Pennsylvania	8.5
18	South Carolina	12.0	39	Virginia	8.5
34	South Dakota	9.3	41	North Dakota	8.3
9	Tennessee	14.2	42	Wisconsin	8.1
5	Texas	15.2	43	New York	7.8
28	Utah	10.5	44	New Hampshire	7.3
38	Vermont	8.9	45	Minnesota	7.2
39	Virginia	8.5	46	Connecticut	6.8
25	Washington	10.8	46	Maryland	6.8
3	West Virginia	16.2	48	Massachusetts	6.5
42	Wisconsin	8.1	49	Hawaii	5.9
10	Wyoming	13.9	50	New Jersey	5.6
				District of Columbia	6.6

Source: U.S. Dept of Health & Human Services, National Center for Health Statistics
(unpublished data)
*Live births to women age 15 to 19 years old by state of residence.

Births to Black Teenage Mothers in 1996

National Total = 130,596 Live Births*

ALPHA ORDER

RANK	STATE	BIRTHS	% of USA
12	Alabama	5,189	4.0%
41	Alaska	58	0.0%
32	Arizona	486	0.4%
21	Arkansas	2,271	1.7%
7	California	6,828	5.2%
31	Colorado	506	0.4%
26	Connecticut	951	0.7%
29	Delaware	638	0.5%
1	Florida	9,202	7.0%
4	Georgia	8,624	6.6%
42	Hawaii	50	0.0%
47	Idaho	10	0.0%
2	Illinois	8,995	6.9%
20	Indiana	2,308	1.8%
35	Iowa	283	0.2%
28	Kansas	704	0.5%
23	Kentucky	1,264	1.0%
6	Louisiana	6,856	5.2%
48	Maine	9	0.0%
16	Maryland	4,012	3.1%
25	Massachusetts	1,070	0.8%
9	Michigan	5,390	4.1%
27	Minnesota	711	0.5%
11	Mississippi	5,307	4.1%
19	Missouri	2,782	2.1%
49	Montana	8	0.0%
34	Nebraska	299	0.2%
33	Nevada	457	0.3%
43	New Hampshire	16	0.0%
18	New Jersey	3,694	2.8%
39	New Mexico	102	0.1%
5	New York	8,559	6.6%
8	North Carolina	6,300	4.8%
45	North Dakota	12	0.0%
10	Ohio	5,339	4.1%
24	Oklahoma	1,115	0.9%
36	Oregon	229	0.2%
13	Pennsylvania	4,591	3.5%
38	Rhode Island	177	0.1%
14	South Carolina	4,404	3.4%
44	South Dakota	15	0.0%
17	Tennessee	3,951	3.0%
3	Texas	8,907	6.8%
40	Utah	62	0.0%
50	Vermont	5	0.0%
15	Virginia	4,055	3.1%
30	Washington	574	0.4%
37	West Virginia	198	0.2%
22	Wisconsin	1,800	1.4%
45	Wyoming	12	0.0%

RANK ORDER

RANK	STATE	BIRTHS	% of USA
1	Florida	9,202	7.0%
2	Illinois	8,995	6.9%
3	Texas	8,907	6.8%
4	Georgia	8,624	6.6%
5	New York	8,559	6.6%
6	Louisiana	6,856	5.2%
7	California	6,828	5.2%
8	North Carolina	6,300	4.8%
9	Michigan	5,390	4.1%
10	Ohio	5,339	4.1%
11	Mississippi	5,307	4.1%
12	Alabama	5,189	4.0%
13	Pennsylvania	4,591	3.5%
14	South Carolina	4,404	3.4%
15	Virginia	4,055	3.1%
16	Maryland	4,012	3.1%
17	Tennessee	3,951	3.0%
18	New Jersey	3,694	2.8%
19	Missouri	2,782	2.1%
20	Indiana	2,308	1.8%
21	Arkansas	2,271	1.7%
22	Wisconsin	1,800	1.4%
23	Kentucky	1,264	1.0%
24	Oklahoma	1,115	0.9%
25	Massachusetts	1,070	0.8%
26	Connecticut	951	0.7%
27	Minnesota	711	0.5%
28	Kansas	704	0.5%
29	Delaware	638	0.5%
30	Washington	574	0.4%
31	Colorado	506	0.4%
32	Arizona	486	0.4%
33	Nevada	457	0.3%
34	Nebraska	299	0.2%
35	Iowa	283	0.2%
36	Oregon	229	0.2%
37	West Virginia	198	0.2%
38	Rhode Island	177	0.1%
39	New Mexico	102	0.1%
40	Utah	62	0.0%
41	Alaska	58	0.0%
42	Hawaii	50	0.0%
43	New Hampshire	16	0.0%
44	South Dakota	15	0.0%
45	North Dakota	12	0.0%
45	Wyoming	12	0.0%
47	Idaho	10	0.0%
48	Maine	9	0.0%
49	Montana	8	0.0%
50	Vermont	5	0.0%
	District of Columbia	1,211	0.9%

Source: U.S. Dept of Health & Human Services, National Center for Health Statistics
(unpublished data)
*Live births to women age 15 to 19 years old by state of residence.

Births to Black Teenage Mothers as a Percent of Black Births in 1996

National Percent = 22.0% of Black Live Births*

ALPHA ORDER				RANK ORDER		
RANK	STATE	PERCENT		RANK	STATE	PERCENT
7	Alabama	26.5		1	Arkansas	28.7
46	Alaska	13.7		2	Mississippi	28.0
32	Arizona	20.8		2	Wisconsin	28.0
1	Arkansas	28.7		4	Iowa	27.0
41	California	17.8		5	Delaware	26.9
33	Colorado	19.6		6	West Virginia	26.7
38	Connecticut	18.1		7	Alabama	26.5
5	Delaware	26.9		8	Vermont	26.3
29	Florida	21.8		9	Indiana	26.1
26	Georgia	22.4		10	Kentucky	26.0
50	Hawaii	9.7		11	Louisiana	25.9
48	Idaho	13.3		12	Oregon	25.6
16	Illinois	24.8		13	Kansas	25.5
9	Indiana	26.1		14	Missouri	25.0
4	Iowa	27.0		15	Oklahoma	24.9
13	Kansas	25.5		16	Illinois	24.8
10	Kentucky	26.0		16	Nebraska	24.8
11	Louisiana	25.9		18	Tennessee	24.7
49	Maine	10.6		19	South Carolina	24.5
42	Maryland	17.5		19	Wyoming	24.5
44	Massachusetts	14.5		21	Ohio	24.2
27	Michigan	22.3		22	Nevada	23.2
24	Minnesota	22.9		22	North Carolina	23.2
2	Mississippi	28.0		24	Minnesota	22.9
14	Missouri	25.0		24	Texas	22.9
31	Montana	21.1		26	Georgia	22.4
16	Nebraska	24.8		27	Michigan	22.3
22	Nevada	23.2		27	Pennsylvania	22.3
45	New Hampshire	14.3		29	Florida	21.8
40	New Jersey	18.0		29	New Mexico	21.8
29	New Mexico	21.8		31	Montana	21.1
43	New York	15.5		32	Arizona	20.8
22	North Carolina	23.2		33	Colorado	19.6
47	North Dakota	13.5		34	Virginia	19.4
21	Ohio	24.2		35	Utah	19.1
15	Oklahoma	24.9		36	Rhode Island	18.7
12	Oregon	25.6		37	Washington	18.4
27	Pennsylvania	22.3		38	Connecticut	18.1
36	Rhode Island	18.7		38	South Dakota	18.1
19	South Carolina	24.5		40	New Jersey	18.0
38	South Dakota	18.1		41	California	17.8
18	Tennessee	24.7		42	Maryland	17.5
24	Texas	22.9		43	New York	15.5
35	Utah	19.1		44	Massachusetts	14.5
8	Vermont	26.3		45	New Hampshire	14.3
34	Virginia	19.4		46	Alaska	13.7
37	Washington	18.4		47	North Dakota	13.5
6	West Virginia	26.7		48	Idaho	13.3
2	Wisconsin	28.0		49	Maine	10.6
19	Wyoming	24.5		50	Hawaii	9.7
					District of Columbia	19.6

Source: U.S. Dept of Health & Human Services, National Center for Health Statistics
(unpublished data)

*Live births to women age 15 to 19 years old by state of residence.

Pregnancy Rate for 15 to 19 Year Old Women in 1995

National Rate = 76.5 Births and Abortions per 1,000 Women 15-19 Years Old*

ALPHA ORDER

RANK	STATE	RATE
7	Alabama	89.8
NA	Alaska**	NA
6	Arizona	90.3
10	Arkansas	88.3
NA	California**	NA
24	Colorado	68.2
27	Connecticut	65.3
NA	Delaware**	NA
NA	Florida**	NA
3	Georgia	98.1
17	Hawaii	78.4
35	Idaho	53.9
NA	Illinois**	NA
22	Indiana	70.0
NA	Iowa**	NA
14	Kansas	80.3
18	Kentucky	75.1
12	Louisiana	83.4
38	Maine	49.8
23	Maryland	69.2
32	Massachusetts	59.5
25	Michigan	67.7
41	Minnesota	47.8
11	Mississippi	87.6
26	Missouri	67.2
29	Montana	61.9
34	Nebraska	54.9
1	Nevada	99.3
NA	New Hampshire**	NA
30	New Jersey	60.9
5	New Mexico	90.7
7	New York	89.8
4	North Carolina	95.0
41	North Dakota	47.8
21	Ohio	70.6
NA	Oklahoma**	NA
16	Oregon	78.6
31	Pennsylvania	60.8
15	Rhode Island	79.4
13	South Carolina	81.0
37	South Dakota	50.1
9	Tennessee	88.8
2	Texas	98.9
40	Utah	48.9
33	Vermont	55.1
20	Virginia	71.5
19	Washington	75.0
28	West Virginia	62.2
36	Wisconsin	50.3
39	Wyoming	49.2

RANK ORDER

RANK	STATE	RATE
1	Nevada	99.3
2	Texas	98.9
3	Georgia	98.1
4	North Carolina	95.0
5	New Mexico	90.7
6	Arizona	90.3
7	Alabama	89.8
7	New York	89.8
9	Tennessee	88.8
10	Arkansas	88.3
11	Mississippi	87.6
12	Louisiana	83.4
13	South Carolina	81.0
14	Kansas	80.3
15	Rhode Island	79.4
16	Oregon	78.6
17	Hawaii	78.4
18	Kentucky	75.1
19	Washington	75.0
20	Virginia	71.5
21	Ohio	70.6
22	Indiana	70.0
23	Maryland	69.2
24	Colorado	68.2
25	Michigan	67.7
26	Missouri	67.2
27	Connecticut	65.3
28	West Virginia	62.2
29	Montana	61.9
30	New Jersey	60.9
31	Pennsylvania	60.8
32	Massachusetts	59.5
33	Vermont	55.1
34	Nebraska	54.9
35	Idaho	53.9
36	Wisconsin	50.3
37	South Dakota	50.1
38	Maine	49.8
39	Wyoming	49.2
40	Utah	48.9
41	Minnesota	47.8
41	North Dakota	47.8
NA	Alaska**	NA
NA	California**	NA
NA	Delaware**	NA
NA	Florida**	NA
NA	Illinois**	NA
NA	Iowa**	NA
NA	New Hampshire**	NA
NA	Oklahoma**	NA

District of Columbia**   NA

Source: Morgan Quitno Press using data from US Dept of Health & Human Serv's, Centers for Disease Control-Prevention
"Abortion Surveillance-United States, 1995" (Morbidity Mortality Weekly Report, Vol. 47, No. SS-2, July 3, 1998)
*The sum of live births and legal induced abortions per 1,000 women aged 15-19 years old. Births by state of
residence, abortions by state of occurrence. National rate includes only states reporting abortions and births.
**Not available.

Percent Change in Pregnancy Rate for 15 to 19 Year Old Women: 1992 to 1995

National Percent Change = 4.0% Decrease*

RANK	STATE	PERCENT CHANGE		RANK	STATE	PERCENT CHANGE
	ALPHA ORDER				**RANK ORDER**	
4	Alabama	(3.6)		1	Arkansas	(2.6)
NA	Alaska**	NA		2	Indiana	(3.0)
30	Arizona	(12.8)		2	Oregon	(3.0)
1	Arkansas	(2.6)		4	Alabama	(3.6)
NA	California**	NA		5	Texas	(4.6)
36	Colorado	(14.5)		6	Ohio	(5.4)
NA	Connecticut**	NA		7	Tennessee	(5.5)
NA	Delaware**	NA		8	West Virginia	(5.9)
NA	Florida**	NA		9	Nevada	(6.3)
14	Georgia	(8.2)		10	New York	(7.0)
17	Hawaii	(9.3)		11	Kansas	(7.7)
19	Idaho	(9.7)		12	South Carolina	(8.0)
NA	Illinois**	NA		13	Kentucky	(8.1)
2	Indiana	(3.0)		14	Georgia	(8.2)
NA	Iowa**	NA		15	Wyoming	(8.4)
11	Kansas	(7.7)		16	North Carolina	(9.2)
13	Kentucky	(8.1)		17	Hawaii	(9.3)
21	Louisiana	(9.9)		18	Virginia	(9.5)
20	Maine	(9.8)		19	Idaho	(9.7)
23	Maryland	(10.0)		20	Maine	(9.8)
35	Massachusetts	(14.4)		21	Louisiana	(9.9)
37	Michigan	(15.1)		21	Rhode Island	(9.9)
32	Minnesota	(13.4)		23	Maryland	(10.0)
31	Mississippi	(13.1)		24	New Mexico	(10.9)
34	Missouri	(13.8)		25	Montana	(11.8)
25	Montana	(11.8)		25	North Dakota	(11.8)
32	Nebraska	(13.4)		27	Washington	(11.9)
9	Nevada	(6.3)		28	Utah	(12.1)
NA	New Hampshire**	NA		29	New Jersey	(12.6)
29	New Jersey	(12.6)		30	Arizona	(12.8)
24	New Mexico	(10.9)		31	Mississippi	(13.1)
10	New York	(7.0)		32	Minnesota	(13.4)
16	North Carolina	(9.2)		32	Nebraska	(13.4)
25	North Dakota	(11.8)		34	Missouri	(13.8)
6	Ohio	(5.4)		35	Massachusetts	(14.4)
NA	Oklahoma**	NA		36	Colorado	(14.5)
2	Oregon	(3.0)		37	Michigan	(15.1)
38	Pennsylvania	(15.2)		38	Pennsylvania	(15.2)
21	Rhode Island	(9.9)		39	South Dakota	(15.7)
12	South Carolina	(8.0)		40	Wisconsin	(17.3)
39	South Dakota	(15.7)		41	Vermont	(19.8)
7	Tennessee	(5.5)		NA	Alaska**	NA
5	Texas	(4.6)		NA	California**	NA
28	Utah	(12.1)		NA	Connecticut**	NA
41	Vermont	(19.8)		NA	Delaware**	NA
18	Virginia	(9.5)		NA	Florida**	NA
27	Washington	(11.9)		NA	Illinois**	NA
8	West Virginia	(5.9)		NA	Iowa**	NA
40	Wisconsin	(17.3)		NA	New Hampshire**	NA
15	Wyoming	(8.4)		NA	Oklahoma**	NA
					District of Columbia**	NA

Source: Morgan Quitno Press using data from US Dept of Health & Human Serv's, Centers for Disease Control-Prevention "Abortion Surveillance-United States, 1995" (Morbidity Mortality Weekly Report, Vol. 47, No. SS-2, July 3, 1998)
*The sum of live births and legal induced abortions per 1,000 women aged 15-19 years old. Births by state of residence, abortions by state of occurrence. National rate includes only states reporting abortions and births.
**Not available.

Births to Teenage Mothers in 1990

National Total = 521,826 Live Births*

ALPHA ORDER

RANK	STATE	BIRTHS	% of USA
15	Alabama	11,252	2.16%
47	Alaska	1,142	0.22%
19	Arizona	9,612	1.84%
27	Arkansas	7,011	1.34%
1	California	69,712	13.36%
28	Colorado	5,975	1.15%
33	Connecticut	4,038	0.77%
44	Delaware	1,277	0.24%
3	Florida	27,017	5.18%
8	Georgia	18,369	3.52%
39	Hawaii	2,122	0.41%
40	Idaho	2,009	0.38%
5	Illinois	24,967	4.78%
12	Indiana	12,335	2.36%
34	Iowa	3,989	0.76%
31	Kansas	4,722	0.90%
20	Kentucky	9,349	1.79%
13	Louisiana	12,270	2.35%
41	Maine	1,857	0.36%
23	Maryland	8,143	1.56%
26	Massachusetts	7,266	1.39%
7	Michigan	20,312	3.89%
29	Minnesota	5,342	1.02%
21	Mississippi	8,909	1.71%
16	Missouri	11,227	2.15%
43	Montana	1,331	0.26%
38	Nebraska	2,352	0.45%
37	Nevada	2,663	0.51%
45	New Hampshire	1,258	0.24%
17	New Jersey	10,068	1.93%
32	New Mexico	4,367	0.84%
4	New York	26,608	5.10%
10	North Carolina	16,506	3.16%
49	North Dakota	793	0.15%
6	Ohio	22,690	4.35%
24	Oklahoma	7,590	1.45%
30	Oregon	5,084	0.97%
9	Pennsylvania	18,216	3.49%
42	Rhode Island	1,564	0.30%
18	South Carolina	9,721	1.86%
46	South Dakota	1,172	0.22%
11	Tennessee	12,928	2.48%
2	Texas	48,302	9.26%
36	Utah	3,707	0.71%
50	Vermont	702	0.13%
14	Virginia	11,353	2.18%
22	Washington	8,397	1.61%
35	West Virginia	3,976	0.76%
25	Wisconsin	7,281	1.40%
48	Wyoming	943	0.18%

RANK ORDER

RANK	STATE	BIRTHS	% of USA
1	California	69,712	13.36%
2	Texas	48,302	9.26%
3	Florida	27,017	5.18%
4	New York	26,608	5.10%
5	Illinois	24,967	4.78%
6	Ohio	22,690	4.35%
7	Michigan	20,312	3.89%
8	Georgia	18,369	3.52%
9	Pennsylvania	18,216	3.49%
10	North Carolina	16,506	3.16%
11	Tennessee	12,928	2.48%
12	Indiana	12,335	2.36%
13	Louisiana	12,270	2.35%
14	Virginia	11,353	2.18%
15	Alabama	11,252	2.16%
16	Missouri	11,227	2.15%
17	New Jersey	10,068	1.93%
18	South Carolina	9,721	1.86%
19	Arizona	9,612	1.84%
20	Kentucky	9,349	1.79%
21	Mississippi	8,909	1.71%
22	Washington	8,397	1.61%
23	Maryland	8,143	1.56%
24	Oklahoma	7,590	1.45%
25	Wisconsin	7,281	1.40%
26	Massachusetts	7,266	1.39%
27	Arkansas	7,011	1.34%
28	Colorado	5,975	1.15%
29	Minnesota	5,342	1.02%
30	Oregon	5,084	0.97%
31	Kansas	4,722	0.90%
32	New Mexico	4,367	0.84%
33	Connecticut	4,038	0.77%
34	Iowa	3,989	0.76%
35	West Virginia	3,976	0.76%
36	Utah	3,707	0.71%
37	Nevada	2,663	0.51%
38	Nebraska	2,352	0.45%
39	Hawaii	2,122	0.41%
40	Idaho	2,009	0.38%
41	Maine	1,857	0.36%
42	Rhode Island	1,564	0.30%
43	Montana	1,331	0.26%
44	Delaware	1,277	0.24%
45	New Hampshire	1,258	0.24%
46	South Dakota	1,172	0.22%
47	Alaska	1,142	0.22%
48	Wyoming	943	0.18%
49	North Dakota	793	0.15%
50	Vermont	702	0.13%
	District of Columbia	2,030	0.39%

Source: U.S. Department of Health and Human Services, Centers for Disease Control and Prevention
    "Surveillance for Pregnancy and Birth Rates Among Teenagers" (MMWR, Vol. 42, No. SS-6, 12/17/93)
*Women aged 15 to 19 years old.

Teenage Birth Rate in 1990

National Rate = 59.9 Live Births per 1,000 Teenage Women*

ALPHA ORDER				RANK ORDER		
RANK	**STATE**	**RATE**		**RANK**	**STATE**	**RATE**
11	Alabama	71.0		1	Mississippi	81.0
17	Alaska	65.3		2	Arkansas	80.1
4	Arizona	75.5		3	New Mexico	78.2
2	Arkansas	80.1		4	Arizona	75.5
12	California	70.6		4	Georgia	75.5
28	Colorado	54.5		6	Texas	75.3
45	Connecticut	38.8		7	Louisiana	74.2
28	Delaware	54.5		8	Nevada	73.3
13	Florida	69.1		9	Tennessee	72.3
4	Georgia	75.5		10	South Carolina	71.3
20	Hawaii	61.2		11	Alabama	71.0
33	Idaho	50.6		12	California	70.6
18	Illinois	62.9		13	Florida	69.1
22	Indiana	58.6		14	Kentucky	67.6
43	Iowa	40.5		14	North Carolina	67.6
26	Kansas	56.1		16	Oklahoma	66.8
14	Kentucky	67.6		17	Alaska	65.3
7	Louisiana	74.2		18	Illinois	62.9
40	Maine	43.0		19	Missouri	62.8
30	Maryland	53.2		20	Hawaii	61.2
48	Massachusetts	35.1		21	Michigan	59.0
21	Michigan	59.0		22	Indiana	58.6
46	Minnesota	36.3		23	Ohio	57.9
1	Mississippi	81.0		24	West Virginia	57.3
19	Missouri	62.8		25	Wyoming	56.3
35	Montana	48.4		26	Kansas	56.1
42	Nebraska	42.3		27	Oregon	54.6
8	Nevada	73.3		28	Colorado	54.5
50	New Hampshire	33.0		28	Delaware	54.5
43	New Jersey	40.5		30	Maryland	53.2
3	New Mexico	78.2		31	Washington	53.1
39	New York	43.6		32	Virginia	52.9
14	North Carolina	67.6		33	Idaho	50.6
47	North Dakota	35.4		34	Utah	48.5
23	Ohio	57.9		35	Montana	48.4
16	Oklahoma	66.8		36	South Dakota	46.8
27	Oregon	54.6		37	Pennsylvania	44.9
37	Pennsylvania	44.9		38	Rhode Island	43.9
38	Rhode Island	43.9		39	New York	43.6
10	South Carolina	71.3		40	Maine	43.0
36	South Dakota	46.8		41	Wisconsin	42.6
9	Tennessee	72.3		42	Nebraska	42.3
6	Texas	75.3		43	Iowa	40.5
34	Utah	48.5		43	New Jersey	40.5
49	Vermont	34.0		45	Connecticut	38.8
32	Virginia	52.9		46	Minnesota	36.3
31	Washington	53.1		47	North Dakota	35.4
24	West Virginia	57.3		48	Massachusetts	35.1
41	Wisconsin	42.6		49	Vermont	34.0
25	Wyoming	56.3		50	New Hampshire	33.0
					District of Columbia	93.1

Source: U.S. Department of Health and Human Services, Centers for Disease Control and Prevention
"Surveillance for Pregnancy and Birth Rates Among Teenagers" (MMWR, Vol. 42, No. SS-6, 12/17/93)
*Women aged 15 to 19 years old.

Percent Change in Teenage Birth Rate: 1990 to 1996

National Percent Change = 9.2% Decrease*

ALPHA ORDER				RANK ORDER		
RANK	STATE	PERCENT CHANGE		RANK	STATE	PERCENT CHANGE
4	Alabama	(2.5)		1	Delaware	4.4
50	Alaska	(28.9)		2	Arizona	(2.1)
2	Arizona	(2.1)		3	Texas	(2.4)
11	Arkansas	(5.9)		4	Alabama	(2.5)
27	California	(11.3)		5	Rhode Island	(3.2)
22	Colorado	(9.2)		6	Connecticut	(3.6)
6	Connecticut	(3.6)		7	New York	(4.1)
1	Delaware	4.4		8	Indiana	(4.3)
42	Florida	(14.8)		9	Nevada	(5.0)
25	Georgia	(9.7)		10	Oklahoma	(5.1)
47	Hawaii	(21.4)		11	Arkansas	(5.9)
13	Idaho	(6.7)		12	North Carolina	(6.1)
22	Illinois	(9.2)		13	Idaho	(6.7)
8	Indiana	(4.3)		13	Iowa	(6.7)
13	Iowa	(6.7)		15	Mississippi	(6.8)
29	Kansas	(11.6)		16	Oregon	(7.0)
21	Kentucky	(9.0)		17	Massachusetts	(8.3)
26	Louisiana	(10.1)		18	Nebraska	(8.5)
49	Maine	(27.0)		19	Tennessee	(8.6)
37	Maryland	(13.3)		20	North Dakota	(8.8)
17	Massachusetts	(8.3)		21	Kentucky	(9.0)
46	Michigan	(21.2)		22	Colorado	(9.2)
29	Minnesota	(11.6)		22	Illinois	(9.2)
15	Mississippi	(6.8)		24	New Mexico	(9.3)
41	Missouri	(14.5)		25	Georgia	(9.7)
45	Montana	(20.2)		26	Louisiana	(10.1)
18	Nebraska	(8.5)		27	California	(11.3)
9	Nevada	(5.0)		28	Vermont	(11.5)
37	New Hampshire	(13.3)		29	Kansas	(11.6)
35	New Jersey	(12.6)		29	Minnesota	(11.6)
24	New Mexico	(9.3)		31	South Carolina	(11.8)
7	New York	(4.1)		31	Utah	(11.8)
12	North Carolina	(6.1)		33	West Virginia	(12.2)
20	North Dakota	(8.8)		34	Pennsylvania	(12.5)
36	Ohio	(13.0)		35	New Jersey	(12.6)
10	Oklahoma	(5.1)		36	Ohio	(13.0)
16	Oregon	(7.0)		37	Maryland	(13.3)
34	Pennsylvania	(12.5)		37	New Hampshire	(13.3)
5	Rhode Island	(3.2)		39	Wisconsin	(13.6)
31	South Carolina	(11.8)		40	Virginia	(14.0)
44	South Dakota	(15.6)		41	Missouri	(14.5)
19	Tennessee	(8.6)		42	Florida	(14.8)
3	Texas	(2.4)		43	Washington	(15.3)
31	Utah	(11.8)		44	South Dakota	(15.6)
28	Vermont	(11.5)		45	Montana	(20.2)
40	Virginia	(14.0)		46	Michigan	(21.2)
43	Washington	(15.3)		47	Hawaii	(21.4)
33	West Virginia	(12.2)		48	Wyoming	(21.8)
39	Wisconsin	(13.6)		49	Maine	(27.0)
48	Wyoming	(21.8)		50	Alaska	(28.9)

District of Columbia   9.7

Source: Morgan Quitno Press using data from U.S. Department of Health and Human Services
   "Monthly Vital Statistics Report" (Vol. 46, No. 11, Supplement, June 30, 1998)
   "Surveillance for Pregnancy and Birth Rates Among Teenagers" (MMWR, Vol. 42, No. SS-6, 12/17/93)
*Women aged 15 to 19 years old.

Births to Teenage Mothers in 1980

National Total = 562,330 Live Births*

ALPHA ORDER

RANK	STATE	BIRTHS	% of USA
15	Alabama	13,096	2.33%
49	Alaska	1,123	0.20%
25	Arizona	8,235	1.46%
26	Arkansas	8,060	1.43%
1	California	56,138	9.98%
29	Colorado	6,592	1.17%
36	Connecticut	4,408	0.78%
45	Delaware	1,572	0.28%
6	Florida	24,042	4.28%
9	Georgia	19,137	3.40%
40	Hawaii	2,085	0.37%
38	Idaho	2,645	0.47%
3	Illinois	29,798	5.30%
12	Indiana	15,331	2.73%
31	Iowa	5,962	1.06%
30	Kansas	6,090	1.08%
16	Kentucky	12,559	2.23%
10	Louisiana	16,504	2.93%
39	Maine	2,522	0.45%
23	Maryland	8,885	1.58%
27	Massachusetts	7,765	1.38%
8	Michigan	20,401	3.63%
28	Minnesota	7,048	1.25%
19	Mississippi	11,079	1.97%
14	Missouri	13,312	2.37%
43	Montana	1,761	0.31%
37	Nebraska	3,313	0.59%
41	Nevada	2,048	0.36%
47	New Hampshire	1,475	0.26%
18	New Jersey	11,904	2.12%
34	New Mexico	4,758	0.85%
4	New York	28,206	5.02%
11	North Carolina	16,192	2.88%
48	North Dakota	1,304	0.23%
5	Ohio	26,567	4.72%
21	Oklahoma	10,206	1.81%
33	Oregon	5,731	1.02%
7	Pennsylvania	22,029	3.92%
46	Rhode Island	1,502	0.27%
20	South Carolina	10,282	1.83%
42	South Dakota	1,797	0.32%
13	Tennessee	13,792	2.45%
2	Texas	50,125	8.91%
35	Utah	4,594	0.82%
50	Vermont	1,024	0.18%
17	Virginia	12,138	2.16%
24	Washington	8,495	1.51%
32	West Virginia	5,911	1.05%
22	Wisconsin	9,220	1.64%
44	Wyoming	1,634	0.29%

RANK ORDER

RANK	STATE	BIRTHS	% of USA
1	California	56,138	9.98%
2	Texas	50,125	8.91%
3	Illinois	29,798	5.30%
4	New York	28,206	5.02%
5	Ohio	26,567	4.72%
6	Florida	24,042	4.28%
7	Pennsylvania	22,029	3.92%
8	Michigan	20,401	3.63%
9	Georgia	19,137	3.40%
10	Louisiana	16,504	2.93%
11	North Carolina	16,192	2.88%
12	Indiana	15,331	2.73%
13	Tennessee	13,792	2.45%
14	Missouri	13,312	2.37%
15	Alabama	13,096	2.33%
16	Kentucky	12,559	2.23%
17	Virginia	12,138	2.16%
18	New Jersey	11,904	2.12%
19	Mississippi	11,079	1.97%
20	South Carolina	10,282	1.83%
21	Oklahoma	10,206	1.81%
22	Wisconsin	9,220	1.64%
23	Maryland	8,885	1.58%
24	Washington	8,495	1.51%
25	Arizona	8,235	1.46%
26	Arkansas	8,060	1.43%
27	Massachusetts	7,765	1.38%
28	Minnesota	7,048	1.25%
29	Colorado	6,592	1.17%
30	Kansas	6,090	1.08%
31	Iowa	5,962	1.06%
32	West Virginia	5,911	1.05%
33	Oregon	5,731	1.02%
34	New Mexico	4,758	0.85%
35	Utah	4,594	0.82%
36	Connecticut	4,408	0.78%
37	Nebraska	3,313	0.59%
38	Idaho	2,645	0.47%
39	Maine	2,522	0.45%
40	Hawaii	2,085	0.37%
41	Nevada	2,048	0.36%
42	South Dakota	1,797	0.32%
43	Montana	1,761	0.31%
44	Wyoming	1,634	0.29%
45	Delaware	1,572	0.28%
46	Rhode Island	1,502	0.27%
47	New Hampshire	1,475	0.26%
48	North Dakota	1,304	0.23%
49	Alaska	1,123	0.20%
50	Vermont	1,024	0.18%
	District of Columbia	1,933	0.34%

Source: U.S. Department of Health and Human Services, National Center for Health Statistics
"Vital Statistics of the United States, 1980" (Vol. I-Natality, issued 1984)
Births to women age 15 to 19 years old.

Teenage Birth Rate in 1980

National Rate = 53.0 Live Births per 1,000 Teenage Women*

ALPHA ORDER

RANK	STATE	RATE
10	Alabama	68.3
15	Alaska	64.4
12	Arizona	65.5
5	Arkansas	74.5
25	California	53.3
31	Colorado	49.9
49	Connecticut	30.5
28	Delaware	51.2
18	Florida	58.5
8	Georgia	71.9
30	Hawaii	50.7
17	Idaho	59.5
24	Illinois	55.8
21	Indiana	57.5
39	Iowa	43.0
23	Kansas	56.8
7	Kentucky	72.3
3	Louisiana	76.0
34	Maine	47.4
38	Maryland	43.4
50	Massachusetts	28.1
37	Michigan	45.0
44	Minnesota	35.4
1	Mississippi	83.7
20	Missouri	57.8
32	Montana	48.5
36	Nebraska	45.1
18	Nevada	58.5
47	New Hampshire	33.6
45	New Jersey	35.2
9	New Mexico	71.8
46	New York	34.8
21	North Carolina	57.5
40	North Dakota	41.7
27	Ohio	52.5
4	Oklahoma	74.6
29	Oregon	50.9
41	Pennsylvania	40.5
48	Rhode Island	33.0
14	South Carolina	64.8
26	South Dakota	52.6
16	Tennessee	64.1
6	Texas	74.3
13	Utah	65.2
42	Vermont	39.5
33	Virginia	48.3
35	Washington	46.7
11	West Virginia	67.8
42	Wisconsin	39.5
2	Wyoming	78.7

RANK ORDER

RANK	STATE	RATE
1	Mississippi	83.7
2	Wyoming	78.7
3	Louisiana	76.0
4	Oklahoma	74.6
5	Arkansas	74.5
6	Texas	74.3
7	Kentucky	72.3
8	Georgia	71.9
9	New Mexico	71.8
10	Alabama	68.3
11	West Virginia	67.8
12	Arizona	65.5
13	Utah	65.2
14	South Carolina	64.8
15	Alaska	64.4
16	Tennessee	64.1
17	Idaho	59.5
18	Florida	58.5
18	Nevada	58.5
20	Missouri	57.8
21	Indiana	57.5
21	North Carolina	57.5
23	Kansas	56.8
24	Illinois	55.8
25	California	53.3
26	South Dakota	52.6
27	Ohio	52.5
28	Delaware	51.2
29	Oregon	50.9
30	Hawaii	50.7
31	Colorado	49.9
32	Montana	48.5
33	Virginia	48.3
34	Maine	47.4
35	Washington	46.7
36	Nebraska	45.1
37	Michigan	45.0
38	Maryland	43.4
39	Iowa	43.0
40	North Dakota	41.7
41	Pennsylvania	40.5
42	Vermont	39.5
42	Wisconsin	39.5
44	Minnesota	35.4
45	New Jersey	35.2
46	New York	34.8
47	New Hampshire	33.6
48	Rhode Island	33.0
49	Connecticut	30.5
50	Massachusetts	28.1
	District of Columbia	62.4

Source: U.S. Department of Health and Human Services, Centers for Disease Control and Prevention "Surveillance for Pregnancy and Birth Rates Among Teenagers" (MMWR, Vol. 42, No. SS-6, 12/17/93)
Women aged 15 to 19 years old.

Births to Women 35 to 49 Years Old in 1996

National Total = 474,359 Live Births*

ALPHA ORDER

RANK	STATE	BIRTHS	% of USA
26	Alabama	4,860	1.0%
44	Alaska	1,335	0.3%
19	Arizona	7,894	1.7%
38	Arkansas	2,450	0.5%
1	California	75,783	16.0%
20	Colorado	7,885	1.7%
18	Connecticut	7,899	1.7%
46	Delaware	1,175	0.2%
4	Florida	23,714	5.0%
12	Georgia	11,623	2.5%
36	Hawaii	2,715	0.6%
41	Idaho	1,719	0.4%
5	Illinois	23,095	4.9%
21	Indiana	7,592	1.6%
31	Iowa	3,726	0.8%
29	Kansas	3,940	0.8%
28	Kentucky	4,213	0.9%
24	Louisiana	5,648	1.2%
42	Maine	1,596	0.3%
13	Maryland	11,187	2.4%
10	Massachusetts	14,577	3.1%
9	Michigan	15,007	3.2%
16	Minnesota	8,695	1.8%
33	Mississippi	2,874	0.6%
22	Missouri	7,538	1.6%
45	Montana	1,316	0.3%
37	Nebraska	2,672	0.6%
35	Nevada	2,791	0.6%
39	New Hampshire	2,254	0.5%
7	New Jersey	20,246	4.3%
34	New Mexico	2,843	0.6%
2	New York	42,515	9.0%
15	North Carolina	9,961	2.1%
49	North Dakota	918	0.2%
8	Ohio	16,110	3.4%
32	Oklahoma	3,697	0.8%
25	Oregon	5,114	1.1%
6	Pennsylvania	20,287	4.3%
40	Rhode Island	1,789	0.4%
27	South Carolina	4,712	1.0%
47	South Dakota	1,083	0.2%
23	Tennessee	6,439	1.4%
3	Texas	31,750	6.7%
30	Utah	3,772	0.8%
48	Vermont	959	0.2%
11	Virginia	12,633	2.7%
14	Washington	10,268	2.2%
43	West Virginia	1,528	0.3%
17	Wisconsin	8,112	1.7%
50	Wyoming	592	0.1%

RANK ORDER

RANK	STATE	BIRTHS	% of USA
1	California	75,783	16.0%
2	New York	42,515	9.0%
3	Texas	31,750	6.7%
4	Florida	23,714	5.0%
5	Illinois	23,095	4.9%
6	Pennsylvania	20,287	4.3%
7	New Jersey	20,246	4.3%
8	Ohio	16,110	3.4%
9	Michigan	15,007	3.2%
10	Massachusetts	14,577	3.1%
11	Virginia	12,633	2.7%
12	Georgia	11,623	2.5%
13	Maryland	11,187	2.4%
14	Washington	10,268	2.2%
15	North Carolina	9,961	2.1%
16	Minnesota	8,695	1.8%
17	Wisconsin	8,112	1.7%
18	Connecticut	7,899	1.7%
19	Arizona	7,894	1.7%
20	Colorado	7,885	1.7%
21	Indiana	7,592	1.6%
22	Missouri	7,538	1.6%
23	Tennessee	6,439	1.4%
24	Louisiana	5,648	1.2%
25	Oregon	5,114	1.1%
26	Alabama	4,860	1.0%
27	South Carolina	4,712	1.0%
28	Kentucky	4,213	0.9%
29	Kansas	3,940	0.8%
30	Utah	3,772	0.8%
31	Iowa	3,726	0.8%
32	Oklahoma	3,697	0.8%
33	Mississippi	2,874	0.6%
34	New Mexico	2,843	0.6%
35	Nevada	2,791	0.6%
36	Hawaii	2,715	0.6%
37	Nebraska	2,672	0.6%
38	Arkansas	2,450	0.5%
39	New Hampshire	2,254	0.5%
40	Rhode Island	1,789	0.4%
41	Idaho	1,719	0.4%
42	Maine	1,596	0.3%
43	West Virginia	1,528	0.3%
44	Alaska	1,335	0.3%
45	Montana	1,316	0.3%
46	Delaware	1,175	0.2%
47	South Dakota	1,083	0.2%
48	Vermont	959	0.2%
49	North Dakota	918	0.2%
50	Wyoming	592	0.1%
	District of Columbia	1,258	0.3%

Source: Morgan Quitno Press using data from U.S. Dept of Health & Human Services, National Center for Health Statistics
(unpublished data)
*By state of residence.

Births to Women 35 to 49 Years Old as a Percent of All Births in 1996

National Percent = 12.2% of Live Births*

ALPHA ORDER				RANK ORDER		
RANK	STATE	PERCENT		RANK	STATE	PERCENT
45	Alabama	8.0		1	Massachusetts	18.2
15	Alaska	13.3		2	Connecticut	17.8
30	Arizona	10.5		3	New Jersey	17.7
50	Arkansas	6.7		4	New York	16.1
11	California	14.0		5	Maryland	15.6
9	Colorado	14.1		6	New Hampshire	15.5
2	Connecticut	17.8		7	Hawaii	14.8
22	Delaware	11.6		8	Vermont	14.2
18	Florida	12.5		9	Colorado	14.1
33	Georgia	10.2		9	Rhode Island	14.1
7	Hawaii	14.8		11	California	14.0
39	Idaho	9.2		12	Pennsylvania	13.7
17	Illinois	12.6		12	Virginia	13.7
41	Indiana	9.1		14	Minnesota	13.6
35	Iowa	10.0		15	Alaska	13.3
27	Kansas	10.8		16	Washington	13.2
45	Kentucky	8.0		17	Illinois	12.6
43	Louisiana	8.7		18	Florida	12.5
22	Maine	11.6		19	Montana	12.1
5	Maryland	15.6		19	Wisconsin	12.1
1	Massachusetts	18.2		21	Oregon	11.7
25	Michigan	11.3		22	Delaware	11.6
14	Minnesota	13.6		22	Maine	11.6
49	Mississippi	7.0		24	Nebraska	11.5
33	Missouri	10.2		25	Michigan	11.3
19	Montana	12.1		26	North Dakota	11.0
24	Nebraska	11.5		27	Kansas	10.8
28	Nevada	10.7		28	Nevada	10.7
6	New Hampshire	15.5		29	Ohio	10.6
3	New Jersey	17.7		30	Arizona	10.5
31	New Mexico	10.4		31	New Mexico	10.4
4	New York	16.1		32	South Dakota	10.3
37	North Carolina	9.5		33	Georgia	10.2
26	North Dakota	11.0		33	Missouri	10.2
29	Ohio	10.6		35	Iowa	10.0
45	Oklahoma	8.0		36	Texas	9.6
21	Oregon	11.7		37	North Carolina	9.5
12	Pennsylvania	13.7		38	Wyoming	9.4
9	Rhode Island	14.1		39	Idaho	9.2
39	South Carolina	9.2		39	South Carolina	9.2
32	South Dakota	10.3		41	Indiana	9.1
43	Tennessee	8.7		42	Utah	9.0
36	Texas	9.6		43	Louisiana	8.7
42	Utah	9.0		43	Tennessee	8.7
8	Vermont	14.2		45	Alabama	8.0
12	Virginia	13.7		45	Kentucky	8.0
16	Washington	13.2		45	Oklahoma	8.0
48	West Virginia	7.4		48	West Virginia	7.4
19	Wisconsin	12.1		49	Mississippi	7.0
38	Wyoming	9.4		50	Arkansas	6.7
					District of Columbia	15.0

Source: Morgan Quitno Press using data from U.S. Dept of Health & Human Services, National Center for Health Statistics
(unpublished data)
*By state of residence.

Births by Vaginal Delivery in 1996

National Total = 3,085,955 Live Births*

ALPHA ORDER

RANK ORDER

RANK	STATE	BIRTHS	% of USA
24	Alabama	46,394	1.5%
45	Alaska	8,361	0.3%
16	Arizona	63,195	2.0%
34	Arkansas	27,169	0.9%
1	California	428,310	13.9%
23	Colorado	47,380	1.5%
29	Connecticut	35,664	1.2%
47	Delaware	8,022	0.3%
4	Florida	148,105	4.8%
9	Georgia	90,208	2.9%
40	Hawaii	15,181	0.5%
39	Idaho	15,645	0.5%
5	Illinois	147,826	4.8%
13	Indiana	66,560	2.2%
31	Iowa	30,231	1.0%
33	Kansas	29,614	1.0%
25	Kentucky	41,480	1.3%
22	Louisiana	47,990	1.6%
42	Maine	10,909	0.4%
20	Maryland	56,082	1.8%
15	Massachusetts	64,381	2.1%
8	Michigan	106,443	3.4%
21	Minnesota	52,935	1.7%
32	Mississippi	30,084	1.0%
17	Missouri	58,770	1.9%
44	Montana	8,783	0.3%
37	Nebraska	18,675	0.6%
36	Nevada	21,083	0.7%
41	New Hampshire	11,572	0.4%
10	New Jersey	86,873	2.8%
35	New Mexico	22,545	0.7%
3	New York	203,515	6.6%
11	North Carolina	82,427	2.7%
48	North Dakota	6,769	0.2%
6	Ohio	122,871	4.0%
28	Oklahoma	35,800	1.2%
27	Oregon	36,280	1.2%
7	Pennsylvania	119,560	3.9%
43	Rhode Island	10,413	0.3%
26	South Carolina	39,565	1.3%
46	South Dakota	8,295	0.3%
18	Tennessee	57,749	1.9%
2	Texas	254,082	8.2%
30	Utah	35,395	1.1%
49	Vermont	5,650	0.2%
12	Virginia	72,867	2.4%
14	Washington	64,850	2.1%
38	West Virginia	16,019	0.5%
19	Wisconsin	56,637	1.8%
50	Wyoming	5,136	0.2%

RANK	STATE	BIRTHS	% of USA
1	California	428,310	13.9%
2	Texas	254,082	8.2%
3	New York	203,515	6.6%
4	Florida	148,105	4.8%
5	Illinois	147,826	4.8%
6	Ohio	122,871	4.0%
7	Pennsylvania	119,560	3.9%
8	Michigan	106,443	3.4%
9	Georgia	90,208	2.9%
10	New Jersey	86,873	2.8%
11	North Carolina	82,427	2.7%
12	Virginia	72,867	2.4%
13	Indiana	66,560	2.2%
14	Washington	64,850	2.1%
15	Massachusetts	64,381	2.1%
16	Arizona	63,195	2.0%
17	Missouri	58,770	1.9%
18	Tennessee	57,749	1.9%
19	Wisconsin	56,637	1.8%
20	Maryland	56,082	1.8%
21	Minnesota	52,935	1.7%
22	Louisiana	47,990	1.6%
23	Colorado	47,380	1.5%
24	Alabama	46,394	1.5%
25	Kentucky	41,480	1.3%
26	South Carolina	39,565	1.3%
27	Oregon	36,280	1.2%
28	Oklahoma	35,800	1.2%
29	Connecticut	35,664	1.2%
30	Utah	35,395	1.1%
31	Iowa	30,231	1.0%
32	Mississippi	30,084	1.0%
33	Kansas	29,614	1.0%
34	Arkansas	27,169	0.9%
35	New Mexico	22,545	0.7%
36	Nevada	21,083	0.7%
37	Nebraska	18,675	0.6%
38	West Virginia	16,019	0.5%
39	Idaho	15,645	0.5%
40	Hawaii	15,181	0.5%
41	New Hampshire	11,572	0.4%
42	Maine	10,909	0.4%
43	Rhode Island	10,413	0.3%
44	Montana	8,783	0.3%
45	Alaska	8,361	0.3%
46	South Dakota	8,295	0.3%
47	Delaware	8,022	0.3%
48	North Dakota	6,769	0.2%
49	Vermont	5,650	0.2%
50	Wyoming	5,136	0.2%

District of Columbia 6,603 0.2%

Source: Morgan Quitno Press using data from U.S. Dept of Health & Human Services, National Center for Health Statistics "Monthly Vital Statistics Report" (Vol. 46, No. 11, Supplement, June 30, 1998)
*By state of residence. Includes VBACs (vaginal births after cesarean).

Percent of Births by Vaginal Delivery in 1996

National Percent = 79.3% of Live Births*

ALPHA ORDER

RANK	STATE	PERCENT
46	Alabama	76.7
7	Alaska	83.3
5	Arizona	83.9
48	Arkansas	74.7
30	California	79.4
1	Colorado	84.9
23	Connecticut	80.2
34	Delaware	79.0
40	Florida	78.2
33	Georgia	79.1
12	Hawaii	82.5
4	Idaho	84.0
20	Illinois	80.7
27	Indiana	79.7
15	Iowa	81.4
19	Kansas	80.8
37	Kentucky	78.7
49	Louisiana	73.6
31	Maine	79.2
38	Maryland	78.4
23	Massachusetts	80.2
26	Michigan	79.8
9	Minnesota	83.1
50	Mississippi	73.4
29	Missouri	79.6
18	Montana	80.9
23	Nebraska	80.2
20	Nevada	80.7
27	New Hampshire	79.7
47	New Jersey	76.0
11	New Mexico	82.8
44	New York	77.1
35	North Carolina	78.9
16	North Dakota	81.1
17	Ohio	81.0
41	Oklahoma	77.5
9	Oregon	83.1
22	Pennsylvania	80.6
13	Rhode Island	82.3
42	South Carolina	77.4
31	South Dakota	79.2
39	Tennessee	78.3
45	Texas	76.9
3	Utah	84.1
6	Vermont	83.5
35	Virginia	78.9
8	Washington	83.2
43	West Virginia	77.2
2	Wisconsin	84.4
14	Wyoming	81.7

RANK ORDER

RANK	STATE	PERCENT
1	Colorado	84.9
2	Wisconsin	84.4
3	Utah	84.1
4	Idaho	84.0
5	Arizona	83.9
6	Vermont	83.5
7	Alaska	83.3
8	Washington	83.2
9	Minnesota	83.1
9	Oregon	83.1
11	New Mexico	82.8
12	Hawaii	82.5
13	Rhode Island	82.3
14	Wyoming	81.7
15	Iowa	81.4
16	North Dakota	81.1
17	Ohio	81.0
18	Montana	80.9
19	Kansas	80.8
20	Illinois	80.7
20	Nevada	80.7
22	Pennsylvania	80.6
23	Connecticut	80.2
23	Massachusetts	80.2
23	Nebraska	80.2
26	Michigan	79.8
27	Indiana	79.7
27	New Hampshire	79.7
29	Missouri	79.6
30	California	79.4
31	Maine	79.2
31	South Dakota	79.2
33	Georgia	79.1
34	Delaware	79.0
35	North Carolina	78.9
35	Virginia	78.9
37	Kentucky	78.7
38	Maryland	78.4
39	Tennessee	78.3
40	Florida	78.2
41	Oklahoma	77.5
42	South Carolina	77.4
43	West Virginia	77.2
44	New York	77.1
45	Texas	76.9
46	Alabama	76.7
47	New Jersey	76.0
48	Arkansas	74.7
49	Louisiana	73.6
50	Mississippi	73.4
	District of Columbia	78.7

Source: Morgan Quitno Press using data from U.S. Dept of Health & Human Services, National Center for Health Statistics "Monthly Vital Statistics Report" (Vol. 46, No. 11, Supplement, June 30, 1998)
*By state of residence. Includes VBACs (vaginal births after cesarean).

Births by Cesarean Delivery in 1996

National Total = 805,539 Live Cesarean Births*

ALPHA ORDER

RANK	STATE	BIRTHS	% of USA
19	Alabama	14,094	1.7%
47	Alaska	1,676	0.2%
21	Arizona	12,127	1.5%
28	Arkansas	9,202	1.1%
1	California	111,123	13.8%
30	Colorado	8,427	1.0%
29	Connecticut	8,805	1.1%
45	Delaware	2,133	0.3%
4	Florida	41,287	5.1%
10	Georgia	23,835	3.0%
39	Hawaii	3,220	0.4%
40	Idaho	2,980	0.4%
5	Illinois	35,354	4.4%
14	Indiana	16,953	2.1%
33	Iowa	6,908	0.9%
32	Kansas	7,037	0.9%
23	Kentucky	11,226	1.4%
13	Louisiana	17,214	2.1%
42	Maine	2,865	0.4%
17	Maryland	15,451	1.9%
16	Massachusetts	15,895	2.0%
9	Michigan	26,944	3.3%
25	Minnesota	10,765	1.3%
24	Mississippi	10,903	1.4%
18	Missouri	15,062	1.9%
46	Montana	2,073	0.3%
38	Nebraska	4,611	0.6%
35	Nevada	5,042	0.6%
41	New Hampshire	2,948	0.4%
8	New Jersey	27,433	3.4%
37	New Mexico	4,683	0.6%
3	New York	60,448	7.5%
11	North Carolina	22,043	2.7%
48	North Dakota	1,578	0.2%
6	Ohio	28,821	3.6%
27	Oklahoma	10,393	1.3%
31	Oregon	7,378	0.9%
7	Pennsylvania	28,778	3.6%
43	Rhode Island	2,239	0.3%
22	South Carolina	11,552	1.4%
44	South Dakota	2,178	0.3%
15	Tennessee	16,005	2.0%
2	Texas	76,324	9.5%
34	Utah	6,692	0.8%
50	Vermont	1,117	0.1%
12	Virginia	19,487	2.4%
20	Washington	13,095	1.6%
36	West Virginia	4,731	0.6%
26	Wisconsin	10,469	1.3%
49	Wyoming	1,150	0.1%

RANK ORDER

RANK	STATE	BIRTHS	% of USA
1	California	111,123	13.8%
2	Texas	76,324	9.5%
3	New York	60,448	7.5%
4	Florida	41,287	5.1%
5	Illinois	35,354	4.4%
6	Ohio	28,821	3.6%
7	Pennsylvania	28,778	3.6%
8	New Jersey	27,433	3.4%
9	Michigan	26,944	3.3%
10	Georgia	23,835	3.0%
11	North Carolina	22,043	2.7%
12	Virginia	19,487	2.4%
13	Louisiana	17,214	2.1%
14	Indiana	16,953	2.1%
15	Tennessee	16,005	2.0%
16	Massachusetts	15,895	2.0%
17	Maryland	15,451	1.9%
18	Missouri	15,062	1.9%
19	Alabama	14,094	1.7%
20	Washington	13,095	1.6%
21	Arizona	12,127	1.5%
22	South Carolina	11,552	1.4%
23	Kentucky	11,226	1.4%
24	Mississippi	10,903	1.4%
25	Minnesota	10,765	1.3%
26	Wisconsin	10,469	1.3%
27	Oklahoma	10,393	1.3%
28	Arkansas	9,202	1.1%
29	Connecticut	8,805	1.1%
30	Colorado	8,427	1.0%
31	Oregon	7,378	0.9%
32	Kansas	7,037	0.9%
33	Iowa	6,908	0.9%
34	Utah	6,692	0.8%
35	Nevada	5,042	0.6%
36	West Virginia	4,731	0.6%
37	New Mexico	4,683	0.6%
38	Nebraska	4,611	0.6%
39	Hawaii	3,220	0.4%
40	Idaho	2,980	0.4%
41	New Hampshire	2,948	0.4%
42	Maine	2,865	0.4%
43	Rhode Island	2,239	0.3%
44	South Dakota	2,178	0.3%
45	Delaware	2,133	0.3%
46	Montana	2,073	0.3%
47	Alaska	1,676	0.2%
48	North Dakota	1,578	0.2%
49	Wyoming	1,150	0.1%
50	Vermont	1,117	0.1%
	District of Columbia	1,787	0.2%

Source: Morgan Quitno Press using data from U.S. Dept of Health & Human Services, National Center for Health Statistics "Monthly Vital Statistics Report" (Vol. 46, No. 11, Supplement, June 30, 1998)
By state of residence.

Percent of Births by Cesarean Delivery in 1996

National Percent = 20.7% of Live Births*

ALPHA ORDER				RANK ORDER		
RANK	STATE	PERCENT		RANK	STATE	PERCENT
5	Alabama	23.3		1	Mississippi	26.6
44	Alaska	16.7		2	Louisiana	26.4
46	Arizona	16.1		3	Arkansas	25.3
3	Arkansas	25.3		4	New Jersey	24.0
21	California	20.6		5	Alabama	23.3
50	Colorado	15.1		6	Texas	23.1
26	Connecticut	19.8		7	New York	22.9
17	Delaware	21.0		8	West Virginia	22.8
12	Florida	21.6		9	South Carolina	22.6
18	Georgia	20.9		10	Oklahoma	22.5
39	Hawaii	17.5		11	Tennessee	21.7
47	Idaho	16.0		12	Florida	21.6
30	Illinois	19.3		12	Maryland	21.6
23	Indiana	20.3		14	Kentucky	21.3
36	Iowa	18.6		15	North Carolina	21.1
32	Kansas	19.2		15	Virginia	21.1
14	Kentucky	21.3		17	Delaware	21.0
2	Louisiana	26.4		18	Georgia	20.9
19	Maine	20.8		19	Maine	20.8
12	Maryland	21.6		19	South Dakota	20.8
26	Massachusetts	19.8		21	California	20.6
25	Michigan	20.2		22	Missouri	20.4
41	Minnesota	16.9		23	Indiana	20.3
1	Mississippi	26.6		23	New Hampshire	20.3
22	Missouri	20.4		25	Michigan	20.2
33	Montana	19.1		26	Connecticut	19.8
26	Nebraska	19.8		26	Massachusetts	19.8
30	Nevada	19.3		26	Nebraska	19.8
23	New Hampshire	20.3		29	Pennsylvania	19.4
4	New Jersey	24.0		30	Illinois	19.3
40	New Mexico	17.2		30	Nevada	19.3
7	New York	22.9		32	Kansas	19.2
15	North Carolina	21.1		33	Montana	19.1
35	North Dakota	18.9		34	Ohio	19.0
34	Ohio	19.0		35	North Dakota	18.9
10	Oklahoma	22.5		36	Iowa	18.6
41	Oregon	16.9		37	Wyoming	18.3
29	Pennsylvania	19.4		38	Rhode Island	17.7
38	Rhode Island	17.7		39	Hawaii	17.5
9	South Carolina	22.6		40	New Mexico	17.2
19	South Dakota	20.8		41	Minnesota	16.9
11	Tennessee	21.7		41	Oregon	16.9
6	Texas	23.1		43	Washington	16.8
48	Utah	15.9		44	Alaska	16.7
45	Vermont	16.5		45	Vermont	16.5
15	Virginia	21.1		46	Arizona	16.1
43	Washington	16.8		47	Idaho	16.0
8	West Virginia	22.8		48	Utah	15.9
49	Wisconsin	15.6		49	Wisconsin	15.6
37	Wyoming	18.3		50	Colorado	15.1
					District of Columbia	21.3

Source: U.S. Department of Health and Human Services, National Center for Health Statistics
"Monthly Vital Statistics Report" (Vol. 46, No. 11, Supplement, June 30, 1998)
*Final data by state of residence.

Percent Change in Rate of Cesarean Births: 1989 to 1996

National Percent Change = 9.2% Decrease*

ALPHA ORDER			RANK ORDER		
RANK	STATE	PERCENT CHANGE	RANK	STATE	PERCENT CHANGE
19	Alabama	(9.0)	1	South Dakota	11.2
2	Alaska	9.9	2	Alaska	9.9
32	Arizona	(13.0)	3	Maine	6.1
11	Arkansas	(6.3)	4	Mississippi	2.7
18	California	(8.8)	5	South Carolina	(0.4)
38	Colorado	(14.2)	6	Indiana	(2.9)
12	Connecticut	(6.6)	7	New York	(3.0)
31	Delaware	(12.5)	8	North Dakota	(3.1)
40	Florida	(15.6)	9	Wyoming	(3.2)
20	Georgia	(9.1)	10	Montana	(5.4)
41	Hawaii	(16.3)	11	Arkansas	(6.3)
43	Idaho	(18.4)	12	Connecticut	(6.6)
39	Illinois	(15.0)	12	New Jersey	(6.6)
6	Indiana	(2.9)	14	Iowa	(7.0)
14	Iowa	(7.0)	15	Texas	(7.6)
44	Kansas	(20.0)	16	New Mexico	(8.0)
37	Kentucky	(14.1)	17	New Hampshire	(8.6)
NA	Louisiana**	NA	18	California	(8.8)
3	Maine	6.1	19	Alabama	(9.0)
NA	Maryland**	NA	20	Georgia	(9.1)
33	Massachusetts	(13.5)	20	Minnesota	(9.1)
27	Michigan	(11.8)	22	North Carolina	(9.4)
20	Minnesota	(9.1)	23	West Virginia	(9.5)
4	Mississippi	2.7	24	Utah	(10.2)
26	Missouri	(11.7)	25	Tennessee	(10.7)
10	Montana	(5.4)	26	Missouri	(11.7)
NA	Nebraska**	NA	27	Michigan	(11.8)
NA	Nevada**	NA	27	Vermont	(11.8)
17	New Hampshire	(8.6)	29	Rhode Island	(11.9)
12	New Jersey	(6.6)	29	Wisconsin	(11.9)
16	New Mexico	(8.0)	31	Delaware	(12.5)
7	New York	(3.0)	32	Arizona	(13.0)
22	North Carolina	(9.4)	33	Massachusetts	(13.5)
8	North Dakota	(3.1)	34	Oregon	(13.8)
45	Ohio	(21.5)	34	Pennsylvania	(13.8)
NA	Oklahoma**	NA	36	Virginia	(13.9)
34	Oregon	(13.8)	37	Kentucky	(14.1)
34	Pennsylvania	(13.8)	38	Colorado	(14.2)
29	Rhode Island	(11.9)	39	Illinois	(15.0)
5	South Carolina	(0.4)	40	Florida	(15.6)
1	South Dakota	11.2	41	Hawaii	(16.3)
25	Tennessee	(10.7)	42	Washington	(16.4)
15	Texas	(7.6)	43	Idaho	(18.4)
24	Utah	(10.2)	44	Kansas	(20.0)
27	Vermont	(11.8)	45	Ohio	(21.5)
36	Virginia	(13.9)	NA	Louisiana**	NA
42	Washington	(16.4)	NA	Maryland**	NA
23	West Virginia	(9.5)	NA	Nebraska**	NA
29	Wisconsin	(11.9)	NA	Nevada**	NA
9	Wyoming	(3.2)	NA	Oklahoma**	NA
				District of Columbia	(21.4)

Source: Morgan Quitno Press using data from US Dept of Health & Human Services, National Center for Health Statistics unpublished data

*Of those births for which delivery data are available.

**Not available.

Births by Vaginal Delivery After a Previous Cesarean Delivery (VBAC) in 1996

National Total = 116,045 Live VBAC Births

ALPHA ORDER

RANK	STATE	BIRTHS	% of USA
24	Alabama	1,449	1.2%
46	Alaska	318	0.3%
23	Arizona	1,510	1.3%
35	Arkansas	867	0.7%
1	California	12,727	11.0%
21	Colorado	1,610	1.4%
28	Connecticut	1,394	1.2%
43	Delaware	422	0.4%
8	Florida	5,041	4.3%
12	Georgia	2,867	2.5%
39	Hawaii	618	0.5%
38	Idaho	652	0.6%
6	Illinois	5,727	4.9%
17	Indiana	2,276	2.0%
26	Iowa	1,411	1.2%
32	Kansas	962	0.8%
25	Kentucky	1,420	1.2%
30	Louisiana	997	0.9%
42	Maine	436	0.4%
15	Maryland	2,485	2.1%
13	Massachusetts	2,767	2.4%
9	Michigan	3,677	3.2%
18	Minnesota	2,103	1.8%
33	Mississippi	955	0.8%
14	Missouri	2,512	2.2%
45	Montana	373	0.3%
36	Nebraska	744	0.6%
37	Nevada	712	0.6%
41	New Hampshire	500	0.4%
7	New Jersey	5,545	4.8%
31	New Mexico	994	0.9%
2	New York	10,071	8.7%
11	North Carolina	2,914	2.5%
48	North Dakota	239	0.2%
5	Ohio	5,855	5.0%
34	Oklahoma	890	0.8%
22	Oregon	1,568	1.4%
4	Pennsylvania	5,883	5.1%
44	Rhode Island	419	0.4%
29	South Carolina	1,213	1.0%
47	South Dakota	243	0.2%
19	Tennessee	2,077	1.8%
3	Texas	8,324	7.2%
27	Utah	1,404	1.2%
49	Vermont	235	0.2%
10	Virginia	3,105	2.7%
16	Washington	2,453	2.1%
40	West Virginia	546	0.5%
20	Wisconsin	2,063	1.8%
50	Wyoming	214	0.2%

RANK ORDER

RANK	STATE	BIRTHS	% of USA
1	California	12,727	11.0%
2	New York	10,071	8.7%
3	Texas	8,324	7.2%
4	Pennsylvania	5,883	5.1%
5	Ohio	5,855	5.0%
6	Illinois	5,727	4.9%
7	New Jersey	5,545	4.8%
8	Florida	5,041	4.3%
9	Michigan	3,677	3.2%
10	Virginia	3,105	2.7%
11	North Carolina	2,914	2.5%
12	Georgia	2,867	2.5%
13	Massachusetts	2,767	2.4%
14	Missouri	2,512	2.2%
15	Maryland	2,485	2.1%
16	Washington	2,453	2.1%
17	Indiana	2,276	2.0%
18	Minnesota	2,103	1.8%
19	Tennessee	2,077	1.8%
20	Wisconsin	2,063	1.8%
21	Colorado	1,610	1.4%
22	Oregon	1,568	1.4%
23	Arizona	1,510	1.3%
24	Alabama	1,449	1.2%
25	Kentucky	1,420	1.2%
26	Iowa	1,411	1.2%
27	Utah	1,404	1.2%
28	Connecticut	1,394	1.2%
29	South Carolina	1,213	1.0%
30	Louisiana	997	0.9%
31	New Mexico	994	0.9%
32	Kansas	962	0.8%
33	Mississippi	955	0.8%
34	Oklahoma	890	0.8%
35	Arkansas	867	0.7%
36	Nebraska	744	0.6%
37	Nevada	712	0.6%
38	Idaho	652	0.6%
39	Hawaii	618	0.5%
40	West Virginia	546	0.5%
41	New Hampshire	500	0.4%
42	Maine	436	0.4%
43	Delaware	422	0.4%
44	Rhode Island	419	0.4%
45	Montana	373	0.3%
46	Alaska	318	0.3%
47	South Dakota	243	0.2%
48	North Dakota	239	0.2%
49	Vermont	235	0.2%
50	Wyoming	214	0.2%
	District of Columbia	177	0.2%

Source: U.S. Department of Health and Human Services, National Center for Health Statistics unpublished data

Percent of Vaginal Births After a Cesarean (VBAC) in 1996

National Percent = 28.3% of Live Births to Women Who Have Had a Cesarean*

ALPHA ORDER

RANK	STATE	PERCENT
45	Alabama	22.4
15	Alaska	34.6
32	Arizona	28.9
48	Arkansas	19.4
43	California	22.8
2	Colorado	40.4
20	Connecticut	33.3
14	Delaware	35.0
38	Florida	25.7
39	Georgia	25.2
12	Hawaii	35.2
5	Idaho	36.8
29	Illinois	30.1
37	Indiana	26.3
8	Iowa	35.7
40	Kansas	25.1
36	Kentucky	26.8
50	Louisiana	12.9
28	Maine	30.4
21	Maryland	33.0
19	Massachusetts	34.0
35	Michigan	27.1
6	Minnesota	36.1
49	Mississippi	18.1
23	Missouri	32.2
22	Montana	32.7
27	Nebraska	30.6
31	Nevada	29.0
25	New Hampshire	31.7
8	New Jersey	35.7
4	New Mexico	36.9
26	New York	31.6
30	North Carolina	29.3
32	North Dakota	28.9
10	Ohio	35.5
46	Oklahoma	22.3
3	Oregon	39.5
16	Pennsylvania	34.5
13	Rhode Island	35.1
42	South Carolina	23.3
43	South Dakota	22.8
34	Tennessee	27.4
47	Texas	21.7
17	Utah	34.3
1	Vermont	41.7
23	Virginia	32.2
7	Washington	35.9
41	West Virginia	23.9
10	Wisconsin	35.5
18	Wyoming	34.2

RANK ORDER

RANK	STATE	PERCENT
1	Vermont	41.7
2	Colorado	40.4
3	Oregon	39.5
4	New Mexico	36.9
5	Idaho	36.8
6	Minnesota	36.1
7	Washington	35.9
8	Iowa	35.7
8	New Jersey	35.7
10	Ohio	35.5
10	Wisconsin	35.5
12	Hawaii	35.2
13	Rhode Island	35.1
14	Delaware	35.0
15	Alaska	34.6
16	Pennsylvania	34.5
17	Utah	34.3
18	Wyoming	34.2
19	Massachusetts	34.0
20	Connecticut	33.3
21	Maryland	33.0
22	Montana	32.7
23	Missouri	32.2
23	Virginia	32.2
25	New Hampshire	31.7
26	New York	31.6
27	Nebraska	30.6
28	Maine	30.4
29	Illinois	30.1
30	North Carolina	29.3
31	Nevada	29.0
32	Arizona	28.9
32	North Dakota	28.9
34	Tennessee	27.4
35	Michigan	27.1
36	Kentucky	26.8
37	Indiana	26.3
38	Florida	25.7
39	Georgia	25.2
40	Kansas	25.1
41	West Virginia	23.9
42	South Carolina	23.3
43	California	22.8
43	South Dakota	22.8
45	Alabama	22.4
46	Oklahoma	22.3
47	Texas	21.7
48	Arkansas	19.4
49	Mississippi	18.1
50	Louisiana	12.9

| | District of Columbia | 21.2 |

Source: U.S. Department of Health and Human Services, National Center for Health Statistics
    "Monthly Vital Statistics Report" (Vol. 46, No. 11, Supplement, June 30, 1998)
Vaginal births after a cesarean delivery as a percent of all births to women with a previous cesarean delivery giving birth in 1996.

Percent of Mothers Beginning Prenatal Care in First Trimester in 1997

National Percent = 82.5% of Mothers*

RANK	STATE	PERCENT
32	Alabama	82.3
39	Alaska	80.9
49	Arizona	75.3
48	Arkansas	75.7
35	California	81.8
27	Colorado	82.9
3	Connecticut	89.3
28	Delaware	82.6
19	Florida	83.9
10	Georgia	85.8
25	Hawaii	83.4
44	Idaho	78.6
31	Illinois	82.5
43	Indiana	78.7
8	Iowa	87.5
12	Kansas	85.6
10	Kentucky	85.8
37	Louisiana	81.3
4	Maine	88.9
6	Maryland	88.8
4	Massachusetts	88.9
17	Michigan	84.2
17	Minnesota	84.2
42	Mississippi	80.0
9	Missouri	86.0
28	Montana	82.6
19	Nebraska	83.9
47	Nevada	76.1
1	New Hampshire	89.6
36	New Jersey	81.4
50	New Mexico	70.2
41	New York	80.6
19	North Carolina	83.9
15	North Dakota	84.8
13	Ohio	85.1
44	Oklahoma	78.6
38	Oregon	81.1
22	Pennsylvania	83.8
2	Rhode Island	89.5
40	South Carolina	80.8
33	South Dakota	82.1
24	Tennessee	83.7
46	Texas	78.5
22	Utah	83.8
7	Vermont	88.1
13	Virginia	85.1
25	Washington	83.4
34	West Virginia	82.0
16	Wisconsin	84.6
28	Wyoming	82.6

RANK	STATE	PERCENT
1	New Hampshire	89.6
2	Rhode Island	89.5
3	Connecticut	89.3
4	Maine	88.9
4	Massachusetts	88.9
6	Maryland	88.8
7	Vermont	88.1
8	Iowa	87.5
9	Missouri	86.0
10	Georgia	85.8
10	Kentucky	85.8
12	Kansas	85.6
13	Ohio	85.1
13	Virginia	85.1
15	North Dakota	84.8
16	Wisconsin	84.6
17	Michigan	84.2
17	Minnesota	84.2
19	Florida	83.9
19	Nebraska	83.9
19	North Carolina	83.9
22	Pennsylvania	83.8
22	Utah	83.8
24	Tennessee	83.7
25	Hawaii	83.4
25	Washington	83.4
27	Colorado	82.9
28	Delaware	82.6
28	Montana	82.6
28	Wyoming	82.6
31	Illinois	82.5
32	Alabama	82.3
33	South Dakota	82.1
34	West Virginia	82.0
35	California	81.8
36	New Jersey	81.4
37	Louisiana	81.3
38	Oregon	81.1
39	Alaska	80.9
40	South Carolina	80.8
41	New York	80.6
42	Mississippi	80.0
43	Indiana	78.7
44	Idaho	78.6
44	Oklahoma	78.6
46	Texas	78.5
47	Nevada	76.1
48	Arkansas	75.7
49	Arizona	75.3
50	New Mexico	70.2
	District of Columbia	66.7

Source: U.S. Department of Health and Human Services, National Center for Health Statistics
"National Vital Statistics Report" (Vol. 47, No. 4, October 7, 1998)
*Preliminary data by state of residence.

Percent of White Mothers Beginning Prenatal Care in First Trimester in 1997

National Percent = 84.7% of White Mothers*

ALPHA ORDER		
RANK	**STATE**	**PERCENT**
15	Alabama	88.1
39	Alaska	83.0
49	Arizona	76.5
45	Arkansas	79.4
41	California	81.8
38	Colorado	83.3
2	Connecticut	90.7
28	Delaware	86.4
20	Florida	87.1
6	Georgia	89.5
9	Hawaii	88.9
46	Idaho	78.9
29	Illinois	85.6
44	Indiana	80.1
15	Iowa	88.1
26	Kansas	86.6
23	Kentucky	86.9
11	Louisiana	88.7
7	Maine	89.3
1	Maryland	92.6
4	Massachusetts	90.4
19	Michigan	87.2
24	Minnesota	86.8
8	Mississippi	89.1
13	Missouri	88.2
33	Montana	84.7
32	Nebraska	85.0
48	Nevada	76.9
5	New Hampshire	89.8
29	New Jersey	85.6
50	New Mexico	72.5
36	New York	84.0
13	North Carolina	88.2
25	North Dakota	86.7
17	Ohio	87.4
43	Oklahoma	81.2
42	Oregon	81.4
26	Pennsylvania	86.6
3	Rhode Island	90.6
20	South Carolina	87.1
31	South Dakota	85.2
20	Tennessee	87.1
47	Texas	78.8
34	Utah	84.6
12	Vermont	88.3
10	Virginia	88.8
35	Washington	84.1
40	West Virginia	82.6
18	Wisconsin	87.3
37	Wyoming	83.4

RANK ORDER		
RANK	**STATE**	**PERCENT**
1	Maryland	92.6
2	Connecticut	90.7
3	Rhode Island	90.6
4	Massachusetts	90.4
5	New Hampshire	89.8
6	Georgia	89.5
7	Maine	89.3
8	Mississippi	89.1
9	Hawaii	88.9
10	Virginia	88.8
11	Louisiana	88.7
12	Vermont	88.3
13	Missouri	88.2
13	North Carolina	88.2
15	Alabama	88.1
15	Iowa	88.1
17	Ohio	87.4
18	Wisconsin	87.3
19	Michigan	87.2
20	Florida	87.1
20	South Carolina	87.1
20	Tennessee	87.1
23	Kentucky	86.9
24	Minnesota	86.8
25	North Dakota	86.7
26	Kansas	86.6
26	Pennsylvania	86.6
28	Delaware	86.4
29	Illinois	85.6
29	New Jersey	85.6
31	South Dakota	85.2
32	Nebraska	85.0
33	Montana	84.7
34	Utah	84.6
35	Washington	84.1
36	New York	84.0
37	Wyoming	83.4
38	Colorado	83.3
39	Alaska	83.0
40	West Virginia	82.6
41	California	81.8
42	Oregon	81.4
43	Oklahoma	81.2
44	Indiana	80.1
45	Arkansas	79.4
46	Idaho	78.9
47	Texas	78.8
48	Nevada	76.9
49	Arizona	76.5
50	New Mexico	72.5
	District of Columbia	81.0

Source: U.S. Department of Health and Human Services, National Center for Health Statistics
   "National Vital Statistics Report" (Vol. 47, No. 4, October 7, 1998)
Preliminary data by state of residence.

Percent of Black Mothers Beginning Prenatal Care in First Trimester in 1997

National Percent = 72.3% of Black Mothers*

ALPHA ORDER

RANK ORDER

RANK	STATE	PERCENT
33	Alabama	70.3
2	Alaska	81.9
31	Arizona	70.8
49	Arkansas	62.8
8	California	78.6
12	Colorado	77.3
4	Connecticut	80.0
28	Delaware	71.4
24	Florida	72.8
9	Georgia	78.5
1	Hawaii	89.2
28	Idaho	71.4
36	Illinois	69.7
45	Indiana	64.4
21	Iowa	73.5
14	Kansas	75.9
16	Kentucky	75.3
30	Louisiana	71.1
7	Maine	79.0
3	Maryland	80.3
10	Massachusetts	78.1
32	Michigan	70.6
45	Minnesota	64.4
37	Mississippi	69.4
20	Missouri	73.6
19	Montana	74.2
26	Nebraska	72.0
43	Nevada	66.6
11	New Hampshire	78.0
48	New Jersey	64.1
47	New Mexico	64.2
35	New York	69.8
23	North Carolina	73.2
17	North Dakota	75.0
25	Ohio	72.2
42	Oklahoma	67.7
6	Oregon	79.3
41	Pennsylvania	68.0
5	Rhode Island	79.7
38	South Carolina	69.2
38	South Dakota	69.2
27	Tennessee	71.8
18	Texas	74.6
33	Utah	70.3
NA	Vermont**	NA
21	Virginia	73.5
13	Washington	77.0
44	West Virginia	65.4
40	Wisconsin	68.9
15	Wyoming	75.8

RANK	STATE	PERCENT
1	Hawaii	89.2
2	Alaska	81.9
3	Maryland	80.3
4	Connecticut	80.0
5	Rhode Island	79.7
6	Oregon	79.3
7	Maine	79.0
8	California	78.6
9	Georgia	78.5
10	Massachusetts	78.1
11	New Hampshire	78.0
12	Colorado	77.3
13	Washington	77.0
14	Kansas	75.9
15	Wyoming	75.8
16	Kentucky	75.3
17	North Dakota	75.0
18	Texas	74.6
19	Montana	74.2
20	Missouri	73.6
21	Iowa	73.5
21	Virginia	73.5
23	North Carolina	73.2
24	Florida	72.8
25	Ohio	72.2
26	Nebraska	72.0
27	Tennessee	71.8
28	Delaware	71.4
28	Idaho	71.4
30	Louisiana	71.1
31	Arizona	70.8
32	Michigan	70.6
33	Alabama	70.3
33	Utah	70.3
35	New York	69.8
36	Illinois	69.7
37	Mississippi	69.4
38	South Carolina	69.2
38	South Dakota	69.2
40	Wisconsin	68.9
41	Pennsylvania	68.0
42	Oklahoma	67.7
43	Nevada	66.6
44	West Virginia	65.4
45	Indiana	64.4
45	Minnesota	64.4
47	New Mexico	64.2
48	New Jersey	64.1
49	Arkansas	62.8
NA	Vermont**	NA
	District of Columbia	61.5

Source: U.S. Department of Health and Human Services, National Center for Health Statistics
   "National Vital Statistics Report" (Vol. 47, No. 4, October 7, 1998)
*Preliminary data by state of residence.
**Insufficient data.

Percent of Mothers Receiving Late or No Prenatal Care in 1996

National Percent = 4.0% of Mothers*

ALPHA ORDER

RANK	STATE	PERCENT
16	Alabama	3.8
27	Alaska	3.3
2	Arizona	7.4
3	Arkansas	6.8
16	California	3.8
10	Colorado	4.5
45	Connecticut	2.3
33	Delaware	3.2
27	Florida	3.3
33	Georgia	3.2
23	Hawaii	3.5
10	Idaho	4.5
12	Illinois	4.2
16	Indiana	3.8
44	Iowa	2.5
42	Kansas	2.6
38	Kentucky	2.9
12	Louisiana	4.2
48	Maine	1.7
40	Maryland	2.7
36	Massachusetts	3.0
36	Michigan	3.0
25	Minnesota	3.4
12	Mississippi	4.2
38	Missouri	2.9
33	Montana	3.2
42	Nebraska	2.6
4	Nevada	6.0
49	New Hampshire	1.5
8	New Jersey	4.6
1	New Mexico	8.0
5	New York	5.4
27	North Carolina	3.3
46	North Dakota	2.0
25	Ohio	3.4
8	Oklahoma	4.6
15	Oregon	3.9
21	Pennsylvania	3.6
49	Rhode Island	1.5
7	South Carolina	4.7
23	South Dakota	3.5
19	Tennessee	3.7
5	Texas	5.4
27	Utah	3.3
46	Vermont	2.0
27	Virginia	3.3
21	Washington	3.6
40	West Virginia	2.7
27	Wisconsin	3.3
19	Wyoming	3.7

RANK ORDER

RANK	STATE	PERCENT
1	New Mexico	8.0
2	Arizona	7.4
3	Arkansas	6.8
4	Nevada	6.0
5	New York	5.4
5	Texas	5.4
7	South Carolina	4.7
8	New Jersey	4.6
8	Oklahoma	4.6
10	Colorado	4.5
10	Idaho	4.5
12	Illinois	4.2
12	Louisiana	4.2
12	Mississippi	4.2
15	Oregon	3.9
16	Alabama	3.8
16	California	3.8
16	Indiana	3.8
19	Tennessee	3.7
19	Wyoming	3.7
21	Pennsylvania	3.6
21	Washington	3.6
23	Hawaii	3.5
23	South Dakota	3.5
25	Minnesota	3.4
25	Ohio	3.4
27	Alaska	3.3
27	Florida	3.3
27	North Carolina	3.3
27	Utah	3.3
27	Virginia	3.3
27	Wisconsin	3.3
33	Delaware	3.2
33	Georgia	3.2
33	Montana	3.2
36	Massachusetts	3.0
36	Michigan	3.0
38	Kentucky	2.9
38	Missouri	2.9
40	Maryland	2.7
40	West Virginia	2.7
42	Kansas	2.6
42	Nebraska	2.6
44	Iowa	2.5
45	Connecticut	2.3
46	North Dakota	2.0
46	Vermont	2.0
48	Maine	1.7
49	New Hampshire	1.5
49	Rhode Island	1.5

	District of Columbia	11.8

Source: U.S. Department of Health and Human Services, National Center for Health Statistics
"Monthly Vital Statistics Report" (Vol. 46, No. 11, Supplement, June 30, 1998)
Final data by state of residence. "Late" means care begun in third trimester.

Percent of White Mothers Receiving Late or No Prenatal Care in 1996

National Percent = 3.3% of White Mothers*

ALPHA ORDER

RANK	STATE	PERCENT
30	Alabama	2.3
30	Alaska	2.3
2	Arizona	7.0
5	Arkansas	5.1
9	California	3.9
7	Colorado	4.3
43	Connecticut	1.9
30	Delaware	2.3
22	Florida	2.5
36	Georgia	2.2
43	Hawaii	1.9
6	Idaho	4.5
15	Illinois	3.0
13	Indiana	3.3
30	Iowa	2.3
26	Kansas	2.4
21	Kentucky	2.6
43	Louisiana	1.9
46	Maine	1.7
47	Maryland	1.6
26	Massachusetts	2.4
30	Michigan	2.3
19	Minnesota	2.7
38	Mississippi	2.1
38	Missouri	2.1
22	Montana	2.5
30	Nebraska	2.3
3	Nevada	5.8
48	New Hampshire	1.5
15	New Jersey	3.0
1	New Mexico	7.5
8	New York	4.2
38	North Carolina	2.1
49	North Dakota	1.4
19	Ohio	2.7
10	Oklahoma	3.8
10	Oregon	3.8
22	Pennsylvania	2.5
50	Rhode Island	1.2
18	South Carolina	2.8
41	South Dakota	2.0
26	Tennessee	2.4
4	Texas	5.4
15	Utah	3.0
41	Vermont	2.0
36	Virginia	2.2
14	Washington	3.2
22	West Virginia	2.5
26	Wisconsin	2.4
12	Wyoming	3.5

RANK ORDER

RANK	STATE	PERCENT
1	New Mexico	7.5
2	Arizona	7.0
3	Nevada	5.8
4	Texas	5.4
5	Arkansas	5.1
6	Idaho	4.5
7	Colorado	4.3
8	New York	4.2
9	California	3.9
10	Oklahoma	3.8
10	Oregon	3.8
12	Wyoming	3.5
13	Indiana	3.3
14	Washington	3.2
15	Illinois	3.0
15	New Jersey	3.0
15	Utah	3.0
18	South Carolina	2.8
19	Minnesota	2.7
19	Ohio	2.7
21	Kentucky	2.6
22	Florida	2.5
22	Montana	2.5
22	Pennsylvania	2.5
22	West Virginia	2.5
26	Kansas	2.4
26	Massachusetts	2.4
26	Tennessee	2.4
26	Wisconsin	2.4
30	Alabama	2.3
30	Alaska	2.3
30	Delaware	2.3
30	Iowa	2.3
30	Michigan	2.3
30	Nebraska	2.3
36	Georgia	2.2
36	Virginia	2.2
38	Mississippi	2.1
38	Missouri	2.1
38	North Carolina	2.1
41	South Dakota	2.0
41	Vermont	2.0
43	Connecticut	1.9
43	Hawaii	1.9
43	Louisiana	1.9
46	Maine	1.7
47	Maryland	1.6
48	New Hampshire	1.5
49	North Dakota	1.4
50	Rhode Island	1.2

| | District of Columbia | 7.2 |

Source: U.S. Department of Health and Human Services, National Center for Health Statistics
"Monthly Vital Statistics Report" (Vol. 46, No. 11, Supplement, June 30, 1998)
Final data by state of residence. "Late" means care begun in third trimester.

Percent of Black Mothers Receiving Late or No Prenatal Care in 1996

National Percent = 7.3% of Black Mothers*

ALPHA ORDER			RANK ORDER		
RANK	STATE	PERCENT	RANK	STATE	PERCENT
22	Alabama	6.9	1	Arkansas	12.7
NA	Alaska**	NA	2	New Jersey	11.6
7	Arizona	9.2	3	Pennsylvania	10.6
1	Arkansas	12.7	4	Minnesota	10.0
40	California	4.3	5	New York	9.3
26	Colorado	6.5	5	Wisconsin	9.3
36	Connecticut	5.1	7	Arizona	9.2
27	Delaware	6.3	8	Nevada	8.9
27	Florida	6.3	9	Illinois	8.8
37	Georgia	5.0	10	Oklahoma	8.6
NA	Hawaii**	NA	11	Indiana	8.4
NA	Idaho**	NA	12	Tennessee	8.3
9	Illinois	8.8	13	Ohio	8.1
11	Indiana	8.4	13	South Carolina	8.1
17	Iowa	7.2	15	Louisiana	7.5
37	Kansas	5.0	16	New Mexico	7.4
34	Kentucky	5.6	17	Iowa	7.2
15	Louisiana	7.5	17	Massachusetts	7.2
NA	Maine**	NA	17	Utah	7.2
35	Maryland	5.3	20	Washington	7.1
17	Massachusetts	7.2	21	Missouri	7.0
29	Michigan	6.2	22	Alabama	6.9
4	Minnesota	10.0	23	Virginia	6.8
25	Mississippi	6.6	24	North Carolina	6.7
21	Missouri	7.0	25	Mississippi	6.6
NA	Montana**	NA	26	Colorado	6.5
32	Nebraska	5.9	27	Delaware	6.3
8	Nevada	8.9	27	Florida	6.3
NA	New Hampshire**	NA	29	Michigan	6.2
2	New Jersey	11.6	29	West Virginia	6.2
16	New Mexico	7.4	31	Texas	6.1
5	New York	9.3	32	Nebraska	5.9
24	North Carolina	6.7	33	Oregon	5.7
NA	North Dakota**	NA	34	Kentucky	5.6
13	Ohio	8.1	35	Maryland	5.3
10	Oklahoma	8.6	36	Connecticut	5.1
33	Oregon	5.7	37	Georgia	5.0
3	Pennsylvania	10.6	37	Kansas	5.0
39	Rhode Island	4.4	39	Rhode Island	4.4
13	South Carolina	8.1	40	California	4.3
NA	South Dakota**	NA	NA	Alaska**	NA
12	Tennessee	8.3	NA	Hawaii**	NA
31	Texas	6.1	NA	Idaho**	NA
17	Utah	7.2	NA	Maine**	NA
NA	Vermont**	NA	NA	Montana**	NA
23	Virginia	6.8	NA	New Hampshire**	NA
20	Washington	7.1	NA	North Dakota**	NA
29	West Virginia	6.2	NA	South Dakota**	NA
5	Wisconsin	9.3	NA	Vermont**	NA
NA	Wyoming**	NA	NA	Wyoming**	NA
				District of Columbia	13.5

Source: U.S. Department of Health and Human Services, National Center for Health Statistics
     "Monthly Vital Statistics Report" (Vol. 46, No. 11, Supplement, June 30, 1998)
Final data by state of residence. "Late" means care begun in third trimester.
**Insufficient data.*

Percent of Births to Women Who Smoked During Pregnancy in 1996

National Percent = 13.6% of Live Births*

RANK	STATE	PERCENT
30	Alabama	13.0
3	Alaska	20.5
42	Arizona	10.3
7	Arkansas	19.3
NA	California***	NA
33	Colorado	12.6
43	Connecticut	10.0
26	Delaware	14.0
35	Florida	12.2
41	Georgia	10.4
45	Hawaii	8.6
24	Idaho	14.3
34	Illinois	12.5
NA	Indiana***	NA
9	Iowa	19.0
31	Kansas	12.9
2	Kentucky	24.5
40	Louisiana	10.7
7	Maine	19.3
38	Maryland	11.3
28	Massachusetts	13.2
16	Michigan	17.6
29	Minnesota	13.1
32	Mississippi	12.8
5	Missouri	19.6
14	Montana	18.0
20	Nebraska	16.5
27	Nevada	13.4
19	New Hampshire	16.8
36	New Jersey	12.1
38	New Mexico	11.3
47	New York**	4.9
23	North Carolina	15.8
11	North Dakota	18.4
6	Ohio	19.5
18	Oklahoma	17.4
15	Oregon	17.8
12	Pennsylvania	18.1
21	Rhode Island	16.4
24	South Carolina	14.3
NA	South Dakota***	NA
16	Tennessee	17.6
46	Texas	7.7
44	Utah	9.3
9	Vermont	19.0
37	Virginia	11.8
22	Washington	16.0
1	West Virginia	25.5
12	Wisconsin	18.1
3	Wyoming	20.5

RANK	STATE	PERCENT
1	West Virginia	25.5
2	Kentucky	24.5
3	Alaska	20.5
3	Wyoming	20.5
5	Missouri	19.6
6	Ohio	19.5
7	Arkansas	19.3
7	Maine	19.3
9	Iowa	19.0
9	Vermont	19.0
11	North Dakota	18.4
12	Pennsylvania	18.1
12	Wisconsin	18.1
14	Montana	18.0
15	Oregon	17.8
16	Michigan	17.6
16	Tennessee	17.6
18	Oklahoma	17.4
19	New Hampshire	16.8
20	Nebraska	16.5
21	Rhode Island	16.4
22	Washington	16.0
23	North Carolina	15.8
24	Idaho	14.3
24	South Carolina	14.3
26	Delaware	14.0
27	Nevada	13.4
28	Massachusetts	13.2
29	Minnesota	13.1
30	Alabama	13.0
31	Kansas	12.9
32	Mississippi	12.8
33	Colorado	12.6
34	Illinois	12.5
35	Florida	12.2
36	New Jersey	12.1
37	Virginia	11.8
38	Maryland	11.3
38	New Mexico	11.3
40	Louisiana	10.7
41	Georgia	10.4
42	Arizona	10.3
43	Connecticut	10.0
44	Utah	9.3
45	Hawaii	8.6
46	Texas	7.7
47	New York**	4.9
NA	California***	NA
NA	Indiana***	NA
NA	South Dakota***	NA
	District of Columbia	7.0

Source: U.S. Department of Health and Human Services, National Center for Health Statistics
"National Vital Statistics Report" (Vol. 47, No. 10, Supplement, November 19, 1998)
*HHS defines "Smoker" as averaging at least one cigarette a day.
**New York's figure is for New York City only.
***Not available.

Percent of Births Attended by Midwives in 1996

National Percent = 6.5% of Live Births*

ALPHA ORDER

RANK	STATE	PERCENT
40	Alabama	3.2
2	Alaska	17.0
14	Arizona	9.0
45	Arkansas	1.8
18	California	7.6
17	Colorado	7.9
22	Connecticut	6.6
6	Delaware	12.0
9	Florida	10.9
5	Georgia	13.7
32	Hawaii	4.5
36	Idaho	3.9
41	Illinois	2.9
43	Indiana	2.4
44	Iowa	2.1
48	Kansas	1.3
42	Kentucky	2.5
50	Louisiana	0.7
10	Maine	10.8
15	Maryland	8.6
7	Massachusetts	11.9
26	Michigan	5.9
18	Minnesota	7.6
46	Mississippi	1.7
49	Missouri	0.8
13	Montana	9.3
47	Nebraska	1.5
22	Nevada	6.6
3	New Hampshire	15.4
29	New Jersey	4.8
1	New Mexico	18.6
11	New York	10.2
27	North Carolina	5.8
28	North Dakota	5.3
36	Ohio	3.9
35	Oklahoma	4.1
4	Oregon	13.9
25	Pennsylvania	6.3
8	Rhode Island	11.5
24	South Carolina	6.5
38	South Dakota	3.6
34	Tennessee	4.2
31	Texas	4.6
20	Utah	7.3
12	Vermont	9.8
38	Virginia	3.6
16	Washington	8.0
21	West Virginia	6.7
29	Wisconsin	4.8
33	Wyoming	4.3

RANK ORDER

RANK	STATE	PERCENT
1	New Mexico	18.6
2	Alaska	17.0
3	New Hampshire	15.4
4	Oregon	13.9
5	Georgia	13.7
6	Delaware	12.0
7	Massachusetts	11.9
8	Rhode Island	11.5
9	Florida	10.9
10	Maine	10.8
11	New York	10.2
12	Vermont	9.8
13	Montana	9.3
14	Arizona	9.0
15	Maryland	8.6
16	Washington	8.0
17	Colorado	7.9
18	California	7.6
18	Minnesota	7.6
20	Utah	7.3
21	West Virginia	6.7
22	Connecticut	6.6
22	Nevada	6.6
24	South Carolina	6.5
25	Pennsylvania	6.3
26	Michigan	5.9
27	North Carolina	5.8
28	North Dakota	5.3
29	New Jersey	4.8
29	Wisconsin	4.8
31	Texas	4.6
32	Hawaii	4.5
33	Wyoming	4.3
34	Tennessee	4.2
35	Oklahoma	4.1
36	Idaho	3.9
36	Ohio	3.9
38	South Dakota	3.6
38	Virginia	3.6
40	Alabama	3.2
41	Illinois	2.9
42	Kentucky	2.5
43	Indiana	2.4
44	Iowa	2.1
45	Arkansas	1.8
46	Mississippi	1.7
47	Nebraska	1.5
48	Kansas	1.3
49	Missouri	0.8
50	Louisiana	0.7

	District of Columbia	3.1

Source: Morgan Quitno Press using data from U.S. Dept of Health & Human Services, National Center for Health Statistics
    (unpublished data)
*Includes certified nurse midwives and other midwives.

Reported Legal Abortions in 1995

National Total = 1,210,883 Abortions*

ALPHA ORDER

RANK	STATE	ABORTIONS	% of USA
17	Alabama	14,221	1.2%
46	Alaska	1,897	0.2%
22	Arizona	11,933	1.0%
33	Arkansas	5,757	0.5%
1	California	289,987	23.9%
28	Colorado	9,384	0.8%
24	Connecticut	11,325	0.9%
38	Delaware	4,295	0.4%
4	Florida	74,749	6.2%
8	Georgia	35,178	2.9%
35	Hawaii	5,533	0.5%
49	Idaho	970	0.1%
5	Illinois	54,092	4.5%
21	Indiana	12,382	1.0%
32	Iowa	5,899	0.5%
26	Kansas	10,767	0.9%
30	Kentucky	7,438	0.6%
23	Louisiana	11,491	0.9%
41	Maine	2,819	0.2%
16	Maryland	16,204	1.3%
12	Massachusetts	29,097	2.4%
11	Michigan	31,091	2.6%
19	Minnesota	14,017	1.2%
40	Mississippi	3,563	0.3%
25	Missouri	11,203	0.9%
43	Montana	2,674	0.2%
36	Nebraska	4,838	0.4%
31	Nevada	6,942	0.6%
42	New Hampshire	2,771	0.2%
10	New Jersey	32,947	2.7%
37	New Mexico	4,811	0.4%
2	New York	139,686	11.5%
9	North Carolina	33,420	2.8%
47	North Dakota	1,334	0.1%
7	Ohio	36,950	3.1%
29	Oklahoma	7,985	0.7%
18	Oregon	14,079	1.2%
6	Pennsylvania	39,050	3.2%
34	Rhode Island	5,707	0.5%
27	South Carolina	9,984	0.8%
48	South Dakota	1,070	0.1%
15	Tennessee	18,023	1.5%
3	Texas	87,308	7.2%
39	Utah	3,705	0.3%
45	Vermont	2,169	0.2%
13	Virginia	25,302	2.1%
14	Washington	25,075	2.1%
44	West Virginia	2,666	0.2%
20	Wisconsin	12,782	1.1%
50	Wyoming	182	0.0%

RANK ORDER

RANK	STATE	ABORTIONS	% of USA
1	California	289,987	23.9%
2	New York	139,686	11.5%
3	Texas	87,308	7.2%
4	Florida	74,749	6.2%
5	Illinois	54,092	4.5%
6	Pennsylvania	39,050	3.2%
7	Ohio	36,950	3.1%
8	Georgia	35,178	2.9%
9	North Carolina	33,420	2.8%
10	New Jersey	32,947	2.7%
11	Michigan	31,091	2.6%
12	Massachusetts	29,097	2.4%
13	Virginia	25,302	2.1%
14	Washington	25,075	2.1%
15	Tennessee	18,023	1.5%
16	Maryland	16,204	1.3%
17	Alabama	14,221	1.2%
18	Oregon	14,079	1.2%
19	Minnesota	14,017	1.2%
20	Wisconsin	12,782	1.1%
21	Indiana	12,382	1.0%
22	Arizona	11,933	1.0%
23	Louisiana	11,491	0.9%
24	Connecticut	11,325	0.9%
25	Missouri	11,203	0.9%
26	Kansas	10,767	0.9%
27	South Carolina	9,984	0.8%
28	Colorado	9,384	0.8%
29	Oklahoma	7,985	0.7%
30	Kentucky	7,438	0.6%
31	Nevada	6,942	0.6%
32	Iowa	5,899	0.5%
33	Arkansas	5,757	0.5%
34	Rhode Island	5,707	0.5%
35	Hawaii	5,533	0.5%
36	Nebraska	4,838	0.4%
37	New Mexico	4,811	0.4%
38	Delaware	4,295	0.4%
39	Utah	3,705	0.3%
40	Mississippi	3,563	0.3%
41	Maine	2,819	0.2%
42	New Hampshire	2,771	0.2%
43	Montana	2,674	0.2%
44	West Virginia	2,666	0.2%
45	Vermont	2,169	0.2%
46	Alaska	1,897	0.2%
47	North Dakota	1,334	0.1%
48	South Dakota	1,070	0.1%
49	Idaho	970	0.1%
50	Wyoming	182	0.0%
	District of Columbia	14,131	1.2%

Source: U.S. Department of Health and Human Services, Centers for Disease Control and Prevention
   "Abortion Surveillance-United States, 1995" (Morbidity Mortality Weekly Report, Vol. 47, No. SS-2, July 3, 1998)
*By state of occurrence.

Reported Legal Abortions per 1,000 Live Births in 1995

National Rate = 311 Abortions per 1,000 Live Births*

ALPHA ORDER			RANK ORDER		
RANK	STATE	RATE	RANK	STATE	RATE
24	Alabama	236	1	California	526
33	Alaska	187	2	New York	525
38	Arizona	165	3	Rhode Island	447
39	Arkansas	164	4	Delaware	419
1	California	526	5	Florida	396
37	Colorado	173	6	Massachusetts	357
20	Connecticut	255	7	Oregon	330
4	Delaware	419	8	North Carolina	329
5	Florida	396	9	Washington	325
11	Georgia	313	10	Vermont	320
12	Hawaii	298	11	Georgia	313
49	Idaho	54	12	Hawaii	298
13	Illinois	291	13	Illinois	291
43	Indiana	149	14	Kansas	290
40	Iowa	160	15	New Jersey	287
14	Kansas	290	16	Nevada	279
44	Kentucky	143	17	Virginia	277
35	Louisiana	175	18	Texas	271
29	Maine	203	19	Pennsylvania	259
26	Maryland	224	20	Connecticut	255
6	Massachusetts	357	21	Tennessee	246
25	Michigan	232	22	Montana	242
27	Minnesota	222	23	Ohio	240
48	Mississippi	86	24	Alabama	236
42	Missouri	154	25	Michigan	232
22	Montana	242	26	Maryland	224
28	Nebraska	208	27	Minnesota	222
16	Nevada	279	28	Nebraska	208
31	New Hampshire	189	29	Maine	203
15	New Jersey	287	30	South Carolina	196
34	New Mexico	179	31	New Hampshire	189
2	New York	525	31	Wisconsin	189
8	North Carolina	329	33	Alaska	187
41	North Dakota	157	34	New Mexico	179
23	Ohio	240	35	Louisiana	175
35	Oklahoma	175	35	Oklahoma	175
7	Oregon	330	37	Colorado	173
19	Pennsylvania	259	38	Arizona	165
3	Rhode Island	447	39	Arkansas	164
30	South Carolina	196	40	Iowa	160
46	South Dakota	102	41	North Dakota	157
21	Tennessee	246	42	Missouri	154
18	Texas	271	43	Indiana	149
47	Utah	94	44	Kentucky	143
10	Vermont	320	45	West Virginia	126
17	Virginia	277	46	South Dakota	102
9	Washington	325	47	Utah	94
45	West Virginia	126	48	Mississippi	86
31	Wisconsin	189	49	Idaho	54
50	Wyoming	29	50	Wyoming	29
				District of Columbia**	NA

Source: U.S. Department of Health and Human Services, Centers for Disease Control and Prevention
    "Abortion Surveillance-United States, 1995" (Morbidity Mortality Weekly Report, Vol. 47, No. SS-2, July 3, 1998)
*By state of occurrence.
**The District of Columbia's ratio was not listed but was noted as being greater than 1,000 abortions per 1,000 live births.

Reported Legal Abortions per 1,000 Women Ages 15 to 44 in 1995

National Rate = 20 Reported Legal Abortions per 1,000 Women Ages 15 to 44*

ALPHA ORDER

RANK ORDER

RANK	STATE	RATE	RANK	STATE	RATE
19	Alabama	15	1	California	40
24	Alaska	14	2	New York	34
29	Arizona	13	3	Delaware	26
41	Arkansas	9	3	Florida	26
1	California	40	3	Rhode Island	26
24	Colorado	14	6	Hawaii	21
17	Connecticut	16	6	Massachusetts	21
3	Delaware	26	6	Nevada	21
3	Florida	26	9	Georgia	20
9	Georgia	20	9	Illinois	20
6	Hawaii	21	9	North Carolina	20
49	Idaho	4	9	Oregon	20
9	Illinois	20	9	Texas	20
41	Indiana	9	9	Washington	20
37	Iowa	10	15	Kansas	19
15	Kansas	19	15	New Jersey	19
44	Kentucky	8	17	Connecticut	16
34	Louisiana	11	17	Vermont	16
37	Maine	10	19	Alabama	15
24	Maryland	14	19	Ohio	15
6	Massachusetts	21	19	Pennsylvania	15
24	Michigan	14	19	Tennessee	15
29	Minnesota	13	19	Virginia	15
48	Mississippi	6	24	Alaska	14
41	Missouri	9	24	Colorado	14
24	Montana	14	24	Maryland	14
29	Nebraska	13	24	Michigan	14
6	Nevada	21	24	Montana	14
37	New Hampshire	10	29	Arizona	13
15	New Jersey	19	29	Minnesota	13
29	New Mexico	13	29	Nebraska	13
2	New York	34	29	New Mexico	13
9	North Carolina	20	33	South Carolina	12
37	North Dakota	10	34	Louisiana	11
19	Ohio	15	34	Oklahoma	11
34	Oklahoma	11	34	Wisconsin	11
9	Oregon	20	37	Iowa	10
19	Pennsylvania	15	37	Maine	10
3	Rhode Island	26	37	New Hampshire	10
33	South Carolina	12	37	North Dakota	10
46	South Dakota	7	41	Arkansas	9
19	Tennessee	15	41	Indiana	9
9	Texas	20	41	Missouri	9
44	Utah	8	44	Kentucky	8
17	Vermont	16	44	Utah	8
19	Virginia	15	46	South Dakota	7
9	Washington	20	46	West Virginia	7
46	West Virginia	7	48	Mississippi	6
34	Wisconsin	11	49	Idaho	4
50	Wyoming	2	50	Wyoming	2
				District of Columbia**	NA

Source: U.S. Department of Health and Human Services, Centers for Disease Control and Prevention
"Abortion Surveillance-United States, 1995" (Morbidity Mortality Weekly Report, Vol. 47, No. SS-2, July 3, 1998)
*By state of occurrence.
**The District of Columbia's rate was not listed but was noted as being greater than 100 abortions per 1,000 women ages 15 to 44 years.

Percent of Legal Abortions Obtained by Out-Of-State Residents in 1995

National Percent = 8.3% of Reported Legal Abortions*

ALPHA ORDER		
RANK	STATE	PERCENT
11	Alabama	12.3
NA	Alaska**	NA
39	Arizona	1.8
21	Arkansas	8.6
NA	California**	NA
19	Colorado	8.9
35	Connecticut	3.7
NA	Delaware**	NA
NA	Florida**	NA
17	Georgia	9.5
40	Hawaii	0.4
25	Idaho	6.8
NA	Illinois**	NA
34	Indiana	3.8
NA	Iowa**	NA
1	Kansas	42.5
4	Kentucky	22.3
NA	Louisiana**	NA
37	Maine	3.0
20	Maryland	8.8
27	Massachusetts	5.6
33	Michigan	4.3
18	Minnesota	9.1
36	Mississippi	3.5
15	Missouri	11.3
9	Montana	16.8
5	Nebraska	20.5
16	Nevada	11.0
NA	New Hampshire**	NA
38	New Jersey	2.0
30	New Mexico	4.9
NA	New York**	NA
12	North Carolina	11.6
2	North Dakota	30.4
22	Ohio	7.8
NA	Oklahoma**	NA
13	Oregon	11.4
31	Pennsylvania	4.8
6	Rhode Island	20.1
24	South Carolina	6.9
7	South Dakota	19.2
8	Tennessee	17.9
32	Texas	4.6
13	Utah	11.4
3	Vermont	22.9
26	Virginia	5.7
29	Washington	5.0
10	West Virginia	13.1
28	Wisconsin	5.1
23	Wyoming	7.7

RANK ORDER		
RANK	STATE	PERCENT
1	Kansas	42.5
2	North Dakota	30.4
3	Vermont	22.9
4	Kentucky	22.3
5	Nebraska	20.5
6	Rhode Island	20.1
7	South Dakota	19.2
8	Tennessee	17.9
9	Montana	16.8
10	West Virginia	13.1
11	Alabama	12.3
12	North Carolina	11.6
13	Oregon	11.4
13	Utah	11.4
15	Missouri	11.3
16	Nevada	11.0
17	Georgia	9.5
18	Minnesota	9.1
19	Colorado	8.9
20	Maryland	8.8
21	Arkansas	8.6
22	Ohio	7.8
23	Wyoming	7.7
24	South Carolina	6.9
25	Idaho	6.8
26	Virginia	5.7
27	Massachusetts	5.6
28	Wisconsin	5.1
29	Washington	5.0
30	New Mexico	4.9
31	Pennsylvania	4.8
32	Texas	4.6
33	Michigan	4.3
34	Indiana	3.8
35	Connecticut	3.7
36	Mississippi	3.5
37	Maine	3.0
38	New Jersey	2.0
39	Arizona	1.8
40	Hawaii	0.4
NA	Alaska**	NA
NA	California**	NA
NA	Delaware**	NA
NA	Florida**	NA
NA	Illinois**	NA
NA	Iowa**	NA
NA	Louisiana**	NA
NA	New Hampshire**	NA
NA	New York**	NA
NA	Oklahoma**	NA

District of Columbia 53.3

Source: U.S. Department of Health and Human Services, Centers for Disease Control and Prevention
"Abortion Surveillance-United States, 1995" (Morbidity Mortality Weekly Report, Vol. 47, No. SS-2, July 3, 1998)
*By state of occurrence.
**Not reported.

Percent of Reported Legal Abortions Obtained by White Women in 1995

Reporting States' Percent = 57.8% of Reported Legal Abortions*

ALPHA ORDER

RANK	STATE	PERCENT
28	Alabama	52.2
NA	Alaska**	NA
15	Arizona	76.8
20	Arkansas	64.0
NA	California**	NA
NA	Colorado**	NA
NA	Connecticut**	NA
NA	Delaware**	NA
NA	Florida**	NA
30	Georgia	45.3
35	Hawaii	29.3
2	Idaho	94.8
NA	Illinois**	NA
18	Indiana	71.7
NA	Iowa**	NA
13	Kansas	77.3
16	Kentucky	76.7
29	Louisiana	47.3
3	Maine	93.9
31	Maryland	43.3
NA	Massachusetts**	NA
NA	Michigan**	NA
14	Minnesota	77.1
33	Mississippi	36.1
21	Missouri	63.2
6	Montana	87.6
NA	Nebraska**	NA
11	Nevada	82.3
NA	New Hampshire**	NA
34	New Jersey	35.7
5	New Mexico	87.7
32	New York**	38.5
26	North Carolina	53.6
4	North Dakota	89.0
22	Ohio	62.2
NA	Oklahoma**	NA
7	Oregon	87.1
24	Pennsylvania	59.1
12	Rhode Island	79.4
27	South Carolina	52.7
8	South Dakota	86.7
23	Tennessee	59.3
19	Texas	71.2
10	Utah	83.8
1	Vermont	97.7
25	Virginia	57.3
NA	Washington**	NA
9	West Virginia	86.6
17	Wisconsin	74.9
NA	Wyoming**	NA

RANK ORDER

RANK	STATE	PERCENT
1	Vermont	97.7
2	Idaho	94.8
3	Maine	93.9
4	North Dakota	89.0
5	New Mexico	87.7
6	Montana	87.6
7	Oregon	87.1
8	South Dakota	86.7
9	West Virginia	86.6
10	Utah	83.8
11	Nevada	82.3
12	Rhode Island	79.4
13	Kansas	77.3
14	Minnesota	77.1
15	Arizona	76.8
16	Kentucky	76.7
17	Wisconsin	74.9
18	Indiana	71.7
19	Texas	71.2
20	Arkansas	64.0
21	Missouri	63.2
22	Ohio	62.2
23	Tennessee	59.3
24	Pennsylvania	59.1
25	Virginia	57.3
26	North Carolina	53.6
27	South Carolina	52.7
28	Alabama	52.2
29	Louisiana	47.3
30	Georgia	45.3
31	Maryland	43.3
32	New York**	38.5
33	Mississippi	36.1
34	New Jersey	35.7
35	Hawaii	29.3
NA	Alaska**	NA
NA	California**	NA
NA	Colorado**	NA
NA	Connecticut**	NA
NA	Delaware**	NA
NA	Florida**	NA
NA	Illinois**	NA
NA	Iowa**	NA
NA	Massachusetts**	NA
NA	Michigan**	NA
NA	Nebraska**	NA
NA	New Hampshire**	NA
NA	Oklahoma**	NA
NA	Washington**	NA
NA	Wyoming**	NA
	District of Columbia	18.2

Source: U.S. Department of Health and Human Services, Centers for Disease Control and Prevention
   "Abortion Surveillance-United States, 1995" (Morbidity Mortality Weekly Report, Vol. 47, No. SS-2, July 3, 1998)
*By state of occurrence. Includes those of Hispanic ethnicity. National percent is for reporting states only.
**Not reported. New York's number is for New York City only.

Percent of Reported Legal Abortions Obtained by Black Women in 1995

Reporting States' Percent = 33.9% of Reported Legal Abortions*

ALPHA ORDER			RANK ORDER		
RANK	STATE	PERCENT	RANK	STATE	PERCENT
6	Alabama	45.2	1	Mississippi	62.8
NA	Alaska**	NA	2	New York**	52.8
26	Arizona	4.7	3	Georgia	50.2
14	Arkansas	32.7	4	Maryland	48.9
NA	California**	NA	5	New Jersey	46.0
NA	Colorado**	NA	6	Alabama	45.2
NA	Connecticut**	NA	7	South Carolina	45.1
NA	Delaware**	NA	8	Louisiana	40.4
NA	Florida**	NA	9	North Carolina	39.9
3	Georgia	50.2	10	Tennessee	38.1
27	Hawaii	2.7	11	Pennsylvania	37.6
34	Idaho	0.5	12	Virginia	36.5
NA	Illinois**	NA	13	Missouri	33.1
16	Indiana	23.7	14	Arkansas	32.7
NA	Iowa**	NA	15	Ohio	31.4
20	Kansas	17.2	16	Indiana	23.7
18	Kentucky	19.4	17	Wisconsin	20.1
8	Louisiana	40.4	18	Kentucky	19.4
32	Maine	1.0	19	Texas	19.1
4	Maryland	48.9	20	Kansas	17.2
NA	Massachusetts**	NA	21	Rhode Island	14.5
NA	Michigan**	NA	22	West Virginia	12.4
23	Minnesota	11.8	23	Minnesota	11.8
1	Mississippi	62.8	24	Nevada	7.6
13	Missouri	33.1	25	Oregon	5.1
35	Montana	0.4	26	Arizona	4.7
NA	Nebraska**	NA	27	Hawaii	2.7
24	Nevada	7.6	28	New Mexico	2.5
NA	New Hampshire**	NA	29	South Dakota	2.2
5	New Jersey	46.0	30	Utah	2.0
28	New Mexico	2.5	31	North Dakota	1.9
2	New York**	52.8	32	Maine	1.0
9	North Carolina	39.9	33	Vermont	0.9
31	North Dakota	1.9	34	Idaho	0.5
15	Ohio	31.4	35	Montana	0.4
NA	Oklahoma**	NA	NA	Alaska**	NA
25	Oregon	5.1	NA	California**	NA
11	Pennsylvania	37.6	NA	Colorado**	NA
21	Rhode Island	14.5	NA	Connecticut**	NA
7	South Carolina	45.1	NA	Delaware**	NA
29	South Dakota	2.2	NA	Florida**	NA
10	Tennessee	38.1	NA	Illinois**	NA
19	Texas	19.1	NA	Iowa**	NA
30	Utah	2.0	NA	Massachusetts**	NA
33	Vermont	0.9	NA	Michigan**	NA
12	Virginia	36.5	NA	Nebraska**	NA
NA	Washington**	NA	NA	New Hampshire**	NA
22	West Virginia	12.4	NA	Oklahoma**	NA
17	Wisconsin	20.1	NA	Washington**	NA
NA	Wyoming**	NA	NA	Wyoming**	NA

District of Columbia   74.9

Source: U.S. Department of Health and Human Services, Centers for Disease Control and Prevention
   "Abortion Surveillance-United States, 1995" (Morbidity Mortality Weekly Report, Vol. 47, No. SS-2, July 3, 1998)
*By state of occurrence. National percent is for reporting states only.
**Not reported. New York's number is for New York City only.

Percent of Reported Legal Abortions Obtained by Married Women in 1995

Reporting States' Percent = 19.3% of Reported Legal Abortions*

ALPHA ORDER

RANK	STATE	PERCENT
31	Alabama	16.0
NA	Alaska**	NA
11	Arizona	20.2
NA	Arkansas**	NA
6	California	21.0
NA	Colorado**	NA
NA	Connecticut**	NA
NA	Delaware**	NA
NA	Florida**	NA
20	Georgia	18.1
14	Hawaii	19.1
5	Idaho	22.2
NA	Illinois**	NA
30	Indiana	16.2
NA	Iowa**	NA
11	Kansas	20.2
26	Kentucky	17.1
NA	Louisiana**	NA
NA	Maine**	NA
18	Maryland	18.6
NA	Massachusetts**	NA
33	Michigan	15.7
16	Minnesota	18.9
29	Mississippi	16.6
9	Missouri	20.3
22	Montana	18.0
NA	Nebraska**	NA
4	Nevada	22.5
NA	New Hampshire**	NA
26	New Jersey	17.1
28	New Mexico	16.8
13	New York**	20.0
NA	North Carolina**	NA
23	North Dakota	17.5
24	Ohio	17.3
NA	Oklahoma**	NA
2	Oregon	23.0
24	Pennsylvania	17.3
7	Rhode Island	20.6
17	South Carolina	18.7
9	South Dakota	20.3
14	Tennessee	19.1
3	Texas	22.6
1	Utah	39.0
8	Vermont	20.5
NA	Virginia**	NA
NA	Washington**	NA
19	West Virginia	18.5
31	Wisconsin	16.0
20	Wyoming	18.1

RANK ORDER

RANK	STATE	PERCENT
1	Utah	39.0
2	Oregon	23.0
3	Texas	22.6
4	Nevada	22.5
5	Idaho	22.2
6	California	21.0
7	Rhode Island	20.6
8	Vermont	20.5
9	Missouri	20.3
9	South Dakota	20.3
11	Arizona	20.2
11	Kansas	20.2
13	New York**	20.0
14	Hawaii	19.1
14	Tennessee	19.1
16	Minnesota	18.9
17	South Carolina	18.7
18	Maryland	18.6
19	West Virginia	18.5
20	Georgia	18.1
20	Wyoming	18.1
22	Montana	18.0
23	North Dakota	17.5
24	Ohio	17.3
24	Pennsylvania	17.3
26	Kentucky	17.1
26	New Jersey	17.1
28	New Mexico	16.8
29	Mississippi	16.6
30	Indiana	16.2
31	Alabama	16.0
31	Wisconsin	16.0
33	Michigan	15.7
NA	Alaska**	NA
NA	Arkansas**	NA
NA	Colorado**	NA
NA	Connecticut**	NA
NA	Delaware**	NA
NA	Florida**	NA
NA	Illinois**	NA
NA	Iowa**	NA
NA	Louisiana**	NA
NA	Maine**	NA
NA	Massachusetts**	NA
NA	Nebraska**	NA
NA	New Hampshire**	NA
NA	North Carolina**	NA
NA	Oklahoma**	NA
NA	Virginia**	NA
NA	Washington**	NA
	District of Columbia**	NA

Source: U.S. Department of Health and Human Services, Centers for Disease Control and Prevention
   "Abortion Surveillance-United States, 1995" (Morbidity Mortality Weekly Report, Vol. 47, No. SS-2, July 3, 1998)
*By state of occurrence. National percent is for reporting states only.
**Not reported. New York's percentage is for New York City only.

Percent of Reported Legal Abortions Obtained by Unmarried Women in 1995

Reporting States' Percent = 78.7% of Reported Legal Abortions*

ALPHA ORDER			RANK ORDER		
RANK	STATE	PERCENT	RANK	STATE	PERCENT
3	Alabama	83.5	1	Michigan	83.6
NA	Alaska**	NA	1	Wisconsin	83.6
20	Arizona	78.6	3	Alabama	83.5
NA	Arkansas**	NA	4	Mississippi	83.3
26	California	77.7	5	Pennsylvania	82.7
NA	Colorado**	NA	6	New Mexico	82.5
NA	Connecticut**	NA	6	North Dakota	82.5
NA	Delaware**	NA	8	New Jersey	82.4
NA	Florida**	NA	9	West Virginia	81.5
10	Georgia	81.4	10	Georgia	81.4
13	Hawaii	80.7	10	Kentucky	81.4
24	Idaho	77.8	12	South Carolina	81.3
NA	Illinois**	NA	13	Hawaii	80.7
24	Indiana	77.8	14	Tennessee	80.5
NA	Iowa**	NA	15	Ohio	80.2
17	Kansas	79.5	15	Wyoming	80.2
10	Kentucky	81.4	17	Kansas	79.5
NA	Louisiana**	NA	18	South Dakota	79.3
NA	Maine**	NA	19	Maryland	78.8
19	Maryland	78.8	20	Arizona	78.6
NA	Massachusetts**	NA	20	Minnesota	78.6
1	Michigan	83.6	22	Rhode Island	78.2
20	Minnesota	78.6	23	Missouri	77.9
4	Mississippi	83.3	24	Idaho	77.8
23	Missouri	77.9	24	Indiana	77.8
28	Montana	77.5	26	California	77.7
NA	Nebraska**	NA	27	New York**	77.6
29	Nevada	75.4	28	Montana	77.5
NA	New Hampshire**	NA	29	Nevada	75.4
8	New Jersey	82.4	29	Oregon	75.4
6	New Mexico	82.5	31	Vermont	73.4
27	New York**	77.6	32	Texas	72.3
NA	North Carolina**	NA	33	Utah	61.0
6	North Dakota	82.5	NA	Alaska**	NA
15	Ohio	80.2	NA	Arkansas**	NA
NA	Oklahoma**	NA	NA	Colorado**	NA
29	Oregon	75.4	NA	Connecticut**	NA
5	Pennsylvania	82.7	NA	Delaware**	NA
22	Rhode Island	78.2	NA	Florida**	NA
12	South Carolina	81.3	NA	Illinois**	NA
18	South Dakota	79.3	NA	Iowa**	NA
14	Tennessee	80.5	NA	Louisiana**	NA
32	Texas	72.3	NA	Maine**	NA
33	Utah	61.0	NA	Massachusetts**	NA
31	Vermont	73.4	NA	Nebraska**	NA
NA	Virginia**	NA	NA	New Hampshire**	NA
NA	Washington**	NA	NA	North Carolina**	NA
9	West Virginia	81.5	NA	Oklahoma**	NA
1	Wisconsin	83.6	NA	Virginia**	NA
15	Wyoming	80.2	NA	Washington**	NA
			District of Columbia**		NA

Source: U.S. Department of Health and Human Services, Centers for Disease Control and Prevention
    "Abortion Surveillance-United States, 1995" (Morbidity Mortality Weekly Report, Vol. 47, No. SS-2, July 3, 1998)
*By state of occurrence. National percent is for reporting states only.
**Not reported. New York's percentage is for New York City only.

Reported Legal Abortions Obtained by Teenagers in 1995

Reporting States' Total = 151,017 Legal Abortions Obtained by Teenagers*

ALPHA ORDER

RANK	STATE	ABORTIONS	% of USA
14	Alabama	3,236	2.1%
NA	Alaska**	NA	NA
22	Arizona	2,328	1.5%
27	Arkansas	1,411	0.9%
NA	California**	NA	NA
25	Colorado	2,164	1.4%
19	Connecticut	2,526	1.7%
NA	Delaware**	NA	NA
NA	Florida**	NA	NA
5	Georgia	7,156	4.7%
28	Hawaii	1,210	0.8%
41	Idaho	252	0.2%
NA	Illinois**	NA	NA
17	Indiana	2,671	1.8%
NA	Iowa**	NA	NA
16	Kansas	2,742	1.8%
26	Kentucky	1,849	1.2%
20	Louisiana	2,474	1.6%
36	Maine	680	0.5%
13	Maryland	3,400	2.3%
11	Massachusetts	4,524	3.0%
7	Michigan	6,638	4.4%
18	Minnesota	2,554	1.7%
33	Mississippi	818	0.5%
23	Missouri	2,296	1.5%
35	Montana	683	0.5%
32	Nebraska	1,070	0.7%
28	Nevada	1,210	0.8%
NA	New Hampshire**	NA	NA
8	New Jersey	5,725	3.8%
31	New Mexico	1,092	0.7%
1	New York	26,793	17.7%
4	North Carolina	7,589	5.0%
39	North Dakota	344	0.2%
6	Ohio	6,799	4.5%
NA	Oklahoma**	NA	NA
15	Oregon	3,100	2.1%
3	Pennsylvania	7,672	5.1%
30	Rhode Island	1,108	0.7%
24	South Carolina	2,220	1.5%
40	South Dakota	298	0.2%
12	Tennessee	3,855	2.6%
2	Texas	16,028	10.6%
34	Utah	706	0.5%
38	Vermont	529	0.4%
10	Virginia	5,020	3.3%
9	Washington	5,175	3.4%
37	West Virginia	675	0.4%
21	Wisconsin	2,360	1.6%
42	Wyoming	37	0.0%

RANK ORDER

RANK	STATE	ABORTIONS	% of USA
1	New York	26,793	17.7%
2	Texas	16,028	10.6%
3	Pennsylvania	7,672	5.1%
4	North Carolina	7,589	5.0%
5	Georgia	7,156	4.7%
6	Ohio	6,799	4.5%
7	Michigan	6,638	4.4%
8	New Jersey	5,725	3.8%
9	Washington	5,175	3.4%
10	Virginia	5,020	3.3%
11	Massachusetts	4,524	3.0%
12	Tennessee	3,855	2.6%
13	Maryland	3,400	2.3%
14	Alabama	3,236	2.1%
15	Oregon	3,100	2.1%
16	Kansas	2,742	1.8%
17	Indiana	2,671	1.8%
18	Minnesota	2,554	1.7%
19	Connecticut	2,526	1.7%
20	Louisiana	2,474	1.6%
21	Wisconsin	2,360	1.6%
22	Arizona	2,328	1.5%
23	Missouri	2,296	1.5%
24	South Carolina	2,220	1.5%
25	Colorado	2,164	1.4%
26	Kentucky	1,849	1.2%
27	Arkansas	1,411	0.9%
28	Hawaii	1,210	0.8%
28	Nevada	1,210	0.8%
30	Rhode Island	1,108	0.7%
31	New Mexico	1,092	0.7%
32	Nebraska	1,070	0.7%
33	Mississippi	818	0.5%
34	Utah	706	0.5%
35	Montana	683	0.5%
36	Maine	680	0.5%
37	West Virginia	675	0.4%
38	Vermont	529	0.4%
39	North Dakota	344	0.2%
40	South Dakota	298	0.2%
41	Idaho	252	0.2%
42	Wyoming	37	0.0%
NA	Alaska**	NA	NA
NA	California**	NA	NA
NA	Delaware**	NA	NA
NA	Florida**	NA	NA
NA	Illinois**	NA	NA
NA	Iowa**	NA	NA
NA	New Hampshire**	NA	NA
NA	Oklahoma**	NA	NA
	District of Columbia**	NA	NA

Source: U.S. Department of Health and Human Services, Centers for Disease Control and Prevention
    "Abortion Surveillance-United States, 1995" (Morbidity Mortality Weekly Report, Vol. 47, No. SS-2, July 3, 1998)
*Nineteen years old and younger by state of occurrence. National total is for reporting states only.
**Not reported.

Percent of Reported Legal Abortions Obtained by Teenagers in 1995

Reporting States' Percent = 12.5% of Legal Abortions*

ALPHA ORDER		
RANK	STATE	PERCENT
13	Alabama	22.8
NA	Alaska**	NA
32	Arizona	19.5
8	Arkansas	24.5
NA	California**	NA
11	Colorado	23.1
16	Connecticut	22.3
NA	Delaware**	NA
NA	Florida**	NA
28	Georgia	20.3
20	Hawaii	21.9
2	Idaho	26.0
NA	Illinois**	NA
21	Indiana	21.6
NA	Iowa**	NA
4	Kansas	25.5
7	Kentucky	24.9
22	Louisiana	21.5
10	Maine	24.1
25	Maryland	21.0
42	Massachusetts	15.5
23	Michigan	21.4
39	Minnesota	18.2
12	Mississippi	23.0
27	Missouri	20.5
4	Montana	25.5
18	Nebraska	22.1
40	Nevada	17.4
NA	New Hampshire**	NA
40	New Jersey	17.4
14	New Mexico	22.7
34	New York	19.2
14	North Carolina	22.7
3	North Dakota	25.8
37	Ohio	18.4
NA	Oklahoma**	NA
19	Oregon	22.0
31	Pennsylvania	19.6
33	Rhode Island	19.4
17	South Carolina	22.2
1	South Dakota	27.9
23	Tennessee	21.4
37	Texas	18.4
35	Utah	19.1
9	Vermont	24.4
30	Virginia	19.8
26	Washington	20.6
6	West Virginia	25.3
36	Wisconsin	18.5
28	Wyoming	20.3

RANK ORDER		
RANK	STATE	PERCENT
1	South Dakota	27.9
2	Idaho	26.0
3	North Dakota	25.8
4	Kansas	25.5
4	Montana	25.5
6	West Virginia	25.3
7	Kentucky	24.9
8	Arkansas	24.5
9	Vermont	24.4
10	Maine	24.1
11	Colorado	23.1
12	Mississippi	23.0
13	Alabama	22.8
14	New Mexico	22.7
14	North Carolina	22.7
16	Connecticut	22.3
17	South Carolina	22.2
18	Nebraska	22.1
19	Oregon	22.0
20	Hawaii	21.9
21	Indiana	21.6
22	Louisiana	21.5
23	Michigan	21.4
23	Tennessee	21.4
25	Maryland	21.0
26	Washington	20.6
27	Missouri	20.5
28	Georgia	20.3
28	Wyoming	20.3
30	Virginia	19.8
31	Pennsylvania	19.6
32	Arizona	19.5
33	Rhode Island	19.4
34	New York	19.2
35	Utah	19.1
36	Wisconsin	18.5
37	Ohio	18.4
37	Texas	18.4
39	Minnesota	18.2
40	Nevada	17.4
40	New Jersey	17.4
42	Massachusetts	15.5
NA	Alaska**	NA
NA	California**	NA
NA	Delaware**	NA
NA	Florida**	NA
NA	Illinois**	NA
NA	Iowa**	NA
NA	New Hampshire**	NA
NA	Oklahoma**	NA
	District of Columbia**	NA

Source: Morgan Quitno Press using data from US Dept of Health & Human Serv's, Centers for Disease Control-Prevention "Abortion Surveillance-United States, 1995" (Morbidity Mortality Weekly Report, Vol. 47, No. SS-2, July 3, 1998)
Nineteen and younger by state of occurrence. National percent is for reporting states only.
**Not reported.*

Reported Legal Abortions Obtained by Teenagers 17 Years and Younger in 1995

Reporting States' Total = 64,391 Reported Legal Abortions*

ALPHA ORDER

RANK	STATE	ABORTIONS	% of USA
14	Alabama	1,385	2.2%
NA	Alaska**	NA	NA
24	Arizona	973	1.5%
27	Arkansas	610	0.9%
NA	California**	NA	NA
19	Colorado	1,059	1.6%
17	Connecticut	1,168	1.8%
NA	Delaware**	NA	NA
NA	Florida**	NA	NA
4	Georgia	3,293	5.1%
29	Hawaii	543	0.8%
41	Idaho	96	0.1%
NA	Illinois**	NA	NA
18	Indiana	1,061	1.6%
NA	Iowa**	NA	NA
16	Kansas	1,305	2.0%
26	Kentucky	794	1.2%
20	Louisiana	1,044	1.6%
34	Maine	311	0.5%
13	Maryland	1,521	2.4%
11	Massachusetts	1,710	2.7%
6	Michigan	2,798	4.3%
21	Minnesota	1,011	1.6%
33	Mississippi	359	0.6%
25	Missouri	930	1.4%
34	Montana	311	0.5%
31	Nebraska	427	0.7%
28	Nevada	576	0.9%
NA	New Hampshire**	NA	NA
9	New Jersey	2,374	3.7%
30	New Mexico	461	0.7%
1	New York	11,774	18.3%
3	North Carolina	3,464	5.4%
40	North Dakota	125	0.2%
7	Ohio	2,777	4.3%
NA	Oklahoma**	NA	NA
15	Oregon	1,375	2.1%
5	Pennsylvania	3,029	4.7%
32	Rhode Island	382	0.6%
23	South Carolina	988	1.5%
39	South Dakota	137	0.2%
12	Tennessee	1,525	2.4%
2	Texas	6,326	9.8%
38	Utah	247	0.4%
37	Vermont	262	0.4%
10	Virginia	2,138	3.3%
8	Washington	2,415	3.8%
36	West Virginia	300	0.5%
22	Wisconsin	991	1.5%
42	Wyoming	16	0.0%

RANK ORDER

RANK	STATE	ABORTIONS	% of USA
1	New York	11,774	18.3%
2	Texas	6,326	9.8%
3	North Carolina	3,464	5.4%
4	Georgia	3,293	5.1%
5	Pennsylvania	3,029	4.7%
6	Michigan	2,798	4.3%
7	Ohio	2,777	4.3%
8	Washington	2,415	3.8%
9	New Jersey	2,374	3.7%
10	Virginia	2,138	3.3%
11	Massachusetts	1,710	2.7%
12	Tennessee	1,525	2.4%
13	Maryland	1,521	2.4%
14	Alabama	1,385	2.2%
15	Oregon	1,375	2.1%
16	Kansas	1,305	2.0%
17	Connecticut	1,168	1.8%
18	Indiana	1,061	1.6%
19	Colorado	1,059	1.6%
20	Louisiana	1,044	1.6%
21	Minnesota	1,011	1.6%
22	Wisconsin	991	1.5%
23	South Carolina	988	1.5%
24	Arizona	973	1.5%
25	Missouri	930	1.4%
26	Kentucky	794	1.2%
27	Arkansas	610	0.9%
28	Nevada	576	0.9%
29	Hawaii	543	0.8%
30	New Mexico	461	0.7%
31	Nebraska	427	0.7%
32	Rhode Island	382	0.6%
33	Mississippi	359	0.6%
34	Maine	311	0.5%
34	Montana	311	0.5%
36	West Virginia	300	0.5%
37	Vermont	262	0.4%
38	Utah	247	0.4%
39	South Dakota	137	0.2%
40	North Dakota	125	0.2%
41	Idaho	96	0.1%
42	Wyoming	16	0.0%
NA	Alaska**	NA	NA
NA	California**	NA	NA
NA	Delaware**	NA	NA
NA	Florida**	NA	NA
NA	Illinois**	NA	NA
NA	Iowa**	NA	NA
NA	New Hampshire**	NA	NA
NA	Oklahoma**	NA	NA
	District of Columbia**	NA	NA

Source: Morgan Quitno Press using data from US Dept of Health & Human Serv's, Centers for Disease Control-Prevention
"Abortion Surveillance-United States, 1995" (Morbidity Mortality Weekly Report, Vol. 47, No. SS-2, July 3, 1998)
*By state of occurrence. National total is for reporting states only.
**Not reported.

Percent of Reported Legal Abortions Obtained
By Teenagers 17 Years and Younger in 1995
Reporting States' Total = 8.5% of Reported Legal Abortions*

ALPHA ORDER

RANK	STATE	PERCENT
17	Alabama	9.7
NA	Alaska**	NA
33	Arizona	8.2
9	Arkansas	10.6
NA	California**	NA
5	Colorado	11.3
11	Connecticut	10.3
NA	Delaware**	NA
NA	Florida**	NA
20	Georgia	9.4
15	Hawaii	9.8
13	Idaho	9.9
NA	Illinois**	NA
27	Indiana	8.6
NA	Iowa**	NA
2	Kansas	12.1
8	Kentucky	10.7
23	Louisiana	9.1
7	Maine	11.0
20	Maryland	9.4
42	Massachusetts	5.9
24	Michigan	9.0
37	Minnesota	7.2
12	Mississippi	10.1
31	Missouri	8.3
4	Montana	11.6
25	Nebraska	8.8
31	Nevada	8.3
NA	New Hampshire**	NA
37	New Jersey	7.2
18	New Mexico	9.6
29	New York	8.4
10	North Carolina	10.4
20	North Dakota	9.4
36	Ohio	7.5
NA	Oklahoma**	NA
15	Oregon	9.8
34	Pennsylvania	7.8
40	Rhode Island	6.7
13	South Carolina	9.9
1	South Dakota	12.8
28	Tennessee	8.5
37	Texas	7.2
40	Utah	6.7
2	Vermont	12.1
29	Virginia	8.4
18	Washington	9.6
5	West Virginia	11.3
34	Wisconsin	7.8
25	Wyoming	8.8

RANK ORDER

RANK	STATE	PERCENT
1	South Dakota	12.8
2	Kansas	12.1
2	Vermont	12.1
4	Montana	11.6
5	Colorado	11.3
5	West Virginia	11.3
7	Maine	11.0
8	Kentucky	10.7
9	Arkansas	10.6
10	North Carolina	10.4
11	Connecticut	10.3
12	Mississippi	10.1
13	Idaho	9.9
13	South Carolina	9.9
15	Hawaii	9.8
15	Oregon	9.8
17	Alabama	9.7
18	New Mexico	9.6
18	Washington	9.6
20	Georgia	9.4
20	Maryland	9.4
20	North Dakota	9.4
23	Louisiana	9.1
24	Michigan	9.0
25	Nebraska	8.8
25	Wyoming	8.8
27	Indiana	8.6
28	Tennessee	8.5
29	New York	8.4
29	Virginia	8.4
31	Missouri	8.3
31	Nevada	8.3
33	Arizona	8.2
34	Pennsylvania	7.8
34	Wisconsin	7.8
36	Ohio	7.5
37	Minnesota	7.2
37	New Jersey	7.2
37	Texas	7.2
40	Rhode Island	6.7
40	Utah	6.7
42	Massachusetts	5.9
NA	Alaska**	NA
NA	California**	NA
NA	Delaware**	NA
NA	Florida**	NA
NA	Illinois**	NA
NA	Iowa**	NA
NA	New Hampshire**	NA
NA	Oklahoma**	NA
	District of Columbia**	NA

Source: Morgan Quitno Press using data from US Dept of Health & Human Serv's, Centers for Disease Control-Prevention "Abortion Surveillance-United States, 1995" (Morbidity Mortality Weekly Report, Vol. 47, No. SS-2, July 3, 1998)
By state of occurrence. National percent is for reporting states only.
***Not reported.*

Percent of Teenage Abortions Obtained
By Teenagers 17 Years and Younger in 1995
Reporting States' Percent = 42.6% of Teenage Abortions*

<u>ALPHA ORDER</u>

RANK	STATE	PERCENT
22	Alabama	42.8
NA	Alaska**	NA
28	Arizona	41.8
19	Arkansas	43.2
NA	California**	NA
2	Colorado	48.9
6	Connecticut	46.2
NA	Delaware**	NA
NA	Florida**	NA
7	Georgia	46.0
12	Hawaii	44.9
38	Idaho	38.1
NA	Illinois**	NA
33	Indiana	39.7
NA	Iowa**	NA
3	Kansas	47.6
21	Kentucky	42.9
24	Louisiana	42.2
9	Maine	45.7
13	Maryland	44.7
39	Massachusetts	37.8
24	Michigan	42.2
34	Minnesota	39.6
17	Mississippi	43.9
31	Missouri	40.5
11	Montana	45.5
32	Nebraska	39.9
3	Nevada	47.6
NA	New Hampshire**	NA
29	New Jersey	41.5
24	New Mexico	42.2
17	New York	43.9
10	North Carolina	45.6
40	North Dakota	36.3
30	Ohio	40.8
NA	Oklahoma**	NA
15	Oregon	44.4
36	Pennsylvania	39.5
42	Rhode Island	34.5
14	South Carolina	44.5
7	South Dakota	46.0
34	Tennessee	39.6
36	Texas	39.5
41	Utah	35.0
1	Vermont	49.5
23	Virginia	42.6
5	Washington	46.7
15	West Virginia	44.4
27	Wisconsin	42.0
19	Wyoming	43.2

<u>RANK ORDER</u>

RANK	STATE	PERCENT
1	Vermont	49.5
2	Colorado	48.9
3	Kansas	47.6
3	Nevada	47.6
5	Washington	46.7
6	Connecticut	46.2
7	Georgia	46.0
7	South Dakota	46.0
9	Maine	45.7
10	North Carolina	45.6
11	Montana	45.5
12	Hawaii	44.9
13	Maryland	44.7
14	South Carolina	44.5
15	Oregon	44.4
15	West Virginia	44.4
17	Mississippi	43.9
17	New York	43.9
19	Arkansas	43.2
19	Wyoming	43.2
21	Kentucky	42.9
22	Alabama	42.8
23	Virginia	42.6
24	Louisiana	42.2
24	Michigan	42.2
24	New Mexico	42.2
27	Wisconsin	42.0
28	Arizona	41.8
29	New Jersey	41.5
30	Ohio	40.8
31	Missouri	40.5
32	Nebraska	39.9
33	Indiana	39.7
34	Minnesota	39.6
34	Tennessee	39.6
36	Pennsylvania	39.5
36	Texas	39.5
38	Idaho	38.1
39	Massachusetts	37.8
40	North Dakota	36.3
41	Utah	35.0
42	Rhode Island	34.5
NA	Alaska**	NA
NA	California**	NA
NA	Delaware**	NA
NA	Florida**	NA
NA	Illinois**	NA
NA	Iowa**	NA
NA	New Hampshire**	NA
NA	Oklahoma**	NA
	District of Columbia**	NA

Source: Morgan Quitno Press using data from US Dept of Health & Human Serv's, Centers for Disease Control-Prevention "Abortion Surveillance-United States, 1995" (Morbidity Mortality Weekly Report, Vol. 47, No. SS-2, July 3, 1998)
*By state of occurrence. National percent is for reporting states only.
**Not reported.

Reported Legal Abortions Performed at 12 Weeks or Less of Gestation in 1995

Reporting States' Total = 587,294 Abortions*

ALPHA ORDER

RANK	STATE	ABORTIONS	% of USA
14	Alabama	12,101	2.1%
NA	Alaska**	NA	NA
17	Arizona	10,256	1.7%
27	Arkansas	4,801	0.8%
NA	California**	NA	NA
23	Colorado	7,966	1.4%
19	Connecticut	9,826	1.7%
NA	Delaware**	NA	NA
NA	Florida**	NA	NA
4	Georgia	29,421	5.0%
28	Hawaii	4,729	0.8%
38	Idaho	920	0.2%
NA	Illinois**	NA	NA
15	Indiana	11,758	2.0%
NA	Iowa**	NA	NA
22	Kansas	8,466	1.4%
25	Kentucky	6,010	1.0%
21	Louisiana	9,393	1.6%
32	Maine	2,573	0.4%
11	Maryland	14,981	2.6%
NA	Massachusetts**	NA	NA
5	Michigan	27,180	4.6%
13	Minnesota	12,158	2.1%
31	Mississippi	3,147	0.5%
18	Missouri	10,029	1.7%
33	Montana	2,402	0.4%
NA	Nebraska**	NA	NA
24	Nevada	6,221	1.1%
NA	New Hampshire**	NA	NA
7	New Jersey	25,538	4.3%
29	New Mexico	3,620	0.6%
1	New York	115,967	19.7%
6	North Carolina	26,134	4.4%
36	North Dakota	1,190	0.2%
NA	Ohio**	NA	NA
NA	Oklahoma**	NA	NA
12	Oregon	12,400	2.1%
3	Pennsylvania	34,342	5.8%
26	Rhode Island	5,173	0.9%
20	South Carolina	9,801	1.7%
37	South Dakota	1,066	0.2%
10	Tennessee	17,070	2.9%
2	Texas	76,211	13.0%
30	Utah	3,389	0.6%
35	Vermont	2,082	0.4%
8	Virginia	24,271	4.1%
9	Washington	21,531	3.7%
34	West Virginia	2,287	0.4%
16	Wisconsin	10,702	1.8%
39	Wyoming	182	0.0%

RANK ORDER

RANK	STATE	ABORTIONS	% of USA
1	New York	115,967	19.7%
2	Texas	76,211	13.0%
3	Pennsylvania	34,342	5.8%
4	Georgia	29,421	5.0%
5	Michigan	27,180	4.6%
6	North Carolina	26,134	4.4%
7	New Jersey	25,538	4.3%
8	Virginia	24,271	4.1%
9	Washington	21,531	3.7%
10	Tennessee	17,070	2.9%
11	Maryland	14,981	2.6%
12	Oregon	12,400	2.1%
13	Minnesota	12,158	2.1%
14	Alabama	12,101	2.1%
15	Indiana	11,758	2.0%
16	Wisconsin	10,702	1.8%
17	Arizona	10,256	1.7%
18	Missouri	10,029	1.7%
19	Connecticut	9,826	1.7%
20	South Carolina	9,801	1.7%
21	Louisiana	9,393	1.6%
22	Kansas	8,466	1.4%
23	Colorado	7,966	1.4%
24	Nevada	6,221	1.1%
25	Kentucky	6,010	1.0%
26	Rhode Island	5,173	0.9%
27	Arkansas	4,801	0.8%
28	Hawaii	4,729	0.8%
29	New Mexico	3,620	0.6%
30	Utah	3,389	0.6%
31	Mississippi	3,147	0.5%
32	Maine	2,573	0.4%
33	Montana	2,402	0.4%
34	West Virginia	2,287	0.4%
35	Vermont	2,082	0.4%
36	North Dakota	1,190	0.2%
37	South Dakota	1,066	0.2%
38	Idaho	920	0.2%
39	Wyoming	182	0.0%
NA	Alaska**	NA	NA
NA	California**	NA	NA
NA	Delaware**	NA	NA
NA	Florida**	NA	NA
NA	Illinois**	NA	NA
NA	Iowa**	NA	NA
NA	Massachusetts**	NA	NA
NA	Nebraska**	NA	NA
NA	New Hampshire**	NA	NA
NA	Ohio**	NA	NA
NA	Oklahoma**	NA	NA
	District of Columbia**	NA	NA

Source: Morgan Quitno Press using data from US Dept of Health & Human Serv's, Centers for Disease Control-Prevention "Abortion Surveillance-United States, 1995" (Morbidity Mortality Weekly Report, Vol. 47, No. SS-2, July 3, 1998)
*By state of occurrence. National total is for reporting states only.
**Not reported.

Percent of Reported Legal Abortions Performed at 12 Weeks
Or Less of Gestation in 1995
Reporting States' Percent = 85.8% of Reported Legal Abortions*

ALPHA ORDER

RANK ORDER

RANK	STATE	PERCENT		RANK	STATE	PERCENT
28	Alabama	85.1		1	Wyoming	100.0
NA	Alaska**	NA		2	South Dakota	99.6
24	Arizona	85.9		3	South Carolina	98.2
32	Arkansas	83.4		4	Vermont	96.0
NA	California**	NA		5	Virginia	95.9
29	Colorado	84.9		6	Indiana	95.0
22	Connecticut	86.8		7	Idaho	94.8
NA	Delaware**	NA		8	Tennessee	94.7
NA	Florida**	NA		9	Maryland	92.5
31	Georgia	83.6		10	Utah	91.5
27	Hawaii	85.5		11	Maine	91.3
7	Idaho	94.8		12	Rhode Island	90.6
NA	Illinois**	NA		13	Montana	89.8
6	Indiana	95.0		14	Nevada	89.6
NA	Iowa**	NA		15	Missouri	89.5
36	Kansas	78.6		16	North Dakota	89.2
35	Kentucky	80.8		17	Mississippi	88.3
34	Louisiana	81.7		18	Oregon	88.1
11	Maine	91.3		19	Pennsylvania	87.9
9	Maryland	92.5		20	Michigan	87.4
NA	Massachusetts**	NA		21	Texas	87.3
20	Michigan	87.4		22	Connecticut	86.8
23	Minnesota	86.7		23	Minnesota	86.7
17	Mississippi	88.3		24	Arizona	85.9
15	Missouri	89.5		24	Washington	85.9
13	Montana	89.8		26	West Virginia	85.8
NA	Nebraska**	NA		27	Hawaii	85.5
14	Nevada	89.6		28	Alabama	85.1
NA	New Hampshire**	NA		29	Colorado	84.9
38	New Jersey	77.5		30	Wisconsin	83.7
39	New Mexico	75.2		31	Georgia	83.6
33	New York	83.0		32	Arkansas	83.4
37	North Carolina	78.2		33	New York	83.0
16	North Dakota	89.2		34	Louisiana	81.7
NA	Ohio**	NA		35	Kentucky	80.8
NA	Oklahoma**	NA		36	Kansas	78.6
18	Oregon	88.1		37	North Carolina	78.2
19	Pennsylvania	87.9		38	New Jersey	77.5
12	Rhode Island	90.6		39	New Mexico	75.2
3	South Carolina	98.2		NA	Alaska**	NA
2	South Dakota	99.6		NA	California**	NA
8	Tennessee	94.7		NA	Delaware**	NA
21	Texas	87.3		NA	Florida**	NA
10	Utah	91.5		NA	Illinois**	NA
4	Vermont	96.0		NA	Iowa**	NA
5	Virginia	95.9		NA	Massachusetts**	NA
24	Washington	85.9		NA	Nebraska**	NA
26	West Virginia	85.8		NA	New Hampshire**	NA
30	Wisconsin	83.7		NA	Ohio**	NA
1	Wyoming	100.0		NA	Oklahoma**	NA
					District of Columbia**	NA

Source: Morgan Quitno Press using data from US Dept of Health & Human Serv's, Centers for Disease Control-Prevention "Abortion Surveillance-United States, 1995" (Morbidity Mortality Weekly Report, Vol. 47, No. SS-2, July 3, 1998)
*By state of occurrence. National percent is for reporting states only.
**Not reported.

Reported Legal Abortions Performed At or After 21 Weeks of Gestation in 1995

Reporting States' Total = 9,685 Abortions*

ALPHA ORDER

RANK	STATE	ABORTIONS	% of USA
15	Alabama	86	0.9%
NA	Alaska**	NA	NA
18	Arizona	78	0.8%
26	Arkansas	15	0.2%
NA	California**	NA	NA
13	Colorado	118	1.2%
30	Connecticut	5	0.1%
NA	Delaware**	NA	NA
NA	Florida**	NA	NA
3	Georgia	1,230	12.7%
17	Hawaii	82	0.8%
30	Idaho	5	0.1%
NA	Illinois**	NA	NA
34	Indiana	2	0.0%
NA	Iowa**	NA	NA
4	Kansas	1,010	10.4%
11	Kentucky	167	1.7%
9	Louisiana	297	3.1%
29	Maine	6	0.1%
32	Maryland	4	0.0%
NA	Massachusetts**	NA	NA
7	Michigan	346	3.6%
15	Minnesota	86	0.9%
25	Mississippi	16	0.2%
20	Missouri	63	0.7%
21	Montana	50	0.5%
NA	Nebraska**	NA	NA
36	Nevada	1	0.0%
NA	New Hampshire**	NA	NA
5	New Jersey	672	6.9%
24	New Mexico	25	0.3%
1	New York	2,550	26.3%
19	North Carolina	77	0.8%
34	North Dakota	2	0.0%
NA	Ohio**	NA	NA
NA	Oklahoma**	NA	NA
10	Oregon	258	2.7%
8	Pennsylvania	332	3.4%
28	Rhode Island	12	0.1%
23	South Carolina	26	0.3%
37	South Dakota	0	0.0%
22	Tennessee	28	0.3%
2	Texas	1,299	13.4%
37	Utah	0	0.0%
33	Vermont	3	0.0%
14	Virginia	97	1.0%
6	Washington	494	5.1%
26	West Virginia	15	0.2%
12	Wisconsin	128	1.3%
37	Wyoming	0	0.0%

RANK ORDER

RANK	STATE	ABORTIONS	% of USA
1	New York	2,550	26.3%
2	Texas	1,299	13.4%
3	Georgia	1,230	12.7%
4	Kansas	1,010	10.4%
5	New Jersey	672	6.9%
6	Washington	494	5.1%
7	Michigan	346	3.6%
8	Pennsylvania	332	3.4%
9	Louisiana	297	3.1%
10	Oregon	258	2.7%
11	Kentucky	167	1.7%
12	Wisconsin	128	1.3%
13	Colorado	118	1.2%
14	Virginia	97	1.0%
15	Alabama	86	0.9%
15	Minnesota	86	0.9%
17	Hawaii	82	0.8%
18	Arizona	78	0.8%
19	North Carolina	77	0.8%
20	Missouri	63	0.7%
21	Montana	50	0.5%
22	Tennessee	28	0.3%
23	South Carolina	26	0.3%
24	New Mexico	25	0.3%
25	Mississippi	16	0.2%
26	Arkansas	15	0.2%
26	West Virginia	15	0.2%
28	Rhode Island	12	0.1%
29	Maine	6	0.1%
30	Connecticut	5	0.1%
30	Idaho	5	0.1%
32	Maryland	4	0.0%
33	Vermont	3	0.0%
34	Indiana	2	0.0%
34	North Dakota	2	0.0%
36	Nevada	1	0.0%
37	South Dakota	0	0.0%
37	Utah	0	0.0%
37	Wyoming	0	0.0%
NA	Alaska**	NA	NA
NA	California**	NA	NA
NA	Delaware**	NA	NA
NA	Florida**	NA	NA
NA	Illinois**	NA	NA
NA	Iowa**	NA	NA
NA	Massachusetts**	NA	NA
NA	Nebraska**	NA	NA
NA	New Hampshire**	NA	NA
NA	Ohio**	NA	NA
NA	Oklahoma**	NA	NA
	District of Columbia**	NA	NA

Source: U.S. Department of Health and Human Services, Centers for Disease Control and Prevention
    "Abortion Surveillance-United States, 1995" (Morbidity Mortality Weekly Report, Vol. 47, No. SS-2, July 3, 1998)
*By state of occurrence. National total is for reporting states only.
**Not reported.

Percent of Reported Legal Abortions Performed At or After
21 Weeks of Gestation in 1995
Reporting States' Percent = 1.4% of Reported Legal Abortions*

ALPHA ORDER

RANK	STATE	PERCENT
17	Alabama	0.6
NA	Alaska**	NA
16	Arizona	0.7
25	Arkansas	0.3
NA	California**	NA
12	Colorado	1.3
33	Connecticut	0.0
NA	Delaware**	NA
NA	Florida**	NA
2	Georgia	3.5
10	Hawaii	1.5
21	Idaho	0.5
NA	Illinois**	NA
33	Indiana	0.0
NA	Iowa**	NA
1	Kansas	9.4
4	Kentucky	2.2
3	Louisiana	2.6
27	Maine	0.2
33	Maryland	0.0
NA	Massachusetts**	NA
13	Michigan	1.1
17	Minnesota	0.6
23	Mississippi	0.4
17	Missouri	0.6
7	Montana	1.9
NA	Nebraska**	NA
33	Nevada	0.0
NA	New Hampshire**	NA
5	New Jersey	2.0
21	New Mexico	0.5
8	New York	1.8
27	North Carolina	0.2
31	North Dakota	0.1
NA	Ohio**	NA
NA	Oklahoma**	NA
8	Oregon	1.8
15	Pennsylvania	0.9
27	Rhode Island	0.2
25	South Carolina	0.3
33	South Dakota	0.0
27	Tennessee	0.2
10	Texas	1.5
33	Utah	0.0
31	Vermont	0.1
23	Virginia	0.4
5	Washington	2.0
17	West Virginia	0.6
13	Wisconsin	1.1
33	Wyoming	0.0

RANK ORDER

RANK	STATE	PERCENT
1	Kansas	9.4
2	Georgia	3.5
3	Louisiana	2.6
4	Kentucky	2.2
5	New Jersey	2.0
5	Washington	2.0
7	Montana	1.9
8	New York	1.8
8	Oregon	1.8
10	Hawaii	1.5
10	Texas	1.5
12	Colorado	1.3
13	Michigan	1.1
13	Wisconsin	1.1
15	Pennsylvania	0.9
16	Arizona	0.7
17	Alabama	0.6
17	Minnesota	0.6
17	Missouri	0.6
17	West Virginia	0.6
21	Idaho	0.5
21	New Mexico	0.5
23	Mississippi	0.4
23	Virginia	0.4
25	Arkansas	0.3
25	South Carolina	0.3
27	Maine	0.2
27	North Carolina	0.2
27	Rhode Island	0.2
27	Tennessee	0.2
31	North Dakota	0.1
31	Vermont	0.1
33	Connecticut	0.0
33	Indiana	0.0
33	Maryland	0.0
33	Nevada	0.0
33	South Dakota	0.0
33	Utah	0.0
33	Wyoming	0.0
NA	Alaska**	NA
NA	California**	NA
NA	Delaware**	NA
NA	Florida**	NA
NA	Illinois**	NA
NA	Iowa**	NA
NA	Massachusetts**	NA
NA	Nebraska**	NA
NA	New Hampshire**	NA
NA	Ohio**	NA
NA	Oklahoma**	NA
	District of Columbia**	NA

Source: Morgan Quitno Press using data from US Dept of Health & Human Serv's, Centers for Disease Control-Prevention
"Abortion Surveillance-United States, 1995" (Morbidity Mortality Weekly Report, Vol. 47, No. SS-2, July 3, 1998)
*By state of occurrence. National percent is for reporting states only.
**Not reported.

II. DEATHS

II. DEATHS (Continued)

Deaths in 1997

National Total = 2,314,738 Deaths*

ALPHA ORDER

RANK	STATE	DEATHS	% of USA
18	Alabama	42,971	1.9%
50	Alaska	2,491	0.1%
23	Arizona	37,215	1.6%
29	Arkansas	27,850	1.2%
1	California**	224,468	9.7%
32	Colorado	25,709	1.1%
27	Connecticut	29,076	1.3%
46	Delaware	6,499	0.3%
3	Florida	154,878	6.7%
11	Georgia	59,349	2.6%
43	Hawaii	7,897	0.3%
42	Idaho	9,013	0.4%
7	Illinois	102,916	4.4%
16	Indiana	48,645	2.1%
30	Iowa	27,709	1.2%
33	Kansas	23,981	1.0%
22	Kentucky	38,157	1.6%
21	Louisiana	40,023	1.7%
38	Maine	11,922	0.5%
20	Maryland	41,810	1.8%
13	Massachusetts	54,582	2.4%
8	Michigan	83,620	3.6%
24	Minnesota	37,191	1.6%
31	Mississippi	27,502	1.2%
12	Missouri	54,589	2.4%
44	Montana	7,780	0.3%
35	Nebraska	15,254	0.7%
36	Nevada	13,361	0.6%
41	New Hampshire	9,518	0.4%
9	New Jersey	72,056	3.1%
37	New Mexico	12,723	0.5%
2	New York	161,155	7.0%
10	North Carolina	66,062	2.9%
47	North Dakota	6,106	0.3%
6	Ohio	105,474	4.6%
25	Oklahoma	33,602	1.5%
28	Oregon	28,830	1.2%
5	Pennsylvania	127,989	5.5%
40	Rhode Island	9,817	0.4%
26	South Carolina	32,986	1.4%
45	South Dakota	7,013	0.3%
15	Tennessee	52,725	2.3%
4	Texas	142,739	6.2%
39	Utah	11,421	0.5%
48	Vermont	5,248	0.2%
14	Virginia	53,885	2.3%
19	Washington	42,916	1.9%
34	West Virginia	20,981	0.9%
17	Wisconsin	45,124	1.9%
49	Wyoming	3,744	0.2%

RANK ORDER

RANK	STATE	DEATHS	% of USA
1	California**	224,468	9.7%
2	New York	161,155	7.0%
3	Florida	154,878	6.7%
4	Texas	142,739	6.2%
5	Pennsylvania	127,989	5.5%
6	Ohio	105,474	4.6%
7	Illinois	102,916	4.4%
8	Michigan	83,620	3.6%
9	New Jersey	72,056	3.1%
10	North Carolina	66,062	2.9%
11	Georgia	59,349	2.6%
12	Missouri	54,589	2.4%
13	Massachusetts	54,582	2.4%
14	Virginia	53,885	2.3%
15	Tennessee	52,725	2.3%
16	Indiana	48,645	2.1%
17	Wisconsin	45,124	1.9%
18	Alabama	42,971	1.9%
19	Washington	42,916	1.9%
20	Maryland	41,810	1.8%
21	Louisiana	40,023	1.7%
22	Kentucky	38,157	1.6%
23	Arizona	37,215	1.6%
24	Minnesota	37,191	1.6%
25	Oklahoma	33,602	1.5%
26	South Carolina	32,986	1.4%
27	Connecticut	29,076	1.3%
28	Oregon	28,830	1.2%
29	Arkansas	27,850	1.2%
30	Iowa	27,709	1.2%
31	Mississippi	27,502	1.2%
32	Colorado	25,709	1.1%
33	Kansas	23,981	1.0%
34	West Virginia	20,981	0.9%
35	Nebraska	15,254	0.7%
36	Nevada	13,361	0.6%
37	New Mexico	12,723	0.5%
38	Maine	11,922	0.5%
39	Utah	11,421	0.5%
40	Rhode Island	9,817	0.4%
41	New Hampshire	9,518	0.4%
42	Idaho	9,013	0.4%
43	Hawaii	7,897	0.3%
44	Montana	7,780	0.3%
45	South Dakota	7,013	0.3%
46	Delaware	6,499	0.3%
47	North Dakota	6,106	0.3%
48	Vermont	5,248	0.2%
49	Wyoming	3,744	0.2%
50	Alaska	2,491	0.1%
	District of Columbia	6,166	0.3%

Source: U.S. Department of Health and Human Services, National Center for Health Statistics
"National Vital Statistics Report" (Vol. 47, No. 4, October 7, 1998)

*Preliminary data by state of residence.

**Due to data processing problems, California's figure is an estimate.

Death Rate in 1997

National Rate = 864.9 Deaths per 100,000 Population*

ALPHA ORDER				RANK ORDER		
RANK	STATE	RATE		RANK	STATE	RATE
8	Alabama	994.9		1	West Virginia	1,155.5
50	Alaska	408.8		2	Arkansas	1,103.9
35	Arizona	817.0		3	Pennsylvania	1,064.8
2	Arkansas	1,103.9		4	Florida	1,056.9
46	California**	697.5		5	Oklahoma	1,013.0
48	Colorado	660.5		6	Missouri	1,010.5
24	Connecticut	889.2		7	Mississippi	1,007.2
27	Delaware	888.4		8	Alabama	994.9
4	Florida	1,056.9		9	Rhode Island	994.2
40	Georgia	792.8		10	Tennessee	982.2
47	Hawaii	665.5		11	Kentucky	976.4
43	Idaho	744.7		12	Iowa	971.4
31	Illinois	865.1		13	Maine	959.9
33	Indiana	829.5		14	North Dakota	952.7
12	Iowa	971.4		15	South Dakota	950.3
17	Kansas	924.2		16	Ohio	942.9
11	Kentucky	976.4		17	Kansas	924.2
19	Louisiana	919.7		18	Nebraska	920.7
13	Maine	959.9		19	Louisiana	919.7
34	Maryland	820.7		20	New Jersey	894.8
21	Massachusetts	892.2		21	Massachusetts	892.2
32	Michigan	855.5		22	Vermont	891.0
39	Minnesota	793.7		23	North Carolina	889.7
7	Mississippi	1,007.2		24	Connecticut	889.2
6	Missouri	1,010.5		25	Oregon	888.9
28	Montana	885.3		26	New York	888.5
18	Nebraska	920.7		27	Delaware	888.4
38	Nevada	796.8		28	Montana	885.3
36	New Hampshire	811.6		29	South Carolina	877.2
20	New Jersey	894.8		30	Wisconsin	872.9
44	New Mexico	735.5		31	Illinois	865.1
26	New York	888.5		32	Michigan	855.5
23	North Carolina	889.7		33	Indiana	829.5
14	North Dakota	952.7		34	Maryland	820.7
16	Ohio	942.9		35	Arizona	817.0
5	Oklahoma	1,013.0		36	New Hampshire	811.6
25	Oregon	888.9		37	Virginia	800.2
3	Pennsylvania	1,064.8		38	Nevada	796.8
9	Rhode Island	994.2		39	Minnesota	793.7
29	South Carolina	877.2		40	Georgia	792.8
15	South Dakota	950.3		41	Wyoming	780.4
10	Tennessee	982.2		42	Washington	764.9
45	Texas	734.3		43	Idaho	744.7
49	Utah	554.6		44	New Mexico	735.5
22	Vermont	891.0		45	Texas	734.3
37	Virginia	800.2		46	California**	697.5
42	Washington	764.9		47	Hawaii	665.5
1	West Virginia	1,155.5		48	Colorado	660.5
30	Wisconsin	872.9		49	Utah	554.6
41	Wyoming	780.4		50	Alaska	408.8
					District of Columbia	1,165.7

Source: U.S. Department of Health and Human Services, National Center for Health Statistics
"National Vital Statistics Report" (Vol. 47, No. 4, October 7, 1998)
*Preliminary data by state of residence. Not age adjusted.
**Due to data processing problems, California's figure is an estimate.

Age-Adjusted Death Rate in 1997

National Rate = 478.1 Deaths per 100,000 Population*

ALPHA ORDER

RANK	STATE	RATE
4	Alabama	564.1
36	Alaska	445.6
22	Arizona	468.4
3	Arkansas	572.1
NA	California**	NA
46	Colorado	417.9
44	Connecticut	423.1
14	Delaware	508.1
26	Florida	464.0
7	Georgia	547.1
49	Hawaii	375.3
41	Idaho	433.1
21	Illinois	486.2
31	Indiana	456.6
45	Iowa	422.1
32	Kansas	455.9
8	Kentucky	547.0
2	Louisiana	582.9
28	Maine	461.7
15	Maryland	503.4
43	Massachusetts	423.8
20	Michigan	486.4
47	Minnesota	402.8
1	Mississippi	609.7
13	Missouri	518.0
30	Montana	457.4
39	Nebraska	438.5
11	Nevada	525.8
37	New Hampshire	443.5
29	New Jersey	460.5
22	New Mexico	468.4
24	New York	467.0
12	North Carolina	520.9
42	North Dakota	426.7
16	Ohio	497.1
10	Oklahoma	537.4
33	Oregon	450.7
17	Pennsylvania	492.2
34	Rhode Island	450.1
9	South Carolina	546.1
35	South Dakota	446.0
5	Tennessee	562.9
18	Texas	489.9
48	Utah	399.0
25	Vermont	465.4
19	Virginia	489.6
38	Washington	438.7
6	West Virginia	553.7
40	Wisconsin	434.8
27	Wyoming	463.9

RANK ORDER

RANK	STATE	RATE
1	Mississippi	609.7
2	Louisiana	582.9
3	Arkansas	572.1
4	Alabama	564.1
5	Tennessee	562.9
6	West Virginia	553.7
7	Georgia	547.1
8	Kentucky	547.0
9	South Carolina	546.1
10	Oklahoma	537.4
11	Nevada	525.8
12	North Carolina	520.9
13	Missouri	518.0
14	Delaware	508.1
15	Maryland	503.4
16	Ohio	497.1
17	Pennsylvania	492.2
18	Texas	489.9
19	Virginia	489.6
20	Michigan	486.4
21	Illinois	486.2
22	Arizona	468.4
22	New Mexico	468.4
24	New York	467.0
25	Vermont	465.4
26	Florida	464.0
27	Wyoming	463.9
28	Maine	461.7
29	New Jersey	460.5
30	Montana	457.4
31	Indiana	456.6
32	Kansas	455.9
33	Oregon	450.7
34	Rhode Island	450.1
35	South Dakota	446.0
36	Alaska	445.6
37	New Hampshire	443.5
38	Washington	438.7
39	Nebraska	438.5
40	Wisconsin	434.8
41	Idaho	433.1
42	North Dakota	426.7
43	Massachusetts	423.8
44	Connecticut	423.1
45	Iowa	422.1
46	Colorado	417.9
47	Minnesota	402.8
48	Utah	399.0
49	Hawaii	375.3
NA	California**	NA
	District of Columbia	719.8

Source: U.S. Department of Health and Human Services, National Center for Health Statistics
"National Vital Statistics Report" (Vol. 47, No. 4, October 7, 1998)
*Preliminary data by state of residence. Age-adjusted rates eliminate the distorting effects of the aging of the population.
**Not available.

Births to Deaths Ratio in 1997

National Ratio = 1.68 Births for Every Death in 1997

ALPHA ORDER				RANK ORDER		
RANK	STATE	RATIO		RANK	STATE	RATIO
37	Alabama	1.42		1	Alaska	3.90
1	Alaska	3.90		2	Utah	3.84
9	Arizona	2.04		3	California	2.34
44	Arkansas	1.32		3	Texas	2.34
3	California	2.34		5	Colorado	2.20
5	Colorado	2.20		5	Hawaii	2.20
32	Connecticut	1.48		7	New Mexico	2.11
23	Delaware	1.58		8	Idaho	2.06
47	Florida	1.24		9	Arizona	2.04
11	Georgia	1.99		10	Nevada	2.02
5	Hawaii	2.20		11	Georgia	1.99
8	Idaho	2.06		12	Washington	1.84
13	Illinois	1.76		13	Illinois	1.76
15	Indiana	1.72		14	Minnesota	1.73
43	Iowa	1.33		15	Indiana	1.72
26	Kansas	1.56		15	Wyoming	1.72
39	Kentucky	1.39		17	Virginia	1.71
19	Louisiana	1.65		18	Maryland	1.68
48	Maine	1.15		19	Louisiana	1.65
18	Maryland	1.68		20	New York	1.63
31	Massachusetts	1.51		21	North Carolina	1.62
22	Michigan	1.60		22	Michigan	1.60
14	Minnesota	1.73		23	Delaware	1.58
27	Mississippi	1.55		24	New Jersey	1.57
41	Missouri	1.37		24	South Carolina	1.57
39	Montana	1.39		26	Kansas	1.56
28	Nebraska	1.53		27	Mississippi	1.55
10	Nevada	2.02		28	Nebraska	1.53
29	New Hampshire	1.52		29	New Hampshire	1.52
24	New Jersey	1.57		29	Oregon	1.52
7	New Mexico	2.11		31	Massachusetts	1.51
20	New York	1.63		32	Connecticut	1.48
21	North Carolina	1.62		32	Wisconsin	1.48
41	North Dakota	1.37		34	South Dakota	1.46
35	Ohio	1.44		35	Ohio	1.44
36	Oklahoma	1.43		36	Oklahoma	1.43
29	Oregon	1.52		37	Alabama	1.42
49	Pennsylvania	1.13		38	Tennessee	1.41
46	Rhode Island	1.26		39	Kentucky	1.39
24	South Carolina	1.57		39	Montana	1.39
34	South Dakota	1.46		41	Missouri	1.37
38	Tennessee	1.41		41	North Dakota	1.37
3	Texas	2.34		43	Iowa	1.33
2	Utah	3.84		44	Arkansas	1.32
45	Vermont	1.27		45	Vermont	1.27
17	Virginia	1.71		46	Rhode Island	1.26
12	Washington	1.84		47	Florida	1.24
50	West Virginia	0.99		48	Maine	1.15
32	Wisconsin	1.48		49	Pennsylvania	1.13
15	Wyoming	1.72		50	West Virginia	0.99
					District of Columbia	1.28

Source: Morgan Quitno Press using data from U.S. Dept. of Health & Human Services, National Center for Health Statistics
"National Vital Statistics Report" (Vol. 47, No. 4, October 7, 1998)
*Preliminary data by state of residence.

Deaths in 1990

National Total = 2,148,463 Deaths*

ALPHA ORDER

RANK	STATE	DEATHS	% of USA
18	Alabama	39,381	1.83%
50	Alaska	2,188	0.10%
26	Arizona	28,789	1.34%
31	Arkansas	24,652	1.15%
1	California	214,369	9.98%
33	Colorado	21,583	1.00%
27	Connecticut	27,607	1.28%
46	Delaware	5,764	0.27%
3	Florida	134,385	6.25%
12	Georgia	51,810	2.41%
44	Hawaii	6,782	0.32%
42	Idaho	7,452	0.35%
6	Illinois	103,006	4.79%
14	Indiana	49,569	2.31%
28	Iowa	26,884	1.25%
32	Kansas	22,279	1.04%
22	Kentucky	35,078	1.63%
20	Louisiana	37,571	1.75%
36	Maine	11,106	0.52%
19	Maryland	38,413	1.79%
11	Massachusetts	53,179	2.48%
8	Michigan	78,744	3.67%
23	Minnesota	34,776	1.62%
30	Mississippi	25,127	1.17%
13	Missouri	50,377	2.34%
43	Montana	6,861	0.32%
35	Nebraska	14,769	0.69%
39	Nevada	9,318	0.43%
41	New Hampshire	8,488	0.40%
9	New Jersey	70,383	3.28%
37	New Mexico	10,625	0.49%
2	New York	168,936	7.86%
10	North Carolina	57,315	2.67%
47	North Dakota	5,678	0.26%
7	Ohio	98,822	4.60%
24	Oklahoma	30,378	1.41%
29	Oregon	25,136	1.17%
5	Pennsylvania	121,951	5.68%
38	Rhode Island	9,576	0.45%
25	South Carolina	29,715	1.38%
45	South Dakota	6,326	0.29%
16	Tennessee	46,315	2.16%
4	Texas	125,479	5.84%
40	Utah	9,192	0.43%
48	Vermont	4,595	0.21%
15	Virginia	48,013	2.23%
21	Washington	37,087	1.73%
34	West Virginia	19,385	0.90%
17	Wisconsin	42,733	1.99%
49	Wyoming	3,203	0.15%

RANK ORDER

RANK	STATE	DEATHS	% of USA
1	California	214,369	9.98%
2	New York	168,936	7.86%
3	Florida	134,385	6.25%
4	Texas	125,479	5.84%
5	Pennsylvania	121,951	5.68%
6	Illinois	103,006	4.79%
7	Ohio	98,822	4.60%
8	Michigan	78,744	3.67%
9	New Jersey	70,383	3.28%
10	North Carolina	57,315	2.67%
11	Massachusetts	53,179	2.48%
12	Georgia	51,810	2.41%
13	Missouri	50,377	2.34%
14	Indiana	49,569	2.31%
15	Virginia	48,013	2.23%
16	Tennessee	46,315	2.16%
17	Wisconsin	42,733	1.99%
18	Alabama	39,381	1.83%
19	Maryland	38,413	1.79%
20	Louisiana	37,571	1.75%
21	Washington	37,087	1.73%
22	Kentucky	35,078	1.63%
23	Minnesota	34,776	1.62%
24	Oklahoma	30,378	1.41%
25	South Carolina	29,715	1.38%
26	Arizona	28,789	1.34%
27	Connecticut	27,607	1.28%
28	Iowa	26,884	1.25%
29	Oregon	25,136	1.17%
30	Mississippi	25,127	1.17%
31	Arkansas	24,652	1.15%
32	Kansas	22,279	1.04%
33	Colorado	21,583	1.00%
34	West Virginia	19,385	0.90%
35	Nebraska	14,769	0.69%
36	Maine	11,106	0.52%
37	New Mexico	10,625	0.49%
38	Rhode Island	9,576	0.45%
39	Nevada	9,318	0.43%
40	Utah	9,192	0.43%
41	New Hampshire	8,488	0.40%
42	Idaho	7,452	0.35%
43	Montana	6,861	0.32%
44	Hawaii	6,782	0.32%
45	South Dakota	6,326	0.29%
46	Delaware	5,764	0.27%
47	North Dakota	5,678	0.26%
48	Vermont	4,595	0.21%
49	Wyoming	3,203	0.15%
50	Alaska	2,188	0.10%
	District of Columbia	7,313	0.34%

Source: U.S. Department of Health and Human Services, National Center for Health Statistics
"Monthly Vital Statistics Report" (Vol. 41, No. 7(S), January 7, 1993)
*Final data by state of residence.

Death Rate in 1990

National Rate = 8.63 Deaths per 1,000 Population*

<u>ALPHA ORDER</u>

RANK	STATE	RATE
7	Alabama	9.74
50	Alaska	3.98
37	Arizona	7.84
2	Arkansas	10.48
44	California	7.19
47	Colorado	6.55
32	Connecticut	8.40
27	Delaware	8.64
3	Florida	10.38
35	Georgia	7.99
48	Hawaii	6.11
42	Idaho	7.40
19	Illinois	9.00
21	Indiana	8.94
8	Iowa	9.68
20	Kansas	8.99
11	Kentucky	9.51
22	Louisiana	8.90
18	Maine	9.05
34	Maryland	8.03
24	Massachusetts	8.84
31	Michigan	8.47
36	Minnesota	7.95
6	Mississippi	9.76
5	Missouri	9.84
29	Montana	8.59
14	Nebraska	9.36
38	Nevada	7.75
40	New Hampshire	7.65
16	New Jersey	9.10
46	New Mexico	7.01
13	New York	9.38
27	North Carolina	8.64
22	North Dakota	8.90
15	Ohio	9.11
9	Oklahoma	9.66
24	Oregon	8.84
4	Pennsylvania	10.26
10	Rhode Island	9.54
30	South Carolina	8.52
17	South Dakota	9.09
12	Tennessee	9.49
43	Texas	7.38
49	Utah	5.33
33	Vermont	8.17
38	Virginia	7.75
41	Washington	7.62
1	West Virginia	10.80
26	Wisconsin	8.74
45	Wyoming	7.06

<u>RANK ORDER</u>

RANK	STATE	RATE
1	West Virginia	10.80
2	Arkansas	10.48
3	Florida	10.38
4	Pennsylvania	10.26
5	Missouri	9.84
6	Mississippi	9.76
7	Alabama	9.74
8	Iowa	9.68
9	Oklahoma	9.66
10	Rhode Island	9.54
11	Kentucky	9.51
12	Tennessee	9.49
13	New York	9.38
14	Nebraska	9.36
15	Ohio	9.11
16	New Jersey	9.10
17	South Dakota	9.09
18	Maine	9.05
19	Illinois	9.00
20	Kansas	8.99
21	Indiana	8.94
22	Louisiana	8.90
22	North Dakota	8.90
24	Massachusetts	8.84
24	Oregon	8.84
26	Wisconsin	8.74
27	Delaware	8.64
27	North Carolina	8.64
29	Montana	8.59
30	South Carolina	8.52
31	Michigan	8.47
32	Connecticut	8.40
33	Vermont	8.17
34	Maryland	8.03
35	Georgia	7.99
36	Minnesota	7.95
37	Arizona	7.84
38	Nevada	7.75
38	Virginia	7.75
40	New Hampshire	7.65
41	Washington	7.62
42	Idaho	7.40
43	Texas	7.38
44	California	7.19
45	Wyoming	7.06
46	New Mexico	7.01
47	Colorado	6.55
48	Hawaii	6.11
49	Utah	5.33
50	Alaska	3.98
	District of Columbia	12.00

Source: U.S. Department of Health and Human Services, National Center for Health Statistics
"Monthly Vital Statistics Report" (Vol. 41, No. 7(S), January 7, 1993)
*Final data by state of residence. Not age adjusted.

Deaths in 1980

National Total = 1,989,841 Deaths*

RANK	STATE	DEATHS	% of USA
19	Alabama	35,542	1.79%
50	Alaska	1,714	0.09%
32	Arizona	21,367	1.07%
29	Arkansas	22,744	1.14%
1	California	186,624	9.38%
34	Colorado	18,956	0.95%
25	Connecticut	27,275	1.37%
46	Delaware	5,044	0.25%
5	Florida	104,670	5.26%
14	Georgia	44,262	2.22%
47	Hawaii	4,981	0.25%
41	Idaho	6,763	0.34%
6	Illinois	102,935	5.17%
13	Indiana	47,345	2.38%
26	Iowa	27,120	1.36%
30	Kansas	22,034	1.11%
21	Kentucky	33,796	1.70%
18	Louisiana	35,651	1.79%
36	Maine	10,800	0.54%
20	Maryland	34,016	1.71%
10	Massachusetts	55,070	2.77%
8	Michigan	75,187	3.78%
22	Minnesota	33,366	1.68%
28	Mississippi	23,656	1.19%
11	Missouri	49,660	2.50%
42	Montana	6,666	0.34%
35	Nebraska	14,474	0.73%
44	Nevada	5,896	0.30%
40	New Hampshire	7,647	0.38%
9	New Jersey	68,943	3.46%
38	New Mexico	9,093	0.46%
2	New York	172,853	8.69%
12	North Carolina	48,440	2.43%
45	North Dakota	5,596	0.28%
7	Ohio	98,421	4.95%
24	Oklahoma	28,234	1.42%
31	Oregon	21,798	1.10%
3	Pennsylvania	123,594	6.21%
37	Rhode Island	9,325	0.47%
27	South Carolina	25,154	1.26%
43	South Dakota	6,556	0.33%
17	Tennessee	40,774	2.05%
4	Texas	108,180	5.44%
39	Utah	8,120	0.41%
48	Vermont	4,582	0.23%
15	Virginia	42,506	2.14%
23	Washington	32,007	1.61%
33	West Virginia	19,237	0.97%
16	Wisconsin	40,838	2.05%
49	Wyoming	3,221	0.16%

RANK	STATE	DEATHS	% of USA
1	California	186,624	9.38%
2	New York	172,853	8.69%
3	Pennsylvania	123,594	6.21%
4	Texas	108,180	5.44%
5	Florida	104,670	5.26%
6	Illinois	102,935	5.17%
7	Ohio	98,421	4.95%
8	Michigan	75,187	3.78%
9	New Jersey	68,943	3.46%
10	Massachusetts	55,070	2.77%
11	Missouri	49,660	2.50%
12	North Carolina	48,440	2.43%
13	Indiana	47,345	2.38%
14	Georgia	44,262	2.22%
15	Virginia	42,506	2.14%
16	Wisconsin	40,838	2.05%
17	Tennessee	40,774	2.05%
18	Louisiana	35,651	1.79%
19	Alabama	35,542	1.79%
20	Maryland	34,016	1.71%
21	Kentucky	33,796	1.70%
22	Minnesota	33,366	1.68%
23	Washington	32,007	1.61%
24	Oklahoma	28,234	1.42%
25	Connecticut	27,275	1.37%
26	Iowa	27,120	1.36%
27	South Carolina	25,154	1.26%
28	Mississippi	23,656	1.19%
29	Arkansas	22,744	1.14%
30	Kansas	22,034	1.11%
31	Oregon	21,798	1.10%
32	Arizona	21,367	1.07%
33	West Virginia	19,237	0.97%
34	Colorado	18,956	0.95%
35	Nebraska	14,474	0.73%
36	Maine	10,800	0.54%
37	Rhode Island	9,325	0.47%
38	New Mexico	9,093	0.46%
39	Utah	8,120	0.41%
40	New Hampshire	7,647	0.38%
41	Idaho	6,763	0.34%
42	Montana	6,666	0.34%
43	South Dakota	6,556	0.33%
44	Nevada	5,896	0.30%
45	North Dakota	5,596	0.28%
46	Delaware	5,044	0.25%
47	Hawaii	4,981	0.25%
48	Vermont	4,582	0.23%
49	Wyoming	3,221	0.16%
50	Alaska	1,714	0.09%
	District of Columbia	7,108	0.36%

Source: U.S. Department of Health and Human Services, National Center for Health Statistics
   "Vital Statistics of the United States 1980" and "Monthly Vital Statistics Report"
*Final data by state of residence.

Death Rate in 1980

National Rate = 8.77 Deaths per 1,000 Population*

ALPHA ORDER			RANK ORDER		
RANK	STATE	RATE	RANK	STATE	RATE
18	Alabama	9.12	1	Florida	10.72
50	Alaska	4.25	2	Pennsylvania	10.41
40	Arizona	7.84	3	Missouri	10.08
4	Arkansas	9.94	4	Arkansas	9.94
39	California	7.86	5	West Virginia	9.87
47	Colorado	6.54	6	New York	9.84
23	Connecticut	8.77	6	Rhode Island	9.84
27	Delaware	8.47	8	Maine	9.60
1	Florida	10.72	9	Massachusetts	9.59
35	Georgia	8.09	10	South Dakota	9.47
49	Hawaii	5.15	11	Mississippi	9.37
44	Idaho	7.15	12	New Jersey	9.36
20	Illinois	8.99	13	Oklahoma	9.32
25	Indiana	8.62	14	Iowa	9.30
14	Iowa	9.30	14	Kansas	9.30
14	Kansas	9.30	16	Kentucky	9.22
16	Kentucky	9.22	17	Nebraska	9.20
28	Louisiana	8.46	18	Alabama	9.12
8	Maine	9.60	19	Ohio	9.11
36	Maryland	8.06	20	Illinois	8.99
9	Massachusetts	9.59	21	Vermont	8.95
34	Michigan	8.11	22	Tennessee	8.87
33	Minnesota	8.17	23	Connecticut	8.77
11	Mississippi	9.37	24	Wisconsin	8.67
3	Missouri	10.08	25	Indiana	8.62
28	Montana	8.46	26	North Dakota	8.56
17	Nebraska	9.20	27	Delaware	8.47
43	Nevada	7.35	28	Louisiana	8.46
30	New Hampshire	8.30	28	Montana	8.46
12	New Jersey	9.36	30	New Hampshire	8.30
45	New Mexico	6.96	31	Oregon	8.27
6	New York	9.84	32	North Carolina	8.23
32	North Carolina	8.23	33	Minnesota	8.17
26	North Dakota	8.56	34	Michigan	8.11
19	Ohio	9.11	35	Georgia	8.09
13	Oklahoma	9.32	36	Maryland	8.06
31	Oregon	8.27	37	South Carolina	8.05
2	Pennsylvania	10.41	38	Virginia	7.94
6	Rhode Island	9.84	39	California	7.86
37	South Carolina	8.05	40	Arizona	7.84
10	South Dakota	9.47	41	Washington	7.73
22	Tennessee	8.87	42	Texas	7.58
42	Texas	7.58	43	Nevada	7.35
48	Utah	5.54	44	Idaho	7.15
21	Vermont	8.95	45	New Mexico	6.96
38	Virginia	7.94	46	Wyoming	6.84
41	Washington	7.73	47	Colorado	6.54
5	West Virginia	9.87	48	Utah	5.54
24	Wisconsin	8.67	49	Hawaii	5.15
46	Wyoming	6.84	50	Alaska	4.25
				District of Columbia	11.09

Source: U.S. Department of Health and Human Services, National Center for Health Statistics
"Vital Statistics of the United States 1980" and "Monthly Vital Statistics Report"
*Final data by state of residence. Not age adjusted.

Infant Deaths in 1998

National Total = 27,600 Infant Deaths*

RANK	STATE	DEATHS	% of USA
16	Alabama	590	2.1%
48	Alaska	57	0.2%
15	Arizona	600	2.2%
32	Arkansas	263	1.0%
1	California	3,333	12.1%
26	Colorado	401	1.5%
30	Connecticut	270	1.0%
42	Delaware	99	0.4%
5	Florida	1,439	5.2%
10	Georgia	969	3.5%
40	Hawaii	108	0.4%
39	Idaho	126	0.5%
3	Illinois	1,536	5.6%
22	Indiana	435	1.6%
34	Iowa	213	0.8%
29	Kansas	296	1.1%
25	Kentucky	407	1.5%
14	Louisiana	612	2.2%
44	Maine	79	0.3%
18	Maryland	574	2.1%
23	Massachusetts	431	1.6%
7	Michigan	1,069	3.9%
28	Minnesota	314	1.1%
21	Mississippi	436	1.6%
17	Missouri	589	2.1%
46	Montana	71	0.3%
38	Nebraska	152	0.6%
35	Nevada	204	0.7%
45	New Hampshire	75	0.3%
11	New Jersey	707	2.6%
36	New Mexico	167	0.6%
4	New York	1,465	5.3%
8	North Carolina	1,055	3.8%
47	North Dakota	60	0.2%
6	Ohio	1,136	4.1%
27	Oklahoma	316	1.1%
33	Oregon	248	0.9%
9	Pennsylvania	1,012	3.7%
43	Rhode Island	91	0.3%
19	South Carolina	475	1.7%
41	South Dakota	101	0.4%
13	Tennessee	652	2.4%
2	Texas	2,257	8.2%
31	Utah	268	1.0%
49	Vermont	43	0.2%
12	Virginia	677	2.5%
24	Washington	429	1.6%
37	West Virginia	157	0.6%
20	Wisconsin	452	1.6%
50	Wyoming	30	0.1%

RANK	STATE	DEATHS	% of USA
1	California	3,333	12.1%
2	Texas	2,257	8.2%
3	Illinois	1,536	5.6%
4	New York	1,465	5.3%
5	Florida	1,439	5.2%
6	Ohio	1,136	4.1%
7	Michigan	1,069	3.9%
8	North Carolina	1,055	3.8%
9	Pennsylvania	1,012	3.7%
10	Georgia	969	3.5%
11	New Jersey	707	2.6%
12	Virginia	677	2.5%
13	Tennessee	652	2.4%
14	Louisiana	612	2.2%
15	Arizona	600	2.2%
16	Alabama	590	2.1%
17	Missouri	589	2.1%
18	Maryland	574	2.1%
19	South Carolina	475	1.7%
20	Wisconsin	452	1.6%
21	Mississippi	436	1.6%
22	Indiana	435	1.6%
23	Massachusetts	431	1.6%
24	Washington	429	1.6%
25	Kentucky	407	1.5%
26	Colorado	401	1.5%
27	Oklahoma	316	1.1%
28	Minnesota	314	1.1%
29	Kansas	296	1.1%
30	Connecticut	270	1.0%
31	Utah	268	1.0%
32	Arkansas	263	1.0%
33	Oregon	248	0.9%
34	Iowa	213	0.8%
35	Nevada	204	0.7%
36	New Mexico	167	0.6%
37	West Virginia	157	0.6%
38	Nebraska	152	0.6%
39	Idaho	126	0.5%
40	Hawaii	108	0.4%
41	South Dakota	101	0.4%
42	Delaware	99	0.4%
43	Rhode Island	91	0.3%
44	Maine	79	0.3%
45	New Hampshire	75	0.3%
46	Montana	71	0.3%
47	North Dakota	60	0.2%
48	Alaska	57	0.2%
49	Vermont	43	0.2%
50	Wyoming	30	0.1%
	District of Columbia	89	0.3%

Source: U.S. Department of Health and Human Services, National Center for Health Statistics (http:www.cdc.gov/nchswww/data/47-15-2.pdf)

*For 12 months ending September 1998. Provisional data. Deaths under 1 year old by state of residence.

Infant Mortality Rate in 1998

National Rate = 7.0 Infant Deaths per 1,000 Live Births*

ALPHA ORDER

RANK	STATE	RATE
5	Alabama	9.5
46	Alaska	5.3
12	Arizona	8.0
26	Arkansas	7.1
37	California	6.1
27	Colorado	7.0
33	Connecticut	6.5
4	Delaware	9.6
21	Florida	7.4
12	Georgia	8.0
36	Hawaii	6.3
35	Idaho	6.4
9	Illinois	8.4
41	Indiana	5.7
12	Iowa	8.0
16	Kansas	7.8
18	Kentucky	7.5
6	Louisiana	9.1
41	Maine	5.7
10	Maryland	8.3
49	Massachusetts	4.8
11	Michigan	8.1
49	Minnesota	4.8
1	Mississippi	10.2
15	Missouri	7.9
28	Montana	6.9
31	Nebraska	6.7
18	Nevada	7.5
45	New Hampshire	5.6
17	New Jersey	7.6
39	New Mexico	6.0
41	New York	5.7
2	North Carolina	9.8
21	North Dakota	7.4
24	Ohio	7.3
37	Oklahoma	6.1
41	Oregon	5.7
28	Pennsylvania	6.9
21	Rhode Island	7.4
7	South Carolina	8.9
2	South Dakota	9.8
8	Tennessee	8.5
33	Texas	6.5
40	Utah	5.9
30	Vermont	6.8
24	Virginia	7.3
46	Washington	5.3
18	West Virginia	7.5
31	Wisconsin	6.7
48	Wyoming	4.9

RANK ORDER

RANK	STATE	RATE
1	Mississippi	10.2
2	North Carolina	9.8
2	South Dakota	9.8
4	Delaware	9.6
5	Alabama	9.5
6	Louisiana	9.1
7	South Carolina	8.9
8	Tennessee	8.5
9	Illinois	8.4
10	Maryland	8.3
11	Michigan	8.1
12	Arizona	8.0
12	Georgia	8.0
12	Iowa	8.0
15	Missouri	7.9
16	Kansas	7.8
17	New Jersey	7.6
18	Kentucky	7.5
18	Nevada	7.5
18	West Virginia	7.5
21	Florida	7.4
21	North Dakota	7.4
21	Rhode Island	7.4
24	Ohio	7.3
24	Virginia	7.3
26	Arkansas	7.1
27	Colorado	7.0
28	Montana	6.9
28	Pennsylvania	6.9
30	Vermont	6.8
31	Nebraska	6.7
31	Wisconsin	6.7
33	Connecticut	6.5
33	Texas	6.5
35	Idaho	6.4
36	Hawaii	6.3
37	California	6.1
37	Oklahoma	6.1
39	New Mexico	6.0
40	Utah	5.9
41	Indiana	5.7
41	Maine	5.7
41	New York	5.7
41	Oregon	5.7
45	New Hampshire	5.6
46	Alaska	5.3
46	Washington	5.3
48	Wyoming	4.9
49	Massachusetts	4.8
49	Minnesota	4.8
	District of Columbia	10.9

Source: U.S. Department of Health and Human Services, National Center for Health Statistics
(http:www.cdc.gov/nchswww/data/47-15-2.pdf)
*For 12 months ending September 1998. Provisional data. Deaths under 1 year old by state of residence.

Infant Deaths in 1997

National Total = 27,000 Infant Deaths*

ALPHA ORDER

RANK	STATE	DEATHS	% of USA
16	Alabama	560	2.1%
47	Alaska	57	0.2%
18	Arizona	540	2.0%
29	Arkansas	312	1.2%
1	California	3,122	11.6%
25	Colorado	395	1.5%
30	Connecticut	301	1.1%
41	Delaware	83	0.3%
5	Florida	1,381	5.1%
10	Georgia	915	3.4%
40	Hawaii	103	0.4%
39	Idaho	109	0.4%
4	Illinois	1,452	5.4%
19	Indiana	509	1.9%
35	Iowa	177	0.7%
31	Kansas	262	1.0%
22	Kentucky	436	1.6%
15	Louisiana	586	2.2%
48	Maine	50	0.2%
14	Maryland	595	2.2%
28	Massachusetts	350	1.3%
7	Michigan	1,078	4.0%
26	Minnesota	380	1.4%
20	Mississippi	464	1.7%
17	Missouri	545	2.0%
44	Montana	72	0.3%
34	Nebraska	184	0.7%
38	Nevada	155	0.6%
45	New Hampshire	64	0.2%
11	New Jersey	709	2.6%
36	New Mexico	169	0.6%
3	New York	1,711	6.3%
9	North Carolina	1,018	3.8%
46	North Dakota	62	0.2%
6	Ohio	1,096	4.1%
27	Oklahoma	367	1.4%
32	Oregon	252	0.9%
8	Pennsylvania	1,056	3.9%
42	Rhode Island	82	0.3%
21	South Carolina	453	1.7%
43	South Dakota	77	0.3%
13	Tennessee	630	2.3%
2	Texas	2,009	7.4%
32	Utah	252	0.9%
49	Vermont	41	0.2%
12	Virginia	661	2.4%
24	Washington	416	1.5%
37	West Virginia	168	0.6%
23	Wisconsin	419	1.6%
50	Wyoming	33	0.1%

RANK ORDER

RANK	STATE	DEATHS	% of USA
1	California	3,122	11.6%
2	Texas	2,009	7.4%
3	New York	1,711	6.3%
4	Illinois	1,452	5.4%
5	Florida	1,381	5.1%
6	Ohio	1,096	4.1%
7	Michigan	1,078	4.0%
8	Pennsylvania	1,056	3.9%
9	North Carolina	1,018	3.8%
10	Georgia	915	3.4%
11	New Jersey	709	2.6%
12	Virginia	661	2.4%
13	Tennessee	630	2.3%
14	Maryland	595	2.2%
15	Louisiana	586	2.2%
16	Alabama	560	2.1%
17	Missouri	545	2.0%
18	Arizona	540	2.0%
19	Indiana	509	1.9%
20	Mississippi	464	1.7%
21	South Carolina	453	1.7%
22	Kentucky	436	1.6%
23	Wisconsin	419	1.6%
24	Washington	416	1.5%
25	Colorado	395	1.5%
26	Minnesota	380	1.4%
27	Oklahoma	367	1.4%
28	Massachusetts	350	1.3%
29	Arkansas	312	1.2%
30	Connecticut	301	1.1%
31	Kansas	262	1.0%
32	Oregon	252	0.9%
32	Utah	252	0.9%
34	Nebraska	184	0.7%
35	Iowa	177	0.7%
36	New Mexico	169	0.6%
37	West Virginia	168	0.6%
38	Nevada	155	0.6%
39	Idaho	109	0.4%
40	Hawaii	103	0.4%
41	Delaware	83	0.3%
42	Rhode Island	82	0.3%
43	South Dakota	77	0.3%
44	Montana	72	0.3%
45	New Hampshire	64	0.2%
46	North Dakota	62	0.2%
47	Alaska	57	0.2%
48	Maine	50	0.2%
49	Vermont	41	0.2%
50	Wyoming	33	0.1%
	District of Columbia	100	0.4%

Source: U.S. Department of Health and Human Services, National Center for Health Statistics "Monthly Vital Statistics Report" (Vol. 46, No. 12, July 28, 1998)
Provisional data. Deaths under 1 year old by state of residence.

Infant Mortality Rate in 1997

National Rate = 7.0 Infant Deaths per 1,000 Live Births*

ALPHA ORDER

RANK ORDER

RANK	STATE	PERCENT	RANK	STATE	PERCENT
3	Alabama	9.2	1	Mississippi	10.9
40	Alaska	5.9	2	North Carolina	9.6
31	Arizona	6.3	3	Alabama	9.2
7	Arkansas	8.4	4	Louisiana	9.1
38	California	6.0	5	Maryland	9.0
16	Colorado	7.6	6	South Carolina	8.8
26	Connecticut	7.0	7	Arkansas	8.4
10	Delaware	8.2	7	Tennessee	8.4
24	Florida	7.2	9	Kentucky	8.3
15	Georgia	7.7	10	Delaware	8.2
38	Hawaii	6.0	10	West Virginia	8.2
35	Idaho	6.1	12	Michigan	8.1
13	Illinois	8.0	13	Illinois	8.0
20	Indiana	7.4	14	Nebraska	7.9
47	Iowa	4.8	15	Georgia	7.7
27	Kansas	6.9	16	Colorado	7.6
9	Kentucky	8.3	16	Oklahoma	7.6
4	Louisiana	9.1	16	South Dakota	7.6
50	Maine	3.7	19	Virginia	7.5
5	Maryland	9.0	20	Indiana	7.4
49	Massachusetts	4.3	20	North Dakota	7.4
12	Michigan	8.1	20	Pennsylvania	7.4
40	Minnesota	5.9	23	Missouri	7.3
1	Mississippi	10.9	24	Florida	7.2
23	Missouri	7.3	24	Ohio	7.2
27	Montana	6.9	26	Connecticut	7.0
14	Nebraska	7.9	27	Kansas	6.9
44	Nevada	5.7	27	Montana	6.9
48	New Hampshire	4.4	29	Rhode Island	6.6
31	New Jersey	6.3	30	New Mexico	6.4
30	New Mexico	6.4	31	Arizona	6.3
35	New York	6.1	31	New Jersey	6.3
2	North Carolina	9.6	31	Texas	6.3
20	North Dakota	7.4	31	Wisconsin	6.3
24	Ohio	7.2	35	Idaho	6.1
16	Oklahoma	7.6	35	New York	6.1
42	Oregon	5.8	35	Vermont	6.1
20	Pennsylvania	7.4	38	California	6.0
29	Rhode Island	6.6	38	Hawaii	6.0
6	South Carolina	8.8	40	Alaska	5.9
16	South Dakota	7.6	40	Minnesota	5.9
7	Tennessee	8.4	42	Oregon	5.8
31	Texas	6.3	42	Utah	5.8
42	Utah	5.8	44	Nevada	5.7
35	Vermont	6.1	45	Washington	5.2
19	Virginia	7.5	45	Wyoming	5.2
45	Washington	5.2	47	Iowa	4.8
10	West Virginia	8.2	48	New Hampshire	4.4
31	Wisconsin	6.3	49	Massachusetts	4.3
45	Wyoming	5.2	50	Maine	3.7
				District of Columbia	12.0

Source: U.S. Department of Health and Human Services, National Center for Health Statistics
"Monthly Vital Statistics Report" (Vol. 46, No. 12, July 28, 1998)
*Provisional data. Deaths under 1 year old by state of residence.

Infant Mortality Rate in 1990

National Rate = 9.22 Infant Deaths per 1,000 Live Births*

ALPHA ORDER

RANK ORDER

RANK	STATE	RATE
5	Alabama	10.84
9	Alaska	10.50
27	Arizona	8.84
22	Arkansas	9.22
42	California	7.91
28	Colorado	8.82
41	Connecticut	7.94
13	Delaware	10.08
17	Florida	9.62
1	Georgia	12.36
48	Hawaii	6.74
29	Idaho	8.70
6	Illinois	10.75
16	Indiana	9.64
37	Iowa	8.09
32	Kansas	8.43
31	Kentucky	8.48
4	Louisiana	11.07
50	Maine	6.22
19	Maryland	9.55
47	Massachusetts	7.02
7	Michigan	10.68
45	Minnesota	7.29
2	Mississippi	12.14
21	Missouri	9.44
24	Montana	9.04
34	Nebraska	8.29
33	Nevada	8.38
46	New Hampshire	7.11
25	New Jersey	9.01
26	New Mexico	8.98
18	New York	9.58
8	North Carolina	10.61
40	North Dakota	8.00
15	Ohio	9.83
23	Oklahoma	9.19
35	Oregon	8.25
19	Pennsylvania	9.55
37	Rhode Island	8.09
3	South Carolina	11.65
12	South Dakota	10.09
10	Tennessee	10.29
39	Texas	8.07
44	Utah	7.47
49	Vermont	6.41
11	Virginia	10.20
43	Washington	7.84
14	West Virginia	9.87
36	Wisconsin	8.20
30	Wyoming	8.59

RANK	STATE	RATE
1	Georgia	12.36
2	Mississippi	12.14
3	South Carolina	11.65
4	Louisiana	11.07
5	Alabama	10.84
6	Illinois	10.75
7	Michigan	10.68
8	North Carolina	10.61
9	Alaska	10.50
10	Tennessee	10.29
11	Virginia	10.20
12	South Dakota	10.09
13	Delaware	10.08
14	West Virginia	9.87
15	Ohio	9.83
16	Indiana	9.64
17	Florida	9.62
18	New York	9.58
19	Maryland	9.55
19	Pennsylvania	9.55
21	Missouri	9.44
22	Arkansas	9.22
23	Oklahoma	9.19
24	Montana	9.04
25	New Jersey	9.01
26	New Mexico	8.98
27	Arizona	8.84
28	Colorado	8.82
29	Idaho	8.70
30	Wyoming	8.59
31	Kentucky	8.48
32	Kansas	8.43
33	Nevada	8.38
34	Nebraska	8.29
35	Oregon	8.25
36	Wisconsin	8.20
37	Iowa	8.09
37	Rhode Island	8.09
39	Texas	8.07
40	North Dakota	8.00
41	Connecticut	7.94
42	California	7.91
43	Washington	7.84
44	Utah	7.47
45	Minnesota	7.29
46	New Hampshire	7.11
47	Massachusetts	7.02
48	Hawaii	6.74
49	Vermont	6.41
50	Maine	6.22

District of Columbia   20.68

Source: U.S. Department of Health and Human Services, National Center for Health Statistics
    "Monthly Vital Statistics Report" (Vol. 41, No. 7(S), January 7, 1993)
Final data by state of residence. Infant deaths are those under 1 year old.

Infant Mortality Rate in 1980

National Rate = 12.60 Infant Deaths per 1,000 Live Births*

ALPHA ORDER

RANK ORDER

RANK	STATE	RATE
3	Alabama	15.15
24	Alaska	12.28
22	Arizona	12.39
18	Arkansas	12.66
35	California	11.05
46	Colorado	10.07
34	Connecticut	11.17
10	Delaware	13.92
5	Florida	14.58
7	Georgia	14.48
44	Hawaii	10.30
39	Idaho	10.71
4	Illinois	14.80
28	Indiana	11.87
29	Iowa	11.82
43	Kansas	10.41
14	Kentucky	12.86
8	Louisiana	14.34
50	Maine	9.23
9	Maryland	14.05
41	Massachusetts	10.51
15	Michigan	12.80
47	Minnesota	10.00
1	Mississippi	17.01
21	Missouri	12.42
22	Montana	12.39
33	Nebraska	11.48
38	Nevada	10.74
48	New Hampshire	9.89
19	New Jersey	12.54
32	New Mexico	11.53
20	New York	12.53
6	North Carolina	14.49
27	North Dakota	12.10
16	Ohio	12.77
17	Oklahoma	12.72
25	Oregon	12.17
13	Pennsylvania	13.23
36	Rhode Island	10.99
2	South Carolina	15.62
37	South Dakota	10.92
12	Tennessee	13.51
26	Texas	12.16
42	Utah	10.43
40	Vermont	10.65
11	Virginia	13.60
31	Washington	11.76
30	West Virginia	11.81
45	Wisconsin	10.29
49	Wyoming	9.75

RANK	STATE	RATE
1	Mississippi	17.01
2	South Carolina	15.62
3	Alabama	15.15
4	Illinois	14.80
5	Florida	14.58
6	North Carolina	14.49
7	Georgia	14.48
8	Louisiana	14.34
9	Maryland	14.05
10	Delaware	13.92
11	Virginia	13.60
12	Tennessee	13.51
13	Pennsylvania	13.23
14	Kentucky	12.86
15	Michigan	12.80
16	Ohio	12.77
17	Oklahoma	12.72
18	Arkansas	12.66
19	New Jersey	12.54
20	New York	12.53
21	Missouri	12.42
22	Arizona	12.39
22	Montana	12.39
24	Alaska	12.28
25	Oregon	12.17
26	Texas	12.16
27	North Dakota	12.10
28	Indiana	11.87
29	Iowa	11.82
30	West Virginia	11.81
31	Washington	11.76
32	New Mexico	11.53
33	Nebraska	11.48
34	Connecticut	11.17
35	California	11.05
36	Rhode Island	10.99
37	South Dakota	10.92
38	Nevada	10.74
39	Idaho	10.71
40	Vermont	10.65
41	Massachusetts	10.51
42	Utah	10.43
43	Kansas	10.41
44	Hawaii	10.30
45	Wisconsin	10.29
46	Colorado	10.07
47	Minnesota	10.00
48	New Hampshire	9.89
49	Wyoming	9.75
50	Maine	9.23
	District of Columbia	25.00

Source: U.S. Department of Health and Human Services, National Center for Health Statistics
   "Monthly Vital Statistics Report"
*Final data by state of residence. Deaths under 1 year old, exclusive of fetal deaths.

Percent Change in Infant Mortality Rate: 1990 to 1997

National Percent Change = 24.1% Decrease*

ALPHA ORDER

RANK ORDER

RANK	STATE	PERCENT CHANGE		RANK	STATE	PERCENT CHANGE
12	Alabama	(15.1)		1	Kentucky	(2.1)
50	Alaska	(43.8)		2	Nebraska	(4.7)
36	Arizona	(28.7)		3	Vermont	(4.8)
6	Arkansas	(8.9)		4	Maryland	(5.8)
28	California	(24.1)		5	North Dakota	(7.5)
11	Colorado	(13.8)		6	Arkansas	(8.9)
10	Connecticut	(11.8)		7	North Carolina	(9.5)
19	Delaware	(18.7)		8	Mississippi	(10.2)
32	Florida	(25.2)		9	Hawaii	(11.0)
44	Georgia	(37.7)		10	Connecticut	(11.8)
9	Hawaii	(11.0)		11	Colorado	(13.8)
39	Idaho	(29.9)		12	Alabama	(15.1)
33	Illinois	(25.6)		13	West Virginia	(16.9)
25	Indiana	(23.2)		14	Oklahoma	(17.3)
49	Iowa	(40.7)		15	Louisiana	(17.8)
16	Kansas	(18.1)		16	Kansas	(18.1)
1	Kentucky	(2.1)		17	Rhode Island	(18.4)
15	Louisiana	(17.8)		17	Tennessee	(18.4)
48	Maine	(40.5)		19	Delaware	(18.7)
4	Maryland	(5.8)		20	Minnesota	(19.1)
46	Massachusetts	(38.7)		21	Texas	(21.9)
29	Michigan	(24.2)		22	Utah	(22.4)
20	Minnesota	(19.1)		23	Pennsylvania	(22.5)
8	Mississippi	(10.2)		24	Missouri	(22.7)
24	Missouri	(22.7)		25	Indiana	(23.2)
27	Montana	(23.7)		25	Wisconsin	(23.2)
2	Nebraska	(4.7)		27	Montana	(23.7)
41	Nevada	(32.0)		28	California	(24.1)
45	New Hampshire	(38.1)		29	Michigan	(24.2)
40	New Jersey	(30.1)		30	South Carolina	(24.5)
36	New Mexico	(28.7)		31	South Dakota	(24.7)
43	New York	(36.3)		32	Florida	(25.2)
7	North Carolina	(9.5)		33	Illinois	(25.6)
5	North Dakota	(7.5)		34	Virginia	(26.5)
35	Ohio	(26.8)		35	Ohio	(26.8)
14	Oklahoma	(17.3)		36	Arizona	(28.7)
38	Oregon	(29.7)		36	New Mexico	(28.7)
23	Pennsylvania	(22.5)		38	Oregon	(29.7)
17	Rhode Island	(18.4)		39	Idaho	(29.9)
30	South Carolina	(24.5)		40	New Jersey	(30.1)
31	South Dakota	(24.7)		41	Nevada	(32.0)
17	Tennessee	(18.4)		42	Washington	(33.7)
21	Texas	(21.9)		43	New York	(36.3)
22	Utah	(22.4)		44	Georgia	(37.7)
3	Vermont	(4.8)		45	New Hampshire	(38.1)
34	Virginia	(26.5)		46	Massachusetts	(38.7)
42	Washington	(33.7)		47	Wyoming	(39.5)
13	West Virginia	(16.9)		48	Maine	(40.5)
25	Wisconsin	(23.2)		49	Iowa	(40.7)
47	Wyoming	(39.5)		50	Alaska	(43.8)

District of Columbia (42.0)

Source: Morgan Quitno Press using data from US Dept of Health & Human Services, National Center for Health Statistics "Monthly Vital Statistics Report" (Vol. 41, No. 7(S), January 7, 1993; Vol. 46, No. 12, July 28, 1998)
*By state of residence. Infant deaths are those under 1 year old.

Percent Change in Infant Mortality Rate: 1980 to 1997

National Percent Change = 44.4% Decrease*

ALPHA ORDER

RANK	STATE	PERCENT CHANGE
18	Alabama	(39.3)
44	Alaska	(52.0)
40	Arizona	(49.2)
5	Arkansas	(33.6)
34	California	(45.7)
1	Colorado	(24.5)
13	Connecticut	(37.3)
22	Delaware	(41.1)
42	Florida	(50.6)
37	Georgia	(46.8)
24	Hawaii	(41.7)
26	Idaho	(43.0)
35	Illinois	(45.9)
14	Indiana	(37.7)
49	Iowa	(59.4)
6	Kansas	(33.7)
8	Kentucky	(35.5)
11	Louisiana	(36.5)
50	Maine	(59.9)
9	Maryland	(35.9)
48	Massachusetts	(59.1)
12	Michigan	(36.7)
21	Minnesota	(41.0)
9	Mississippi	(35.9)
23	Missouri	(41.2)
30	Montana	(44.3)
4	Nebraska	(31.2)
38	Nevada	(46.9)
46	New Hampshire	(55.5)
41	New Jersey	(49.8)
32	New Mexico	(44.5)
43	New York	(51.3)
6	North Carolina	(33.7)
16	North Dakota	(38.8)
27	Ohio	(43.6)
20	Oklahoma	(40.3)
45	Oregon	(52.3)
29	Pennsylvania	(44.1)
19	Rhode Island	(39.9)
28	South Carolina	(43.7)
2	South Dakota	(30.4)
15	Tennessee	(37.8)
39	Texas	(48.2)
31	Utah	(44.4)
25	Vermont	(42.7)
33	Virginia	(44.9)
47	Washington	(55.8)
3	West Virginia	(30.6)
16	Wisconsin	(38.8)
36	Wyoming	(46.7)

RANK ORDER

RANK	STATE	PERCENT CHANGE
1	Colorado	(24.5)
2	South Dakota	(30.4)
3	West Virginia	(30.6)
4	Nebraska	(31.2)
5	Arkansas	(33.6)
6	Kansas	(33.7)
6	North Carolina	(33.7)
8	Kentucky	(35.5)
9	Maryland	(35.9)
9	Mississippi	(35.9)
11	Louisiana	(36.5)
12	Michigan	(36.7)
13	Connecticut	(37.3)
14	Indiana	(37.7)
15	Tennessee	(37.8)
16	North Dakota	(38.8)
16	Wisconsin	(38.8)
18	Alabama	(39.3)
19	Rhode Island	(39.9)
20	Oklahoma	(40.3)
21	Minnesota	(41.0)
22	Delaware	(41.1)
23	Missouri	(41.2)
24	Hawaii	(41.7)
25	Vermont	(42.7)
26	Idaho	(43.0)
27	Ohio	(43.6)
28	South Carolina	(43.7)
29	Pennsylvania	(44.1)
30	Montana	(44.3)
31	Utah	(44.4)
32	New Mexico	(44.5)
33	Virginia	(44.9)
34	California	(45.7)
35	Illinois	(45.9)
36	Wyoming	(46.7)
37	Georgia	(46.8)
38	Nevada	(46.9)
39	Texas	(48.2)
40	Arizona	(49.2)
41	New Jersey	(49.8)
42	Florida	(50.6)
43	New York	(51.3)
44	Alaska	(52.0)
45	Oregon	(52.3)
46	New Hampshire	(55.5)
47	Washington	(55.8)
48	Massachusetts	(59.1)
49	Iowa	(59.4)
50	Maine	(59.9)

District of Columbia (52.0)

Source: Morgan Quitno Press using data from US Dept of Health & Human Services, National Center for Health Statistics
"Monthly Vital Statistics Report" (Vol. 46, No. 12, July 28, 1998)
"Vital Statistics of the United States, 1980" (Vol. I-Natality, issued 1984) and unpublished data
*Final data by state of residence. Infant deaths are those occurring under 1 year, exclusive of fetal deaths.

White Infant Deaths in 1996

National Total = 18,761 Deaths*

ALPHA ORDER

RANK	STATE	DEATHS	% of USA
19	Alabama	330	1.8%
46	Alaska	39	0.2%
11	Arizona	472	2.5%
30	Arkansas	225	1.2%
1	California	2,415	12.9%
21	Colorado	326	1.7%
32	Connecticut	201	1.1%
45	Delaware	45	0.2%
5	Florida	832	4.4%
12	Georgia	460	2.5%
50	Hawaii	21	0.1%
38	Idaho	133	0.7%
4	Illinois	899	4.8%
9	Indiana	555	3.0%
29	Iowa	230	1.2%
27	Kansas	236	1.3%
21	Kentucky	326	1.7%
26	Louisiana	242	1.3%
42	Maine	59	0.3%
25	Maryland	260	1.4%
20	Massachusetts	329	1.8%
8	Michigan	628	3.3%
23	Minnesota	291	1.6%
35	Mississippi	171	0.9%
15	Missouri	383	2.0%
41	Montana	65	0.3%
34	Nebraska	180	1.0%
39	Nevada	120	0.6%
40	New Hampshire	71	0.4%
13	New Jersey	456	2.4%
36	New Mexico	141	0.8%
3	New York	1,093	5.8%
10	North Carolina	521	2.8%
48	North Dakota	37	0.2%
6	Ohio	801	4.3%
24	Oklahoma	282	1.5%
31	Oregon	215	1.1%
7	Pennsylvania	799	4.3%
43	Rhode Island	57	0.3%
33	South Carolina	182	1.0%
46	South Dakota	39	0.2%
17	Tennessee	379	2.0%
2	Texas	1,599	8.5%
28	Utah	235	1.3%
44	Vermont	46	0.2%
14	Virginia	409	2.2%
16	Washington	381	2.0%
37	West Virginia	137	0.7%
18	Wisconsin	356	1.9%
48	Wyoming	37	0.2%

RANK ORDER

RANK	STATE	DEATHS	% of USA
1	California	2,415	12.9%
2	Texas	1,599	8.5%
3	New York	1,093	5.8%
4	Illinois	899	4.8%
5	Florida	832	4.4%
6	Ohio	801	4.3%
7	Pennsylvania	799	4.3%
8	Michigan	628	3.3%
9	Indiana	555	3.0%
10	North Carolina	521	2.8%
11	Arizona	472	2.5%
12	Georgia	460	2.5%
13	New Jersey	456	2.4%
14	Virginia	409	2.2%
15	Missouri	383	2.0%
16	Washington	381	2.0%
17	Tennessee	379	2.0%
18	Wisconsin	356	1.9%
19	Alabama	330	1.8%
20	Massachusetts	329	1.8%
21	Colorado	326	1.7%
21	Kentucky	326	1.7%
23	Minnesota	291	1.6%
24	Oklahoma	282	1.5%
25	Maryland	260	1.4%
26	Louisiana	242	1.3%
27	Kansas	236	1.3%
28	Utah	235	1.3%
29	Iowa	230	1.2%
30	Arkansas	225	1.2%
31	Oregon	215	1.1%
32	Connecticut	201	1.1%
33	South Carolina	182	1.0%
34	Nebraska	180	1.0%
35	Mississippi	171	0.9%
36	New Mexico	141	0.8%
37	West Virginia	137	0.7%
38	Idaho	133	0.7%
39	Nevada	120	0.6%
40	New Hampshire	71	0.4%
41	Montana	65	0.3%
42	Maine	59	0.3%
43	Rhode Island	57	0.3%
44	Vermont	46	0.2%
45	Delaware	45	0.2%
46	Alaska	39	0.2%
46	South Dakota	39	0.2%
48	North Dakota	37	0.2%
48	Wyoming	37	0.2%
50	Hawaii	21	0.1%
	District of Columbia	15	0.1%

Source: U.S. Department of Health and Human Services, National Center for Health Statistics
"National Vital Statistics Report" (Vol. 47, No. 9, November 10, 1998)
*Final data. Deaths of infants under 1 year old, exclusive of fetal deaths. Based on race of the mother.

White Infant Mortality Rate in 1996

National Rate = 6.1 White Infant Deaths per 1,000 White Live Births*

ALPHA ORDER

RANK ORDER

RANK	STATE	RATE	RANK	STATE	RATE
2	Alabama	8.2	1	Nebraska	8.4
31	Alaska	5.8	2	Alabama	8.2
9	Arizona	7.1	3	Arkansas	8.1
3	Arkansas	8.1	4	Mississippi	8.0
38	California	5.5	5	Oklahoma	7.7
18	Colorado	6.4	6	Indiana	7.5
40	Connecticut	5.3	7	Idaho	7.4
28	Delaware	6.0	8	Kansas	7.2
31	Florida	5.8	9	Arizona	7.1
21	Georgia	6.3	9	North Carolina	7.1
49	Hawaii	4.4	11	Kentucky	6.9
7	Idaho	7.4	11	Vermont	6.9
18	Illinois	6.4	11	West Virginia	6.9
6	Indiana	7.5	14	Montana	6.8
16	Iowa	6.5	15	Tennessee	6.7
8	Kansas	7.2	16	Iowa	6.5
11	Kentucky	6.9	16	Louisiana	6.5
16	Louisiana	6.5	18	Colorado	6.4
49	Maine	4.4	18	Illinois	6.4
33	Maryland	5.7	18	Pennsylvania	6.4
47	Massachusetts	4.8	21	Georgia	6.3
29	Michigan	5.9	21	Ohio	6.3
43	Minnesota	5.1	23	Missouri	6.2
4	Mississippi	8.0	23	Wyoming	6.2
23	Missouri	6.2	25	New Mexico	6.1
14	Montana	6.8	25	Virginia	6.1
1	Nebraska	8.4	25	Wisconsin	6.1
39	Nevada	5.4	28	Delaware	6.0
45	New Hampshire	5.0	29	Michigan	5.9
40	New Jersey	5.3	29	Utah	5.9
25	New Mexico	6.1	31	Alaska	5.8
33	New York	5.7	31	Florida	5.8
9	North Carolina	7.1	33	Maryland	5.7
45	North Dakota	5.0	33	New York	5.7
21	Ohio	6.3	33	Texas	5.7
5	Oklahoma	7.7	36	South Carolina	5.6
40	Oregon	5.3	36	Washington	5.6
18	Pennsylvania	6.4	38	California	5.5
43	Rhode Island	5.1	39	Nevada	5.4
36	South Carolina	5.6	40	Connecticut	5.3
48	South Dakota	4.5	40	New Jersey	5.3
15	Tennessee	6.7	40	Oregon	5.3
33	Texas	5.7	43	Minnesota	5.1
29	Utah	5.9	43	Rhode Island	5.1
11	Vermont	6.9	45	New Hampshire	5.0
25	Virginia	6.1	45	North Dakota	5.0
36	Washington	5.6	47	Massachusetts	4.8
11	West Virginia	6.9	48	South Dakota	4.5
25	Wisconsin	6.1	49	Hawaii	4.4
23	Wyoming	6.2	49	Maine	4.4
				District of Columbia**	NA

Source: U.S. Department of Health and Human Services, National Center for Health Statistics
"National Vital Statistics Report" (Vol. 47, No. 9, November 10, 1998)
*Final data. Deaths of infants under 1 year old, exclusive of fetal deaths. Based on race of the mother.
**Not available, fewer than 20 white infant deaths.

Black Infant Deaths in 1996

National Total = 8,730 Deaths*

ALPHA ORDER

RANK	STATE	DEATHS	% of USA
14	Alabama	303	3.5%
38	Alaska	7	0.1%
29	Arizona	48	0.5%
22	Arkansas	111	1.3%
5	California	535	6.1%
31	Colorado	38	0.4%
24	Connecticut	78	0.9%
32	Delaware	30	0.3%
4	Florida	564	6.5%
3	Georgia	572	6.6%
38	Hawaii	7	0.1%
45	Idaho	0	0.0%
2	Illinois	659	7.5%
20	Indiana	162	1.9%
34	Iowa	24	0.3%
27	Kansas	64	0.7%
25	Kentucky	66	0.8%
11	Louisiana	339	3.9%
43	Maine	2	0.0%
12	Maryland	332	3.8%
26	Massachusetts	65	0.7%
7	Michigan	426	4.9%
30	Minnesota	45	0.5%
16	Mississippi	277	3.2%
19	Missouri	175	2.0%
45	Montana	0	0.0%
35	Nebraska	17	0.2%
33	Nevada	27	0.3%
45	New Hampshire	0	0.0%
13	New Jersey	306	3.5%
40	New Mexico	6	0.1%
1	New York	687	7.9%
8	North Carolina	416	4.8%
45	North Dakota	0	0.0%
9	Ohio	358	4.1%
23	Oklahoma	79	0.9%
37	Oregon	14	0.2%
10	Pennsylvania	348	4.0%
40	Rhode Island	6	0.1%
17	South Carolina	247	2.8%
44	South Dakota	1	0.0%
17	Tennessee	247	2.8%
6	Texas	453	5.2%
42	Utah	5	0.1%
45	Vermont	0	0.0%
15	Virginia	289	3.3%
28	Washington	49	0.6%
36	West Virginia	16	0.2%
21	Wisconsin	121	1.4%
45	Wyoming	0	0.0%

RANK ORDER

RANK	STATE	DEATHS	% of USA
1	New York	687	7.9%
2	Illinois	659	7.5%
3	Georgia	572	6.6%
4	Florida	564	6.5%
5	California	535	6.1%
6	Texas	453	5.2%
7	Michigan	426	4.9%
8	North Carolina	416	4.8%
9	Ohio	358	4.1%
10	Pennsylvania	348	4.0%
11	Louisiana	339	3.9%
12	Maryland	332	3.8%
13	New Jersey	306	3.5%
14	Alabama	303	3.5%
15	Virginia	289	3.3%
16	Mississippi	277	3.2%
17	South Carolina	247	2.8%
17	Tennessee	247	2.8%
19	Missouri	175	2.0%
20	Indiana	162	1.9%
21	Wisconsin	121	1.4%
22	Arkansas	111	1.3%
23	Oklahoma	79	0.9%
24	Connecticut	78	0.9%
25	Kentucky	66	0.8%
26	Massachusetts	65	0.7%
27	Kansas	64	0.7%
28	Washington	49	0.6%
29	Arizona	48	0.5%
30	Minnesota	45	0.5%
31	Colorado	38	0.4%
32	Delaware	30	0.3%
33	Nevada	27	0.3%
34	Iowa	24	0.3%
35	Nebraska	17	0.2%
36	West Virginia	16	0.2%
37	Oregon	14	0.2%
38	Alaska	7	0.1%
38	Hawaii	7	0.1%
40	New Mexico	6	0.1%
40	Rhode Island	6	0.1%
42	Utah	5	0.1%
43	Maine	2	0.0%
44	South Dakota	1	0.0%
45	Idaho	0	0.0%
45	Montana	0	0.0%
45	New Hampshire	0	0.0%
45	North Dakota	0	0.0%
45	Vermont	0	0.0%
45	Wyoming	0	0.0%
	District of Columbia	109	1.2%

Source: U.S. Department of Health and Human Services, National Center for Health Statistics
"National Vital Statistics Report" (Vol. 47, No. 9, November 10, 1998)
*Final data. Deaths of infants under 1 year old, exclusive of fetal deaths. Based on race of the mother.

Black Infant Mortality Rate in 1996

National Rate = 14.7 Black Infant Deaths per 1,000 Black Live Births*

ALPHA ORDER			RANK ORDER		
RANK	STATE	RATE	RANK	STATE	RATE
13	Alabama	15.5	1	Kansas	23.1
NA	Alaska**	NA	2	Iowa	22.9
3	Arizona	20.5	3	Arizona	20.5
23	Arkansas	14.0	4	Wisconsin	18.8
24	California	13.9	5	Indiana	18.4
19	Colorado	14.7	6	Illinois	18.2
16	Connecticut	14.9	7	Michigan	17.6
31	Delaware	12.7	7	Oklahoma	17.6
29	Florida	13.3	9	Pennsylvania	16.9
16	Georgia	14.9	10	Ohio	16.2
NA	Hawaii**	NA	11	Missouri	15.7
NA	Idaho**	NA	11	Washington	15.7
6	Illinois	18.2	13	Alabama	15.5
5	Indiana	18.4	14	Tennessee	15.4
2	Iowa	22.9	15	North Carolina	15.3
1	Kansas	23.1	16	Connecticut	14.9
28	Kentucky	13.6	16	Georgia	14.9
30	Louisiana	12.8	16	New Jersey	14.9
NA	Maine**	NA	19	Colorado	14.7
21	Maryland	14.5	20	Mississippi	14.6
34	Massachusetts	8.8	21	Maryland	14.5
7	Michigan	17.6	21	Minnesota	14.5
21	Minnesota	14.5	23	Arkansas	14.0
20	Mississippi	14.6	24	California	13.9
11	Missouri	15.7	25	Virginia	13.8
NA	Montana**	NA	26	Nevada	13.7
NA	Nebraska**	NA	26	South Carolina	13.7
26	Nevada	13.7	28	Kentucky	13.6
NA	New Hampshire**	NA	29	Florida	13.3
16	New Jersey	14.9	30	Louisiana	12.8
NA	New Mexico**	NA	31	Delaware	12.7
32	New York	12.4	32	New York	12.4
15	North Carolina	15.3	33	Texas	11.7
NA	North Dakota**	NA	34	Massachusetts	8.8
10	Ohio	16.2	NA	Alaska**	NA
7	Oklahoma	17.6	NA	Hawaii**	NA
NA	Oregon**	NA	NA	Idaho**	NA
9	Pennsylvania	16.9	NA	Maine**	NA
NA	Rhode Island**	NA	NA	Montana**	NA
26	South Carolina	13.7	NA	Nebraska**	NA
NA	South Dakota**	NA	NA	New Hampshire**	NA
14	Tennessee	15.4	NA	New Mexico**	NA
33	Texas	11.7	NA	North Dakota**	NA
NA	Utah**	NA	NA	Oregon**	NA
NA	Vermont**	NA	NA	Rhode Island**	NA
25	Virginia	13.8	NA	South Dakota**	NA
11	Washington	15.7	NA	Utah**	NA
NA	West Virginia**	NA	NA	Vermont**	NA
4	Wisconsin	18.8	NA	West Virginia**	NA
NA	Wyoming**	NA	NA	Wyoming**	NA
				District of Columbia	17.6

Source: U.S. Department of Health and Human Services, National Center for Health Statistics
"National Vital Statistics Report" (Vol. 47, No. 9, November 10, 1998)
*Final data. Deaths of infants under 1 year old, exclusive of fetal deaths. Based on race of the mother.
**Not available, fewer than 20 black infant deaths.

White Infant Mortality Rate in 1990

National Rate = 7.7 White Infant Deaths per 1,000 Live Births*

<table>
<tr><td colspan="3">ALPHA ORDER</td><td colspan="3">RANK ORDER</td></tr>
<tr><td>RANK</td><td>STATE</td><td>RATE</td><td>RANK</td><td>STATE</td><td>RATE</td></tr>
<tr><td>13</td><td>Alabama</td><td>8.3</td><td>1</td><td>West Virginia</td><td>9.6</td></tr>
<tr><td>10</td><td>Alaska</td><td>8.5</td><td>2</td><td>Oklahoma</td><td>9.4</td></tr>
<tr><td>17</td><td>Arizona</td><td>8.2</td><td>3</td><td>New Mexico</td><td>9.3</td></tr>
<tr><td>21</td><td>Arkansas</td><td>8.0</td><td>4</td><td>Georgia</td><td>9.1</td></tr>
<tr><td>32</td><td>California</td><td>7.6</td><td>5</td><td>Indiana</td><td>8.9</td></tr>
<tr><td>12</td><td>Colorado</td><td>8.4</td><td>6</td><td>Wyoming</td><td>8.8</td></tr>
<tr><td>46</td><td>Connecticut</td><td>6.6</td><td>7</td><td>Idaho</td><td>8.7</td></tr>
<tr><td>37</td><td>Delaware</td><td>7.3</td><td>8</td><td>Montana</td><td>8.6</td></tr>
<tr><td>32</td><td>Florida</td><td>7.6</td><td>8</td><td>South Dakota</td><td>8.6</td></tr>
<tr><td>4</td><td>Georgia</td><td>9.1</td><td>10</td><td>Alaska</td><td>8.5</td></tr>
<tr><td>50</td><td>Hawaii</td><td>5.1</td><td>10</td><td>Mississippi</td><td>8.5</td></tr>
<tr><td>7</td><td>Idaho</td><td>8.7</td><td>12</td><td>Colorado</td><td>8.4</td></tr>
<tr><td>29</td><td>Illinois</td><td>7.7</td><td>13</td><td>Alabama</td><td>8.3</td></tr>
<tr><td>5</td><td>Indiana</td><td>8.9</td><td>13</td><td>North Carolina</td><td>8.3</td></tr>
<tr><td>26</td><td>Iowa</td><td>7.8</td><td>13</td><td>Rhode Island</td><td>8.3</td></tr>
<tr><td>29</td><td>Kansas</td><td>7.7</td><td>13</td><td>South Carolina</td><td>8.3</td></tr>
<tr><td>21</td><td>Kentucky</td><td>8.0</td><td>17</td><td>Arizona</td><td>8.2</td></tr>
<tr><td>37</td><td>Louisiana</td><td>7.3</td><td>17</td><td>Ohio</td><td>8.2</td></tr>
<tr><td>49</td><td>Maine</td><td>6.2</td><td>19</td><td>Nevada</td><td>8.1</td></tr>
<tr><td>47</td><td>Maryland</td><td>6.5</td><td>19</td><td>Oregon</td><td>8.1</td></tr>
<tr><td>44</td><td>Massachusetts</td><td>6.7</td><td>21</td><td>Arkansas</td><td>8.0</td></tr>
<tr><td>24</td><td>Michigan</td><td>7.9</td><td>21</td><td>Kentucky</td><td>8.0</td></tr>
<tr><td>44</td><td>Minnesota</td><td>6.7</td><td>21</td><td>Tennessee</td><td>8.0</td></tr>
<tr><td>10</td><td>Mississippi</td><td>8.5</td><td>24</td><td>Michigan</td><td>7.9</td></tr>
<tr><td>26</td><td>Missouri</td><td>7.8</td><td>24</td><td>North Dakota</td><td>7.9</td></tr>
<tr><td>8</td><td>Montana</td><td>8.6</td><td>26</td><td>Iowa</td><td>7.8</td></tr>
<tr><td>39</td><td>Nebraska</td><td>7.2</td><td>26</td><td>Missouri</td><td>7.8</td></tr>
<tr><td>19</td><td>Nevada</td><td>8.1</td><td>26</td><td>Pennsylvania</td><td>7.8</td></tr>
<tr><td>39</td><td>New Hampshire</td><td>7.2</td><td>29</td><td>Illinois</td><td>7.7</td></tr>
<tr><td>43</td><td>New Jersey</td><td>6.8</td><td>29</td><td>Kansas</td><td>7.7</td></tr>
<tr><td>3</td><td>New Mexico</td><td>9.3</td><td>29</td><td>New York</td><td>7.7</td></tr>
<tr><td>29</td><td>New York</td><td>7.7</td><td>32</td><td>California</td><td>7.6</td></tr>
<tr><td>13</td><td>North Carolina</td><td>8.3</td><td>32</td><td>Florida</td><td>7.6</td></tr>
<tr><td>24</td><td>North Dakota</td><td>7.9</td><td>32</td><td>Washington</td><td>7.6</td></tr>
<tr><td>17</td><td>Ohio</td><td>8.2</td><td>35</td><td>Virginia</td><td>7.5</td></tr>
<tr><td>2</td><td>Oklahoma</td><td>9.4</td><td>36</td><td>Utah</td><td>7.4</td></tr>
<tr><td>19</td><td>Oregon</td><td>8.1</td><td>37</td><td>Delaware</td><td>7.3</td></tr>
<tr><td>26</td><td>Pennsylvania</td><td>7.8</td><td>37</td><td>Louisiana</td><td>7.3</td></tr>
<tr><td>13</td><td>Rhode Island</td><td>8.3</td><td>39</td><td>Nebraska</td><td>7.2</td></tr>
<tr><td>13</td><td>South Carolina</td><td>8.3</td><td>39</td><td>New Hampshire</td><td>7.2</td></tr>
<tr><td>8</td><td>South Dakota</td><td>8.6</td><td>39</td><td>Wisconsin</td><td>7.2</td></tr>
<tr><td>21</td><td>Tennessee</td><td>8.0</td><td>42</td><td>Texas</td><td>7.1</td></tr>
<tr><td>42</td><td>Texas</td><td>7.1</td><td>43</td><td>New Jersey</td><td>6.8</td></tr>
<tr><td>36</td><td>Utah</td><td>7.4</td><td>44</td><td>Massachusetts</td><td>6.7</td></tr>
<tr><td>47</td><td>Vermont</td><td>6.5</td><td>44</td><td>Minnesota</td><td>6.7</td></tr>
<tr><td>35</td><td>Virginia</td><td>7.5</td><td>46</td><td>Connecticut</td><td>6.6</td></tr>
<tr><td>32</td><td>Washington</td><td>7.6</td><td>47</td><td>Maryland</td><td>6.5</td></tr>
<tr><td>1</td><td>West Virginia</td><td>9.6</td><td>47</td><td>Vermont</td><td>6.5</td></tr>
<tr><td>39</td><td>Wisconsin</td><td>7.2</td><td>49</td><td>Maine</td><td>6.2</td></tr>
<tr><td>6</td><td>Wyoming</td><td>8.8</td><td>50</td><td>Hawaii</td><td>5.1</td></tr>
<tr><td></td><td></td><td></td><td></td><td>District of Columbia</td><td>12.1</td></tr>
</table>

Source: U.S. Department of Health and Human Services, National Center for Health Statistics,
    "Vital Statistics of the United States"
*Deaths of infants under 1 year old, exclusive of fetal deaths. Final data by state of residence.

96

Black Infant Mortality Rate in 1990

National Rate = 17.0 Black Infant Deaths per 1,000 Live Births*

ALPHA ORDER				RANK ORDER		
RANK	STATE	RATE		RANK	STATE	RATE
27	Alabama	15.9		1	Illinois	21.5
41	Alaska	11.2		2	Michigan	21.0
17	Arizona	16.7		3	Minnesota	19.7
33	Arkansas	13.6		4	Delaware	19.4
31	California	14.2		5	Pennsylvania	18.8
19	Colorado	16.5		5	Virginia	18.8
24	Connecticut	16.0		7	Ohio	18.3
4	Delaware	19.4		8	Wisconsin	18.1
22	Florida	16.2		9	Georgia	18.0
9	Georgia	18.0		9	Iowa	18.0
40	Hawaii	11.5		11	Missouri	17.5
42	Idaho	10.9		11	Tennessee	17.5
1	Illinois	21.5		13	New Jersey	17.3
24	Indiana	16.0		13	New York	17.3
9	Iowa	18.0		15	South Carolina	17.1
28	Kansas	15.4		16	Nebraska	16.8
33	Kentucky	13.6		17	Arizona	16.7
19	Louisiana	16.5		18	West Virginia	16.6
46	Maine	6.1		19	Colorado	16.5
21	Maryland	16.3		19	Louisiana	16.5
43	Massachusetts	10.4		21	Maryland	16.3
2	Michigan	21.0		22	Florida	16.2
3	Minnesota	19.7		23	Mississippi	16.1
23	Mississippi	16.1		24	Connecticut	16.0
11	Missouri	17.5		24	Indiana	16.0
35	Montana	13.3		24	North Carolina	16.0
16	Nebraska	16.8		27	Alabama	15.9
39	Nevada	12.5		28	Kansas	15.4
47	New Hampshire	5.4		29	Oregon	15.1
13	New Jersey	17.3		30	Washington	14.5
38	New Mexico	12.8		31	California	14.2
13	New York	17.3		32	Texas	13.9
24	North Carolina	16.0		33	Arkansas	13.6
NA	North Dakota**	NA		33	Kentucky	13.6
7	Ohio	18.3		35	Montana	13.3
36	Oklahoma	13.2		36	Oklahoma	13.2
29	Oregon	15.1		37	Utah	13.0
5	Pennsylvania	18.8		38	New Mexico	12.8
44	Rhode Island	9.7		39	Nevada	12.5
15	South Carolina	17.1		40	Hawaii	11.5
45	South Dakota	7.4		41	Alaska	11.2
11	Tennessee	17.5		42	Idaho	10.9
32	Texas	13.9		43	Massachusetts	10.4
37	Utah	13.0		44	Rhode Island	9.7
NA	Vermont**	NA		45	South Dakota	7.4
5	Virginia	18.8		46	Maine	6.1
30	Washington	14.5		47	New Hampshire	5.4
18	West Virginia	16.6		NA	North Dakota**	NA
8	Wisconsin	18.1		NA	Vermont**	NA
NA	Wyoming**	NA		NA	Wyoming**	NA
					District of Columbia	24.4

Source: U.S. Department of Health and Human Services, National Center for Health Statistics,
*   "Vital Statistics of the United States"*
Deaths of infants under 1 year old, exclusive of fetal deaths. Final data by state of residence.
**Not available.*

Neonatal Deaths in 1996

National Total = 18,572 Deaths*

ALPHA ORDER					RANK ORDER			
RANK	STATE	DEATHS	% of USA		RANK	STATE	DEATHS	% of USA
15	Alabama	415	2.2%		1	California	2,053	11.1%
46	Alaska	35	0.2%		2	New York	1,260	6.8%
17	Arizona	383	2.1%		3	Texas	1,259	6.8%
29	Arkansas	204	1.1%		4	Illinois	1,036	5.6%
1	California	2,053	11.1%		5	Florida	897	4.8%
26	Colorado	245	1.3%		6	Pennsylvania	806	4.3%
29	Connecticut	204	1.1%		7	Ohio	769	4.1%
41	Delaware	52	0.3%		8	Michigan	709	3.8%
5	Florida	897	4.8%		9	Georgia	705	3.8%
9	Georgia	705	3.8%		10	North Carolina	637	3.4%
40	Hawaii	66	0.4%		11	New Jersey	547	2.9%
39	Idaho	82	0.4%		12	Virginia	489	2.6%
4	Illinois	1,036	5.6%		13	Indiana	466	2.5%
13	Indiana	466	2.5%		14	Maryland	418	2.3%
32	Iowa	182	1.0%		15	Alabama	415	2.2%
31	Kansas	203	1.1%		16	Tennessee	386	2.1%
25	Kentucky	256	1.4%		17	Arizona	383	2.1%
18	Louisiana	367	2.0%		18	Louisiana	367	2.0%
45	Maine	47	0.3%		19	Missouri	358	1.9%
14	Maryland	418	2.3%		20	Wisconsin	313	1.7%
23	Massachusetts	291	1.6%		21	Mississippi	294	1.6%
8	Michigan	709	3.8%		22	South Carolina	292	1.6%
27	Minnesota	231	1.2%		23	Massachusetts	291	1.6%
21	Mississippi	294	1.6%		23	Washington	291	1.6%
19	Missouri	358	1.9%		25	Kentucky	256	1.4%
44	Montana	48	0.3%		26	Colorado	245	1.3%
35	Nebraska	136	0.7%		27	Minnesota	231	1.2%
38	Nevada	88	0.5%		28	Oklahoma	230	1.2%
42	New Hampshire	51	0.3%		29	Arkansas	204	1.1%
11	New Jersey	547	2.9%		29	Connecticut	204	1.1%
36	New Mexico	107	0.6%		31	Kansas	203	1.1%
2	New York	1,260	6.8%		32	Iowa	182	1.0%
10	North Carolina	637	3.4%		33	Utah	167	0.9%
47	North Dakota	31	0.2%		34	Oregon	144	0.8%
7	Ohio	769	4.1%		35	Nebraska	136	0.7%
28	Oklahoma	230	1.2%		36	New Mexico	107	0.6%
34	Oregon	144	0.8%		37	West Virginia	101	0.5%
6	Pennsylvania	806	4.3%		38	Nevada	88	0.5%
43	Rhode Island	50	0.3%		39	Idaho	82	0.4%
22	South Carolina	292	1.6%		40	Hawaii	66	0.4%
47	South Dakota	31	0.2%		41	Delaware	52	0.3%
16	Tennessee	386	2.1%		42	New Hampshire	51	0.3%
3	Texas	1,259	6.8%		43	Rhode Island	50	0.3%
33	Utah	167	0.9%		44	Montana	48	0.3%
47	Vermont	31	0.2%		45	Maine	47	0.3%
12	Virginia	489	2.6%		46	Alaska	35	0.2%
23	Washington	291	1.6%		47	North Dakota	31	0.2%
37	West Virginia	101	0.5%		47	South Dakota	31	0.2%
20	Wisconsin	313	1.7%		47	Vermont	31	0.2%
50	Wyoming	25	0.1%		50	Wyoming	25	0.1%

	District of Columbia	84	0.5%

Source: U.S. Department of Health and Human Services, National Center for Health Statistics
"National Vital Statistics Report" (Vol. 47, No. 9, November 10, 1998)
*Final data. Deaths of infants under 28 days, exclusive of fetal deaths.

Neonatal Death Rate in 1996

National Rate = 4.8 Neonatal Deaths per 1,000 Live Births*

ALPHA ORDER			RANK ORDER		
RANK	STATE	RATE	RANK	STATE	RATE
2	Alabama	6.9	1	Mississippi	7.2
45	Alaska	3.5	2	Alabama	6.9
17	Arizona	5.1	3	Georgia	6.2
9	Arkansas	5.6	4	North Carolina	6.1
38	California	3.8	5	Maryland	5.8
31	Colorado	4.4	5	Nebraska	5.8
29	Connecticut	4.6	7	Illinois	5.7
17	Delaware	5.1	7	South Carolina	5.7
27	Florida	4.7	9	Arkansas	5.6
3	Georgia	6.2	9	Indiana	5.6
42	Hawaii	3.6	9	Louisiana	5.6
31	Idaho	4.4	12	Kansas	5.5
7	Illinois	5.7	13	Pennsylvania	5.4
9	Indiana	5.6	14	Michigan	5.3
21	Iowa	4.9	14	Virginia	5.3
12	Kansas	5.5	16	Tennessee	5.2
21	Kentucky	4.9	17	Arizona	5.1
9	Louisiana	5.6	17	Delaware	5.1
47	Maine	3.4	17	Ohio	5.1
5	Maryland	5.8	20	Oklahoma	5.0
42	Massachusetts	3.6	21	Iowa	4.9
14	Michigan	5.3	21	Kentucky	4.9
42	Minnesota	3.6	21	West Virginia	4.9
1	Mississippi	7.2	24	Missouri	4.8
24	Missouri	4.8	24	New Jersey	4.8
31	Montana	4.4	24	New York	4.8
5	Nebraska	5.8	27	Florida	4.7
47	Nevada	3.4	27	Wisconsin	4.7
45	New Hampshire	3.5	29	Connecticut	4.6
24	New Jersey	4.8	29	Vermont	4.6
37	New Mexico	3.9	31	Colorado	4.4
24	New York	4.8	31	Idaho	4.4
4	North Carolina	6.1	31	Montana	4.4
40	North Dakota	3.7	34	Rhode Island	4.0
17	Ohio	5.1	34	Utah	4.0
20	Oklahoma	5.0	34	Wyoming	4.0
49	Oregon	3.3	37	New Mexico	3.9
13	Pennsylvania	5.4	38	California	3.8
34	Rhode Island	4.0	38	Texas	3.8
7	South Carolina	5.7	40	North Dakota	3.7
50	South Dakota	3.0	40	Washington	3.7
16	Tennessee	5.2	42	Hawaii	3.6
38	Texas	3.8	42	Massachusetts	3.6
34	Utah	4.0	42	Minnesota	3.6
29	Vermont	4.6	45	Alaska	3.5
14	Virginia	5.3	45	New Hampshire	3.5
40	Washington	3.7	47	Maine	3.4
21	West Virginia	4.9	47	Nevada	3.4
27	Wisconsin	4.7	49	Oregon	3.3
34	Wyoming	4.0	50	South Dakota	3.0
				District of Columbia	10.0

Source: U.S. Department of Health and Human Services, National Center for Health Statistics
"National Vital Statistics Report" (Vol. 47, No. 9, November 10, 1998)
Final data. Deaths of infants under 28 days, exclusive of fetal deaths.

White Neonatal Deaths in 1996

National Total = 12,293 Deaths*

ALPHA ORDER

RANK	STATE	DEATHS	% of USA
22	Alabama	205	1.7%
48	Alaska	22	0.2%
12	Arizona	323	2.6%
31	Arkansas	139	1.1%
1	California	1,576	12.8%
20	Colorado	216	1.8%
30	Connecticut	144	1.2%
45	Delaware	29	0.2%
7	Florida	523	4.3%
13	Georgia	292	2.4%
50	Hawaii	14	0.1%
38	Idaho	79	0.6%
4	Illinois	615	5.0%
9	Indiana	368	3.0%
25	Iowa	164	1.3%
28	Kansas	155	1.3%
21	Kentucky	212	1.7%
29	Louisiana	148	1.2%
41	Maine	46	0.4%
26	Maryland	162	1.3%
15	Massachusetts	251	2.0%
8	Michigan	413	3.4%
23	Minnesota	182	1.5%
35	Mississippi	105	0.9%
17	Missouri	243	2.0%
43	Montana	40	0.3%
33	Nebraska	123	1.0%
39	Nevada	61	0.5%
40	New Hampshire	51	0.4%
11	New Jersey	337	2.7%
36	New Mexico	93	0.8%
3	New York	776	6.3%
10	North Carolina	348	2.8%
46	North Dakota	27	0.2%
6	Ohio	525	4.3%
24	Oklahoma	168	1.4%
32	Oregon	126	1.0%
5	Pennsylvania	563	4.6%
42	Rhode Island	44	0.4%
34	South Carolina	114	0.9%
49	South Dakota	20	0.2%
18	Tennessee	237	1.9%
2	Texas	959	7.8%
27	Utah	157	1.3%
44	Vermont	30	0.2%
14	Virginia	270	2.2%
16	Washington	245	2.0%
37	West Virginia	89	0.7%
19	Wisconsin	231	1.9%
47	Wyoming	24	0.2%

RANK ORDER

RANK	STATE	DEATHS	% of USA
1	California	1,576	12.8%
2	Texas	959	7.8%
3	New York	776	6.3%
4	Illinois	615	5.0%
5	Pennsylvania	563	4.6%
6	Ohio	525	4.3%
7	Florida	523	4.3%
8	Michigan	413	3.4%
9	Indiana	368	3.0%
10	North Carolina	348	2.8%
11	New Jersey	337	2.7%
12	Arizona	323	2.6%
13	Georgia	292	2.4%
14	Virginia	270	2.2%
15	Massachusetts	251	2.0%
16	Washington	245	2.0%
17	Missouri	243	2.0%
18	Tennessee	237	1.9%
19	Wisconsin	231	1.9%
20	Colorado	216	1.8%
21	Kentucky	212	1.7%
22	Alabama	205	1.7%
23	Minnesota	182	1.5%
24	Oklahoma	168	1.4%
25	Iowa	164	1.3%
26	Maryland	162	1.3%
27	Utah	157	1.3%
28	Kansas	155	1.3%
29	Louisiana	148	1.2%
30	Connecticut	144	1.2%
31	Arkansas	139	1.1%
32	Oregon	126	1.0%
33	Nebraska	123	1.0%
34	South Carolina	114	0.9%
35	Mississippi	105	0.9%
36	New Mexico	93	0.8%
37	West Virginia	89	0.7%
38	Idaho	79	0.6%
39	Nevada	61	0.5%
40	New Hampshire	51	0.4%
41	Maine	46	0.4%
42	Rhode Island	44	0.4%
43	Montana	40	0.3%
44	Vermont	30	0.2%
45	Delaware	29	0.2%
46	North Dakota	27	0.2%
47	Wyoming	24	0.2%
48	Alaska	22	0.2%
49	South Dakota	20	0.2%
50	Hawaii	14	0.1%
	District of Columbia	9	0.1%

Source: U.S. Department of Health and Human Services, National Center for Health Statistics
"National Vital Statistics Report" (Vol. 47, No. 9, November 10, 1998)
*Final data. Deaths of infants under 28 days, exclusive of fetal deaths. Based on race of the mother.

White Neonatal Death Rate in 1996

National Rate = 4.0 White Neonatal Deaths per 1,000 White Live Births*

ALPHA ORDER

RANK	STATE	RATE
2	Alabama	5.1
45	Alaska	3.2
5	Arizona	4.9
3	Arkansas	5.0
36	California	3.6
17	Colorado	4.2
33	Connecticut	3.8
33	Delaware	3.8
35	Florida	3.7
21	Georgia	4.0
NA	Hawaii**	NA
15	Idaho	4.4
15	Illinois	4.4
3	Indiana	5.0
7	Iowa	4.7
7	Kansas	4.7
11	Kentucky	4.5
21	Louisiana	4.0
43	Maine	3.4
41	Maryland	3.5
36	Massachusetts	3.6
29	Michigan	3.9
45	Minnesota	3.2
5	Mississippi	4.9
21	Missouri	4.0
17	Montana	4.2
1	Nebraska	5.8
48	Nevada	2.7
36	New Hampshire	3.6
29	New Jersey	3.9
21	New Mexico	4.0
21	New York	4.0
7	North Carolina	4.7
36	North Dakota	3.6
20	Ohio	4.1
10	Oklahoma	4.6
47	Oregon	3.1
11	Pennsylvania	4.5
29	Rhode Island	3.9
41	South Carolina	3.5
49	South Dakota	2.3
17	Tennessee	4.2
43	Texas	3.4
29	Utah	3.9
11	Vermont	4.5
21	Virginia	4.0
36	Washington	3.6
11	West Virginia	4.5
21	Wisconsin	4.0
21	Wyoming	4.0

RANK ORDER

RANK	STATE	RATE
1	Nebraska	5.8
2	Alabama	5.1
3	Arkansas	5.0
3	Indiana	5.0
5	Arizona	4.9
5	Mississippi	4.9
7	Iowa	4.7
7	Kansas	4.7
7	North Carolina	4.7
10	Oklahoma	4.6
11	Kentucky	4.5
11	Pennsylvania	4.5
11	Vermont	4.5
11	West Virginia	4.5
15	Idaho	4.4
15	Illinois	4.4
17	Colorado	4.2
17	Montana	4.2
17	Tennessee	4.2
20	Ohio	4.1
21	Georgia	4.0
21	Louisiana	4.0
21	Missouri	4.0
21	New Mexico	4.0
21	New York	4.0
21	Virginia	4.0
21	Wisconsin	4.0
21	Wyoming	4.0
29	Michigan	3.9
29	New Jersey	3.9
29	Rhode Island	3.9
29	Utah	3.9
33	Connecticut	3.8
33	Delaware	3.8
35	Florida	3.7
36	California	3.6
36	Massachusetts	3.6
36	New Hampshire	3.6
36	North Dakota	3.6
36	Washington	3.6
41	Maryland	3.5
41	South Carolina	3.5
43	Maine	3.4
43	Texas	3.4
45	Alaska	3.2
45	Minnesota	3.2
47	Oregon	3.1
48	Nevada	2.7
49	South Dakota	2.3
NA	Hawaii**	NA
	District of Columbia**	NA

Source: U.S. Department of Health and Human Services, National Center for Health Statistics
"National Vital Statistics Report" (Vol. 47, No. 9, November 10, 1998)
*Final data. Deaths of infants under 28 days, exclusive of fetal deaths. Based on race of the mother.
**Not available. Fewer than 20 white neonatal deaths.

Black Neonatal Deaths in 1996

National Total = 5,688 Deaths*

ALPHA ORDER

RANK	STATE	DEATHS	% of USA
14	Alabama	208	3.7%
42	Alaska	3	0.1%
28	Arizona	30	0.5%
22	Arkansas	64	1.1%
5	California	314	5.5%
31	Colorado	25	0.4%
23	Connecticut	56	1.0%
32	Delaware	22	0.4%
4	Florida	362	6.4%
2	Georgia	405	7.1%
39	Hawaii	4	0.1%
44	Idaho	0	0.0%
3	Illinois	403	7.1%
20	Indiana	94	1.7%
34	Iowa	12	0.2%
25	Kansas	44	0.8%
26	Kentucky	42	0.7%
12	Louisiana	213	3.7%
43	Maine	1	0.0%
9	Maryland	246	4.3%
27	Massachusetts	35	0.6%
6	Michigan	281	4.9%
28	Minnesota	30	0.5%
16	Mississippi	188	3.3%
19	Missouri	114	2.0%
44	Montana	0	0.0%
35	Nebraska	11	0.2%
33	Nevada	16	0.3%
44	New Hampshire	0	0.0%
15	New Jersey	197	3.5%
38	New Mexico	5	0.1%
1	New York	447	7.9%
7	North Carolina	280	4.9%
44	North Dakota	0	0.0%
10	Ohio	238	4.2%
24	Oklahoma	50	0.9%
37	Oregon	8	0.1%
11	Pennsylvania	233	4.1%
39	Rhode Island	4	0.1%
17	South Carolina	178	3.1%
44	South Dakota	0	0.0%
18	Tennessee	149	2.6%
8	Texas	277	4.9%
39	Utah	4	0.1%
44	Vermont	0	0.0%
13	Virginia	209	3.7%
30	Washington	28	0.5%
35	West Virginia	11	0.2%
21	Wisconsin	73	1.3%
44	Wyoming	0	0.0%

RANK ORDER

RANK	STATE	DEATHS	% of USA
1	New York	447	7.9%
2	Georgia	405	7.1%
3	Illinois	403	7.1%
4	Florida	362	6.4%
5	California	314	5.5%
6	Michigan	281	4.9%
7	North Carolina	280	4.9%
8	Texas	277	4.9%
9	Maryland	246	4.3%
10	Ohio	238	4.2%
11	Pennsylvania	233	4.1%
12	Louisiana	213	3.7%
13	Virginia	209	3.7%
14	Alabama	208	3.7%
15	New Jersey	197	3.5%
16	Mississippi	188	3.3%
17	South Carolina	178	3.1%
18	Tennessee	149	2.6%
19	Missouri	114	2.0%
20	Indiana	94	1.7%
21	Wisconsin	73	1.3%
22	Arkansas	64	1.1%
23	Connecticut	56	1.0%
24	Oklahoma	50	0.9%
25	Kansas	44	0.8%
26	Kentucky	42	0.7%
27	Massachusetts	35	0.6%
28	Arizona	30	0.5%
28	Minnesota	30	0.5%
30	Washington	28	0.5%
31	Colorado	25	0.4%
32	Delaware	22	0.4%
33	Nevada	16	0.3%
34	Iowa	12	0.2%
35	Nebraska	11	0.2%
35	West Virginia	11	0.2%
37	Oregon	8	0.1%
38	New Mexico	5	0.1%
39	Hawaii	4	0.1%
39	Rhode Island	4	0.1%
39	Utah	4	0.1%
42	Alaska	3	0.1%
43	Maine	1	0.0%
44	Idaho	0	0.0%
44	Montana	0	0.0%
44	New Hampshire	0	0.0%
44	North Dakota	0	0.0%
44	South Dakota	0	0.0%
44	Vermont	0	0.0%
44	Wyoming	0	0.0%
	District of Columbia	74	1.3%

Source: U.S. Department of Health and Human Services, National Center for Health Statistics
"National Vital Statistics Report" (Vol. 47, No. 9, November 10, 1998)
*Final data. Deaths of infants under 28 days, exclusive of fetal deaths. Based on race of the mother.

Black Neonatal Death Rate in 1996

National Rate = 9.6 Black Neonatal Deaths per 1,000 Black Live Births*

ALPHA ORDER

RANK	STATE	RATE
11	Alabama	10.6
NA	Alaska**	NA
2	Arizona	12.8
28	Arkansas	8.1
27	California	8.2
19	Colorado	9.7
9	Connecticut	10.7
22	Delaware	9.3
25	Florida	8.6
13	Georgia	10.5
NA	Hawaii**	NA
NA	Idaho**	NA
7	Illinois	11.1
11	Indiana	10.6
NA	Iowa**	NA
1	Kansas	15.9
25	Kentucky	8.6
30	Louisiana	8.0
NA	Maine**	NA
9	Maryland	10.7
32	Massachusetts	4.7
3	Michigan	11.6
20	Minnesota	9.6
17	Mississippi	9.9
14	Missouri	10.3
NA	Montana**	NA
NA	Nebraska**	NA
NA	Nevada**	NA
NA	New Hampshire**	NA
20	New Jersey	9.6
NA	New Mexico**	NA
28	New York	8.1
14	North Carolina	10.3
NA	North Dakota**	NA
8	Ohio	10.8
6	Oklahoma	11.2
NA	Oregon**	NA
5	Pennsylvania	11.3
NA	Rhode Island**	NA
17	South Carolina	9.9
NA	South Dakota**	NA
22	Tennessee	9.3
31	Texas	7.1
NA	Utah**	NA
NA	Vermont**	NA
16	Virginia	10.0
24	Washington	9.0
NA	West Virginia**	NA
4	Wisconsin	11.4
NA	Wyoming**	NA

RANK ORDER

RANK	STATE	RATE
1	Kansas	15.9
2	Arizona	12.8
3	Michigan	11.6
4	Wisconsin	11.4
5	Pennsylvania	11.3
6	Oklahoma	11.2
7	Illinois	11.1
8	Ohio	10.8
9	Connecticut	10.7
9	Maryland	10.7
11	Alabama	10.6
11	Indiana	10.6
13	Georgia	10.5
14	Missouri	10.3
14	North Carolina	10.3
16	Virginia	10.0
17	Mississippi	9.9
17	South Carolina	9.9
19	Colorado	9.7
20	Minnesota	9.6
20	New Jersey	9.6
22	Delaware	9.3
22	Tennessee	9.3
24	Washington	9.0
25	Florida	8.6
25	Kentucky	8.6
27	California	8.2
28	Arkansas	8.1
28	New York	8.1
30	Louisiana	8.0
31	Texas	7.1
32	Massachusetts	4.7
NA	Alaska**	NA
NA	Hawaii**	NA
NA	Idaho**	NA
NA	Iowa**	NA
NA	Maine**	NA
NA	Montana**	NA
NA	Nebraska**	NA
NA	Nevada**	NA
NA	New Hampshire**	NA
NA	New Mexico**	NA
NA	North Dakota**	NA
NA	Oregon**	NA
NA	Rhode Island**	NA
NA	South Dakota**	NA
NA	Utah**	NA
NA	Vermont**	NA
NA	West Virginia**	NA
NA	Wyoming**	NA
	District of Columbia	12.0

Source: U.S. Department of Health and Human Services, National Center for Health Statistics
"National Vital Statistics Report" (Vol. 47, No. 9, November 10, 1998)
*Final data. Deaths of infants under 28 days, exclusive of fetal deaths. Based on race of the mother.
**Not available. Fewer than 20 black neonatal deaths.

Deaths by AIDS Through 1996

National Total = 294,087 Deaths*

ALPHA ORDER

RANK	STATE	DEATHS	% of USA
23	Alabama	2,378	0.8%
46	Alaska	160	0.1%
21	Arizona	2,976	1.0%
32	Arkansas	959	0.3%
2	California	50,529	17.2%
20	Colorado	2,977	1.0%
17	Connecticut	3,718	1.3%
36	Delaware	800	0.3%
3	Florida	27,792	9.5%
6	Georgia	9,962	3.4%
34	Hawaii	904	0.3%
44	Idaho	228	0.1%
7	Illinois	9,675	3.3%
24	Indiana	2,223	0.8%
39	Iowa	577	0.2%
33	Kansas	958	0.3%
31	Kentucky	1,173	0.4%
15	Louisiana	4,778	1.6%
40	Maine	451	0.2%
9	Maryland	7,313	2.5%
10	Massachusetts	6,023	2.0%
14	Michigan	4,897	1.7%
26	Minnesota	1,660	0.6%
28	Mississippi	1,599	0.5%
19	Missouri	3,251	1.1%
47	Montana	146	0.0%
42	Nebraska	448	0.2%
30	Nevada	1,281	0.4%
43	New Hampshire	314	0.1%
5	New Jersey	17,814	6.1%
35	New Mexico	880	0.3%
1	New York	57,957	19.7%
11	North Carolina	5,910	2.0%
50	North Dakota	56	0.0%
12	Ohio	5,371	1.8%
27	Oklahoma	1,610	0.5%
25	Oregon	1,959	0.7%
8	Pennsylvania	8,943	3.0%
37	Rhode Island	735	0.2%
18	South Carolina	3,438	1.2%
48	South Dakota	81	0.0%
22	Tennessee	2,772	0.9%
4	Texas	20,063	6.8%
38	Utah	585	0.2%
45	Vermont	177	0.1%
13	Virginia	5,022	1.7%
16	Washington	3,958	1.3%
41	West Virginia	449	0.2%
29	Wisconsin	1,522	0.5%
49	Wyoming	77	0.0%

RANK ORDER

RANK	STATE	DEATHS	% of USA
1	New York	57,957	19.7%
2	California	50,529	17.2%
3	Florida	27,792	9.5%
4	Texas	20,063	6.8%
5	New Jersey	17,814	6.1%
6	Georgia	9,962	3.4%
7	Illinois	9,675	3.3%
8	Pennsylvania	8,943	3.0%
9	Maryland	7,313	2.5%
10	Massachusetts	6,023	2.0%
11	North Carolina	5,910	2.0%
12	Ohio	5,371	1.8%
13	Virginia	5,022	1.7%
14	Michigan	4,897	1.7%
15	Louisiana	4,778	1.6%
16	Washington	3,958	1.3%
17	Connecticut	3,718	1.3%
18	South Carolina	3,438	1.2%
19	Missouri	3,251	1.1%
20	Colorado	2,977	1.0%
21	Arizona	2,976	1.0%
22	Tennessee	2,772	0.9%
23	Alabama	2,378	0.8%
24	Indiana	2,223	0.8%
25	Oregon	1,959	0.7%
26	Minnesota	1,660	0.6%
27	Oklahoma	1,610	0.5%
28	Mississippi	1,599	0.5%
29	Wisconsin	1,522	0.5%
30	Nevada	1,281	0.4%
31	Kentucky	1,173	0.4%
32	Arkansas	959	0.3%
33	Kansas	958	0.3%
34	Hawaii	904	0.3%
35	New Mexico	880	0.3%
36	Delaware	800	0.3%
37	Rhode Island	735	0.2%
38	Utah	585	0.2%
39	Iowa	577	0.2%
40	Maine	451	0.2%
41	West Virginia	449	0.2%
42	Nebraska	448	0.2%
43	New Hampshire	314	0.1%
44	Idaho	228	0.1%
45	Vermont	177	0.1%
46	Alaska	160	0.1%
47	Montana	146	0.0%
48	South Dakota	81	0.0%
49	Wyoming	77	0.0%
50	North Dakota	56	0.0%
	District of Columbia	4,558	1.5%

Source: U.S. Department of Health and Human Services, National Center for Health Statistics (http://wonder.cdc.gov/WONDER/)

*Cumulative deaths through 1996. However, due to reporting delays, these totals should increase. AIDS is Acquired Immunodeficiency Syndrome. The definition of what is AIDS was expanded in 1985, 1987 and 1993.

Deaths by AIDS in 1996

National Total = 31,130 Deaths*

ALPHA ORDER

RANK	STATE	DEATHS	% of USA
20	Alabama	355	1.1%
45	Alaska	16	0.1%
21	Arizona	334	1.1%
33	Arkansas	126	0.4%
2	California	4,219	13.6%
23	Colorado	244	0.8%
18	Connecticut	393	1.3%
32	Delaware	133	0.4%
3	Florida	3,097	9.9%
6	Georgia	1,271	4.1%
36	Hawaii	72	0.2%
44	Idaho	22	0.1%
7	Illinois	1,127	3.6%
24	Indiana	232	0.7%
37	Iowa	71	0.2%
34	Kansas	94	0.3%
30	Kentucky	141	0.5%
13	Louisiana	601	1.9%
42	Maine	42	0.1%
9	Maryland	1,059	3.4%
12	Massachusetts	609	2.0%
16	Michigan	509	1.6%
28	Minnesota	177	0.6%
25	Mississippi	231	0.7%
22	Missouri	321	1.0%
48	Montana	9	0.0%
40	Nebraska	61	0.2%
30	Nevada	141	0.5%
42	New Hampshire	42	0.1%
5	New Jersey	1,757	5.6%
35	New Mexico	85	0.3%
1	New York	5,688	18.3%
10	North Carolina	826	2.7%
50	North Dakota	4	0.0%
11	Ohio	664	2.1%
27	Oklahoma	180	0.6%
26	Oregon	205	0.7%
8	Pennsylvania	1,066	3.4%
38	Rhode Island	67	0.2%
15	South Carolina	534	1.7%
47	South Dakota	10	0.0%
19	Tennessee	390	1.3%
4	Texas	2,073	6.7%
39	Utah	65	0.2%
46	Vermont	13	0.0%
14	Virginia	589	1.9%
17	Washington	397	1.3%
41	West Virginia	57	0.2%
29	Wisconsin	161	0.5%
48	Wyoming	9	0.0%

RANK ORDER

RANK	STATE	DEATHS	% of USA
1	New York	5,688	18.3%
2	California	4,219	13.6%
3	Florida	3,097	9.9%
4	Texas	2,073	6.7%
5	New Jersey	1,757	5.6%
6	Georgia	1,271	4.1%
7	Illinois	1,127	3.6%
8	Pennsylvania	1,066	3.4%
9	Maryland	1,059	3.4%
10	North Carolina	826	2.7%
11	Ohio	664	2.1%
12	Massachusetts	609	2.0%
13	Louisiana	601	1.9%
14	Virginia	589	1.9%
15	South Carolina	534	1.7%
16	Michigan	509	1.6%
17	Washington	397	1.3%
18	Connecticut	393	1.3%
19	Tennessee	390	1.3%
20	Alabama	355	1.1%
21	Arizona	334	1.1%
22	Missouri	321	1.0%
23	Colorado	244	0.8%
24	Indiana	232	0.7%
25	Mississippi	231	0.7%
26	Oregon	205	0.7%
27	Oklahoma	180	0.6%
28	Minnesota	177	0.6%
29	Wisconsin	161	0.5%
30	Kentucky	141	0.5%
30	Nevada	141	0.5%
32	Delaware	133	0.4%
33	Arkansas	126	0.4%
34	Kansas	94	0.3%
35	New Mexico	85	0.3%
36	Hawaii	72	0.2%
37	Iowa	71	0.2%
38	Rhode Island	67	0.2%
39	Utah	65	0.2%
40	Nebraska	61	0.2%
41	West Virginia	57	0.2%
42	Maine	42	0.1%
42	New Hampshire	42	0.1%
44	Idaho	22	0.1%
45	Alaska	16	0.1%
46	Vermont	13	0.0%
47	South Dakota	10	0.0%
48	Montana	9	0.0%
48	Wyoming	9	0.0%
50	North Dakota	4	0.0%
	District of Columbia	541	1.7%

Source: U.S. Department of Health and Human Services, National Center for Health Statistics
     "National Vital Statistics Report" (Vol. 47, No. 9, November 10, 1998)
*AIDS is Acquired Immunodeficiency Syndrome. It is a specific group of diseases or conditions which are indicative
of severe immunosuppression related to infection with the Human Immunodeficiency Virus (HIV).

Death Rate by AIDS in 1996

National Rate = 11.7 Deaths per 100,000 Population*

ALPHA ORDER

RANK	STATE	RATE
19	Alabama	8.3
43	Alaska	2.6
20	Arizona	7.5
31	Arkansas	5.0
9	California	13.3
24	Colorado	6.4
10	Connecticut	12.0
5	Delaware	18.3
3	Florida	21.5
6	Georgia	17.3
26	Hawaii	6.1
46	Idaho	1.9
14	Illinois	9.4
33	Indiana	4.0
44	Iowa	2.5
36	Kansas	3.6
36	Kentucky	3.6
8	Louisiana	13.8
39	Maine	3.4
4	Maryland	20.9
13	Massachusetts	10.0
30	Michigan	5.2
34	Minnesota	3.8
18	Mississippi	8.5
27	Missouri	6.0
49	Montana	1.0
35	Nebraska	3.7
16	Nevada	8.8
36	New Hampshire	3.6
2	New Jersey	21.9
31	New Mexico	5.0
1	New York	31.4
11	North Carolina	11.3
50	North Dakota	0.6
28	Ohio	5.9
29	Oklahoma	5.5
24	Oregon	6.4
15	Pennsylvania	8.9
23	Rhode Island	6.8
7	South Carolina	14.3
48	South Dakota	1.4
21	Tennessee	7.3
12	Texas	10.9
40	Utah	3.2
45	Vermont	2.2
16	Virginia	8.8
22	Washington	7.2
41	West Virginia	3.1
41	Wisconsin	3.1
46	Wyoming	1.9

RANK ORDER

RANK	STATE	RATE
1	New York	31.4
2	New Jersey	21.9
3	Florida	21.5
4	Maryland	20.9
5	Delaware	18.3
6	Georgia	17.3
7	South Carolina	14.3
8	Louisiana	13.8
9	California	13.3
10	Connecticut	12.0
11	North Carolina	11.3
12	Texas	10.9
13	Massachusetts	10.0
14	Illinois	9.4
15	Pennsylvania	8.9
16	Nevada	8.8
16	Virginia	8.8
18	Mississippi	8.5
19	Alabama	8.3
20	Arizona	7.5
21	Tennessee	7.3
22	Washington	7.2
23	Rhode Island	6.8
24	Colorado	6.4
24	Oregon	6.4
26	Hawaii	6.1
27	Missouri	6.0
28	Ohio	5.9
29	Oklahoma	5.5
30	Michigan	5.2
31	Arkansas	5.0
31	New Mexico	5.0
33	Indiana	4.0
34	Minnesota	3.8
35	Nebraska	3.7
36	Kansas	3.6
36	Kentucky	3.6
36	New Hampshire	3.6
39	Maine	3.4
40	Utah	3.2
41	West Virginia	3.1
41	Wisconsin	3.1
43	Alaska	2.6
44	Iowa	2.5
45	Vermont	2.2
46	Idaho	1.9
46	Wyoming	1.9
48	South Dakota	1.4
49	Montana	1.0
50	North Dakota	0.6

District of Columbia	100.3

Source: Morgan Quitno Press using data from U.S. Dept of Health & Human Serv's, Nat'l Center for Health Statistics "National Vital Statistics Report" (Vol. 41, No. 7(S), January 7, 1993)

*AIDS is Acquired Immunodeficiency Syndrome. It is a specific group of diseases or conditions which are indicative of severe immunosuppression related to infection with the Human Immunodeficiency Virus (HIV). Not age-adjusted.

Age-Adjusted Death Rate by AIDS in 1996

National Rate = 11.1 Deaths per 100,000 Population*

ALPHA ORDER				RANK ORDER		
RANK	STATE	RATE		RANK	STATE	RATE
17	Alabama	8.1		1	New York	29.0
NA	Alaska**	NA		2	Florida	21.4
20	Arizona	7.3		3	New Jersey	20.0
30	Arkansas	5.2		4	Maryland	18.4
9	California	12.4		5	Delaware	16.5
26	Colorado	5.7		6	Georgia	15.8
10	Connecticut	10.9		7	Louisiana	13.7
5	Delaware	16.5		7	South Carolina	13.7
2	Florida	21.4		9	California	12.4
6	Georgia	15.8		10	Connecticut	10.9
26	Hawaii	5.7		11	North Carolina	10.6
44	Idaho	1.8		12	Texas	10.4
13	Illinois	9.0		13	Illinois	9.0
33	Indiana	3.8		14	Massachusetts	8.9
43	Iowa	2.4		15	Mississippi	8.8
35	Kansas	3.7		16	Pennsylvania	8.5
36	Kentucky	3.5		17	Alabama	8.1
7	Louisiana	13.7		18	Nevada	7.9
40	Maine	3.2		19	Virginia	7.8
4	Maryland	18.4		20	Arizona	7.3
14	Massachusetts	8.9		21	Tennessee	7.0
31	Michigan	5.0		22	Rhode Island	6.4
36	Minnesota	3.5		22	Washington	6.4
15	Mississippi	8.8		24	Oregon	6.1
25	Missouri	5.8		25	Missouri	5.8
NA	Montana**	NA		26	Colorado	5.7
33	Nebraska	3.8		26	Hawaii	5.7
18	Nevada	7.9		26	Ohio	5.7
41	New Hampshire	3.1		29	Oklahoma	5.6
3	New Jersey	20.0		30	Arkansas	5.2
32	New Mexico	4.9		31	Michigan	5.0
1	New York	29.0		32	New Mexico	4.9
11	North Carolina	10.6		33	Indiana	3.8
NA	North Dakota**	NA		33	Nebraska	3.8
26	Ohio	5.7		35	Kansas	3.7
29	Oklahoma	5.6		36	Kentucky	3.5
24	Oregon	6.1		36	Minnesota	3.5
16	Pennsylvania	8.5		36	Utah	3.5
22	Rhode Island	6.4		39	West Virginia	3.3
7	South Carolina	13.7		40	Maine	3.2
NA	South Dakota**	NA		41	New Hampshire	3.1
21	Tennessee	7.0		42	Wisconsin	3.0
12	Texas	10.4		43	Iowa	2.4
36	Utah	3.5		44	Idaho	1.8
NA	Vermont**	NA		NA	Alaska**	NA
19	Virginia	7.8		NA	Montana**	NA
22	Washington	6.4		NA	North Dakota**	NA
39	West Virginia	3.3		NA	South Dakota**	NA
42	Wisconsin	3.0		NA	Vermont**	NA
NA	Wyoming**	NA		NA	Wyoming**	NA
					District of Columbia	87.6

Source: U.S. Department of Health and Human Services, National Center for Health Statistics
   "National Vital Statistics Report" (Vol. 47, No. 9, November 10, 1998)
*AIDS is Acquired Immunodeficiency Syndrome. It is a specific group of diseases or conditions which are indicative
of severe immunosuppression related to infection with the Human Immunodeficiency Virus (HIV).

Estimated Deaths by Cancer in 1999

National Estimated Total = 563,100 Deaths

ALPHA ORDER

RANK	STATE	DEATHS	% of USA
20	Alabama	9,700	1.7%
50	Alaska	600	0.1%
23	Arizona	9,200	1.6%
30	Arkansas	6,400	1.1%
1	California	51,700	9.2%
31	Colorado	6,200	1.1%
28	Connecticut	7,000	1.2%
45	Delaware	1,800	0.3%
2	Florida	40,600	7.2%
12	Georgia	13,400	2.4%
43	Hawaii	2,000	0.4%
42	Idaho	2,100	0.4%
6	Illinois	26,200	4.7%
14	Indiana	12,900	2.3%
29	Iowa	6,600	1.2%
33	Kansas	5,600	1.0%
21	Kentucky	9,500	1.7%
22	Louisiana	9,400	1.7%
37	Maine	3,200	0.6%
19	Maryland	10,400	1.8%
11	Massachusetts	14,200	2.5%
8	Michigan	20,400	3.6%
24	Minnesota	9,000	1.6%
32	Mississippi	6,000	1.1%
14	Missouri	12,900	2.3%
44	Montana	1,900	0.3%
36	Nebraska	3,400	0.6%
35	Nevada	3,800	0.7%
39	New Hampshire	2,500	0.4%
9	New Jersey	18,400	3.3%
38	New Mexico	3,000	0.5%
3	New York	38,300	6.8%
10	North Carolina	16,300	2.9%
47	North Dakota	1,400	0.2%
7	Ohio	26,000	4.6%
26	Oklahoma	7,300	1.3%
26	Oregon	7,300	1.3%
5	Pennsylvania	30,700	5.5%
40	Rhode Island	2,400	0.4%
25	South Carolina	8,200	1.5%
46	South Dakota	1,600	0.3%
16	Tennessee	12,300	2.2%
4	Texas	35,700	6.3%
40	Utah	2,400	0.4%
48	Vermont	1,200	0.2%
13	Virginia	13,300	2.4%
17	Washington	11,000	2.0%
34	West Virginia	4,900	0.9%
18	Wisconsin	10,900	1.9%
49	Wyoming	900	0.2%

RANK ORDER

RANK	STATE	DEATHS	% of USA
1	California	51,700	9.2%
2	Florida	40,600	7.2%
3	New York	38,300	6.8%
4	Texas	35,700	6.3%
5	Pennsylvania	30,700	5.5%
6	Illinois	26,200	4.7%
7	Ohio	26,000	4.6%
8	Michigan	20,400	3.6%
9	New Jersey	18,400	3.3%
10	North Carolina	16,300	2.9%
11	Massachusetts	14,200	2.5%
12	Georgia	13,400	2.4%
13	Virginia	13,300	2.4%
14	Indiana	12,900	2.3%
14	Missouri	12,900	2.3%
16	Tennessee	12,300	2.2%
17	Washington	11,000	2.0%
18	Wisconsin	10,900	1.9%
19	Maryland	10,400	1.8%
20	Alabama	9,700	1.7%
21	Kentucky	9,500	1.7%
22	Louisiana	9,400	1.7%
23	Arizona	9,200	1.6%
24	Minnesota	9,000	1.6%
25	South Carolina	8,200	1.5%
26	Oklahoma	7,300	1.3%
26	Oregon	7,300	1.3%
28	Connecticut	7,000	1.2%
29	Iowa	6,600	1.2%
30	Arkansas	6,400	1.1%
31	Colorado	6,200	1.1%
32	Mississippi	6,000	1.1%
33	Kansas	5,600	1.0%
34	West Virginia	4,900	0.9%
35	Nevada	3,800	0.7%
36	Nebraska	3,400	0.6%
37	Maine	3,200	0.6%
38	New Mexico	3,000	0.5%
39	New Hampshire	2,500	0.4%
40	Rhode Island	2,400	0.4%
40	Utah	2,400	0.4%
42	Idaho	2,100	0.4%
43	Hawaii	2,000	0.4%
44	Montana	1,900	0.3%
45	Delaware	1,800	0.3%
46	South Dakota	1,600	0.3%
47	North Dakota	1,400	0.2%
48	Vermont	1,200	0.2%
49	Wyoming	900	0.2%
50	Alaska	600	0.1%
	District of Columbia	1,400	0.2%

Source: American Cancer Society
"1999 Facts & Figures" (Copyright 1999, Reprinted with permission from the American Cancer Society)

Estimated Death Rate by Cancer in 1999

National Estimated Rate = 208.3 Deaths per 100,000 Population*

ALPHA ORDER

RANK	STATE	RATE
15	Alabama	222.9
50	Alaska	97.7
37	Arizona	197.1
5	Arkansas	252.1
47	California	158.3
48	Colorado	156.1
27	Connecticut	213.8
7	Delaware	242.1
1	Florida	272.2
43	Georgia	175.3
46	Hawaii	167.6
45	Idaho	170.9
21	Illinois	217.5
18	Indiana	218.7
12	Iowa	230.6
29	Kansas	213.0
8	Kentucky	241.3
26	Louisiana	215.2
3	Maine	257.2
36	Maryland	202.5
11	Massachusetts	231.0
33	Michigan	207.8
40	Minnesota	190.5
20	Mississippi	218.0
9	Missouri	237.2
25	Montana	215.8
34	Nebraska	204.5
21	Nevada	217.5
30	New Hampshire	211.0
13	New Jersey	226.7
44	New Mexico	172.7
31	New York	210.7
24	North Carolina	216.0
17	North Dakota	219.4
10	Ohio	231.9
19	Oklahoma	218.1
16	Oregon	222.4
4	Pennsylvania	255.8
6	Rhode Island	242.8
27	South Carolina	213.8
23	South Dakota	216.8
14	Tennessee	226.5
42	Texas	180.7
49	Utah	114.3
35	Vermont	203.1
38	Virginia	195.8
39	Washington	193.3
2	West Virginia	270.5
32	Wisconsin	208.7
41	Wyoming	187.1

RANK ORDER

RANK	STATE	RATE
1	Florida	272.2
2	West Virginia	270.5
3	Maine	257.2
4	Pennsylvania	255.8
5	Arkansas	252.1
6	Rhode Island	242.8
7	Delaware	242.1
8	Kentucky	241.3
9	Missouri	237.2
10	Ohio	231.9
11	Massachusetts	231.0
12	Iowa	230.6
13	New Jersey	226.7
14	Tennessee	226.5
15	Alabama	222.9
16	Oregon	222.4
17	North Dakota	219.4
18	Indiana	218.7
19	Oklahoma	218.1
20	Mississippi	218.0
21	Illinois	217.5
21	Nevada	217.5
23	South Dakota	216.8
24	North Carolina	216.0
25	Montana	215.8
26	Louisiana	215.2
27	Connecticut	213.8
27	South Carolina	213.8
29	Kansas	213.0
30	New Hampshire	211.0
31	New York	210.7
32	Wisconsin	208.7
33	Michigan	207.8
34	Nebraska	204.5
35	Vermont	203.1
36	Maryland	202.5
37	Arizona	197.1
38	Virginia	195.8
39	Washington	193.3
40	Minnesota	190.5
41	Wyoming	187.1
42	Texas	180.7
43	Georgia	175.3
44	New Mexico	172.7
45	Idaho	170.9
46	Hawaii	167.6
47	California	158.3
48	Colorado	156.1
49	Utah	114.3
50	Alaska	97.7
	District of Columbia	267.6

Source: Morgan Quitno Press using data from American Cancer Society
"1999 Facts & Figures" (Copyright 1999, Reprinted with permission from the American Cancer Society)
Rates calculated using 1998 Census resident population estimates. Not age-adjusted.

Estimated Deaths by Female Breast Cancer in 1999

National Estimated Total = 43,300 Deaths

ALPHA ORDER

RANK ORDER

RANK	STATE	DEATHS	% of USA		RANK	STATE	DEATHS	% of USA
24	Alabama	600	1.4%		1	California	4,200	9.7%
44	Alaska	100	0.2%		2	New York	3,200	7.4%
21	Arizona	700	1.6%		3	Florida	2,900	6.7%
31	Arkansas	400	0.9%		4	Texas	2,800	6.5%
1	California	4,200	9.7%		5	Pennsylvania	2,500	5.8%
27	Colorado	500	1.2%		6	Illinois	2,100	4.8%
27	Connecticut	500	1.2%		6	Ohio	2,100	4.8%
44	Delaware	100	0.2%		8	Michigan	1,600	3.7%
3	Florida	2,900	6.7%		9	New Jersey	1,500	3.5%
12	Georgia	1,000	2.3%		10	North Carolina	1,200	2.8%
44	Hawaii	100	0.2%		11	Massachusetts	1,100	2.5%
37	Idaho	200	0.5%		12	Georgia	1,000	2.3%
6	Illinois	2,100	4.8%		12	Indiana	1,000	2.3%
12	Indiana	1,000	2.3%		12	Tennessee	1,000	2.3%
27	Iowa	500	1.2%		12	Virginia	1,000	2.3%
31	Kansas	400	0.9%		16	Maryland	900	2.1%
21	Kentucky	700	1.6%		16	Missouri	900	2.1%
18	Louisiana	800	1.8%		18	Louisiana	800	1.8%
37	Maine	200	0.5%		18	Washington	800	1.8%
16	Maryland	900	2.1%		18	Wisconsin	800	1.8%
11	Massachusetts	1,100	2.5%		21	Arizona	700	1.6%
8	Michigan	1,600	3.7%		21	Kentucky	700	1.6%
21	Minnesota	700	1.6%		21	Minnesota	700	1.6%
31	Mississippi	400	0.9%		24	Alabama	600	1.4%
16	Missouri	900	2.1%		24	Oklahoma	600	1.4%
37	Montana	200	0.5%		24	South Carolina	600	1.4%
34	Nebraska	300	0.7%		27	Colorado	500	1.2%
34	Nevada	300	0.7%		27	Connecticut	500	1.2%
37	New Hampshire	200	0.5%		27	Iowa	500	1.2%
9	New Jersey	1,500	3.5%		27	Oregon	500	1.2%
37	New Mexico	200	0.5%		31	Arkansas	400	0.9%
2	New York	3,200	7.4%		31	Kansas	400	0.9%
10	North Carolina	1,200	2.8%		31	Mississippi	400	0.9%
44	North Dakota	100	0.2%		34	Nebraska	300	0.7%
6	Ohio	2,100	4.8%		34	Nevada	300	0.7%
24	Oklahoma	600	1.4%		34	West Virginia	300	0.7%
27	Oregon	500	1.2%		37	Idaho	200	0.5%
5	Pennsylvania	2,500	5.8%		37	Maine	200	0.5%
37	Rhode Island	200	0.5%		37	Montana	200	0.5%
24	South Carolina	600	1.4%		37	New Hampshire	200	0.5%
44	South Dakota	100	0.2%		37	New Mexico	200	0.5%
12	Tennessee	1,000	2.3%		37	Rhode Island	200	0.5%
4	Texas	2,800	6.5%		37	Utah	200	0.5%
37	Utah	200	0.5%		44	Alaska	100	0.2%
44	Vermont	100	0.2%		44	Delaware	100	0.2%
12	Virginia	1,000	2.3%		44	Hawaii	100	0.2%
18	Washington	800	1.8%		44	North Dakota	100	0.2%
34	West Virginia	300	0.7%		44	South Dakota	100	0.2%
18	Wisconsin	800	1.8%		44	Vermont	100	0.2%
44	Wyoming	100	0.2%		44	Wyoming	100	0.2%
						District of Columbia	100	0.2%

Source: American Cancer Society
   "1999 Facts & Figures" (Copyright 1999, Reprinted with permission from the American Cancer Society)

Estimated Death Rate by Female Breast Cancer in 1999

National Estimated Rate = 31.7 Deaths per 100,000 Female Population*

ALPHA ORDER

RANK	STATE	RATE
42	Alabama	26.8
15	Alaska	34.6
32	Arizona	30.5
31	Arkansas	30.7
45	California	26.1
47	Colorado	25.5
36	Connecticut	29.8
43	Delaware	26.7
5	Florida	38.5
45	Georgia	26.1
50	Hawaii	17.0
23	Idaho	33.1
16	Illinois	34.5
22	Indiana	33.3
18	Iowa	34.2
35	Kansas	30.4
13	Kentucky	34.9
10	Louisiana	35.5
27	Maine	31.5
17	Maryland	34.4
14	Massachusetts	34.8
25	Michigan	31.9
37	Minnesota	29.5
41	Mississippi	28.2
24	Missouri	32.4
1	Montana	45.4
10	Nebraska	35.5
6	Nevada	36.5
20	New Hampshire	33.6
8	New Jersey	36.2
48	New Mexico	22.8
19	New York	34.1
27	North Carolina	31.5
29	North Dakota	31.1
7	Ohio	36.4
12	Oklahoma	35.4
32	Oregon	30.5
3	Pennsylvania	40.1
4	Rhode Island	39.1
30	South Carolina	30.9
43	South Dakota	26.7
9	Tennessee	36.1
39	Texas	28.5
49	Utah	19.4
21	Vermont	33.5
38	Virginia	29.1
40	Washington	28.4
25	West Virginia	31.9
32	Wisconsin	30.5
2	Wyoming	42.0

RANK ORDER

RANK	STATE	RATE
1	Montana	45.4
2	Wyoming	42.0
3	Pennsylvania	40.1
4	Rhode Island	39.1
5	Florida	38.5
6	Nevada	36.5
7	Ohio	36.4
8	New Jersey	36.2
9	Tennessee	36.1
10	Louisiana	35.5
10	Nebraska	35.5
12	Oklahoma	35.4
13	Kentucky	34.9
14	Massachusetts	34.8
15	Alaska	34.6
16	Illinois	34.5
17	Maryland	34.4
18	Iowa	34.2
19	New York	34.1
20	New Hampshire	33.6
21	Vermont	33.5
22	Indiana	33.3
23	Idaho	33.1
24	Missouri	32.4
25	Michigan	31.9
25	West Virginia	31.9
27	Maine	31.5
27	North Carolina	31.5
29	North Dakota	31.1
30	South Carolina	30.9
31	Arkansas	30.7
32	Arizona	30.5
32	Oregon	30.5
32	Wisconsin	30.5
35	Kansas	30.4
36	Connecticut	29.8
37	Minnesota	29.5
38	Virginia	29.1
39	Texas	28.5
40	Washington	28.4
41	Mississippi	28.2
42	Alabama	26.8
43	Delaware	26.7
43	South Dakota	26.7
45	California	26.1
45	Georgia	26.1
47	Colorado	25.5
48	New Mexico	22.8
49	Utah	19.4
50	Hawaii	17.0
	District of Columbia	35.6

Source: Morgan Quitno Press using data from American Cancer Society
    "1999 Facts & Figures" (Copyright 1999, Reprinted with permission from the American Cancer Society)
*Rates calculated using 1997 Census resident female population estimates. Not age-adjusted.

Estimated Deaths by Colon and Rectum Cancer in 1999

National Estimated Total = 56,600 Deaths

RANK	STATE	DEATHS	% of USA
26	Alabama	700	1.2%
47	Alaska	100	0.2%
21	Arizona	900	1.6%
30	Arkansas	600	1.1%
1	California	4,900	8.7%
30	Colorado	600	1.1%
26	Connecticut	700	1.2%
42	Delaware	200	0.4%
3	Florida	3,900	6.9%
15	Georgia	1,200	2.1%
42	Hawaii	200	0.4%
42	Idaho	200	0.4%
6	Illinois	2,700	4.8%
12	Indiana	1,300	2.3%
25	Iowa	800	1.4%
33	Kansas	500	0.9%
21	Kentucky	900	1.6%
19	Louisiana	1,000	1.8%
36	Maine	300	0.5%
17	Maryland	1,100	1.9%
11	Massachusetts	1,600	2.8%
8	Michigan	2,100	3.7%
21	Minnesota	900	1.6%
30	Mississippi	600	1.1%
12	Missouri	1,300	2.3%
42	Montana	200	0.4%
35	Nebraska	400	0.7%
36	Nevada	300	0.5%
36	New Hampshire	300	0.5%
9	New Jersey	2,000	3.5%
36	New Mexico	300	0.5%
2	New York	4,100	7.2%
10	North Carolina	1,700	3.0%
42	North Dakota	200	0.4%
6	Ohio	2,700	4.8%
26	Oklahoma	700	1.2%
26	Oregon	700	1.2%
5	Pennsylvania	3,400	6.0%
36	Rhode Island	300	0.5%
21	South Carolina	900	1.6%
47	South Dakota	100	0.2%
15	Tennessee	1,200	2.1%
4	Texas	3,700	6.5%
36	Utah	300	0.5%
47	Vermont	100	0.2%
12	Virginia	1,300	2.3%
19	Washington	1,000	1.8%
33	West Virginia	500	0.9%
17	Wisconsin	1,100	1.9%
47	Wyoming	100	0.2%

RANK	STATE	DEATHS	% of USA
1	California	4,900	8.7%
2	New York	4,100	7.2%
3	Florida	3,900	6.9%
4	Texas	3,700	6.5%
5	Pennsylvania	3,400	6.0%
6	Illinois	2,700	4.8%
6	Ohio	2,700	4.8%
8	Michigan	2,100	3.7%
9	New Jersey	2,000	3.5%
10	North Carolina	1,700	3.0%
11	Massachusetts	1,600	2.8%
12	Indiana	1,300	2.3%
12	Missouri	1,300	2.3%
12	Virginia	1,300	2.3%
15	Georgia	1,200	2.1%
15	Tennessee	1,200	2.1%
17	Maryland	1,100	1.9%
17	Wisconsin	1,100	1.9%
19	Louisiana	1,000	1.8%
19	Washington	1,000	1.8%
21	Arizona	900	1.6%
21	Kentucky	900	1.6%
21	Minnesota	900	1.6%
21	South Carolina	900	1.6%
25	Iowa	800	1.4%
26	Alabama	700	1.2%
26	Connecticut	700	1.2%
26	Oklahoma	700	1.2%
26	Oregon	700	1.2%
30	Arkansas	600	1.1%
30	Colorado	600	1.1%
30	Mississippi	600	1.1%
33	Kansas	500	0.9%
33	West Virginia	500	0.9%
35	Nebraska	400	0.7%
36	Maine	300	0.5%
36	Nevada	300	0.5%
36	New Hampshire	300	0.5%
36	New Mexico	300	0.5%
36	Rhode Island	300	0.5%
36	Utah	300	0.5%
42	Delaware	200	0.4%
42	Hawaii	200	0.4%
42	Idaho	200	0.4%
42	Montana	200	0.4%
42	North Dakota	200	0.4%
47	Alaska	100	0.2%
47	South Dakota	100	0.2%
47	Vermont	100	0.2%
47	Wyoming	100	0.2%
	District of Columbia	100	0.2%

Source: American Cancer Society
"1999 Facts & Figures" (Copyright 1999, Reprinted with permission from the American Cancer Society)

Estimated Death Rate by Colon and Rectum Cancer in 1999

National Rate = 20.9 Deaths per 100,000 Population*

ALPHA ORDER			RANK ORDER		
RANK	STATE	RATE	RANK	STATE	RATE
45	Alabama	16.1	1	North Dakota	31.3
43	Alaska	16.3	2	Rhode Island	30.3
33	Arizona	19.3	3	Pennsylvania	28.3
15	Arkansas	23.6	4	Iowa	27.9
48	California	15.0	5	West Virginia	27.6
47	Colorado	15.1	6	Delaware	26.9
26	Connecticut	21.4	7	Florida	26.1
6	Delaware	26.9	8	Massachusetts	26.0
7	Florida	26.1	9	New Hampshire	25.3
46	Georgia	15.7	10	New Jersey	24.6
42	Hawaii	16.8	11	Maine	24.1
43	Idaho	16.3	11	Nebraska	24.1
22	Illinois	22.4	11	Ohio	24.1
24	Indiana	22.0	14	Missouri	23.9
4	Iowa	27.9	15	Arkansas	23.6
35	Kansas	19.0	16	South Carolina	23.5
17	Kentucky	22.9	17	Kentucky	22.9
17	Louisiana	22.9	17	Louisiana	22.9
11	Maine	24.1	19	Montana	22.7
26	Maryland	21.4	20	New York	22.6
8	Massachusetts	26.0	21	North Carolina	22.5
26	Michigan	21.4	22	Illinois	22.4
35	Minnesota	19.0	23	Tennessee	22.1
25	Mississippi	21.8	24	Indiana	22.0
14	Missouri	23.9	25	Mississippi	21.8
19	Montana	22.7	26	Connecticut	21.4
11	Nebraska	24.1	26	Maryland	21.4
40	Nevada	17.2	26	Michigan	21.4
9	New Hampshire	25.3	29	Oregon	21.3
10	New Jersey	24.6	30	Wisconsin	21.1
39	New Mexico	17.3	31	Oklahoma	20.9
20	New York	22.6	32	Wyoming	20.8
21	North Carolina	22.5	33	Arizona	19.3
1	North Dakota	31.3	34	Virginia	19.1
11	Ohio	24.1	35	Kansas	19.0
31	Oklahoma	20.9	35	Minnesota	19.0
29	Oregon	21.3	37	Texas	18.7
3	Pennsylvania	28.3	38	Washington	17.6
2	Rhode Island	30.3	39	New Mexico	17.3
16	South Carolina	23.5	40	Nevada	17.2
50	South Dakota	13.5	41	Vermont	16.9
23	Tennessee	22.1	42	Hawaii	16.8
37	Texas	18.7	43	Alaska	16.3
49	Utah	14.3	43	Idaho	16.3
41	Vermont	16.9	45	Alabama	16.1
34	Virginia	19.1	46	Georgia	15.7
38	Washington	17.6	47	Colorado	15.1
5	West Virginia	27.6	48	California	15.0
30	Wisconsin	21.1	49	Utah	14.3
32	Wyoming	20.8	50	South Dakota	13.5
				District of Columbia	19.1

Source: Morgan Quitno Press using data from American Cancer Society
"1999 Facts & Figures" (Copyright 1999, Reprinted with permission from the American Cancer Society)
*Rates calculated using 1998 Census resident population estimates. Not age-adjusted.

Estimated Deaths by Esophagus Cancer in 1999

National Estimated Total = 12,200 Deaths

RANK	STATE	DEATHS	% of USA
17	Alabama	200	1.6%
NA	Alaska*	NA	NA
17	Arizona	200	1.6%
27	Arkansas	100	0.8%
1	California	1,100	9.0%
27	Colorado	100	0.8%
17	Connecticut	200	1.6%
27	Delaware	100	0.8%
2	Florida	900	7.4%
17	Georgia	200	1.6%
NA	Hawaii*	NA	NA
27	Idaho	100	0.8%
4	Illinois	700	5.7%
10	Indiana	300	2.5%
27	Iowa	100	0.8%
27	Kansas	100	0.8%
17	Kentucky	200	1.6%
27	Louisiana	100	0.8%
27	Maine	100	0.8%
17	Maryland	200	1.6%
10	Massachusetts	300	2.5%
8	Michigan	500	4.1%
17	Minnesota	200	1.6%
27	Mississippi	100	0.8%
10	Missouri	300	2.5%
NA	Montana*	NA	NA
27	Nebraska	100	0.8%
27	Nevada	100	0.8%
27	New Hampshire	100	0.8%
9	New Jersey	400	3.3%
27	New Mexico	100	0.8%
2	New York	900	7.4%
10	North Carolina	300	2.5%
NA	North Dakota*	NA	NA
7	Ohio	600	4.9%
27	Oklahoma	100	0.8%
17	Oregon	200	1.6%
4	Pennsylvania	700	5.7%
NA	Rhode Island*	NA	NA
17	South Carolina	200	1.6%
NA	South Dakota*	NA	NA
17	Tennessee	200	1.6%
4	Texas	700	5.7%
NA	Utah*	NA	NA
NA	Vermont*	NA	NA
10	Virginia	300	2.5%
10	Washington	300	2.5%
27	West Virginia	100	0.8%
10	Wisconsin	300	2.5%
NA	Wyoming*	NA	NA

RANK	STATE	DEATHS	% of USA
1	California	1,100	9.0%
2	Florida	900	7.4%
2	New York	900	7.4%
4	Illinois	700	5.7%
4	Pennsylvania	700	5.7%
4	Texas	700	5.7%
7	Ohio	600	4.9%
8	Michigan	500	4.1%
9	New Jersey	400	3.3%
10	Indiana	300	2.5%
10	Massachusetts	300	2.5%
10	Missouri	300	2.5%
10	North Carolina	300	2.5%
10	Virginia	300	2.5%
10	Washington	300	2.5%
10	Wisconsin	300	2.5%
17	Alabama	200	1.6%
17	Arizona	200	1.6%
17	Connecticut	200	1.6%
17	Georgia	200	1.6%
17	Kentucky	200	1.6%
17	Maryland	200	1.6%
17	Minnesota	200	1.6%
17	Oregon	200	1.6%
17	South Carolina	200	1.6%
17	Tennessee	200	1.6%
27	Arkansas	100	0.8%
27	Colorado	100	0.8%
27	Delaware	100	0.8%
27	Idaho	100	0.8%
27	Iowa	100	0.8%
27	Kansas	100	0.8%
27	Louisiana	100	0.8%
27	Maine	100	0.8%
27	Mississippi	100	0.8%
27	Nebraska	100	0.8%
27	Nevada	100	0.8%
27	New Hampshire	100	0.8%
27	New Mexico	100	0.8%
27	Oklahoma	100	0.8%
27	West Virginia	100	0.8%
NA	Alaska*	NA	NA
NA	Hawaii*	NA	NA
NA	Montana*	NA	NA
NA	North Dakota*	NA	NA
NA	Rhode Island*	NA	NA
NA	South Dakota*	NA	NA
NA	Utah*	NA	NA
NA	Vermont*	NA	NA
NA	Wyoming*	NA	NA
	District of Columbia*	NA	NA

Source: American Cancer Society
"1999 Facts & Figures" (Copyright 1999, Reprinted with permission from the American Cancer Society)
*Fewer than 50 deaths.

Estimated Death Rate by Esophagus Cancer in 1999

National Estimated Rate = 4.5 Deaths per 100,000 Population*

ALPHA ORDER			RANK ORDER		
RANK	STATE	RATE	RANK	STATE	RATE
25	Alabama	4.6	1	Delaware	13.4
NA	Alaska**	NA	2	New Hampshire	8.4
27	Arizona	4.3	3	Idaho	8.1
30	Arkansas	3.9	4	Maine	8.0
37	California	3.4	5	Connecticut	6.1
40	Colorado	2.5	5	Oregon	6.1
5	Connecticut	6.1	7	Florida	6.0
1	Delaware	13.4	7	Nebraska	6.0
7	Florida	6.0	9	Illinois	5.8
39	Georgia	2.6	9	New Mexico	5.8
NA	Hawaii**	NA	9	Pennsylvania	5.8
3	Idaho	8.1	12	Nevada	5.7
9	Illinois	5.8	12	Wisconsin	5.7
19	Indiana	5.1	14	Missouri	5.5
35	Iowa	3.5	14	West Virginia	5.5
32	Kansas	3.8	16	Ohio	5.4
19	Kentucky	5.1	17	Washington	5.3
41	Louisiana	2.3	18	South Carolina	5.2
4	Maine	8.0	19	Indiana	5.1
30	Maryland	3.9	19	Kentucky	5.1
23	Massachusetts	4.9	19	Michigan	5.1
19	Michigan	5.1	22	New York	5.0
28	Minnesota	4.2	23	Massachusetts	4.9
34	Mississippi	3.6	23	New Jersey	4.9
14	Missouri	5.5	25	Alabama	4.6
NA	Montana**	NA	26	Virginia	4.4
7	Nebraska	6.0	27	Arizona	4.3
12	Nevada	5.7	28	Minnesota	4.2
2	New Hampshire	8.4	29	North Carolina	4.0
23	New Jersey	4.9	30	Arkansas	3.9
9	New Mexico	5.8	30	Maryland	3.9
22	New York	5.0	32	Kansas	3.8
29	North Carolina	4.0	33	Tennessee	3.7
NA	North Dakota**	NA	34	Mississippi	3.6
16	Ohio	5.4	35	Iowa	3.5
38	Oklahoma	3.0	35	Texas	3.5
5	Oregon	6.1	37	California	3.4
9	Pennsylvania	5.8	38	Oklahoma	3.0
NA	Rhode Island**	NA	39	Georgia	2.6
18	South Carolina	5.2	40	Colorado	2.5
NA	South Dakota**	NA	41	Louisiana	2.3
33	Tennessee	3.7	NA	Alaska**	NA
35	Texas	3.5	NA	Hawaii**	NA
NA	Utah**	NA	NA	Montana**	NA
NA	Vermont**	NA	NA	North Dakota**	NA
26	Virginia	4.4	NA	Rhode Island**	NA
17	Washington	5.3	NA	South Dakota**	NA
14	West Virginia	5.5	NA	Utah**	NA
12	Wisconsin	5.7	NA	Vermont**	NA
NA	Wyoming**	NA	NA	Wyoming**	NA
			District of Columbia**		NA

Source: Morgan Quitno Press using data from American Cancer Society
"1999 Facts & Figures" (Copyright 1999, Reprinted with permission from the American Cancer Society)
*Rates calculated using 1998 Census resident population estimates. Not age-adjusted.
**Fewer than 50 deaths.

Estimated Deaths by Leukemia in 1999

National Estimated Total = 22,100 Deaths

ALPHA ORDER

RANK	STATE	DEATHS	% of USA
20	Alabama	400	1.8%
NA	Alaska*	NA	NA
20	Arizona	400	1.8%
23	Arkansas	300	1.4%
1	California	2,100	9.5%
23	Colorado	300	1.4%
23	Connecticut	300	1.4%
36	Delaware	100	0.5%
2	Florida	1,500	6.8%
10	Georgia	600	2.7%
36	Hawaii	100	0.5%
36	Idaho	100	0.5%
6	Illinois	1,100	5.0%
12	Indiana	500	2.3%
23	Iowa	300	1.4%
32	Kansas	200	0.9%
23	Kentucky	300	1.4%
20	Louisiana	400	1.8%
36	Maine	100	0.5%
23	Maryland	300	1.4%
12	Massachusetts	500	2.3%
9	Michigan	700	3.2%
12	Minnesota	500	2.3%
32	Mississippi	200	0.9%
12	Missouri	500	2.3%
36	Montana	100	0.5%
32	Nebraska	200	0.9%
36	Nevada	100	0.5%
36	New Hampshire	100	0.5%
8	New Jersey	800	3.6%
36	New Mexico	100	0.5%
3	New York	1,400	6.3%
10	North Carolina	600	2.7%
NA	North Dakota*	NA	NA
7	Ohio	1,000	4.5%
23	Oklahoma	300	1.4%
23	Oregon	300	1.4%
5	Pennsylvania	1,200	5.4%
36	Rhode Island	100	0.5%
23	South Carolina	300	1.4%
36	South Dakota	100	0.5%
12	Tennessee	500	2.3%
3	Texas	1,400	6.3%
36	Utah	100	0.5%
NA	Vermont*	NA	NA
12	Virginia	500	2.3%
12	Washington	500	2.3%
32	West Virginia	200	0.9%
12	Wisconsin	500	2.3%
NA	Wyoming*	NA	NA

RANK ORDER

RANK	STATE	DEATHS	% of USA
1	California	2,100	9.5%
2	Florida	1,500	6.8%
3	New York	1,400	6.3%
3	Texas	1,400	6.3%
5	Pennsylvania	1,200	5.4%
6	Illinois	1,100	5.0%
7	Ohio	1,000	4.5%
8	New Jersey	800	3.6%
9	Michigan	700	3.2%
10	Georgia	600	2.7%
10	North Carolina	600	2.7%
12	Indiana	500	2.3%
12	Massachusetts	500	2.3%
12	Minnesota	500	2.3%
12	Missouri	500	2.3%
12	Tennessee	500	2.3%
12	Virginia	500	2.3%
12	Washington	500	2.3%
12	Wisconsin	500	2.3%
20	Alabama	400	1.8%
20	Arizona	400	1.8%
20	Louisiana	400	1.8%
23	Arkansas	300	1.4%
23	Colorado	300	1.4%
23	Connecticut	300	1.4%
23	Iowa	300	1.4%
23	Kentucky	300	1.4%
23	Maryland	300	1.4%
23	Oklahoma	300	1.4%
23	Oregon	300	1.4%
23	South Carolina	300	1.4%
32	Kansas	200	0.9%
32	Mississippi	200	0.9%
32	Nebraska	200	0.9%
32	West Virginia	200	0.9%
36	Delaware	100	0.5%
36	Hawaii	100	0.5%
36	Idaho	100	0.5%
36	Maine	100	0.5%
36	Montana	100	0.5%
36	Nevada	100	0.5%
36	New Hampshire	100	0.5%
36	New Mexico	100	0.5%
36	Rhode Island	100	0.5%
36	South Dakota	100	0.5%
36	Utah	100	0.5%
NA	Alaska*	NA	NA
NA	North Dakota*	NA	NA
NA	Vermont*	NA	NA
NA	Wyoming*	NA	NA
	District of Columbia*	NA	NA

Source: American Cancer Society
   "1999 Facts & Figures" (Copyright 1999, Reprinted with permission from the American Cancer Society)
*Fewer than 50 deaths.

Estimated Death Rate by Leukemia in 1999

National Estimated Rate = 8.2 Deaths per 100,000 Population*

<u>ALPHA ORDER</u>

RANK	STATE	RATE
14	Alabama	9.2
NA	Alaska**	NA
24	Arizona	8.6
4	Arkansas	11.8
42	California	6.4
35	Colorado	7.6
14	Connecticut	9.2
2	Delaware	13.4
9	Florida	10.1
32	Georgia	7.9
26	Hawaii	8.4
28	Idaho	8.1
19	Illinois	9.1
25	Indiana	8.5
8	Iowa	10.5
35	Kansas	7.6
35	Kentucky	7.6
14	Louisiana	9.2
30	Maine	8.0
43	Maryland	5.8
28	Massachusetts	8.1
40	Michigan	7.1
7	Minnesota	10.6
39	Mississippi	7.3
14	Missouri	9.2
5	Montana	11.4
3	Nebraska	12.0
45	Nevada	5.7
26	New Hampshire	8.4
12	New Jersey	9.9
43	New Mexico	5.8
34	New York	7.7
30	North Carolina	8.0
NA	North Dakota**	NA
22	Ohio	8.9
21	Oklahoma	9.0
19	Oregon	9.1
11	Pennsylvania	10.0
9	Rhode Island	10.1
33	South Carolina	7.8
1	South Dakota	13.5
14	Tennessee	9.2
40	Texas	7.1
46	Utah	4.8
NA	Vermont**	NA
38	Virginia	7.4
23	Washington	8.8
6	West Virginia	11.0
13	Wisconsin	9.6
NA	Wyoming**	NA

<u>RANK ORDER</u>

RANK	STATE	RATE
1	South Dakota	13.5
2	Delaware	13.4
3	Nebraska	12.0
4	Arkansas	11.8
5	Montana	11.4
6	West Virginia	11.0
7	Minnesota	10.6
8	Iowa	10.5
9	Florida	10.1
9	Rhode Island	10.1
11	Pennsylvania	10.0
12	New Jersey	9.9
13	Wisconsin	9.6
14	Alabama	9.2
14	Connecticut	9.2
14	Louisiana	9.2
14	Missouri	9.2
14	Tennessee	9.2
19	Illinois	9.1
19	Oregon	9.1
21	Oklahoma	9.0
22	Ohio	8.9
23	Washington	8.8
24	Arizona	8.6
25	Indiana	8.5
26	Hawaii	8.4
26	New Hampshire	8.4
28	Idaho	8.1
28	Massachusetts	8.1
30	Maine	8.0
30	North Carolina	8.0
32	Georgia	7.9
33	South Carolina	7.8
34	New York	7.7
35	Colorado	7.6
35	Kansas	7.6
35	Kentucky	7.6
38	Virginia	7.4
39	Mississippi	7.3
40	Michigan	7.1
40	Texas	7.1
42	California	6.4
43	Maryland	5.8
43	New Mexico	5.8
45	Nevada	5.7
46	Utah	4.8
NA	Alaska**	NA
NA	North Dakota**	NA
NA	Vermont**	NA
NA	Wyoming**	NA
	District of Columbia**	NA

Source: Morgan Quitno Press using data from American Cancer Society
"1999 Facts & Figures" (Copyright 1999, Reprinted with permission from the American Cancer Society)
Rates calculated using 1998 Census resident population estimates. Not age-adjusted.
**Fewer than 50 deaths.*

Estimated Deaths by Lung Cancer in 1999

National Estimated Total = 158,900 Deaths

ALPHA ORDER

RANK	STATE	DEATHS	% of USA
20	Alabama	2,700	1.7%
50	Alaska	200	0.1%
22	Arizona	2,600	1.6%
26	Arkansas	2,200	1.4%
1	California	13,500	8.5%
33	Colorado	1,500	0.9%
29	Connecticut	1,800	1.1%
41	Delaware	600	0.4%
2	Florida	12,100	7.6%
11	Georgia	4,100	2.6%
42	Hawaii	500	0.3%
42	Idaho	500	0.3%
7	Illinois	7,300	4.6%
12	Indiana	4,000	2.5%
29	Iowa	1,800	1.1%
33	Kansas	1,500	0.9%
17	Kentucky	3,300	2.1%
20	Louisiana	2,700	1.7%
36	Maine	1,000	0.6%
19	Maryland	3,000	1.9%
15	Massachusetts	3,800	2.4%
8	Michigan	5,900	3.7%
26	Minnesota	2,200	1.4%
31	Mississippi	1,700	1.1%
12	Missouri	4,000	2.5%
42	Montana	500	0.3%
37	Nebraska	900	0.6%
35	Nevada	1,100	0.7%
38	New Hampshire	700	0.4%
10	New Jersey	4,500	2.8%
38	New Mexico	700	0.4%
4	New York	9,900	6.2%
9	North Carolina	4,900	3.1%
47	North Dakota	300	0.2%
6	Ohio	7,700	4.8%
24	Oklahoma	2,300	1.4%
28	Oregon	2,100	1.3%
5	Pennsylvania	8,400	5.3%
38	Rhode Island	700	0.4%
24	South Carolina	2,300	1.4%
45	South Dakota	400	0.3%
14	Tennessee	3,900	2.5%
3	Texas	10,600	6.7%
45	Utah	400	0.3%
47	Vermont	300	0.2%
15	Virginia	3,800	2.4%
18	Washington	3,100	2.0%
32	West Virginia	1,600	1.0%
22	Wisconsin	2,600	1.6%
47	Wyoming	300	0.2%

RANK ORDER

RANK	STATE	DEATHS	% of USA
1	California	13,500	8.5%
2	Florida	12,100	7.6%
3	Texas	10,600	6.7%
4	New York	9,900	6.2%
5	Pennsylvania	8,400	5.3%
6	Ohio	7,700	4.8%
7	Illinois	7,300	4.6%
8	Michigan	5,900	3.7%
9	North Carolina	4,900	3.1%
10	New Jersey	4,500	2.8%
11	Georgia	4,100	2.6%
12	Indiana	4,000	2.5%
12	Missouri	4,000	2.5%
14	Tennessee	3,900	2.5%
15	Massachusetts	3,800	2.4%
15	Virginia	3,800	2.4%
17	Kentucky	3,300	2.1%
18	Washington	3,100	2.0%
19	Maryland	3,000	1.9%
20	Alabama	2,700	1.7%
20	Louisiana	2,700	1.7%
22	Arizona	2,600	1.6%
22	Wisconsin	2,600	1.6%
24	Oklahoma	2,300	1.4%
24	South Carolina	2,300	1.4%
26	Arkansas	2,200	1.4%
26	Minnesota	2,200	1.4%
28	Oregon	2,100	1.3%
29	Connecticut	1,800	1.1%
29	Iowa	1,800	1.1%
31	Mississippi	1,700	1.1%
32	West Virginia	1,600	1.0%
33	Colorado	1,500	0.9%
33	Kansas	1,500	0.9%
35	Nevada	1,100	0.7%
36	Maine	1,000	0.6%
37	Nebraska	900	0.6%
38	New Hampshire	700	0.4%
38	New Mexico	700	0.4%
38	Rhode Island	700	0.4%
41	Delaware	600	0.4%
42	Hawaii	500	0.3%
42	Idaho	500	0.3%
42	Montana	500	0.3%
45	South Dakota	400	0.3%
45	Utah	400	0.3%
47	North Dakota	300	0.2%
47	Vermont	300	0.2%
47	Wyoming	300	0.2%
50	Alaska	200	0.1%
	District of Columbia	300	0.2%

Source: American Cancer Society
"1999 Facts & Figures" (Copyright 1999, Reprinted with permission from the American Cancer Society)

Estimated Death Rate by Lung Cancer in 1999

National Estimated Rate = 58.8 Deaths per 100,000 Population*

ALPHA ORDER

RANK	STATE	RATE
19	Alabama	62.0
49	Alaska	32.6
31	Arizona	55.7
2	Arkansas	86.7
45	California	41.3
48	Colorado	37.8
33	Connecticut	55.0
5	Delaware	80.7
4	Florida	81.1
38	Georgia	53.6
44	Hawaii	41.9
46	Idaho	40.7
23	Illinois	60.6
13	Indiana	67.8
17	Iowa	62.9
28	Kansas	57.1
3	Kentucky	83.8
20	Louisiana	61.8
6	Maine	80.4
27	Maryland	58.4
20	Massachusetts	61.8
24	Michigan	60.1
43	Minnesota	46.6
20	Mississippi	61.8
7	Missouri	73.5
29	Montana	56.8
37	Nebraska	54.1
16	Nevada	63.0
26	New Hampshire	59.1
32	New Jersey	55.5
47	New Mexico	40.3
34	New York	54.5
14	North Carolina	64.9
42	North Dakota	47.0
11	Ohio	68.7
11	Oklahoma	68.7
15	Oregon	64.0
10	Pennsylvania	70.0
9	Rhode Island	70.8
25	South Carolina	60.0
36	South Dakota	54.2
8	Tennessee	71.8
38	Texas	53.6
50	Utah	19.0
40	Vermont	50.8
30	Virginia	56.0
34	Washington	54.5
1	West Virginia	88.3
41	Wisconsin	49.8
18	Wyoming	62.4

RANK ORDER

RANK	STATE	RATE
1	West Virginia	88.3
2	Arkansas	86.7
3	Kentucky	83.8
4	Florida	81.1
5	Delaware	80.7
6	Maine	80.4
7	Missouri	73.5
8	Tennessee	71.8
9	Rhode Island	70.8
10	Pennsylvania	70.0
11	Ohio	68.7
11	Oklahoma	68.7
13	Indiana	67.8
14	North Carolina	64.9
15	Oregon	64.0
16	Nevada	63.0
17	Iowa	62.9
18	Wyoming	62.4
19	Alabama	62.0
20	Louisiana	61.8
20	Massachusetts	61.8
20	Mississippi	61.8
23	Illinois	60.6
24	Michigan	60.1
25	South Carolina	60.0
26	New Hampshire	59.1
27	Maryland	58.4
28	Kansas	57.1
29	Montana	56.8
30	Virginia	56.0
31	Arizona	55.7
32	New Jersey	55.5
33	Connecticut	55.0
34	New York	54.5
34	Washington	54.5
36	South Dakota	54.2
37	Nebraska	54.1
38	Georgia	53.6
38	Texas	53.6
40	Vermont	50.8
41	Wisconsin	49.8
42	North Dakota	47.0
43	Minnesota	46.6
44	Hawaii	41.9
45	California	41.3
46	Idaho	40.7
47	New Mexico	40.3
48	Colorado	37.8
49	Alaska	32.6
50	Utah	19.0

| District of Columbia | 57.3 |

Source: Morgan Quitno Press using data from American Cancer Society
    "1999 Facts & Figures" (Copyright 1999, Reprinted with permission from the American Cancer Society)
*Rates calculated using 1998 Census resident population estimates. Not age-adjusted.

Estimated Deaths by Non-Hodgkin's Lymphoma in 1999

National Estimated Total = 25,700 Deaths

ALPHA ORDER

RANK	STATE	DEATHS	% of USA
20	Alabama	400	1.6%
NA	Alaska*	NA	NA
20	Arizona	400	1.6%
32	Arkansas	200	0.8%
1	California	2,300	8.9%
27	Colorado	300	1.2%
27	Connecticut	300	1.2%
38	Delaware	100	0.4%
2	Florida	1,800	7.0%
15	Georgia	500	1.9%
38	Hawaii	100	0.4%
38	Idaho	100	0.4%
7	Illinois	1,200	4.7%
12	Indiana	600	2.3%
27	Iowa	300	1.2%
27	Kansas	300	1.2%
20	Kentucky	400	1.6%
20	Louisiana	400	1.6%
32	Maine	200	0.8%
20	Maryland	400	1.6%
10	Massachusetts	700	2.7%
8	Michigan	900	3.5%
15	Minnesota	500	1.9%
32	Mississippi	200	0.8%
15	Missouri	500	1.9%
38	Montana	100	0.4%
38	Nebraska	100	0.4%
32	Nevada	200	0.8%
38	New Hampshire	100	0.4%
8	New Jersey	900	3.5%
38	New Mexico	100	0.4%
2	New York	1,800	7.0%
10	North Carolina	700	2.7%
38	North Dakota	100	0.4%
6	Ohio	1,300	5.1%
20	Oklahoma	400	1.6%
20	Oregon	400	1.6%
5	Pennsylvania	1,500	5.8%
38	Rhode Island	100	0.4%
27	South Carolina	300	1.2%
38	South Dakota	100	0.4%
15	Tennessee	500	1.9%
4	Texas	1,700	6.6%
32	Utah	200	0.8%
38	Vermont	100	0.4%
12	Virginia	600	2.3%
15	Washington	500	1.9%
32	West Virginia	200	0.8%
12	Wisconsin	600	2.3%
NA	Wyoming*	NA	NA

RANK ORDER

RANK	STATE	DEATHS	% of USA
1	California	2,300	8.9%
2	Florida	1,800	7.0%
2	New York	1,800	7.0%
4	Texas	1,700	6.6%
5	Pennsylvania	1,500	5.8%
6	Ohio	1,300	5.1%
7	Illinois	1,200	4.7%
8	Michigan	900	3.5%
8	New Jersey	900	3.5%
10	Massachusetts	700	2.7%
10	North Carolina	700	2.7%
12	Indiana	600	2.3%
12	Virginia	600	2.3%
12	Wisconsin	600	2.3%
15	Georgia	500	1.9%
15	Minnesota	500	1.9%
15	Missouri	500	1.9%
15	Tennessee	500	1.9%
15	Washington	500	1.9%
20	Alabama	400	1.6%
20	Arizona	400	1.6%
20	Kentucky	400	1.6%
20	Louisiana	400	1.6%
20	Maryland	400	1.6%
20	Oklahoma	400	1.6%
20	Oregon	400	1.6%
27	Colorado	300	1.2%
27	Connecticut	300	1.2%
27	Iowa	300	1.2%
27	Kansas	300	1.2%
27	South Carolina	300	1.2%
32	Arkansas	200	0.8%
32	Maine	200	0.8%
32	Mississippi	200	0.8%
32	Nevada	200	0.8%
32	Utah	200	0.8%
32	West Virginia	200	0.8%
38	Delaware	100	0.4%
38	Hawaii	100	0.4%
38	Idaho	100	0.4%
38	Montana	100	0.4%
38	Nebraska	100	0.4%
38	New Hampshire	100	0.4%
38	New Mexico	100	0.4%
38	North Dakota	100	0.4%
38	Rhode Island	100	0.4%
38	South Dakota	100	0.4%
38	Vermont	100	0.4%
NA	Alaska*	NA	NA
NA	Wyoming*	NA	NA
	District of Columbia*	NA	NA

Source: American Cancer Society
   "1999 Facts & Figures" (Copyright 1999, Reprinted with permission from the American Cancer Society)
*Fewer than 50 deaths.

Estimated Death Rate by Non-Hodgkin's Lymphoma in 1999

National Estimated Rate = 9.5 Deaths per 100,000 Population*

ALPHA ORDER

RANK	STATE	RATE
27	Alabama	9.2
NA	Alaska**	NA
35	Arizona	8.6
40	Arkansas	7.9
45	California	7.0
43	Colorado	7.6
27	Connecticut	9.2
5	Delaware	13.4
8	Florida	12.1
46	Georgia	6.5
37	Hawaii	8.4
39	Idaho	8.1
23	Illinois	10.0
20	Indiana	10.2
19	Iowa	10.5
12	Kansas	11.4
20	Kentucky	10.2
27	Louisiana	9.2
2	Maine	16.1
41	Maryland	7.8
12	Massachusetts	11.4
27	Michigan	9.2
18	Minnesota	10.6
44	Mississippi	7.3
27	Missouri	9.2
12	Montana	11.4
47	Nebraska	6.0
12	Nevada	11.4
37	New Hampshire	8.4
16	New Jersey	11.1
48	New Mexico	5.8
24	New York	9.9
26	North Carolina	9.3
3	North Dakota	15.7
10	Ohio	11.6
9	Oklahoma	12.0
7	Oregon	12.2
6	Pennsylvania	12.5
22	Rhode Island	10.1
41	South Carolina	7.8
4	South Dakota	13.5
27	Tennessee	9.2
35	Texas	8.6
25	Utah	9.5
1	Vermont	16.9
33	Virginia	8.8
33	Washington	8.8
17	West Virginia	11.0
11	Wisconsin	11.5
NA	Wyoming**	NA

RANK ORDER

RANK	STATE	RATE
1	Vermont	16.9
2	Maine	16.1
3	North Dakota	15.7
4	South Dakota	13.5
5	Delaware	13.4
6	Pennsylvania	12.5
7	Oregon	12.2
8	Florida	12.1
9	Oklahoma	12.0
10	Ohio	11.6
11	Wisconsin	11.5
12	Kansas	11.4
12	Massachusetts	11.4
12	Montana	11.4
12	Nevada	11.4
16	New Jersey	11.1
17	West Virginia	11.0
18	Minnesota	10.6
19	Iowa	10.5
20	Indiana	10.2
20	Kentucky	10.2
22	Rhode Island	10.1
23	Illinois	10.0
24	New York	9.9
25	Utah	9.5
26	North Carolina	9.3
27	Alabama	9.2
27	Connecticut	9.2
27	Louisiana	9.2
27	Michigan	9.2
27	Missouri	9.2
27	Tennessee	9.2
33	Virginia	8.8
33	Washington	8.8
35	Arizona	8.6
35	Texas	8.6
37	Hawaii	8.4
37	New Hampshire	8.4
39	Idaho	8.1
40	Arkansas	7.9
41	Maryland	7.8
41	South Carolina	7.8
43	Colorado	7.6
44	Mississippi	7.3
45	California	7.0
46	Georgia	6.5
47	Nebraska	6.0
48	New Mexico	5.8
NA	Alaska**	NA
NA	Wyoming**	NA
	District of Columbia**	NA

Source: Morgan Quitno Press using data from American Cancer Society
    "1999 Facts & Figures" (Copyright 1999, Reprinted with permission from the American Cancer Society)
*Rates calculated using 1998 Census resident population estimates. Not age-adjusted.
**Fewer than 50 deaths.

Estimated Deaths by Pancreatic Cancer in 1999

National Estimated Total = 28,600 Deaths

ALPHA ORDER

RANK	STATE	DEATHS	% of USA
17	Alabama	500	1.7%
NA	Alaska*	NA	NA
17	Arizona	500	1.7%
28	Arkansas	300	1.0%
1	California	2,700	9.4%
28	Colorado	300	1.0%
24	Connecticut	400	1.4%
39	Delaware	100	0.3%
2	Florida	2,200	7.7%
11	Georgia	700	2.4%
39	Hawaii	100	0.3%
39	Idaho	100	0.3%
7	Illinois	1,200	4.2%
11	Indiana	700	2.4%
28	Iowa	300	1.0%
28	Kansas	300	1.0%
24	Kentucky	400	1.4%
17	Louisiana	500	1.7%
34	Maine	200	0.7%
17	Maryland	500	1.7%
11	Massachusetts	700	2.4%
9	Michigan	1,000	3.5%
17	Minnesota	500	1.7%
28	Mississippi	300	1.0%
14	Missouri	600	2.1%
39	Montana	100	0.3%
34	Nebraska	200	0.7%
34	Nevada	200	0.7%
39	New Hampshire	100	0.3%
8	New Jersey	1,100	3.8%
34	New Mexico	200	0.7%
2	New York	2,200	7.7%
10	North Carolina	800	2.8%
39	North Dakota	100	0.3%
6	Ohio	1,300	4.5%
28	Oklahoma	300	1.0%
24	Oregon	400	1.4%
5	Pennsylvania	1,500	5.2%
39	Rhode Island	100	0.3%
24	South Carolina	400	1.4%
39	South Dakota	100	0.3%
17	Tennessee	500	1.7%
4	Texas	1,900	6.6%
39	Utah	100	0.3%
NA	Vermont*	NA	NA
14	Virginia	600	2.1%
17	Washington	500	1.7%
34	West Virginia	200	0.7%
14	Wisconsin	600	2.1%
39	Wyoming	100	0.3%

RANK ORDER

RANK	STATE	DEATHS	% of USA
1	California	2,700	9.4%
2	Florida	2,200	7.7%
2	New York	2,200	7.7%
4	Texas	1,900	6.6%
5	Pennsylvania	1,500	5.2%
6	Ohio	1,300	4.5%
7	Illinois	1,200	4.2%
8	New Jersey	1,100	3.8%
9	Michigan	1,000	3.5%
10	North Carolina	800	2.8%
11	Georgia	700	2.4%
11	Indiana	700	2.4%
11	Massachusetts	700	2.4%
14	Missouri	600	2.1%
14	Virginia	600	2.1%
14	Wisconsin	600	2.1%
17	Alabama	500	1.7%
17	Arizona	500	1.7%
17	Louisiana	500	1.7%
17	Maryland	500	1.7%
17	Minnesota	500	1.7%
17	Tennessee	500	1.7%
17	Washington	500	1.7%
24	Connecticut	400	1.4%
24	Kentucky	400	1.4%
24	Oregon	400	1.4%
24	South Carolina	400	1.4%
28	Arkansas	300	1.0%
28	Colorado	300	1.0%
28	Iowa	300	1.0%
28	Kansas	300	1.0%
28	Mississippi	300	1.0%
28	Oklahoma	300	1.0%
34	Maine	200	0.7%
34	Nebraska	200	0.7%
34	Nevada	200	0.7%
34	New Mexico	200	0.7%
34	West Virginia	200	0.7%
39	Delaware	100	0.3%
39	Hawaii	100	0.3%
39	Idaho	100	0.3%
39	Montana	100	0.3%
39	New Hampshire	100	0.3%
39	North Dakota	100	0.3%
39	Rhode Island	100	0.3%
39	South Dakota	100	0.3%
39	Utah	100	0.3%
39	Wyoming	100	0.3%
NA	Alaska*	NA	NA
NA	Vermont*	NA	NA
	District of Columbia	100	0.3%

Source: American Cancer Society
    "1999 Facts & Figures" (Copyright 1999, Reprinted with permission from the American Cancer Society)
Fewer than 50 deaths.

Estimated Death Rate by Pancreatic Cancer in 1999

National Estimated Rate = 10.6 Deaths per 100,000 Population*

ALPHA ORDER

RANK	STATE	RATE
16	Alabama	11.5
NA	Alaska**	NA
27	Arizona	10.7
14	Arkansas	11.8
45	California	8.3
47	Colorado	7.6
9	Connecticut	12.2
7	Delaware	13.4
4	Florida	14.7
38	Georgia	9.2
43	Hawaii	8.4
46	Idaho	8.1
35	Illinois	10.0
13	Indiana	11.9
30	Iowa	10.5
19	Kansas	11.4
32	Kentucky	10.2
19	Louisiana	11.4
2	Maine	16.1
36	Maryland	9.7
19	Massachusetts	11.4
32	Michigan	10.2
28	Minnesota	10.6
26	Mississippi	10.9
24	Missouri	11.0
19	Montana	11.4
12	Nebraska	12.0
19	Nevada	11.4
43	New Hampshire	8.4
5	New Jersey	13.6
16	New Mexico	11.5
11	New York	12.1
28	North Carolina	10.6
3	North Dakota	15.7
15	Ohio	11.6
40	Oklahoma	9.0
9	Oregon	12.2
8	Pennsylvania	12.5
34	Rhode Island	10.1
31	South Carolina	10.4
6	South Dakota	13.5
38	Tennessee	9.2
37	Texas	9.6
48	Utah	4.8
NA	Vermont**	NA
41	Virginia	8.8
41	Washington	8.8
24	West Virginia	11.0
16	Wisconsin	11.5
1	Wyoming	20.8

RANK ORDER

RANK	STATE	RATE
1	Wyoming	20.8
2	Maine	16.1
3	North Dakota	15.7
4	Florida	14.7
5	New Jersey	13.6
6	South Dakota	13.5
7	Delaware	13.4
8	Pennsylvania	12.5
9	Connecticut	12.2
9	Oregon	12.2
11	New York	12.1
12	Nebraska	12.0
13	Indiana	11.9
14	Arkansas	11.8
15	Ohio	11.6
16	Alabama	11.5
16	New Mexico	11.5
16	Wisconsin	11.5
19	Kansas	11.4
19	Louisiana	11.4
19	Massachusetts	11.4
19	Montana	11.4
19	Nevada	11.4
24	Missouri	11.0
24	West Virginia	11.0
26	Mississippi	10.9
27	Arizona	10.7
28	Minnesota	10.6
28	North Carolina	10.6
30	Iowa	10.5
31	South Carolina	10.4
32	Kentucky	10.2
32	Michigan	10.2
34	Rhode Island	10.1
35	Illinois	10.0
36	Maryland	9.7
37	Texas	9.6
38	Georgia	9.2
38	Tennessee	9.2
40	Oklahoma	9.0
41	Virginia	8.8
41	Washington	8.8
43	Hawaii	8.4
43	New Hampshire	8.4
45	California	8.3
46	Idaho	8.1
47	Colorado	7.6
48	Utah	4.8
NA	Alaska**	NA
NA	Vermont**	NA

District of Columbia   19.1

Source: Morgan Quitno Press using data from American Cancer Society
"1999 Facts & Figures" (Copyright 1999, Reprinted with permission from the American Cancer Society)
Rates calculated using 1998 Census resident population estimates. Not age-adjusted.
**Fewer than 50 deaths.*

Estimated Deaths by Prostate Cancer in 1999

National Estimated Total = 37,000 Deaths

ALPHA ORDER

RANK	STATE	DEATHS	% of USA
22	Alabama	600	1.6%
NA	Alaska*	NA	NA
17	Arizona	700	1.9%
25	Arkansas	500	1.4%
1	California	3,400	9.2%
29	Colorado	400	1.1%
29	Connecticut	400	1.1%
41	Delaware	100	0.3%
2	Florida	2,800	7.6%
11	Georgia	900	2.4%
41	Hawaii	100	0.3%
35	Idaho	200	0.5%
6	Illinois	1,600	4.3%
13	Indiana	800	2.2%
29	Iowa	400	1.1%
29	Kansas	400	1.1%
25	Kentucky	500	1.4%
22	Louisiana	600	1.6%
35	Maine	200	0.5%
17	Maryland	700	1.9%
13	Massachusetts	800	2.2%
8	Michigan	1,300	3.5%
17	Minnesota	700	1.9%
25	Mississippi	500	1.4%
13	Missouri	800	2.2%
41	Montana	100	0.3%
35	Nebraska	200	0.5%
35	Nevada	200	0.5%
41	New Hampshire	100	0.3%
9	New Jersey	1,200	3.2%
35	New Mexico	200	0.5%
3	New York	2,400	6.5%
10	North Carolina	1,100	3.0%
41	North Dakota	100	0.3%
6	Ohio	1,600	4.3%
29	Oklahoma	400	1.1%
25	Oregon	500	1.4%
5	Pennsylvania	2,000	5.4%
41	Rhode Island	100	0.3%
22	South Carolina	600	1.6%
41	South Dakota	100	0.3%
17	Tennessee	700	1.9%
3	Texas	2,400	6.5%
35	Utah	200	0.5%
41	Vermont	100	0.3%
11	Virginia	900	2.4%
17	Washington	700	1.9%
34	West Virginia	300	0.8%
13	Wisconsin	800	2.2%
41	Wyoming	100	0.3%

RANK ORDER

RANK	STATE	DEATHS	% of USA
1	California	3,400	9.2%
2	Florida	2,800	7.6%
3	New York	2,400	6.5%
3	Texas	2,400	6.5%
5	Pennsylvania	2,000	5.4%
6	Illinois	1,600	4.3%
6	Ohio	1,600	4.3%
8	Michigan	1,300	3.5%
9	New Jersey	1,200	3.2%
10	North Carolina	1,100	3.0%
11	Georgia	900	2.4%
11	Virginia	900	2.4%
13	Indiana	800	2.2%
13	Massachusetts	800	2.2%
13	Missouri	800	2.2%
13	Wisconsin	800	2.2%
17	Arizona	700	1.9%
17	Maryland	700	1.9%
17	Minnesota	700	1.9%
17	Tennessee	700	1.9%
17	Washington	700	1.9%
22	Alabama	600	1.6%
22	Louisiana	600	1.6%
22	South Carolina	600	1.6%
25	Arkansas	500	1.4%
25	Kentucky	500	1.4%
25	Mississippi	500	1.4%
25	Oregon	500	1.4%
29	Colorado	400	1.1%
29	Connecticut	400	1.1%
29	Iowa	400	1.1%
29	Kansas	400	1.1%
29	Oklahoma	400	1.1%
34	West Virginia	300	0.8%
35	Idaho	200	0.5%
35	Maine	200	0.5%
35	Nebraska	200	0.5%
35	Nevada	200	0.5%
35	New Mexico	200	0.5%
35	Utah	200	0.5%
41	Delaware	100	0.3%
41	Hawaii	100	0.3%
41	Montana	100	0.3%
41	New Hampshire	100	0.3%
41	North Dakota	100	0.3%
41	Rhode Island	100	0.3%
41	South Dakota	100	0.3%
41	Vermont	100	0.3%
41	Wyoming	100	0.3%
NA	Alaska*	NA	NA
	District of Columbia	100	0.3%

Source: American Cancer Society
 "1999 Facts & Figures" (Copyright 1999, Reprinted with permission from the American Cancer Society)
Fewer than 50 deaths.

Estimated Death Rate by Prostate Cancer in 1999

National Estimated Rate = 28.2 Deaths per 100,000 Male Population*

ALPHA ORDER

RANK	STATE	RATE
21	Alabama	28.9
NA	Alaska**	NA
15	Arizona	31.0
2	Arkansas	40.9
44	California	21.0
46	Colorado	20.7
35	Connecticut	25.2
25	Delaware	28.0
3	Florida	39.3
38	Georgia	24.7
49	Hawaii	16.8
8	Idaho	33.0
27	Illinois	27.5
25	Indiana	28.0
22	Iowa	28.7
12	Kansas	31.3
34	Kentucky	26.3
23	Louisiana	28.6
8	Maine	33.0
24	Maryland	28.2
32	Massachusetts	27.1
30	Michigan	27.3
19	Minnesota	30.3
4	Mississippi	38.1
17	Missouri	30.5
43	Montana	22.8
39	Nebraska	24.6
41	Nevada	23.4
48	New Hampshire	17.3
16	New Jersey	30.7
41	New Mexico	23.4
27	New York	27.5
17	North Carolina	30.5
12	North Dakota	31.3
20	Ohio	29.5
39	Oklahoma	24.6
14	Oregon	31.2
5	Pennsylvania	34.6
44	Rhode Island	21.0
8	South Carolina	33.0
27	South Dakota	27.5
33	Tennessee	27.0
36	Texas	25.0
47	Utah	19.5
6	Vermont	34.5
30	Virginia	27.3
36	Washington	25.0
7	West Virginia	34.2
11	Wisconsin	31.4
1	Wyoming	41.4

RANK ORDER

RANK	STATE	RATE
1	Wyoming	41.4
2	Arkansas	40.9
3	Florida	39.3
4	Mississippi	38.1
5	Pennsylvania	34.6
6	Vermont	34.5
7	West Virginia	34.2
8	Idaho	33.0
8	Maine	33.0
8	South Carolina	33.0
11	Wisconsin	31.4
12	Kansas	31.3
12	North Dakota	31.3
14	Oregon	31.2
15	Arizona	31.0
16	New Jersey	30.7
17	Missouri	30.5
17	North Carolina	30.5
19	Minnesota	30.3
20	Ohio	29.5
21	Alabama	28.9
22	Iowa	28.7
23	Louisiana	28.6
24	Maryland	28.2
25	Delaware	28.0
25	Indiana	28.0
27	Illinois	27.5
27	New York	27.5
27	South Dakota	27.5
30	Michigan	27.3
30	Virginia	27.3
32	Massachusetts	27.1
33	Tennessee	27.0
34	Kentucky	26.3
35	Connecticut	25.2
36	Texas	25.0
36	Washington	25.0
38	Georgia	24.7
39	Nebraska	24.6
39	Oklahoma	24.6
41	Nevada	23.4
41	New Mexico	23.4
43	Montana	22.8
44	California	21.0
44	Rhode Island	21.0
46	Colorado	20.7
47	Utah	19.5
48	New Hampshire	17.3
49	Hawaii	16.8
NA	Alaska**	NA
	District of Columbia	40.3

Source: Morgan Quitno Press using data from American Cancer Society
"1999 Facts & Figures" (Copyright 1999, Reprinted with permission from the American Cancer Society)
*Rates calculated using 1997 Census resident male population estimates. Not age-adjusted.
**Fewer than 50 deaths.

Estimated Deaths by Ovarian Cancer in 1999

National Estimated Total = 14,500 Deaths

ALPHA ORDER

RANK	STATE	DEATHS	% of USA
20	Alabama	200	1.4%
NA	Alaska*	NA	NA
13	Arizona	300	2.1%
20	Arkansas	200	1.4%
1	California	1,500	10.3%
31	Colorado	100	0.7%
20	Connecticut	200	1.4%
NA	Delaware*	NA	NA
2	Florida	1,000	6.9%
10	Georgia	400	2.8%
NA	Hawaii*	NA	NA
31	Idaho	100	0.7%
6	Illinois	600	4.1%
10	Indiana	400	2.8%
31	Iowa	100	0.7%
20	Kansas	200	1.4%
20	Kentucky	200	1.4%
20	Louisiana	200	1.4%
31	Maine	100	0.7%
20	Maryland	200	1.4%
13	Massachusetts	300	2.1%
8	Michigan	500	3.4%
20	Minnesota	200	1.4%
31	Mississippi	100	0.7%
13	Missouri	300	2.1%
31	Montana	100	0.7%
31	Nebraska	100	0.7%
31	Nevada	100	0.7%
31	New Hampshire	100	0.7%
8	New Jersey	500	3.4%
31	New Mexico	100	0.7%
2	New York	1,000	6.9%
10	North Carolina	400	2.8%
31	North Dakota	100	0.7%
6	Ohio	600	4.1%
20	Oklahoma	200	1.4%
20	Oregon	200	1.4%
5	Pennsylvania	800	5.5%
NA	Rhode Island*	NA	NA
20	South Carolina	200	1.4%
NA	South Dakota*	NA	NA
13	Tennessee	300	2.1%
4	Texas	900	6.2%
31	Utah	100	0.7%
NA	Vermont*	NA	NA
13	Virginia	300	2.1%
13	Washington	300	2.1%
31	West Virginia	100	0.7%
13	Wisconsin	300	2.1%
NA	Wyoming*	NA	NA

RANK ORDER

RANK	STATE	DEATHS	% of USA
1	California	1,500	10.3%
2	Florida	1,000	6.9%
2	New York	1,000	6.9%
4	Texas	900	6.2%
5	Pennsylvania	800	5.5%
6	Illinois	600	4.1%
6	Ohio	600	4.1%
8	Michigan	500	3.4%
8	New Jersey	500	3.4%
10	Georgia	400	2.8%
10	Indiana	400	2.8%
10	North Carolina	400	2.8%
13	Arizona	300	2.1%
13	Massachusetts	300	2.1%
13	Missouri	300	2.1%
13	Tennessee	300	2.1%
13	Virginia	300	2.1%
13	Washington	300	2.1%
13	Wisconsin	300	2.1%
20	Alabama	200	1.4%
20	Arkansas	200	1.4%
20	Connecticut	200	1.4%
20	Kansas	200	1.4%
20	Kentucky	200	1.4%
20	Louisiana	200	1.4%
20	Maryland	200	1.4%
20	Minnesota	200	1.4%
20	Oklahoma	200	1.4%
20	Oregon	200	1.4%
20	South Carolina	200	1.4%
31	Colorado	100	0.7%
31	Idaho	100	0.7%
31	Iowa	100	0.7%
31	Maine	100	0.7%
31	Mississippi	100	0.7%
31	Montana	100	0.7%
31	Nebraska	100	0.7%
31	Nevada	100	0.7%
31	New Hampshire	100	0.7%
31	New Mexico	100	0.7%
31	North Dakota	100	0.7%
31	Utah	100	0.7%
31	West Virginia	100	0.7%
NA	Alaska*	NA	NA
NA	Delaware*	NA	NA
NA	Hawaii*	NA	NA
NA	Rhode Island*	NA	NA
NA	South Dakota*	NA	NA
NA	Vermont*	NA	NA
NA	Wyoming*	NA	NA
	District of Columbia*	NA	NA

Source: American Cancer Society
"1999 Facts & Figures" (Copyright 1999, Reprinted with permission from the American Cancer Society)
*Fewer than 50 deaths.

Estimated Death Rate by Ovarian Cancer in 1999

National Estimated Rate = 10.6 Deaths per 100,000 Female Population*

ALPHA ORDER

RANK	STATE	RATE
36	Alabama	8.9
NA	Alaska**	NA
10	Arizona	13.1
6	Arkansas	15.4
34	California	9.3
43	Colorado	5.1
15	Connecticut	11.9
NA	Delaware**	NA
8	Florida	13.3
26	Georgia	10.4
NA	Hawaii**	NA
4	Idaho	16.5
31	Illinois	9.9
8	Indiana	13.3
42	Iowa	6.8
7	Kansas	15.2
29	Kentucky	10.0
36	Louisiana	8.9
5	Maine	15.7
40	Maryland	7.7
33	Massachusetts	9.5
29	Michigan	10.0
39	Minnesota	8.4
41	Mississippi	7.0
20	Missouri	10.8
2	Montana	22.7
16	Nebraska	11.8
12	Nevada	12.2
3	New Hampshire	16.8
14	New Jersey	12.1
18	New Mexico	11.4
23	New York	10.6
25	North Carolina	10.5
1	North Dakota	31.1
26	Ohio	10.4
16	Oklahoma	11.8
12	Oregon	12.2
11	Pennsylvania	12.8
NA	Rhode Island**	NA
28	South Carolina	10.3
NA	South Dakota**	NA
20	Tennessee	10.8
35	Texas	9.2
32	Utah	9.7
NA	Vermont**	NA
38	Virginia	8.7
22	Washington	10.7
23	West Virginia	10.6
18	Wisconsin	11.4
NA	Wyoming**	NA

RANK ORDER

RANK	STATE	RATE
1	North Dakota	31.1
2	Montana	22.7
3	New Hampshire	16.8
4	Idaho	16.5
5	Maine	15.7
6	Arkansas	15.4
7	Kansas	15.2
8	Florida	13.3
8	Indiana	13.3
10	Arizona	13.1
11	Pennsylvania	12.8
12	Nevada	12.2
12	Oregon	12.2
14	New Jersey	12.1
15	Connecticut	11.9
16	Nebraska	11.8
16	Oklahoma	11.8
18	New Mexico	11.4
18	Wisconsin	11.4
20	Missouri	10.8
20	Tennessee	10.8
22	Washington	10.7
23	New York	10.6
23	West Virginia	10.6
25	North Carolina	10.5
26	Georgia	10.4
26	Ohio	10.4
28	South Carolina	10.3
29	Kentucky	10.0
29	Michigan	10.0
31	Illinois	9.9
32	Utah	9.7
33	Massachusetts	9.5
34	California	9.3
35	Texas	9.2
36	Alabama	8.9
36	Louisiana	8.9
38	Virginia	8.7
39	Minnesota	8.4
40	Maryland	7.7
41	Mississippi	7.0
42	Iowa	6.8
43	Colorado	5.1
NA	Alaska**	NA
NA	Delaware**	NA
NA	Hawaii**	NA
NA	Rhode Island**	NA
NA	South Dakota**	NA
NA	Vermont**	NA
NA	Wyoming**	NA
	District of Columbia**	NA

*Source: Morgan Quitno Press using data from American Cancer Society
"1999 Facts & Figures" (Copyright 1999, Reprinted with permission from the American Cancer Society)*
Rates calculated using 1997 Census resident female population estimates. Not age-adjusted.
**Fewer than 50 deaths.*

Estimated Deaths by Stomach Cancer in 1999

National Estimated Total = 13,500 Deaths

<table>
<tr><td colspan="4">ALPHA ORDER</td><td colspan="4">RANK ORDER</td></tr>
<tr><th>RANK</th><th>STATE</th><th>DEATHS</th><th>% of USA</th><th>RANK</th><th>STATE</th><th>DEATHS</th><th>% of USA</th></tr>
<tr><td>17</td><td>Alabama</td><td>200</td><td>1.5%</td><td>1</td><td>California</td><td>1,600</td><td>11.9%</td></tr>
<tr><td>NA</td><td>Alaska*</td><td>NA</td><td>NA</td><td>2</td><td>New York</td><td>1,300</td><td>9.6%</td></tr>
<tr><td>17</td><td>Arizona</td><td>200</td><td>1.5%</td><td>3</td><td>Texas</td><td>1,000</td><td>7.4%</td></tr>
<tr><td>27</td><td>Arkansas</td><td>100</td><td>0.7%</td><td>4</td><td>Florida</td><td>900</td><td>6.7%</td></tr>
<tr><td>1</td><td>California</td><td>1,600</td><td>11.9%</td><td>5</td><td>Pennsylvania</td><td>700</td><td>5.2%</td></tr>
<tr><td>27</td><td>Colorado</td><td>100</td><td>0.7%</td><td>6</td><td>Illinois</td><td>600</td><td>4.4%</td></tr>
<tr><td>17</td><td>Connecticut</td><td>200</td><td>1.5%</td><td>7</td><td>New Jersey</td><td>500</td><td>3.7%</td></tr>
<tr><td>NA</td><td>Delaware*</td><td>NA</td><td>NA</td><td>7</td><td>Ohio</td><td>500</td><td>3.7%</td></tr>
<tr><td>4</td><td>Florida</td><td>900</td><td>6.7%</td><td>9</td><td>Michigan</td><td>400</td><td>3.0%</td></tr>
<tr><td>11</td><td>Georgia</td><td>300</td><td>2.2%</td><td>9</td><td>North Carolina</td><td>400</td><td>3.0%</td></tr>
<tr><td>27</td><td>Hawaii</td><td>100</td><td>0.7%</td><td>11</td><td>Georgia</td><td>300</td><td>2.2%</td></tr>
<tr><td>27</td><td>Idaho</td><td>100</td><td>0.7%</td><td>11</td><td>Louisiana</td><td>300</td><td>2.2%</td></tr>
<tr><td>6</td><td>Illinois</td><td>600</td><td>4.4%</td><td>11</td><td>Maryland</td><td>300</td><td>2.2%</td></tr>
<tr><td>17</td><td>Indiana</td><td>200</td><td>1.5%</td><td>11</td><td>Massachusetts</td><td>300</td><td>2.2%</td></tr>
<tr><td>27</td><td>Iowa</td><td>100</td><td>0.7%</td><td>11</td><td>Missouri</td><td>300</td><td>2.2%</td></tr>
<tr><td>27</td><td>Kansas</td><td>100</td><td>0.7%</td><td>11</td><td>Virginia</td><td>300</td><td>2.2%</td></tr>
<tr><td>17</td><td>Kentucky</td><td>200</td><td>1.5%</td><td>17</td><td>Alabama</td><td>200</td><td>1.5%</td></tr>
<tr><td>11</td><td>Louisiana</td><td>300</td><td>2.2%</td><td>17</td><td>Arizona</td><td>200</td><td>1.5%</td></tr>
<tr><td>27</td><td>Maine</td><td>100</td><td>0.7%</td><td>17</td><td>Connecticut</td><td>200</td><td>1.5%</td></tr>
<tr><td>11</td><td>Maryland</td><td>300</td><td>2.2%</td><td>17</td><td>Indiana</td><td>200</td><td>1.5%</td></tr>
<tr><td>11</td><td>Massachusetts</td><td>300</td><td>2.2%</td><td>17</td><td>Kentucky</td><td>200</td><td>1.5%</td></tr>
<tr><td>9</td><td>Michigan</td><td>400</td><td>3.0%</td><td>17</td><td>Minnesota</td><td>200</td><td>1.5%</td></tr>
<tr><td>17</td><td>Minnesota</td><td>200</td><td>1.5%</td><td>17</td><td>South Carolina</td><td>200</td><td>1.5%</td></tr>
<tr><td>27</td><td>Mississippi</td><td>100</td><td>0.7%</td><td>17</td><td>Tennessee</td><td>200</td><td>1.5%</td></tr>
<tr><td>11</td><td>Missouri</td><td>300</td><td>2.2%</td><td>17</td><td>Washington</td><td>200</td><td>1.5%</td></tr>
<tr><td>NA</td><td>Montana*</td><td>NA</td><td>NA</td><td>17</td><td>Wisconsin</td><td>200</td><td>1.5%</td></tr>
<tr><td>27</td><td>Nebraska</td><td>100</td><td>0.7%</td><td>27</td><td>Arkansas</td><td>100</td><td>0.7%</td></tr>
<tr><td>27</td><td>Nevada</td><td>100</td><td>0.7%</td><td>27</td><td>Colorado</td><td>100</td><td>0.7%</td></tr>
<tr><td>NA</td><td>New Hampshire*</td><td>NA</td><td>NA</td><td>27</td><td>Hawaii</td><td>100</td><td>0.7%</td></tr>
<tr><td>7</td><td>New Jersey</td><td>500</td><td>3.7%</td><td>27</td><td>Idaho</td><td>100</td><td>0.7%</td></tr>
<tr><td>27</td><td>New Mexico</td><td>100</td><td>0.7%</td><td>27</td><td>Iowa</td><td>100</td><td>0.7%</td></tr>
<tr><td>2</td><td>New York</td><td>1,300</td><td>9.6%</td><td>27</td><td>Kansas</td><td>100</td><td>0.7%</td></tr>
<tr><td>9</td><td>North Carolina</td><td>400</td><td>3.0%</td><td>27</td><td>Maine</td><td>100</td><td>0.7%</td></tr>
<tr><td>NA</td><td>North Dakota*</td><td>NA</td><td>NA</td><td>27</td><td>Mississippi</td><td>100</td><td>0.7%</td></tr>
<tr><td>7</td><td>Ohio</td><td>500</td><td>3.7%</td><td>27</td><td>Nebraska</td><td>100</td><td>0.7%</td></tr>
<tr><td>27</td><td>Oklahoma</td><td>100</td><td>0.7%</td><td>27</td><td>Nevada</td><td>100</td><td>0.7%</td></tr>
<tr><td>27</td><td>Oregon</td><td>100</td><td>0.7%</td><td>27</td><td>New Mexico</td><td>100</td><td>0.7%</td></tr>
<tr><td>5</td><td>Pennsylvania</td><td>700</td><td>5.2%</td><td>27</td><td>Oklahoma</td><td>100</td><td>0.7%</td></tr>
<tr><td>27</td><td>Rhode Island</td><td>100</td><td>0.7%</td><td>27</td><td>Oregon</td><td>100</td><td>0.7%</td></tr>
<tr><td>17</td><td>South Carolina</td><td>200</td><td>1.5%</td><td>27</td><td>Rhode Island</td><td>100</td><td>0.7%</td></tr>
<tr><td>NA</td><td>South Dakota*</td><td>NA</td><td>NA</td><td>27</td><td>West Virginia</td><td>100</td><td>0.7%</td></tr>
<tr><td>17</td><td>Tennessee</td><td>200</td><td>1.5%</td><td>NA</td><td>Alaska*</td><td>NA</td><td>NA</td></tr>
<tr><td>3</td><td>Texas</td><td>1,000</td><td>7.4%</td><td>NA</td><td>Delaware*</td><td>NA</td><td>NA</td></tr>
<tr><td>NA</td><td>Utah*</td><td>NA</td><td>NA</td><td>NA</td><td>Montana*</td><td>NA</td><td>NA</td></tr>
<tr><td>NA</td><td>Vermont*</td><td>NA</td><td>NA</td><td>NA</td><td>New Hampshire*</td><td>NA</td><td>NA</td></tr>
<tr><td>11</td><td>Virginia</td><td>300</td><td>2.2%</td><td>NA</td><td>North Dakota*</td><td>NA</td><td>NA</td></tr>
<tr><td>17</td><td>Washington</td><td>200</td><td>1.5%</td><td>NA</td><td>South Dakota*</td><td>NA</td><td>NA</td></tr>
<tr><td>27</td><td>West Virginia</td><td>100</td><td>0.7%</td><td>NA</td><td>Utah*</td><td>NA</td><td>NA</td></tr>
<tr><td>17</td><td>Wisconsin</td><td>200</td><td>1.5%</td><td>NA</td><td>Vermont*</td><td>NA</td><td>NA</td></tr>
<tr><td>NA</td><td>Wyoming*</td><td>NA</td><td>NA</td><td>NA</td><td>Wyoming*</td><td>NA</td><td>NA</td></tr>
<tr><td></td><td></td><td></td><td></td><td></td><td>District of Columbia</td><td>100</td><td>0.7%</td></tr>
</table>

Source: American Cancer Society
   "1999 Facts & Figures" (Copyright 1999, Reprinted with permission from the American Cancer Society)
*Fewer than 50 deaths.

Estimated Death Rate by Stomach Cancer in 1999

National Estimated Rate = 5.0 Deaths per 100,000 Population*

ALPHA ORDER

RANK	STATE	RATE
24	Alabama	4.6
NA	Alaska**	NA
27	Arizona	4.3
30	Arkansas	3.9
22	California	4.9
41	Colorado	2.5
8	Connecticut	6.1
NA	Delaware**	NA
9	Florida	6.0
30	Georgia	3.9
2	Hawaii	8.4
3	Idaho	8.1
21	Illinois	5.0
38	Indiana	3.4
36	Iowa	3.5
32	Kansas	3.8
19	Kentucky	5.1
6	Louisiana	6.9
4	Maine	8.0
11	Maryland	5.8
22	Massachusetts	4.9
29	Michigan	4.1
28	Minnesota	4.2
35	Mississippi	3.6
15	Missouri	5.5
NA	Montana**	NA
9	Nebraska	6.0
14	Nevada	5.7
NA	New Hampshire**	NA
7	New Jersey	6.2
11	New Mexico	5.8
5	New York	7.2
17	North Carolina	5.3
NA	North Dakota**	NA
25	Ohio	4.5
39	Oklahoma	3.0
39	Oregon	3.0
11	Pennsylvania	5.8
1	Rhode Island	10.1
18	South Carolina	5.2
NA	South Dakota**	NA
34	Tennessee	3.7
19	Texas	5.1
NA	Utah**	NA
NA	Vermont**	NA
26	Virginia	4.4
36	Washington	3.5
15	West Virginia	5.5
32	Wisconsin	3.8
NA	Wyoming**	NA

RANK ORDER

RANK	STATE	RATE
1	Rhode Island	10.1
2	Hawaii	8.4
3	Idaho	8.1
4	Maine	8.0
5	New York	7.2
6	Louisiana	6.9
7	New Jersey	6.2
8	Connecticut	6.1
9	Florida	6.0
9	Nebraska	6.0
11	Maryland	5.8
11	New Mexico	5.8
11	Pennsylvania	5.8
14	Nevada	5.7
15	Missouri	5.5
15	West Virginia	5.5
17	North Carolina	5.3
18	South Carolina	5.2
19	Kentucky	5.1
19	Texas	5.1
21	Illinois	5.0
22	California	4.9
22	Massachusetts	4.9
24	Alabama	4.6
25	Ohio	4.5
26	Virginia	4.4
27	Arizona	4.3
28	Minnesota	4.2
29	Michigan	4.1
30	Arkansas	3.9
30	Georgia	3.9
32	Kansas	3.8
32	Wisconsin	3.8
34	Tennessee	3.7
35	Mississippi	3.6
36	Iowa	3.5
36	Washington	3.5
38	Indiana	3.4
39	Oklahoma	3.0
39	Oregon	3.0
41	Colorado	2.5
NA	Alaska**	NA
NA	Delaware**	NA
NA	Montana**	NA
NA	New Hampshire**	NA
NA	North Dakota**	NA
NA	South Dakota**	NA
NA	Utah**	NA
NA	Vermont**	NA
NA	Wyoming**	NA

District of Columbia	19.1

Source: Morgan Quitno Press using data from American Cancer Society
    "1999 Facts & Figures" (Copyright 1999, Reprinted with permission from the American Cancer Society)
*Rates calculated using 1998 Census resident population estimates. Not age-adjusted.
**Fewer than 50 deaths.

Deaths by Alzheimer's Disease in 1996

National Total = 21,397 Deaths*

ALPHA ORDER

RANK	STATE	DEATHS	% of USA
21	Alabama	437	2.0%
50	Alaska	25	0.1%
19	Arizona	449	2.1%
33	Arkansas	189	0.9%
1	California	1,969	9.2%
28	Colorado	295	1.4%
31	Connecticut	240	1.1%
48	Delaware	47	0.2%
3	Florida	1,480	6.9%
9	Georgia	601	2.8%
46	Hawaii	61	0.3%
39	Idaho	111	0.5%
4	Illinois	1,043	4.9%
12	Indiana	590	2.8%
26	Iowa	354	1.7%
29	Kansas	255	1.2%
24	Kentucky	382	1.8%
23	Louisiana	409	1.9%
35	Maine	178	0.8%
25	Maryland	363	1.7%
8	Massachusetts	631	2.9%
11	Michigan	599	2.8%
17	Minnesota	459	2.1%
36	Mississippi	162	0.8%
20	Missouri	446	2.1%
43	Montana	94	0.4%
32	Nebraska	209	1.0%
42	Nevada	96	0.4%
37	New Hampshire	135	0.6%
9	New Jersey	601	2.8%
40	New Mexico	101	0.5%
13	New York	575	2.7%
7	North Carolina	683	3.2%
48	North Dakota	47	0.2%
5	Ohio	981	4.6%
30	Oklahoma	250	1.2%
22	Oregon	420	2.0%
6	Pennsylvania	937	4.4%
41	Rhode Island	100	0.5%
27	South Carolina	344	1.6%
44	South Dakota	78	0.4%
18	Tennessee	451	2.1%
2	Texas	1,503	7.0%
38	Utah	118	0.6%
45	Vermont	76	0.4%
15	Virginia	512	2.4%
14	Washington	536	2.5%
33	West Virginia	189	0.9%
16	Wisconsin	496	2.3%
47	Wyoming	50	0.2%

RANK ORDER

RANK	STATE	DEATHS	% of USA
1	California	1,969	9.2%
2	Texas	1,503	7.0%
3	Florida	1,480	6.9%
4	Illinois	1,043	4.9%
5	Ohio	981	4.6%
6	Pennsylvania	937	4.4%
7	North Carolina	683	3.2%
8	Massachusetts	631	2.9%
9	Georgia	601	2.8%
9	New Jersey	601	2.8%
11	Michigan	599	2.8%
12	Indiana	590	2.8%
13	New York	575	2.7%
14	Washington	536	2.5%
15	Virginia	512	2.4%
16	Wisconsin	496	2.3%
17	Minnesota	459	2.1%
18	Tennessee	451	2.1%
19	Arizona	449	2.1%
20	Missouri	446	2.1%
21	Alabama	437	2.0%
22	Oregon	420	2.0%
23	Louisiana	409	1.9%
24	Kentucky	382	1.8%
25	Maryland	363	1.7%
26	Iowa	354	1.7%
27	South Carolina	344	1.6%
28	Colorado	295	1.4%
29	Kansas	255	1.2%
30	Oklahoma	250	1.2%
31	Connecticut	240	1.1%
32	Nebraska	209	1.0%
33	Arkansas	189	0.9%
33	West Virginia	189	0.9%
35	Maine	178	0.8%
36	Mississippi	162	0.8%
37	New Hampshire	135	0.6%
38	Utah	118	0.6%
39	Idaho	111	0.5%
40	New Mexico	101	0.5%
41	Rhode Island	100	0.5%
42	Nevada	96	0.4%
43	Montana	94	0.4%
44	South Dakota	78	0.4%
45	Vermont	76	0.4%
46	Hawaii	61	0.3%
47	Wyoming	50	0.2%
48	Delaware	47	0.2%
48	North Dakota	47	0.2%
50	Alaska	25	0.1%
	District of Columbia	40	0.2%

Source: U.S. Department of Health and Human Services, National Center for Health Statistics
    "National Vital Statistics Report" (Vol. 47, No. 9, November 10, 1998)
*Final data by state of residence. A degenerative disease of the brain cells producing loss of memory and general intellectual impairment. It usually affects people over age 65. As the disease progresses, a variety of symptoms may become apparent, including confusion, irritability, and restlessness, as well as disorientation and impaired judgment and concentration.

Death Rate by Alzheimer's Disease in 1996

National Rate = 8.1 Deaths per 100,000 Population*

ALPHA ORDER

RANK	STATE	RATE
13	Alabama	10.2
49	Alaska	4.1
14	Arizona	10.1
36	Arkansas	7.5
42	California	6.2
33	Colorado	7.7
38	Connecticut	7.4
41	Delaware	6.5
12	Florida	10.3
30	Georgia	8.2
48	Hawaii	5.1
22	Idaho	9.4
27	Illinois	8.7
14	Indiana	10.1
5	Iowa	12.4
17	Kansas	9.9
19	Kentucky	9.8
22	Louisiana	9.4
1	Maine	14.4
40	Maryland	7.2
9	Massachusetts	10.4
42	Michigan	6.2
17	Minnesota	9.9
44	Mississippi	6.0
29	Missouri	8.3
7	Montana	10.7
4	Nebraska	12.7
44	Nevada	6.0
6	New Hampshire	11.6
36	New Jersey	7.5
46	New Mexico	5.9
50	New York	3.2
24	North Carolina	9.3
39	North Dakota	7.3
26	Ohio	8.8
35	Oklahoma	7.6
2	Oregon	13.1
32	Pennsylvania	7.8
14	Rhode Island	10.1
25	South Carolina	9.2
8	South Dakota	10.6
28	Tennessee	8.5
31	Texas	7.9
47	Utah	5.8
3	Vermont	13.0
33	Virginia	7.7
20	Washington	9.7
9	West Virginia	10.4
21	Wisconsin	9.6
9	Wyoming	10.4

RANK ORDER

RANK	STATE	RATE
1	Maine	14.4
2	Oregon	13.1
3	Vermont	13.0
4	Nebraska	12.7
5	Iowa	12.4
6	New Hampshire	11.6
7	Montana	10.7
8	South Dakota	10.6
9	Massachusetts	10.4
9	West Virginia	10.4
9	Wyoming	10.4
12	Florida	10.3
13	Alabama	10.2
14	Arizona	10.1
14	Indiana	10.1
14	Rhode Island	10.1
17	Kansas	9.9
17	Minnesota	9.9
19	Kentucky	9.8
20	Washington	9.7
21	Wisconsin	9.6
22	Idaho	9.4
22	Louisiana	9.4
24	North Carolina	9.3
25	South Carolina	9.2
26	Ohio	8.8
27	Illinois	8.7
28	Tennessee	8.5
29	Missouri	8.3
30	Georgia	8.2
31	Texas	7.9
32	Pennsylvania	7.8
33	Colorado	7.7
33	Virginia	7.7
35	Oklahoma	7.6
36	Arkansas	7.5
36	New Jersey	7.5
38	Connecticut	7.4
39	North Dakota	7.3
40	Maryland	7.2
41	Delaware	6.5
42	California	6.2
42	Michigan	6.2
44	Mississippi	6.0
44	Nevada	6.0
46	New Mexico	5.9
47	Utah	5.8
48	Hawaii	5.1
49	Alaska	4.1
50	New York	3.2

| District of Columbia | 7.4 |

Source: Morgan Quitno Press using data from U.S. Dept of Health & Human Serv's, Nat'l Center for Health Statistics
"National Vital Statistics Report" (Vol. 47, No. 9, November 10, 1998)
*Final data by state of residence. A degenerative disease of the brain cells producing loss of memory and general intellectual impairment. It usually affects people over age 65. As the disease progresses, a variety of symptoms may become apparent, including confusion, irritability, and restlessness, as well as disorientation and impaired judgment and concentration. Not age-adjusted.

Age-Adjusted Death Rate by Alzheimer's Disease in 1996

National Rate = 2.7 Deaths per 100,000 Population*

ALPHA ORDER

RANK	STATE	RATE
10	Alabama	3.6
1	Alaska	4.8
17	Arizona	3.2
37	Arkansas	2.4
37	California	2.4
17	Colorado	3.2
46	Connecticut	2.1
37	Delaware	2.4
37	Florida	2.4
6	Georgia	3.8
48	Hawaii	1.7
17	Idaho	3.2
25	Illinois	2.9
11	Indiana	3.5
22	Iowa	3.1
25	Kansas	2.9
16	Kentucky	3.3
9	Louisiana	3.7
4	Maine	4.0
33	Maryland	2.7
25	Massachusetts	2.9
43	Michigan	2.3
23	Minnesota	3.0
45	Mississippi	2.2
36	Missouri	2.5
17	Montana	3.2
12	Nebraska	3.4
25	Nevada	2.9
3	New Hampshire	4.1
37	New Jersey	2.4
37	New Mexico	2.4
50	New York	1.0
12	North Carolina	3.4
49	North Dakota	1.6
31	Ohio	2.8
43	Oklahoma	2.3
4	Oregon	4.0
46	Pennsylvania	2.1
35	Rhode Island	2.6
6	South Carolina	3.8
33	South Dakota	2.7
23	Tennessee	3.0
12	Texas	3.4
31	Utah	2.8
2	Vermont	4.3
17	Virginia	3.2
12	Washington	3.4
25	West Virginia	2.9
25	Wisconsin	2.9
6	Wyoming	3.8

RANK ORDER

RANK	STATE	RATE
1	Alaska	4.8
2	Vermont	4.3
3	New Hampshire	4.1
4	Maine	4.0
4	Oregon	4.0
6	Georgia	3.8
6	South Carolina	3.8
6	Wyoming	3.8
9	Louisiana	3.7
10	Alabama	3.6
11	Indiana	3.5
12	Nebraska	3.4
12	North Carolina	3.4
12	Texas	3.4
12	Washington	3.4
16	Kentucky	3.3
17	Arizona	3.2
17	Colorado	3.2
17	Idaho	3.2
17	Montana	3.2
17	Virginia	3.2
22	Iowa	3.1
23	Minnesota	3.0
23	Tennessee	3.0
25	Illinois	2.9
25	Kansas	2.9
25	Massachusetts	2.9
25	Nevada	2.9
25	West Virginia	2.9
25	Wisconsin	2.9
31	Ohio	2.8
31	Utah	2.8
33	Maryland	2.7
33	South Dakota	2.7
35	Rhode Island	2.6
36	Missouri	2.5
37	Arkansas	2.4
37	California	2.4
37	Delaware	2.4
37	Florida	2.4
37	New Jersey	2.4
37	New Mexico	2.4
43	Michigan	2.3
43	Oklahoma	2.3
45	Mississippi	2.2
46	Connecticut	2.1
46	Pennsylvania	2.1
48	Hawaii	1.7
49	North Dakota	1.6
50	New York	1.0
	District of Columbia	2.1

Source: U.S. Department of Health and Human Services, National Center for Health Statistics
"National Vital Statistics Report" (Vol. 47, No. 9, November 10, 1998)
*Final data by state of residence. A degenerative disease of the brain cells producing loss of memory and general intellectual impairment. It usually affects people over age 65. As the disease progresses, a variety of symptoms may become apparent, including confusion, irritability, and restlessness, as well as disorientation and impaired judgment and concentration.

Deaths by Atherosclerosis in 1996

National Total = 16,740 Deaths*

ALPHA ORDER

RANK	STATE	DEATHS	% of USA
27	Alabama	239	1.4%
50	Alaska	17	0.1%
23	Arizona	306	1.8%
31	Arkansas	162	1.0%
1	California	1,890	11.3%
16	Colorado	382	2.3%
29	Connecticut	209	1.2%
46	Delaware	28	0.2%
2	Florida	1,133	6.8%
9	Georgia	557	3.3%
49	Hawaii	18	0.1%
43	Idaho	64	0.4%
8	Illinois	694	4.1%
11	Indiana	450	2.7%
14	Iowa	401	2.4%
21	Kansas	314	1.9%
30	Kentucky	170	1.0%
24	Louisiana	277	1.7%
37	Maine	87	0.5%
33	Maryland	149	0.9%
17	Massachusetts	371	2.2%
5	Michigan	757	4.5%
25	Minnesota	250	1.5%
35	Mississippi	107	0.6%
20	Missouri	322	1.9%
42	Montana	69	0.4%
28	Nebraska	216	1.3%
41	Nevada	79	0.5%
38	New Hampshire	84	0.5%
10	New Jersey	480	2.9%
36	New Mexico	103	0.6%
5	New York	757	4.5%
15	North Carolina	385	2.3%
39	North Dakota	81	0.5%
7	Ohio	714	4.3%
12	Oklahoma	422	2.5%
26	Oregon	243	1.5%
4	Pennsylvania	775	4.6%
45	Rhode Island	47	0.3%
34	South Carolina	134	0.8%
44	South Dakota	57	0.3%
13	Tennessee	403	2.4%
3	Texas	978	5.8%
39	Utah	81	0.5%
48	Vermont	22	0.1%
19	Virginia	366	2.2%
18	Washington	370	2.2%
31	West Virginia	162	1.0%
22	Wisconsin	307	1.8%
47	Wyoming	23	0.1%

RANK ORDER

RANK	STATE	DEATHS	% of USA
1	California	1,890	11.3%
2	Florida	1,133	6.8%
3	Texas	978	5.8%
4	Pennsylvania	775	4.6%
5	Michigan	757	4.5%
5	New York	757	4.5%
7	Ohio	714	4.3%
8	Illinois	694	4.1%
9	Georgia	557	3.3%
10	New Jersey	480	2.9%
11	Indiana	450	2.7%
12	Oklahoma	422	2.5%
13	Tennessee	403	2.4%
14	Iowa	401	2.4%
15	North Carolina	385	2.3%
16	Colorado	382	2.3%
17	Massachusetts	371	2.2%
18	Washington	370	2.2%
19	Virginia	366	2.2%
20	Missouri	322	1.9%
21	Kansas	314	1.9%
22	Wisconsin	307	1.8%
23	Arizona	306	1.8%
24	Louisiana	277	1.7%
25	Minnesota	250	1.5%
26	Oregon	243	1.5%
27	Alabama	239	1.4%
28	Nebraska	216	1.3%
29	Connecticut	209	1.2%
30	Kentucky	170	1.0%
31	Arkansas	162	1.0%
31	West Virginia	162	1.0%
33	Maryland	149	0.9%
34	South Carolina	134	0.8%
35	Mississippi	107	0.6%
36	New Mexico	103	0.6%
37	Maine	87	0.5%
38	New Hampshire	84	0.5%
39	North Dakota	81	0.5%
39	Utah	81	0.5%
41	Nevada	79	0.5%
42	Montana	69	0.4%
43	Idaho	64	0.4%
44	South Dakota	57	0.3%
45	Rhode Island	47	0.3%
46	Delaware	28	0.2%
47	Wyoming	23	0.1%
48	Vermont	22	0.1%
49	Hawaii	18	0.1%
50	Alaska	17	0.1%
	District of Columbia	28	0.2%

Source: U.S. Department of Health and Human Services, National Center for Health Statistics
(http://wonder.cdc.gov/WONDER/)
*Final data by state of residence. Atherosclerosis is a form of hardening of the arteries.

Death Rate by Atherosclerosis in 1996

National Rate = 6.3 Deaths per 100,000 Population*

ALPHA ORDER				RANK ORDER		
RANK	STATE	RATE		RANK	STATE	RATE
32	Alabama	5.6		1	Iowa	14.1
49	Alaska**	2.8		2	Nebraska	13.1
18	Arizona	6.9		3	Oklahoma	12.8
20	Arkansas	6.5		4	North Dakota	12.6
26	California	6.0		5	Kansas	12.1
6	Colorado	10.0		6	Colorado	10.0
21	Connecticut	6.4		7	West Virginia	8.9
44	Delaware	3.9		8	Florida	7.9
8	Florida	7.9		8	Montana	7.9
13	Georgia	7.6		10	Michigan	7.8
50	Hawaii**	1.5		11	Indiana	7.7
34	Idaho	5.4		11	South Dakota	7.7
31	Illinois	5.8		13	Georgia	7.6
11	Indiana	7.7		13	Oregon	7.6
1	Iowa	14.1		13	Tennessee	7.6
5	Kansas	12.1		16	New Hampshire	7.2
41	Kentucky	4.4		17	Maine	7.0
21	Louisiana	6.4		18	Arizona	6.9
17	Maine	7.0		19	Washington	6.7
48	Maryland	2.9		20	Arkansas	6.5
25	Massachusetts	6.1		21	Connecticut	6.4
10	Michigan	7.8		21	Louisiana	6.4
34	Minnesota	5.4		21	Ohio	6.4
44	Mississippi	3.9		21	Pennsylvania	6.4
26	Missouri	6.0		25	Massachusetts	6.1
8	Montana	7.9		26	California	6.0
2	Nebraska	13.1		26	Missouri	6.0
38	Nevada	4.9		26	New Jersey	6.0
16	New Hampshire	7.2		26	New Mexico	6.0
26	New Jersey	6.0		30	Wisconsin	5.9
26	New Mexico	6.0		31	Illinois	5.8
42	New York	4.2		32	Alabama	5.6
36	North Carolina	5.3		33	Virginia	5.5
4	North Dakota	12.6		34	Idaho	5.4
21	Ohio	6.4		34	Minnesota	5.4
3	Oklahoma	12.8		36	North Carolina	5.3
13	Oregon	7.6		37	Texas	5.1
21	Pennsylvania	6.4		38	Nevada	4.9
39	Rhode Island	4.8		39	Rhode Island	4.8
47	South Carolina	3.6		39	Wyoming	4.8
11	South Dakota	7.7		41	Kentucky	4.4
13	Tennessee	7.6		42	New York	4.2
37	Texas	5.1		43	Utah	4.0
43	Utah	4.0		44	Delaware	3.9
46	Vermont	3.8		44	Mississippi	3.9
33	Virginia	5.5		46	Vermont	3.8
19	Washington	6.7		47	South Carolina	3.6
7	West Virginia	8.9		48	Maryland	2.9
30	Wisconsin	5.9		49	Alaska**	2.8
39	Wyoming	4.8		50	Hawaii**	1.5

District of Columbia   5.2

Source: Morgan Quitno Press using data from U.S. Dept of Health & Human Serv's, Nat'l Center for Health Statistics
(http://wonder.cdc.gov/WONDER/)
*Final data by state of residence. Atherosclerosis is a form of hardening of the arteries. Not age-adjusted.
**Due to low numbers of deaths, rates for these states should be interpreted with caution.

Age-Adjusted Death Rate by Atherosclerosis in 1996

National Rate = 2.2 Deaths per 100,000 Population*

ALPHA ORDER

RANK	STATE	RATE
17	Alabama	2.5
4	Alaska**	3.3
15	Arizona	2.6
29	Arkansas	2.0
22	California	2.4
2	Colorado	3.9
35	Connecticut	1.8
48	Delaware	1.3
32	Florida	1.9
3	Georgia	3.8
50	Hawaii**	0.6
35	Idaho	1.8
32	Illinois	1.9
17	Indiana	2.5
4	Iowa	3.3
7	Kansas	3.1
45	Kentucky	1.4
15	Louisiana	2.6
25	Maine	2.2
49	Maryland	1.0
35	Massachusetts	1.8
10	Michigan	2.9
41	Minnesota	1.7
43	Mississippi	1.5
35	Missouri	1.8
13	Montana	2.7
7	Nebraska	3.1
17	Nevada	2.5
11	New Hampshire	2.8
26	New Jersey	2.1
17	New Mexico	2.5
43	New York	1.5
26	North Carolina	2.1
9	North Dakota	3.0
26	Ohio	2.1
1	Oklahoma	4.3
22	Oregon	2.4
35	Pennsylvania	1.8
45	Rhode Island	1.4
45	South Carolina	1.4
29	South Dakota	2.0
6	Tennessee	3.2
24	Texas	2.3
32	Utah	1.9
42	Vermont	1.6
17	Virginia	2.5
13	Washington	2.7
11	West Virginia	2.8
35	Wisconsin	1.8
29	Wyoming	2.0

RANK ORDER

RANK	STATE	RATE
1	Oklahoma	4.3
2	Colorado	3.9
3	Georgia	3.8
4	Alaska**	3.3
4	Iowa	3.3
6	Tennessee	3.2
7	Kansas	3.1
7	Nebraska	3.1
9	North Dakota	3.0
10	Michigan	2.9
11	New Hampshire	2.8
11	West Virginia	2.8
13	Montana	2.7
13	Washington	2.7
15	Arizona	2.6
15	Louisiana	2.6
17	Alabama	2.5
17	Indiana	2.5
17	Nevada	2.5
17	New Mexico	2.5
17	Virginia	2.5
22	California	2.4
22	Oregon	2.4
24	Texas	2.3
25	Maine	2.2
26	New Jersey	2.1
26	North Carolina	2.1
26	Ohio	2.1
29	Arkansas	2.0
29	South Dakota	2.0
29	Wyoming	2.0
32	Florida	1.9
32	Illinois	1.9
32	Utah	1.9
35	Connecticut	1.8
35	Idaho	1.8
35	Massachusetts	1.8
35	Missouri	1.8
35	Pennsylvania	1.8
35	Wisconsin	1.8
41	Minnesota	1.7
42	Vermont	1.6
43	Mississippi	1.5
43	New York	1.5
45	Kentucky	1.4
45	Rhode Island	1.4
45	South Carolina	1.4
48	Delaware	1.3
49	Maryland	1.0
50	Hawaii**	0.6

	District of Columbia	1.7

Source: U.S. Department of Health and Human Services, National Center for Health Statistics
(http://wonder.cdc.gov/WONDER/)
*Final data by state of residence. Atherosclerosis is a form of hardening of the arteries.
**Due to low numbers of deaths, rates for these states should be interpreted with caution.

Deaths by Cerebrovascular Diseases in 1996

National Total = 159,942 Deaths*

ALPHA ORDER

RANK	STATE	DEATHS	% of USA
20	Alabama	2,860	1.8%
50	Alaska	142	0.1%
27	Arizona	2,347	1.5%
28	Arkansas	2,295	1.4%
1	California	16,545	10.3%
33	Colorado	1,680	1.1%
30	Connecticut	1,954	1.2%
47	Delaware	346	0.2%
2	Florida	9,872	6.2%
11	Georgia	4,254	2.7%
42	Hawaii	617	0.4%
40	Idaho	687	0.4%
6	Illinois	7,428	4.6%
13	Indiana	3,951	2.5%
29	Iowa	2,274	1.4%
31	Kansas	1,878	1.2%
24	Kentucky	2,584	1.6%
25	Louisiana	2,576	1.6%
39	Maine	731	0.5%
22	Maryland	2,649	1.7%
18	Massachusetts	3,358	2.1%
8	Michigan	5,755	3.6%
19	Minnesota	3,028	1.9%
32	Mississippi	1,708	1.1%
15	Missouri	3,780	2.4%
44	Montana	550	0.3%
35	Nebraska	1,140	0.7%
37	Nevada	796	0.5%
41	New Hampshire	686	0.4%
10	New Jersey	4,298	2.7%
38	New Mexico	792	0.5%
5	New York	8,258	5.2%
9	North Carolina	5,332	3.3%
45	North Dakota	508	0.3%
7	Ohio	6,766	4.2%
26	Oklahoma	2,418	1.5%
23	Oregon	2,621	1.6%
4	Pennsylvania	8,656	5.4%
43	Rhode Island	585	0.4%
21	South Carolina	2,853	1.8%
46	South Dakota	483	0.3%
12	Tennessee	4,010	2.5%
3	Texas	9,854	6.2%
36	Utah	844	0.5%
48	Vermont	321	0.2%
14	Virginia	3,856	2.4%
17	Washington	3,480	2.2%
34	West Virginia	1,219	0.8%
16	Wisconsin	3,685	2.3%
49	Wyoming	265	0.2%

RANK ORDER

RANK	STATE	DEATHS	% of USA
1	California	16,545	10.3%
2	Florida	9,872	6.2%
3	Texas	9,854	6.2%
4	Pennsylvania	8,656	5.4%
5	New York	8,258	5.2%
6	Illinois	7,428	4.6%
7	Ohio	6,766	4.2%
8	Michigan	5,755	3.6%
9	North Carolina	5,332	3.3%
10	New Jersey	4,298	2.7%
11	Georgia	4,254	2.7%
12	Tennessee	4,010	2.5%
13	Indiana	3,951	2.5%
14	Virginia	3,856	2.4%
15	Missouri	3,780	2.4%
16	Wisconsin	3,685	2.3%
17	Washington	3,480	2.2%
18	Massachusetts	3,358	2.1%
19	Minnesota	3,028	1.9%
20	Alabama	2,860	1.8%
21	South Carolina	2,853	1.8%
22	Maryland	2,649	1.7%
23	Oregon	2,621	1.6%
24	Kentucky	2,584	1.6%
25	Louisiana	2,576	1.6%
26	Oklahoma	2,418	1.5%
27	Arizona	2,347	1.5%
28	Arkansas	2,295	1.4%
29	Iowa	2,274	1.4%
30	Connecticut	1,954	1.2%
31	Kansas	1,878	1.2%
32	Mississippi	1,708	1.1%
33	Colorado	1,680	1.1%
34	West Virginia	1,219	0.8%
35	Nebraska	1,140	0.7%
36	Utah	844	0.5%
37	Nevada	796	0.5%
38	New Mexico	792	0.5%
39	Maine	731	0.5%
40	Idaho	687	0.4%
41	New Hampshire	686	0.4%
42	Hawaii	617	0.4%
43	Rhode Island	585	0.4%
44	Montana	550	0.3%
45	North Dakota	508	0.3%
46	South Dakota	483	0.3%
47	Delaware	346	0.2%
48	Vermont	321	0.2%
49	Wyoming	265	0.2%
50	Alaska	142	0.1%
	District of Columbia	367	0.2%

Source: U.S. Department of Health and Human Services, National Center for Health Statistics
    "National Vital Statistics Report" (Vol. 47, No. 9, November 10, 1998)
Final data by state of residence. Cerebrovascular diseases include stroke and other disorders of the blood vessels of the brain.

Death Rate by Cerebrovascular Diseases in 1996

National Rate = 60.3 Deaths per 100,000 Population*

ALPHA ORDER

RANK	STATE	RATE
17	Alabama	66.6
50	Alaska	23.5
39	Arizona	53.0
1	Arkansas	91.6
41	California	52.1
48	Colorado	44.1
26	Connecticut	59.9
45	Delaware	47.6
14	Florida	68.4
32	Georgia	58.0
42	Hawaii	52.0
33	Idaho	57.9
24	Illinois	62.2
15	Indiana	67.8
3	Iowa	79.8
9	Kansas	72.7
17	Kentucky	66.6
27	Louisiana	59.4
31	Maine	59.0
40	Maryland	52.4
35	Massachusetts	55.2
30	Michigan	59.1
20	Minnesota	65.1
22	Mississippi	63.0
12	Missouri	70.4
23	Montana	62.7
13	Nebraska	69.2
44	Nevada	49.7
28	New Hampshire	59.2
38	New Jersey	53.7
46	New Mexico	46.4
47	New York	45.5
8	North Carolina	73.0
4	North Dakota	79.0
25	Ohio	60.6
7	Oklahoma	73.4
2	Oregon	82.0
10	Pennsylvania	71.9
28	Rhode Island	59.2
5	South Carolina	76.3
19	South Dakota	65.5
6	Tennessee	75.6
43	Texas	51.8
49	Utah	41.7
37	Vermont	54.7
34	Virginia	57.8
21	Washington	63.1
16	West Virginia	67.0
11	Wisconsin	71.2
35	Wyoming	55.2

RANK ORDER

RANK	STATE	RATE
1	Arkansas	91.6
2	Oregon	82.0
3	Iowa	79.8
4	North Dakota	79.0
5	South Carolina	76.3
6	Tennessee	75.6
7	Oklahoma	73.4
8	North Carolina	73.0
9	Kansas	72.7
10	Pennsylvania	71.9
11	Wisconsin	71.2
12	Missouri	70.4
13	Nebraska	69.2
14	Florida	68.4
15	Indiana	67.8
16	West Virginia	67.0
17	Alabama	66.6
17	Kentucky	66.6
19	South Dakota	65.5
20	Minnesota	65.1
21	Washington	63.1
22	Mississippi	63.0
23	Montana	62.7
24	Illinois	62.2
25	Ohio	60.6
26	Connecticut	59.9
27	Louisiana	59.4
28	New Hampshire	59.2
28	Rhode Island	59.2
30	Michigan	59.1
31	Maine	59.0
32	Georgia	58.0
33	Idaho	57.9
34	Virginia	57.8
35	Massachusetts	55.2
35	Wyoming	55.2
37	Vermont	54.7
38	New Jersey	53.7
39	Arizona	53.0
40	Maryland	52.4
41	California	52.1
42	Hawaii	52.0
43	Texas	51.8
44	Nevada	49.7
45	Delaware	47.6
46	New Mexico	46.4
47	New York	45.5
48	Colorado	44.1
49	Utah	41.7
50	Alaska	23.5

District of Columbia   68.0

Source: Morgan Quitno Press using data from U.S. Dept of Health & Human Serv's, Nat'l Center for Health Statistics
     "National Vital Statistics Report" (Vol. 47, No. 9, November 10, 1998)
*Final data by state of residence. Cerebrovascular diseases include stroke and other disorders of the blood
vessels of the brain. Not age-adjusted.

Age-Adjusted Death Rate by Cerebrovascular Diseases in 1996

National Rate = 26.4 Deaths per 100,000 Population*

ALPHA ORDER

RANK	STATE	RATE
7	Alabama	31.8
27	Alaska	25.6
40	Arizona	22.9
2	Arkansas	35.7
22	California	26.3
46	Colorado	22.0
46	Connecticut	22.0
37	Delaware	23.9
41	Florida	22.8
3	Georgia	34.8
34	Hawaii	24.4
29	Idaho	25.5
16	Illinois	27.5
13	Indiana	28.5
30	Iowa	25.2
24	Kansas	26.0
11	Kentucky	29.5
8	Louisiana	31.7
42	Maine	22.7
23	Maryland	26.2
48	Massachusetts	19.9
19	Michigan	27.2
32	Minnesota	24.6
6	Mississippi	32.1
17	Missouri	27.4
36	Montana	24.0
35	Nebraska	24.1
14	Nevada	27.9
33	New Hampshire	24.5
39	New Jersey	23.0
42	New Mexico	22.7
49	New York	19.7
5	North Carolina	34.1
20	North Dakota	26.8
27	Ohio	25.6
10	Oklahoma	30.0
9	Oregon	30.5
26	Pennsylvania	25.7
50	Rhode Island	19.4
1	South Carolina	39.4
44	South Dakota	22.6
4	Tennessee	34.4
15	Texas	27.7
38	Utah	23.8
45	Vermont	22.2
12	Virginia	29.0
17	Washington	27.4
25	West Virginia	25.9
21	Wisconsin	26.5
31	Wyoming	24.9

RANK ORDER

RANK	STATE	RATE
1	South Carolina	39.4
2	Arkansas	35.7
3	Georgia	34.8
4	Tennessee	34.4
5	North Carolina	34.1
6	Mississippi	32.1
7	Alabama	31.8
8	Louisiana	31.7
9	Oregon	30.5
10	Oklahoma	30.0
11	Kentucky	29.5
12	Virginia	29.0
13	Indiana	28.5
14	Nevada	27.9
15	Texas	27.7
16	Illinois	27.5
17	Missouri	27.4
17	Washington	27.4
19	Michigan	27.2
20	North Dakota	26.8
21	Wisconsin	26.5
22	California	26.3
23	Maryland	26.2
24	Kansas	26.0
25	West Virginia	25.9
26	Pennsylvania	25.7
27	Alaska	25.6
27	Ohio	25.6
29	Idaho	25.5
30	Iowa	25.2
31	Wyoming	24.9
32	Minnesota	24.6
33	New Hampshire	24.5
34	Hawaii	24.4
35	Nebraska	24.1
36	Montana	24.0
37	Delaware	23.9
38	Utah	23.8
39	New Jersey	23.0
40	Arizona	22.9
41	Florida	22.8
42	Maine	22.7
42	New Mexico	22.7
44	South Dakota	22.6
45	Vermont	22.2
46	Colorado	22.0
46	Connecticut	22.0
48	Massachusetts	19.9
49	New York	19.7
50	Rhode Island	19.4

| | District of Columbia | 33.6 |

Source: U.S. Department of Health and Human Services, National Center for Health Statistics
"National Vital Statistics Report" (Vol. 47, No. 9, November 10, 1998)
*Final data by state of residence. Cerebrovascular diseases include stroke and other disorders of the blood vessels of the brain.

Deaths by Chronic Liver Disease and Cirrhosis in 1996

National Total = 25,047 Deaths*

ALPHA ORDER

RANK ORDER

RANK	STATE	DEATHS	% of USA
20	Alabama	408	1.6%
47	Alaska	54	0.2%
13	Arizona	546	2.2%
33	Arkansas	196	0.8%
1	California	3,534	14.1%
25	Colorado	342	1.4%
27	Connecticut	303	1.2%
42	Delaware	81	0.3%
3	Florida	1,831	7.3%
11	Georgia	596	2.4%
44	Hawaii	78	0.3%
45	Idaho	71	0.3%
5	Illinois	1,129	4.5%
17	Indiana	439	1.8%
35	Iowa	177	0.7%
36	Kansas	164	0.7%
24	Kentucky	345	1.4%
21	Louisiana	369	1.5%
37	Maine	123	0.5%
18	Maryland	426	1.7%
12	Massachusetts	574	2.3%
7	Michigan	968	3.9%
28	Minnesota	293	1.2%
30	Mississippi	255	1.0%
19	Missouri	419	1.7%
41	Montana	84	0.3%
42	Nebraska	81	0.3%
32	Nevada	212	0.8%
38	New Hampshire	107	0.4%
9	New Jersey	792	3.2%
31	New Mexico	249	1.0%
4	New York	1,712	6.8%
10	North Carolina	688	2.7%
48	North Dakota	52	0.2%
8	Ohio	922	3.7%
29	Oklahoma	290	1.2%
26	Oregon	315	1.3%
6	Pennsylvania	1,103	4.4%
39	Rhode Island	102	0.4%
23	South Carolina	347	1.4%
46	South Dakota	64	0.3%
14	Tennessee	516	2.1%
2	Texas	1,945	7.8%
40	Utah	88	0.4%
50	Vermont	31	0.1%
15	Virginia	480	1.9%
16	Washington	461	1.8%
34	West Virginia	194	0.8%
22	Wisconsin	358	1.4%
49	Wyoming	37	0.1%

RANK	STATE	DEATHS	% of USA
1	California	3,534	14.1%
2	Texas	1,945	7.8%
3	Florida	1,831	7.3%
4	New York	1,712	6.8%
5	Illinois	1,129	4.5%
6	Pennsylvania	1,103	4.4%
7	Michigan	968	3.9%
8	Ohio	922	3.7%
9	New Jersey	792	3.2%
10	North Carolina	688	2.7%
11	Georgia	596	2.4%
12	Massachusetts	574	2.3%
13	Arizona	546	2.2%
14	Tennessee	516	2.1%
15	Virginia	480	1.9%
16	Washington	461	1.8%
17	Indiana	439	1.8%
18	Maryland	426	1.7%
19	Missouri	419	1.7%
20	Alabama	408	1.6%
21	Louisiana	369	1.5%
22	Wisconsin	358	1.4%
23	South Carolina	347	1.4%
24	Kentucky	345	1.4%
25	Colorado	342	1.4%
26	Oregon	315	1.3%
27	Connecticut	303	1.2%
28	Minnesota	293	1.2%
29	Oklahoma	290	1.2%
30	Mississippi	255	1.0%
31	New Mexico	249	1.0%
32	Nevada	212	0.8%
33	Arkansas	196	0.8%
34	West Virginia	194	0.8%
35	Iowa	177	0.7%
36	Kansas	164	0.7%
37	Maine	123	0.5%
38	New Hampshire	107	0.4%
39	Rhode Island	102	0.4%
40	Utah	88	0.4%
41	Montana	84	0.3%
42	Delaware	81	0.3%
42	Nebraska	81	0.3%
44	Hawaii	78	0.3%
45	Idaho	71	0.3%
46	South Dakota	64	0.3%
47	Alaska	54	0.2%
48	North Dakota	52	0.2%
49	Wyoming	37	0.1%
50	Vermont	31	0.1%
	District of Columbia	96	0.4%

Source: U.S. Department of Health and Human Services, National Center for Health Statistics
   "National Vital Statistics Report" (Vol. 47, No. 9, November 10, 1998)
*Final data by state of residence. Cirrhosis of the liver is characterized by the replacement of normal tissue with fibrous tissue and the loss of functional liver cells. It can result from alcohol abuse, nutritional deprivation, or infection especially by the hepatitis virus.

Death Rate by Chronic Liver Disease and Cirrhosis in 1996

National Rate = 9.4 Deaths per 100,000 Population*

ALPHA ORDER		
RANK	STATE	RATE
16	Alabama	9.5
27	Alaska	8.9
4	Arizona	12.3
37	Arkansas	7.8
5	California	11.1
26	Colorado	9.0
22	Connecticut	9.3
5	Delaware	11.1
3	Florida	12.7
35	Georgia	8.1
43	Hawaii	6.6
47	Idaho	6.0
16	Illinois	9.5
40	Indiana	7.5
46	Iowa	6.2
44	Kansas	6.3
27	Kentucky	8.9
31	Louisiana	8.5
10	Maine	9.9
32	Maryland	8.4
18	Massachusetts	9.4
10	Michigan	9.9
44	Minnesota	6.3
18	Mississippi	9.4
37	Missouri	7.8
15	Montana	9.6
49	Nebraska	4.9
2	Nevada	13.2
24	New Hampshire	9.2
10	New Jersey	9.9
1	New Mexico	14.6
18	New York	9.4
18	North Carolina	9.4
35	North Dakota	8.1
34	Ohio	8.3
29	Oklahoma	8.8
10	Oregon	9.9
24	Pennsylvania	9.2
8	Rhode Island	10.3
22	South Carolina	9.3
30	South Dakota	8.7
14	Tennessee	9.7
9	Texas	10.2
50	Utah	4.4
48	Vermont	5.3
41	Virginia	7.2
32	Washington	8.4
7	West Virginia	10.7
42	Wisconsin	6.9
39	Wyoming	7.7

RANK ORDER		
RANK	STATE	RATE
1	New Mexico	14.6
2	Nevada	13.2
3	Florida	12.7
4	Arizona	12.3
5	California	11.1
5	Delaware	11.1
7	West Virginia	10.7
8	Rhode Island	10.3
9	Texas	10.2
10	Maine	9.9
10	Michigan	9.9
10	New Jersey	9.9
10	Oregon	9.9
14	Tennessee	9.7
15	Montana	9.6
16	Alabama	9.5
16	Illinois	9.5
18	Massachusetts	9.4
18	Mississippi	9.4
18	New York	9.4
18	North Carolina	9.4
22	Connecticut	9.3
22	South Carolina	9.3
24	New Hampshire	9.2
24	Pennsylvania	9.2
26	Colorado	9.0
27	Alaska	8.9
27	Kentucky	8.9
29	Oklahoma	8.8
30	South Dakota	8.7
31	Louisiana	8.5
32	Maryland	8.4
32	Washington	8.4
34	Ohio	8.3
35	Georgia	8.1
35	North Dakota	8.1
37	Arkansas	7.8
37	Missouri	7.8
39	Wyoming	7.7
40	Indiana	7.5
41	Virginia	7.2
42	Wisconsin	6.9
43	Hawaii	6.6
44	Kansas	6.3
44	Minnesota	6.3
46	Iowa	6.2
47	Idaho	6.0
48	Vermont	5.3
49	Nebraska	4.9
50	Utah	4.4
	District of Columbia	17.8

Source: Morgan Quitno Press using data from U.S. Dept of Health & Human Serv's, Nat'l Center for Health Statistics
"National Vital Statistics Report" (Vol. 47, No. 9, November 10, 1998)
*Final data by state of residence. Cirrhosis of the liver is characterized by the replacement of normal tissue with
fibrous tissue and the loss of functional liver cells. It can result from alcohol abuse, nutritional deprivation, or
infection especially by the hepatitis virus. Not age-adjusted.

Age-Adjusted Death Rate by Chronic Liver Disease and Cirrhosis in 1996

National Rate = 7.5 Deaths per 100,000 Population*

ALPHA ORDER				RANK ORDER		
RANK	STATE	RATE		RANK	STATE	RATE
19	Alabama	7.3		1	New Mexico	12.8
7	Alaska	8.8		2	Nevada	11.0
3	Arizona	10.0		3	Arizona	10.0
37	Arkansas	5.8		4	California	9.9
4	California	9.9		5	Delaware	9.1
19	Colorado	7.3		6	Texas	8.9
33	Connecticut	6.7		7	Alaska	8.8
5	Delaware	9.1		8	Florida	8.5
8	Florida	8.5		9	Michigan	8.0
26	Georgia	7.0		9	Mississippi	8.0
45	Hawaii	4.9		11	Rhode Island	7.7
45	Idaho	4.9		12	Illinois	7.6
12	Illinois	7.6		12	Oregon	7.6
36	Indiana	5.9		12	South Carolina	7.6
48	Iowa	4.2		12	Tennessee	7.6
43	Kansas	5.0		16	New Jersey	7.4
29	Kentucky	6.9		16	North Carolina	7.4
24	Louisiana	7.1		16	West Virginia	7.4
26	Maine	7.0		19	Alabama	7.3
29	Maryland	6.9		19	Colorado	7.3
26	Massachusetts	7.0		19	New York	7.3
9	Michigan	8.0		22	New Hampshire	7.2
43	Minnesota	5.0		22	South Dakota	7.2
9	Mississippi	8.0		24	Louisiana	7.1
37	Missouri	5.8		24	Montana	7.1
24	Montana	7.1		26	Georgia	7.0
50	Nebraska	3.7		26	Maine	7.0
2	Nevada	11.0		26	Massachusetts	7.0
22	New Hampshire	7.2		29	Kentucky	6.9
16	New Jersey	7.4		29	Maryland	6.9
1	New Mexico	12.8		31	Oklahoma	6.8
19	New York	7.3		31	Washington	6.8
16	North Carolina	7.4		33	Connecticut	6.7
40	North Dakota	5.7		34	Pennsylvania	6.2
35	Ohio	6.1		35	Ohio	6.1
31	Oklahoma	6.8		36	Indiana	5.9
12	Oregon	7.6		37	Arkansas	5.8
34	Pennsylvania	6.2		37	Missouri	5.8
11	Rhode Island	7.7		37	Virginia	5.8
12	South Carolina	7.6		40	North Dakota	5.7
22	South Dakota	7.2		40	Wyoming	5.7
12	Tennessee	7.6		42	Wisconsin	5.3
6	Texas	8.9		43	Kansas	5.0
47	Utah	4.3		43	Minnesota	5.0
48	Vermont	4.2		45	Hawaii	4.9
37	Virginia	5.8		45	Idaho	4.9
31	Washington	6.8		47	Utah	4.3
16	West Virginia	7.4		48	Iowa	4.2
42	Wisconsin	5.3		48	Vermont	4.2
40	Wyoming	5.7		50	Nebraska	3.7
					District of Columbia	14.3

Source: U.S. Department of Health and Human Services, National Center for Health Statistics
"National Vital Statistics Report" (Vol. 47, No. 9, November 10, 1998)
*Final data by state of residence. Cirrhosis of the liver is characterized by the replacement of normal tissue with fibrous tissue and the loss of functional liver cells. It can result from alcohol abuse, nutritional deprivation, or infection especially by the hepatitis virus.

Deaths by Chronic Obstructive Pulmonary Diseases in 1996

National Total = 106,027 Deaths*

ALPHA ORDER

RANK	STATE	DEATHS	% of USA
22	Alabama	1,741	1.6%
50	Alaska	113	0.1%
18	Arizona	2,130	2.0%
32	Arkansas	1,117	1.1%
1	California	11,416	10.8%
24	Colorado	1,654	1.6%
30	Connecticut	1,212	1.1%
45	Delaware	279	0.3%
2	Florida	7,707	7.3%
12	Georgia	2,533	2.4%
49	Hawaii	239	0.2%
41	Idaho	477	0.4%
7	Illinois	4,361	4.1%
11	Indiana	2,607	2.5%
29	Iowa	1,346	1.3%
31	Kansas	1,132	1.1%
20	Kentucky	1,946	1.8%
28	Louisiana	1,439	1.4%
37	Maine	659	0.6%
21	Maryland	1,762	1.7%
14	Massachusetts	2,442	2.3%
8	Michigan	3,682	3.5%
23	Minnesota	1,681	1.6%
34	Mississippi	1,007	0.9%
13	Missouri	2,504	2.4%
39	Montana	544	0.5%
36	Nebraska	783	0.7%
35	Nevada	889	0.8%
40	New Hampshire	493	0.5%
10	New Jersey	2,809	2.6%
38	New Mexico	653	0.6%
4	New York	6,112	5.8%
9	North Carolina	3,009	2.8%
45	North Dakota	279	0.3%
6	Ohio	5,123	4.8%
26	Oklahoma	1,566	1.5%
25	Oregon	1,640	1.5%
5	Pennsylvania	5,414	5.1%
43	Rhode Island	410	0.4%
27	South Carolina	1,459	1.4%
44	South Dakota	294	0.3%
15	Tennessee	2,300	2.2%
3	Texas	6,378	6.0%
42	Utah	460	0.4%
48	Vermont	243	0.2%
16	Virginia	2,263	2.1%
17	Washington	2,211	2.1%
33	West Virginia	1,100	1.0%
19	Wisconsin	2,002	1.9%
47	Wyoming	245	0.2%

RANK ORDER

RANK	STATE	DEATHS	% of USA
1	California	11,416	10.8%
2	Florida	7,707	7.3%
3	Texas	6,378	6.0%
4	New York	6,112	5.8%
5	Pennsylvania	5,414	5.1%
6	Ohio	5,123	4.8%
7	Illinois	4,361	4.1%
8	Michigan	3,682	3.5%
9	North Carolina	3,009	2.8%
10	New Jersey	2,809	2.6%
11	Indiana	2,607	2.5%
12	Georgia	2,533	2.4%
13	Missouri	2,504	2.4%
14	Massachusetts	2,442	2.3%
15	Tennessee	2,300	2.2%
16	Virginia	2,263	2.1%
17	Washington	2,211	2.1%
18	Arizona	2,130	2.0%
19	Wisconsin	2,002	1.9%
20	Kentucky	1,946	1.8%
21	Maryland	1,762	1.7%
22	Alabama	1,741	1.6%
23	Minnesota	1,681	1.6%
24	Colorado	1,654	1.6%
25	Oregon	1,640	1.5%
26	Oklahoma	1,566	1.5%
27	South Carolina	1,459	1.4%
28	Louisiana	1,439	1.4%
29	Iowa	1,346	1.3%
30	Connecticut	1,212	1.1%
31	Kansas	1,132	1.1%
32	Arkansas	1,117	1.1%
33	West Virginia	1,100	1.0%
34	Mississippi	1,007	0.9%
35	Nevada	889	0.8%
36	Nebraska	783	0.7%
37	Maine	659	0.6%
38	New Mexico	653	0.6%
39	Montana	544	0.5%
40	New Hampshire	493	0.5%
41	Idaho	477	0.4%
42	Utah	460	0.4%
43	Rhode Island	410	0.4%
44	South Dakota	294	0.3%
45	Delaware	279	0.3%
45	North Dakota	279	0.3%
47	Wyoming	245	0.2%
48	Vermont	243	0.2%
49	Hawaii	239	0.2%
50	Alaska	113	0.1%
	District of Columbia	162	0.2%

Source: U.S. Department of Health and Human Services, National Center for Health Statistics
   "National Vital Statistics Report" (Vol. 47, No. 9, November 10, 1998)
*Final data by state of residence. Chronic obstructive pulmonary diseases are diseases of the lungs including bronchitis, emphysema and asthma. Includes allied conditions.

Death Rate by Chronic Obstructive Pulmonary Diseases in 1996

National Rate = 40.0 Deaths per 100,000 Population*

ALPHA ORDER

RANK	STATE	RATE
26	Alabama	40.6
50	Alaska	18.7
9	Arizona	48.1
17	Arkansas	44.6
40	California	35.9
19	Colorado	43.4
37	Connecticut	37.1
33	Delaware	38.4
4	Florida	53.4
43	Georgia	34.5
49	Hawaii	20.1
27	Idaho	40.2
38	Illinois	36.5
16	Indiana	44.7
12	Iowa	47.3
18	Kansas	43.8
8	Kentucky	50.1
47	Louisiana	33.2
5	Maine	53.2
42	Maryland	34.8
28	Massachusetts	40.1
35	Michigan	37.8
39	Minnesota	36.2
36	Mississippi	37.2
13	Missouri	46.6
1	Montana	62.0
10	Nebraska	47.5
3	Nevada	55.6
22	New Hampshire	42.5
41	New Jersey	35.1
34	New Mexico	38.2
45	New York	33.7
25	North Carolina	41.2
19	North Dakota	43.4
14	Ohio	45.9
10	Oklahoma	47.5
6	Oregon	51.3
15	Pennsylvania	45.0
23	Rhode Island	41.5
31	South Carolina	39.0
30	South Dakota	39.9
21	Tennessee	43.3
46	Texas	33.5
48	Utah	22.7
24	Vermont	41.4
44	Virginia	33.9
28	Washington	40.1
2	West Virginia	60.4
32	Wisconsin	38.7
7	Wyoming	51.0

RANK ORDER

RANK	STATE	RATE
1	Montana	62.0
2	West Virginia	60.4
3	Nevada	55.6
4	Florida	53.4
5	Maine	53.2
6	Oregon	51.3
7	Wyoming	51.0
8	Kentucky	50.1
9	Arizona	48.1
10	Nebraska	47.5
10	Oklahoma	47.5
12	Iowa	47.3
13	Missouri	46.6
14	Ohio	45.9
15	Pennsylvania	45.0
16	Indiana	44.7
17	Arkansas	44.6
18	Kansas	43.8
19	Colorado	43.4
19	North Dakota	43.4
21	Tennessee	43.3
22	New Hampshire	42.5
23	Rhode Island	41.5
24	Vermont	41.4
25	North Carolina	41.2
26	Alabama	40.6
27	Idaho	40.2
28	Massachusetts	40.1
28	Washington	40.1
30	South Dakota	39.9
31	South Carolina	39.0
32	Wisconsin	38.7
33	Delaware	38.4
34	New Mexico	38.2
35	Michigan	37.8
36	Mississippi	37.2
37	Connecticut	37.1
38	Illinois	36.5
39	Minnesota	36.2
40	California	35.9
41	New Jersey	35.1
42	Maryland	34.8
43	Georgia	34.5
44	Virginia	33.9
45	New York	33.7
46	Texas	33.5
47	Louisiana	33.2
48	Utah	22.7
49	Hawaii	20.1
50	Alaska	18.7
	District of Columbia	30.0

Source: Morgan Quitno Press using data from U.S. Dept of Health & Human Serv's, Nat'l Center for Health Statistics
"National Vital Statistics Report" (Vol. 47, No. 9, November 10, 1998)
*Final data by state of residence. Chronic obstructive pulmonary diseases are diseases of the lungs including
bronchitis, emphysema and asthma. Includes allied conditions. Not age-adjusted.

Age-Adjusted Death Rate by Chronic Obstructive Pulmonary Diseases in 1996

National Rate = 21.0 Deaths per 100,000 Population*

ALPHA ORDER

RANK	STATE	RATE
28	Alabama	21.5
16	Alaska	22.9
10	Arizona	24.5
25	Arkansas	21.8
30	California	21.1
5	Colorado	27.1
48	Connecticut	16.4
33	Delaware	20.9
34	Florida	20.1
13	Georgia	23.8
50	Hawaii	10.6
19	Idaho	22.7
37	Illinois	19.9
12	Indiana	24.0
32	Iowa	21.0
23	Kansas	22.0
4	Kentucky	27.9
37	Louisiana	19.9
9	Maine	24.6
34	Maryland	20.1
43	Massachusetts	18.1
30	Michigan	21.1
42	Minnesota	18.3
24	Mississippi	21.9
18	Missouri	22.8
2	Montana	30.5
21	Nebraska	22.4
1	Nevada	33.7
25	New Hampshire	21.8
46	New Jersey	16.8
20	New Mexico	22.5
47	New York	16.6
16	North Carolina	22.9
40	North Dakota	18.8
15	Ohio	23.1
8	Oklahoma	24.7
7	Oregon	25.5
39	Pennsylvania	19.0
49	Rhode Island	16.1
14	South Carolina	23.3
44	South Dakota	17.4
11	Tennessee	24.3
28	Texas	21.5
45	Utah	17.0
22	Vermont	22.2
36	Virginia	20.0
25	Washington	21.8
6	West Virginia	27.0
41	Wisconsin	18.4
3	Wyoming	29.4

RANK ORDER

RANK	STATE	RATE
1	Nevada	33.7
2	Montana	30.5
3	Wyoming	29.4
4	Kentucky	27.9
5	Colorado	27.1
6	West Virginia	27.0
7	Oregon	25.5
8	Oklahoma	24.7
9	Maine	24.6
10	Arizona	24.5
11	Tennessee	24.3
12	Indiana	24.0
13	Georgia	23.8
14	South Carolina	23.3
15	Ohio	23.1
16	Alaska	22.9
16	North Carolina	22.9
18	Missouri	22.8
19	Idaho	22.7
20	New Mexico	22.5
21	Nebraska	22.4
22	Vermont	22.2
23	Kansas	22.0
24	Mississippi	21.9
25	Arkansas	21.8
25	New Hampshire	21.8
25	Washington	21.8
28	Alabama	21.5
28	Texas	21.5
30	California	21.1
30	Michigan	21.1
32	Iowa	21.0
33	Delaware	20.9
34	Florida	20.1
34	Maryland	20.1
36	Virginia	20.0
37	Illinois	19.9
37	Louisiana	19.9
39	Pennsylvania	19.0
40	North Dakota	18.8
41	Wisconsin	18.4
42	Minnesota	18.3
43	Massachusetts	18.1
44	South Dakota	17.4
45	Utah	17.0
46	New Jersey	16.8
47	New York	16.6
48	Connecticut	16.4
49	Rhode Island	16.1
50	Hawaii	10.6
	District of Columbia	15.8

Source: U.S. Department of Health and Human Services, National Center for Health Statistics
   "National Vital Statistics Report" (Vol. 47, No. 9, November 10, 1998)
*Final data by state of residence. Chronic obstructive pulmonary diseases are diseases of the lungs including bronchitis, emphysema and asthma. Includes allied conditions.

Deaths by Diabetes Mellitus in 1996

National Total = 61,767 Deaths*

ALPHA ORDER

RANK	STATE	DEATHS	% of USA
21	Alabama	1,135	1.8%
50	Alaska	65	0.1%
25	Arizona	899	1.5%
32	Arkansas	577	0.9%
1	California	5,406	8.8%
33	Colorado	552	0.9%
28	Connecticut	712	1.2%
44	Delaware	192	0.3%
3	Florida	3,803	6.2%
15	Georgia	1,291	2.1%
43	Hawaii	214	0.3%
42	Idaho	243	0.4%
7	Illinois	2,730	4.4%
12	Indiana	1,490	2.4%
30	Iowa	605	1.0%
31	Kansas	603	1.0%
23	Kentucky	977	1.6%
11	Louisiana	1,624	2.6%
38	Maine	303	0.5%
13	Maryland	1,413	2.3%
14	Massachusetts	1,354	2.2%
9	Michigan	2,352	3.8%
22	Minnesota	1,109	1.8%
34	Mississippi	538	0.9%
16	Missouri	1,274	2.1%
45	Montana	188	0.3%
37	Nebraska	333	0.5%
41	Nevada	263	0.4%
39	New Hampshire	286	0.5%
8	New Jersey	2,362	3.8%
35	New Mexico	432	0.7%
6	New York	3,520	5.7%
10	North Carolina	1,819	2.9%
47	North Dakota	164	0.3%
4	Ohio	3,611	5.8%
26	Oklahoma	722	1.2%
27	Oregon	713	1.2%
5	Pennsylvania	3,565	5.8%
40	Rhode Island	266	0.4%
24	South Carolina	937	1.5%
46	South Dakota	179	0.3%
18	Tennessee	1,252	2.0%
2	Texas	4,585	7.4%
36	Utah	418	0.7%
48	Vermont	154	0.2%
17	Virginia	1,260	2.0%
20	Washington	1,152	1.9%
29	West Virginia	669	1.1%
19	Wisconsin	1,170	1.9%
49	Wyoming	84	0.1%

RANK ORDER

RANK	STATE	DEATHS	% of USA
1	California	5,406	8.8%
2	Texas	4,585	7.4%
3	Florida	3,803	6.2%
4	Ohio	3,611	5.8%
5	Pennsylvania	3,565	5.8%
6	New York	3,520	5.7%
7	Illinois	2,730	4.4%
8	New Jersey	2,362	3.8%
9	Michigan	2,352	3.8%
10	North Carolina	1,819	2.9%
11	Louisiana	1,624	2.6%
12	Indiana	1,490	2.4%
13	Maryland	1,413	2.3%
14	Massachusetts	1,354	2.2%
15	Georgia	1,291	2.1%
16	Missouri	1,274	2.1%
17	Virginia	1,260	2.0%
18	Tennessee	1,252	2.0%
19	Wisconsin	1,170	1.9%
20	Washington	1,152	1.9%
21	Alabama	1,135	1.8%
22	Minnesota	1,109	1.8%
23	Kentucky	977	1.6%
24	South Carolina	937	1.5%
25	Arizona	899	1.5%
26	Oklahoma	722	1.2%
27	Oregon	713	1.2%
28	Connecticut	712	1.2%
29	West Virginia	669	1.1%
30	Iowa	605	1.0%
31	Kansas	603	1.0%
32	Arkansas	577	0.9%
33	Colorado	552	0.9%
34	Mississippi	538	0.9%
35	New Mexico	432	0.7%
36	Utah	418	0.7%
37	Nebraska	333	0.5%
38	Maine	303	0.5%
39	New Hampshire	286	0.5%
40	Rhode Island	266	0.4%
41	Nevada	263	0.4%
42	Idaho	243	0.4%
43	Hawaii	214	0.3%
44	Delaware	192	0.3%
45	Montana	188	0.3%
46	South Dakota	179	0.3%
47	North Dakota	164	0.3%
48	Vermont	154	0.2%
49	Wyoming	84	0.1%
50	Alaska	65	0.1%
	District of Columbia	202	0.3%

Source: U.S. Department of Health and Human Services, National Center for Health Statistics
"National Vital Statistics Report" (Vol. 47, No. 9, November 10, 1998)

*Final data by state of residence. A severe, chronic form of diabetes caused by insufficient production of insulin and resulting in abnormal metabolism of carbohydrates, fats, and proteins. The disease, which typically appears in childhood or adolescence, is characterized by increased sugar levels in the blood and urine, excessive thirst and frequent urination.

Death Rate by Diabetes Mellitus in 1996

National Rate = 23.3 Deaths per 100,000 Population*

ALPHA ORDER

RANK	STATE	RATE
8	Alabama	26.5
50	Alaska	10.7
39	Arizona	20.3
27	Arkansas	23.0
47	California	17.0
49	Colorado	14.5
33	Connecticut	21.8
9	Delaware	26.4
9	Florida	26.4
45	Georgia	17.6
44	Hawaii	18.0
38	Idaho	20.5
28	Illinois	22.9
12	Indiana	25.6
35	Iowa	21.2
26	Kansas	23.3
15	Kentucky	25.2
1	Louisiana	37.4
19	Maine	24.5
6	Maryland	27.9
30	Massachusetts	22.3
21	Michigan	24.2
23	Minnesota	23.9
41	Mississippi	19.9
24	Missouri	23.7
34	Montana	21.4
40	Nebraska	20.2
48	Nevada	16.4
18	New Hampshire	24.7
5	New Jersey	29.5
14	New Mexico	25.3
42	New York	19.4
17	North Carolina	24.9
13	North Dakota	25.5
3	Ohio	32.3
32	Oklahoma	21.9
30	Oregon	22.3
4	Pennsylvania	29.6
7	Rhode Island	26.9
16	South Carolina	25.1
20	South Dakota	24.3
25	Tennessee	23.6
22	Texas	24.1
37	Utah	20.7
11	Vermont	26.3
43	Virginia	18.9
36	Washington	20.9
2	West Virginia	36.8
29	Wisconsin	22.6
46	Wyoming	17.5

RANK ORDER

RANK	STATE	RATE
1	Louisiana	37.4
2	West Virginia	36.8
3	Ohio	32.3
4	Pennsylvania	29.6
5	New Jersey	29.5
6	Maryland	27.9
7	Rhode Island	26.9
8	Alabama	26.5
9	Delaware	26.4
9	Florida	26.4
11	Vermont	26.3
12	Indiana	25.6
13	North Dakota	25.5
14	New Mexico	25.3
15	Kentucky	25.2
16	South Carolina	25.1
17	North Carolina	24.9
18	New Hampshire	24.7
19	Maine	24.5
20	South Dakota	24.3
21	Michigan	24.2
22	Texas	24.1
23	Minnesota	23.9
24	Missouri	23.7
25	Tennessee	23.6
26	Kansas	23.3
27	Arkansas	23.0
28	Illinois	22.9
29	Wisconsin	22.6
30	Massachusetts	22.3
30	Oregon	22.3
32	Oklahoma	21.9
33	Connecticut	21.8
34	Montana	21.4
35	Iowa	21.2
36	Washington	20.9
37	Utah	20.7
38	Idaho	20.5
39	Arizona	20.3
40	Nebraska	20.2
41	Mississippi	19.9
42	New York	19.4
43	Virginia	18.9
44	Hawaii	18.0
45	Georgia	17.6
46	Wyoming	17.5
47	California	17.0
48	Nevada	16.4
49	Colorado	14.5
50	Alaska	10.7

District of Columbia	37.4

Source: Morgan Quitno Press using data from U.S. Dept of Health & Human Serv's, Nat'l Center for Health Statistics
   "National Vital Statistics Report" (Vol. 47, No. 9, November 10, 1998)
*Final data by state of residence. A severe, chronic form of diabetes caused by insufficient production of insulin and resulting in abnormal metabolism of carbohydrates, fats, and proteins. The disease, which typically appears in childhood or adolescence, is characterized by increased sugar levels in the blood and urine, excessive thirst and frequent urination. Not age-adjusted.

Age-Adjusted Death Rate by Diabetes Mellitus in 1996

National Rate = 13.6 Deaths per 100,000 Population*

<table>
<tr><td colspan="3">ALPHA ORDER</td><td colspan="3">RANK ORDER</td></tr>
<tr><td>RANK</td><td>STATE</td><td>RATE</td><td>RANK</td><td>STATE</td><td>RATE</td></tr>
<tr><td>13</td><td>Alabama</td><td>15.1</td><td>1</td><td>Louisiana</td><td>23.8</td></tr>
<tr><td>21</td><td>Alaska</td><td>12.9</td><td>2</td><td>West Virginia</td><td>18.8</td></tr>
<tr><td>27</td><td>Arizona</td><td>12.6</td><td>3</td><td>Ohio</td><td>17.8</td></tr>
<tr><td>35</td><td>Arkansas</td><td>12.2</td><td>4</td><td>Maryland</td><td>17.5</td></tr>
<tr><td>39</td><td>California</td><td>11.7</td><td>5</td><td>Texas</td><td>16.9</td></tr>
<tr><td>50</td><td>Colorado</td><td>9.6</td><td>6</td><td>New Mexico</td><td>16.7</td></tr>
<tr><td>43</td><td>Connecticut</td><td>11.2</td><td>7</td><td>South Carolina</td><td>16.5</td></tr>
<tr><td>10</td><td>Delaware</td><td>15.8</td><td>8</td><td>New Jersey</td><td>16.3</td></tr>
<tr><td>36</td><td>Florida</td><td>12.1</td><td>9</td><td>Utah</td><td>16.1</td></tr>
<tr><td>26</td><td>Georgia</td><td>12.7</td><td>10</td><td>Delaware</td><td>15.8</td></tr>
<tr><td>46</td><td>Hawaii</td><td>10.8</td><td>11</td><td>Vermont</td><td>15.6</td></tr>
<tr><td>32</td><td>Idaho</td><td>12.5</td><td>12</td><td>North Carolina</td><td>15.3</td></tr>
<tr><td>20</td><td>Illinois</td><td>13.5</td><td>13</td><td>Alabama</td><td>15.1</td></tr>
<tr><td>16</td><td>Indiana</td><td>14.5</td><td>14</td><td>New Hampshire</td><td>14.8</td></tr>
<tr><td>48</td><td>Iowa</td><td>9.9</td><td>15</td><td>Kentucky</td><td>14.6</td></tr>
<tr><td>27</td><td>Kansas</td><td>12.6</td><td>16</td><td>Indiana</td><td>14.5</td></tr>
<tr><td>15</td><td>Kentucky</td><td>14.6</td><td>16</td><td>Pennsylvania</td><td>14.5</td></tr>
<tr><td>1</td><td>Louisiana</td><td>23.8</td><td>18</td><td>Michigan</td><td>14.3</td></tr>
<tr><td>27</td><td>Maine</td><td>12.6</td><td>19</td><td>Tennessee</td><td>13.9</td></tr>
<tr><td>4</td><td>Maryland</td><td>17.5</td><td>20</td><td>Illinois</td><td>13.5</td></tr>
<tr><td>40</td><td>Massachusetts</td><td>11.4</td><td>21</td><td>Alaska</td><td>12.9</td></tr>
<tr><td>18</td><td>Michigan</td><td>14.3</td><td>21</td><td>Minnesota</td><td>12.9</td></tr>
<tr><td>21</td><td>Minnesota</td><td>12.9</td><td>21</td><td>Missouri</td><td>12.9</td></tr>
<tr><td>27</td><td>Mississippi</td><td>12.6</td><td>21</td><td>Washington</td><td>12.9</td></tr>
<tr><td>21</td><td>Missouri</td><td>12.9</td><td>25</td><td>Rhode Island</td><td>12.8</td></tr>
<tr><td>42</td><td>Montana</td><td>11.3</td><td>26</td><td>Georgia</td><td>12.7</td></tr>
<tr><td>49</td><td>Nebraska</td><td>9.7</td><td>27</td><td>Arizona</td><td>12.6</td></tr>
<tr><td>46</td><td>Nevada</td><td>10.8</td><td>27</td><td>Kansas</td><td>12.6</td></tr>
<tr><td>14</td><td>New Hampshire</td><td>14.8</td><td>27</td><td>Maine</td><td>12.6</td></tr>
<tr><td>8</td><td>New Jersey</td><td>16.3</td><td>27</td><td>Mississippi</td><td>12.6</td></tr>
<tr><td>6</td><td>New Mexico</td><td>16.7</td><td>27</td><td>Virginia</td><td>12.6</td></tr>
<tr><td>44</td><td>New York</td><td>10.9</td><td>32</td><td>Idaho</td><td>12.5</td></tr>
<tr><td>12</td><td>North Carolina</td><td>15.3</td><td>32</td><td>Oklahoma</td><td>12.5</td></tr>
<tr><td>44</td><td>North Dakota</td><td>10.9</td><td>34</td><td>South Dakota</td><td>12.4</td></tr>
<tr><td>3</td><td>Ohio</td><td>17.8</td><td>35</td><td>Arkansas</td><td>12.2</td></tr>
<tr><td>32</td><td>Oklahoma</td><td>12.5</td><td>36</td><td>Florida</td><td>12.1</td></tr>
<tr><td>38</td><td>Oregon</td><td>11.8</td><td>37</td><td>Wisconsin</td><td>12.0</td></tr>
<tr><td>16</td><td>Pennsylvania</td><td>14.5</td><td>38</td><td>Oregon</td><td>11.8</td></tr>
<tr><td>25</td><td>Rhode Island</td><td>12.8</td><td>39</td><td>California</td><td>11.7</td></tr>
<tr><td>7</td><td>South Carolina</td><td>16.5</td><td>40</td><td>Massachusetts</td><td>11.4</td></tr>
<tr><td>34</td><td>South Dakota</td><td>12.4</td><td>40</td><td>Wyoming</td><td>11.4</td></tr>
<tr><td>19</td><td>Tennessee</td><td>13.9</td><td>42</td><td>Montana</td><td>11.3</td></tr>
<tr><td>5</td><td>Texas</td><td>16.9</td><td>43</td><td>Connecticut</td><td>11.2</td></tr>
<tr><td>9</td><td>Utah</td><td>16.1</td><td>44</td><td>New York</td><td>10.9</td></tr>
<tr><td>11</td><td>Vermont</td><td>15.6</td><td>44</td><td>North Dakota</td><td>10.9</td></tr>
<tr><td>27</td><td>Virginia</td><td>12.6</td><td>46</td><td>Hawaii</td><td>10.8</td></tr>
<tr><td>21</td><td>Washington</td><td>12.9</td><td>46</td><td>Nevada</td><td>10.8</td></tr>
<tr><td>2</td><td>West Virginia</td><td>18.8</td><td>48</td><td>Iowa</td><td>9.9</td></tr>
<tr><td>37</td><td>Wisconsin</td><td>12.0</td><td>49</td><td>Nebraska</td><td>9.7</td></tr>
<tr><td>40</td><td>Wyoming</td><td>11.4</td><td>50</td><td>Colorado</td><td>9.6</td></tr>
<tr><td></td><td></td><td></td><td></td><td>District of Columbia</td><td>22.3</td></tr>
</table>

Source: U.S. Department of Health and Human Services, National Center for Health Statistics
"National Vital Statistics Report" (Vol. 47, No. 9, November 10, 1998)
*Final data by state of residence. A severe, chronic form of diabetes caused by insufficient production of insulin and resulting in abnormal metabolism of carbohydrates, fats, and proteins. The disease, which typically appears in childhood or adolescence, is characterized by increased sugar levels in the blood and urine, excessive thirst and frequent urination.

Deaths by Diseases of the Heart in 1996

National Total = 733,361 Deaths*

ALPHA ORDER

RANK	STATE	DEATHS	% of USA
18	Alabama	13,497	1.8%
50	Alaska	516	0.1%
24	Arizona	10,242	1.4%
30	Arkansas	8,323	1.1%
1	California	68,228	9.3%
34	Colorado	6,599	0.9%
27	Connecticut	9,927	1.4%
46	Delaware	2,014	0.3%
3	Florida	49,735	6.8%
12	Georgia	17,513	2.4%
42	Hawaii	2,445	0.3%
43	Idaho	2,384	0.3%
6	Illinois	34,334	4.7%
14	Indiana	16,815	2.3%
29	Iowa	9,183	1.3%
32	Kansas	7,239	1.0%
20	Kentucky	11,911	1.6%
21	Louisiana	11,765	1.6%
37	Maine	3,541	0.5%
19	Maryland	11,944	1.6%
13	Massachusetts	16,843	2.3%
8	Michigan	28,020	3.8%
26	Minnesota	10,034	1.4%
28	Mississippi	9,538	1.3%
11	Missouri	18,224	2.5%
45	Montana	2,143	0.3%
35	Nebraska	5,003	0.7%
36	Nevada	3,863	0.5%
40	New Hampshire	2,918	0.4%
9	New Jersey	23,864	3.3%
39	New Mexico	3,195	0.4%
2	New York	62,737	8.6%
10	North Carolina	19,865	2.7%
47	North Dakota	1,877	0.3%
7	Ohio	34,213	4.7%
23	Oklahoma	11,315	1.5%
31	Oregon	7,669	1.0%
4	Pennsylvania	43,663	6.0%
38	Rhode Island	3,265	0.4%
25	South Carolina	10,097	1.4%
44	South Dakota	2,197	0.3%
15	Tennessee	16,240	2.2%
5	Texas	42,417	5.8%
41	Utah	2,886	0.4%
48	Vermont	1,487	0.2%
16	Virginia	16,074	2.2%
22	Washington	11,734	1.6%
33	West Virginia	7,055	1.0%
17	Wisconsin	14,202	1.9%
49	Wyoming	949	0.1%

RANK ORDER

RANK	STATE	DEATHS	% of USA
1	California	68,228	9.3%
2	New York	62,737	8.6%
3	Florida	49,735	6.8%
4	Pennsylvania	43,663	6.0%
5	Texas	42,417	5.8%
6	Illinois	34,334	4.7%
7	Ohio	34,213	4.7%
8	Michigan	28,020	3.8%
9	New Jersey	23,864	3.3%
10	North Carolina	19,865	2.7%
11	Missouri	18,224	2.5%
12	Georgia	17,513	2.4%
13	Massachusetts	16,843	2.3%
14	Indiana	16,815	2.3%
15	Tennessee	16,240	2.2%
16	Virginia	16,074	2.2%
17	Wisconsin	14,202	1.9%
18	Alabama	13,497	1.8%
19	Maryland	11,944	1.6%
20	Kentucky	11,911	1.6%
21	Louisiana	11,765	1.6%
22	Washington	11,734	1.6%
23	Oklahoma	11,315	1.5%
24	Arizona	10,242	1.4%
25	South Carolina	10,097	1.4%
26	Minnesota	10,034	1.4%
27	Connecticut	9,927	1.4%
28	Mississippi	9,538	1.3%
29	Iowa	9,183	1.3%
30	Arkansas	8,323	1.1%
31	Oregon	7,669	1.0%
32	Kansas	7,239	1.0%
33	West Virginia	7,055	1.0%
34	Colorado	6,599	0.9%
35	Nebraska	5,003	0.7%
36	Nevada	3,863	0.5%
37	Maine	3,541	0.5%
38	Rhode Island	3,265	0.4%
39	New Mexico	3,195	0.4%
40	New Hampshire	2,918	0.4%
41	Utah	2,886	0.4%
42	Hawaii	2,445	0.3%
43	Idaho	2,384	0.3%
44	South Dakota	2,197	0.3%
45	Montana	2,143	0.3%
46	Delaware	2,014	0.3%
47	North Dakota	1,877	0.3%
48	Vermont	1,487	0.2%
49	Wyoming	949	0.1%
50	Alaska	516	0.1%
	District of Columbia	1,619	0.2%

Source: U.S. Department of Health and Human Services, National Center for Health Statistics
"National Vital Statistics Report" (Vol. 47, No. 9, November 10, 1998)
*Final data by state of residence.

Death Rate by Diseases of the Heart in 1996

National Rate = 276.5 Deaths per 100,000 Population*

ALPHA ORDER			RANK ORDER		
RANK	**STATE**	**RATE**	**RANK**	**STATE**	**RATE**
11	Alabama	314.5	1	West Virginia	387.6
50	Alaska	85.3	2	Pennsylvania	362.8
39	Arizona	231.1	3	Mississippi	352.0
8	Arkansas	332.2	4	New York	345.8
42	California	214.8	5	Florida	344.8
48	Colorado	173.0	6	Oklahoma	343.3
15	Connecticut	304.1	7	Missouri	339.4
25	Delaware	277.0	8	Arkansas	332.2
5	Florida	344.8	9	Rhode Island	330.4
37	Georgia	238.8	10	Iowa	322.4
44	Hawaii	205.9	11	Alabama	314.5
45	Idaho	201.0	12	Kentucky	306.8
22	Illinois	287.7	13	Ohio	306.3
20	Indiana	288.5	14	Tennessee	306.0
10	Iowa	322.4	15	Connecticut	304.1
24	Kansas	280.1	16	Nebraska	303.6
12	Kentucky	306.8	17	New Jersey	298.0
29	Louisiana	271.1	17	South Dakota	298.0
23	Maine	286.0	19	North Dakota	292.0
38	Maryland	236.1	20	Indiana	288.5
26	Massachusetts	276.9	21	Michigan	287.9
21	Michigan	287.9	22	Illinois	287.7
41	Minnesota	215.9	23	Maine	286.0
3	Mississippi	352.0	24	Kansas	280.1
7	Missouri	339.4	25	Delaware	277.0
33	Montana	244.4	26	Massachusetts	276.9
16	Nebraska	303.6	27	Wisconsin	274.5
34	Nevada	241.4	28	North Carolina	271.8
32	New Hampshire	251.7	29	Louisiana	271.1
17	New Jersey	298.0	30	South Carolina	270.2
47	New Mexico	187.1	31	Vermont	253.6
4	New York	345.8	32	New Hampshire	251.7
28	North Carolina	271.8	33	Montana	244.4
19	North Dakota	292.0	34	Nevada	241.4
13	Ohio	306.3	35	Virginia	241.1
6	Oklahoma	343.3	36	Oregon	240.0
36	Oregon	240.0	37	Georgia	238.8
2	Pennsylvania	362.8	38	Maryland	236.1
9	Rhode Island	330.4	39	Arizona	231.1
30	South Carolina	270.2	40	Texas	222.9
17	South Dakota	298.0	41	Minnesota	215.9
14	Tennessee	306.0	42	California	214.8
40	Texas	222.9	43	Washington	212.6
49	Utah	142.7	44	Hawaii	205.9
31	Vermont	253.6	45	Idaho	201.0
35	Virginia	241.1	46	Wyoming	197.7
43	Washington	212.6	47	New Mexico	187.1
1	West Virginia	387.6	48	Colorado	173.0
27	Wisconsin	274.5	49	Utah	142.7
46	Wyoming	197.7	50	Alaska	85.3
				District of Columbia	300.0

Source: Morgan Quitno Press using data from U.S. Dept of Health & Human Serv's, Nat'l Center for Health Statistics "National Vital Statistics Report" (Vol. 47, No. 9, November 10, 1998)
*Final data by state of residence. Not age-adjusted.

Age-Adjusted Death Rate by Diseases of the Heart in 1996

National Rate = 134.5 Deaths per 100,000 Population*

ALPHA ORDER

RANK	STATE	RATE
3	Alabama	161.3
49	Alaska	96.8
38	Arizona	114.5
12	Arkansas	147.8
36	California	117.1
48	Colorado	98.2
25	Connecticut	126.0
20	Delaware	141.9
29	Florida	123.1
9	Georgia	152.5
42	Hawaii	108.4
45	Idaho	104.9
18	Illinois	142.7
18	Indiana	142.7
32	Iowa	121.9
35	Kansas	119.6
6	Kentucky	155.7
8	Louisiana	154.6
28	Maine	123.3
23	Maryland	131.6
37	Massachusetts	116.4
13	Michigan	147.0
47	Minnesota	98.4
1	Mississippi	187.4
11	Missouri	149.0
40	Montana	111.7
30	Nebraska	122.7
14	Nevada	146.9
31	New Hampshire	122.3
24	New Jersey	131.0
46	New Mexico	103.6
10	New York	151.0
16	North Carolina	144.9
39	North Dakota	114.4
17	Ohio	144.5
4	Oklahoma	158.9
44	Oregon	105.3
15	Pennsylvania	145.7
26	Rhode Island	125.5
5	South Carolina	156.0
27	South Dakota	123.8
7	Tennessee	155.6
22	Texas	134.0
50	Utah	95.3
34	Vermont	120.4
21	Virginia	136.4
43	Washington	107.7
2	West Virginia	167.8
33	Wisconsin	121.8
41	Wyoming	109.0

RANK ORDER

RANK	STATE	RATE
1	Mississippi	187.4
2	West Virginia	167.8
3	Alabama	161.3
4	Oklahoma	158.9
5	South Carolina	156.0
6	Kentucky	155.7
7	Tennessee	155.6
8	Louisiana	154.6
9	Georgia	152.5
10	New York	151.0
11	Missouri	149.0
12	Arkansas	147.8
13	Michigan	147.0
14	Nevada	146.9
15	Pennsylvania	145.7
16	North Carolina	144.9
17	Ohio	144.5
18	Illinois	142.7
18	Indiana	142.7
20	Delaware	141.9
21	Virginia	136.4
22	Texas	134.0
23	Maryland	131.6
24	New Jersey	131.0
25	Connecticut	126.0
26	Rhode Island	125.5
27	South Dakota	123.8
28	Maine	123.3
29	Florida	123.1
30	Nebraska	122.7
31	New Hampshire	122.3
32	Iowa	121.9
33	Wisconsin	121.8
34	Vermont	120.4
35	Kansas	119.6
36	California	117.1
37	Massachusetts	116.4
38	Arizona	114.5
39	North Dakota	114.4
40	Montana	111.7
41	Wyoming	109.0
42	Hawaii	108.4
43	Washington	107.7
44	Oregon	105.3
45	Idaho	104.9
46	New Mexico	103.6
47	Minnesota	98.4
48	Colorado	98.2
49	Alaska	96.8
50	Utah	95.3
	District of Columbia	154.2

Source: U.S. Department of Health and Human Services, National Center for Health Statistics
  "National Vital Statistics Report" (Vol. 47, No. 9, November 10, 1998)
*Final data by state of residence.

Deaths by Malignant Neoplasms in 1996

National Total = 539,533 Deaths*

<u>ALPHA ORDER</u>

RANK	STATE	DEATHS	% of USA
20	Alabama	9,502	1.8%
50	Alaska	646	0.1%
24	Arizona	8,319	1.5%
30	Arkansas	5,962	1.1%
1	California	51,055	9.5%
32	Colorado	5,655	1.0%
26	Connecticut	7,146	1.3%
45	Delaware	1,688	0.3%
3	Florida	37,694	7.0%
14	Georgia	12,432	2.3%
43	Hawaii	1,861	0.3%
42	Idaho	1,987	0.4%
7	Illinois	24,783	4.6%
13	Indiana	12,487	2.3%
29	Iowa	6,493	1.2%
33	Kansas	5,344	1.0%
22	Kentucky	9,025	1.7%
21	Louisiana	9,314	1.7%
37	Maine	2,952	0.5%
18	Maryland	10,161	1.9%
11	Massachusetts	13,952	2.6%
8	Michigan	19,585	3.6%
23	Minnesota	8,846	1.6%
31	Mississippi	5,757	1.1%
15	Missouri	11,960	2.2%
44	Montana	1,768	0.3%
35	Nebraska	3,326	0.6%
36	Nevada	3,192	0.6%
40	New Hampshire	2,387	0.4%
9	New Jersey	18,315	3.4%
38	New Mexico	2,740	0.5%
2	New York	38,149	7.1%
10	North Carolina	15,192	2.8%
47	North Dakota	1,392	0.3%
6	Ohio	25,326	4.7%
27	Oklahoma	7,128	1.3%
28	Oregon	6,711	1.2%
5	Pennsylvania	30,511	5.7%
39	Rhode Island	2,516	0.5%
25	South Carolina	7,619	1.4%
46	South Dakota	1,541	0.3%
16	Tennessee	11,617	2.2%
4	Texas	32,007	5.9%
41	Utah	2,105	0.4%
48	Vermont	1,207	0.2%
12	Virginia	12,710	2.4%
19	Washington	10,063	1.9%
34	West Virginia	4,673	0.9%
17	Wisconsin	10,483	1.9%
49	Wyoming	869	0.2%

<u>RANK ORDER</u>

RANK	STATE	DEATHS	% of USA
1	California	51,055	9.5%
2	New York	38,149	7.1%
3	Florida	37,694	7.0%
4	Texas	32,007	5.9%
5	Pennsylvania	30,511	5.7%
6	Ohio	25,326	4.7%
7	Illinois	24,783	4.6%
8	Michigan	19,585	3.6%
9	New Jersey	18,315	3.4%
10	North Carolina	15,192	2.8%
11	Massachusetts	13,952	2.6%
12	Virginia	12,710	2.4%
13	Indiana	12,487	2.3%
14	Georgia	12,432	2.3%
15	Missouri	11,960	2.2%
16	Tennessee	11,617	2.2%
17	Wisconsin	10,483	1.9%
18	Maryland	10,161	1.9%
19	Washington	10,063	1.9%
20	Alabama	9,502	1.8%
21	Louisiana	9,314	1.7%
22	Kentucky	9,025	1.7%
23	Minnesota	8,846	1.6%
24	Arizona	8,319	1.5%
25	South Carolina	7,619	1.4%
26	Connecticut	7,146	1.3%
27	Oklahoma	7,128	1.3%
28	Oregon	6,711	1.2%
29	Iowa	6,493	1.2%
30	Arkansas	5,962	1.1%
31	Mississippi	5,757	1.1%
32	Colorado	5,655	1.0%
33	Kansas	5,344	1.0%
34	West Virginia	4,673	0.9%
35	Nebraska	3,326	0.6%
36	Nevada	3,192	0.6%
37	Maine	2,952	0.5%
38	New Mexico	2,740	0.5%
39	Rhode Island	2,516	0.5%
40	New Hampshire	2,387	0.4%
41	Utah	2,105	0.4%
42	Idaho	1,987	0.4%
43	Hawaii	1,861	0.3%
44	Montana	1,768	0.3%
45	Delaware	1,688	0.3%
46	South Dakota	1,541	0.3%
47	North Dakota	1,392	0.3%
48	Vermont	1,207	0.2%
49	Wyoming	869	0.2%
50	Alaska	646	0.1%
	District of Columbia	1,380	0.3%

*Source: U.S. Department of Health and Human Services, National Center for Health Statistics
"National Vital Statistics Report" (Vol. 47, No. 9, November 10, 1998)*
Final data by state of residence. Neoplasms are abnormal tissue, tumors. Includes many cancers.

Death Rate by Malignant Neoplasms in 1996

National Rate = 203.5 Deaths per 100,000 Population*

<u>ALPHA ORDER</u>

RANK	STATE	RATE
14	Alabama	221.4
49	Alaska	106.7
39	Arizona	187.7
6	Arkansas	238.0
45	California	160.7
48	Colorado	148.3
15	Connecticut	218.9
8	Delaware	232.2
1	Florida	261.3
42	Georgia	169.5
47	Hawaii	156.7
44	Idaho	167.5
26	Illinois	207.7
20	Indiana	214.3
11	Iowa	227.9
27	Kansas	206.8
7	Kentucky	232.5
19	Louisiana	214.6
5	Maine	238.4
35	Maryland	200.9
9	Massachusetts	229.4
34	Michigan	201.2
38	Minnesota	190.3
21	Mississippi	212.4
13	Missouri	222.8
33	Montana	201.7
32	Nebraska	201.8
36	Nevada	199.5
28	New Hampshire	205.9
10	New Jersey	228.7
46	New Mexico	160.4
22	New York	210.3
25	North Carolina	207.9
17	North Dakota	216.6
12	Ohio	226.7
18	Oklahoma	216.3
23	Oregon	210.0
4	Pennsylvania	253.5
3	Rhode Island	254.6
30	South Carolina	203.9
24	South Dakota	209.0
15	Tennessee	218.9
43	Texas	168.2
50	Utah	104.1
28	Vermont	205.9
37	Virginia	190.6
40	Washington	182.3
2	West Virginia	256.7
31	Wisconsin	202.6
41	Wyoming	181.0

<u>RANK ORDER</u>

RANK	STATE	RATE
1	Florida	261.3
2	West Virginia	256.7
3	Rhode Island	254.6
4	Pennsylvania	253.5
5	Maine	238.4
6	Arkansas	238.0
7	Kentucky	232.5
8	Delaware	232.2
9	Massachusetts	229.4
10	New Jersey	228.7
11	Iowa	227.9
12	Ohio	226.7
13	Missouri	222.8
14	Alabama	221.4
15	Connecticut	218.9
15	Tennessee	218.9
17	North Dakota	216.6
18	Oklahoma	216.3
19	Louisiana	214.6
20	Indiana	214.3
21	Mississippi	212.4
22	New York	210.3
23	Oregon	210.0
24	South Dakota	209.0
25	North Carolina	207.9
26	Illinois	207.7
27	Kansas	206.8
28	New Hampshire	205.9
28	Vermont	205.9
30	South Carolina	203.9
31	Wisconsin	202.6
32	Nebraska	201.8
33	Montana	201.7
34	Michigan	201.2
35	Maryland	200.9
36	Nevada	199.5
37	Virginia	190.6
38	Minnesota	190.3
39	Arizona	187.7
40	Washington	182.3
41	Wyoming	181.0
42	Georgia	169.5
43	Texas	168.2
44	Idaho	167.5
45	California	160.7
46	New Mexico	160.4
47	Hawaii	156.7
48	Colorado	148.3
49	Alaska	106.7
50	Utah	104.1

District of Columbia   255.7

Source: Morgan Quitno Press using data from U.S. Dept of Health & Human Serv's, Nat'l Center for Health Statistics
    "National Vital Statistics Report" (Vol. 47, No. 9, November 10, 1998)
*Final data by state of residence. Neoplasms are abnormal tissue, tumors. Includes many cancers. Not age-adjusted.

Age-Adjusted Death Rate by Malignant Neoplasms in 1996

National Rate = 127.9 Deaths per 100,000 Population*

ALPHA ORDER			RANK ORDER		
RANK	STATE	RATE	RANK	STATE	RATE
6	Alabama	138.5	1	Kentucky	149.0
30	Alaska	125.1	2	Louisiana	148.5
45	Arizona	114.6	3	Delaware	147.4
8	Arkansas	137.7	4	Mississippi	141.4
44	California	114.9	5	Tennessee	139.3
48	Colorado	105.9	6	Alabama	138.5
33	Connecticut	122.9	7	South Carolina	137.8
3	Delaware	147.4	8	Arkansas	137.7
28	Florida	127.5	8	West Virginia	137.7
25	Georgia	129.7	10	Rhode Island	137.4
49	Hawaii	100.5	11	Nevada	136.7
46	Idaho	109.4	12	Ohio	136.4
19	Illinois	133.3	13	Maryland	136.3
16	Indiana	134.9	14	New Hampshire	136.1
36	Iowa	120.2	15	Maine	135.5
34	Kansas	121.9	16	Indiana	134.9
1	Kentucky	149.0	17	North Carolina	133.8
2	Louisiana	148.5	18	New Jersey	133.7
15	Maine	135.5	19	Illinois	133.3
13	Maryland	136.3	19	Pennsylvania	133.3
24	Massachusetts	130.9	21	Missouri	132.6
23	Michigan	131.7	22	Virginia	132.0
41	Minnesota	118.3	23	Michigan	131.7
4	Mississippi	141.4	24	Massachusetts	130.9
21	Missouri	132.6	25	Georgia	129.7
42	Montana	116.0	26	Oklahoma	129.6
43	Nebraska	115.8	27	Vermont	128.3
11	Nevada	136.7	28	Florida	127.5
14	New Hampshire	136.1	29	New York	126.6
18	New Jersey	133.7	30	Alaska	125.1
47	New Mexico	108.8	31	Texas	124.7
29	New York	126.6	32	Oregon	123.5
17	North Carolina	133.8	33	Connecticut	122.9
39	North Dakota	118.8	34	Kansas	121.9
12	Ohio	136.4	35	Wisconsin	121.4
26	Oklahoma	129.6	36	Iowa	120.2
32	Oregon	123.5	37	Washington	119.6
19	Pennsylvania	133.3	38	South Dakota	119.5
10	Rhode Island	137.4	39	North Dakota	118.8
7	South Carolina	137.8	40	Wyoming	118.7
38	South Dakota	119.5	41	Minnesota	118.3
5	Tennessee	139.3	42	Montana	116.0
31	Texas	124.7	43	Nebraska	115.8
50	Utah	89.8	44	California	114.9
27	Vermont	128.3	45	Arizona	114.6
22	Virginia	132.0	46	Idaho	109.4
37	Washington	119.6	47	New Mexico	108.8
8	West Virginia	137.7	48	Colorado	105.9
35	Wisconsin	121.4	49	Hawaii	100.5
40	Wyoming	118.7	50	Utah	89.8
				District of Columbia	153.1

Source: U.S. Department of Health and Human Services, National Center for Health Statistics
"National Vital Statistics Report" (Vol. 47, No. 9, November 10, 1998)
*Final data by state of residence. Neoplasms are abnormal tissue, tumors. Includes many cancers.

Deaths by Pneumonia and Influenza in 1996

National Total = 83,727 Deaths*

ALPHA ORDER

RANK	STATE	DEATHS	% of USA
21	Alabama	1,329	1.6%
50	Alaska	36	0.0%
23	Arizona	1,273	1.5%
31	Arkansas	947	1.1%
1	California	11,170	13.3%
29	Colorado	981	1.2%
25	Connecticut	1,143	1.4%
47	Delaware	199	0.2%
6	Florida	3,812	4.6%
13	Georgia	2,101	2.5%
40	Hawaii	334	0.4%
42	Idaho	310	0.4%
5	Illinois	3,942	4.7%
17	Indiana	1,704	2.0%
26	Iowa	1,142	1.4%
32	Kansas	910	1.1%
22	Kentucky	1,316	1.6%
28	Louisiana	1,046	1.2%
38	Maine	401	0.5%
19	Maryland	1,442	1.7%
9	Massachusetts	2,797	3.3%
8	Michigan	3,013	3.6%
24	Minnesota	1,245	1.5%
33	Mississippi	888	1.1%
12	Missouri	2,164	2.6%
44	Montana	248	0.3%
35	Nebraska	572	0.7%
39	Nevada	374	0.4%
46	New Hampshire	204	0.2%
11	New Jersey	2,440	2.9%
37	New Mexico	419	0.5%
2	New York	6,553	7.8%
10	North Carolina	2,529	3.0%
45	North Dakota	242	0.3%
7	Ohio	3,330	4.0%
20	Oklahoma	1,357	1.6%
30	Oregon	965	1.2%
3	Pennsylvania	4,408	5.3%
41	Rhode Island	323	0.4%
27	South Carolina	1,104	1.3%
43	South Dakota	285	0.3%
15	Tennessee	1,840	2.2%
4	Texas	4,046	4.8%
36	Utah	472	0.6%
48	Vermont	169	0.2%
14	Virginia	1,880	2.2%
18	Washington	1,623	1.9%
34	West Virginia	617	0.7%
16	Wisconsin	1,758	2.1%
49	Wyoming	121	0.1%

RANK ORDER

RANK	STATE	DEATHS	% of USA
1	California	11,170	13.3%
2	New York	6,553	7.8%
3	Pennsylvania	4,408	5.3%
4	Texas	4,046	4.8%
5	Illinois	3,942	4.7%
6	Florida	3,812	4.6%
7	Ohio	3,330	4.0%
8	Michigan	3,013	3.6%
9	Massachusetts	2,797	3.3%
10	North Carolina	2,529	3.0%
11	New Jersey	2,440	2.9%
12	Missouri	2,164	2.6%
13	Georgia	2,101	2.5%
14	Virginia	1,880	2.2%
15	Tennessee	1,840	2.2%
16	Wisconsin	1,758	2.1%
17	Indiana	1,704	2.0%
18	Washington	1,623	1.9%
19	Maryland	1,442	1.7%
20	Oklahoma	1,357	1.6%
21	Alabama	1,329	1.6%
22	Kentucky	1,316	1.6%
23	Arizona	1,273	1.5%
24	Minnesota	1,245	1.5%
25	Connecticut	1,143	1.4%
26	Iowa	1,142	1.4%
27	South Carolina	1,104	1.3%
28	Louisiana	1,046	1.2%
29	Colorado	981	1.2%
30	Oregon	965	1.2%
31	Arkansas	947	1.1%
32	Kansas	910	1.1%
33	Mississippi	888	1.1%
34	West Virginia	617	0.7%
35	Nebraska	572	0.7%
36	Utah	472	0.6%
37	New Mexico	419	0.5%
38	Maine	401	0.5%
39	Nevada	374	0.4%
40	Hawaii	334	0.4%
41	Rhode Island	323	0.4%
42	Idaho	310	0.4%
43	South Dakota	285	0.3%
44	Montana	248	0.3%
45	North Dakota	242	0.3%
46	New Hampshire	204	0.2%
47	Delaware	199	0.2%
48	Vermont	169	0.2%
49	Wyoming	121	0.1%
50	Alaska	36	0.0%
	District of Columbia	203	0.2%

Source: U.S. Department of Health and Human Services, National Center for Health Statistics
   "National Vital Statistics Report" (Vol. 47, No. 9, November 10, 1998)
*Final data by state of residence.

Death Rate by Pneumonia and Influenza in 1996

National Rate = 31.6 Deaths per 100,000 Population*

ALPHA ORDER

RANK	STATE	RATE
23	Alabama	31.0
50	Alaska	5.9
32	Arizona	28.7
6	Arkansas	37.8
10	California	35.2
42	Colorado	25.7
12	Connecticut	35.0
38	Delaware	27.4
40	Florida	26.4
33	Georgia	28.6
37	Hawaii	28.1
41	Idaho	26.1
19	Illinois	33.0
30	Indiana	29.2
4	Iowa	40.1
10	Kansas	35.2
17	Kentucky	33.9
45	Louisiana	24.1
22	Maine	32.4
34	Maryland	28.5
1	Massachusetts	46.0
23	Michigan	31.0
39	Minnesota	26.8
20	Mississippi	32.8
3	Missouri	40.3
35	Montana	28.3
13	Nebraska	34.7
46	Nevada	23.4
49	New Hampshire	17.6
25	New Jersey	30.5
44	New Mexico	24.5
9	New York	36.1
15	North Carolina	34.6
7	North Dakota	37.6
27	Ohio	29.8
2	Oklahoma	41.2
26	Oregon	30.2
8	Pennsylvania	36.6
21	Rhode Island	32.7
28	South Carolina	29.5
5	South Dakota	38.7
13	Tennessee	34.7
48	Texas	21.3
47	Utah	23.3
31	Vermont	28.8
36	Virginia	28.2
29	Washington	29.4
17	West Virginia	33.9
16	Wisconsln	34.0
43	Wyoming	25.2

RANK ORDER

RANK	STATE	RATE
1	Massachusetts	46.0
2	Oklahoma	41.2
3	Missouri	40.3
4	Iowa	40.1
5	South Dakota	38.7
6	Arkansas	37.8
7	North Dakota	37.6
8	Pennsylvania	36.6
9	New York	36.1
10	California	35.2
10	Kansas	35.2
12	Connecticut	35.0
13	Nebraska	34.7
13	Tennessee	34.7
15	North Carolina	34.6
16	Wisconsin	34.0
17	Kentucky	33.9
17	West Virginia	33.9
19	Illinois	33.0
20	Mississippi	32.8
21	Rhode Island	32.7
22	Maine	32.4
23	Alabama	31.0
23	Michigan	31.0
25	New Jersey	30.5
26	Oregon	30.2
27	Ohio	29.8
28	South Carolina	29.5
29	Washington	29.4
30	Indiana	29.2
31	Vermont	28.8
32	Arizona	28.7
33	Georgia	28.6
34	Maryland	28.5
35	Montana	28.3
36	Virginia	28.2
37	Hawaii	28.1
38	Delaware	27.4
39	Minnesota	26.8
40	Florida	26.4
41	Idaho	26.1
42	Colorado	25.7
43	Wyoming	25.2
44	New Mexico	24.5
45	Louisiana	24.1
46	Nevada	23.4
47	Utah	23.3
48	Texas	21.3
49	New Hampshire	17.6
50	Alaska	5.9
	District of Columbia	37.6

Source: Morgan Quitno Press using data from U.S. Dept of Health & Human Serv's, Nat'l Center for Health Statistics
    "National Vital Statistics Report" (Vol. 47, No. 9, November 10, 1998)
*Final data by state of residence. Not age-adjusted.

Age-Adjusted Death Rate by Pneumonia and Influenza in 1996

National Rate = 12.8 Deaths per 100,000 Population*

ALPHA ORDER

RANK	STATE	RATE
17	Alabama	12.9
50	Alaska	6.2
20	Arizona	12.6
11	Arkansas	13.8
1	California	15.9
21	Colorado	12.5
33	Connecticut	11.7
35	Delaware	11.6
47	Florida	8.9
1	Georgia	15.9
27	Hawaii	11.9
35	Idaho	11.6
11	Illinois	13.8
26	Indiana	12.0
23	Iowa	12.1
30	Kansas	11.8
16	Kentucky	13.4
37	Louisiana	11.4
43	Maine	10.5
15	Maryland	13.5
7	Massachusetts	14.5
11	Michigan	13.8
47	Minnesota	8.9
5	Mississippi	14.8
10	Missouri	14.0
46	Montana	9.9
38	Nebraska	10.8
14	Nevada	13.7
49	New Hampshire	6.4
23	New Jersey	12.1
33	New Mexico	11.7
9	New York	14.1
4	North Carolina	14.9
38	North Dakota	10.8
27	Ohio	11.9
3	Oklahoma	15.5
41	Oregon	10.7
23	Pennsylvania	12.1
44	Rhode Island	10.3
7	South Carolina	14.5
21	South Dakota	12.5
6	Tennessee	14.7
38	Texas	10.8
18	Utah	12.8
41	Vermont	10.7
18	Virginia	12.8
27	Washington	11.9
30	West Virginia	11.8
30	Wisconsin	11.8
44	Wyoming	10.3

RANK ORDER

RANK	STATE	RATE
1	California	15.9
1	Georgia	15.9
3	Oklahoma	15.5
4	North Carolina	14.9
5	Mississippi	14.8
6	Tennessee	14.7
7	Massachusetts	14.5
7	South Carolina	14.5
9	New York	14.1
10	Missouri	14.0
11	Arkansas	13.8
11	Illinois	13.8
11	Michigan	13.8
14	Nevada	13.7
15	Maryland	13.5
16	Kentucky	13.4
17	Alabama	12.9
18	Utah	12.8
18	Virginia	12.8
20	Arizona	12.6
21	Colorado	12.5
21	South Dakota	12.5
23	Iowa	12.1
23	New Jersey	12.1
23	Pennsylvania	12.1
26	Indiana	12.0
27	Hawaii	11.9
27	Ohio	11.9
27	Washington	11.9
30	Kansas	11.8
30	West Virginia	11.8
30	Wisconsin	11.8
33	Connecticut	11.7
33	New Mexico	11.7
35	Delaware	11.6
35	Idaho	11.6
37	Louisiana	11.4
38	Nebraska	10.8
38	North Dakota	10.8
38	Texas	10.8
41	Oregon	10.7
41	Vermont	10.7
43	Maine	10.5
44	Rhode Island	10.3
44	Wyoming	10.3
46	Montana	9.9
47	Florida	8.9
47	Minnesota	8.9
49	New Hampshire	6.4
50	Alaska	6.2
	District of Columbia	17.0

Source: U.S. Department of Health and Human Services, National Center for Health Statistics
    "National Vital Statistics Report" (Vol. 47, No. 9, November 10, 1998)
Final data by state of residence.

Deaths by Complications of Pregnancy and Childbirth in 1996

National Total = 294 Deaths*

ALPHA ORDER

RANK ORDER

RANK	STATE	DEATHS	% of USA
16	Alabama	6	2.0%
34	Alaska	1	0.3%
12	Arizona	9	3.1%
34	Arkansas	1	0.3%
1	California	33	11.2%
17	Colorado	5	1.7%
34	Connecticut	1	0.3%
44	Delaware	0	0.0%
3	Florida	21	7.1%
6	Georgia	15	5.1%
34	Hawaii	1	0.3%
28	Idaho	2	0.7%
5	Illinois	18	6.1%
20	Indiana	4	1.4%
34	Iowa	1	0.3%
28	Kansas	2	0.7%
20	Kentucky	4	1.4%
13	Louisiana	8	2.7%
34	Maine	1	0.3%
7	Maryland	13	4.4%
15	Massachusetts	7	2.4%
17	Michigan	5	1.7%
24	Minnesota	3	1.0%
34	Mississippi	1	0.3%
9	Missouri	11	3.7%
34	Montana	1	0.3%
44	Nebraska	0	0.0%
34	Nevada	1	0.3%
44	New Hampshire	0	0.0%
13	New Jersey	8	2.7%
28	New Mexico	2	0.7%
2	New York	25	8.5%
9	North Carolina	11	3.7%
28	North Dakota	2	0.7%
17	Ohio	5	1.7%
24	Oklahoma	3	1.0%
28	Oregon	2	0.7%
8	Pennsylvania	12	4.1%
44	Rhode Island	0	0.0%
20	South Carolina	4	1.4%
44	South Dakota	0	0.0%
9	Tennessee	11	3.7%
4	Texas	20	6.8%
28	Utah	2	0.7%
44	Vermont	0	0.0%
20	Virginia	4	1.4%
24	Washington	3	1.0%
34	West Virginia	1	0.3%
24	Wisconsin	3	1.0%
44	Wyoming	0	0.0%

RANK	STATE	DEATHS	% of USA
1	California	33	11.2%
2	New York	25	8.5%
3	Florida	21	7.1%
4	Texas	20	6.8%
5	Illinois	18	6.1%
6	Georgia	15	5.1%
7	Maryland	13	4.4%
8	Pennsylvania	12	4.1%
9	Missouri	11	3.7%
9	North Carolina	11	3.7%
9	Tennessee	11	3.7%
12	Arizona	9	3.1%
13	Louisiana	8	2.7%
13	New Jersey	8	2.7%
15	Massachusetts	7	2.4%
16	Alabama	6	2.0%
17	Colorado	5	1.7%
17	Michigan	5	1.7%
17	Ohio	5	1.7%
20	Indiana	4	1.4%
20	Kentucky	4	1.4%
20	South Carolina	4	1.4%
20	Virginia	4	1.4%
24	Minnesota	3	1.0%
24	Oklahoma	3	1.0%
24	Washington	3	1.0%
24	Wisconsin	3	1.0%
28	Idaho	2	0.7%
28	Kansas	2	0.7%
28	New Mexico	2	0.7%
28	North Dakota	2	0.7%
28	Oregon	2	0.7%
28	Utah	2	0.7%
34	Alaska	1	0.3%
34	Arkansas	1	0.3%
34	Connecticut	1	0.3%
34	Hawaii	1	0.3%
34	Iowa	1	0.3%
34	Maine	1	0.3%
34	Mississippi	1	0.3%
34	Montana	1	0.3%
34	Nevada	1	0.3%
34	West Virginia	1	0.3%
44	Delaware	0	0.0%
44	Nebraska	0	0.0%
44	New Hampshire	0	0.0%
44	Rhode Island	0	0.0%
44	South Dakota	0	0.0%
44	Vermont	0	0.0%
44	Wyoming	0	0.0%
	District of Columbia	1	0.3%

Source: U.S. Department of Health and Human Services, National Center for Health Statistics
(http://wonder.cdc.gov/WONDER/)
*By state of residence.

Death Rate by Complications of Pregnancy and Childbirth in 1996

National Rate = 0.22 Deaths per 100,000 Female Population*

ALPHA ORDER

RANK	STATE	RATE
13	Alabama	0.27
8	Alaska	0.35
3	Arizona	0.40
40	Arkansas	0.08
19	California	0.21
15	Colorado	0.26
43	Connecticut	0.06
44	Delaware	0.00
12	Florida	0.28
3	Georgia	0.40
27	Hawaii	0.17
9	Idaho	0.34
10	Illinois	0.30
30	Indiana	0.13
41	Iowa	0.07
29	Kansas	0.15
22	Kentucky	0.20
7	Louisiana	0.36
28	Maine	0.16
2	Maryland	0.50
18	Massachusetts	0.22
38	Michigan	0.10
30	Minnesota	0.13
41	Mississippi	0.07
3	Missouri	0.40
16	Montana	0.23
44	Nebraska	0.00
30	Nevada	0.13
44	New Hampshire	0.00
24	New Jersey	0.19
16	New Mexico	0.23
13	New York	0.27
11	North Carolina	0.29
1	North Dakota	0.62
39	Ohio	0.09
26	Oklahoma	0.18
33	Oregon	0.12
24	Pennsylvania	0.19
44	Rhode Island	0.00
19	South Carolina	0.21
44	South Dakota	0.00
3	Tennessee	0.40
19	Texas	0.21
22	Utah	0.20
44	Vermont	0.00
33	Virginia	0.12
35	Washington	0.11
35	West Virginia	0.11
35	Wisconsin	0.11
44	Wyoming	0.00

RANK ORDER

RANK	STATE	RATE
1	North Dakota	0.62
2	Maryland	0.50
3	Arizona	0.40
3	Georgia	0.40
3	Missouri	0.40
3	Tennessee	0.40
7	Louisiana	0.36
8	Alaska	0.35
9	Idaho	0.34
10	Illinois	0.30
11	North Carolina	0.29
12	Florida	0.28
13	Alabama	0.27
13	New York	0.27
15	Colorado	0.26
16	Montana	0.23
16	New Mexico	0.23
18	Massachusetts	0.22
19	California	0.21
19	South Carolina	0.21
19	Texas	0.21
22	Kentucky	0.20
22	Utah	0.20
24	New Jersey	0.19
24	Pennsylvania	0.19
26	Oklahoma	0.18
27	Hawaii	0.17
28	Maine	0.16
29	Kansas	0.15
30	Indiana	0.13
30	Minnesota	0.13
30	Nevada	0.13
33	Oregon	0.12
33	Virginia	0.12
35	Washington	0.11
35	West Virginia	0.11
35	Wisconsin	0.11
38	Michigan	0.10
39	Ohio	0.09
40	Arkansas	0.08
41	Iowa	0.07
41	Mississippi	0.07
43	Connecticut	0.06
44	Delaware	0.00
44	Nebraska	0.00
44	New Hampshire	0.00
44	Rhode Island	0.00
44	South Dakota	0.00
44	Vermont	0.00
44	Wyoming	0.00

District of Columbia 0.35

Source: Morgan Quitno Press using data from U.S. Dept of Health & Human Serv's, Nat'l Center for Health Statistics
    (http://wonder.cdc.gov/WONDER/)
*By state of residence. Not-age adjusted. Due to low numbers of deaths, rates for all states should be interpreted with caution.

Age-Adjusted Death Rate by Complications of Pregnancy and Childbirth in 1996

National Rate = 0.3 Deaths per 100,000

ALPHA ORDER			RANK ORDER		
RANK	STATE	RATE	RANK	STATE	RATE
11	Alabama	0.3	1	North Dakota	0.7
11	Alaska	0.3	2	Maryland	0.6
3	Arizona	0.4	3	Arizona	0.4
30	Arkansas	0.1	3	Florida	0.4
18	California	0.2	3	Georgia	0.4
11	Colorado	0.3	3	Idaho	0.4
30	Connecticut	0.1	3	Illinois	0.4
44	Delaware	0.0	3	Louisiana	0.4
3	Florida	0.4	3	Missouri	0.4
3	Georgia	0.4	3	Tennessee	0.4
18	Hawaii	0.2	11	Alabama	0.3
3	Idaho	0.4	11	Alaska	0.3
3	Illinois	0.4	11	Colorado	0.3
30	Indiana	0.1	11	Montana	0.3
30	Iowa	0.1	11	New York	0.3
30	Kansas	0.1	11	North Carolina	0.3
18	Kentucky	0.2	11	Pennsylvania	0.3
3	Louisiana	0.4	18	California	0.2
18	Maine	0.2	18	Hawaii	0.2
2	Maryland	0.6	18	Kentucky	0.2
18	Massachusetts	0.2	18	Maine	0.2
30	Michigan	0.1	18	Massachusetts	0.2
30	Minnesota	0.1	18	New Jersey	0.2
30	Mississippi	0.1	18	New Mexico	0.2
3	Missouri	0.4	18	Oklahoma	0.2
11	Montana	0.3	18	South Carolina	0.2
44	Nebraska	0.0	18	Texas	0.2
30	Nevada	0.1	18	Utah	0.2
44	New Hampshire	0.0	18	Virginia	0.2
18	New Jersey	0.2	30	Arkansas	0.1
18	New Mexico	0.2	30	Connecticut	0.1
11	New York	0.3	30	Indiana	0.1
11	North Carolina	0.3	30	Iowa	0.1
1	North Dakota	0.7	30	Kansas	0.1
30	Ohio	0.1	30	Michigan	0.1
18	Oklahoma	0.2	30	Minnesota	0.1
30	Oregon	0.1	30	Mississippi	0.1
11	Pennsylvania	0.3	30	Nevada	0.1
44	Rhode Island	0.0	30	Ohio	0.1
18	South Carolina	0.2	30	Oregon	0.1
44	South Dakota	0.0	30	Washington	0.1
3	Tennessee	0.4	30	West Virginia	0.1
18	Texas	0.2	30	Wisconsin	0.1
18	Utah	0.2	44	Delaware	0.0
44	Vermont	0.0	44	Nebraska	0.0
18	Virginia	0.2	44	New Hampshire	0.0
30	Washington	0.1	44	Rhode Island	0.0
30	West Virginia	0.1	44	South Dakota	0.0
30	Wisconsin	0.1	44	Vermont	0.0
44	Wyoming	0.0	44	Wyoming	0.0
				District of Columbia	0.6

Source: U.S. Department of Health and Human Services, National Center for Health Statistics
   (http://wonder.cdc.gov/WONDER/)
By state of residence. Due to low numbers of deaths, rates for all states should be interpreted with caution.

Deaths by Tuberculosis in 1996

National Total = 1,202 Deaths*

ALPHA ORDER

ALPHA ORDER

RANK	STATE	DEATHS	% of USA
11	Alabama	32	2.7%
41	Alaska	3	0.2%
20	Arizona	18	1.5%
31	Arkansas	8	0.7%
1	California	185	15.4%
27	Colorado	12	1.0%
29	Connecticut	9	0.7%
43	Delaware	2	0.2%
4	Florida	90	7.5%
6	Georgia	40	3.3%
37	Hawaii	5	0.4%
46	Idaho	1	0.1%
5	Illinois	62	5.2%
19	Indiana	20	1.7%
37	Iowa	5	0.4%
35	Kansas	7	0.6%
23	Kentucky	16	1.3%
13	Louisiana	30	2.5%
31	Maine	8	0.7%
24	Maryland	15	1.2%
18	Massachusetts	22	1.8%
14	Michigan	28	2.3%
31	Minnesota	8	0.7%
15	Mississippi	25	2.1%
21	Missouri	17	1.4%
46	Montana	1	0.1%
43	Nebraska	2	0.2%
27	Nevada	12	1.0%
40	New Hampshire	4	0.3%
10	New Jersey	33	2.7%
31	New Mexico	8	0.7%
3	New York	97	8.1%
7	North Carolina	38	3.2%
43	North Dakota	2	0.2%
8	Ohio	36	3.0%
24	Oklahoma	15	1.2%
29	Oregon	9	0.7%
8	Pennsylvania	36	3.0%
37	Rhode Island	5	0.4%
16	South Carolina	23	1.9%
41	South Dakota	3	0.2%
16	Tennessee	23	1.9%
2	Texas	104	8.7%
49	Utah	0	0.0%
46	Vermont	1	0.1%
11	Virginia	32	2.7%
21	Washington	17	1.4%
35	West Virginia	7	0.6%
24	Wisconsin	15	1.2%
49	Wyoming	0	0.0%

RANK ORDER

RANK	STATE	DEATHS	% of USA
1	California	185	15.4%
2	Texas	104	8.7%
3	New York	97	8.1%
4	Florida	90	7.5%
5	Illinois	62	5.2%
6	Georgia	40	3.3%
7	North Carolina	38	3.2%
8	Ohio	36	3.0%
8	Pennsylvania	36	3.0%
10	New Jersey	33	2.7%
11	Alabama	32	2.7%
11	Virginia	32	2.7%
13	Louisiana	30	2.5%
14	Michigan	28	2.3%
15	Mississippi	25	2.1%
16	South Carolina	23	1.9%
16	Tennessee	23	1.9%
18	Massachusetts	22	1.8%
19	Indiana	20	1.7%
20	Arizona	18	1.5%
21	Missouri	17	1.4%
21	Washington	17	1.4%
23	Kentucky	16	1.3%
24	Maryland	15	1.2%
24	Oklahoma	15	1.2%
24	Wisconsin	15	1.2%
27	Colorado	12	1.0%
27	Nevada	12	1.0%
29	Connecticut	9	0.7%
29	Oregon	9	0.7%
31	Arkansas	8	0.7%
31	Maine	8	0.7%
31	Minnesota	8	0.7%
31	New Mexico	8	0.7%
35	Kansas	7	0.6%
35	West Virginia	7	0.6%
37	Hawaii	5	0.4%
37	Iowa	5	0.4%
37	Rhode Island	5	0.4%
40	New Hampshire	4	0.3%
41	Alaska	3	0.2%
41	South Dakota	3	0.2%
43	Delaware	2	0.2%
43	Nebraska	2	0.2%
43	North Dakota	2	0.2%
46	Idaho	1	0.1%
46	Montana	1	0.1%
46	Vermont	1	0.1%
49	Utah	0	0.0%
49	Wyoming	0	0.0%
	District of Columbia	11	0.9%

Source: U.S. Department of Health and Human Services, National Center for Health Statistics
    (http://wonder.cdc.gov/WONDER/)
*By state of residence.

Death Rate by Tuberculosis in 1996

National Rate = 0.45 Deaths per 100,000 Population*

ALPHA ORDER

RANK	STATE	RATE
2	Alabama	0.75
15	Alaska	0.50
21	Arizona	0.41
29	Arkansas	0.32
8	California	0.58
32	Colorado	0.31
39	Connecticut	0.28
39	Delaware	0.28
6	Florida	0.62
9	Georgia	0.55
20	Hawaii	0.42
48	Idaho	0.08
12	Illinois	0.52
27	Indiana	0.34
43	Iowa	0.18
42	Kansas	0.27
21	Kentucky	0.41
4	Louisiana	0.69
5	Maine	0.65
35	Maryland	0.30
26	Massachusetts	0.36
37	Michigan	0.29
44	Minnesota	0.17
1	Mississippi	0.92
29	Missouri	0.32
47	Montana	0.11
46	Nebraska	0.12
2	Nevada	0.75
27	New Hampshire	0.34
21	New Jersey	0.41
17	New Mexico	0.47
11	New York	0.53
12	North Carolina	0.52
32	North Dakota	0.31
29	Ohio	0.32
18	Oklahoma	0.46
39	Oregon	0.28
35	Pennsylvania	0.30
14	Rhode Island	0.51
6	South Carolina	0.62
21	South Dakota	0.41
19	Tennessee	0.43
9	Texas	0.55
49	Utah	0.00
44	Vermont	0.17
16	Virginia	0.48
32	Washington	0.31
25	West Virginia	0.38
37	Wisconsin	0.29
49	Wyoming	0.00

RANK ORDER

RANK	STATE	RATE
1	Mississippi	0.92
2	Alabama	0.75
2	Nevada	0.75
4	Louisiana	0.69
5	Maine	0.65
6	Florida	0.62
6	South Carolina	0.62
8	California	0.58
9	Georgia	0.55
9	Texas	0.55
11	New York	0.53
12	Illinois	0.52
12	North Carolina	0.52
14	Rhode Island	0.51
15	Alaska	0.50
16	Virginia	0.48
17	New Mexico	0.47
18	Oklahoma	0.46
19	Tennessee	0.43
20	Hawaii	0.42
21	Arizona	0.41
21	Kentucky	0.41
21	New Jersey	0.41
21	South Dakota	0.41
25	West Virginia	0.38
26	Massachusetts	0.36
27	Indiana	0.34
27	New Hampshire	0.34
29	Arkansas	0.32
29	Missouri	0.32
29	Ohio	0.32
32	Colorado	0.31
32	North Dakota	0.31
32	Washington	0.31
35	Maryland	0.30
35	Pennsylvania	0.30
37	Michigan	0.29
37	Wisconsin	0.29
39	Connecticut	0.28
39	Delaware	0.28
39	Oregon	0.28
42	Kansas	0.27
43	Iowa	0.18
44	Minnesota	0.17
44	Vermont	0.17
46	Nebraska	0.12
47	Montana	0.11
48	Idaho	0.08
49	Utah	0.00
49	Wyoming	0.00

District of Columbia 2.04

Source: Morgan Quitno Press using data from U.S. Dept of Health & Human Serv's, Nat'l Center for Health Statistics (http://wonder.cdc.gov/WONDER/)

*By state of residence. Not age-adjusted. Due to low numbers of deaths, rates for all states should be interpreted with caution.

Age-Adjusted Death Rate by Tuberculosis in 1997

National Rate = 0.2 Deaths per 100,000 Population*

ALPHA ORDER

RANK	STATE	RATE
12	Alabama	0.3
3	Alaska	0.5
12	Arizona	0.3
12	Arkansas	0.3
5	California	0.4
26	Colorado	0.1
39	Connecticut	0.0
26	Delaware	0.1
12	Florida	0.3
5	Georgia	0.4
5	Hawaii	0.4
39	Idaho	0.0
12	Illinois	0.3
26	Indiana	0.1
26	Iowa	0.1
39	Kansas	0.0
26	Kentucky	0.1
1	Louisiana	0.6
12	Maine	0.3
26	Maryland	0.1
26	Massachusetts	0.1
39	Michigan	0.0
39	Minnesota	0.0
5	Mississippi	0.4
39	Missouri	0.0
39	Montana	0.0
26	Nebraska	0.1
1	Nevada	0.6
20	New Hampshire	0.2
20	New Jersey	0.2
12	New Mexico	0.3
5	New York	0.4
5	North Carolina	0.4
26	North Dakota	0.1
26	Ohio	0.1
20	Oklahoma	0.2
26	Oregon	0.1
39	Pennsylvania	0.0
12	Rhode Island	0.3
5	South Carolina	0.4
20	South Dakota	0.2
20	Tennessee	0.2
3	Texas	0.5
39	Utah	0.0
26	Vermont	0.1
20	Virginia	0.2
39	Washington	0.0
26	West Virginia	0.1
39	Wisconsin	0.0
39	Wyoming	0.0

RANK ORDER

RANK	STATE	RATE
1	Louisiana	0.6
1	Nevada	0.6
3	Alaska	0.5
3	Texas	0.5
5	California	0.4
5	Georgia	0.4
5	Hawaii	0.4
5	Mississippi	0.4
5	New York	0.4
5	North Carolina	0.4
5	South Carolina	0.4
12	Alabama	0.3
12	Arizona	0.3
12	Arkansas	0.3
12	Florida	0.3
12	Illinois	0.3
12	Maine	0.3
12	New Mexico	0.3
12	Rhode Island	0.3
20	New Hampshire	0.2
20	New Jersey	0.2
20	Oklahoma	0.2
20	South Dakota	0.2
20	Tennessee	0.2
20	Virginia	0.2
26	Colorado	0.1
26	Delaware	0.1
26	Indiana	0.1
26	Iowa	0.1
26	Kentucky	0.1
26	Maryland	0.1
26	Massachusetts	0.1
26	Nebraska	0.1
26	North Dakota	0.1
26	Ohio	0.1
26	Oregon	0.1
26	Vermont	0.1
26	West Virginia	0.1
39	Connecticut	0.0
39	Idaho	0.0
39	Kansas	0.0
39	Michigan	0.0
39	Minnesota	0.0
39	Missouri	0.0
39	Montana	0.0
39	Pennsylvania	0.0
39	Utah	0.0
39	Washington	0.0
39	Wisconsin	0.0
39	Wyoming	0.0

District of Columbia   1.3

Source: U.S. Department of Health and Human Services, National Center for Health Statistics
    (http://wonder.cdc.gov/WONDER/)
*By state of residence. Due to low numbers of deaths, rates for all states should be interpreted with caution.

Deaths by Injury in 1996

National Total = 150,298 Deaths*

Source: U.S. Department of Health and Human Services, National Center for Health Statistics
(http://wonder.cdc.gov/WONDER/)
*By state of residence. Injury as used here includes Accidents (including motor vehicle), Suicides, Homicides and
"Other" undetermined.

Death Rate by Injury

National Rate = 57.6 Deaths by Injury per 100,000 Population*

RANK	STATE	RATE
4	Alabama	76.8
3	Alaska	79.8
6	Arizona	75.5
7	Arkansas	74.5
39	California	50.9
22	Colorado	62.8
44	Connecticut	47.2
30	Delaware	55.3
23	Florida	61.3
19	Georgia	63.9
43	Hawaii	48.3
15	Idaho	66.8
38	Illinois	51.2
27	Indiana	56.6
35	Iowa	52.6
24	Kansas	60.9
20	Kentucky	63.8
10	Louisiana	73.8
41	Maine	48.8
26	Maryland	58.9
49	Massachusetts	37.7
34	Michigan	52.8
40	Minnesota	50.5
2	Mississippi	82.2
14	Missouri	68.3
11	Montana	71.7
31	Nebraska	55.2
5	Nevada	75.8
48	New Hampshire	40.4
46	New Jersey	42.2
1	New Mexico	85.9
47	New York	41.6
17	North Carolina	64.9
37	North Dakota	52.0
45	Ohio	45.0
12	Oklahoma	71.3
18	Oregon	64.7
28	Pennsylvania	56.2
50	Rhode Island	36.9
13	South Carolina	70.1
16	South Dakota	66.2
9	Tennessee	73.9
25	Texas	59.2
31	Utah	55.2
42	Vermont	48.6
33	Virginia	54.6
29	Washington	56.0
21	West Virginia	63.1
36	Wisconsin	52.3
8	Wyoming	74.2

RANK	STATE	RATE
1	New Mexico	85.9
2	Mississippi	82.2
3	Alaska	79.8
4	Alabama	76.8
5	Nevada	75.8
6	Arizona	75.5
7	Arkansas	74.5
8	Wyoming	74.2
9	Tennessee	73.9
10	Louisiana	73.8
11	Montana	71.7
12	Oklahoma	71.3
13	South Carolina	70.1
14	Missouri	68.3
15	Idaho	66.8
16	South Dakota	66.2
17	North Carolina	64.9
18	Oregon	64.7
19	Georgia	63.9
20	Kentucky	63.8
21	West Virginia	63.1
22	Colorado	62.8
23	Florida	61.3
24	Kansas	60.9
25	Texas	59.2
26	Maryland	58.9
27	Indiana	56.6
28	Pennsylvania	56.2
29	Washington	56.0
30	Delaware	55.3
31	Nebraska	55.2
31	Utah	55.2
33	Virginia	54.6
34	Michigan	52.8
35	Iowa	52.6
36	Wisconsin	52.3
37	North Dakota	52.0
38	Illinois	51.2
39	California	50.9
40	Minnesota	50.5
41	Maine	48.8
42	Vermont	48.6
43	Hawaii	48.3
44	Connecticut	47.2
45	Ohio	45.0
46	New Jersey	42.2
47	New York	41.6
48	New Hampshire	40.4
49	Massachusetts	37.7
50	Rhode Island	36.9

| | District of Columbia | 102.7 |

*Source: Morgan Quitno Press using data from U.S. Dept of Health & Human Serv's, Nat'l Center for Health Statistics
    (http://wonder.cdc.gov/WONDER/)*
**By state of residence. Injury as used here includes Accidents (including motor vehicle), Suicides, Homicides and
"Other" undetermined. Not age-adjusted.*

Age-Adjusted Death Rate by Injury in 1996

National Age-Adjusted Rate = 50.8 Deaths per 100,000 Population*

ALPHA ORDER				RANK ORDER		
RANK	STATE	RATE		RANK	STATE	RATE
7	Alabama	69.8		1	Alaska	81.9
1	Alaska	81.9		2	New Mexico	80.8
6	Arizona	69.9		3	Mississippi	76.8
8	Arkansas	68.3		4	Nevada	72.2
32	California	48.0		5	Louisiana	70.4
19	Colorado	56.5		6	Arizona	69.9
43	Connecticut	40.3		7	Alabama	69.8
30	Delaware	48.7		8	Arkansas	68.3
24	Florida	54.3		9	Wyoming	67.7
15	Georgia	59.9		10	Tennessee	66.5
40	Hawaii	42.2		11	South Carolina	65.0
15	Idaho	59.9		12	Oklahoma	64.1
34	Illinois	47.4		13	Montana	63.4
28	Indiana	49.9		14	Missouri	60.0
39	Iowa	42.9		15	Georgia	59.9
27	Kansas	52.6		15	Idaho	59.9
21	Kentucky	55.8		17	North Carolina	57.9
5	Louisiana	70.4		18	South Dakota	57.1
44	Maine	39.8		19	Colorado	56.5
25	Maryland	54.0		19	Oregon	56.5
49	Massachusetts	30.8		21	Kentucky	55.8
35	Michigan	47.3		22	Texas	55.0
41	Minnesota	41.3		23	West Virginia	54.6
3	Mississippi	76.8		24	Florida	54.3
14	Missouri	60.0		25	Maryland	54.0
13	Montana	63.4		26	Utah	53.2
36	Nebraska	45.2		27	Kansas	52.6
4	Nevada	72.2		28	Indiana	49.9
48	New Hampshire	35.1		29	Washington	49.5
47	New Jersey	36.4		30	Delaware	48.7
2	New Mexico	80.8		31	Pennsylvania	48.2
46	New York	37.1		32	California	48.0
17	North Carolina	57.9		33	Virginia	47.9
38	North Dakota	43.9		34	Illinois	47.4
45	Ohio	38.7		35	Michigan	47.3
12	Oklahoma	64.1		36	Nebraska	45.2
19	Oregon	56.5		37	Wisconsin	44.1
31	Pennsylvania	48.2		38	North Dakota	43.9
50	Rhode Island	29.6		39	Iowa	42.9
11	South Carolina	65.0		40	Hawaii	42.2
18	South Dakota	57.1		41	Minnesota	41.3
10	Tennessee	66.5		42	Vermont	40.9
22	Texas	55.0		43	Connecticut	40.3
26	Utah	53.2		44	Maine	39.8
42	Vermont	40.9		45	Ohio	38.7
33	Virginia	47.9		46	New York	37.1
29	Washington	49.5		47	New Jersey	36.4
23	West Virginia	54.6		48	New Hampshire	35.1
37	Wisconsin	44.1		49	Massachusetts	30.8
9	Wyoming	67.7		50	Rhode Island	29.6
					District of Columbia	108.7

Source: U.S. Department of Health and Human Services, National Center for Health Statistics
        (http://wonder.cdc.gov/WONDER/)
*By state of residence. Injury as used here includes Accidents (including motor vehicle), Suicides, Homicides and "Other" undetermined.

Deaths by Accidents in 1996

National Total = 94,948 Deaths*

ALPHA ORDER

RANK	STATE	DEATHS	% of USA
15	Alabama	2,198	2.3%
44	Alaska	317	0.3%
16	Arizona	2,123	2.2%
30	Arkansas	1,262	1.3%
1	California	9,487	10.0%
26	Colorado	1,431	1.5%
33	Connecticut	1,046	1.1%
48	Delaware	241	0.3%
3	Florida	5,407	5.7%
10	Georgia	2,995	3.2%
42	Hawaii	368	0.4%
39	Idaho	562	0.6%
6	Illinois	3,683	3.9%
17	Indiana	2,092	2.2%
31	Iowa	1,091	1.1%
32	Kansas	1,075	1.1%
21	Kentucky	1,737	1.8%
20	Louisiana	1,815	1.9%
41	Maine	395	0.4%
27	Maryland	1,420	1.5%
29	Massachusetts	1,279	1.3%
9	Michigan	3,081	3.2%
23	Minnesota	1,642	1.7%
25	Mississippi	1,509	1.6%
12	Missouri	2,392	2.5%
40	Montana	398	0.4%
36	Nebraska	648	0.7%
38	Nevada	604	0.6%
45	New Hampshire	285	0.3%
13	New Jersey	2,289	2.4%
34	New Mexico	958	1.0%
4	New York	4,738	5.0%
8	North Carolina	3,132	3.3%
47	North Dakota	243	0.3%
7	Ohio	3,407	3.6%
24	Oklahoma	1,580	1.7%
28	Oregon	1,353	1.4%
5	Pennsylvania	4,436	4.7%
49	Rhode Island	208	0.2%
22	South Carolina	1,717	1.8%
43	South Dakota	342	0.4%
11	Tennessee	2,637	2.8%
2	Texas	7,269	7.7%
37	Utah	644	0.7%
50	Vermont	194	0.2%
14	Virginia	2,237	2.4%
18	Washington	1,949	2.1%
35	West Virginia	763	0.8%
19	Wisconsin	1,845	1.9%
46	Wyoming	245	0.3%

RANK ORDER

RANK	STATE	DEATHS	% of USA
1	California	9,487	10.0%
2	Texas	7,269	7.7%
3	Florida	5,407	5.7%
4	New York	4,738	5.0%
5	Pennsylvania	4,436	4.7%
6	Illinois	3,683	3.9%
7	Ohio	3,407	3.6%
8	North Carolina	3,132	3.3%
9	Michigan	3,081	3.2%
10	Georgia	2,995	3.2%
11	Tennessee	2,637	2.8%
12	Missouri	2,392	2.5%
13	New Jersey	2,289	2.4%
14	Virginia	2,237	2.4%
15	Alabama	2,198	2.3%
16	Arizona	2,123	2.2%
17	Indiana	2,092	2.2%
18	Washington	1,949	2.1%
19	Wisconsin	1,845	1.9%
20	Louisiana	1,815	1.9%
21	Kentucky	1,737	1.8%
22	South Carolina	1,717	1.8%
23	Minnesota	1,642	1.7%
24	Oklahoma	1,580	1.7%
25	Mississippi	1,509	1.6%
26	Colorado	1,431	1.5%
27	Maryland	1,420	1.5%
28	Oregon	1,353	1.4%
29	Massachusetts	1,279	1.3%
30	Arkansas	1,262	1.3%
31	Iowa	1,091	1.1%
32	Kansas	1,075	1.1%
33	Connecticut	1,046	1.1%
34	New Mexico	958	1.0%
35	West Virginia	763	0.8%
36	Nebraska	648	0.7%
37	Utah	644	0.7%
38	Nevada	604	0.6%
39	Idaho	562	0.6%
40	Montana	398	0.4%
41	Maine	395	0.4%
42	Hawaii	368	0.4%
43	South Dakota	342	0.4%
44	Alaska	317	0.3%
45	New Hampshire	285	0.3%
46	Wyoming	245	0.3%
47	North Dakota	243	0.3%
48	Delaware	241	0.3%
49	Rhode Island	208	0.2%
50	Vermont	194	0.2%
	District of Columbia	179	0.2%

Source: U.S. Department of Health and Human Services, National Center for Health Statistics
"National Vital Statistics Report" (Vol. 47, No. 9, November 10, 1998)
Final data by state of residence. Includes motor vehicle deaths, poisoning, falls, drowning and other accidents.

Death Rate by Accidents in 1996

National Rate = 35.8 Deaths per 100,000 Population*

ALPHA ORDER				RANK ORDER		
RANK	STATE	RATE		RANK	STATE	RATE
4	Alabama	51.2		1	New Mexico	56.1
3	Alaska	52.4		2	Mississippi	55.7
8	Arizona	47.9		3	Alaska	52.4
6	Arkansas	50.4		4	Alabama	51.2
44	California	29.9		5	Wyoming	51.0
27	Colorado	37.5		6	Arkansas	50.4
37	Connecticut	32.0		7	Tennessee	49.7
35	Delaware	33.1		8	Arizona	47.9
27	Florida	37.5		8	Oklahoma	47.9
21	Georgia	40.8		10	Idaho	47.4
41	Hawaii	31.0		11	South Dakota	46.4
10	Idaho	47.4		12	South Carolina	45.9
42	Illinois	30.9		13	Montana	45.4
30	Indiana	35.9		14	Kentucky	44.7
23	Iowa	38.3		15	Missouri	44.6
20	Kansas	41.6		16	North Carolina	42.9
14	Kentucky	44.7		17	Oregon	42.3
19	Louisiana	41.8		18	West Virginia	41.9
38	Maine	31.9		19	Louisiana	41.8
46	Maryland	28.1		20	Kansas	41.6
49	Massachusetts	21.0		21	Georgia	40.8
40	Michigan	31.7		22	Nebraska	39.3
32	Minnesota	35.3		23	Iowa	38.3
2	Mississippi	55.7		24	Texas	38.2
15	Missouri	44.6		25	North Dakota	37.8
13	Montana	45.4		26	Nevada	37.7
22	Nebraska	39.3		27	Colorado	37.5
26	Nevada	37.7		27	Florida	37.5
48	New Hampshire	24.6		29	Pennsylvania	36.9
45	New Jersey	28.6		30	Indiana	35.9
1	New Mexico	56.1		31	Wisconsin	35.7
47	New York	26.1		32	Minnesota	35.3
16	North Carolina	42.9		32	Washington	35.3
25	North Dakota	37.8		34	Virginia	33.6
43	Ohio	30.5		35	Delaware	33.1
8	Oklahoma	47.9		35	Vermont	33.1
17	Oregon	42.3		37	Connecticut	32.0
29	Pennsylvania	36.9		38	Maine	31.9
49	Rhode Island	21.0		39	Utah	31.8
12	South Carolina	45.9		40	Michigan	31.7
11	South Dakota	46.4		41	Hawaii	31.0
7	Tennessee	49.7		42	Illinois	30.9
24	Texas	38.2		43	Ohio	30.5
39	Utah	31.8		44	California	29.9
35	Vermont	33.1		45	New Jersey	28.6
34	Virginia	33.6		46	Maryland	28.1
32	Washington	35.3		47	New York	26.1
18	West Virginia	41.9		48	New Hampshire	24.6
31	Wisconsin	35.7		49	Massachusetts	21.0
5	Wyoming	51.0		49	Rhode Island	21.0
				District of Columbia		33.2

Source: Morgan Quitno Press using data from U.S. Dept of Health & Human Serv's, Nat'l Center for Health Statistics
"National Vital Statistics Report" (Vol. 47, No. 9, November 10, 1998)
*Final data by state of residence. Includes motor vehicle deaths, poisoning, falls, drowning and other accidents.
Not age-adjusted.

Age-Adjusted Death Rate by Accidents in 1996

National Rate = 30.4 Deaths per 100,000 Population*

ALPHA ORDER

RANK	STATE	RATE
5	Alabama	45.0
1	Alaska	53.1
8	Arizona	41.6
6	Arkansas	43.9
36	California	27.1
24	Colorado	32.5
42	Connecticut	25.1
33	Delaware	28.5
25	Florida	31.5
16	Georgia	37.1
41	Hawaii	25.6
10	Idaho	41.5
38	Illinois	26.3
28	Indiana	29.6
31	Iowa	29.1
23	Kansas	33.9
12	Kentucky	38.2
15	Louisiana	37.7
43	Maine	24.7
45	Maryland	23.4
49	Massachusetts	14.7
36	Michigan	27.1
38	Minnesota	26.3
3	Mississippi	50.2
17	Missouri	36.7
12	Montana	38.2
30	Nebraska	29.5
20	Nevada	34.9
48	New Hampshire	20.0
46	New Jersey	23.0
2	New Mexico	51.2
47	New York	21.4
18	North Carolina	36.3
26	North Dakota	29.9
43	Ohio	24.7
11	Oklahoma	41.1
19	Oregon	35.5
32	Pennsylvania	28.8
50	Rhode Island	14.3
8	South Carolina	41.6
12	South Dakota	38.2
7	Tennessee	42.9
22	Texas	34.3
28	Utah	29.6
40	Vermont	26.2
35	Virginia	27.7
27	Washington	29.7
21	West Virginia	34.8
34	Wisconsin	27.8
4	Wyoming	46.4

RANK ORDER

RANK	STATE	RATE
1	Alaska	53.1
2	New Mexico	51.2
3	Mississippi	50.2
4	Wyoming	46.4
5	Alabama	45.0
6	Arkansas	43.9
7	Tennessee	42.9
8	Arizona	41.6
8	South Carolina	41.6
10	Idaho	41.5
11	Oklahoma	41.1
12	Kentucky	38.2
12	Montana	38.2
12	South Dakota	38.2
15	Louisiana	37.7
16	Georgia	37.1
17	Missouri	36.7
18	North Carolina	36.3
19	Oregon	35.5
20	Nevada	34.9
21	West Virginia	34.8
22	Texas	34.3
23	Kansas	33.9
24	Colorado	32.5
25	Florida	31.5
26	North Dakota	29.9
27	Washington	29.7
28	Indiana	29.6
28	Utah	29.6
30	Nebraska	29.5
31	Iowa	29.1
32	Pennsylvania	28.8
33	Delaware	28.5
34	Wisconsin	27.8
35	Virginia	27.7
36	California	27.1
36	Michigan	27.1
38	Illinois	26.3
38	Minnesota	26.3
40	Vermont	26.2
41	Hawaii	25.6
42	Connecticut	25.1
43	Maine	24.7
43	Ohio	24.7
45	Maryland	23.4
46	New Jersey	23.0
47	New York	21.4
48	New Hampshire	20.0
49	Massachusetts	14.7
50	Rhode Island	14.3

	District of Columbia	26.7

Source: U.S. Department of Health and Human Services, National Center for Health Statistics
   "National Vital Statistics Report" (Vol. 47, No. 9, November 10, 1998)
*Final data by state of residence. Includes motor vehicle deaths, poisoning, falls, drowning and other accidents.

Deaths by Motor Vehicle Accidents in 1996

National Total = 43,649 Deaths*

ALPHA ORDER

RANK	STATE	DEATHS	% of USA
12	Alabama	1,176	2.7%
48	Alaska	98	0.2%
14	Arizona	996	2.3%
27	Arkansas	636	1.5%
1	California	4,224	9.7%
25	Colorado	669	1.5%
37	Connecticut	326	0.7%
47	Delaware	105	0.2%
3	Florida	2,809	6.4%
7	Georgia	1,588	3.6%
43	Hawaii	139	0.3%
39	Idaho	282	0.6%
5	Illinois	1,600	3.7%
15	Indiana	969	2.2%
31	Iowa	490	1.1%
30	Kansas	521	1.2%
22	Kentucky	808	1.9%
16	Louisiana	911	2.1%
41	Maine	177	0.4%
26	Maryland	652	1.5%
32	Massachusetts	458	1.0%
8	Michigan	1,579	3.6%
28	Minnesota	634	1.5%
19	Mississippi	867	2.0%
13	Missouri	1,127	2.6%
40	Montana	191	0.4%
38	Nebraska	301	0.7%
36	Nevada	328	0.8%
44	New Hampshire	134	0.3%
20	New Jersey	834	1.9%
33	New Mexico	443	1.0%
4	New York	1,761	4.0%
9	North Carolina	1,511	3.5%
46	North Dakota	108	0.2%
10	Ohio	1,429	3.3%
21	Oklahoma	809	1.9%
29	Oregon	533	1.2%
6	Pennsylvania	1,594	3.7%
50	Rhode Island	78	0.2%
17	South Carolina	901	2.1%
42	South Dakota	172	0.4%
11	Tennessee	1,308	3.0%
2	Texas	3,956	9.1%
34	Utah	342	0.8%
49	Vermont	84	0.2%
18	Virginia	886	2.0%
24	Washington	793	1.8%
35	West Virginia	337	0.8%
23	Wisconsin	798	1.8%
45	Wyoming	118	0.3%

RANK ORDER

RANK	STATE	DEATHS	% of USA
1	California	4,224	9.7%
2	Texas	3,956	9.1%
3	Florida	2,809	6.4%
4	New York	1,761	4.0%
5	Illinois	1,600	3.7%
6	Pennsylvania	1,594	3.7%
7	Georgia	1,588	3.6%
8	Michigan	1,579	3.6%
9	North Carolina	1,511	3.5%
10	Ohio	1,429	3.3%
11	Tennessee	1,308	3.0%
12	Alabama	1,176	2.7%
13	Missouri	1,127	2.6%
14	Arizona	996	2.3%
15	Indiana	969	2.2%
16	Louisiana	911	2.1%
17	South Carolina	901	2.1%
18	Virginia	886	2.0%
19	Mississippi	867	2.0%
20	New Jersey	834	1.9%
21	Oklahoma	809	1.9%
22	Kentucky	808	1.9%
23	Wisconsin	798	1.8%
24	Washington	793	1.8%
25	Colorado	669	1.5%
26	Maryland	652	1.5%
27	Arkansas	636	1.5%
28	Minnesota	634	1.5%
29	Oregon	533	1.2%
30	Kansas	521	1.2%
31	Iowa	490	1.1%
32	Massachusetts	458	1.0%
33	New Mexico	443	1.0%
34	Utah	342	0.8%
35	West Virginia	337	0.8%
36	Nevada	328	0.8%
37	Connecticut	326	0.7%
38	Nebraska	301	0.7%
39	Idaho	282	0.6%
40	Montana	191	0.4%
41	Maine	177	0.4%
42	South Dakota	172	0.4%
43	Hawaii	139	0.3%
44	New Hampshire	134	0.3%
45	Wyoming	118	0.3%
46	North Dakota	108	0.2%
47	Delaware	105	0.2%
48	Alaska	98	0.2%
49	Vermont	84	0.2%
50	Rhode Island	78	0.2%
	District of Columbia	59	0.1%

Source: U.S. Department of Health and Human Services, National Center for Health Statistics
"National Vital Statistics Report" (Vol. 47, No. 9, November 10, 1998)
Final data by state of residence. These numbers are compiled from death certificates by the Centers for Disease Control and Prevention. They may differ from motor vehicle deaths collected by the U.S. Department of Transportation from other sources.

Death Rate by Motor Vehicle Accidents in 1996

National Rate = 16.5 Deaths per 100,000 Population*

ALPHA ORDER		
RANK	STATE	RATE
2	Alabama	27.4
30	Alaska	16.2
11	Arizona	22.5
4	Arkansas	25.4
39	California	13.3
24	Colorado	17.5
47	Connecticut	10.0
33	Delaware	14.4
21	Florida	19.5
13	Georgia	21.7
44	Hawaii	11.7
9	Idaho	23.8
38	Illinois	13.4
29	Indiana	16.6
25	Iowa	17.2
20	Kansas	20.2
16	Kentucky	20.8
14	Louisiana	21.0
35	Maine	14.3
42	Maryland	12.9
50	Massachusetts	7.5
30	Michigan	16.2
37	Minnesota	13.6
1	Mississippi	32.0
14	Missouri	21.0
12	Montana	21.8
23	Nebraska	18.3
19	Nevada	20.5
45	New Hampshire	11.6
46	New Jersey	10.4
3	New Mexico	25.9
48	New York	9.7
18	North Carolina	20.7
27	North Dakota	16.8
43	Ohio	12.8
7	Oklahoma	24.5
28	Oregon	16.7
41	Pennsylvania	13.2
49	Rhode Island	7.9
8	South Carolina	24.1
10	South Dakota	23.3
5	Tennessee	24.6
16	Texas	20.8
26	Utah	16.9
35	Vermont	14.3
39	Virginia	13.3
33	Washington	14.4
22	West Virginia	18.5
32	Wisconsin	15.4
5	Wyoming	24.6

RANK ORDER		
RANK	STATE	RATE
1	Mississippi	32.0
2	Alabama	27.4
3	New Mexico	25.9
4	Arkansas	25.4
5	Tennessee	24.6
5	Wyoming	24.6
7	Oklahoma	24.5
8	South Carolina	24.1
9	Idaho	23.8
10	South Dakota	23.3
11	Arizona	22.5
12	Montana	21.8
13	Georgia	21.7
14	Louisiana	21.0
14	Missouri	21.0
16	Kentucky	20.8
16	Texas	20.8
18	North Carolina	20.7
19	Nevada	20.5
20	Kansas	20.2
21	Florida	19.5
22	West Virginia	18.5
23	Nebraska	18.3
24	Colorado	17.5
25	Iowa	17.2
26	Utah	16.9
27	North Dakota	16.8
28	Oregon	16.7
29	Indiana	16.6
30	Alaska	16.2
30	Michigan	16.2
32	Wisconsin	15.4
33	Delaware	14.4
33	Washington	14.4
35	Maine	14.3
35	Vermont	14.3
37	Minnesota	13.6
38	Illinois	13.4
39	California	13.3
39	Virginia	13.3
41	Pennsylvania	13.2
42	Maryland	12.9
43	Ohio	12.8
44	Hawaii	11.7
45	New Hampshire	11.6
46	New Jersey	10.4
47	Connecticut	10.0
48	New York	9.7
49	Rhode Island	7.9
50	Massachusetts	7.5
	District of Columbia	10.9

Source: Morgan Quitno Press using data from U.S. Dept of Health & Human Serv's, Nat'l Center for Health Statistics "National Vital Statistics Report" (Vol. 47, No. 9, November 10, 1998)

Final data by state of residence. These numbers are compiled from death certificates by the Centers for Disease Control and Prevention. They may differ from motor vehicle deaths collected by the U.S. Department of Transportation from other sources. Not age-adjusted.

Age-Adjusted Death Rate by Motor Vehicle Accidents in 1996

National Rate = 16.2 Deaths per 100,000 Population*

ALPHA ORDER

RANK ORDER

RANK	STATE	RATE		RANK	STATE	RATE
2	Alabama	27.2		1	Mississippi	31.6
28	Alaska	16.5		2	Alabama	27.2
10	Arizona	22.1		3	New Mexico	26.3
4	Arkansas	25.7		4	Arkansas	25.7
39	California	13.0		5	Wyoming	25.2
23	Colorado	17.6		6	Tennessee	24.2
46	Connecticut	10.1		7	South Carolina	24.1
33	Delaware	14.5		8	Oklahoma	24.0
21	Florida	18.8		9	Idaho	23.0
12	Georgia	21.7		10	Arizona	22.1
44	Hawaii	11.5		10	South Dakota	22.1
9	Idaho	23.0		12	Georgia	21.7
37	Illinois	13.5		13	Montana	21.5
30	Indiana	16.4		14	Louisiana	20.9
26	Iowa	16.8		14	Missouri	20.9
19	Kansas	20.2		16	Kentucky	20.5
16	Kentucky	20.5		16	Texas	20.5
14	Louisiana	20.9		18	North Carolina	20.4
35	Maine	14.0		19	Kansas	20.2
40	Maryland	12.8		20	Nevada	19.9
50	Massachusetts	7.2		21	Florida	18.8
31	Michigan	16.1		22	West Virginia	18.6
37	Minnesota	13.5		23	Colorado	17.6
1	Mississippi	31.6		24	Nebraska	17.5
14	Missouri	20.9		25	Utah	16.9
13	Montana	21.5		26	Iowa	16.8
24	Nebraska	17.5		27	Oregon	16.7
20	Nevada	19.9		28	Alaska	16.5
44	New Hampshire	11.5		28	North Dakota	16.5
47	New Jersey	9.8		30	Indiana	16.4
3	New Mexico	26.3		31	Michigan	16.1
48	New York	9.3		32	Wisconsin	15.2
18	North Carolina	20.4		33	Delaware	14.5
28	North Dakota	16.5		34	Washington	14.2
43	Ohio	12.6		35	Maine	14.0
8	Oklahoma	24.0		36	Vermont	13.9
27	Oregon	16.7		37	Illinois	13.5
42	Pennsylvania	12.7		37	Minnesota	13.5
49	Rhode Island	7.5		39	California	13.0
7	South Carolina	24.1		40	Maryland	12.8
10	South Dakota	22.1		40	Virginia	12.8
6	Tennessee	24.2		42	Pennsylvania	12.7
16	Texas	20.5		43	Ohio	12.6
25	Utah	16.9		44	Hawaii	11.5
36	Vermont	13.9		44	New Hampshire	11.5
40	Virginia	12.8		46	Connecticut	10.1
34	Washington	14.2		47	New Jersey	9.8
22	West Virginia	18.6		48	New York	9.3
32	Wisconsin	15.2		49	Rhode Island	7.5
5	Wyoming	25.2		50	Massachusetts	7.2
					District of Columbia	10.5

Source: U.S. Department of Health and Human Services, National Center for Health Statistics
 "National Vital Statistics Report" (Vol. 47, No. 9, November 10, 1998)
*Final data by state of residence. These numbers are compiled from death certificates by the Centers for Disease Control and Prevention. They may differ from motor vehicle deaths collected by the U.S. Department of Transportation from other sources.

Deaths by Homicide in 1996

National Total = 20,971 Homicides*

ALPHA ORDER

RANK	STATE	HOMICIDES	% of USA
14	Alabama	529	2.5%
41	Alaska	42	0.2%
17	Arizona	446	2.1%
24	Arkansas	239	1.1%
1	California	3,056	14.6%
26	Colorado	214	1.0%
32	Connecticut	173	0.8%
38	Delaware	57	0.3%
5	Florida	1,189	5.7%
8	Georgia	736	3.5%
42	Hawaii	41	0.2%
39	Idaho	50	0.2%
4	Illinois	1,267	6.0%
18	Indiana	400	1.9%
36	Iowa	71	0.3%
34	Kansas	144	0.7%
25	Kentucky	233	1.1%
7	Louisiana	798	3.8%
44	Maine	29	0.1%
11	Maryland	605	2.9%
29	Massachusetts	191	0.9%
6	Michigan	808	3.9%
31	Minnesota	177	0.8%
21	Mississippi	376	1.8%
16	Missouri	467	2.2%
43	Montana	37	0.2%
39	Nebraska	50	0.2%
28	Nevada	206	1.0%
46	New Hampshire	22	0.1%
19	New Jersey	388	1.9%
30	New Mexico	187	0.9%
3	New York	1,369	6.5%
10	North Carolina	675	3.2%
49	North Dakota	12	0.1%
15	Ohio	502	2.4%
22	Oklahoma	269	1.3%
33	Oregon	150	0.7%
9	Pennsylvania	715	3.4%
45	Rhode Island	28	0.1%
20	South Carolina	379	1.8%
47	South Dakota	16	0.1%
12	Tennessee	536	2.6%
2	Texas	1,584	7.6%
37	Utah	66	0.3%
50	Vermont	9	0.0%
13	Virginia	531	2.5%
23	Washington	260	1.2%
35	West Virginia	88	0.4%
26	Wisconsin	214	1.0%
48	Wyoming	15	0.1%

RANK ORDER

RANK	STATE	HOMICIDES	% of USA
1	California	3,056	14.6%
2	Texas	1,584	7.6%
3	New York	1,369	6.5%
4	Illinois	1,267	6.0%
5	Florida	1,189	5.7%
6	Michigan	808	3.9%
7	Louisiana	798	3.8%
8	Georgia	736	3.5%
9	Pennsylvania	715	3.4%
10	North Carolina	675	3.2%
11	Maryland	605	2.9%
12	Tennessee	536	2.6%
13	Virginia	531	2.5%
14	Alabama	529	2.5%
15	Ohio	502	2.4%
16	Missouri	467	2.2%
17	Arizona	446	2.1%
18	Indiana	400	1.9%
19	New Jersey	388	1.9%
20	South Carolina	379	1.8%
21	Mississippi	376	1.8%
22	Oklahoma	269	1.3%
23	Washington	260	1.2%
24	Arkansas	239	1.1%
25	Kentucky	233	1.1%
26	Colorado	214	1.0%
26	Wisconsin	214	1.0%
28	Nevada	206	1.0%
29	Massachusetts	191	0.9%
30	New Mexico	187	0.9%
31	Minnesota	177	0.8%
32	Connecticut	173	0.8%
33	Oregon	150	0.7%
34	Kansas	144	0.7%
35	West Virginia	88	0.4%
36	Iowa	71	0.3%
37	Utah	66	0.3%
38	Delaware	57	0.3%
39	Idaho	50	0.2%
39	Nebraska	50	0.2%
41	Alaska	42	0.2%
42	Hawaii	41	0.2%
43	Montana	37	0.2%
44	Maine	29	0.1%
45	Rhode Island	28	0.1%
46	New Hampshire	22	0.1%
47	South Dakota	16	0.1%
48	Wyoming	15	0.1%
49	North Dakota	12	0.1%
50	Vermont	9	0.0%
	District of Columbia	325	1.5%

Source: U.S. Department of Health and Human Services, National Center for Health Statistics
"National Vital Statistics Report" (Vol. 47, No. 9, November 10, 1998)
By state of residence. Includes legal intervention. Homicide data shown here are collected by the Centers for Disease Control and Prevention based on death certificates and differ from murder data collected by the F.B.I. from other sources.

Death Rate by Homicide in 1996

National Rate = 7.9 Deaths by Homicide per 100,000 Population*

ALPHA ORDER

RANK	STATE	RATE
4	Alabama	12.3
23	Alaska	6.9
8	Arizona	10.1
13	Arkansas	9.5
12	California	9.6
27	Colorado	5.6
29	Connecticut	5.3
21	Delaware	7.8
18	Florida	8.2
11	Georgia	10.0
39	Hawaii	3.5
35	Idaho	4.2
7	Illinois	10.6
23	Indiana	6.9
45	Iowa	2.5
27	Kansas	5.6
25	Kentucky	6.0
1	Louisiana	18.4
46	Maine	2.3
5	Maryland	12.0
41	Massachusetts	3.1
16	Michigan	8.3
38	Minnesota	3.8
2	Mississippi	13.9
15	Missouri	8.7
35	Montana	4.2
43	Nebraska	3.0
3	Nevada	12.9
48	New Hampshire	1.9
30	New Jersey	4.8
6	New Mexico	10.9
22	New York	7.5
14	North Carolina	9.2
48	North Dakota	1.9
34	Ohio	4.5
18	Oklahoma	8.2
32	Oregon	4.7
26	Pennsylvania	5.9
44	Rhode Island	2.8
8	South Carolina	10.1
47	South Dakota	2.2
8	Tennessee	10.1
16	Texas	8.3
40	Utah	3.3
50	Vermont	1.5
20	Virginia	8.0
32	Washington	4.7
30	West Virginia	4.8
37	Wisconsin	4.1
41	Wyoming	3.1

RANK ORDER

RANK	STATE	RATE
1	Louisiana	18.4
2	Mississippi	13.9
3	Nevada	12.9
4	Alabama	12.3
5	Maryland	12.0
6	New Mexico	10.9
7	Illinois	10.6
8	Arizona	10.1
8	South Carolina	10.1
8	Tennessee	10.1
11	Georgia	10.0
12	California	9.6
13	Arkansas	9.5
14	North Carolina	9.2
15	Missouri	8.7
16	Michigan	8.3
16	Texas	8.3
18	Florida	8.2
18	Oklahoma	8.2
20	Virginia	8.0
21	Delaware	7.8
22	New York	7.5
23	Alaska	6.9
23	Indiana	6.9
25	Kentucky	6.0
26	Pennsylvania	5.9
27	Colorado	5.6
27	Kansas	5.6
29	Connecticut	5.3
30	New Jersey	4.8
30	West Virginia	4.8
32	Oregon	4.7
32	Washington	4.7
34	Ohio	4.5
35	Idaho	4.2
35	Montana	4.2
37	Wisconsin	4.1
38	Minnesota	3.8
39	Hawaii	3.5
40	Utah	3.3
41	Massachusetts	3.1
41	Wyoming	3.1
43	Nebraska	3.0
44	Rhode Island	2.8
45	Iowa	2.5
46	Maine	2.3
47	South Dakota	2.2
48	New Hampshire	1.9
48	North Dakota	1.9
50	Vermont	1.5

| | District of Columbia | 60.2 |

Source: Morgan Quitno Press using data from U.S. Dept of Health & Human Serv's, Nat'l Center for Health Statistics "National Vital Statistics Report" (Vol. 47, No. 9, November 10, 1998)

*By state of residence. Includes legal intervention. Homicide data shown here are collected by the Centers for Disease Control and Prevention based on death certificates and differ from murder data collected by the F.B.I. from other sources. Not age-adjusted.

Age-Adjusted Death Rate by Homicide in 1996

National Rate = 8.5 Deaths by Homicide per 100,000 Population*

ALPHA ORDER			RANK ORDER		
RANK	STATE	RATE	RANK	STATE	RATE
5	Alabama	13.0	1	Louisiana	19.5
24	Alaska	7.0	2	Mississippi	14.1
8	Arizona	10.9	3	Nevada	13.5
13	Arkansas	9.9	4	Maryland	13.4
11	California	10.3	5	Alabama	13.0
29	Colorado	5.9	6	Illinois	12.0
27	Connecticut	6.0	7	New Mexico	11.6
22	Delaware	7.5	8	Arizona	10.9
16	Florida	9.2	9	Tennessee	10.5
12	Georgia	10.2	10	South Carolina	10.4
39	Hawaii	3.7	11	California	10.3
37	Idaho	4.3	12	Georgia	10.2
6	Illinois	12.0	13	Arkansas	9.9
23	Indiana	7.4	14	North Carolina	9.7
44	Iowa	2.8	15	Missouri	9.3
26	Kansas	6.1	16	Florida	9.2
27	Kentucky	6.0	17	Michigan	9.0
1	Louisiana	19.5	18	Oklahoma	8.6
45	Maine	2.3	19	Texas	8.5
4	Maryland	13.4	20	New York	8.3
40	Massachusetts	3.6	21	Virginia	8.1
17	Michigan	9.0	22	Delaware	7.5
38	Minnesota	4.0	23	Indiana	7.4
2	Mississippi	14.1	24	Alaska	7.0
15	Missouri	9.3	25	Pennsylvania	6.8
36	Montana	4.4	26	Kansas	6.1
41	Nebraska	3.4	27	Connecticut	6.0
3	Nevada	13.5	27	Kentucky	6.0
46	New Hampshire	1.8	29	Colorado	5.9
30	New Jersey	5.5	30	New Jersey	5.5
7	New Mexico	11.6	31	West Virginia	5.1
20	New York	8.3	32	Oregon	5.0
14	North Carolina	9.7	33	Washington	4.9
NA	North Dakota*	NA	34	Ohio	4.8
34	Ohio	4.8	35	Wisconsin	4.5
18	Oklahoma	8.6	36	Montana	4.4
32	Oregon	5.0	37	Idaho	4.3
25	Pennsylvania	6.8	38	Minnesota	4.0
43	Rhode Island	3.1	39	Hawaii	3.7
10	South Carolina	10.4	40	Massachusetts	3.6
NA	South Dakota*	NA	41	Nebraska	3.4
9	Tennessee	10.5	42	Utah	3.3
19	Texas	8.5	43	Rhode Island	3.1
42	Utah	3.3	44	Iowa	2.8
NA	Vermont*	NA	45	Maine	2.3
21	Virginia	8.1	46	New Hampshire	1.8
33	Washington	4.9	NA	North Dakota*	NA
31	West Virginia	5.1	NA	South Dakota*	NA
35	Wisconsin	4.5	NA	Vermont*	NA
NA	Wyoming*	NA	NA	Wyoming*	NA
			District of Columbia		72.9

Source: U.S. Department of Health and Human Services, National Center for Health Statistics
    "National Vital Statistics Report" (Vol. 47, No. 9, November 10, 1998)
*By state of residence. Includes legal intervention. Homicide data shown here are collected by the Centers for Disease Control and Prevention based on death certificates and differ from murder data collected by the F.B.I. from other sources.
**Insufficient number for a valid rate.

Deaths by Suicide in 1996

National Total = 30,903 Suicides*

ALPHA ORDER

RANK	STATE	SUICIDES	% of USA
22	Alabama	513	1.7%
45	Alaska	120	0.4%
15	Arizona	726	2.3%
31	Arkansas	323	1.0%
1	California	3,408	11.0%
16	Colorado	694	2.2%
35	Connecticut	292	0.9%
46	Delaware	97	0.3%
3	Florida	2,153	7.0%
10	Georgia	867	2.8%
43	Hawaii	127	0.4%
39	Idaho	177	0.6%
7	Illinois	1,061	3.4%
14	Indiana	738	2.4%
32	Iowa	321	1.0%
30	Kansas	334	1.1%
27	Kentucky	488	1.6%
20	Louisiana	531	1.7%
41	Maine	171	0.6%
23	Maryland	501	1.6%
26	Massachusetts	490	1.6%
6	Michigan	1,114	3.6%
25	Minnesota	491	1.6%
34	Mississippi	310	1.0%
13	Missouri	760	2.5%
40	Montana	174	0.6%
38	Nebraska	189	0.6%
29	Nevada	335	1.1%
42	New Hampshire	137	0.4%
19	New Jersey	586	1.9%
33	New Mexico	318	1.0%
5	New York	1,327	4.3%
9	North Carolina	908	2.9%
49	North Dakota	77	0.2%
8	Ohio	1,054	3.4%
28	Oklahoma	467	1.5%
21	Oregon	520	1.7%
4	Pennsylvania	1,428	4.6%
48	Rhode Island	83	0.3%
24	South Carolina	497	1.6%
44	South Dakota	124	0.4%
17	Tennessee	691	2.2%
2	Texas	2,223	7.2%
36	Utah	287	0.9%
50	Vermont	66	0.2%
11	Virginia	829	2.7%
12	Washington	773	2.5%
37	West Virginia	279	0.9%
18	Wisconsin	601	1.9%
47	Wyoming	88	0.3%

RANK ORDER

RANK	STATE	SUICIDES	% of USA
1	California	3,408	11.0%
2	Texas	2,223	7.2%
3	Florida	2,153	7.0%
4	Pennsylvania	1,428	4.6%
5	New York	1,327	4.3%
6	Michigan	1,114	3.6%
7	Illinois	1,061	3.4%
8	Ohio	1,054	3.4%
9	North Carolina	908	2.9%
10	Georgia	867	2.8%
11	Virginia	829	2.7%
12	Washington	773	2.5%
13	Missouri	760	2.5%
14	Indiana	738	2.4%
15	Arizona	726	2.3%
16	Colorado	694	2.2%
17	Tennessee	691	2.2%
18	Wisconsin	601	1.9%
19	New Jersey	586	1.9%
20	Louisiana	531	1.7%
21	Oregon	520	1.7%
22	Alabama	513	1.7%
23	Maryland	501	1.6%
24	South Carolina	497	1.6%
25	Minnesota	491	1.6%
26	Massachusetts	490	1.6%
27	Kentucky	488	1.6%
28	Oklahoma	467	1.5%
29	Nevada	335	1.1%
30	Kansas	334	1.1%
31	Arkansas	323	1.0%
32	Iowa	321	1.0%
33	New Mexico	318	1.0%
34	Mississippi	310	1.0%
35	Connecticut	292	0.9%
36	Utah	287	0.9%
37	West Virginia	279	0.9%
38	Nebraska	189	0.6%
39	Idaho	177	0.6%
40	Montana	174	0.6%
41	Maine	171	0.6%
42	New Hampshire	137	0.4%
43	Hawaii	127	0.4%
44	South Dakota	124	0.4%
45	Alaska	120	0.4%
46	Delaware	97	0.3%
47	Wyoming	88	0.3%
48	Rhode Island	83	0.3%
49	North Dakota	77	0.2%
50	Vermont	66	0.2%
	District of Columbia	35	0.1%

Source: U.S. Department of Health and Human Services, National Center for Health Statistics
"National Vital Statistics Report" (Vol. 47, No. 9, November 10, 1998)
Final data by state of residence.

Death Rate by Suicide in 1996

National Rate = 11.7 Suicides per 100,000 Population*

RANK	STATE	RATE
28	Alabama	12.0
2	Alaska	19.8
8	Arizona	16.4
21	Arkansas	12.9
40	California	10.7
6	Colorado	18.2
45	Connecticut	8.9
18	Delaware	13.3
11	Florida	14.9
31	Georgia	11.8
40	Hawaii	10.7
11	Idaho	14.9
45	Illinois	8.9
23	Indiana	12.7
38	Iowa	11.3
21	Kansas	12.9
24	Kentucky	12.6
27	Louisiana	12.2
17	Maine	13.8
43	Maryland	9.9
48	Massachusetts	8.1
36	Michigan	11.4
42	Minnesota	10.6
36	Mississippi	11.4
13	Missouri	14.2
2	Montana	19.8
35	Nebraska	11.5
1	Nevada	20.9
31	New Hampshire	11.8
49	New Jersey	7.3
4	New Mexico	18.6
49	New York	7.3
25	North Carolina	12.4
28	North Dakota	12.0
44	Ohio	9.4
13	Oklahoma	14.2
9	Oregon	16.3
30	Pennsylvania	11.9
47	Rhode Island	8.4
18	South Carolina	13.3
7	South Dakota	16.8
20	Tennessee	13.0
33	Texas	11.7
13	Utah	14.2
38	Vermont	11.3
25	Virginia	12.4
16	Washington	14.0
10	West Virginia	15.3
34	Wisconsin	11.6
5	Wyoming	18.3

RANK	STATE	RATE
1	Nevada	20.9
2	Alaska	19.8
2	Montana	19.8
4	New Mexico	18.6
5	Wyoming	18.3
6	Colorado	18.2
7	South Dakota	16.8
8	Arizona	16.4
9	Oregon	16.3
10	West Virginia	15.3
11	Florida	14.9
11	Idaho	14.9
13	Missouri	14.2
13	Oklahoma	14.2
13	Utah	14.2
16	Washington	14.0
17	Maine	13.8
18	Delaware	13.3
18	South Carolina	13.3
20	Tennessee	13.0
21	Arkansas	12.9
21	Kansas	12.9
23	Indiana	12.7
24	Kentucky	12.6
25	North Carolina	12.4
25	Virginia	12.4
27	Louisiana	12.2
28	Alabama	12.0
28	North Dakota	12.0
30	Pennsylvania	11.9
31	Georgia	11.8
31	New Hampshire	11.8
33	Texas	11.7
34	Wisconsin	11.6
35	Nebraska	11.5
36	Michigan	11.4
36	Mississippi	11.4
38	Iowa	11.3
38	Vermont	11.3
40	California	10.7
40	Hawaii	10.7
42	Minnesota	10.6
43	Maryland	9.9
44	Ohio	9.4
45	Connecticut	8.9
45	Illinois	8.9
47	Rhode Island	8.4
48	Massachusetts	8.1
49	New Jersey	7.3
49	New York	7.3
	District of Columbia	6.5

Source: Morgan Quitno Press using data from U.S. Dept of Health & Human Serv's, Nat'l Center for Health Statistics "National Vital Statistics Report" (Vol. 47, No. 9, November 10, 1998)

Final data by state of residence. Not age-adjusted.

Age-Adjusted Death Rate by Suicide in 1996

National Rate = 10.8 Suicides per 100,000 Population*

<table>
<tr><td colspan="3">ALPHA ORDER</td><td colspan="3">RANK ORDER</td></tr>
<tr><td>RANK</td><td>STATE</td><td>RATE</td><td>RANK</td><td>STATE</td><td>RATE</td></tr>
<tr><td>34</td><td>Alabama</td><td>11.0</td><td>1</td><td>Alaska</td><td>20.5</td></tr>
<tr><td>1</td><td>Alaska</td><td>20.5</td><td>2</td><td>Nevada</td><td>19.8</td></tr>
<tr><td>8</td><td>Arizona</td><td>15.3</td><td>3</td><td>Montana</td><td>18.6</td></tr>
<tr><td>17</td><td>Arkansas</td><td>12.6</td><td>4</td><td>New Mexico</td><td>17.9</td></tr>
<tr><td>42</td><td>California</td><td>10.0</td><td>5</td><td>Colorado</td><td>16.8</td></tr>
<tr><td>5</td><td>Colorado</td><td>16.8</td><td>6</td><td>South Dakota</td><td>16.4</td></tr>
<tr><td>44</td><td>Connecticut</td><td>8.6</td><td>7</td><td>Wyoming</td><td>16.1</td></tr>
<tr><td>21</td><td>Delaware</td><td>11.9</td><td>8</td><td>Arizona</td><td>15.3</td></tr>
<tr><td>15</td><td>Florida</td><td>13.1</td><td>9</td><td>Oregon</td><td>14.7</td></tr>
<tr><td>29</td><td>Georgia</td><td>11.2</td><td>9</td><td>Utah</td><td>14.7</td></tr>
<tr><td>39</td><td>Hawaii</td><td>10.4</td><td>11</td><td>Idaho</td><td>13.8</td></tr>
<tr><td>11</td><td>Idaho</td><td>13.8</td><td>12</td><td>West Virginia</td><td>13.7</td></tr>
<tr><td>46</td><td>Illinois</td><td>8.4</td><td>13</td><td>Oklahoma</td><td>13.6</td></tr>
<tr><td>25</td><td>Indiana</td><td>11.7</td><td>14</td><td>Missouri</td><td>13.2</td></tr>
<tr><td>38</td><td>Iowa</td><td>10.6</td><td>15</td><td>Florida</td><td>13.1</td></tr>
<tr><td>19</td><td>Kansas</td><td>12.1</td><td>16</td><td>Washington</td><td>12.9</td></tr>
<tr><td>27</td><td>Kentucky</td><td>11.4</td><td>17</td><td>Arkansas</td><td>12.6</td></tr>
<tr><td>21</td><td>Louisiana</td><td>11.9</td><td>17</td><td>South Carolina</td><td>12.6</td></tr>
<tr><td>23</td><td>Maine</td><td>11.8</td><td>19</td><td>Kansas</td><td>12.1</td></tr>
<tr><td>43</td><td>Maryland</td><td>9.2</td><td>20</td><td>Tennessee</td><td>12.0</td></tr>
<tr><td>48</td><td>Massachusetts</td><td>7.5</td><td>21</td><td>Delaware</td><td>11.9</td></tr>
<tr><td>37</td><td>Michigan</td><td>10.8</td><td>21</td><td>Louisiana</td><td>11.9</td></tr>
<tr><td>41</td><td>Minnesota</td><td>10.1</td><td>23</td><td>Maine</td><td>11.8</td></tr>
<tr><td>29</td><td>Mississippi</td><td>11.2</td><td>23</td><td>North Dakota</td><td>11.8</td></tr>
<tr><td>14</td><td>Missouri</td><td>13.2</td><td>25</td><td>Indiana</td><td>11.7</td></tr>
<tr><td>3</td><td>Montana</td><td>18.6</td><td>26</td><td>North Carolina</td><td>11.5</td></tr>
<tr><td>31</td><td>Nebraska</td><td>11.1</td><td>27</td><td>Kentucky</td><td>11.4</td></tr>
<tr><td>2</td><td>Nevada</td><td>19.8</td><td>27</td><td>Virginia</td><td>11.4</td></tr>
<tr><td>31</td><td>New Hampshire</td><td>11.1</td><td>29</td><td>Georgia</td><td>11.2</td></tr>
<tr><td>49</td><td>New Jersey</td><td>6.7</td><td>29</td><td>Mississippi</td><td>11.2</td></tr>
<tr><td>4</td><td>New Mexico</td><td>17.9</td><td>31</td><td>Nebraska</td><td>11.1</td></tr>
<tr><td>49</td><td>New York</td><td>6.7</td><td>31</td><td>New Hampshire</td><td>11.1</td></tr>
<tr><td>26</td><td>North Carolina</td><td>11.5</td><td>31</td><td>Texas</td><td>11.1</td></tr>
<tr><td>23</td><td>North Dakota</td><td>11.8</td><td>34</td><td>Alabama</td><td>11.0</td></tr>
<tr><td>44</td><td>Ohio</td><td>8.6</td><td>34</td><td>Pennsylvania</td><td>11.0</td></tr>
<tr><td>13</td><td>Oklahoma</td><td>13.6</td><td>36</td><td>Wisconsin</td><td>10.9</td></tr>
<tr><td>9</td><td>Oregon</td><td>14.7</td><td>37</td><td>Michigan</td><td>10.8</td></tr>
<tr><td>34</td><td>Pennsylvania</td><td>11.0</td><td>38</td><td>Iowa</td><td>10.6</td></tr>
<tr><td>47</td><td>Rhode Island</td><td>7.8</td><td>39</td><td>Hawaii</td><td>10.4</td></tr>
<tr><td>17</td><td>South Carolina</td><td>12.6</td><td>40</td><td>Vermont</td><td>10.3</td></tr>
<tr><td>6</td><td>South Dakota</td><td>16.4</td><td>41</td><td>Minnesota</td><td>10.1</td></tr>
<tr><td>20</td><td>Tennessee</td><td>12.0</td><td>42</td><td>California</td><td>10.0</td></tr>
<tr><td>31</td><td>Texas</td><td>11.1</td><td>43</td><td>Maryland</td><td>9.2</td></tr>
<tr><td>9</td><td>Utah</td><td>14.7</td><td>44</td><td>Connecticut</td><td>8.6</td></tr>
<tr><td>40</td><td>Vermont</td><td>10.3</td><td>44</td><td>Ohio</td><td>8.6</td></tr>
<tr><td>27</td><td>Virginia</td><td>11.4</td><td>46</td><td>Illinois</td><td>8.4</td></tr>
<tr><td>16</td><td>Washington</td><td>12.9</td><td>47</td><td>Rhode Island</td><td>7.8</td></tr>
<tr><td>12</td><td>West Virginia</td><td>13.7</td><td>48</td><td>Massachusetts</td><td>7.5</td></tr>
<tr><td>36</td><td>Wisconsin</td><td>10.9</td><td>49</td><td>New Jersey</td><td>6.7</td></tr>
<tr><td>7</td><td>Wyoming</td><td>16.1</td><td>49</td><td>New York</td><td>6.7</td></tr>
<tr><td></td><td></td><td></td><td></td><td>District of Columbia</td><td>5.7</td></tr>
</table>

Source: U.S. Department of Health and Human Services, National Center for Health Statistics
    "National Vital Statistics Report" (Vol. 47, No. 9, November 10, 1998)
*Final data by state of residence.

Years Lost by Premature Death in 1996

National Average = 7,742.6 Years Lost per 100,000 Population*

ALPHA ORDER

RANK	STATE	YEARS
3	Alabama	9,958.3
21	Alaska	7,795.0
13	Arizona	8,298.6
5	Arkansas	9,225.4
32	California	7,041.2
38	Colorado	6,569.1
36	Connecticut	6,741.1
16	Delaware	8,188.3
12	Florida	8,367.9
6	Georgia	9,201.1
42	Hawaii	6,266.9
37	Idaho	6,602.9
19	Illinois	8,065.2
23	Indiana	7,652.6
41	Iowa	6,391.4
29	Kansas	7,301.8
15	Kentucky	8,246.4
2	Louisiana	10,051.5
46	Maine	6,111.0
11	Maryland	8,475.1
45	Massachusetts	6,126.9
25	Michigan	7,584.0
50	Minnesota	5,839.0
1	Mississippi	10,738.1
17	Missouri	8,150.6
31	Montana	7,096.0
35	Nebraska	6,766.3
8	Nevada	8,776.1
49	New Hampshire	5,866.1
26	New Jersey	7,403.5
18	New Mexico	8,136.9
20	New York	7,822.4
9	North Carolina	8,692.2
48	North Dakota	5,913.1
28	Ohio	7,353.5
10	Oklahoma	8,632.3
33	Oregon	7,025.7
24	Pennsylvania	7,604.0
47	Rhode Island	6,038.6
4	South Carolina	9,692.2
34	South Dakota	6,933.4
7	Tennessee	9,041.2
22	Texas	7,723.3
44	Utah	6,189.4
43	Vermont	6,241.0
27	Virginia	7,403.1
39	Washington	6,550.0
14	West Virginia	8,264.9
40	Wisconsin	6,433.7
30	Wyoming	7,195.3

RANK ORDER

RANK	STATE	YEARS
1	Mississippi	10,738.1
2	Louisiana	10,051.5
3	Alabama	9,958.3
4	South Carolina	9,692.2
5	Arkansas	9,225.4
6	Georgia	9,201.1
7	Tennessee	9,041.2
8	Nevada	8,776.1
9	North Carolina	8,692.2
10	Oklahoma	8,632.3
11	Maryland	8,475.1
12	Florida	8,367.9
13	Arizona	8,298.6
14	West Virginia	8,264.9
15	Kentucky	8,246.4
16	Delaware	8,188.3
17	Missouri	8,150.6
18	New Mexico	8,136.9
19	Illinois	8,065.2
20	New York	7,822.4
21	Alaska	7,795.0
22	Texas	7,723.3
23	Indiana	7,652.6
24	Pennsylvania	7,604.0
25	Michigan	7,584.0
26	New Jersey	7,403.5
27	Virginia	7,403.1
28	Ohio	7,353.5
29	Kansas	7,301.8
30	Wyoming	7,195.3
31	Montana	7,096.0
32	California	7,041.2
33	Oregon	7,025.7
34	South Dakota	6,933.4
35	Nebraska	6,766.3
36	Connecticut	6,741.1
37	Idaho	6,602.9
38	Colorado	6,569.1
39	Washington	6,550.0
40	Wisconsin	6,433.7
41	Iowa	6,391.4
42	Hawaii	6,266.9
43	Vermont	6,241.0
44	Utah	6,189.4
45	Massachusetts	6,126.9
46	Maine	6,111.0
47	Rhode Island	6,038.6
48	North Dakota	5,913.1
49	New Hampshire	5,866.1
50	Minnesota	5,839.0
	District of Columbia	18,478.1

Source: U.S. Department of Health and Human Services, National Center for Health Statistics unpublished data

*Age-adjusted years of potential life lost due to death before age 75.

Years Lost by Premature Death from Cancer in 1996

National Average = 1,554.5 Years Lost per 100,000 Population*

ALPHA ORDER

RANK	STATE	YEARS
8	Alabama	1,724.4
43	Alaska	1,337.2
41	Arizona	1,384.5
5	Arkansas	1,752.4
37	California	1,398.7
49	Colorado	1,188.6
30	Connecticut	1,491.5
4	Delaware	1,794.7
13	Florida	1,639.9
15	Georgia	1,617.8
47	Hawaii	1,271.8
48	Idaho	1,209.3
19	Illinois	1,605.2
21	Indiana	1,592.7
35	Iowa	1,426.2
32	Kansas	1,466.2
2	Kentucky	1,855.3
1	Louisiana	1,855.8
25	Maine	1,576.3
20	Maryland	1,602.8
28	Massachusetts	1,549.3
27	Michigan	1,560.4
38	Minnesota	1,395.0
3	Mississippi	1,843.2
12	Missouri	1,655.3
44	Montana	1,325.2
39	Nebraska	1,392.5
22	Nevada	1,591.0
17	New Hampshire	1,611.1
16	New Jersey	1,617.6
45	New Mexico	1,299.7
23	New York	1,585.2
11	North Carolina	1,666.5
42	North Dakota	1,350.0
14	Ohio	1,634.9
18	Oklahoma	1,609.7
33	Oregon	1,458.0
24	Pennsylvania	1,582.0
9	Rhode Island	1,681.2
6	South Carolina	1,746.4
36	South Dakota	1,422.0
7	Tennessee	1,729.1
29	Texas	1,512.2
50	Utah	1,116.1
31	Vermont	1,480.7
26	Virginia	1,570.4
40	Washington	1,387.3
10	West Virginia	1,679.6
34	Wisconsin	1,444.8
46	Wyoming	1,296.0

RANK ORDER

RANK	STATE	YEARS
1	Louisiana	1,855.8
2	Kentucky	1,855.3
3	Mississippi	1,843.2
4	Delaware	1,794.7
5	Arkansas	1,752.4
6	South Carolina	1,746.4
7	Tennessee	1,729.1
8	Alabama	1,724.4
9	Rhode Island	1,681.2
10	West Virginia	1,679.6
11	North Carolina	1,666.5
12	Missouri	1,655.3
13	Florida	1,639.9
14	Ohio	1,634.9
15	Georgia	1,617.8
16	New Jersey	1,617.6
17	New Hampshire	1,611.1
18	Oklahoma	1,609.7
19	Illinois	1,605.2
20	Maryland	1,602.8
21	Indiana	1,592.7
22	Nevada	1,591.0
23	New York	1,585.2
24	Pennsylvania	1,582.0
25	Maine	1,576.3
26	Virginia	1,570.4
27	Michigan	1,560.4
28	Massachusetts	1,549.3
29	Texas	1,512.2
30	Connecticut	1,491.5
31	Vermont	1,480.7
32	Kansas	1,466.2
33	Oregon	1,458.0
34	Wisconsin	1,444.8
35	Iowa	1,426.2
36	South Dakota	1,422.0
37	California	1,398.7
38	Minnesota	1,395.0
39	Nebraska	1,392.5
40	Washington	1,387.3
41	Arizona	1,384.5
42	North Dakota	1,350.0
43	Alaska	1,337.2
44	Montana	1,325.2
45	New Mexico	1,299.7
46	Wyoming	1,296.0
47	Hawaii	1,271.8
48	Idaho	1,209.3
49	Colorado	1,188.6
50	Utah	1,116.1

| | District of Columbia | 2,066.1 |

Source: U.S. Department of Health and Human Services, National Center for Health Statistics
    unpublished data
*Age-adjusted years of potential life lost due to death before age 75.

179

Years Lost by Premature Death from Heart Disease in 1996

National Average = 1,222.7 Years Lost per 100,000 Population*

ALPHA ORDER

RANK	STATE	YEARS
2	Alabama	1,721.4
48	Alaska	832.9
28	Arizona	1,086.0
10	Arkansas	1,457.3
39	California	999.0
49	Colorado	772.2
25	Connecticut	1,144.9
14	Delaware	1,352.2
24	Florida	1,185.8
9	Georgia	1,508.8
26	Hawaii	1,129.0
43	Idaho	906.6
16	Illinois	1,320.9
15	Indiana	1,334.5
32	Iowa	1,055.9
33	Kansas	1,042.4
8	Kentucky	1,511.3
5	Louisiana	1,572.9
35	Maine	1,019.1
22	Maryland	1,234.2
36	Massachusetts	1,017.9
18	Michigan	1,299.8
47	Minnesota	854.9
1	Mississippi	1,967.8
13	Missouri	1,357.9
37	Montana	1,004.7
30	Nebraska	1,076.4
12	Nevada	1,376.5
41	New Hampshire	959.6
29	New Jersey	1,084.1
46	New Mexico	876.5
23	New York	1,223.0
11	North Carolina	1,440.2
40	North Dakota	982.0
19	Ohio	1,295.1
6	Oklahoma	1,533.6
45	Oregon	892.3
17	Pennsylvania	1,320.4
31	Rhode Island	1,074.0
3	South Carolina	1,624.7
27	South Dakota	1,111.3
7	Tennessee	1,519.6
21	Texas	1,237.1
50	Utah	740.8
42	Vermont	957.7
20	Virginia	1,258.3
44	Washington	895.2
4	West Virginia	1,615.2
34	Wisconsin	1,038.6
38	Wyoming	999.3

RANK ORDER

RANK	STATE	YEARS
1	Mississippi	1,967.8
2	Alabama	1,721.4
3	South Carolina	1,624.7
4	West Virginia	1,615.2
5	Louisiana	1,572.9
6	Oklahoma	1,533.6
7	Tennessee	1,519.6
8	Kentucky	1,511.3
9	Georgia	1,508.8
10	Arkansas	1,457.3
11	North Carolina	1,440.2
12	Nevada	1,376.5
13	Missouri	1,357.9
14	Delaware	1,352.2
15	Indiana	1,334.5
16	Illinois	1,320.9
17	Pennsylvania	1,320.4
18	Michigan	1,299.8
19	Ohio	1,295.1
20	Virginia	1,258.3
21	Texas	1,237.1
22	Maryland	1,234.2
23	New York	1,223.0
24	Florida	1,185.8
25	Connecticut	1,144.9
26	Hawaii	1,129.0
27	South Dakota	1,111.3
28	Arizona	1,086.0
29	New Jersey	1,084.1
30	Nebraska	1,076.4
31	Rhode Island	1,074.0
32	Iowa	1,055.9
33	Kansas	1,042.4
34	Wisconsin	1,038.6
35	Maine	1,019.1
36	Massachusetts	1,017.9
37	Montana	1,004.7
38	Wyoming	999.3
39	California	999.0
40	North Dakota	982.0
41	New Hampshire	959.6
42	Vermont	957.7
43	Idaho	906.6
44	Washington	895.2
45	Oregon	892.3
46	New Mexico	876.5
47	Minnesota	854.9
48	Alaska	832.9
49	Colorado	772.2
50	Utah	740.8
	District of Columbia	1,943.6

Source: U.S. Department of Health and Human Services, National Center for Health Statistics
 unpublished data

*Age-adjusted years of potential life lost due to death before age 75.

Years Lost by Premature Death from HIV Infection in 1996

National Average = 402.2 Years Lost per 100,000 Population*

ALPHA ORDER

RANK ORDER

RANK	STATE	YEARS
17	Alabama	309.4
NA	Alaska**	NA
20	Arizona	273.5
29	Arkansas	204.4
9	California	429.4
26	Colorado	217.6
11	Connecticut	393.3
5	Delaware	590.6
2	Florida	781.4
6	Georgia	588.5
30	Hawaii	188.9
44	Idaho	65.3
15	Illinois	324.1
34	Indiana	147.5
43	Iowa	89.9
35	Kansas	145.3
37	Kentucky	131.6
8	Louisiana	511.8
40	Maine	118.2
4	Maryland	676.4
14	Massachusetts	330.0
31	Michigan	184.0
38	Minnesota	130.6
13	Mississippi	350.1
27	Missouri	216.0
NA	Montana**	NA
33	Nebraska	151.3
19	Nevada	288.2
41	New Hampshire	112.4
3	New Jersey	719.5
32	New Mexico	179.0
1	New York	1,021.8
10	North Carolina	397.5
NA	North Dakota**	NA
25	Ohio	218.1
28	Oklahoma	214.7
24	Oregon	224.7
16	Pennsylvania	313.8
23	Rhode Island	224.9
7	South Carolina	517.2
NA	South Dakota**	NA
21	Tennessee	265.9
12	Texas	391.4
39	Utah	125.5
NA	Vermont**	NA
18	Virginia	288.3
22	Washington	235.3
36	West Virginia	136.1
42	Wisconsin	108.5
NA	Wyoming**	NA

RANK	STATE	YEARS
1	New York	1,021.8
2	Florida	781.4
3	New Jersey	719.5
4	Maryland	676.4
5	Delaware	590.6
6	Georgia	588.5
7	South Carolina	517.2
8	Louisiana	511.8
9	California	429.4
10	North Carolina	397.5
11	Connecticut	393.3
12	Texas	391.4
13	Mississippi	350.1
14	Massachusetts	330.0
15	Illinois	324.1
16	Pennsylvania	313.8
17	Alabama	309.4
18	Virginia	288.3
19	Nevada	288.2
20	Arizona	273.5
21	Tennessee	265.9
22	Washington	235.3
23	Rhode Island	224.9
24	Oregon	224.7
25	Ohio	218.1
26	Colorado	217.6
27	Missouri	216.0
28	Oklahoma	214.7
29	Arkansas	204.4
30	Hawaii	188.9
31	Michigan	184.0
32	New Mexico	179.0
33	Nebraska	151.3
34	Indiana	147.5
35	Kansas	145.3
36	West Virginia	136.1
37	Kentucky	131.6
38	Minnesota	130.6
39	Utah	125.5
40	Maine	118.2
41	New Hampshire	112.4
42	Wisconsin	108.5
43	Iowa	89.9
44	Idaho	65.3
NA	Alaska**	NA
NA	Montana**	NA
NA	North Dakota**	NA
NA	South Dakota**	NA
NA	Vermont**	NA
NA	Wyoming**	NA

District of Columbia   3,194.2

Source: U.S. Department of Health and Human Services, National Center for Health Statistics unpublished data

*Age-adjusted years of potential life lost due to death before age 75.

**Data for states with fewer than 20 deaths from HIV infection for persons under 75 years of age are considered unreliable and are not shown.

Years Lost by Premature Death from Homicide and Suicide in 1996

National Average = 389.3 Years Lost per 100,000 Population*

ALPHA ORDER

RANK	STATE	YEARS
6	Alabama	579.4
23	Alaska	322.6
8	Arizona	494.1
14	Arkansas	434.0
9	California	480.0
28	Colorado	265.1
27	Connecticut	276.8
26	Delaware	282.7
16	Florida	414.0
11	Georgia	450.4
42	Hawaii	153.7
38	Idaho	175.2
5	Illinois	583.6
22	Indiana	349.4
44	Iowa	133.4
25	Kansas	285.7
30	Kentucky	253.2
1	Louisiana	909.4
45	Maine	97.9
2	Maryland	640.9
37	Massachusetts	175.6
17	Michigan	410.2
36	Minnesota	183.4
3	Mississippi	620.4
15	Missouri	419.4
39	Montana	173.4
40	Nebraska	159.4
4	Nevada	614.5
NA	New Hampshire**	NA
29	New Jersey	259.2
7	New Mexico	531.0
18	New York	388.3
13	North Carolina	440.1
NA	North Dakota**	NA
33	Ohio	223.9
20	Oklahoma	361.5
31	Oregon	229.7
24	Pennsylvania	317.0
41	Rhode Island	158.7
12	South Carolina	446.7
NA	South Dakota**	NA
10	Tennessee	466.5
19	Texas	379.7
43	Utah	136.5
NA	Vermont**	NA
21	Virginia	353.3
34	Washington	222.2
32	West Virginia	224.3
35	Wisconsin	215.3
NA	Wyoming**	NA

RANK ORDER

RANK	STATE	YEARS
1	Louisiana	909.4
2	Maryland	640.9
3	Mississippi	620.4
4	Nevada	614.5
5	Illinois	583.6
6	Alabama	579.4
7	New Mexico	531.0
8	Arizona	494.1
9	California	480.0
10	Tennessee	466.5
11	Georgia	450.4
12	South Carolina	446.7
13	North Carolina	440.1
14	Arkansas	434.0
15	Missouri	419.4
16	Florida	414.0
17	Michigan	410.2
18	New York	388.3
19	Texas	379.7
20	Oklahoma	361.5
21	Virginia	353.3
22	Indiana	349.4
23	Alaska	322.6
24	Pennsylvania	317.0
25	Kansas	285.7
26	Delaware	282.7
27	Connecticut	276.8
28	Colorado	265.1
29	New Jersey	259.2
30	Kentucky	253.2
31	Oregon	229.7
32	West Virginia	224.3
33	Ohio	223.9
34	Washington	222.2
35	Wisconsin	215.3
36	Minnesota	183.4
37	Massachusetts	175.6
38	Idaho	175.2
39	Montana	173.4
40	Nebraska	159.4
41	Rhode Island	158.7
42	Hawaii	153.7
43	Utah	136.5
44	Iowa	133.4
45	Maine	97.9
NA	New Hampshire**	NA
NA	North Dakota**	NA
NA	South Dakota**	NA
NA	Vermont**	NA
NA	Wyoming**	NA

District of Columbia   3,782.9

Source: U.S. Department of Health and Human Services, National Center for Health Statistics
    unpublished data

*Age-adjusted years of potential life lost due to death before age 75.

**Data for states with fewer than 20 deaths from HIV infection for persons under 75 years of age are considered unreliable and are not shown.

Years Lost by Premature Death from Unintentional Injuries in 1996

National Average = 1,137.0 Years Lost per 100,000 Population*

<table>
<tr><td colspan="3">ALPHA ORDER</td><td colspan="3">RANK ORDER</td></tr>
<tr><th>RANK</th><th>STATE</th><th>YEARS</th><th>RANK</th><th>STATE</th><th>YEARS</th></tr>
<tr><td>5</td><td>Alabama</td><td>1,727.5</td><td>1</td><td>Alaska</td><td>2,040.7</td></tr>
<tr><td>1</td><td>Alaska</td><td>2,040.7</td><td>2</td><td>Mississippi</td><td>1,995.9</td></tr>
<tr><td>9</td><td>Arizona</td><td>1,617.2</td><td>3</td><td>New Mexico</td><td>1,984.9</td></tr>
<tr><td>6</td><td>Arkansas</td><td>1,715.0</td><td>4</td><td>Wyoming</td><td>1,947.1</td></tr>
<tr><td>37</td><td>California</td><td>994.9</td><td>5</td><td>Alabama</td><td>1,727.5</td></tr>
<tr><td>25</td><td>Colorado</td><td>1,207.0</td><td>6</td><td>Arkansas</td><td>1,715.0</td></tr>
<tr><td>44</td><td>Connecticut</td><td>890.5</td><td>7</td><td>Tennessee</td><td>1,653.7</td></tr>
<tr><td>26</td><td>Delaware</td><td>1,114.6</td><td>8</td><td>South Carolina</td><td>1,620.5</td></tr>
<tr><td>24</td><td>Florida</td><td>1,237.8</td><td>9</td><td>Arizona</td><td>1,617.2</td></tr>
<tr><td>15</td><td>Georgia</td><td>1,418.8</td><td>10</td><td>Idaho</td><td>1,548.3</td></tr>
<tr><td>40</td><td>Hawaii</td><td>936.4</td><td>11</td><td>Oklahoma</td><td>1,541.9</td></tr>
<tr><td>10</td><td>Idaho</td><td>1,548.3</td><td>12</td><td>Montana</td><td>1,463.3</td></tr>
<tr><td>38</td><td>Illinois</td><td>968.2</td><td>13</td><td>Louisiana</td><td>1,457.0</td></tr>
<tr><td>27</td><td>Indiana</td><td>1,109.4</td><td>14</td><td>Kentucky</td><td>1,453.3</td></tr>
<tr><td>28</td><td>Iowa</td><td>1,108.1</td><td>15</td><td>Georgia</td><td>1,418.8</td></tr>
<tr><td>22</td><td>Kansas</td><td>1,314.3</td><td>16</td><td>South Dakota</td><td>1,409.5</td></tr>
<tr><td>14</td><td>Kentucky</td><td>1,453.3</td><td>17</td><td>Missouri</td><td>1,395.9</td></tr>
<tr><td>13</td><td>Louisiana</td><td>1,457.0</td><td>18</td><td>Oregon</td><td>1,380.2</td></tr>
<tr><td>41</td><td>Maine</td><td>927.9</td><td>19</td><td>West Virginia</td><td>1,363.3</td></tr>
<tr><td>46</td><td>Maryland</td><td>806.7</td><td>20</td><td>North Carolina</td><td>1,354.9</td></tr>
<tr><td>49</td><td>Massachusetts</td><td>494.7</td><td>21</td><td>Nevada</td><td>1,353.4</td></tr>
<tr><td>36</td><td>Michigan</td><td>1,001.9</td><td>22</td><td>Kansas</td><td>1,314.3</td></tr>
<tr><td>42</td><td>Minnesota</td><td>904.6</td><td>23</td><td>Texas</td><td>1,304.3</td></tr>
<tr><td>2</td><td>Mississippi</td><td>1,995.9</td><td>24</td><td>Florida</td><td>1,237.8</td></tr>
<tr><td>17</td><td>Missouri</td><td>1,395.9</td><td>25</td><td>Colorado</td><td>1,207.0</td></tr>
<tr><td>12</td><td>Montana</td><td>1,463.3</td><td>26</td><td>Delaware</td><td>1,114.6</td></tr>
<tr><td>31</td><td>Nebraska</td><td>1,091.4</td><td>27</td><td>Indiana</td><td>1,109.4</td></tr>
<tr><td>21</td><td>Nevada</td><td>1,353.4</td><td>28</td><td>Iowa</td><td>1,108.1</td></tr>
<tr><td>48</td><td>New Hampshire</td><td>700.7</td><td>29</td><td>North Dakota</td><td>1,101.6</td></tr>
<tr><td>45</td><td>New Jersey</td><td>817.3</td><td>30</td><td>Washington</td><td>1,095.7</td></tr>
<tr><td>3</td><td>New Mexico</td><td>1,984.9</td><td>31</td><td>Nebraska</td><td>1,091.4</td></tr>
<tr><td>47</td><td>New York</td><td>760.1</td><td>32</td><td>Utah</td><td>1,077.0</td></tr>
<tr><td>20</td><td>North Carolina</td><td>1,354.9</td><td>33</td><td>Pennsylvania</td><td>1,051.0</td></tr>
<tr><td>29</td><td>North Dakota</td><td>1,101.6</td><td>34</td><td>Vermont</td><td>1,025.8</td></tr>
<tr><td>43</td><td>Ohio</td><td>903.4</td><td>35</td><td>Wisconsin</td><td>1,020.9</td></tr>
<tr><td>11</td><td>Oklahoma</td><td>1,541.9</td><td>36</td><td>Michigan</td><td>1,001.9</td></tr>
<tr><td>18</td><td>Oregon</td><td>1,380.2</td><td>37</td><td>California</td><td>994.9</td></tr>
<tr><td>33</td><td>Pennsylvania</td><td>1,051.0</td><td>38</td><td>Illinois</td><td>968.2</td></tr>
<tr><td>50</td><td>Rhode Island</td><td>467.4</td><td>39</td><td>Virginia</td><td>961.5</td></tr>
<tr><td>8</td><td>South Carolina</td><td>1,620.5</td><td>40</td><td>Hawaii</td><td>936.4</td></tr>
<tr><td>16</td><td>South Dakota</td><td>1,409.5</td><td>41</td><td>Maine</td><td>927.9</td></tr>
<tr><td>7</td><td>Tennessee</td><td>1,653.7</td><td>42</td><td>Minnesota</td><td>904.6</td></tr>
<tr><td>23</td><td>Texas</td><td>1,304.3</td><td>43</td><td>Ohio</td><td>903.4</td></tr>
<tr><td>32</td><td>Utah</td><td>1,077.0</td><td>44</td><td>Connecticut</td><td>890.5</td></tr>
<tr><td>34</td><td>Vermont</td><td>1,025.8</td><td>45</td><td>New Jersey</td><td>817.3</td></tr>
<tr><td>39</td><td>Virginia</td><td>961.5</td><td>46</td><td>Maryland</td><td>806.7</td></tr>
<tr><td>30</td><td>Washington</td><td>1,095.7</td><td>47</td><td>New York</td><td>760.1</td></tr>
<tr><td>19</td><td>West Virginia</td><td>1,363.3</td><td>48</td><td>New Hampshire</td><td>700.7</td></tr>
<tr><td>35</td><td>Wisconsin</td><td>1,020.9</td><td>49</td><td>Massachusetts</td><td>494.7</td></tr>
<tr><td>4</td><td>Wyoming</td><td>1,947.1</td><td>50</td><td>Rhode Island</td><td>467.4</td></tr>
<tr><td></td><td></td><td></td><td></td><td>District of Columbia</td><td>922.0</td></tr>
</table>

Source: U.S. Department of Health and Human Services, National Center for Health Statistics
   unpublished data
*Age-adjusted years of potential life lost due to death before age 75. Includes such subcategories as falls, drowning, fires/burns, poisonings and motor vehicle injuries.

Average Annual Years of Potential Life Lost Due to Smoking: 1990-94

National Total = 5,721,206 Years*

<u>ALPHA ORDER</u>

RANK	STATE	YEARS	% of USA
21	Alabama	101,953	1.8%
50	Alaska	7,228	0.1%
25	Arizona	77,939	1.4%
27	Arkansas	71,690	1.3%
1	California	554,042	9.7%
32	Colorado	58,838	1.0%
29	Connecticut	67,551	1.2%
43	Delaware	17,669	0.3%
3	Florida	376,988	6.6%
11	Georgia	146,318	2.6%
44	Hawaii	16,545	0.3%
42	Idaho	17,993	0.3%
7	Illinois	265,561	4.6%
12	Indiana	141,056	2.5%
31	Iowa	61,275	1.1%
34	Kansas	52,749	0.9%
17	Kentucky	112,695	2.0%
18	Louisiana	104,813	1.8%
37	Maine	30,556	0.5%
20	Maryland	102,119	1.8%
16	Massachusetts	132,751	2.3%
8	Michigan	223,229	3.9%
26	Minnesota	77,654	1.4%
28	Mississippi	68,818	1.2%
15	Missouri	134,994	2.4%
41	Montana	18,025	0.3%
36	Nebraska	32,866	0.6%
35	Nevada	38,269	0.7%
40	New Hampshire	23,416	0.4%
9	New Jersey	172,539	3.0%
38	New Mexico	24,569	0.4%
2	New York	417,206	7.3%
10	North Carolina	170,621	3.0%
47	North Dakota	12,032	0.2%
6	Ohio	270,475	4.7%
24	Oklahoma	85,650	1.5%
30	Oregon	67,351	1.2%
5	Pennsylvania	307,829	5.4%
39	Rhode Island	24,067	0.4%
23	South Carolina	90,122	1.6%
46	South Dakota	14,705	0.3%
14	Tennessee	135,175	2.4%
4	Texas	347,215	6.1%
45	Utah	15,158	0.3%
48	Vermont	12,019	0.2%
13	Virginia	135,385	2.4%
19	Washington	102,769	1.8%
33	West Virginia	57,678	1.0%
22	Wisconsin	100,624	1.8%
49	Wyoming	9,271	0.2%

<u>RANK ORDER</u>

RANK	STATE	YEARS	% of USA
1	California	554,042	9.7%
2	New York	417,206	7.3%
3	Florida	376,988	6.6%
4	Texas	347,215	6.1%
5	Pennsylvania	307,829	5.4%
6	Ohio	270,475	4.7%
7	Illinois	265,561	4.6%
8	Michigan	223,229	3.9%
9	New Jersey	172,539	3.0%
10	North Carolina	170,621	3.0%
11	Georgia	146,318	2.6%
12	Indiana	141,056	2.5%
13	Virginia	135,385	2.4%
14	Tennessee	135,175	2.4%
15	Missouri	134,994	2.4%
16	Massachusetts	132,751	2.3%
17	Kentucky	112,695	2.0%
18	Louisiana	104,813	1.8%
19	Washington	102,769	1.8%
20	Maryland	102,119	1.8%
21	Alabama	101,953	1.8%
22	Wisconsin	100,624	1.8%
23	South Carolina	90,122	1.6%
24	Oklahoma	85,650	1.5%
25	Arizona	77,939	1.4%
26	Minnesota	77,654	1.4%
27	Arkansas	71,690	1.3%
28	Mississippi	68,818	1.2%
29	Connecticut	67,551	1.2%
30	Oregon	67,351	1.2%
31	Iowa	61,275	1.1%
32	Colorado	58,838	1.0%
33	West Virginia	57,678	1.0%
34	Kansas	52,749	0.9%
35	Nevada	38,269	0.7%
36	Nebraska	32,866	0.6%
37	Maine	30,556	0.5%
38	New Mexico	24,569	0.4%
39	Rhode Island	24,067	0.4%
40	New Hampshire	23,416	0.4%
41	Montana	18,025	0.3%
42	Idaho	17,993	0.3%
43	Delaware	17,669	0.3%
44	Hawaii	16,545	0.3%
45	Utah	15,158	0.3%
46	South Dakota	14,705	0.3%
47	North Dakota	12,032	0.2%
48	Vermont	12,019	0.2%
49	Wyoming	9,271	0.2%
50	Alaska	7,228	0.1%
	District of Columbia	15,184	0.3%

Source: Centers for Disease Control and Prevention, Office on Smoking and Health
   "State and National Tobacco Control Highlights" (http://www.cdc.gov/nccdphp/osh/statehi/statehi.htm)
*Estimates. Calculated by using life expectancy at age of death.

Average Annual Deaths Due to Smoking: 1990-1994

National Estimated Total = 430,741 Deaths*

ALPHA ORDER

RANK	STATE	DEATHS	% of USA
22	Alabama	7,055	1.6%
50	Alaska	421	0.1%
25	Arizona	5,912	1.4%
27	Arkansas	5,271	1.2%
1	California	41,883	9.7%
32	Colorado	4,467	1.0%
28	Connecticut	5,251	1.2%
43	Delaware	1,248	0.3%
3	Florida	29,060	6.7%
14	Georgia	9,666	2.2%
45	Hawaii	1,163	0.3%
42	Idaho	1,404	0.3%
7	Illinois	19,016	4.4%
11	Indiana	10,373	2.4%
30	Iowa	4,962	1.2%
34	Kansas	4,215	1.0%
17	Kentucky	7,953	1.8%
21	Louisiana	7,075	1.6%
37	Maine	2,326	0.5%
20	Maryland	7,180	1.7%
12	Massachusetts	10,242	2.4%
8	Michigan	15,786	3.7%
24	Minnesota	6,150	1.4%
31	Mississippi	4,762	1.1%
13	Missouri	9,960	2.3%
41	Montana	1,434	0.3%
36	Nebraska	2,623	0.6%
35	Nevada	2,665	0.6%
40	New Hampshire	1,777	0.4%
9	New Jersey	12,831	3.0%
38	New Mexico	1,871	0.4%
2	New York	30,741	7.1%
10	North Carolina	11,642	2.7%
47	North Dakota	968	0.2%
6	Ohio	19,527	4.5%
23	Oklahoma	6,255	1.5%
29	Oregon	5,210	1.2%
5	Pennsylvania	23,170	5.4%
39	Rhode Island	1,849	0.4%
26	South Carolina	5,887	1.4%
44	South Dakota	1,198	0.3%
16	Tennessee	9,359	2.2%
4	Texas	24,789	5.8%
46	Utah	1,133	0.3%
48	Vermont	914	0.2%
15	Virginia	9,530	2.2%
18	Washington	7,892	1.8%
33	West Virginia	4,229	1.0%
19	Wisconsin	7,853	1.8%
49	Wyoming	712	0.2%

RANK ORDER

RANK	STATE	DEATHS	% of USA
1	California	41,883	9.7%
2	New York	30,741	7.1%
3	Florida	29,060	6.7%
4	Texas	24,789	5.8%
5	Pennsylvania	23,170	5.4%
6	Ohio	19,527	4.5%
7	Illinois	19,016	4.4%
8	Michigan	15,786	3.7%
9	New Jersey	12,831	3.0%
10	North Carolina	11,642	2.7%
11	Indiana	10,373	2.4%
12	Massachusetts	10,242	2.4%
13	Missouri	9,960	2.3%
14	Georgia	9,666	2.2%
15	Virginia	9,530	2.2%
16	Tennessee	9,359	2.2%
17	Kentucky	7,953	1.8%
18	Washington	7,892	1.8%
19	Wisconsin	7,853	1.8%
20	Maryland	7,180	1.7%
21	Louisiana	7,075	1.6%
22	Alabama	7,055	1.6%
23	Oklahoma	6,255	1.5%
24	Minnesota	6,150	1.4%
25	Arizona	5,912	1.4%
26	South Carolina	5,887	1.4%
27	Arkansas	5,271	1.2%
28	Connecticut	5,251	1.2%
29	Oregon	5,210	1.2%
30	Iowa	4,962	1.2%
31	Mississippi	4,762	1.1%
32	Colorado	4,467	1.0%
33	West Virginia	4,229	1.0%
34	Kansas	4,215	1.0%
35	Nevada	2,665	0.6%
36	Nebraska	2,623	0.6%
37	Maine	2,326	0.5%
38	New Mexico	1,871	0.4%
39	Rhode Island	1,849	0.4%
40	New Hampshire	1,777	0.4%
41	Montana	1,434	0.3%
42	Idaho	1,404	0.3%
43	Delaware	1,248	0.3%
44	South Dakota	1,198	0.3%
45	Hawaii	1,163	0.3%
46	Utah	1,133	0.3%
47	North Dakota	968	0.2%
48	Vermont	914	0.2%
49	Wyoming	712	0.2%
50	Alaska	421	0.1%
	District of Columbia	929	0.2%

Source: Centers for Disease Control and Prevention, Office on Smoking and Health
"State and National Tobacco Control Highlights" (http://www.cdc.gov/nccdphp/osh/statehi/statehi.htm)
*Estimates.

Average Annual Death Rate Due to Smoking: 1990-1994

National Rate = 358 Deaths per 100,000 Population*

<table>
<tr><td colspan="3">ALPHA ORDER</td><td colspan="3">RANK ORDER</td></tr>
<tr><td>RANK</td><td>STATE</td><td>RATE</td><td>RANK</td><td>STATE</td><td>RATE</td></tr>
<tr><td>23</td><td>Alabama</td><td>353</td><td>1</td><td>Nevada</td><td>469</td></tr>
<tr><td>15</td><td>Alaska</td><td>367</td><td>2</td><td>Kentucky</td><td>444</td></tr>
<tr><td>38</td><td>Arizona</td><td>325</td><td>3</td><td>West Virginia</td><td>424</td></tr>
<tr><td>4</td><td>Arkansas</td><td>405</td><td>4</td><td>Arkansas</td><td>405</td></tr>
<tr><td>32</td><td>California</td><td>343</td><td>5</td><td>Delaware</td><td>400</td></tr>
<tr><td>35</td><td>Colorado</td><td>331</td><td>6</td><td>Mississippi</td><td>392</td></tr>
<tr><td>41</td><td>Connecticut</td><td>310</td><td>7</td><td>Tennessee</td><td>390</td></tr>
<tr><td>5</td><td>Delaware</td><td>400</td><td>8</td><td>Louisiana</td><td>388</td></tr>
<tr><td>27</td><td>Florida</td><td>350</td><td>9</td><td>Indiana</td><td>387</td></tr>
<tr><td>17</td><td>Georgia</td><td>364</td><td>9</td><td>Oklahoma</td><td>387</td></tr>
<tr><td>49</td><td>Hawaii</td><td>237</td><td>11</td><td>South Carolina</td><td>378</td></tr>
<tr><td>45</td><td>Idaho</td><td>296</td><td>12</td><td>Maine</td><td>371</td></tr>
<tr><td>30</td><td>Illinois</td><td>347</td><td>13</td><td>Michigan</td><td>368</td></tr>
<tr><td>9</td><td>Indiana</td><td>387</td><td>13</td><td>North Carolina</td><td>368</td></tr>
<tr><td>43</td><td>Iowa</td><td>308</td><td>15</td><td>Alaska</td><td>367</td></tr>
<tr><td>39</td><td>Kansas</td><td>319</td><td>15</td><td>Missouri</td><td>367</td></tr>
<tr><td>2</td><td>Kentucky</td><td>444</td><td>17</td><td>Georgia</td><td>364</td></tr>
<tr><td>8</td><td>Louisiana</td><td>388</td><td>17</td><td>Ohio</td><td>364</td></tr>
<tr><td>12</td><td>Maine</td><td>371</td><td>19</td><td>New Hampshire</td><td>361</td></tr>
<tr><td>24</td><td>Maryland</td><td>351</td><td>20</td><td>Virginia</td><td>360</td></tr>
<tr><td>35</td><td>Massachusetts</td><td>331</td><td>21</td><td>Texas</td><td>358</td></tr>
<tr><td>13</td><td>Michigan</td><td>368</td><td>22</td><td>Wyoming</td><td>357</td></tr>
<tr><td>47</td><td>Minnesota</td><td>287</td><td>23</td><td>Alabama</td><td>353</td></tr>
<tr><td>6</td><td>Mississippi</td><td>392</td><td>24</td><td>Maryland</td><td>351</td></tr>
<tr><td>15</td><td>Missouri</td><td>367</td><td>24</td><td>Vermont</td><td>351</td></tr>
<tr><td>28</td><td>Montana</td><td>348</td><td>24</td><td>Washington</td><td>351</td></tr>
<tr><td>43</td><td>Nebraska</td><td>308</td><td>27</td><td>Florida</td><td>350</td></tr>
<tr><td>1</td><td>Nevada</td><td>469</td><td>28</td><td>Montana</td><td>348</td></tr>
<tr><td>19</td><td>New Hampshire</td><td>361</td><td>28</td><td>Oregon</td><td>348</td></tr>
<tr><td>37</td><td>New Jersey</td><td>327</td><td>30</td><td>Illinois</td><td>347</td></tr>
<tr><td>46</td><td>New Mexico</td><td>289</td><td>31</td><td>Pennsylvania</td><td>346</td></tr>
<tr><td>32</td><td>New York</td><td>343</td><td>32</td><td>California</td><td>343</td></tr>
<tr><td>13</td><td>North Carolina</td><td>368</td><td>32</td><td>New York</td><td>343</td></tr>
<tr><td>48</td><td>North Dakota</td><td>280</td><td>34</td><td>Rhode Island</td><td>340</td></tr>
<tr><td>17</td><td>Ohio</td><td>364</td><td>35</td><td>Colorado</td><td>331</td></tr>
<tr><td>9</td><td>Oklahoma</td><td>387</td><td>35</td><td>Massachusetts</td><td>331</td></tr>
<tr><td>28</td><td>Oregon</td><td>348</td><td>37</td><td>New Jersey</td><td>327</td></tr>
<tr><td>31</td><td>Pennsylvania</td><td>346</td><td>38</td><td>Arizona</td><td>325</td></tr>
<tr><td>34</td><td>Rhode Island</td><td>340</td><td>39</td><td>Kansas</td><td>319</td></tr>
<tr><td>11</td><td>South Carolina</td><td>378</td><td>40</td><td>Wisconsin</td><td>313</td></tr>
<tr><td>42</td><td>South Dakota</td><td>309</td><td>41</td><td>Connecticut</td><td>310</td></tr>
<tr><td>7</td><td>Tennessee</td><td>390</td><td>42</td><td>South Dakota</td><td>309</td></tr>
<tr><td>21</td><td>Texas</td><td>358</td><td>43</td><td>Iowa</td><td>308</td></tr>
<tr><td>50</td><td>Utah</td><td>188</td><td>43</td><td>Nebraska</td><td>308</td></tr>
<tr><td>24</td><td>Vermont</td><td>351</td><td>45</td><td>Idaho</td><td>296</td></tr>
<tr><td>20</td><td>Virginia</td><td>360</td><td>46</td><td>New Mexico</td><td>289</td></tr>
<tr><td>24</td><td>Washington</td><td>351</td><td>47</td><td>Minnesota</td><td>287</td></tr>
<tr><td>3</td><td>West Virginia</td><td>424</td><td>48</td><td>North Dakota</td><td>280</td></tr>
<tr><td>40</td><td>Wisconsin</td><td>313</td><td>49</td><td>Hawaii</td><td>237</td></tr>
<tr><td>22</td><td>Wyoming</td><td>357</td><td>50</td><td>Utah</td><td>188</td></tr>
<tr><td></td><td></td><td></td><td></td><td>District of Columbia</td><td>327</td></tr>
</table>

Source: Centers for Disease Control and Prevention, Office on Smoking and Health
   "State and National Tobacco Control Highlights" (http://www.cdc.gov/nccdphp/osh/statehi/statehi.htm)
*Estimates.

Alcohol-Induced Deaths in 1996

National Total = 19,770 Deaths*

ALPHA ORDER

ALPHA ORDER

RANK	STATE	DEATHS	% of USA
26	Alabama	275	1.4%
37	Alaska	109	0.6%
12	Arizona	485	2.5%
36	Arkansas	119	0.6%
1	California	3,370	17.0%
16	Colorado	372	1.9%
32	Connecticut	179	0.9%
45	Delaware	63	0.3%
3	Florida	1,253	6.3%
9	Georgia	564	2.9%
48	Hawaii	50	0.3%
44	Idaho	69	0.3%
5	Illinois	715	3.6%
22	Indiana	318	1.6%
35	Iowa	124	0.6%
34	Kansas	126	0.6%
28	Kentucky	242	1.2%
27	Louisiana	263	1.3%
38	Maine	108	0.5%
23	Maryland	308	1.6%
21	Massachusetts	323	1.6%
7	Michigan	678	3.4%
24	Minnesota	299	1.5%
31	Mississippi	186	0.9%
17	Missouri	366	1.9%
41	Montana	83	0.4%
43	Nebraska	72	0.4%
30	Nevada	214	1.1%
40	New Hampshire	86	0.4%
10	New Jersey	540	2.7%
25	New Mexico	288	1.5%
2	New York	1,489	7.5%
6	North Carolina	690	3.5%
47	North Dakota	52	0.3%
8	Ohio	574	2.9%
28	Oklahoma	242	1.2%
20	Oregon	358	1.8%
11	Pennsylvania	491	2.5%
45	Rhode Island	63	0.3%
14	South Carolina	405	2.0%
42	South Dakota	76	0.4%
15	Tennessee	392	2.0%
4	Texas	1,153	5.8%
39	Utah	99	0.5%
50	Vermont	25	0.1%
18	Virginia	361	1.8%
13	Washington	447	2.3%
33	West Virginia	127	0.6%
19	Wisconsin	359	1.8%
49	Wyoming	46	0.2%

RANK ORDER

RANK	STATE	DEATHS	% of USA
1	California	3,370	17.0%
2	New York	1,489	7.5%
3	Florida	1,253	6.3%
4	Texas	1,153	5.8%
5	Illinois	715	3.6%
6	North Carolina	690	3.5%
7	Michigan	678	3.4%
8	Ohio	574	2.9%
9	Georgia	564	2.9%
10	New Jersey	540	2.7%
11	Pennsylvania	491	2.5%
12	Arizona	485	2.5%
13	Washington	447	2.3%
14	South Carolina	405	2.0%
15	Tennessee	392	2.0%
16	Colorado	372	1.9%
17	Missouri	366	1.9%
18	Virginia	361	1.8%
19	Wisconsin	359	1.8%
20	Oregon	358	1.8%
21	Massachusetts	323	1.6%
22	Indiana	318	1.6%
23	Maryland	308	1.6%
24	Minnesota	299	1.5%
25	New Mexico	288	1.5%
26	Alabama	275	1.4%
27	Louisiana	263	1.3%
28	Kentucky	242	1.2%
28	Oklahoma	242	1.2%
30	Nevada	214	1.1%
31	Mississippi	186	0.9%
32	Connecticut	179	0.9%
33	West Virginia	127	0.6%
34	Kansas	126	0.6%
35	Iowa	124	0.6%
36	Arkansas	119	0.6%
37	Alaska	109	0.6%
38	Maine	108	0.5%
39	Utah	99	0.5%
40	New Hampshire	86	0.4%
41	Montana	83	0.4%
42	South Dakota	76	0.4%
43	Nebraska	72	0.4%
44	Idaho	69	0.3%
45	Delaware	63	0.3%
45	Rhode Island	63	0.3%
47	North Dakota	52	0.3%
48	Hawaii	50	0.3%
49	Wyoming	46	0.2%
50	Vermont	25	0.1%
	District of Columbia	74	0.4%

Source: U.S. Department of Health and Human Services, National Center for Health Statistics
(http://wonder.cdc.gov/WONDER/)

*By state of residence. Includes excessive blood level of alcohol, accidental poisoning by alcohol and the following alcohol-related causes: psychoses, dependence syndrome, polyneuropathy, cardiomyopathy, gastritis, chronic liver disease and cirrhosis. Excludes accidents, homicides and other causes indirectly related to alcohol use.

Death Rate from Alcohol-Induced Deaths in 1996

National Rate = 7.5 Deaths per 100,000 Population*

ALPHA ORDER

RANK	STATE	RATE
29	Alabama	6.4
1	Alaska	18.0
5	Arizona	10.9
45	Arkansas	4.8
7	California	10.6
9	Colorado	9.8
38	Connecticut	5.5
13	Delaware	8.7
13	Florida	8.7
19	Georgia	7.7
49	Hawaii	4.2
37	Idaho	5.8
36	Illinois	6.0
38	Indiana	5.5
46	Iowa	4.4
43	Kansas	4.9
32	Kentucky	6.2
33	Louisiana	6.1
13	Maine	8.7
33	Maryland	6.1
41	Massachusetts	5.3
23	Michigan	7.0
29	Minnesota	6.4
25	Mississippi	6.9
27	Missouri	6.8
11	Montana	9.5
46	Nebraska	4.4
3	Nevada	13.4
20	New Hampshire	7.4
28	New Jersey	6.7
2	New Mexico	16.9
16	New York	8.2
12	North Carolina	9.4
17	North Dakota	8.1
42	Ohio	5.1
22	Oklahoma	7.3
4	Oregon	11.2
50	Pennsylvania	4.1
29	Rhode Island	6.4
6	South Carolina	10.8
8	South Dakota	10.3
20	Tennessee	7.4
33	Texas	6.1
43	Utah	4.9
48	Vermont	4.3
40	Virginia	5.4
17	Washington	8.1
23	West Virginia	7.0
25	Wisconsin	6.9
10	Wyoming	9.6

RANK ORDER

RANK	STATE	RATE
1	Alaska	18.0
2	New Mexico	16.9
3	Nevada	13.4
4	Oregon	11.2
5	Arizona	10.9
6	South Carolina	10.8
7	California	10.6
8	South Dakota	10.3
9	Colorado	9.8
10	Wyoming	9.6
11	Montana	9.5
12	North Carolina	9.4
13	Delaware	8.7
13	Florida	8.7
13	Maine	8.7
16	New York	8.2
17	North Dakota	8.1
17	Washington	8.1
19	Georgia	7.7
20	New Hampshire	7.4
20	Tennessee	7.4
22	Oklahoma	7.3
23	Michigan	7.0
23	West Virginia	7.0
25	Mississippi	6.9
25	Wisconsin	6.9
27	Missouri	6.8
28	New Jersey	6.7
29	Alabama	6.4
29	Minnesota	6.4
29	Rhode Island	6.4
32	Kentucky	6.2
33	Louisiana	6.1
33	Maryland	6.1
33	Texas	6.1
36	Illinois	6.0
37	Idaho	5.8
38	Connecticut	5.5
38	Indiana	5.5
40	Virginia	5.4
41	Massachusetts	5.3
42	Ohio	5.1
43	Kansas	4.9
43	Utah	4.9
45	Arkansas	4.8
46	Iowa	4.4
46	Nebraska	4.4
48	Vermont	4.3
49	Hawaii	4.2
50	Pennsylvania	4.1

District of Columbia	13.7

Source: Morgan Quitno Press using data from U.S. Dept of Health & Human Serv's, Nat'l Center for Health Statistics (http://wonder.cdc.gov/WONDER/)

By state of residence. Includes excessive blood level of alcohol, accidental poisoning by alcohol and the following alcohol-related causes: psychoses, dependence syndrome, polyneuropathy, cardiomyopathy, gastritis, chronic liver disease and cirrhosis. Excludes accidents, homicides and other causes indirectly related to alcohol use. Not age-adjusted.

Age-Adjusted Death Rate from Alcohol-Induced Deaths in 1996

National Rate = 6.4 Deaths per 100,000 Population*

ALPHA ORDER

RANK	STATE	RATE
31	Alabama	5.4
1	Alaska	18.2
4	Arizona	10.0
45	Arkansas	4.0
5	California	9.8
9	Colorado	8.4
42	Connecticut	4.4
11	Delaware	7.9
18	Florida	6.8
14	Georgia	7.2
47	Hawaii	3.5
38	Idaho	4.9
31	Illinois	5.4
40	Indiana	4.6
47	Iowa	3.5
44	Kansas	4.1
31	Kentucky	5.4
31	Louisiana	5.4
15	Maine	6.9
35	Maryland	5.3
39	Massachusetts	4.7
24	Michigan	5.9
27	Minnesota	5.7
23	Mississippi	6.0
24	Missouri	5.9
13	Montana	7.6
46	Nebraska	3.6
3	Nevada	11.1
21	New Hampshire	6.2
29	New Jersey	5.6
2	New Mexico	15.6
15	New York	6.9
10	North Carolina	8.1
19	North Dakota	6.4
43	Ohio	4.3
22	Oklahoma	6.1
8	Oregon	8.9
49	Pennsylvania	3.4
37	Rhode Island	5.0
6	South Carolina	9.5
7	South Dakota	9.1
19	Tennessee	6.4
30	Texas	5.5
36	Utah	5.2
49	Vermont	3.4
40	Virginia	4.6
15	Washington	6.9
27	West Virginia	5.7
24	Wisconsin	5.9
12	Wyoming	7.8

RANK ORDER

RANK	STATE	RATE
1	Alaska	18.2
2	New Mexico	15.6
3	Nevada	11.1
4	Arizona	10.0
5	California	9.8
6	South Carolina	9.5
7	South Dakota	9.1
8	Oregon	8.9
9	Colorado	8.4
10	North Carolina	8.1
11	Delaware	7.9
12	Wyoming	7.8
13	Montana	7.6
14	Georgia	7.2
15	Maine	6.9
15	New York	6.9
15	Washington	6.9
18	Florida	6.8
19	North Dakota	6.4
19	Tennessee	6.4
21	New Hampshire	6.2
22	Oklahoma	6.1
23	Mississippi	6.0
24	Michigan	5.9
24	Missouri	5.9
24	Wisconsin	5.9
27	Minnesota	5.7
27	West Virginia	5.7
29	New Jersey	5.6
30	Texas	5.5
31	Alabama	5.4
31	Illinois	5.4
31	Kentucky	5.4
31	Louisiana	5.4
35	Maryland	5.3
36	Utah	5.2
37	Rhode Island	5.0
38	Idaho	4.9
39	Massachusetts	4.7
40	Indiana	4.6
40	Virginia	4.6
42	Connecticut	4.4
43	Ohio	4.3
44	Kansas	4.1
45	Arkansas	4.0
46	Nebraska	3.6
47	Hawaii	3.5
47	Iowa	3.5
49	Pennsylvania	3.4
49	Vermont	3.4
	District of Columbia	11.9

Source: U.S. Department of Health and Human Services, National Center for Health Statistics
     (http://wonder.cdc.gov/WONDER/)
*By state of residence. Includes excessive blood level of alcohol, accidental poisoning by alcohol and the following alcohol-related causes: psychoses, dependence syndrome, polyneuropathy, cardiomyopathy, gastritis, chronic liver disease and cirrhosis. Excludes accidents, homicides and other causes indirectly related to alcohol use.

Drug-Induced Deaths in 1996

National Total = 14,843 Deaths*

RANK	STATE	DEATHS	% of USA
31	Alabama	119	0.8%
42	Alaska	45	0.3%
11	Arizona	413	2.8%
34	Arkansas	77	0.5%
1	California	2,875	19.4%
18	Colorado	235	1.6%
17	Connecticut	245	1.7%
37	Delaware	53	0.4%
5	Florida	706	4.8%
14	Georgia	297	2.0%
33	Hawaii	79	0.5%
43	Idaho	39	0.3%
7	Illinois	504	3.4%
23	Indiana	183	1.2%
39	Iowa	52	0.4%
36	Kansas	61	0.4%
28	Kentucky	142	1.0%
24	Louisiana	167	1.1%
44	Maine	38	0.3%
10	Maryland	479	3.2%
12	Massachusetts	404	2.7%
8	Michigan	494	3.3%
32	Minnesota	110	0.7%
35	Mississippi	73	0.5%
20	Missouri	226	1.5%
45	Montana	28	0.2%
46	Nebraska	25	0.2%
27	Nevada	148	1.0%
39	New Hampshire	52	0.4%
6	New Jersey	700	4.7%
22	New Mexico	199	1.3%
2	New York	1,092	7.4%
20	North Carolina	226	1.5%
50	North Dakota	9	0.1%
13	Ohio	345	2.3%
26	Oklahoma	154	1.0%
14	Oregon	297	2.0%
4	Pennsylvania	922	6.2%
37	Rhode Island	53	0.4%
30	South Carolina	134	0.9%
47	South Dakota	23	0.2%
16	Tennessee	261	1.8%
3	Texas	930	6.3%
25	Utah	159	1.1%
48	Vermont	19	0.1%
19	Virginia	228	1.5%
9	Washington	481	3.2%
41	West Virginia	51	0.3%
29	Wisconsin	139	0.9%
49	Wyoming	17	0.1%

RANK	STATE	DEATHS	% of USA
1	California	2,875	19.4%
2	New York	1,092	7.4%
3	Texas	930	6.3%
4	Pennsylvania	922	6.2%
5	Florida	706	4.8%
6	New Jersey	700	4.7%
7	Illinois	504	3.4%
8	Michigan	494	3.3%
9	Washington	481	3.2%
10	Maryland	479	3.2%
11	Arizona	413	2.8%
12	Massachusetts	404	2.7%
13	Ohio	345	2.3%
14	Georgia	297	2.0%
14	Oregon	297	2.0%
16	Tennessee	261	1.8%
17	Connecticut	245	1.7%
18	Colorado	235	1.6%
19	Virginia	228	1.5%
20	Missouri	226	1.5%
20	North Carolina	226	1.5%
22	New Mexico	199	1.3%
23	Indiana	183	1.2%
24	Louisiana	167	1.1%
25	Utah	159	1.1%
26	Oklahoma	154	1.0%
27	Nevada	148	1.0%
28	Kentucky	142	1.0%
29	Wisconsin	139	0.9%
30	South Carolina	134	0.9%
31	Alabama	119	0.8%
32	Minnesota	110	0.7%
33	Hawaii	79	0.5%
34	Arkansas	77	0.5%
35	Mississippi	73	0.5%
36	Kansas	61	0.4%
37	Delaware	53	0.4%
37	Rhode Island	53	0.4%
39	Iowa	52	0.4%
39	New Hampshire	52	0.4%
41	West Virginia	51	0.3%
42	Alaska	45	0.3%
43	Idaho	39	0.3%
44	Maine	38	0.3%
45	Montana	28	0.2%
46	Nebraska	25	0.2%
47	South Dakota	23	0.2%
48	Vermont	19	0.1%
49	Wyoming	17	0.1%
50	North Dakota	9	0.1%
	District of Columbia	35	0.2%

Source: U.S. Department of Health and Human Services, National Center for Health Statistics (http://wonder.cdc.gov/WONDER/)

By state of residence. Includes drug psychoses, drug dependence, nondependent use excluding alcohol and tobacco, accidental poisoning or suicide by drugs, medicaments and biologicals. Excludes accidents, homicides and other causes indirectly related to drug use.

Death Rate from Drug-Induced Deaths in 1996

National Rate = 5.6 Deaths per 100,000 Population*

ALPHA ORDER

RANK	STATE	RATE
42	Alabama	2.8
12	Alaska	7.4
3	Arizona	9.3
36	Arkansas	3.1
6	California	9.1
16	Colorado	6.2
11	Connecticut	7.5
13	Delaware	7.3
20	Florida	4.9
27	Georgia	4.0
14	Hawaii	6.7
33	Idaho	3.3
25	Illinois	4.2
36	Indiana	3.1
48	Iowa	1.8
46	Kansas	2.4
29	Kentucky	3.7
28	Louisiana	3.8
36	Maine	3.1
2	Maryland	9.5
15	Massachusetts	6.6
19	Michigan	5.1
46	Minnesota	2.4
44	Mississippi	2.7
25	Missouri	4.2
34	Montana	3.2
49	Nebraska	1.5
5	Nevada	9.2
24	New Hampshire	4.5
7	New Jersey	8.7
1	New Mexico	11.7
17	New York	6.0
36	North Carolina	3.1
50	North Dakota	1.4
36	Ohio	3.1
23	Oklahoma	4.7
3	Oregon	9.3
10	Pennsylvania	7.7
18	Rhode Island	5.4
30	South Carolina	3.6
36	South Dakota	3.1
20	Tennessee	4.9
20	Texas	4.9
9	Utah	7.9
34	Vermont	3.2
32	Virginia	3.4
7	Washington	8.7
42	West Virginia	2.8
44	Wisconsin	2.7
31	Wyoming	3.5

RANK ORDER

RANK	STATE	RATE
1	New Mexico	11.7
2	Maryland	9.5
3	Arizona	9.3
3	Oregon	9.3
5	Nevada	9.2
6	California	9.1
7	New Jersey	8.7
7	Washington	8.7
9	Utah	7.9
10	Pennsylvania	7.7
11	Connecticut	7.5
12	Alaska	7.4
13	Delaware	7.3
14	Hawaii	6.7
15	Massachusetts	6.6
16	Colorado	6.2
17	New York	6.0
18	Rhode Island	5.4
19	Michigan	5.1
20	Florida	4.9
20	Tennessee	4.9
20	Texas	4.9
23	Oklahoma	4.7
24	New Hampshire	4.5
25	Illinois	4.2
25	Missouri	4.2
27	Georgia	4.0
28	Louisiana	3.8
29	Kentucky	3.7
30	South Carolina	3.6
31	Wyoming	3.5
32	Virginia	3.4
33	Idaho	3.3
34	Montana	3.2
34	Vermont	3.2
36	Arkansas	3.1
36	Indiana	3.1
36	Maine	3.1
36	North Carolina	3.1
36	Ohio	3.1
36	South Dakota	3.1
42	Alabama	2.8
42	West Virginia	2.8
44	Mississippi	2.7
44	Wisconsin	2.7
46	Kansas	2.4
46	Minnesota	2.4
48	Iowa	1.8
49	Nebraska	1.5
50	North Dakota	1.4

District of Columbia 6.5

Source: Morgan Quitno Press using data from U.S. Dept of Health & Human Serv's, Nat'l Center for Health Statistics
(http://wonder.cdc.gov/WONDER/)
*By state of residence. Includes drug psychoses, drug dependence, nondependent use excluding alcohol and
tobacco, accidental poisoning or suicide by drugs, medicaments and biologicals. Excludes accidents, homicides
and other causes indirectly related to drug use. Not age-adjusted.

Age-Adjusted Death Rate from Drug-Induced Deaths in 1996

National Rate = 5.3 Deaths per 100,000 Population*

ALPHA ORDER

RANK	STATE	RATE
42	Alabama	2.4
11	Alaska	7.1
2	Arizona	9.1
33	Arkansas	3.0
3	California	8.6
17	Colorado	5.4
11	Connecticut	7.1
13	Delaware	6.6
19	Florida	4.7
28	Georgia	3.5
14	Hawaii	6.0
30	Idaho	3.3
24	Illinois	4.0
36	Indiana	2.8
48	Iowa	1.6
47	Kansas	2.0
28	Kentucky	3.5
27	Louisiana	3.7
39	Maine	2.7
6	Maryland	8.3
14	Massachusetts	6.0
22	Michigan	4.4
45	Minnesota	2.2
41	Mississippi	2.5
24	Missouri	4.0
30	Montana	3.3
50	Nebraska	1.3
3	Nevada	8.6
26	New Hampshire	3.9
6	New Jersey	8.3
1	New Mexico	11.7
16	New York	5.5
36	North Carolina	2.8
49	North Dakota**	1.4
36	Ohio	2.8
20	Oklahoma	4.6
5	Oregon	8.5
10	Pennsylvania	7.2
18	Rhode Island	5.0
30	South Carolina	3.3
39	South Dakota	2.7
22	Tennessee	4.4
20	Texas	4.6
6	Utah	8.3
42	Vermont**	2.4
33	Virginia	3.0
9	Washington	7.7
42	West Virginia	2.4
45	Wisconsin	2.2
33	Wyoming**	3.0

RANK ORDER

RANK	STATE	RATE
1	New Mexico	11.7
2	Arizona	9.1
3	California	8.6
3	Nevada	8.6
5	Oregon	8.5
6	Maryland	8.3
6	New Jersey	8.3
6	Utah	8.3
9	Washington	7.7
10	Pennsylvania	7.2
11	Alaska	7.1
11	Connecticut	7.1
13	Delaware	6.6
14	Hawaii	6.0
14	Massachusetts	6.0
16	New York	5.5
17	Colorado	5.4
18	Rhode Island	5.0
19	Florida	4.7
20	Oklahoma	4.6
20	Texas	4.6
22	Michigan	4.4
22	Tennessee	4.4
24	Illinois	4.0
24	Missouri	4.0
26	New Hampshire	3.9
27	Louisiana	3.7
28	Georgia	3.5
28	Kentucky	3.5
30	Idaho	3.3
30	Montana	3.3
30	South Carolina	3.3
33	Arkansas	3.0
33	Virginia	3.0
33	Wyoming**	3.0
36	Indiana	2.8
36	North Carolina	2.8
36	Ohio	2.8
39	Maine	2.7
39	South Dakota	2.7
41	Mississippi	2.5
42	Alabama	2.4
42	Vermont**	2.4
42	West Virginia	2.4
45	Minnesota	2.2
45	Wisconsin	2.2
47	Kansas	2.0
48	Iowa	1.6
49	North Dakota**	1.4
50	Nebraska	1.3
	District of Columbia	5.5

Source: Morgan Quitno Press using data from U.S. Dept of Health & Human Serv's, Nat'l Center for Health Statistics
(http://wonder.cdc.gov/WONDER/)

*By state of residence. Includes drug psychoses, drug dependence, nondependent use excluding alcohol and tobacco, accidental poisoning or suicide by drugs, medicaments and biologicals. Excludes accidents, homicides and other causes indirectly related to drug use.

**Due to low numbers of deaths, rates for these states should be interpreted with caution.

Occupational Fatalities in 1997

National Total = 6,218 Deaths

ALPHA ORDER

RANK ORDER

RANK	STATE	DEATHS	% of USA
15	Alabama	139	2.2%
38	Alaska	51	0.8%
33	Arizona	58	0.9%
24	Arkansas	102	1.6%
1	California	636	10.2%
19	Colorado	120	1.9%
42	Connecticut	32	0.5%
48	Delaware	17	0.3%
3	Florida	366	5.9%
6	Georgia	241	3.9%
46	Hawaii	19	0.3%
34	Idaho	56	0.9%
7	Illinois	240	3.9%
10	Indiana	190	3.1%
29	Iowa	80	1.3%
26	Kansas	93	1.5%
14	Kentucky	143	2.3%
16	Louisiana	137	2.2%
46	Maine	19	0.3%
28	Maryland	82	1.3%
31	Massachusetts	69	1.1%
11	Michigan	174	2.8%
30	Minnesota	72	1.2%
22	Mississippi	104	1.7%
18	Missouri	123	2.0%
34	Montana	56	0.9%
40	Nebraska	46	0.7%
36	Nevada	55	0.9%
44	New Hampshire	23	0.4%
25	New Jersey	101	1.6%
39	New Mexico	50	0.8%
4	New York	264	4.2%
8	North Carolina	210	3.4%
41	North Dakota	35	0.6%
9	Ohio	201	3.2%
22	Oklahoma	104	1.7%
27	Oregon	84	1.4%
5	Pennsylvania	259	4.2%
49	Rhode Island	10	0.2%
17	South Carolina	129	2.1%
44	South Dakota	23	0.4%
12	Tennessee	168	2.7%
2	Texas	460	7.4%
32	Utah	66	1.1%
50	Vermont	9	0.1%
13	Virginia	166	2.7%
21	Washington	112	1.8%
37	West Virginia	53	0.9%
20	Wisconsin	114	1.8%
43	Wyoming	29	0.5%

RANK	STATE	DEATHS	% of USA
1	California	636	10.2%
2	Texas	460	7.4%
3	Florida	366	5.9%
4	New York	264	4.2%
5	Pennsylvania	259	4.2%
6	Georgia	241	3.9%
7	Illinois	240	3.9%
8	North Carolina	210	3.4%
9	Ohio	201	3.2%
10	Indiana	190	3.1%
11	Michigan	174	2.8%
12	Tennessee	168	2.7%
13	Virginia	166	2.7%
14	Kentucky	143	2.3%
15	Alabama	139	2.2%
16	Louisiana	137	2.2%
17	South Carolina	129	2.1%
18	Missouri	123	2.0%
19	Colorado	120	1.9%
20	Wisconsin	114	1.8%
21	Washington	112	1.8%
22	Mississippi	104	1.7%
22	Oklahoma	104	1.7%
24	Arkansas	102	1.6%
25	New Jersey	101	1.6%
26	Kansas	93	1.5%
27	Oregon	84	1.4%
28	Maryland	82	1.3%
29	Iowa	80	1.3%
30	Minnesota	72	1.2%
31	Massachusetts	69	1.1%
32	Utah	66	1.1%
33	Arizona	58	0.9%
34	Idaho	56	0.9%
34	Montana	56	0.9%
36	Nevada	55	0.9%
37	West Virginia	53	0.9%
38	Alaska	51	0.8%
39	New Mexico	50	0.8%
40	Nebraska	46	0.7%
41	North Dakota	35	0.6%
42	Connecticut	32	0.5%
43	Wyoming	29	0.5%
44	New Hampshire	23	0.4%
44	South Dakota	23	0.4%
46	Hawaii	19	0.3%
46	Maine	19	0.3%
48	Delaware	17	0.3%
49	Rhode Island	10	0.2%
50	Vermont	9	0.1%
	District of Columbia	23	0.4%

Source: U.S. Department of Labor, Bureau of Labor Statistics
  "National Census of Fatal Occupational Injuries, 1997" (press release, August 12, 1998)

Occupational Fatalities per 100,000 Workers in 1997

National Rate = 4.8 Deaths per 100,000 Workers

ALPHA ORDER				RANK ORDER		
RANK	STATE	RATE		RANK	STATE	RATE
14	Alabama	6.7		1	Alaska	17.5
1	Alaska	17.5		2	Montana	13.0
45	Arizona	2.8		3	Wyoming	12.2
6	Arkansas	8.9		4	North Dakota	10.3
33	California	4.2		5	Idaho	9.3
22	Colorado	5.7		6	Arkansas	8.9
50	Connecticut	2.0		7	Mississippi	8.7
30	Delaware	4.7		8	Kentucky	7.8
24	Florida	5.4		9	Louisiana	7.2
16	Georgia	6.5		10	Kansas	7.1
40	Hawaii	3.4		10	South Carolina	7.1
5	Idaho	9.3		10	West Virginia	7.1
34	Illinois	4.1		13	Oklahoma	6.8
20	Indiana	6.4		14	Alabama	6.7
25	Iowa	5.2		15	Tennessee	6.6
10	Kansas	7.1		16	Georgia	6.5
8	Kentucky	7.8		16	Nevada	6.5
9	Louisiana	7.2		16	New Mexico	6.5
43	Maine	3.0		16	Utah	6.5
42	Maryland	3.1		20	Indiana	6.4
48	Massachusetts	2.2		21	South Dakota	6.0
39	Michigan	3.6		22	Colorado	5.7
45	Minnesota	2.8		22	North Carolina	5.7
7	Mississippi	8.7		24	Florida	5.4
32	Missouri	4.4		25	Iowa	5.2
2	Montana	13.0		25	Nebraska	5.2
25	Nebraska	5.2		25	Oregon	5.2
16	Nevada	6.5		28	Virginia	5.1
37	New Hampshire	3.7		29	Texas	4.9
47	New Jersey	2.5		30	Delaware	4.7
16	New Mexico	6.5		31	Pennsylvania	4.6
41	New York	3.2		32	Missouri	4.4
22	North Carolina	5.7		33	California	4.2
4	North Dakota	10.3		34	Illinois	4.1
37	Ohio	3.7		35	Wisconsin	4.0
13	Oklahoma	6.8		36	Washington	3.9
25	Oregon	5.2		37	New Hampshire	3.7
31	Pennsylvania	4.6		37	Ohio	3.7
49	Rhode Island	2.1		39	Michigan	3.6
10	South Carolina	7.1		40	Hawaii	3.4
21	South Dakota	6.0		41	New York	3.2
15	Tennessee	6.6		42	Maryland	3.1
29	Texas	4.9		43	Maine	3.0
16	Utah	6.5		44	Vermont	2.9
44	Vermont	2.9		45	Arizona	2.8
28	Virginia	5.1		45	Minnesota	2.8
36	Washington	3.9		47	New Jersey	2.5
10	West Virginia	7.1		48	Massachusetts	2.2
35	Wisconsin	4.0		49	Rhode Island	2.1
3	Wyoming	12.2		50	Connecticut	2.0
					District of Columbia	9.7

Source: Morgan Quitno Press using data from U.S. Department of Labor, Bureau of Labor Statistics
"National Census of Fatal Occupational Injuries, 1997" (press release, August 12, 1998)

III. FACILITIES

Community Hospitals in 1997

National total = 5,057 Hospitals*

ALPHA ORDER

RANK	STATE	HOSPITALS	% of USA
19	Alabama	111	2.2%
47	Alaska	17	0.3%
31	Arizona	63	1.2%
28	Arkansas	82	1.6%
1	California	414	8.2%
29	Colorado	67	1.3%
42	Connecticut	34	0.7%
50	Delaware	6	0.1%
5	Florida	206	4.1%
8	Georgia	158	3.1%
45	Hawaii	19	0.4%
37	Idaho	42	0.8%
6	Illinois	202	4.0%
18	Indiana	112	2.2%
17	Iowa	115	2.3%
11	Kansas	130	2.6%
21	Kentucky	105	2.1%
12	Louisiana	127	2.5%
40	Maine	38	0.8%
35	Maryland	51	1.0%
27	Massachusetts	84	1.7%
9	Michigan	154	3.0%
10	Minnesota	137	2.7%
22	Mississippi	97	1.9%
15	Missouri	123	2.4%
34	Montana	54	1.1%
25	Nebraska	87	1.7%
45	Nevada	19	0.4%
43	New Hampshire	28	0.6%
26	New Jersey	85	1.7%
41	New Mexico	36	0.7%
3	New York	225	4.4%
16	North Carolina	118	2.3%
38	North Dakota	41	0.8%
7	Ohio	170	3.4%
19	Oklahoma	111	2.2%
32	Oregon	61	1.2%
4	Pennsylvania	217	4.3%
49	Rhode Island	11	0.2%
30	South Carolina	65	1.3%
36	South Dakota	49	1.0%
13	Tennessee	124	2.5%
2	Texas	407	8.0%
38	Utah	41	0.8%
48	Vermont	14	0.3%
23	Virginia	93	1.8%
24	Washington	88	1.7%
33	West Virginia	58	1.1%
13	Wisconsin	124	2.5%
44	Wyoming	25	0.5%

RANK ORDER

RANK	STATE	HOSPITALS	% of USA
1	California	414	8.2%
2	Texas	407	8.0%
3	New York	225	4.4%
4	Pennsylvania	217	4.3%
5	Florida	206	4.1%
6	Illinois	202	4.0%
7	Ohio	170	3.4%
8	Georgia	158	3.1%
9	Michigan	154	3.0%
10	Minnesota	137	2.7%
11	Kansas	130	2.6%
12	Louisiana	127	2.5%
13	Tennessee	124	2.5%
13	Wisconsin	124	2.5%
15	Missouri	123	2.4%
16	North Carolina	118	2.3%
17	Iowa	115	2.3%
18	Indiana	112	2.2%
19	Alabama	111	2.2%
19	Oklahoma	111	2.2%
21	Kentucky	105	2.1%
22	Mississippi	97	1.9%
23	Virginia	93	1.8%
24	Washington	88	1.7%
25	Nebraska	87	1.7%
26	New Jersey	85	1.7%
27	Massachusetts	84	1.7%
28	Arkansas	82	1.6%
29	Colorado	67	1.3%
30	South Carolina	65	1.3%
31	Arizona	63	1.2%
32	Oregon	61	1.2%
33	West Virginia	58	1.1%
34	Montana	54	1.1%
35	Maryland	51	1.0%
36	South Dakota	49	1.0%
37	Idaho	42	0.8%
38	North Dakota	41	0.8%
38	Utah	41	0.8%
40	Maine	38	0.8%
41	New Mexico	36	0.7%
42	Connecticut	34	0.7%
43	New Hampshire	28	0.6%
44	Wyoming	25	0.5%
45	Hawaii	19	0.4%
45	Nevada	19	0.4%
47	Alaska	17	0.3%
48	Vermont	14	0.3%
49	Rhode Island	11	0.2%
50	Delaware	6	0.1%
	District of Columbia	12	0.2%

Source: American Hospital Association (Chicago, IL)
"Hospital Statistics" (1999 edition)
*Community hospitals are all nonfederal, short-term, general and special hospitals whose facilities and services are available to the public.

Rate of Community Hospitals in 1997

National Rate = 1.9 Community Hospitals per 100,000 Population*

ALPHA ORDER

RANK	STATE	RATE
18	Alabama	2.6
16	Alaska	2.8
39	Arizona	1.4
11	Arkansas	3.2
43	California	1.3
31	Colorado	1.7
48	Connecticut	1.0
50	Delaware	0.8
39	Florida	1.4
24	Georgia	2.1
34	Hawaii	1.6
9	Idaho	3.5
31	Illinois	1.7
28	Indiana	1.9
7	Iowa	4.0
6	Kansas	5.0
17	Kentucky	2.7
14	Louisiana	2.9
13	Maine	3.1
48	Maryland	1.0
39	Massachusetts	1.4
34	Michigan	1.6
14	Minnesota	2.9
8	Mississippi	3.6
22	Missouri	2.3
3	Montana	6.1
4	Nebraska	5.3
45	Nevada	1.1
19	New Hampshire	2.4
45	New Jersey	1.1
24	New Mexico	2.1
44	New York	1.2
34	North Carolina	1.6
2	North Dakota	6.4
38	Ohio	1.5
10	Oklahoma	3.3
28	Oregon	1.9
30	Pennsylvania	1.8
45	Rhode Island	1.1
31	South Carolina	1.7
1	South Dakota	6.6
22	Tennessee	2.3
24	Texas	2.1
27	Utah	2.0
19	Vermont	2.4
39	Virginia	1.4
34	Washington	1.6
11	West Virginia	3.2
19	Wisconsin	2.4
5	Wyoming	5.2

RANK ORDER

RANK	STATE	RATE
1	South Dakota	6.6
2	North Dakota	6.4
3	Montana	6.1
4	Nebraska	5.3
5	Wyoming	5.2
6	Kansas	5.0
7	Iowa	4.0
8	Mississippi	3.6
9	Idaho	3.5
10	Oklahoma	3.3
11	Arkansas	3.2
11	West Virginia	3.2
13	Maine	3.1
14	Louisiana	2.9
14	Minnesota	2.9
16	Alaska	2.8
17	Kentucky	2.7
18	Alabama	2.6
19	New Hampshire	2.4
19	Vermont	2.4
19	Wisconsin	2.4
22	Missouri	2.3
22	Tennessee	2.3
24	Georgia	2.1
24	New Mexico	2.1
24	Texas	2.1
27	Utah	2.0
28	Indiana	1.9
28	Oregon	1.9
30	Pennsylvania	1.8
31	Colorado	1.7
31	Illinois	1.7
31	South Carolina	1.7
34	Hawaii	1.6
34	Michigan	1.6
34	North Carolina	1.6
34	Washington	1.6
38	Ohio	1.5
39	Arizona	1.4
39	Florida	1.4
39	Massachusetts	1.4
39	Virginia	1.4
43	California	1.3
44	New York	1.2
45	Nevada	1.1
45	New Jersey	1.1
45	Rhode Island	1.1
48	Connecticut	1.0
48	Maryland	1.0
50	Delaware	0.8
	District of Columbia	2.3

Source: Morgan Quitno Press using data from American Hospital Association (Chicago, IL) "Hospital Statistics" (1999 edition)

Community hospitals are all nonfederal, short-term, general and special hospitals whose facilities and services are available to the public.

Community Hospitals per 1,000 Square Miles in 1997

National Rate = 1.4 Community Hospitals*

ALPHA ORDER

RANK ORDER

RANK	STATE	RATE	RANK	STATE	RATE
23	Alabama	2.1	1	New Jersey	10.3
50	Alaska**	0.0	2	Massachusetts	9.1
39	Arizona	0.6	3	Rhode Island	8.9
33	Arkansas	1.5	4	Connecticut	6.1
16	California	2.6	5	Pennsylvania	4.7
39	Colorado	0.6	6	New York	4.2
4	Connecticut	6.1	7	Maryland	4.1
19	Delaware	2.5	8	Ohio	3.8
10	Florida	3.4	9	Illinois	3.5
15	Georgia	2.7	10	Florida	3.4
13	Hawaii	2.9	11	Indiana	3.1
44	Idaho	0.5	12	New Hampshire	3.0
9	Illinois	3.5	13	Hawaii	2.9
11	Indiana	3.1	13	Tennessee	2.9
25	Iowa	2.0	15	Georgia	2.7
29	Kansas	1.6	16	California	2.6
16	Kentucky	2.6	16	Kentucky	2.6
16	Louisiana	2.6	16	Louisiana	2.6
37	Maine	1.1	19	Delaware	2.5
7	Maryland	4.1	20	West Virginia	2.4
2	Massachusetts	9.1	21	North Carolina	2.2
29	Michigan	1.6	21	Virginia	2.2
29	Minnesota	1.6	23	Alabama	2.1
25	Mississippi	2.0	23	South Carolina	2.1
28	Missouri	1.8	25	Iowa	2.0
46	Montana	0.4	25	Mississippi	2.0
37	Nebraska	1.1	27	Wisconsin	1.9
49	Nevada	0.2	28	Missouri	1.8
12	New Hampshire	3.0	29	Kansas	1.6
1	New Jersey	10.3	29	Michigan	1.6
47	New Mexico	0.3	29	Minnesota	1.6
6	New York	4.2	29	Oklahoma	1.6
21	North Carolina	2.2	33	Arkansas	1.5
39	North Dakota	0.6	33	Texas	1.5
8	Ohio	3.8	33	Vermont	1.5
29	Oklahoma	1.6	36	Washington	1.2
39	Oregon	0.6	37	Maine	1.1
5	Pennsylvania	4.7	37	Nebraska	1.1
3	Rhode Island	8.9	39	Arizona	0.6
23	South Carolina	2.1	39	Colorado	0.6
39	South Dakota	0.6	39	North Dakota	0.6
13	Tennessee	2.9	39	Oregon	0.6
33	Texas	1.5	39	South Dakota	0.6
44	Utah	0.5	44	Idaho	0.5
33	Vermont	1.5	44	Utah	0.5
21	Virginia	2.2	46	Montana	0.4
36	Washington	1.2	47	New Mexico	0.3
20	West Virginia	2.4	47	Wyoming	0.3
27	Wisconsin	1.9	49	Nevada	0.2
47	Wyoming	0.3	50	Alaska**	0.0

District of Columbia***   NA

Source: Morgan Quitno Press using data from American Hospital Association (Chicago, IL)
      "Hospital Statistics" (1999 edition)
*Based on 1990 Census land and water area figures. Community hospitals are nonfederal short-term general and other special hospitals, whose facilities and services are available to the public.
**Alaska has 17 community hospitals for its 615,230 square miles.
***The District of Columbia has 12 community hospitals for its 68 square miles.

Community Hospitals in Urban Areas in 1997

National Total = 2,852 Hospitals*

ALPHA ORDER

RANK	STATE	HOSPITALS	% of USA
16	Alabama	58	2.0%
48	Alaska	2	0.1%
21	Arizona	48	1.7%
29	Arkansas	27	0.9%
1	California	373	13.1%
27	Colorado	32	1.1%
28	Connecticut	28	1.0%
46	Delaware	4	0.1%
4	Florida	175	6.1%
12	Georgia	70	2.5%
38	Hawaii	11	0.4%
43	Idaho	7	0.2%
6	Illinois	129	4.5%
13	Indiana	65	2.3%
32	Iowa	21	0.7%
31	Kansas	25	0.9%
26	Kentucky	33	1.2%
10	Louisiana	78	2.7%
42	Maine	9	0.3%
23	Maryland	42	1.5%
11	Massachusetts	75	2.6%
8	Michigan	95	3.3%
22	Minnesota	47	1.6%
33	Mississippi	20	0.7%
14	Missouri	64	2.2%
47	Montana	3	0.1%
36	Nebraska	13	0.5%
38	Nevada	11	0.4%
40	New Hampshire	10	0.4%
9	New Jersey	85	3.0%
36	New Mexico	13	0.5%
3	New York	189	6.6%
19	North Carolina	54	1.9%
44	North Dakota	5	0.2%
7	Ohio	117	4.1%
23	Oklahoma	42	1.5%
29	Oregon	27	0.9%
5	Pennsylvania	172	6.0%
40	Rhode Island	10	0.4%
25	South Carolina	37	1.3%
44	South Dakota	5	0.2%
15	Tennessee	61	2.1%
2	Texas	244	8.6%
34	Utah	19	0.7%
48	Vermont	2	0.1%
17	Virginia	57	2.0%
20	Washington	49	1.7%
35	West Virginia	18	0.6%
17	Wisconsin	57	2.0%
48	Wyoming	2	0.1%

RANK ORDER

RANK	STATE	HOSPITALS	% of USA
1	California	373	13.1%
2	Texas	244	8.6%
3	New York	189	6.6%
4	Florida	175	6.1%
5	Pennsylvania	172	6.0%
6	Illinois	129	4.5%
7	Ohio	117	4.1%
8	Michigan	95	3.3%
9	New Jersey	85	3.0%
10	Louisiana	78	2.7%
11	Massachusetts	75	2.6%
12	Georgia	70	2.5%
13	Indiana	65	2.3%
14	Missouri	64	2.2%
15	Tennessee	61	2.1%
16	Alabama	58	2.0%
17	Virginia	57	2.0%
17	Wisconsin	57	2.0%
19	North Carolina	54	1.9%
20	Washington	49	1.7%
21	Arizona	48	1.7%
22	Minnesota	47	1.6%
23	Maryland	42	1.5%
23	Oklahoma	42	1.5%
25	South Carolina	37	1.3%
26	Kentucky	33	1.2%
27	Colorado	32	1.1%
28	Connecticut	28	1.0%
29	Arkansas	27	0.9%
29	Oregon	27	0.9%
31	Kansas	25	0.9%
32	Iowa	21	0.7%
33	Mississippi	20	0.7%
34	Utah	19	0.7%
35	West Virginia	18	0.6%
36	Nebraska	13	0.5%
36	New Mexico	13	0.5%
38	Hawaii	11	0.4%
38	Nevada	11	0.4%
40	New Hampshire	10	0.4%
40	Rhode Island	10	0.4%
42	Maine	9	0.3%
43	Idaho	7	0.2%
44	North Dakota	5	0.2%
44	South Dakota	5	0.2%
46	Delaware	4	0.1%
47	Montana	3	0.1%
48	Alaska	2	0.1%
48	Vermont	2	0.1%
48	Wyoming	2	0.1%
	District of Columbia	12	0.4%

Source: American Hospital Association (Chicago, IL)
     "Hospital Statistics" (1999 edition)
*Community hospitals are all nonfederal, short-term, general and special hospitals whose facilities and services are available to the public. Urban is defined as any area inside a metropolitan statistical area as defined by the U.S. Office of Management and Budget.

Percent of Community Hospitals in Urban Areas in 1997

National Percent = 56.4% of Community Hospitals*

ALPHA ORDER

ALPHA ORDER

RANK ORDER

RANK	STATE	PERCENT		RANK	STATE	PERCENT
23	Alabama	52.3		1	New Jersey	100.0
47	Alaska	11.8		2	Rhode Island	90.9
10	Arizona	76.2		3	California	90.1
36	Arkansas	32.9		4	Massachusetts	89.3
3	California	90.1		5	Florida	85.0
26	Colorado	47.8		6	New York	84.0
7	Connecticut	82.4		7	Connecticut	82.4
12	Delaware	66.7		7	Maryland	82.4
5	Florida	85.0		9	Pennsylvania	79.3
30	Georgia	44.3		10	Arizona	76.2
19	Hawaii	57.9		11	Ohio	68.8
43	Idaho	16.7		12	Delaware	66.7
13	Illinois	63.9		13	Illinois	63.9
18	Indiana	58.0		14	Michigan	61.7
42	Iowa	18.3		15	Louisiana	61.4
41	Kansas	19.2		16	Virginia	61.3
37	Kentucky	31.4		17	Texas	60.0
15	Louisiana	61.4		18	Indiana	58.0
39	Maine	23.7		19	Hawaii	57.9
7	Maryland	82.4		19	Nevada	57.9
4	Massachusetts	89.3		21	South Carolina	56.9
14	Michigan	61.7		22	Washington	55.7
35	Minnesota	34.3		23	Alabama	52.3
40	Mississippi	20.6		24	Missouri	52.0
24	Missouri	52.0		25	Tennessee	49.2
50	Montana	5.6		26	Colorado	47.8
44	Nebraska	14.9		27	Utah	46.3
19	Nevada	57.9		28	Wisconsin	46.0
34	New Hampshire	35.7		29	North Carolina	45.8
1	New Jersey	100.0		30	Georgia	44.3
33	New Mexico	36.1		30	Oregon	44.3
6	New York	84.0		32	Oklahoma	37.8
29	North Carolina	45.8		33	New Mexico	36.1
46	North Dakota	12.2		34	New Hampshire	35.7
11	Ohio	68.8		35	Minnesota	34.3
32	Oklahoma	37.8		36	Arkansas	32.9
30	Oregon	44.3		37	Kentucky	31.4
9	Pennsylvania	79.3		38	West Virginia	31.0
2	Rhode Island	90.9		39	Maine	23.7
21	South Carolina	56.9		40	Mississippi	20.6
48	South Dakota	10.2		41	Kansas	19.2
25	Tennessee	49.2		42	Iowa	18.3
17	Texas	60.0		43	Idaho	16.7
27	Utah	46.3		44	Nebraska	14.9
45	Vermont	14.3		45	Vermont	14.3
16	Virginia	61.3		46	North Dakota	12.2
22	Washington	55.7		47	Alaska	11.8
38	West Virginia	31.0		48	South Dakota	10.2
28	Wisconsin	46.0		49	Wyoming	8.0
49	Wyoming	8.0		50	Montana	5.6

District of Columbia 100.0

Source: Morgan Quitno Press using data from American Hospital Association (Chicago, IL)
"Hospital Statistics" (1999 edition)
*Community hospitals are all nonfederal, short-term, general and special hospitals whose facilities and services are available to the public. Urban is defined as any area inside a metropolitan statistical area as defined by the U.S. Office of Management and Budget.

Community Hospitals in Rural Areas in 1997

National Total = 2,205 Hospitals*

ALPHA ORDER

RANK	STATE	HOSPITALS	% of USA
17	Alabama	53	2.4%
40	Alaska	15	0.7%
40	Arizona	15	0.7%
16	Arkansas	55	2.5%
24	California	41	1.9%
30	Colorado	35	1.6%
47	Connecticut	6	0.3%
48	Delaware	2	0.1%
33	Florida	31	1.4%
5	Georgia	88	4.0%
45	Hawaii	8	0.4%
30	Idaho	35	1.6%
8	Illinois	73	3.3%
21	Indiana	47	2.1%
3	Iowa	94	4.3%
2	Kansas	105	4.8%
9	Kentucky	72	3.3%
20	Louisiana	49	2.2%
34	Maine	29	1.3%
43	Maryland	9	0.4%
43	Massachusetts	9	0.4%
14	Michigan	59	2.7%
4	Minnesota	90	4.1%
6	Mississippi	77	3.5%
14	Missouri	59	2.7%
19	Montana	51	2.3%
7	Nebraska	74	3.4%
45	Nevada	8	0.4%
39	New Hampshire	18	0.8%
50	New Jersey	0	0.0%
36	New Mexico	23	1.0%
27	New York	36	1.6%
12	North Carolina	64	2.9%
27	North Dakota	36	1.6%
17	Ohio	53	2.4%
10	Oklahoma	69	3.1%
32	Oregon	34	1.5%
22	Pennsylvania	45	2.0%
49	Rhode Island	1	0.0%
35	South Carolina	28	1.3%
23	South Dakota	44	2.0%
13	Tennessee	63	2.9%
1	Texas	163	7.4%
38	Utah	22	1.0%
42	Vermont	12	0.5%
27	Virginia	36	1.6%
26	Washington	39	1.8%
25	West Virginia	40	1.8%
11	Wisconsin	67	3.0%
36	Wyoming	23	1.0%

RANK ORDER

RANK	STATE	HOSPITALS	% of USA
1	Texas	163	7.4%
2	Kansas	105	4.8%
3	Iowa	94	4.3%
4	Minnesota	90	4.1%
5	Georgia	88	4.0%
6	Mississippi	77	3.5%
7	Nebraska	74	3.4%
8	Illinois	73	3.3%
9	Kentucky	72	3.3%
10	Oklahoma	69	3.1%
11	Wisconsin	67	3.0%
12	North Carolina	64	2.9%
13	Tennessee	63	2.9%
14	Michigan	59	2.7%
14	Missouri	59	2.7%
16	Arkansas	55	2.5%
17	Alabama	53	2.4%
17	Ohio	53	2.4%
19	Montana	51	2.3%
20	Louisiana	49	2.2%
21	Indiana	47	2.1%
22	Pennsylvania	45	2.0%
23	South Dakota	44	2.0%
24	California	41	1.9%
25	West Virginia	40	1.8%
26	Washington	39	1.8%
27	New York	36	1.6%
27	North Dakota	36	1.6%
27	Virginia	36	1.6%
30	Colorado	35	1.6%
30	Idaho	35	1.6%
32	Oregon	34	1.5%
33	Florida	31	1.4%
34	Maine	29	1.3%
35	South Carolina	28	1.3%
36	New Mexico	23	1.0%
36	Wyoming	23	1.0%
38	Utah	22	1.0%
39	New Hampshire	18	0.8%
40	Alaska	15	0.7%
40	Arizona	15	0.7%
42	Vermont	12	0.5%
43	Maryland	9	0.4%
43	Massachusetts	9	0.4%
45	Hawaii	8	0.4%
45	Nevada	8	0.4%
47	Connecticut	6	0.3%
48	Delaware	2	0.1%
49	Rhode Island	1	0.0%
50	New Jersey	0	0.0%
	District of Columbia	0	0.0%

Source: American Hospital Association (Chicago, IL)
    "Hospital Statistics" (1999 edition)
*Community hospitals are all nonfederal, short-term, general and special hospitals whose facilities and services are available to the public. Rural is defined as any area outside a metropolitan statistical area as defined by the U.S. Office of Management and Budget.

Percent of Community Hospitals in Rural Areas in 1997

National Percent = 43.6% of Community Hospitals*

ALPHA ORDER				RANK ORDER		
RANK	STATE	PERCENT		RANK	STATE	PERCENT
28	Alabama	47.7		1	Montana	94.4
4	Alaska	88.2		2	Wyoming	92.0
41	Arizona	23.8		3	South Dakota	89.8
15	Arkansas	67.1		4	Alaska	88.2
48	California	9.9		5	North Dakota	87.8
25	Colorado	52.2		6	Vermont	85.7
43	Connecticut	17.6		7	Nebraska	85.1
39	Delaware	33.3		8	Idaho	83.3
46	Florida	15.0		9	Iowa	81.7
20	Georgia	55.7		10	Kansas	80.8
31	Hawaii	42.1		11	Mississippi	79.4
8	Idaho	83.3		12	Maine	76.3
38	Illinois	36.1		13	West Virginia	69.0
33	Indiana	42.0		14	Kentucky	68.6
9	Iowa	81.7		15	Arkansas	67.1
10	Kansas	80.8		16	Minnesota	65.7
14	Kentucky	68.6		17	New Hampshire	64.3
36	Louisiana	38.6		18	New Mexico	63.9
12	Maine	76.3		19	Oklahoma	62.2
43	Maryland	17.6		20	Georgia	55.7
47	Massachusetts	10.7		20	Oregon	55.7
37	Michigan	38.3		22	North Carolina	54.2
16	Minnesota	65.7		23	Wisconsin	54.0
11	Mississippi	79.4		24	Utah	53.7
27	Missouri	48.0		25	Colorado	52.2
1	Montana	94.4		26	Tennessee	50.8
7	Nebraska	85.1		27	Missouri	48.0
31	Nevada	42.1		28	Alabama	47.7
17	New Hampshire	64.3		29	Washington	44.3
50	New Jersey	0.0		30	South Carolina	43.1
18	New Mexico	63.9		31	Hawaii	42.1
45	New York	16.0		31	Nevada	42.1
22	North Carolina	54.2		33	Indiana	42.0
5	North Dakota	87.8		34	Texas	40.0
40	Ohio	31.2		35	Virginia	38.7
19	Oklahoma	62.2		36	Louisiana	38.6
20	Oregon	55.7		37	Michigan	38.3
42	Pennsylvania	20.7		38	Illinois	36.1
49	Rhode Island	9.1		39	Delaware	33.3
30	South Carolina	43.1		40	Ohio	31.2
3	South Dakota	89.8		41	Arizona	23.8
26	Tennessee	50.8		42	Pennsylvania	20.7
34	Texas	40.0		43	Connecticut	17.6
24	Utah	53.7		43	Maryland	17.6
6	Vermont	85.7		45	New York	16.0
35	Virginia	38.7		46	Florida	15.0
29	Washington	44.3		47	Massachusetts	10.7
13	West Virginia	69.0		48	California	9.9
23	Wisconsin	54.0		49	Rhode Island	9.1
2	Wyoming	92.0		50	New Jersey	0.0
					District of Columbia	0.0

Source: Morgan Quitno Press using data from American Hospital Association (Chicago, IL)
   "Hospital Statistics" (1999 edition)
*Community hospitals are all nonfederal, short-term, general and special hospitals whose facilities and services are available to the public. Rural is defined as any area outside a metropolitan statistical area as defined by the U.S. Office of Management and Budget.

Nongovernment Not-For-Profit Hospitals in 1997

National Total = 3,000 Hospitals*

ALPHA ORDER

RANK	STATE	HOSPITALS	% of USA
32	Alabama	36	1.2%
47	Alaska	8	0.3%
28	Arizona	41	1.4%
23	Arkansas	46	1.5%
1	California	224	7.5%
35	Colorado	32	1.1%
36	Connecticut	31	1.0%
49	Delaware	6	0.2%
9	Florida	87	2.9%
19	Georgia	54	1.8%
45	Hawaii	12	0.4%
44	Idaho	13	0.4%
4	Illinois	156	5.2%
17	Indiana	57	1.9%
20	Iowa	53	1.8%
18	Kansas	56	1.9%
16	Kentucky	69	2.3%
38	Louisiana	29	1.0%
33	Maine	34	1.1%
22	Maryland	49	1.6%
13	Massachusetts	72	2.4%
7	Michigan	130	4.3%
10	Minnesota	84	2.8%
37	Mississippi	30	1.0%
12	Missouri	73	2.4%
31	Montana	39	1.3%
25	Nebraska	43	1.4%
49	Nevada	6	0.2%
39	New Hampshire	24	0.8%
11	New Jersey	80	2.7%
41	New Mexico	20	0.7%
3	New York	187	6.2%
14	North Carolina	70	2.3%
29	North Dakota	40	1.3%
5	Ohio	138	4.6%
29	Oklahoma	40	1.3%
26	Oregon	42	1.4%
2	Pennsylvania	208	6.9%
46	Rhode Island	11	0.4%
40	South Carolina	22	0.7%
26	South Dakota	42	1.4%
21	Tennessee	50	1.7%
6	Texas	137	4.6%
41	Utah	20	0.7%
43	Vermont	14	0.5%
14	Virginia	70	2.3%
24	Washington	44	1.5%
34	West Virginia	33	1.1%
8	Wisconsin	121	4.0%
48	Wyoming	7	0.2%

RANK ORDER

RANK	STATE	HOSPITALS	% of USA
1	California	224	7.5%
2	Pennsylvania	208	6.9%
3	New York	187	6.2%
4	Illinois	156	5.2%
5	Ohio	138	4.6%
6	Texas	137	4.6%
7	Michigan	130	4.3%
8	Wisconsin	121	4.0%
9	Florida	87	2.9%
10	Minnesota	84	2.8%
11	New Jersey	80	2.7%
12	Missouri	73	2.4%
13	Massachusetts	72	2.4%
14	North Carolina	70	2.3%
14	Virginia	70	2.3%
16	Kentucky	69	2.3%
17	Indiana	57	1.9%
18	Kansas	56	1.9%
19	Georgia	54	1.8%
20	Iowa	53	1.8%
21	Tennessee	50	1.7%
22	Maryland	49	1.6%
23	Arkansas	46	1.5%
24	Washington	44	1.5%
25	Nebraska	43	1.4%
26	Oregon	42	1.4%
26	South Dakota	42	1.4%
28	Arizona	41	1.4%
29	North Dakota	40	1.3%
29	Oklahoma	40	1.3%
31	Montana	39	1.3%
32	Alabama	36	1.2%
33	Maine	34	1.1%
34	West Virginia	33	1.1%
35	Colorado	32	1.1%
36	Connecticut	31	1.0%
37	Mississippi	30	1.0%
38	Louisiana	29	1.0%
39	New Hampshire	24	0.8%
40	South Carolina	22	0.7%
41	New Mexico	20	0.7%
41	Utah	20	0.7%
43	Vermont	14	0.5%
44	Idaho	13	0.4%
45	Hawaii	12	0.4%
46	Rhode Island	11	0.4%
47	Alaska	8	0.3%
48	Wyoming	7	0.2%
49	Delaware	6	0.2%
49	Nevada	6	0.2%
	District of Columbia	10	0.3%

Source: American Hospital Association (Chicago, IL)
"Hospital Statistics" (1999 edition)

Nongovernment not-for-profit hospitals are a subset of community hospitals.

Investor-Owned (For-Profit) Hospitals in 1997

National Total = 797 Hospitals*

ALPHA ORDER

RANK	STATE	HOSPITALS	% of USA
7	Alabama	34	4.3%
38	Alaska	1	0.1%
13	Arizona	17	2.1%
10	Arkansas	19	2.4%
2	California	109	13.7%
22	Colorado	9	1.1%
38	Connecticut	1	0.1%
46	Delaware	0	0.0%
3	Florida	95	11.9%
6	Georgia	39	4.9%
38	Hawaii	1	0.1%
32	Idaho	3	0.4%
18	Illinois	12	1.5%
21	Indiana	10	1.3%
34	Iowa	2	0.3%
22	Kansas	9	1.1%
8	Kentucky	22	2.8%
5	Louisiana	41	5.1%
38	Maine	1	0.1%
34	Maryland	2	0.3%
26	Massachusetts	6	0.8%
32	Michigan	3	0.4%
46	Minnesota	0	0.0%
11	Mississippi	18	2.3%
16	Missouri	14	1.8%
38	Montana	1	0.1%
34	Nebraska	2	0.3%
27	Nevada	5	0.6%
29	New Hampshire	4	0.5%
38	New Jersey	1	0.1%
27	New Mexico	5	0.6%
20	New York	11	1.4%
17	North Carolina	13	1.6%
38	North Dakota	1	0.1%
22	Ohio	9	1.1%
11	Oklahoma	18	2.3%
29	Oregon	4	0.5%
25	Pennsylvania	8	1.0%
46	Rhode Island	0	0.0%
9	South Carolina	20	2.5%
46	South Dakota	0	0.0%
4	Tennessee	43	5.4%
1	Texas	132	16.6%
18	Utah	12	1.5%
46	Vermont	0	0.0%
13	Virginia	17	2.1%
29	Washington	4	0.5%
15	West Virginia	15	1.9%
38	Wisconsin	1	0.1%
34	Wyoming	2	0.3%

RANK ORDER

RANK	STATE	HOSPITALS	% of USA
1	Texas	132	16.6%
2	California	109	13.7%
3	Florida	95	11.9%
4	Tennessee	43	5.4%
5	Louisiana	41	5.1%
6	Georgia	39	4.9%
7	Alabama	34	4.3%
8	Kentucky	22	2.8%
9	South Carolina	20	2.5%
10	Arkansas	19	2.4%
11	Mississippi	18	2.3%
11	Oklahoma	18	2.3%
13	Arizona	17	2.1%
13	Virginia	17	2.1%
15	West Virginia	15	1.9%
16	Missouri	14	1.8%
17	North Carolina	13	1.6%
18	Illinois	12	1.5%
18	Utah	12	1.5%
20	New York	11	1.4%
21	Indiana	10	1.3%
22	Colorado	9	1.1%
22	Kansas	9	1.1%
22	Ohio	9	1.1%
25	Pennsylvania	8	1.0%
26	Massachusetts	6	0.8%
27	Nevada	5	0.6%
27	New Mexico	5	0.6%
29	New Hampshire	4	0.5%
29	Oregon	4	0.5%
29	Washington	4	0.5%
32	Idaho	3	0.4%
32	Michigan	3	0.4%
34	Iowa	2	0.3%
34	Maryland	2	0.3%
34	Nebraska	2	0.3%
34	Wyoming	2	0.3%
38	Alaska	1	0.1%
38	Connecticut	1	0.1%
38	Hawaii	1	0.1%
38	Maine	1	0.1%
38	Montana	1	0.1%
38	New Jersey	1	0.1%
38	North Dakota	1	0.1%
38	Wisconsin	1	0.1%
46	Delaware	0	0.0%
46	Minnesota	0	0.0%
46	Rhode Island	0	0.0%
46	South Dakota	0	0.0%
46	Vermont	0	0.0%
	District of Columbia	1	0.1%

Source: American Hospital Association (Chicago, IL)
    "Hospital Statistics" (1999 edition)
*Investor-owned (for-profit) hospitals are a subset of community hospitals.

State and Local Government-Owned Hospitals in 1997

National Total = 1,260 Hospitals*

ALPHA ORDER

RANK	STATE	HOSPITALS	% of USA
12	Alabama	41	3.3%
33	Alaska	8	0.6%
39	Arizona	5	0.4%
25	Arkansas	17	1.3%
2	California	81	6.4%
19	Colorado	26	2.1%
42	Connecticut	2	0.2%
45	Delaware	0	0.0%
21	Florida	24	1.9%
3	Georgia	65	5.2%
36	Hawaii	6	0.5%
19	Idaho	26	2.1%
16	Illinois	34	2.7%
10	Indiana	45	3.6%
5	Iowa	60	4.8%
3	Kansas	65	5.2%
28	Kentucky	14	1.1%
6	Louisiana	57	4.5%
41	Maine	3	0.2%
45	Maryland	0	0.0%
36	Massachusetts	6	0.5%
24	Michigan	21	1.7%
7	Minnesota	53	4.2%
9	Mississippi	49	3.9%
14	Missouri	36	2.9%
28	Montana	14	1.1%
11	Nebraska	42	3.3%
33	Nevada	8	0.6%
45	New Hampshire	0	0.0%
40	New Jersey	4	0.3%
30	New Mexico	11	0.9%
18	New York	27	2.1%
15	North Carolina	35	2.8%
45	North Dakota	0	0.0%
22	Ohio	23	1.8%
7	Oklahoma	53	4.2%
27	Oregon	15	1.2%
44	Pennsylvania	1	0.1%
45	Rhode Island	0	0.0%
22	South Carolina	23	1.8%
35	South Dakota	7	0.6%
17	Tennessee	31	2.5%
1	Texas	138	11.0%
32	Utah	9	0.7%
45	Vermont	0	0.0%
36	Virginia	6	0.5%
13	Washington	40	3.2%
31	West Virginia	10	0.8%
42	Wisconsin	2	0.2%
26	Wyoming	16	1.3%

RANK ORDER

RANK	STATE	HOSPITALS	% of USA
1	Texas	138	11.0%
2	California	81	6.4%
3	Georgia	65	5.2%
3	Kansas	65	5.2%
5	Iowa	60	4.8%
6	Louisiana	57	4.5%
7	Minnesota	53	4.2%
7	Oklahoma	53	4.2%
9	Mississippi	49	3.9%
10	Indiana	45	3.6%
11	Nebraska	42	3.3%
12	Alabama	41	3.3%
13	Washington	40	3.2%
14	Missouri	36	2.9%
15	North Carolina	35	2.8%
16	Illinois	34	2.7%
17	Tennessee	31	2.5%
18	New York	27	2.1%
19	Colorado	26	2.1%
19	Idaho	26	2.1%
21	Florida	24	1.9%
22	Ohio	23	1.8%
22	South Carolina	23	1.8%
24	Michigan	21	1.7%
25	Arkansas	17	1.3%
26	Wyoming	16	1.3%
27	Oregon	15	1.2%
28	Kentucky	14	1.1%
28	Montana	14	1.1%
30	New Mexico	11	0.9%
31	West Virginia	10	0.8%
32	Utah	9	0.7%
33	Alaska	8	0.6%
33	Nevada	8	0.6%
35	South Dakota	7	0.6%
36	Hawaii	6	0.5%
36	Massachusetts	6	0.5%
36	Virginia	6	0.5%
39	Arizona	5	0.4%
40	New Jersey	4	0.3%
41	Maine	3	0.2%
42	Connecticut	2	0.2%
42	Wisconsin	2	0.2%
44	Pennsylvania	1	0.1%
45	Delaware	0	0.0%
45	Maryland	0	0.0%
45	New Hampshire	0	0.0%
45	North Dakota	0	0.0%
45	Rhode Island	0	0.0%
45	Vermont	0	0.0%
	District of Columbia	1	0.1%

Source: American Hospital Association (Chicago, IL)
   "Hospital Statistics" (1999 edition)
*State and local government-owned hospitals are a subset of community hospitals.

Beds in Community Hospitals in 1997

National total = 853,287 Beds*

ALPHA ORDER

RANK	STATE	BEDS	% of USA
16	Alabama	18,599	2.2%
50	Alaska	1,440	0.2%
29	Arizona	10,624	1.2%
30	Arkansas	10,111	1.2%
1	California	74,119	8.7%
31	Colorado	9,122	1.1%
34	Connecticut	7,238	0.8%
48	Delaware	1,888	0.2%
4	Florida	49,762	5.8%
10	Georgia	25,735	3.0%
45	Hawaii	2,783	0.3%
43	Idaho	3,467	0.4%
6	Illinois	40,254	4.7%
14	Indiana	19,406	2.3%
24	Iowa	12,248	1.4%
28	Kansas	10,829	1.3%
21	Kentucky	15,351	1.8%
15	Louisiana	18,605	2.2%
40	Maine	3,691	0.4%
23	Maryland	12,680	1.5%
18	Massachusetts	17,431	2.0%
9	Michigan	27,923	3.3%
19	Minnesota	17,076	2.0%
22	Mississippi	12,904	1.5%
13	Missouri	20,867	2.4%
36	Montana	4,482	0.5%
33	Nebraska	7,750	0.9%
42	Nevada	3,539	0.4%
44	New Hampshire	2,951	0.3%
8	New Jersey	28,089	3.3%
41	New Mexico	3,607	0.4%
2	New York	70,973	8.3%
11	North Carolina	23,244	2.7%
39	North Dakota	3,900	0.5%
7	Ohio	36,079	4.2%
26	Oklahoma	10,882	1.3%
35	Oregon	6,986	0.8%
5	Pennsylvania	45,723	5.4%
46	Rhode Island	2,544	0.3%
25	South Carolina	11,974	1.4%
37	South Dakota	4,416	0.5%
12	Tennessee	21,077	2.5%
3	Texas	55,759	6.5%
38	Utah	4,134	0.5%
49	Vermont	1,565	0.2%
17	Virginia	18,179	2.1%
27	Washington	10,845	1.3%
32	West Virginia	8,155	1.0%
20	Wisconsin	16,695	2.0%
47	Wyoming	1,966	0.2%

RANK ORDER

RANK	STATE	BEDS	% of USA
1	California	74,119	8.7%
2	New York	70,973	8.3%
3	Texas	55,759	6.5%
4	Florida	49,762	5.8%
5	Pennsylvania	45,723	5.4%
6	Illinois	40,254	4.7%
7	Ohio	36,079	4.2%
8	New Jersey	28,089	3.3%
9	Michigan	27,923	3.3%
10	Georgia	25,735	3.0%
11	North Carolina	23,244	2.7%
12	Tennessee	21,077	2.5%
13	Missouri	20,867	2.4%
14	Indiana	19,406	2.3%
15	Louisiana	18,605	2.2%
16	Alabama	18,599	2.2%
17	Virginia	18,179	2.1%
18	Massachusetts	17,431	2.0%
19	Minnesota	17,076	2.0%
20	Wisconsin	16,695	2.0%
21	Kentucky	15,351	1.8%
22	Mississippi	12,904	1.5%
23	Maryland	12,680	1.5%
24	Iowa	12,248	1.4%
25	South Carolina	11,974	1.4%
26	Oklahoma	10,882	1.3%
27	Washington	10,845	1.3%
28	Kansas	10,829	1.3%
29	Arizona	10,624	1.2%
30	Arkansas	10,111	1.2%
31	Colorado	9,122	1.1%
32	West Virginia	8,155	1.0%
33	Nebraska	7,750	0.9%
34	Connecticut	7,238	0.8%
35	Oregon	6,986	0.8%
36	Montana	4,482	0.5%
37	South Dakota	4,416	0.5%
38	Utah	4,134	0.5%
39	North Dakota	3,900	0.5%
40	Maine	3,691	0.4%
41	New Mexico	3,607	0.4%
42	Nevada	3,539	0.4%
43	Idaho	3,467	0.4%
44	New Hampshire	2,951	0.3%
45	Hawaii	2,783	0.3%
46	Rhode Island	2,544	0.3%
47	Wyoming	1,966	0.2%
48	Delaware	1,888	0.2%
49	Vermont	1,565	0.2%
50	Alaska	1,440	0.2%
	District of Columbia	3,620	0.4%

Source: American Hospital Association (Chicago, IL)
   "Hospital Statistics" (1999 edition)
All nonfederal short-term general and other special hospitals, whose facilities and services are available to the public. Includes beds in hospital and nursing home units.

Rate of Beds in Community Hospitals in 1997

National Rate = 319 Beds per 100,000 Population*

ALPHA ORDER				RANK ORDER		
RANK	STATE	RATE		RANK	STATE	RATE
7	Alabama	430		1	North Dakota	608
40	Alaska	236		2	South Dakota	599
42	Arizona	233		3	Montana	510
12	Arkansas	401		4	Mississippi	472
44	California	230		5	Nebraska	468
41	Colorado	234		6	West Virginia	449
45	Connecticut	222		7	Alabama	430
37	Delaware	257		8	Iowa	429
21	Florida	339		9	Louisiana	427
20	Georgia	344		10	Kansas	416
42	Hawaii	233		11	Wyoming	410
31	Idaho	287		12	Arkansas	401
22	Illinois	336		13	Kentucky	393
23	Indiana	331		14	Tennessee	392
8	Iowa	429		15	New York	391
10	Kansas	416		16	Missouri	386
13	Kentucky	393		17	Pennsylvania	381
9	Louisiana	427		18	Minnesota	364
29	Maine	297		19	New Jersey	349
39	Maryland	249		20	Georgia	344
33	Massachusetts	285		21	Florida	339
32	Michigan	286		22	Illinois	336
18	Minnesota	364		23	Indiana	331
4	Mississippi	472		24	Oklahoma	328
16	Missouri	386		25	Ohio	322
3	Montana	510		26	Wisconsin	321
5	Nebraska	468		27	South Carolina	316
47	Nevada	211		28	North Carolina	313
38	New Hampshire	252		29	Maine	297
19	New Jersey	349		30	Texas	288
48	New Mexico	209		31	Idaho	287
15	New York	391		32	Michigan	286
28	North Carolina	313		33	Massachusetts	285
1	North Dakota	608		34	Virginia	270
25	Ohio	322		35	Vermont	266
24	Oklahoma	328		36	Rhode Island	258
46	Oregon	215		37	Delaware	257
17	Pennsylvania	381		38	New Hampshire	252
36	Rhode Island	258		39	Maryland	249
27	South Carolina	316		40	Alaska	236
2	South Dakota	599		41	Colorado	234
14	Tennessee	392		42	Arizona	233
30	Texas	288		42	Hawaii	233
49	Utah	200		44	California	230
35	Vermont	266		45	Connecticut	222
34	Virginia	270		46	Oregon	215
50	Washington	193		47	Nevada	211
6	West Virginia	449		48	New Mexico	209
26	Wisconsin	321		49	Utah	200
11	Wyoming	410		50	Washington	193
					District of Columbia	683

Source: Morgan Quitno Press using data from American Hospital Association (Chicago, IL)
    "Hospital Statistics" (1999 edition)
*All nonfederal short-term general and other special hospitals, whose facilities and services are available to the public. Includes beds in hospital and nursing home units.

Average Number of Beds per Community Hospital in 1997

National Average = 169 Beds per Community Hospital*

ALPHA ORDER				RANK ORDER		
RANK	STATE	BEDS		RANK	STATE	BEDS
22	Alabama	168		1	New Jersey	330
46	Alaska	85		2	Delaware	315
21	Arizona	169		2	New York	315
33	Arkansas	123		4	Maryland	249
17	California	179		5	Florida	242
29	Colorado	136		6	Rhode Island	231
7	Connecticut	213		7	Connecticut	213
2	Delaware	315		8	Ohio	212
5	Florida	242		9	Pennsylvania	211
23	Georgia	163		10	Massachusetts	208
24	Hawaii	146		11	Illinois	199
47	Idaho	83		12	North Carolina	197
11	Illinois	199		13	Virginia	195
18	Indiana	173		14	Nevada	186
37	Iowa	107		15	South Carolina	184
47	Kansas	83		16	Michigan	181
24	Kentucky	146		17	California	179
24	Louisiana	146		18	Indiana	173
42	Maine	97		19	Missouri	170
4	Maryland	249		19	Tennessee	170
10	Massachusetts	208		21	Arizona	169
16	Michigan	181		22	Alabama	168
32	Minnesota	125		23	Georgia	163
31	Mississippi	133		24	Hawaii	146
19	Missouri	170		24	Kentucky	146
47	Montana	83		24	Louisiana	146
45	Nebraska	89		27	West Virginia	141
14	Nevada	186		28	Texas	137
38	New Hampshire	105		29	Colorado	136
1	New Jersey	330		30	Wisconsin	135
40	New Mexico	100		31	Mississippi	133
2	New York	315		32	Minnesota	125
12	North Carolina	197		33	Arkansas	123
43	North Dakota	95		33	Washington	123
8	Ohio	212		35	Oregon	115
41	Oklahoma	98		36	Vermont	112
35	Oregon	115		37	Iowa	107
9	Pennsylvania	211		38	New Hampshire	105
6	Rhode Island	231		39	Utah	101
15	South Carolina	184		40	New Mexico	100
44	South Dakota	90		41	Oklahoma	98
19	Tennessee	170		42	Maine	97
28	Texas	137		43	North Dakota	95
39	Utah	101		44	South Dakota	90
36	Vermont	112		45	Nebraska	89
13	Virginia	195		46	Alaska	85
33	Washington	123		47	Idaho	83
27	West Virginia	141		47	Kansas	83
30	Wisconsin	135		47	Montana	83
50	Wyoming	79		50	Wyoming	79
					District of Columbia	302

Source: Morgan Quitno Press using data from American Hospital Association (Chicago, IL)
     "Hospital Statistics" (1999 edition)
*All nonfederal short-term general and other special hospitals, whose facilities and services are available to the public. Includes beds in hospital and nursing home units.

Admissions to Community Hospitals in 1997

National Total = 31,576,960 Admissions*

ALPHA ORDER

RANK	STATE	ADMISSIONS	% of USA
17	Alabama	684,823	2.2%
50	Alaska	40,493	0.1%
24	Arizona	476,329	1.5%
30	Arkansas	346,426	1.1%
1	California	3,110,316	9.8%
29	Colorado	366,494	1.2%
31	Connecticut	338,108	1.1%
47	Delaware	80,602	0.3%
4	Florida	1,882,928	6.0%
11	Georgia	856,076	2.7%
44	Hawaii	96,743	0.3%
42	Idaho	108,440	0.3%
6	Illinois	1,442,514	4.6%
16	Indiana	695,279	2.2%
28	Iowa	366,703	1.2%
33	Kansas	298,451	0.9%
21	Kentucky	542,640	1.7%
18	Louisiana	650,104	2.1%
39	Maine	143,351	0.5%
19	Maryland	570,234	1.8%
12	Massachusetts	764,322	2.4%
8	Michigan	1,111,527	3.5%
22	Minnesota	526,742	1.7%
26	Mississippi	413,472	1.3%
14	Missouri	729,914	2.3%
43	Montana	98,788	0.3%
35	Nebraska	190,960	0.6%
38	Nevada	160,770	0.5%
41	New Hampshire	110,193	0.3%
9	New Jersey	1,095,897	3.5%
37	New Mexico	163,372	0.5%
2	New York	2,371,164	7.5%
10	North Carolina	874,389	2.8%
46	North Dakota	83,688	0.3%
7	Ohio	1,376,291	4.4%
27	Oklahoma	377,776	1.2%
32	Oregon	308,512	1.0%
5	Pennsylvania	1,756,446	5.6%
40	Rhode Island	116,354	0.4%
25	South Carolina	443,355	1.4%
45	South Dakota	94,101	0.3%
13	Tennessee	762,758	2.4%
3	Texas	2,125,610	6.7%
36	Utah	186,393	0.6%
48	Vermont	52,275	0.2%
15	Virginia	705,038	2.2%
23	Washington	477,874	1.5%
34	West Virginia	277,257	0.9%
20	Wisconsin	551,436	1.7%
49	Wyoming	44,170	0.1%

RANK ORDER

RANK	STATE	ADMISSIONS	% of USA
1	California	3,110,316	9.8%
2	New York	2,371,164	7.5%
3	Texas	2,125,610	6.7%
4	Florida	1,882,928	6.0%
5	Pennsylvania	1,756,446	5.6%
6	Illinois	1,442,514	4.6%
7	Ohio	1,376,291	4.4%
8	Michigan	1,111,527	3.5%
9	New Jersey	1,095,897	3.5%
10	North Carolina	874,389	2.8%
11	Georgia	856,076	2.7%
12	Massachusetts	764,322	2.4%
13	Tennessee	762,758	2.4%
14	Missouri	729,914	2.3%
15	Virginia	705,038	2.2%
16	Indiana	695,279	2.2%
17	Alabama	684,823	2.2%
18	Louisiana	650,104	2.1%
19	Maryland	570,234	1.8%
20	Wisconsin	551,436	1.7%
21	Kentucky	542,640	1.7%
22	Minnesota	526,742	1.7%
23	Washington	477,874	1.5%
24	Arizona	476,329	1.5%
25	South Carolina	443,355	1.4%
26	Mississippi	413,472	1.3%
27	Oklahoma	377,776	1.2%
28	Iowa	366,703	1.2%
29	Colorado	366,494	1.2%
30	Arkansas	346,426	1.1%
31	Connecticut	338,108	1.1%
32	Oregon	308,512	1.0%
33	Kansas	298,451	0.9%
34	West Virginia	277,257	0.9%
35	Nebraska	190,960	0.6%
36	Utah	186,393	0.6%
37	New Mexico	163,372	0.5%
38	Nevada	160,770	0.5%
39	Maine	143,351	0.5%
40	Rhode Island	116,354	0.4%
41	New Hampshire	110,193	0.3%
42	Idaho	108,440	0.3%
43	Montana	98,788	0.3%
44	Hawaii	96,743	0.3%
45	South Dakota	94,101	0.3%
46	North Dakota	83,688	0.3%
47	Delaware	80,602	0.3%
48	Vermont	52,275	0.2%
49	Wyoming	44,170	0.1%
50	Alaska	40,493	0.1%
	District of Columbia	129,062	0.4%

Source: American Hospital Association (Chicago, IL)
        "Hospital Statistics" (1999 edition)
*Admissions to all nonfederal short-term general and other special hospitals, whose facilities and services are available to the public. Includes admissions to hospital and nursing home units.

Inpatient Days in Community Hospitals in 1997

National Total = 192,504,015 Inpatient Days*

<u>ALPHA ORDER</u>

RANK	STATE	DAYS	% of USA
18	Alabama	3,926,995	2.0%
49	Alaska	383,646	0.2%
26	Arizona	2,400,418	1.2%
29	Arkansas	2,126,384	1.1%
2	California	16,117,513	8.4%
31	Colorado	1,829,756	1.0%
32	Connecticut	1,815,702	0.9%
47	Delaware	488,879	0.3%
5	Florida	10,659,344	5.5%
11	Georgia	5,529,715	2.9%
41	Hawaii	829,757	0.4%
45	Idaho	679,075	0.4%
6	Illinois	8,542,006	4.4%
17	Indiana	4,077,184	2.1%
25	Iowa	2,508,509	1.3%
30	Kansas	2,095,243	1.1%
21	Kentucky	3,187,922	1.7%
19	Louisiana	3,682,678	1.9%
40	Maine	857,274	0.4%
22	Maryland	3,129,218	1.6%
14	Massachusetts	4,283,021	2.2%
9	Michigan	6,591,143	3.4%
15	Minnesota	4,254,912	2.2%
23	Mississippi	2,946,321	1.5%
13	Missouri	4,311,021	2.2%
37	Montana	1,014,709	0.5%
34	Nebraska	1,683,706	0.9%
39	Nevada	869,239	0.5%
44	New Hampshire	682,841	0.4%
8	New Jersey	6,969,448	3.6%
43	New Mexico	761,888	0.4%
1	New York	19,652,565	10.2%
10	North Carolina	5,783,489	3.0%
38	North Dakota	877,085	0.5%
7	Ohio	7,674,238	4.0%
28	Oklahoma	2,148,426	1.1%
35	Oregon	1,347,809	0.7%
4	Pennsylvania	11,165,571	5.8%
46	Rhode Island	658,143	0.3%
24	South Carolina	2,802,382	1.5%
36	South Dakota	1,047,494	0.5%
12	Tennessee	4,523,889	2.4%
3	Texas	11,355,612	5.9%
42	Utah	820,872	0.4%
48	Vermont	406,985	0.2%
16	Virginia	4,216,773	2.2%
27	Washington	2,254,232	1.2%
33	West Virginia	1,745,689	0.9%
20	Wisconsin	3,471,636	1.8%
50	Wyoming	376,111	0.2%

<u>RANK ORDER</u>

RANK	STATE	DAYS	% of USA
1	New York	19,652,565	10.2%
2	California	16,117,513	8.4%
3	Texas	11,355,612	5.9%
4	Pennsylvania	11,165,571	5.8%
5	Florida	10,659,344	5.5%
6	Illinois	8,542,006	4.4%
7	Ohio	7,674,238	4.0%
8	New Jersey	6,969,448	3.6%
9	Michigan	6,591,143	3.4%
10	North Carolina	5,783,489	3.0%
11	Georgia	5,529,715	2.9%
12	Tennessee	4,523,889	2.4%
13	Missouri	4,311,021	2.2%
14	Massachusetts	4,283,021	2.2%
15	Minnesota	4,254,912	2.2%
16	Virginia	4,216,773	2.2%
17	Indiana	4,077,184	2.1%
18	Alabama	3,926,995	2.0%
19	Louisiana	3,682,678	1.9%
20	Wisconsin	3,471,636	1.8%
21	Kentucky	3,187,922	1.7%
22	Maryland	3,129,218	1.6%
23	Mississippi	2,946,321	1.5%
24	South Carolina	2,802,382	1.5%
25	Iowa	2,508,509	1.3%
26	Arizona	2,400,418	1.2%
27	Washington	2,254,232	1.2%
28	Oklahoma	2,148,426	1.1%
29	Arkansas	2,126,384	1.1%
30	Kansas	2,095,243	1.1%
31	Colorado	1,829,756	1.0%
32	Connecticut	1,815,702	0.9%
33	West Virginia	1,745,689	0.9%
34	Nebraska	1,683,706	0.9%
35	Oregon	1,347,809	0.7%
36	South Dakota	1,047,494	0.5%
37	Montana	1,014,709	0.5%
38	North Dakota	877,085	0.5%
39	Nevada	869,239	0.5%
40	Maine	857,274	0.4%
41	Hawaii	829,757	0.4%
42	Utah	820,872	0.4%
43	New Mexico	761,888	0.4%
44	New Hampshire	682,841	0.4%
45	Idaho	679,075	0.4%
46	Rhode Island	658,143	0.3%
47	Delaware	488,879	0.3%
48	Vermont	406,985	0.2%
49	Alaska	383,646	0.2%
50	Wyoming	376,111	0.2%
	District of Columbia	939,547	0.5%

Source: American Hospital Association (Chicago, IL)
 "Hospital Statistics" (1999 edition)
*Inpatient days in all nonfederal short-term general and other special hospitals, whose facilities and services are available to the public. Includes days in hospital and nursing home units.

Average Daily Census in Community Hospitals in 1997

National Average = 527,408 Inpatients*

ALPHA ORDER

RANK	STATE	INPATIENTS	RANK	STATE	INPATIENTS
18	Alabama	10,759	1	New York	53,843
49	Alaska	1,051	2	California	44,158
26	Arizona	6,576	3	Texas	31,111
29	Arkansas	5,826	4	Pennsylvania	30,591
2	California	44,158	5	Florida	29,204
31	Colorado	5,013	6	Illinois	23,403
32	Connecticut	4,975	7	Ohio	21,025
47	Delaware	1,339	8	New Jersey	19,094
5	Florida	29,204	9	Michigan	18,058
11	Georgia	15,150	10	North Carolina	15,845
41	Hawaii	2,273	11	Georgia	15,150
45	Idaho	1,860	12	Tennessee	12,394
6	Illinois	23,403	13	Missouri	11,811
17	Indiana	11,170	14	Massachusetts	11,734
25	Iowa	6,873	15	Minnesota	11,657
30	Kansas	5,740	16	Virginia	11,553
21	Kentucky	8,734	17	Indiana	11,170
19	Louisiana	10,090	18	Alabama	10,759
40	Maine	2,349	19	Louisiana	10,090
22	Maryland	8,573	20	Wisconsin	9,511
14	Massachusetts	11,734	21	Kentucky	8,734
9	Michigan	18,058	22	Maryland	8,573
15	Minnesota	11,657	23	Mississippi	8,072
23	Mississippi	8,072	24	South Carolina	7,678
13	Missouri	11,811	25	Iowa	6,873
37	Montana	2,780	26	Arizona	6,576
34	Nebraska	4,613	27	Washington	6,176
39	Nevada	2,381	28	Oklahoma	5,886
44	New Hampshire	1,871	29	Arkansas	5,826
8	New Jersey	19,094	30	Kansas	5,740
43	New Mexico	2,087	31	Colorado	5,013
1	New York	53,843	32	Connecticut	4,975
10	North Carolina	15,845	33	West Virginia	4,783
38	North Dakota	2,403	34	Nebraska	4,613
7	Ohio	21,025	35	Oregon	3,693
28	Oklahoma	5,886	36	South Dakota	2,870
35	Oregon	3,693	37	Montana	2,780
4	Pennsylvania	30,591	38	North Dakota	2,403
46	Rhode Island	1,803	39	Nevada	2,381
24	South Carolina	7,678	40	Maine	2,349
36	South Dakota	2,870	41	Hawaii	2,273
12	Tennessee	12,394	42	Utah	2,249
3	Texas	31,111	43	New Mexico	2,087
42	Utah	2,249	44	New Hampshire	1,871
48	Vermont	1,115	45	Idaho	1,860
16	Virginia	11,553	46	Rhode Island	1,803
27	Washington	6,176	47	Delaware	1,339
33	West Virginia	4,783	48	Vermont	1,115
20	Wisconsin	9,511	49	Alaska	1,051
50	Wyoming	1,030	50	Wyoming	1,030
				District of Columbia	2,574

Source: Morgan Quitno Press using data from American Hospital Association (Chicago, IL)
      "Hospital Statistics" (1999 edition)
*Average total of inpatients receiving care in all nonfederal short-term general and other special hospitals, whose facilities and services are available to the public. Excludes newborns.

Average Stay in Community Hospitals in 1997

National Average = 6.1 Days*

<table>
<tr><td colspan="3">ALPHA ORDER</td><td colspan="3">RANK ORDER</td></tr>
<tr><td>RANK</td><td>STATE</td><td>DAYS</td><td>RANK</td><td>STATE</td><td>DAYS</td></tr>
<tr><td>33</td><td>Alabama</td><td>5.7</td><td>1</td><td>South Dakota</td><td>11.1</td></tr>
<tr><td>4</td><td>Alaska</td><td>9.5</td><td>2</td><td>North Dakota</td><td>10.5</td></tr>
<tr><td>45</td><td>Arizona</td><td>5.0</td><td>3</td><td>Montana</td><td>10.3</td></tr>
<tr><td>23</td><td>Arkansas</td><td>6.1</td><td>4</td><td>Alaska</td><td>9.5</td></tr>
<tr><td>44</td><td>California</td><td>5.2</td><td>5</td><td>Nebraska</td><td>8.8</td></tr>
<tr><td>45</td><td>Colorado</td><td>5.0</td><td>6</td><td>Hawaii</td><td>8.6</td></tr>
<tr><td>41</td><td>Connecticut</td><td>5.4</td><td>7</td><td>Wyoming</td><td>8.5</td></tr>
<tr><td>23</td><td>Delaware</td><td>6.1</td><td>8</td><td>New York</td><td>8.3</td></tr>
<tr><td>33</td><td>Florida</td><td>5.7</td><td>9</td><td>Minnesota</td><td>8.1</td></tr>
<tr><td>15</td><td>Georgia</td><td>6.5</td><td>10</td><td>Vermont</td><td>7.8</td></tr>
<tr><td>6</td><td>Hawaii</td><td>8.6</td><td>11</td><td>Mississippi</td><td>7.1</td></tr>
<tr><td>18</td><td>Idaho</td><td>6.3</td><td>12</td><td>Kansas</td><td>7.0</td></tr>
<tr><td>27</td><td>Illinois</td><td>5.9</td><td>13</td><td>Iowa</td><td>6.8</td></tr>
<tr><td>27</td><td>Indiana</td><td>5.9</td><td>14</td><td>North Carolina</td><td>6.6</td></tr>
<tr><td>13</td><td>Iowa</td><td>6.8</td><td>15</td><td>Georgia</td><td>6.5</td></tr>
<tr><td>12</td><td>Kansas</td><td>7.0</td><td>16</td><td>New Jersey</td><td>6.4</td></tr>
<tr><td>27</td><td>Kentucky</td><td>5.9</td><td>16</td><td>Pennsylvania</td><td>6.4</td></tr>
<tr><td>33</td><td>Louisiana</td><td>5.7</td><td>18</td><td>Idaho</td><td>6.3</td></tr>
<tr><td>25</td><td>Maine</td><td>6.0</td><td>18</td><td>South Carolina</td><td>6.3</td></tr>
<tr><td>40</td><td>Maryland</td><td>5.5</td><td>18</td><td>West Virginia</td><td>6.3</td></tr>
<tr><td>38</td><td>Massachusetts</td><td>5.6</td><td>18</td><td>Wisconsin</td><td>6.3</td></tr>
<tr><td>27</td><td>Michigan</td><td>5.9</td><td>22</td><td>New Hampshire</td><td>6.2</td></tr>
<tr><td>9</td><td>Minnesota</td><td>8.1</td><td>23</td><td>Arkansas</td><td>6.1</td></tr>
<tr><td>11</td><td>Mississippi</td><td>7.1</td><td>23</td><td>Delaware</td><td>6.1</td></tr>
<tr><td>27</td><td>Missouri</td><td>5.9</td><td>25</td><td>Maine</td><td>6.0</td></tr>
<tr><td>3</td><td>Montana</td><td>10.3</td><td>25</td><td>Virginia</td><td>6.0</td></tr>
<tr><td>5</td><td>Nebraska</td><td>8.8</td><td>27</td><td>Illinois</td><td>5.9</td></tr>
<tr><td>41</td><td>Nevada</td><td>5.4</td><td>27</td><td>Indiana</td><td>5.9</td></tr>
<tr><td>22</td><td>New Hampshire</td><td>6.2</td><td>27</td><td>Kentucky</td><td>5.9</td></tr>
<tr><td>16</td><td>New Jersey</td><td>6.4</td><td>27</td><td>Michigan</td><td>5.9</td></tr>
<tr><td>47</td><td>New Mexico</td><td>4.7</td><td>27</td><td>Missouri</td><td>5.9</td></tr>
<tr><td>8</td><td>New York</td><td>8.3</td><td>27</td><td>Tennessee</td><td>5.9</td></tr>
<tr><td>14</td><td>North Carolina</td><td>6.6</td><td>33</td><td>Alabama</td><td>5.7</td></tr>
<tr><td>2</td><td>North Dakota</td><td>10.5</td><td>33</td><td>Florida</td><td>5.7</td></tr>
<tr><td>38</td><td>Ohio</td><td>5.6</td><td>33</td><td>Louisiana</td><td>5.7</td></tr>
<tr><td>33</td><td>Oklahoma</td><td>5.7</td><td>33</td><td>Oklahoma</td><td>5.7</td></tr>
<tr><td>49</td><td>Oregon</td><td>4.4</td><td>33</td><td>Rhode Island</td><td>5.7</td></tr>
<tr><td>16</td><td>Pennsylvania</td><td>6.4</td><td>38</td><td>Massachusetts</td><td>5.6</td></tr>
<tr><td>33</td><td>Rhode Island</td><td>5.7</td><td>38</td><td>Ohio</td><td>5.6</td></tr>
<tr><td>18</td><td>South Carolina</td><td>6.3</td><td>40</td><td>Maryland</td><td>5.5</td></tr>
<tr><td>1</td><td>South Dakota</td><td>11.1</td><td>41</td><td>Connecticut</td><td>5.4</td></tr>
<tr><td>27</td><td>Tennessee</td><td>5.9</td><td>41</td><td>Nevada</td><td>5.4</td></tr>
<tr><td>43</td><td>Texas</td><td>5.3</td><td>43</td><td>Texas</td><td>5.3</td></tr>
<tr><td>49</td><td>Utah</td><td>4.4</td><td>44</td><td>California</td><td>5.2</td></tr>
<tr><td>10</td><td>Vermont</td><td>7.8</td><td>45</td><td>Arizona</td><td>5.0</td></tr>
<tr><td>25</td><td>Virginia</td><td>6.0</td><td>45</td><td>Colorado</td><td>5.0</td></tr>
<tr><td>47</td><td>Washington</td><td>4.7</td><td>47</td><td>New Mexico</td><td>4.7</td></tr>
<tr><td>18</td><td>West Virginia</td><td>6.3</td><td>47</td><td>Washington</td><td>4.7</td></tr>
<tr><td>18</td><td>Wisconsin</td><td>6.3</td><td>49</td><td>Oregon</td><td>4.4</td></tr>
<tr><td>7</td><td>Wyoming</td><td>8.5</td><td>49</td><td>Utah</td><td>4.4</td></tr>
<tr><td></td><td></td><td></td><td></td><td>District of Columbia</td><td>7.3</td></tr>
</table>

Source: American Hospital Association (Chicago, IL)
    "Hospital Statistics" (1999 edition)
*All nonfederal short-term general and other special hospitals, whose facilities and services are available to the public.

Occupancy Rate in Community Hospitals in 1997

National Rate = 61.8% of Community Hospital Beds Occupied*

ALPHA ORDER

RANK ORDER

RANK	STATE	PERCENT		RANK	STATE	PERCENT
34	Alabama	57.8		1	Hawaii	81.7
3	Alaska	73.0		2	New York	75.9
23	Arizona	61.9		3	Alaska	73.0
35	Arkansas	57.6		4	Vermont	71.2
25	California	59.6		5	Delaware	70.9
43	Colorado	55.0		5	Rhode Island	70.9
7	Connecticut	68.7		7	Connecticut	68.7
5	Delaware	70.9		8	Minnesota	68.3
29	Florida	58.7		9	North Carolina	68.2
27	Georgia	58.9		10	New Jersey	68.0
1	Hawaii	81.7		11	Maryland	67.6
47	Idaho	53.6		12	Massachusetts	67.3
32	Illinois	58.1		12	Nevada	67.3
35	Indiana	57.6		14	Pennsylvania	66.9
41	Iowa	56.1		15	South Dakota	65.0
48	Kansas	53.0		16	Michigan	64.7
38	Kentucky	56.9		17	South Carolina	64.1
45	Louisiana	54.2		18	Maine	63.6
18	Maine	63.6		18	Virginia	63.6
11	Maryland	67.6		20	New Hampshire	63.4
12	Massachusetts	67.3		21	Mississippi	62.6
16	Michigan	64.7		22	Montana	62.0
8	Minnesota	68.3		23	Arizona	61.9
21	Mississippi	62.6		24	North Dakota	61.6
40	Missouri	56.6		25	California	59.6
22	Montana	62.0		26	Nebraska	59.5
26	Nebraska	59.5		27	Georgia	58.9
12	Nevada	67.3		28	Tennessee	58.8
20	New Hampshire	63.4		29	Florida	58.7
10	New Jersey	68.0		29	West Virginia	58.7
33	New Mexico	57.9		31	Ohio	58.3
2	New York	75.9		32	Illinois	58.1
9	North Carolina	68.2		33	New Mexico	57.9
24	North Dakota	61.6		34	Alabama	57.8
31	Ohio	58.3		35	Arkansas	57.6
46	Oklahoma	54.1		35	Indiana	57.6
49	Oregon	52.9		37	Wisconsin	57.0
14	Pennsylvania	66.9		38	Kentucky	56.9
5	Rhode Island	70.9		38	Washington	56.9
17	South Carolina	64.1		40	Missouri	56.6
15	South Dakota	65.0		41	Iowa	56.1
28	Tennessee	58.8		42	Texas	55.8
42	Texas	55.8		43	Colorado	55.0
44	Utah	54.4		44	Utah	54.4
4	Vermont	71.2		45	Louisiana	54.2
18	Virginia	63.6		46	Oklahoma	54.1
38	Washington	56.9		47	Idaho	53.6
29	West Virginia	58.7		48	Kansas	53.0
37	Wisconsin	57.0		49	Oregon	52.9
50	Wyoming	52.4		50	Wyoming	52.4

District of Columbia   71.1

*Source: Morgan Quitno Press using data from American Hospital Association (Chicago, IL)
    "Hospital Statistics" (1999 edition)*
Average daily census compared to number of community hospital beds.

Outpatient Visits to Community Hospitals in 1997

National Total = 450,140,010 Visits*

ALPHA ORDER

RANK	STATE	VISITS	% of USA
22	Alabama	6,982,267	1.6%
48	Alaska	937,793	0.2%
31	Arizona	4,439,956	1.0%
32	Arkansas	4,176,670	0.9%
1	California	43,638,606	9.7%
24	Colorado	6,188,121	1.4%
21	Connecticut	7,225,265	1.6%
47	Delaware	1,226,463	0.3%
8	Florida	18,672,887	4.1%
12	Georgia	10,205,456	2.3%
39	Hawaii	2,439,337	0.5%
41	Idaho	2,123,991	0.5%
6	Illinois	22,007,152	4.9%
11	Indiana	12,399,340	2.8%
20	Iowa	7,451,973	1.7%
29	Kansas	4,718,713	1.0%
23	Kentucky	6,804,345	1.5%
16	Louisiana	8,594,671	1.9%
37	Maine	2,661,645	0.6%
28	Maryland	5,418,623	1.2%
10	Massachusetts	13,624,662	3.0%
7	Michigan	21,191,292	4.7%
26	Minnesota	5,768,971	1.3%
34	Mississippi	3,887,192	0.9%
14	Missouri	9,563,201	2.1%
43	Montana	1,479,242	0.3%
38	Nebraska	2,546,017	0.6%
44	Nevada	1,360,256	0.3%
40	New Hampshire	2,131,381	0.5%
9	New Jersey	14,123,117	3.1%
36	New Mexico	2,899,100	0.6%
2	New York	40,919,779	9.1%
13	North Carolina	10,056,808	2.2%
45	North Dakota	1,339,570	0.3%
5	Ohio	23,982,975	5.3%
33	Oklahoma	4,165,004	0.9%
27	Oregon	5,582,132	1.2%
3	Pennsylvania	27,667,730	6.1%
42	Rhode Island	1,985,486	0.4%
25	South Carolina	5,895,709	1.3%
46	South Dakota	1,256,237	0.3%
17	Tennessee	8,420,489	1.9%
4	Texas	25,857,374	5.7%
35	Utah	3,564,265	0.8%
49	Vermont	863,588	0.2%
18	Virginia	8,030,769	1.8%
19	Washington	7,731,625	1.7%
30	West Virginia	4,556,664	1.0%
15	Wisconsin	9,314,725	2.1%
50	Wyoming	829,705	0.2%

RANK ORDER

RANK	STATE	VISITS	% of USA
1	California	43,638,606	9.7%
2	New York	40,919,779	9.1%
3	Pennsylvania	27,667,730	6.1%
4	Texas	25,857,374	5.7%
5	Ohio	23,982,975	5.3%
6	Illinois	22,007,152	4.9%
7	Michigan	21,191,292	4.7%
8	Florida	18,672,887	4.1%
9	New Jersey	14,123,117	3.1%
10	Massachusetts	13,624,662	3.0%
11	Indiana	12,399,340	2.8%
12	Georgia	10,205,456	2.3%
13	North Carolina	10,056,808	2.2%
14	Missouri	9,563,201	2.1%
15	Wisconsin	9,314,725	2.1%
16	Louisiana	8,594,671	1.9%
17	Tennessee	8,420,489	1.9%
18	Virginia	8,030,769	1.8%
19	Washington	7,731,625	1.7%
20	Iowa	7,451,973	1.7%
21	Connecticut	7,225,265	1.6%
22	Alabama	6,982,267	1.6%
23	Kentucky	6,804,345	1.5%
24	Colorado	6,188,121	1.4%
25	South Carolina	5,895,709	1.3%
26	Minnesota	5,768,971	1.3%
27	Oregon	5,582,132	1.2%
28	Maryland	5,418,623	1.2%
29	Kansas	4,718,713	1.0%
30	West Virginia	4,556,664	1.0%
31	Arizona	4,439,956	1.0%
32	Arkansas	4,176,670	0.9%
33	Oklahoma	4,165,004	0.9%
34	Mississippi	3,887,192	0.9%
35	Utah	3,564,265	0.8%
36	New Mexico	2,899,100	0.6%
37	Maine	2,661,645	0.6%
38	Nebraska	2,546,017	0.6%
39	Hawaii	2,439,337	0.5%
40	New Hampshire	2,131,381	0.5%
41	Idaho	2,123,991	0.5%
42	Rhode Island	1,985,486	0.4%
43	Montana	1,479,242	0.3%
44	Nevada	1,360,256	0.3%
45	North Dakota	1,339,570	0.3%
46	South Dakota	1,256,237	0.3%
47	Delaware	1,226,463	0.3%
48	Alaska	937,793	0.2%
49	Vermont	863,588	0.2%
50	Wyoming	829,705	0.2%
	District of Columbia	1,231,671	0.3%

Source: American Hospital Association (Chicago, IL)
   "Hospital Statistics" (1999 edition)
*All nonfederal short-term general and other special hospitals, whose facilities and services are available to the public. Includes emergency and other visits.

Emergency Outpatient Visits to Community Hospitals in 1997

National Total = 92,819,892 Visits*

ALPHA ORDER

RANK	STATE	VISITS	% of USA
18	Alabama	1,987,378	2.1%
50	Alaska	152,725	0.2%
25	Arizona	1,213,179	1.3%
30	Arkansas	996,491	1.1%
1	California	9,006,700	9.7%
32	Colorado	951,705	1.0%
27	Connecticut	1,164,834	1.3%
44	Delaware	255,986	0.3%
4	Florida	5,041,372	5.4%
10	Georgia	2,705,906	2.9%
43	Hawaii	295,946	0.3%
42	Idaho	361,189	0.4%
7	Illinois	4,207,882	4.5%
15	Indiana	2,148,386	2.3%
29	Iowa	999,586	1.1%
34	Kansas	787,809	0.8%
19	Kentucky	1,645,843	1.8%
14	Louisiana	2,198,306	2.4%
36	Maine	603,070	0.6%
20	Maryland	1,611,360	1.7%
11	Massachusetts	2,559,125	2.8%
8	Michigan	3,422,070	3.7%
26	Minnesota	1,195,116	1.3%
24	Mississippi	1,442,454	1.6%
17	Missouri	2,036,674	2.2%
45	Montana	254,728	0.3%
40	Nebraska	421,382	0.5%
39	Nevada	431,476	0.5%
38	New Hampshire	450,857	0.5%
12	New Jersey	2,443,630	2.6%
37	New Mexico	489,745	0.5%
2	New York	6,768,851	7.3%
9	North Carolina	2,816,826	3.0%
47	North Dakota	201,721	0.2%
5	Ohio	4,732,151	5.1%
28	Oklahoma	1,037,970	1.1%
33	Oregon	928,641	1.0%
6	Pennsylvania	4,620,241	5.0%
41	Rhode Island	415,173	0.4%
23	South Carolina	1,466,495	1.6%
48	South Dakota	175,193	0.2%
13	Tennessee	2,325,632	2.5%
3	Texas	6,296,427	6.8%
35	Utah	632,366	0.7%
46	Vermont	221,636	0.2%
16	Virginia	2,126,854	2.3%
22	Washington	1,493,542	1.6%
31	West Virginia	994,710	1.1%
21	Wisconsin	1,604,779	1.7%
49	Wyoming	165,863	0.2%

RANK ORDER

RANK	STATE	VISITS	% of USA
1	California	9,006,700	9.7%
2	New York	6,768,851	7.3%
3	Texas	6,296,427	6.8%
4	Florida	5,041,372	5.4%
5	Ohio	4,732,151	5.1%
6	Pennsylvania	4,620,241	5.0%
7	Illinois	4,207,882	4.5%
8	Michigan	3,422,070	3.7%
9	North Carolina	2,816,826	3.0%
10	Georgia	2,705,906	2.9%
11	Massachusetts	2,559,125	2.8%
12	New Jersey	2,443,630	2.6%
13	Tennessee	2,325,632	2.5%
14	Louisiana	2,198,306	2.4%
15	Indiana	2,148,386	2.3%
16	Virginia	2,126,854	2.3%
17	Missouri	2,036,674	2.2%
18	Alabama	1,987,378	2.1%
19	Kentucky	1,645,843	1.8%
20	Maryland	1,611,360	1.7%
21	Wisconsin	1,604,779	1.7%
22	Washington	1,493,542	1.6%
23	South Carolina	1,466,495	1.6%
24	Mississippi	1,442,454	1.6%
25	Arizona	1,213,179	1.3%
26	Minnesota	1,195,116	1.3%
27	Connecticut	1,164,834	1.3%
28	Oklahoma	1,037,970	1.1%
29	Iowa	999,586	1.1%
30	Arkansas	996,491	1.1%
31	West Virginia	994,710	1.1%
32	Colorado	951,705	1.0%
33	Oregon	928,641	1.0%
34	Kansas	787,809	0.8%
35	Utah	632,366	0.7%
36	Maine	603,070	0.6%
37	New Mexico	489,745	0.5%
38	New Hampshire	450,857	0.5%
39	Nevada	431,476	0.5%
40	Nebraska	421,382	0.5%
41	Rhode Island	415,173	0.4%
42	Idaho	361,189	0.4%
43	Hawaii	295,946	0.3%
44	Delaware	255,986	0.3%
45	Montana	254,728	0.3%
46	Vermont	221,636	0.2%
47	North Dakota	201,721	0.2%
48	South Dakota	175,193	0.2%
49	Wyoming	165,863	0.2%
50	Alaska	152,725	0.2%
	District of Columbia	311,911	0.3%

Source: American Hospital Association (Chicago, IL)
    "Hospital Statistics" (1999 edition)
*All nonfederal short-term general and other special hospitals, whose facilities and services are available to the public.

Surgical Operations in Community Hospitals in 1997

National Total = 24,187,371 Surgical Operations*

ALPHA ORDER

RANK ORDER

RANK	STATE	OPERATIONS	% of USA	RANK	STATE	OPERATIONS	% of USA
18	Alabama	500,801	2.1%	1	California	2,032,937	8.4%
50	Alaska	32,726	0.1%	2	New York	1,763,607	7.3%
27	Arizona	301,521	1.2%	3	Pennsylvania	1,526,670	6.3%
31	Arkansas	254,721	1.1%	4	Texas	1,511,929	6.3%
1	California	2,032,937	8.4%	5	Florida	1,286,472	5.3%
26	Colorado	303,927	1.3%	6	Ohio	1,228,996	5.1%
28	Connecticut	288,442	1.2%	7	Illinois	1,034,349	4.3%
43	Delaware	84,730	0.4%	8	Michigan	977,475	4.0%
5	Florida	1,286,472	5.3%	9	New Jersey	676,427	2.8%
10	Georgia	671,539	2.8%	10	Georgia	671,539	2.8%
44	Hawaii	75,400	0.3%	11	North Carolina	665,185	2.8%
41	Idaho	95,325	0.4%	12	Massachusetts	601,436	2.5%
7	Illinois	1,034,349	4.3%	13	Indiana	595,436	2.5%
13	Indiana	595,436	2.5%	14	Tennessee	570,375	2.4%
24	Iowa	353,000	1.5%	15	Virginia	558,357	2.3%
33	Kansas	252,680	1.0%	16	Missouri	553,503	2.3%
20	Kentucky	437,186	1.8%	17	Maryland	509,504	2.1%
21	Louisiana	423,880	1.8%	18	Alabama	500,801	2.1%
39	Maine	117,868	0.5%	19	Wisconsin	493,087	2.0%
17	Maryland	509,504	2.1%	20	Kentucky	437,186	1.8%
12	Massachusetts	601,436	2.5%	21	Louisiana	423,880	1.8%
8	Michigan	977,475	4.0%	22	Minnesota	420,960	1.7%
22	Minnesota	420,960	1.7%	23	Washington	383,423	1.6%
32	Mississippi	253,279	1.0%	24	Iowa	353,000	1.5%
16	Missouri	553,503	2.3%	25	South Carolina	346,723	1.4%
47	Montana	72,964	0.3%	26	Colorado	303,927	1.3%
35	Nebraska	189,334	0.8%	27	Arizona	301,521	1.2%
38	Nevada	119,725	0.5%	28	Connecticut	288,442	1.2%
42	New Hampshire	87,311	0.4%	29	Oklahoma	270,122	1.1%
9	New Jersey	676,427	2.8%	30	Oregon	264,259	1.1%
37	New Mexico	135,622	0.6%	31	Arkansas	254,721	1.1%
2	New York	1,763,607	7.3%	32	Mississippi	253,279	1.0%
11	North Carolina	665,185	2.8%	33	Kansas	252,680	1.0%
46	North Dakota	75,026	0.3%	34	West Virginia	242,433	1.0%
6	Ohio	1,228,996	5.1%	35	Nebraska	189,334	0.8%
29	Oklahoma	270,122	1.1%	36	Utah	167,780	0.7%
30	Oregon	264,259	1.1%	37	New Mexico	135,622	0.6%
3	Pennsylvania	1,526,670	6.3%	38	Nevada	119,725	0.5%
40	Rhode Island	111,052	0.5%	39	Maine	117,868	0.5%
25	South Carolina	346,723	1.4%	40	Rhode Island	111,052	0.5%
45	South Dakota	75,067	0.3%	41	Idaho	95,325	0.4%
14	Tennessee	570,375	2.4%	42	New Hampshire	87,311	0.4%
4	Texas	1,511,929	6.3%	43	Delaware	84,730	0.4%
36	Utah	167,780	0.7%	44	Hawaii	75,400	0.3%
48	Vermont	48,247	0.2%	45	South Dakota	75,067	0.3%
15	Virginia	558,357	2.3%	46	North Dakota	75,026	0.3%
23	Washington	383,423	1.6%	47	Montana	72,964	0.3%
34	West Virginia	242,433	1.0%	48	Vermont	48,247	0.2%
19	Wisconsin	493,087	2.0%	49	Wyoming	35,855	0.1%
49	Wyoming	35,855	0.1%	50	Alaska	32,726	0.1%
					District of Columbia	108,698	0.4%

Source: American Hospital Association (Chicago, IL)
  "Hospital Statistics" (1999 edition)
*Includes inpatient and outpatient surgeries.

Medicare and Medicaid Certified Facilities in 1999

National Total = 225,167 Facilities*

ALPHA ORDER

RANK	STATE	FACILITIES	% of USA
20	Alabama	3,889	1.7%
50	Alaska	487	0.2%
28	Arizona	3,119	1.4%
31	Arkansas	2,684	1.2%
1	California	21,856	9.7%
30	Colorado	2,905	1.3%
29	Connecticut	3,115	1.4%
47	Delaware	642	0.3%
3	Florida	13,791	6.1%
9	Georgia	6,251	2.8%
45	Hawaii	893	0.4%
40	Idaho	1,027	0.5%
6	Illinois	9,709	4.3%
11	Indiana	6,065	2.7%
23	Iowa	3,420	1.5%
27	Kansas	3,191	1.4%
25	Kentucky	3,336	1.5%
14	Louisiana	5,199	2.3%
38	Maine	1,299	0.6%
18	Maryland	4,021	1.8%
17	Massachusetts	4,692	2.1%
8	Michigan	7,773	3.5%
21	Minnesota	3,599	1.6%
32	Mississippi	2,485	1.1%
13	Missouri	5,509	2.4%
42	Montana	927	0.4%
35	Nebraska	1,725	0.8%
39	Nevada	1,058	0.5%
41	New Hampshire	1,022	0.5%
12	New Jersey	5,535	2.5%
36	New Mexico	1,450	0.6%
4	New York	12,312	5.5%
10	North Carolina	6,183	2.7%
46	North Dakota	826	0.4%
5	Ohio	10,874	4.8%
19	Oklahoma	3,929	1.7%
33	Oregon	2,444	1.1%
7	Pennsylvania	9,509	4.2%
42	Rhode Island	927	0.4%
26	South Carolina	3,276	1.5%
44	South Dakota	907	0.4%
16	Tennessee	4,855	2.2%
2	Texas	19,459	8.6%
37	Utah	1,311	0.6%
48	Vermont	514	0.2%
15	Virginia	5,089	2.3%
24	Washington	3,377	1.5%
34	West Virginia	2,003	0.9%
22	Wisconsin	3,484	1.5%
49	Wyoming	500	0.2%

RANK ORDER

RANK	STATE	FACILITIES	% of USA
1	California	21,856	9.7%
2	Texas	19,459	8.6%
3	Florida	13,791	6.1%
4	New York	12,312	5.5%
5	Ohio	10,874	4.8%
6	Illinois	9,709	4.3%
7	Pennsylvania	9,509	4.2%
8	Michigan	7,773	3.5%
9	Georgia	6,251	2.8%
10	North Carolina	6,183	2.7%
11	Indiana	6,065	2.7%
12	New Jersey	5,535	2.5%
13	Missouri	5,509	2.4%
14	Louisiana	5,199	2.3%
15	Virginia	5,089	2.3%
16	Tennessee	4,855	2.2%
17	Massachusetts	4,692	2.1%
18	Maryland	4,021	1.8%
19	Oklahoma	3,929	1.7%
20	Alabama	3,889	1.7%
21	Minnesota	3,599	1.6%
22	Wisconsin	3,484	1.5%
23	Iowa	3,420	1.5%
24	Washington	3,377	1.5%
25	Kentucky	3,336	1.5%
26	South Carolina	3,276	1.5%
27	Kansas	3,191	1.4%
28	Arizona	3,119	1.4%
29	Connecticut	3,115	1.4%
30	Colorado	2,905	1.3%
31	Arkansas	2,684	1.2%
32	Mississippi	2,485	1.1%
33	Oregon	2,444	1.1%
34	West Virginia	2,003	0.9%
35	Nebraska	1,725	0.8%
36	New Mexico	1,450	0.6%
37	Utah	1,311	0.6%
38	Maine	1,299	0.6%
39	Nevada	1,058	0.5%
40	Idaho	1,027	0.5%
41	New Hampshire	1,022	0.5%
42	Montana	927	0.4%
42	Rhode Island	927	0.4%
44	South Dakota	907	0.4%
45	Hawaii	893	0.4%
46	North Dakota	826	0.4%
47	Delaware	642	0.3%
48	Vermont	514	0.2%
49	Wyoming	500	0.2%
50	Alaska	487	0.2%
	District of Columbia	714	0.3%

Source: U.S. Department of Health and Human Services, Health Care Financing Administration
   OSCAR Report 10 (January 25, 1999)

*Certified by HCFA to participate in the Medicare/Medicaid programs. All provider groups including hospitals, home health agencies, rural health centers, community mental health centers, nursing facilities, outpatient physical therapy facilities and hospices. Also includes 166,372 laboratories. National total does not include 1,214 certified facilities in U.S. territories.

Medicare and Medicaid Certified Hospitals in 1999

National Total = 6,103 Hospitals*

ALPHA ORDER

RANK	STATE	HOSPITALS	% of USA
19	Alabama	128	2.1%
47	Alaska	24	0.4%
29	Arizona	90	1.5%
28	Arkansas	95	1.6%
2	California	481	7.9%
30	Colorado	85	1.4%
40	Connecticut	47	0.8%
50	Delaware	10	0.2%
5	Florida	255	4.2%
8	Georgia	198	3.2%
46	Hawaii	27	0.4%
40	Idaho	47	0.8%
6	Illinois	224	3.7%
11	Indiana	159	2.6%
21	Iowa	121	2.0%
14	Kansas	148	2.4%
22	Kentucky	120	2.0%
10	Louisiana	174	2.9%
42	Maine	42	0.7%
32	Maryland	70	1.1%
20	Massachusetts	127	2.1%
9	Michigan	178	2.9%
12	Minnesota	151	2.5%
25	Mississippi	109	1.8%
15	Missouri	147	2.4%
35	Montana	60	1.0%
27	Nebraska	97	1.6%
43	Nevada	40	0.7%
44	New Hampshire	31	0.5%
24	New Jersey	113	1.9%
37	New Mexico	53	0.9%
3	New York	266	4.4%
17	North Carolina	144	2.4%
38	North Dakota	50	0.8%
7	Ohio	202	3.3%
16	Oklahoma	146	2.4%
34	Oregon	62	1.0%
4	Pennsylvania	257	4.2%
48	Rhode Island	17	0.3%
31	South Carolina	74	1.2%
33	South Dakota	63	1.0%
13	Tennessee	149	2.4%
1	Texas	492	8.1%
39	Utah	49	0.8%
49	Vermont	16	0.3%
22	Virginia	120	2.0%
26	Washington	98	1.6%
35	West Virginia	60	1.0%
18	Wisconsin	142	2.3%
45	Wyoming	29	0.5%

RANK ORDER

RANK	STATE	HOSPITALS	% of USA
1	Texas	492	8.1%
2	California	481	7.9%
3	New York	266	4.4%
4	Pennsylvania	257	4.2%
5	Florida	255	4.2%
6	Illinois	224	3.7%
7	Ohio	202	3.3%
8	Georgia	198	3.2%
9	Michigan	178	2.9%
10	Louisiana	174	2.9%
11	Indiana	159	2.6%
12	Minnesota	151	2.5%
13	Tennessee	149	2.4%
14	Kansas	148	2.4%
15	Missouri	147	2.4%
16	Oklahoma	146	2.4%
17	North Carolina	144	2.4%
18	Wisconsin	142	2.3%
19	Alabama	128	2.1%
20	Massachusetts	127	2.1%
21	Iowa	121	2.0%
22	Kentucky	120	2.0%
22	Virginia	120	2.0%
24	New Jersey	113	1.9%
25	Mississippi	109	1.8%
26	Washington	98	1.6%
27	Nebraska	97	1.6%
28	Arkansas	95	1.6%
29	Arizona	90	1.5%
30	Colorado	85	1.4%
31	South Carolina	74	1.2%
32	Maryland	70	1.1%
33	South Dakota	63	1.0%
34	Oregon	62	1.0%
35	Montana	60	1.0%
35	West Virginia	60	1.0%
37	New Mexico	53	0.9%
38	North Dakota	50	0.8%
39	Utah	49	0.8%
40	Connecticut	47	0.8%
40	Idaho	47	0.8%
42	Maine	42	0.7%
43	Nevada	40	0.7%
44	New Hampshire	31	0.5%
45	Wyoming	29	0.5%
46	Hawaii	27	0.4%
47	Alaska	24	0.4%
48	Rhode Island	17	0.3%
49	Vermont	16	0.3%
50	Delaware	10	0.2%
	District of Columbia	16	0.3%

Source: U.S. Department of Health and Human Services, Health Care Financing Administration
OSCAR Report 10 (January 25, 1999)
*Certified by HCFA to participate in the Medicare/Medicaid programs. Excludes licensed facilities that do not accept federal funding and facilities managed by the Department of Veterans Affairs. National total does not include 61 certified hospitals in U.S. territories.

Beds in Medicare and Medicaid Certified Hospitals in 1999

National Total = 1,000,020 Beds*

ALPHA ORDER

RANK	STATE	BEDS	% of USA
18	Alabama	21,162	2.1%
50	Alaska	1,564	0.2%
31	Arizona	11,409	1.1%
29	Arkansas	12,144	1.2%
1	California	85,836	8.6%
30	Colorado	11,634	1.2%
32	Connecticut	10,030	1.0%
47	Delaware	2,290	0.2%
4	Florida	56,281	5.6%
10	Georgia	28,038	2.8%
46	Hawaii	2,874	0.3%
44	Idaho	2,979	0.3%
5	Illinois	51,206	5.1%
14	Indiana	23,691	2.4%
25	Iowa	12,857	1.3%
27	Kansas	12,594	1.3%
20	Kentucky	17,992	1.8%
19	Louisiana	20,003	2.0%
40	Maine	4,211	0.4%
22	Maryland	17,257	1.7%
16	Massachusetts	21,625	2.2%
9	Michigan	33,211	3.3%
21	Minnesota	17,643	1.8%
28	Mississippi	12,576	1.3%
12	Missouri	27,100	2.7%
45	Montana	2,977	0.3%
35	Nebraska	7,622	0.8%
38	Nevada	4,432	0.4%
42	New Hampshire	3,580	0.4%
8	New Jersey	33,504	3.4%
37	New Mexico	5,084	0.5%
2	New York	82,912	8.3%
11	North Carolina	27,342	2.7%
41	North Dakota	3,650	0.4%
6	Ohio	50,107	5.0%
23	Oklahoma	15,508	1.6%
34	Oregon	8,163	0.8%
7	Pennsylvania	46,086	4.6%
39	Rhode Island	4,244	0.4%
26	South Carolina	12,611	1.3%
43	South Dakota	3,359	0.3%
13	Tennessee	26,885	2.7%
3	Texas	60,856	6.1%
36	Utah	5,359	0.5%
48	Vermont	2,026	0.2%
15	Virginia	23,104	2.3%
24	Washington	14,685	1.5%
33	West Virginia	9,671	1.0%
17	Wisconsin	21,283	2.1%
49	Wyoming	1,658	0.2%

RANK ORDER

RANK	STATE	BEDS	% of USA
1	California	85,836	8.6%
2	New York	82,912	8.3%
3	Texas	60,856	6.1%
4	Florida	56,281	5.6%
5	Illinois	51,206	5.1%
6	Ohio	50,107	5.0%
7	Pennsylvania	46,086	4.6%
8	New Jersey	33,504	3.4%
9	Michigan	33,211	3.3%
10	Georgia	28,038	2.8%
11	North Carolina	27,342	2.7%
12	Missouri	27,100	2.7%
13	Tennessee	26,885	2.7%
14	Indiana	23,691	2.4%
15	Virginia	23,104	2.3%
16	Massachusetts	21,625	2.2%
17	Wisconsin	21,283	2.1%
18	Alabama	21,162	2.1%
19	Louisiana	20,003	2.0%
20	Kentucky	17,992	1.8%
21	Minnesota	17,643	1.8%
22	Maryland	17,257	1.7%
23	Oklahoma	15,508	1.6%
24	Washington	14,685	1.5%
25	Iowa	12,857	1.3%
26	South Carolina	12,611	1.3%
27	Kansas	12,594	1.3%
28	Mississippi	12,576	1.3%
29	Arkansas	12,144	1.2%
30	Colorado	11,634	1.2%
31	Arizona	11,409	1.1%
32	Connecticut	10,030	1.0%
33	West Virginia	9,671	1.0%
34	Oregon	8,163	0.8%
35	Nebraska	7,622	0.8%
36	Utah	5,359	0.5%
37	New Mexico	5,084	0.5%
38	Nevada	4,432	0.4%
39	Rhode Island	4,244	0.4%
40	Maine	4,211	0.4%
41	North Dakota	3,650	0.4%
42	New Hampshire	3,580	0.4%
43	South Dakota	3,359	0.3%
44	Idaho	2,979	0.3%
45	Montana	2,977	0.3%
46	Hawaii	2,874	0.3%
47	Delaware	2,290	0.2%
48	Vermont	2,026	0.2%
49	Wyoming	1,658	0.2%
50	Alaska	1,564	0.2%
	District of Columbia	5,105	0.5%

Source: U.S. Department of Health and Human Services, Health Care Financing Administration
    OSCAR Report 10 (January 25, 1999)
*Beds in hospitals certified by HCFA to participate in the Medicare/Medicaid programs. Excludes licensed facilities that do not accept federal funding and facilities managed by the Department of Veterans Affairs. National total does not include 11,209 beds in U.S. territories.

Medicare and Medicaid Certified Children's Hospitals in 1999

National Total = 70 Hospitals*

ALPHA ORDER					RANK ORDER			
RANK	STATE	HOSPITALS	% of USA		RANK	STATE	HOSPITALS	% of USA
17	Alabama	1	1.4%		1	California	8	11.4%
33	Alaska	0	0.0%		1	Ohio	8	11.4%
17	Arizona	1	1.4%		3	Texas	7	10.0%
17	Arkansas	1	1.4%		4	Pennsylvania	5	7.1%
1	California	8	11.4%		5	Minnesota	3	4.3%
17	Colorado	1	1.4%		6	Florida	2	2.9%
17	Connecticut	1	1.4%		6	Georgia	2	2.9%
17	Delaware	1	1.4%		6	Illinois	2	2.9%
6	Florida	2	2.9%		6	Maryland	2	2.9%
6	Georgia	2	2.9%		6	Massachusetts	2	2.9%
17	Hawaii	1	1.4%		6	Missouri	2	2.9%
33	Idaho	0	0.0%		6	Nebraska	2	2.9%
6	Illinois	2	2.9%		6	Oklahoma	2	2.9%
17	Indiana	1	1.4%		6	Tennessee	2	2.9%
33	Iowa	0	0.0%		6	Virginia	2	2.9%
17	Kansas	1	1.4%		6	Washington	2	2.9%
33	Kentucky	0	0.0%		17	Alabama	1	1.4%
17	Louisiana	1	1.4%		17	Arizona	1	1.4%
33	Maine	0	0.0%		17	Arkansas	1	1.4%
6	Maryland	2	2.9%		17	Colorado	1	1.4%
6	Massachusetts	2	2.9%		17	Connecticut	1	1.4%
17	Michigan	1	1.4%		17	Delaware	1	1.4%
5	Minnesota	3	4.3%		17	Hawaii	1	1.4%
33	Mississippi	0	0.0%		17	Indiana	1	1.4%
6	Missouri	2	2.9%		17	Kansas	1	1.4%
33	Montana	0	0.0%		17	Louisiana	1	1.4%
6	Nebraska	2	2.9%		17	Michigan	1	1.4%
33	Nevada	0	0.0%		17	New Jersey	1	1.4%
33	New Hampshire	0	0.0%		17	New Mexico	1	1.4%
17	New Jersey	1	1.4%		17	New York	1	1.4%
17	New Mexico	1	1.4%		17	Utah	1	1.4%
17	New York	1	1.4%		17	Wisconsin	1	1.4%
33	North Carolina	0	0.0%		33	Alaska	0	0.0%
33	North Dakota	0	0.0%		33	Idaho	0	0.0%
1	Ohio	8	11.4%		33	Iowa	0	0.0%
6	Oklahoma	2	2.9%		33	Kentucky	0	0.0%
33	Oregon	0	0.0%		33	Maine	0	0.0%
4	Pennsylvania	5	7.1%		33	Mississippi	0	0.0%
33	Rhode Island	0	0.0%		33	Montana	0	0.0%
33	South Carolina	0	0.0%		33	Nevada	0	0.0%
33	South Dakota	0	0.0%		33	New Hampshire	0	0.0%
6	Tennessee	2	2.9%		33	North Carolina	0	0.0%
3	Texas	7	10.0%		33	North Dakota	0	0.0%
17	Utah	1	1.4%		33	Oregon	0	0.0%
33	Vermont	0	0.0%		33	Rhode Island	0	0.0%
6	Virginia	2	2.9%		33	South Carolina	0	0.0%
6	Washington	2	2.9%		33	South Dakota	0	0.0%
33	West Virginia	0	0.0%		33	Vermont	0	0.0%
17	Wisconsin	1	1.4%		33	West Virginia	0	0.0%
33	Wyoming	0	0.0%		33	Wyoming	0	0.0%
						District of Columbia	1	1.4%

Source: U.S. Department of Health and Human Services, Health Care Financing Administration
    OSCAR Report 10 (January 25, 1999)
*Certified by HCFA to participate in the Medicare/Medicaid programs. National total does not include one facility in U.S. territories. Excludes licensed facilities that do not accept federal funding and facilities managed by the Department of Veterans Affairs.

Beds in Medicare and Medicaid Certified Children's Hospitals in 1999

National Total = 11,142 Beds*

ALPHA ORDER

RANK	STATE	BEDS	% of USA
18	Alabama	225	2.0%
33	Alaska	0	0.0%
32	Arizona	15	0.1%
12	Arkansas	280	2.5%
2	California	1,277	11.5%
14	Colorado	253	2.3%
25	Connecticut	97	0.9%
25	Delaware	97	0.9%
9	Florida	376	3.4%
8	Georgia	400	3.6%
17	Hawaii	232	2.1%
33	Idaho	0	0.0%
10	Illinois	351	3.2%
31	Indiana	20	0.2%
33	Iowa	0	0.0%
30	Kansas	34	0.3%
33	Kentucky	0	0.0%
20	Louisiana	188	1.7%
33	Maine	0	0.0%
23	Maryland	165	1.5%
5	Massachusetts	425	3.8%
16	Michigan	245	2.2%
11	Minnesota	329	3.0%
33	Mississippi	0	0.0%
7	Missouri	402	3.6%
33	Montana	0	0.0%
24	Nebraska	142	1.3%
33	Nevada	0	0.0%
33	New Hampshire	0	0.0%
28	New Jersey	60	0.5%
29	New Mexico	37	0.3%
6	New York	405	3.6%
33	North Carolina	0	0.0%
33	North Dakota	0	0.0%
1	Ohio	1,809	16.2%
27	Oklahoma	68	0.6%
33	Oregon	0	0.0%
4	Pennsylvania	641	5.8%
33	Rhode Island	0	0.0%
33	South Carolina	0	0.0%
33	South Dakota	0	0.0%
22	Tennessee	175	1.6%
3	Texas	1,245	11.2%
19	Utah	194	1.7%
33	Vermont	0	0.0%
15	Virginia	250	2.2%
13	Washington	276	2.5%
33	West Virginia	0	0.0%
21	Wisconsin	186	1.7%
33	Wyoming	0	0.0%

RANK ORDER

RANK	STATE	BEDS	% of USA
1	Ohio	1,809	16.2%
2	California	1,277	11.5%
3	Texas	1,245	11.2%
4	Pennsylvania	641	5.8%
5	Massachusetts	425	3.8%
6	New York	405	3.6%
7	Missouri	402	3.6%
8	Georgia	400	3.6%
9	Florida	376	3.4%
10	Illinois	351	3.2%
11	Minnesota	329	3.0%
12	Arkansas	280	2.5%
13	Washington	276	2.5%
14	Colorado	253	2.3%
15	Virginia	250	2.2%
16	Michigan	245	2.2%
17	Hawaii	232	2.1%
18	Alabama	225	2.0%
19	Utah	194	1.7%
20	Louisiana	188	1.7%
21	Wisconsin	186	1.7%
22	Tennessee	175	1.6%
23	Maryland	165	1.5%
24	Nebraska	142	1.3%
25	Connecticut	97	0.9%
25	Delaware	97	0.9%
27	Oklahoma	68	0.6%
28	New Jersey	60	0.5%
29	New Mexico	37	0.3%
30	Kansas	34	0.3%
31	Indiana	20	0.2%
32	Arizona	15	0.1%
33	Alaska	0	0.0%
33	Idaho	0	0.0%
33	Iowa	0	0.0%
33	Kentucky	0	0.0%
33	Maine	0	0.0%
33	Mississippi	0	0.0%
33	Montana	0	0.0%
33	Nevada	0	0.0%
33	New Hampshire	0	0.0%
33	North Carolina	0	0.0%
33	North Dakota	0	0.0%
33	Oregon	0	0.0%
33	Rhode Island	0	0.0%
33	South Carolina	0	0.0%
33	South Dakota	0	0.0%
33	Vermont	0	0.0%
33	West Virginia	0	0.0%
33	Wyoming	0	0.0%
	District of Columbia	243	2.2%

Source: U.S. Department of Health and Human Services, Health Care Financing Administration OSCAR Report 10 (January 25, 1999)

Beds in hospitals certified by HCFA to participate in the Medicare/Medicaid programs. Excludes licensed facilities that do not accept federal funding and facilities managed by the Department of Veterans Affairs. National total does not include 215 beds in U.S. territories.

Medicare and Medicaid Certified Rehabilitation Hospitals in 1999

National Total = 199 Hospitals*

ALPHA ORDER					RANK ORDER			
RANK	STATE		HOSPITALS	% of USA	RANK	STATE	HOSPITALS	% of USA
11	Alabama		5	2.5%	1	Texas	34	17.1%
43	Alaska		0	0.0%	2	Pennsylvania	17	8.5%
16	Arizona		4	2.0%	3	Florida	14	7.0%
7	Arkansas		6	3.0%	4	California	11	5.5%
4	California		11	5.5%	4	Louisiana	11	5.5%
25	Colorado		2	1.0%	6	Massachusetts	7	3.5%
31	Connecticut		1	0.5%	7	Arkansas	6	3.0%
31	Delaware		1	0.5%	7	Michigan	6	3.0%
3	Florida		14	7.0%	7	New Jersey	6	3.0%
25	Georgia		2	1.0%	7	West Virginia	6	3.0%
31	Hawaii		1	0.5%	11	Alabama	5	2.5%
31	Idaho		1	0.5%	11	Indiana	5	2.5%
20	Illinois		3	1.5%	11	Kansas	5	2.5%
11	Indiana		5	2.5%	11	Tennessee	5	2.5%
43	Iowa		0	0.0%	11	Virginia	5	2.5%
11	Kansas		5	2.5%	16	Arizona	4	2.0%
16	Kentucky		4	2.0%	16	Kentucky	4	2.0%
4	Louisiana		11	5.5%	16	New Mexico	4	2.0%
31	Maine		1	0.5%	16	New York	4	2.0%
25	Maryland		2	1.0%	20	Illinois	3	1.5%
6	Massachusetts		7	3.5%	20	Missouri	3	1.5%
7	Michigan		6	3.0%	20	Nevada	3	1.5%
43	Minnesota		0	0.0%	20	Oklahoma	3	1.5%
31	Mississippi		1	0.5%	20	South Carolina	3	1.5%
20	Missouri		3	1.5%	25	Colorado	2	1.0%
43	Montana		0	0.0%	25	Georgia	2	1.0%
31	Nebraska		1	0.5%	25	Maryland	2	1.0%
20	Nevada		3	1.5%	25	New Hampshire	2	1.0%
25	New Hampshire		2	1.0%	25	North Carolina	2	1.0%
7	New Jersey		6	3.0%	25	Ohio	2	1.0%
16	New Mexico		4	2.0%	31	Connecticut	1	0.5%
16	New York		4	2.0%	31	Delaware	1	0.5%
25	North Carolina		2	1.0%	31	Hawaii	1	0.5%
43	North Dakota		0	0.0%	31	Idaho	1	0.5%
25	Ohio		2	1.0%	31	Maine	1	0.5%
20	Oklahoma		3	1.5%	31	Mississippi	1	0.5%
43	Oregon		0	0.0%	31	Nebraska	1	0.5%
2	Pennsylvania		17	8.5%	31	Rhode Island	1	0.5%
31	Rhode Island		1	0.5%	31	Utah	1	0.5%
20	South Carolina		3	1.5%	31	Washington	1	0.5%
43	South Dakota		0	0.0%	31	Wisconsin	1	0.5%
11	Tennessee		5	2.5%	31	Wyoming	1	0.5%
1	Texas		34	17.1%	43	Alaska	0	0.0%
31	Utah		1	0.5%	43	Iowa	0	0.0%
43	Vermont		0	0.0%	43	Minnesota	0	0.0%
11	Virginia		5	2.5%	43	Montana	0	0.0%
31	Washington		1	0.5%	43	North Dakota	0	0.0%
7	West Virginia		6	3.0%	43	Oregon	0	0.0%
31	Wisconsin		1	0.5%	43	South Dakota	0	0.0%
31	Wyoming		1	0.5%	43	Vermont	0	0.0%
						District of Columbia	1	0.5%

Source: U.S. Department of Health and Human Services, Health Care Financing Administration
   OSCAR Report 10 (January 25, 1999)
*Certified by HCFA to participate in the Medicare/Medicaid programs. Excludes licensed facilities that do not accept federal funding and facilities managed by the Department of Veterans Affairs.

Beds in Medicare and Medicaid Certified Rehabilitation Hospitals in 1999

National Total = 13,301 Beds*

ALPHA ORDER					RANK ORDER			
RANK	STATE		BEDS	% of USA	RANK	STATE	BEDS	% of USA
14	Alabama		289	2.2%	1	Texas	1,780	13.4%
43	Alaska		0	0.0%	2	Pennsylvania	1,588	11.9%
21	Arizona		208	1.6%	3	Florida	863	6.5%
8	Arkansas		442	3.3%	4	Massachusetts	699	5.3%
6	California		576	4.3%	5	New Jersey	650	4.9%
23	Colorado		196	1.5%	6	California	576	4.3%
37	Connecticut		60	0.5%	7	Louisiana	523	3.9%
37	Delaware		60	0.5%	8	Arkansas	442	3.3%
3	Florida		863	6.5%	9	New York	428	3.2%
30	Georgia		108	0.8%	10	Michigan	406	3.1%
32	Hawaii		100	0.8%	11	Illinois	371	2.8%
40	Idaho		54	0.4%	12	Tennessee	350	2.6%
11	Illinois		371	2.8%	13	Indiana	307	2.3%
13	Indiana		307	2.3%	14	Alabama	289	2.2%
43	Iowa		0	0.0%	15	Virginia	281	2.1%
16	Kansas		267	2.0%	16	Kansas	267	2.0%
18	Kentucky		225	1.7%	17	West Virginia	246	1.8%
7	Louisiana		523	3.9%	18	Kentucky	225	1.7%
32	Maine		100	0.8%	19	North Carolina	223	1.7%
36	Maryland		66	0.5%	20	South Carolina	213	1.6%
4	Massachusetts		699	5.3%	21	Arizona	208	1.6%
10	Michigan		406	3.1%	22	Oklahoma	197	1.5%
43	Minnesota		0	0.0%	23	Colorado	196	1.5%
29	Mississippi		124	0.9%	24	Missouri	180	1.4%
24	Missouri		180	1.4%	25	New Hampshire	152	1.1%
43	Montana		0	0.0%	26	Nevada	144	1.1%
37	Nebraska		60	0.5%	27	New Mexico	143	1.1%
26	Nevada		144	1.1%	28	Ohio	132	1.0%
25	New Hampshire		152	1.1%	29	Mississippi	124	0.9%
5	New Jersey		650	4.9%	30	Georgia	108	0.8%
27	New Mexico		143	1.1%	31	Washington	102	0.8%
9	New York		428	3.2%	32	Hawaii	100	0.8%
19	North Carolina		223	1.7%	32	Maine	100	0.8%
43	North Dakota		0	0.0%	34	Rhode Island	82	0.6%
28	Ohio		132	1.0%	35	Wisconsin	81	0.6%
22	Oklahoma		197	1.5%	36	Maryland	66	0.5%
43	Oregon		0	0.0%	37	Connecticut	60	0.5%
2	Pennsylvania		1,588	11.9%	37	Delaware	60	0.5%
34	Rhode Island		82	0.6%	37	Nebraska	60	0.5%
20	South Carolina		213	1.6%	40	Idaho	54	0.4%
43	South Dakota		0	0.0%	41	Utah	50	0.4%
12	Tennessee		350	2.6%	42	Wyoming	15	0.1%
1	Texas		1,780	13.4%	43	Alaska	0	0.0%
41	Utah		50	0.4%	43	Iowa	0	0.0%
43	Vermont		0	0.0%	43	Minnesota	0	0.0%
15	Virginia		281	2.1%	43	Montana	0	0.0%
31	Washington		102	0.8%	43	North Dakota	0	0.0%
17	West Virginia		246	1.8%	43	Oregon	0	0.0%
35	Wisconsin		81	0.6%	43	South Dakota	0	0.0%
42	Wyoming		15	0.1%	43	Vermont	0	0.0%
						District of Columbia	160	1.2%

Source: U.S. Department of Health and Human Services, Health Care Financing Administration
OSCAR Report 10 (January 25, 1999)

*Beds in hospitals certified by HCFA to participate in the Medicare/Medicaid programs. Excludes licensed facilities that do not accept federal funding and facilities managed by the Department of Veterans Affairs.

Medicare and Medicaid Certified Psychiatric Hospitals in 1999

National Total = 597 Psychiatric Hospitals*

ALPHA ORDER

ALPHA ORDER

RANK ORDER

RANK	STATE	HOSPITALS	% of USA		RANK	STATE	HOSPITALS	% of USA
22	Alabama	11	1.8%		1	California	46	7.7%
44	Alaska	2	0.3%		2	Texas	41	6.9%
24	Arizona	9	1.5%		3	New York	35	5.9%
23	Arkansas	10	1.7%		4	Florida	32	5.4%
1	California	46	7.7%		5	Pennsylvania	29	4.9%
24	Colorado	9	1.5%		6	Indiana	27	4.5%
24	Connecticut	9	1.5%		7	Georgia	25	4.2%
40	Delaware	3	0.5%		8	Louisiana	22	3.7%
4	Florida	32	5.4%		9	Massachusetts	18	3.0%
7	Georgia	25	4.2%		9	Virginia	18	3.0%
49	Hawaii	1	0.2%		11	Illinois	17	2.8%
34	Idaho	4	0.7%		11	Missouri	17	2.8%
11	Illinois	17	2.8%		11	New Jersey	17	2.8%
6	Indiana	27	4.5%		14	Ohio	16	2.7%
34	Iowa	4	0.7%		15	Wisconsin	15	2.5%
24	Kansas	9	1.5%		16	North Carolina	14	2.3%
17	Kentucky	13	2.2%		17	Kentucky	13	2.2%
8	Louisiana	22	3.7%		17	Michigan	13	2.2%
34	Maine	4	0.7%		17	Oklahoma	13	2.2%
21	Maryland	12	2.0%		17	Tennessee	13	2.2%
9	Massachusetts	18	3.0%		21	Maryland	12	2.0%
17	Michigan	13	2.2%		22	Alabama	11	1.8%
29	Minnesota	7	1.2%		23	Arkansas	10	1.7%
34	Mississippi	4	0.7%		24	Arizona	9	1.5%
11	Missouri	17	2.8%		24	Colorado	9	1.5%
44	Montana	2	0.3%		24	Connecticut	9	1.5%
34	Nebraska	4	0.7%		24	Kansas	9	1.5%
31	Nevada	5	0.8%		28	South Carolina	8	1.3%
40	New Hampshire	3	0.5%		29	Minnesota	7	1.2%
11	New Jersey	17	2.8%		30	Utah	6	1.0%
31	New Mexico	5	0.8%		31	Nevada	5	0.8%
3	New York	35	5.9%		31	New Mexico	5	0.8%
16	North Carolina	14	2.3%		31	Washington	5	0.8%
44	North Dakota	2	0.3%		34	Idaho	4	0.7%
14	Ohio	16	2.7%		34	Iowa	4	0.7%
17	Oklahoma	13	2.2%		34	Maine	4	0.7%
40	Oregon	3	0.5%		34	Mississippi	4	0.7%
5	Pennsylvania	29	4.9%		34	Nebraska	4	0.7%
40	Rhode Island	3	0.5%		34	West Virginia	4	0.7%
28	South Carolina	8	1.3%		40	Delaware	3	0.5%
49	South Dakota	1	0.2%		40	New Hampshire	3	0.5%
17	Tennessee	13	2.2%		40	Oregon	3	0.5%
2	Texas	41	6.9%		40	Rhode Island	3	0.5%
30	Utah	6	1.0%		44	Alaska	2	0.3%
44	Vermont	2	0.3%		44	Montana	2	0.3%
9	Virginia	18	3.0%		44	North Dakota	2	0.3%
31	Washington	5	0.8%		44	Vermont	2	0.3%
34	West Virginia	4	0.7%		44	Wyoming	2	0.3%
15	Wisconsin	15	2.5%		49	Hawaii	1	0.2%
44	Wyoming	2	0.3%		49	South Dakota	1	0.2%
						District of Columbia	3	0.5%

Source: U.S. Department of Health and Human Services, Health Care Financing Administration
    OSCAR Report 10 (January 25, 1999)
*Certified by HCFA to participate in the Medicare/Medicaid programs. Excludes licensed facilities that do not accept federal funding and facilities managed by the Department of Veterans Affairs. National total does not include three certified psychiatric hospitals in U.S. territories.

Beds in Medicare and Medicaid Certified Psychiatric Hospitals in 1999

National Total = 76,738 Beds*

ALPHA ORDER

RANK	STATE	BEDS	% of USA
28	Alabama	857	1.1%
45	Alaska	188	0.2%
35	Arizona	420	0.5%
29	Arkansas	771	1.0%
4	California	3,368	4.4%
22	Colorado	1,305	1.7%
24	Connecticut	1,197	1.6%
42	Delaware	241	0.3%
10	Florida	2,571	3.4%
8	Georgia	2,698	3.5%
48	Hawaii	88	0.1%
46	Idaho	145	0.2%
12	Illinois	1,820	2.4%
19	Indiana	1,447	1.9%
34	Iowa	427	0.6%
26	Kansas	1,086	1.4%
13	Kentucky	1,715	2.2%
11	Louisiana	2,184	2.8%
40	Maine	306	0.4%
6	Maryland	2,954	3.8%
20	Massachusetts	1,383	1.8%
9	Michigan	2,576	3.4%
18	Minnesota	1,466	1.9%
39	Mississippi	316	0.4%
23	Missouri	1,208	1.6%
50	Montana	50	0.1%
31	Nebraska	592	0.8%
33	Nevada	437	0.6%
36	New Hampshire	416	0.5%
3	New Jersey	3,587	4.7%
37	New Mexico	373	0.5%
1	New York	13,377	17.4%
5	North Carolina	3,273	4.3%
38	North Dakota	369	0.5%
17	Ohio	1,471	1.9%
25	Oklahoma	1,140	1.5%
41	Oregon	302	0.4%
2	Pennsylvania	6,169	8.0%
43	Rhode Island	219	0.3%
27	South Carolina	876	1.1%
47	South Dakota	95	0.1%
21	Tennessee	1,313	1.7%
7	Texas	2,929	3.8%
30	Utah	625	0.8%
44	Vermont	211	0.3%
15	Virginia	1,624	2.1%
16	Washington	1,566	2.0%
32	West Virginia	494	0.6%
14	Wisconsin	1,680	2.2%
49	Wyoming	80	0.1%

RANK ORDER

RANK	STATE	BEDS	% of USA
1	New York	13,377	17.4%
2	Pennsylvania	6,169	8.0%
3	New Jersey	3,587	4.7%
4	California	3,368	4.4%
5	North Carolina	3,273	4.3%
6	Maryland	2,954	3.8%
7	Texas	2,929	3.8%
8	Georgia	2,698	3.5%
9	Michigan	2,576	3.4%
10	Florida	2,571	3.4%
11	Louisiana	2,184	2.8%
12	Illinois	1,820	2.4%
13	Kentucky	1,715	2.2%
14	Wisconsin	1,680	2.2%
15	Virginia	1,624	2.1%
16	Washington	1,566	2.0%
17	Ohio	1,471	1.9%
18	Minnesota	1,466	1.9%
19	Indiana	1,447	1.9%
20	Massachusetts	1,383	1.8%
21	Tennessee	1,313	1.7%
22	Colorado	1,305	1.7%
23	Missouri	1,208	1.6%
24	Connecticut	1,197	1.6%
25	Oklahoma	1,140	1.5%
26	Kansas	1,086	1.4%
27	South Carolina	876	1.1%
28	Alabama	857	1.1%
29	Arkansas	771	1.0%
30	Utah	625	0.8%
31	Nebraska	592	0.8%
32	West Virginia	494	0.6%
33	Nevada	437	0.6%
34	Iowa	427	0.6%
35	Arizona	420	0.5%
36	New Hampshire	416	0.5%
37	New Mexico	373	0.5%
38	North Dakota	369	0.5%
39	Mississippi	316	0.4%
40	Maine	306	0.4%
41	Oregon	302	0.4%
42	Delaware	241	0.3%
43	Rhode Island	219	0.3%
44	Vermont	211	0.3%
45	Alaska	188	0.2%
46	Idaho	145	0.2%
47	South Dakota	95	0.1%
48	Hawaii	88	0.1%
49	Wyoming	80	0.1%
50	Montana	50	0.1%
	District of Columbia	733	1.0%

Source: U.S. Department of Health and Human Services, Health Care Financing Administration
   OSCAR Report 10 (January 25, 1999)
*Beds in hospitals certified by HCFA to participate in the Medicare/Medicaid programs. Excludes licensed facilities that do not accept federal funding and facilities managed by the Department of Veterans Affairs. National total does not include 703 beds in U.S. territories.

Medicare and Medicaid Certified Community Mental Health Centers in 1999

National Total = 1,013 Centers*

ALPHA ORDER

RANK	STATE	CENTERS	% of USA
3	Alabama	90	8.9%
45	Alaska	0	0.0%
29	Arizona	7	0.7%
21	Arkansas	14	1.4%
10	California	28	2.8%
16	Colorado	17	1.7%
29	Connecticut	7	0.7%
45	Delaware	0	0.0%
1	Florida	189	18.7%
29	Georgia	7	0.7%
45	Hawaii	0	0.0%
42	Idaho	1	0.1%
12	Illinois	22	2.2%
23	Indiana	13	1.3%
25	Iowa	12	1.2%
13	Kansas	20	2.0%
21	Kentucky	14	1.4%
4	Louisiana	49	4.8%
36	Maine	4	0.4%
27	Maryland	10	1.0%
16	Massachusetts	17	1.7%
15	Michigan	18	1.8%
20	Minnesota	16	1.6%
29	Mississippi	7	0.7%
11	Missouri	24	2.4%
36	Montana	4	0.4%
42	Nebraska	1	0.1%
41	Nevada	2	0.2%
35	New Hampshire	5	0.5%
6	New Jersey	39	3.8%
16	New Mexico	17	1.7%
23	New York	13	1.3%
9	North Carolina	32	3.2%
45	North Dakota	0	0.0%
7	Ohio	34	3.4%
28	Oklahoma	9	0.9%
16	Oregon	17	1.7%
5	Pennsylvania	46	4.5%
45	Rhode Island	0	0.0%
25	South Carolina	12	1.2%
39	South Dakota	3	0.3%
13	Tennessee	20	2.0%
2	Texas	117	11.5%
29	Utah	7	0.7%
45	Vermont	0	0.0%
29	Virginia	7	0.7%
7	Washington	34	3.4%
36	West Virginia	4	0.4%
42	Wisconsin	1	0.1%
39	Wyoming	3	0.3%

RANK ORDER

RANK	STATE	CENTERS	% of USA
1	Florida	189	18.7%
2	Texas	117	11.5%
3	Alabama	90	8.9%
4	Louisiana	49	4.8%
5	Pennsylvania	46	4.5%
6	New Jersey	39	3.8%
7	Ohio	34	3.4%
7	Washington	34	3.4%
9	North Carolina	32	3.2%
10	California	28	2.8%
11	Missouri	24	2.4%
12	Illinois	22	2.2%
13	Kansas	20	2.0%
13	Tennessee	20	2.0%
15	Michigan	18	1.8%
16	Colorado	17	1.7%
16	Massachusetts	17	1.7%
16	New Mexico	17	1.7%
16	Oregon	17	1.7%
20	Minnesota	16	1.6%
21	Arkansas	14	1.4%
21	Kentucky	14	1.4%
23	Indiana	13	1.3%
23	New York	13	1.3%
25	Iowa	12	1.2%
25	South Carolina	12	1.2%
27	Maryland	10	1.0%
28	Oklahoma	9	0.9%
29	Arizona	7	0.7%
29	Connecticut	7	0.7%
29	Georgia	7	0.7%
29	Mississippi	7	0.7%
29	Utah	7	0.7%
29	Virginia	7	0.7%
35	New Hampshire	5	0.5%
36	Maine	4	0.4%
36	Montana	4	0.4%
36	West Virginia	4	0.4%
39	South Dakota	3	0.3%
39	Wyoming	3	0.3%
41	Nevada	2	0.2%
42	Idaho	1	0.1%
42	Nebraska	1	0.1%
42	Wisconsin	1	0.1%
45	Alaska	0	0.0%
45	Delaware	0	0.0%
45	Hawaii	0	0.0%
45	North Dakota	0	0.0%
45	Rhode Island	0	0.0%
45	Vermont	0	0.0%
	District of Columbia	0	0.0%

Source: U.S. Department of Health and Human Services, Health Care Financing Administration
OSCAR Report 10 (January 25, 1999)
*Certified by HCFA to participate in the Medicare/Medicaid programs. Excludes licensed facilities that do not accept federal funding and facilities managed by the Department of Veterans Affairs. National total does not include 14 certified mental health centers in U.S. territories.

Medicare and Medicaid Certified Outpatient Physical Therapy Facilities in 1999

National Total = 2,982 Facilities*

ALPHA ORDER				RANK ORDER			
RANK	STATE	FACILITIES	% of USA	RANK	STATE	FACILITIES	% of USA
31	Alabama	27	0.9%	1	Florida	305	10.2%
36	Alaska	18	0.6%	2	California	238	8.0%
26	Arizona	39	1.3%	3	Texas	203	6.8%
29	Arkansas	32	1.1%	4	Michigan	192	6.4%
2	California	238	8.0%	5	Pennsylvania	153	5.1%
16	Colorado	58	1.9%	6	Georgia	152	5.1%
24	Connecticut	41	1.4%	7	Ohio	124	4.2%
34	Delaware	21	0.7%	8	Virginia	120	4.0%
1	Florida	305	10.2%	9	New Jersey	111	3.7%
6	Georgia	152	5.1%	10	Tennessee	93	3.1%
42	Hawaii	10	0.3%	11	Maryland	85	2.9%
39	Idaho	15	0.5%	12	Illinois	76	2.5%
12	Illinois	76	2.5%	13	Missouri	67	2.2%
14	Indiana	62	2.1%	14	Indiana	62	2.1%
22	Iowa	42	1.4%	15	Wisconsin	60	2.0%
28	Kansas	33	1.1%	16	Colorado	58	1.9%
21	Kentucky	54	1.8%	17	South Carolina	57	1.9%
18	Louisiana	56	1.9%	18	Louisiana	56	1.9%
35	Maine	19	0.6%	18	Minnesota	56	1.9%
11	Maryland	85	2.9%	20	North Carolina	55	1.8%
37	Massachusetts	17	0.6%	21	Kentucky	54	1.8%
4	Michigan	192	6.4%	22	Iowa	42	1.4%
18	Minnesota	56	1.9%	22	Oklahoma	42	1.4%
25	Mississippi	40	1.3%	24	Connecticut	41	1.4%
13	Missouri	67	2.2%	25	Mississippi	40	1.3%
42	Montana	10	0.3%	26	Arizona	39	1.3%
37	Nebraska	17	0.6%	27	Washington	37	1.2%
41	Nevada	12	0.4%	28	Kansas	33	1.1%
40	New Hampshire	13	0.4%	29	Arkansas	32	1.1%
9	New Jersey	111	3.7%	30	New Mexico	31	1.0%
30	New Mexico	31	1.0%	31	Alabama	27	0.9%
32	New York	25	0.8%	32	New York	25	0.8%
20	North Carolina	55	1.8%	33	Oregon	22	0.7%
45	North Dakota	8	0.3%	34	Delaware	21	0.7%
7	Ohio	124	4.2%	35	Maine	19	0.6%
22	Oklahoma	42	1.4%	36	Alaska	18	0.6%
33	Oregon	22	0.7%	37	Massachusetts	17	0.6%
5	Pennsylvania	153	5.1%	37	Nebraska	17	0.6%
49	Rhode Island	3	0.1%	39	Idaho	15	0.5%
17	South Carolina	57	1.9%	40	New Hampshire	13	0.4%
48	South Dakota	5	0.2%	41	Nevada	12	0.4%
10	Tennessee	93	3.1%	42	Hawaii	10	0.3%
3	Texas	203	6.8%	42	Montana	10	0.3%
42	Utah	10	0.3%	42	Utah	10	0.3%
50	Vermont	2	0.1%	45	North Dakota	8	0.3%
8	Virginia	120	4.0%	46	West Virginia	7	0.2%
27	Washington	37	1.2%	47	Wyoming	6	0.2%
46	West Virginia	7	0.2%	48	South Dakota	5	0.2%
15	Wisconsin	60	2.0%	49	Rhode Island	3	0.1%
47	Wyoming	6	0.2%	50	Vermont	2	0.1%
					District of Columbia	1	0.0%

Source: U.S. Department of Health and Human Services, Health Care Financing Administration
    OSCAR Report 10 (January 25, 1999)
*Certified by HCFA to participate in the Medicare/Medicaid programs. Excludes licensed facilities that do not
accept federal funding and facilities managed by the Department of Veterans Affairs. National total does not
include three certified outpatient physical therapy facilities in U.S. territories.

Medicare and Medicaid Certified Rural Health Clinics in 1999

National Total = 3,537 Rural Health Clinics*

ALPHA ORDER					RANK ORDER			
RANK	STATE		CLINICS	% of USA	RANK	STATE	CLINICS	% of USA
17	Alabama		74	2.1%	1	Texas	475	13.4%
40	Alaska		12	0.3%	2	California	210	5.9%
41	Arizona		11	0.3%	3	Illinois	187	5.3%
12	Arkansas		98	2.8%	4	Kansas	177	5.0%
2	California		210	5.9%	4	Missouri	177	5.0%
30	Colorado		39	1.1%	6	Michigan	164	4.6%
46	Connecticut		0	0.0%	7	Mississippi	161	4.6%
46	Delaware		0	0.0%	8	Georgia	142	4.0%
9	Florida		136	3.8%	9	Florida	136	3.8%
8	Georgia		142	4.0%	10	North Carolina	134	3.8%
44	Hawaii		1	0.0%	11	Iowa	129	3.6%
31	Idaho		28	0.8%	12	Arkansas	98	2.8%
3	Illinois		187	5.3%	13	South Carolina	93	2.6%
28	Indiana		48	1.4%	14	Oklahoma	79	2.2%
11	Iowa		129	3.6%	15	Kentucky	77	2.2%
4	Kansas		177	5.0%	16	Nebraska	75	2.1%
15	Kentucky		77	2.2%	17	Alabama	74	2.1%
21	Louisiana		60	1.7%	17	North Dakota	74	2.1%
27	Maine		49	1.4%	19	Virginia	68	1.9%
46	Maryland		0	0.0%	20	West Virginia	67	1.9%
46	Massachusetts		0	0.0%	21	Louisiana	60	1.7%
6	Michigan		164	4.6%	21	Minnesota	60	1.7%
21	Minnesota		60	1.7%	23	Wisconsin	59	1.7%
7	Mississippi		161	4.6%	24	South Dakota	55	1.6%
4	Missouri		177	5.0%	25	Washington	54	1.5%
32	Montana		25	0.7%	26	Pennsylvania	53	1.5%
16	Nebraska		75	2.1%	27	Maine	49	1.4%
43	Nevada		3	0.1%	28	Indiana	48	1.4%
35	New Hampshire		21	0.6%	29	Tennessee	46	1.3%
46	New Jersey		0	0.0%	30	Colorado	39	1.1%
36	New Mexico		16	0.5%	31	Idaho	28	0.8%
42	New York		10	0.3%	32	Montana	25	0.7%
10	North Carolina		134	3.8%	33	Vermont	23	0.7%
17	North Dakota		74	2.1%	34	Oregon	22	0.6%
38	Ohio		14	0.4%	35	New Hampshire	21	0.6%
14	Oklahoma		79	2.2%	36	New Mexico	16	0.5%
34	Oregon		22	0.6%	36	Wyoming	16	0.5%
26	Pennsylvania		53	1.5%	38	Ohio	14	0.4%
44	Rhode Island		1	0.0%	38	Utah	14	0.4%
13	South Carolina		93	2.6%	40	Alaska	12	0.3%
24	South Dakota		55	1.6%	41	Arizona	11	0.3%
29	Tennessee		46	1.3%	42	New York	10	0.3%
1	Texas		475	13.4%	43	Nevada	3	0.1%
38	Utah		14	0.4%	44	Hawaii	1	0.0%
33	Vermont		23	0.7%	44	Rhode Island	1	0.0%
19	Virginia		68	1.9%	46	Connecticut	0	0.0%
25	Washington		54	1.5%	46	Delaware	0	0.0%
20	West Virginia		67	1.9%	46	Maryland	0	0.0%
23	Wisconsin		59	1.7%	46	Massachusetts	0	0.0%
36	Wyoming		16	0.5%	46	New Jersey	0	0.0%
						District of Columbia	0	0.0%

Source: U.S. Department of Health and Human Services, Health Care Financing Administration
      OSCAR Report 10 (January 25, 1999)
*Certified by HCFA to participate in the Medicare/Medicaid programs. Excludes licensed facilities that do not accept federal funding and facilities managed by the Department of Veterans Affairs. There are no certified rural health centers in U.S. territories.

Medicare and Medicaid Certified Home Health Agencies in 1999

National Total = 9,258 Home Health Agencies*

ALPHA ORDER

RANK	STATE	AGENCIES	% of USA
19	Alabama	181	2.0%
48	Alaska	18	0.2%
25	Arizona	112	1.2%
16	Arkansas	195	2.1%
2	California	710	7.7%
23	Colorado	161	1.7%
27	Connecticut	100	1.1%
48	Delaware	18	0.2%
6	Florida	366	4.0%
26	Georgia	103	1.1%
47	Hawaii	21	0.2%
37	Idaho	62	0.7%
7	Illinois	362	3.9%
10	Indiana	247	2.7%
16	Iowa	195	2.1%
18	Kansas	193	2.1%
24	Kentucky	116	1.3%
4	Louisiana	405	4.4%
42	Maine	45	0.5%
31	Maryland	77	0.8%
19	Massachusetts	181	2.0%
13	Michigan	221	2.4%
9	Minnesota	261	2.8%
35	Mississippi	69	0.7%
13	Missouri	221	2.4%
38	Montana	60	0.6%
32	Nebraska	76	0.8%
44	Nevada	41	0.4%
43	New Hampshire	43	0.5%
40	New Jersey	55	0.6%
28	New Mexico	95	1.0%
12	New York	223	2.4%
21	North Carolina	175	1.9%
45	North Dakota	35	0.4%
3	Ohio	426	4.6%
8	Oklahoma	304	3.3%
33	Oregon	74	0.8%
5	Pennsylvania	374	4.0%
46	Rhode Island	29	0.3%
30	South Carolina	78	0.8%
41	South Dakota	51	0.6%
15	Tennessee	207	2.2%
1	Texas	1,563	16.9%
34	Utah	72	0.8%
50	Vermont	13	0.1%
11	Virginia	226	2.4%
36	Washington	66	0.7%
29	West Virginia	88	1.0%
22	Wisconsin	166	1.8%
39	Wyoming	56	0.6%

RANK ORDER

RANK	STATE	AGENCIES	% of USA
1	Texas	1,563	16.9%
2	California	710	7.7%
3	Ohio	426	4.6%
4	Louisiana	405	4.4%
5	Pennsylvania	374	4.0%
6	Florida	366	4.0%
7	Illinois	362	3.9%
8	Oklahoma	304	3.3%
9	Minnesota	261	2.8%
10	Indiana	247	2.7%
11	Virginia	226	2.4%
12	New York	223	2.4%
13	Michigan	221	2.4%
13	Missouri	221	2.4%
15	Tennessee	207	2.2%
16	Arkansas	195	2.1%
16	Iowa	195	2.1%
18	Kansas	193	2.1%
19	Alabama	181	2.0%
19	Massachusetts	181	2.0%
21	North Carolina	175	1.9%
22	Wisconsin	166	1.8%
23	Colorado	161	1.7%
24	Kentucky	116	1.3%
25	Arizona	112	1.2%
26	Georgia	103	1.1%
27	Connecticut	100	1.1%
28	New Mexico	95	1.0%
29	West Virginia	88	1.0%
30	South Carolina	78	0.8%
31	Maryland	77	0.8%
32	Nebraska	76	0.8%
33	Oregon	74	0.8%
34	Utah	72	0.8%
35	Mississippi	69	0.7%
36	Washington	66	0.7%
37	Idaho	62	0.7%
38	Montana	60	0.6%
39	Wyoming	56	0.6%
40	New Jersey	55	0.6%
41	South Dakota	51	0.6%
42	Maine	45	0.5%
43	New Hampshire	43	0.5%
44	Nevada	41	0.4%
45	North Dakota	35	0.4%
46	Rhode Island	29	0.3%
47	Hawaii	21	0.2%
48	Alaska	18	0.2%
48	Delaware	18	0.2%
50	Vermont	13	0.1%
	District of Columbia	22	0.2%

Source: U.S. Department of Health and Human Services, Health Care Financing Administration
OSCAR Report 10 (January 25, 1999)

Certified by HCFA to participate in the Medicare/Medicaid programs. Excludes agencies that do not accept federal funding. National total does not include 50 certified home health agencies in U.S. territories. A home health agency provides health services to individuals in their homes for the purpose of promoting, maintaining or restoring health or maximizing the level of independence, while minimizing the effects of disability and illness.

Medicare and Medicaid Certified Hospices in 1999

National Total = 2,261 Hospices*

ALPHA ORDER					RANK ORDER			
RANK	STATE	HOSPICES	% of USA		RANK	STATE	HOSPICES	% of USA
8	Alabama	69	3.1%		1	California	188	8.3%
50	Alaska	2	0.1%		2	Texas	145	6.4%
27	Arizona	37	1.6%		3	Pennsylvania	119	5.3%
15	Arkansas	56	2.5%		4	Ohio	92	4.1%
1	California	188	8.3%		5	Illinois	89	3.9%
22	Colorado	40	1.8%		6	Michigan	77	3.4%
34	Connecticut	28	1.2%		7	North Carolina	71	3.1%
49	Delaware	5	0.2%		8	Alabama	69	3.1%
22	Florida	40	1.8%		9	Missouri	67	3.0%
10	Georgia	65	2.9%		10	Georgia	65	2.9%
46	Hawaii	8	0.4%		10	Tennessee	65	2.9%
34	Idaho	28	1.2%		12	Minnesota	62	2.7%
5	Illinois	89	3.9%		13	Indiana	60	2.7%
13	Indiana	60	2.7%		14	Iowa	57	2.5%
14	Iowa	57	2.5%		15	Arkansas	56	2.5%
29	Kansas	33	1.5%		16	New York	55	2.4%
31	Kentucky	29	1.3%		17	Oklahoma	53	2.3%
22	Louisiana	40	1.8%		17	Wisconsin	53	2.3%
41	Maine	15	0.7%		19	Virginia	46	2.0%
28	Maryland	34	1.5%		20	New Jersey	45	2.0%
21	Massachusetts	43	1.9%		21	Massachusetts	43	1.9%
6	Michigan	77	3.4%		22	Colorado	40	1.8%
12	Minnesota	62	2.7%		22	Florida	40	1.8%
26	Mississippi	39	1.7%		22	Louisiana	40	1.8%
9	Missouri	67	3.0%		22	Oregon	40	1.8%
39	Montana	18	0.8%		26	Mississippi	39	1.7%
34	Nebraska	28	1.2%		27	Arizona	37	1.6%
46	Nevada	8	0.4%		28	Maryland	34	1.5%
37	New Hampshire	21	0.9%		29	Kansas	33	1.5%
20	New Jersey	45	2.0%		29	South Carolina	33	1.5%
31	New Mexico	29	1.3%		31	Kentucky	29	1.3%
16	New York	55	2.4%		31	New Mexico	29	1.3%
7	North Carolina	71	3.1%		31	Washington	29	1.3%
42	North Dakota	14	0.6%		34	Connecticut	28	1.2%
4	Ohio	92	4.1%		34	Idaho	28	1.2%
17	Oklahoma	53	2.3%		34	Nebraska	28	1.2%
22	Oregon	40	1.8%		37	New Hampshire	21	0.9%
3	Pennsylvania	119	5.3%		37	West Virginia	21	0.9%
48	Rhode Island	7	0.3%		39	Montana	18	0.8%
29	South Carolina	33	1.5%		39	Utah	18	0.8%
42	South Dakota	14	0.6%		41	Maine	15	0.7%
10	Tennessee	65	2.9%		42	North Dakota	14	0.6%
2	Texas	145	6.4%		42	South Dakota	14	0.6%
39	Utah	18	0.8%		44	Wyoming	13	0.6%
45	Vermont	9	0.4%		45	Vermont	9	0.4%
19	Virginia	46	2.0%		46	Hawaii	8	0.4%
31	Washington	29	1.3%		46	Nevada	8	0.4%
37	West Virginia	21	0.9%		48	Rhode Island	7	0.3%
17	Wisconsin	53	2.3%		49	Delaware	5	0.2%
44	Wyoming	13	0.6%		50	Alaska	2	0.1%
					District of Columbia		4	0.2%

Source: U.S. Department of Health and Human Services, Health Care Financing Administration
OSCAR Report 10 (January 25, 1999)

*Certified by HCFA to participate in the Medicare/Medicaid programs. Excludes licensed facilities that do not accept federal funding and facilities managed by the Department of Veterans Affairs. National total does not include 33 certified hospices in U.S. territories. An hospice provides specialized services for terminally ill people and their families.

Hospice Patients in Residential Facilities in 1999

National Total = 9,905 Patients*

ALPHA ORDER

RANK	STATE	PATIENTS	% of USA
43	Alabama	6	0.1%
48	Alaska	0	0.0%
26	Arizona	65	0.7%
24	Arkansas	108	1.1%
2	California	862	8.7%
16	Colorado	215	2.2%
29	Connecticut	54	0.5%
42	Delaware	7	0.1%
1	Florida	1,322	13.3%
19	Georgia	167	1.7%
45	Hawaii	3	0.0%
34	Idaho	18	0.2%
6	Illinois	562	5.7%
14	Indiana	280	2.8%
20	Iowa	142	1.4%
26	Kansas	65	0.7%
13	Kentucky	290	2.9%
34	Louisiana	18	0.2%
37	Maine	12	0.1%
21	Maryland	128	1.3%
18	Massachusetts	180	1.8%
12	Michigan	302	3.0%
23	Minnesota	116	1.2%
37	Mississippi	12	0.1%
11	Missouri	340	3.4%
28	Montana	57	0.6%
22	Nebraska	124	1.3%
31	Nevada	46	0.5%
48	New Hampshire	0	0.0%
15	New Jersey	274	2.8%
37	New Mexico	12	0.1%
10	New York	343	3.5%
17	North Carolina	197	2.0%
41	North Dakota	9	0.1%
7	Ohio	425	4.3%
5	Oklahoma	612	6.2%
8	Oregon	352	3.6%
3	Pennsylvania	799	8.1%
48	Rhode Island	0	0.0%
30	South Carolina	52	0.5%
44	South Dakota	4	0.0%
32	Tennessee	37	0.4%
4	Texas	788	8.0%
40	Utah	10	0.1%
36	Vermont	13	0.1%
33	Virginia	22	0.2%
9	Washington	348	3.5%
46	West Virginia	2	0.0%
25	Wisconsin	86	0.9%
46	Wyoming	2	0.0%

RANK ORDER

RANK	STATE	PATIENTS	% of USA
1	Florida	1,322	13.3%
2	California	862	8.7%
3	Pennsylvania	799	8.1%
4	Texas	788	8.0%
5	Oklahoma	612	6.2%
6	Illinois	562	5.7%
7	Ohio	425	4.3%
8	Oregon	352	3.6%
9	Washington	348	3.5%
10	New York	343	3.5%
11	Missouri	340	3.4%
12	Michigan	302	3.0%
13	Kentucky	290	2.9%
14	Indiana	280	2.8%
15	New Jersey	274	2.8%
16	Colorado	215	2.2%
17	North Carolina	197	2.0%
18	Massachusetts	180	1.8%
19	Georgia	167	1.7%
20	Iowa	142	1.4%
21	Maryland	128	1.3%
22	Nebraska	124	1.3%
23	Minnesota	116	1.2%
24	Arkansas	108	1.1%
25	Wisconsin	86	0.9%
26	Arizona	65	0.7%
26	Kansas	65	0.7%
28	Montana	57	0.6%
29	Connecticut	54	0.5%
30	South Carolina	52	0.5%
31	Nevada	46	0.5%
32	Tennessee	37	0.4%
33	Virginia	22	0.2%
34	Idaho	18	0.2%
34	Louisiana	18	0.2%
36	Vermont	13	0.1%
37	Maine	12	0.1%
37	Mississippi	12	0.1%
37	New Mexico	12	0.1%
40	Utah	10	0.1%
41	North Dakota	9	0.1%
42	Delaware	7	0.1%
43	Alabama	6	0.1%
44	South Dakota	4	0.0%
45	Hawaii	3	0.0%
46	West Virginia	2	0.0%
46	Wyoming	2	0.0%
48	Alaska	0	0.0%
48	New Hampshire	0	0.0%
48	Rhode Island	0	0.0%
	District of Columbia	20	0.2%

Source: U.S. Department of Health and Human Services, Health Care Financing Administration
OSCAR Report 10 (January 25, 1999)

Patients in facilities certified by HCFA to participate in the Medicare/Medicaid programs. Excludes licensed facilities that do not accept federal funding and facilities managed by the Department of Veterans Affairs. National total does not include five patients in U.S. territories. An hospice provides specialized services for terminally ill people and their families.

Medicare and Medicaid Certified Nursing Care Facilities in 1999

National Total = 17,287 Nursing Care Facilities*

ALPHA ORDER

RANK	STATE	FACILITIES	% of USA
30	Alabama	224	1.3%
50	Alaska	15	0.1%
33	Arizona	169	1.0%
25	Arkansas	275	1.6%
1	California	1,420	8.2%
29	Colorado	229	1.3%
27	Connecticut	259	1.5%
47	Delaware	44	0.3%
6	Florida	748	4.3%
18	Georgia	361	2.1%
47	Hawaii	44	0.3%
42	Idaho	84	0.5%
4	Illinois	880	5.1%
8	Indiana	572	3.3%
11	Iowa	470	2.7%
16	Kansas	405	2.3%
22	Kentucky	315	1.8%
21	Louisiana	323	1.9%
36	Maine	131	0.8%
26	Maryland	264	1.5%
9	Massachusetts	563	3.3%
12	Michigan	447	2.6%
13	Minnesota	445	2.6%
31	Mississippi	200	1.2%
9	Missouri	563	3.3%
38	Montana	105	0.6%
28	Nebraska	240	1.4%
45	Nevada	48	0.3%
42	New Hampshire	84	0.5%
19	New Jersey	357	2.1%
44	New Mexico	81	0.5%
7	New York	662	3.8%
17	North Carolina	404	2.3%
41	North Dakota	88	0.5%
3	Ohio	1,013	5.9%
15	Oklahoma	412	2.4%
34	Oregon	162	0.9%
5	Pennsylvania	805	4.7%
39	Rhode Island	101	0.6%
32	South Carolina	175	1.0%
37	South Dakota	114	0.7%
20	Tennessee	356	2.1%
2	Texas	1,293	7.5%
40	Utah	93	0.5%
46	Vermont	45	0.3%
24	Virginia	282	1.6%
23	Washington	283	1.6%
35	West Virginia	149	0.9%
14	Wisconsin	424	2.5%
49	Wyoming	40	0.2%

RANK ORDER

RANK	STATE	FACILITIES	% of USA
1	California	1,420	8.2%
2	Texas	1,293	7.5%
3	Ohio	1,013	5.9%
4	Illinois	880	5.1%
5	Pennsylvania	805	4.7%
6	Florida	748	4.3%
7	New York	662	3.8%
8	Indiana	572	3.3%
9	Massachusetts	563	3.3%
9	Missouri	563	3.3%
11	Iowa	470	2.7%
12	Michigan	447	2.6%
13	Minnesota	445	2.6%
14	Wisconsin	424	2.5%
15	Oklahoma	412	2.4%
16	Kansas	405	2.3%
17	North Carolina	404	2.3%
18	Georgia	361	2.1%
19	New Jersey	357	2.1%
20	Tennessee	356	2.1%
21	Louisiana	323	1.9%
22	Kentucky	315	1.8%
23	Washington	283	1.6%
24	Virginia	282	1.6%
25	Arkansas	275	1.6%
26	Maryland	264	1.5%
27	Connecticut	259	1.5%
28	Nebraska	240	1.4%
29	Colorado	229	1.3%
30	Alabama	224	1.3%
31	Mississippi	200	1.2%
32	South Carolina	175	1.0%
33	Arizona	169	1.0%
34	Oregon	162	0.9%
35	West Virginia	149	0.9%
36	Maine	131	0.8%
37	South Dakota	114	0.7%
38	Montana	105	0.6%
39	Rhode Island	101	0.6%
40	Utah	93	0.5%
41	North Dakota	88	0.5%
42	Idaho	84	0.5%
42	New Hampshire	84	0.5%
44	New Mexico	81	0.5%
45	Nevada	48	0.3%
46	Vermont	45	0.3%
47	Delaware	44	0.3%
47	Hawaii	44	0.3%
49	Wyoming	40	0.2%
50	Alaska	15	0.1%
	District of Columbia	21	0.1%

Source: U.S. Department of Health and Human Services, Health Care Financing Administration
    OSCAR Report 10 (January 25, 1999)

*Certified by HCFA to participate in the Medicare/Medicaid programs. Excludes licensed facilities that do not accept federal funding and facilities managed by the Department of Veterans Affairs. National total does not include nine certified nursing facilities in U.S. territories.

Beds in Medicare and Medicaid Certified Nursing Care Facilities in 1999

National Total = 1,731,333 Beds*

RANK	STATE	BEDS	% of USA
27	Alabama	24,697	1.4%
50	Alaska	720	0.0%
31	Arizona	17,355	1.0%
24	Arkansas	26,523	1.5%
1	California	127,550	7.4%
29	Colorado	19,245	1.1%
21	Connecticut	31,729	1.8%
45	Delaware	4,545	0.3%
7	Florida	78,152	4.5%
16	Georgia	38,772	2.2%
47	Hawaii	3,797	0.2%
44	Idaho	5,656	0.3%
4	Illinois	100,752	5.8%
9	Indiana	54,498	3.1%
18	Iowa	35,000	2.0%
25	Kansas	26,519	1.5%
28	Kentucky	24,324	1.4%
19	Louisiana	34,897	2.0%
37	Maine	9,001	0.5%
23	Maryland	29,894	1.7%
8	Massachusetts	57,191	3.3%
12	Michigan	49,535	2.9%
14	Minnesota	44,333	2.6%
32	Mississippi	16,762	1.0%
10	Missouri	50,339	2.9%
40	Montana	7,582	0.4%
30	Nebraska	17,388	1.0%
46	Nevada	4,334	0.3%
39	New Hampshire	7,675	0.4%
11	New Jersey	49,978	2.9%
42	New Mexico	7,127	0.4%
2	New York	118,455	6.8%
15	North Carolina	39,390	2.3%
43	North Dakota	6,997	0.4%
6	Ohio	95,164	5.5%
20	Oklahoma	33,717	1.9%
34	Oregon	13,680	0.8%
5	Pennsylvania	95,818	5.5%
36	Rhode Island	10,224	0.6%
33	South Carolina	16,629	1.0%
38	South Dakota	7,996	0.5%
17	Tennessee	38,620	2.2%
3	Texas	115,579	6.7%
41	Utah	7,389	0.4%
48	Vermont	3,694	0.2%
22	Virginia	30,239	1.7%
26	Washington	26,022	1.5%
35	West Virginia	12,127	0.7%
13	Wisconsin	47,460	2.7%
49	Wyoming	3,144	0.2%

RANK	STATE	BEDS	% of USA
1	California	127,550	7.4%
2	New York	118,455	6.8%
3	Texas	115,579	6.7%
4	Illinois	100,752	5.8%
5	Pennsylvania	95,818	5.5%
6	Ohio	95,164	5.5%
7	Florida	78,152	4.5%
8	Massachusetts	57,191	3.3%
9	Indiana	54,498	3.1%
10	Missouri	50,339	2.9%
11	New Jersey	49,978	2.9%
12	Michigan	49,535	2.9%
13	Wisconsin	47,460	2.7%
14	Minnesota	44,333	2.6%
15	North Carolina	39,390	2.3%
16	Georgia	38,772	2.2%
17	Tennessee	38,620	2.2%
18	Iowa	35,000	2.0%
19	Louisiana	34,897	2.0%
20	Oklahoma	33,717	1.9%
21	Connecticut	31,729	1.8%
22	Virginia	30,239	1.7%
23	Maryland	29,894	1.7%
24	Arkansas	26,523	1.5%
25	Kansas	26,519	1.5%
26	Washington	26,022	1.5%
27	Alabama	24,697	1.4%
28	Kentucky	24,324	1.4%
29	Colorado	19,245	1.1%
30	Nebraska	17,388	1.0%
31	Arizona	17,355	1.0%
32	Mississippi	16,762	1.0%
33	South Carolina	16,629	1.0%
34	Oregon	13,680	0.8%
35	West Virginia	12,127	0.7%
36	Rhode Island	10,224	0.6%
37	Maine	9,001	0.5%
38	South Dakota	7,996	0.5%
39	New Hampshire	7,675	0.4%
40	Montana	7,582	0.4%
41	Utah	7,389	0.4%
42	New Mexico	7,127	0.4%
43	North Dakota	6,997	0.4%
44	Idaho	5,656	0.3%
45	Delaware	4,545	0.3%
46	Nevada	4,334	0.3%
47	Hawaii	3,797	0.2%
48	Vermont	3,694	0.2%
49	Wyoming	3,144	0.2%
50	Alaska	720	0.0%
	District of Columbia	3,119	0.2%

Source: U.S. Department of Health and Human Services, Health Care Financing Administration
    OSCAR Report 10 (January 25, 1999)
*Beds in nursing care facilities certified by HCFA to participate in the Medicare/Medicaid programs. National total does not include 363 beds in U.S. territories.

Rate of Beds in Medicare and Medicaid Certified Nursing Care Facilities in 1999

National Rate = 447 Beds per 1,000 Population 85 Years and Older*

ALPHA ORDER

RANK	STATE	RATE
35	Alabama	403
44	Alaska	346
47	Arizona	295
3	Arkansas	627
45	California	328
27	Colorado	440
11	Connecticut	538
23	Delaware	494
49	Florida	267
22	Georgia	501
50	Hawaii	246
42	Idaho	357
7	Illinois	570
2	Indiana	646
6	Iowa	571
9	Kansas	545
28	Kentucky	438
1	Louisiana	656
30	Maine	421
24	Maryland	486
18	Massachusetts	523
39	Michigan	374
8	Minnesota	560
29	Mississippi	426
14	Missouri	531
14	Montana	531
16	Nebraska	528
46	Nevada	313
25	New Hampshire	462
34	New Jersey	404
41	New Mexico	360
33	New York	408
31	North Carolina	417
21	North Dakota	507
5	Ohio	578
4	Oklahoma	616
48	Oregon	268
26	Pennsylvania	449
20	Rhode Island	517
38	South Carolina	388
13	South Dakota	534
19	Tennessee	518
12	Texas	535
40	Utah	373
32	Vermont	409
37	Virginia	389
43	Washington	347
35	West Virginia	403
10	Wisconsin	539
17	Wyoming	525

RANK ORDER

RANK	STATE	RATE
1	Louisiana	656
2	Indiana	646
3	Arkansas	627
4	Oklahoma	616
5	Ohio	578
6	Iowa	571
7	Illinois	570
8	Minnesota	560
9	Kansas	545
10	Wisconsin	539
11	Connecticut	538
12	Texas	535
13	South Dakota	534
14	Missouri	531
14	Montana	531
16	Nebraska	528
17	Wyoming	525
18	Massachusetts	523
19	Tennessee	518
20	Rhode Island	517
21	North Dakota	507
22	Georgia	501
23	Delaware	494
24	Maryland	486
25	New Hampshire	462
26	Pennsylvania	449
27	Colorado	440
28	Kentucky	438
29	Mississippi	426
30	Maine	421
31	North Carolina	417
32	Vermont	409
33	New York	408
34	New Jersey	404
35	Alabama	403
35	West Virginia	403
37	Virginia	389
38	South Carolina	388
39	Michigan	374
40	Utah	373
41	New Mexico	360
42	Idaho	357
43	Washington	347
44	Alaska	346
45	California	328
46	Nevada	313
47	Arizona	295
48	Oregon	268
49	Florida	267
50	Hawaii	246

District of Columbia — 356

Source: Morgan Quitno Press using data from U.S. Dept. of Health & Human Services, Health Care Financing Admin. OSCAR Report 10 (January 25, 1999)

*Beds in nursing care facilities certified by HCFA to participate in the Medicare/Medicaid programs. National rate does not include beds or population in U.S. territories. Calculated using 1997 Census population estimates.

Nursing Home Occupancy Rate in 1996

National Rate = 82.7% of Beds in Nursing Homes Occupied

ALPHA ORDER

RANK	STATE	RATE
15	Alabama	90.9
NA	Alaska*	NA
41	Arizona	77.4
48	Arkansas	65.9
40	California	77.6
25	Colorado	86.9
6	Connecticut	93.4
37	Delaware	80.0
32	Florida	83.7
12	Georgia	91.6
NA	Hawaii*	NA
38	Idaho	78.7
38	Illinois	78.7
44	Indiana	73.2
47	Iowa	66.4
35	Kansas	81.0
24	Kentucky	87.2
33	Louisiana	81.3
21	Maine	88.3
28	Maryland	85.6
19	Massachusetts	89.8
26	Michigan	86.7
10	Minnesota	92.4
9	Mississippi	92.7
43	Missouri	73.3
27	Montana	86.0
23	Nebraska	87.3
20	Nevada	88.5
13	New Hampshire	91.5
11	New Jersey	92.1
30	New Mexico	84.3
3	New York	94.6
5	North Carolina	93.8
2	North Dakota	95.5
46	Ohio	69.0
42	Oklahoma	74.9
34	Oregon	81.2
16	Pennsylvania	90.2
8	Rhode Island	93.1
22	South Carolina	87.9
4	South Dakota	94.0
18	Tennessee	89.9
45	Texas	70.6
36	Utah	80.1
1	Vermont	95.9
14	Virginia	91.1
29	Washington	84.5
7	West Virginia	93.2
17	Wisconsin	90.1
31	Wyoming	83.9

RANK ORDER

RANK	STATE	RATE
1	Vermont	95.9
2	North Dakota	95.5
3	New York	94.6
4	South Dakota	94.0
5	North Carolina	93.8
6	Connecticut	93.4
7	West Virginia	93.2
8	Rhode Island	93.1
9	Mississippi	92.7
10	Minnesota	92.4
11	New Jersey	92.1
12	Georgia	91.6
13	New Hampshire	91.5
14	Virginia	91.1
15	Alabama	90.9
16	Pennsylvania	90.2
17	Wisconsin	90.1
18	Tennessee	89.9
19	Massachusetts	89.8
20	Nevada	88.5
21	Maine	88.3
22	South Carolina	87.9
23	Nebraska	87.3
24	Kentucky	87.2
25	Colorado	86.9
26	Michigan	86.7
27	Montana	86.0
28	Maryland	85.6
29	Washington	84.5
30	New Mexico	84.3
31	Wyoming	83.9
32	Florida	83.7
33	Louisiana	81.3
34	Oregon	81.2
35	Kansas	81.0
36	Utah	80.1
37	Delaware	80.0
38	Idaho	78.7
38	Illinois	78.7
40	California	77.6
41	Arizona	77.4
42	Oklahoma	74.9
43	Missouri	73.3
44	Indiana	73.2
45	Texas	70.6
46	Ohio	69.0
47	Iowa	66.4
48	Arkansas	65.9
NA	Alaska*	NA
NA	Hawaii*	NA
	District of Columbia*	NA

Source: U.S. Department of Health and Human Services, Health Care Financing Administration
    "Health, United States, 1998" (July 1998)
*Not available.

Nursing Home Resident Rate in 1996

National Rate = 407.0 Residents per 1,000 Population Age 85 and Older*

ALPHA ORDER

RANK ORDER

RANK	STATE	RATE		RANK	STATE	RATE
36	Alabama	367.8		1	Louisiana	608.7
NA	Alaska**	NA		2	Indiana	549.0
46	Arizona	243.2		3	Minnesota	547.5
5	Arkansas	527.4		4	Connecticut	532.1
45	California	291.0		5	Arkansas	527.4
27	Colorado	416.6		6	South Dakota	525.6
4	Connecticut	532.1		7	Ohio	516.9
23	Delaware	443.6		8	Kansas	513.8
47	Florida	236.2		9	Iowa	506.1
18	Georgia	480.1		10	North Dakota	504.1
NA	Hawaii**	NA		11	Oklahoma	501.3
43	Idaho	319.2		12	Wisconsin	496.7
13	Illinois	494.5		13	Illinois	494.5
2	Indiana	549.0		14	Rhode Island	493.3
9	Iowa	506.1		15	Nebraska	490.2
8	Kansas	513.8		16	Massachusetts	485.7
28	Kentucky	411.8		17	Tennessee	483.8
1	Louisiana	608.7		18	Georgia	480.1
32	Maine	400.8		19	Montana	471.6
20	Maryland	464.6		20	Maryland	464.6
16	Massachusetts	485.7		21	New Hampshire	455.1
39	Michigan	353.0		22	Missouri	452.8
3	Minnesota	547.5		23	Delaware	443.6
29	Mississippi	409.8		24	Wyoming	439.1
22	Missouri	452.8		25	Texas	423.3
19	Montana	471.6		26	Pennsylvania	416.9
15	Nebraska	490.2		27	Colorado	416.6
44	Nevada	293.7		28	Kentucky	411.8
21	New Hampshire	455.1		29	Mississippi	409.8
34	New Jersey	378.6		30	Vermont	404.7
41	New Mexico	325.3		31	North Carolina	401.5
33	New York	386.7		32	Maine	400.8
31	North Carolina	401.5		33	New York	386.7
10	North Dakota	504.1		34	New Jersey	378.6
7	Ohio	516.9		35	Virginia	376.0
11	Oklahoma	501.3		36	Alabama	367.8
48	Oregon	231.4		37	South Carolina	364.9
26	Pennsylvania	416.9		38	West Virginia	363.9
14	Rhode Island	493.3		39	Michigan	353.0
37	South Carolina	364.9		40	Washington	325.4
6	South Dakota	525.6		41	New Mexico	325.3
17	Tennessee	483.8		42	Utah	324.6
25	Texas	423.3		43	Idaho	319.2
42	Utah	324.6		44	Nevada	293.7
30	Vermont	404.7		45	California	291.0
35	Virginia	376.0		46	Arizona	243.2
40	Washington	325.4		47	Florida	236.2
38	West Virginia	363.9		48	Oregon	231.4
12	Wisconsin	496.7		NA	Alaska**	NA
24	Wyoming	439.1		NA	Hawaii**	NA
					District of Columbia**	NA

Source: U.S. Department of Health and Human Services, Health Care Financing Administration
   "Health, United States, 1998" (July 1998)
*Number of nursing home residents (all ages) per 1,000 resident population 85 years of age and over.
**Not available.

Nursing Home Population in 1991

National Total = 1,478,903 Persons in Nursing Homes*

ALPHA ORDER

RANK	STATE	POPULATION	% of USA
27	Alabama	21,675	1.47%
50	Alaska	808	0.05%
34	Arizona	12,103	0.82%
28	Arkansas	20,298	1.37%
2	California	98,885	6.69%
30	Colorado	15,871	1.07%
20	Connecticut	27,921	1.89%
45	Delaware	4,308	0.29%
7	Florida	59,878	4.05%
15	Georgia	34,728	2.35%
48	Hawaii	2,840	0.19%
44	Idaho	4,871	0.33%
4	Illinois	87,540	5.92%
10	Indiana	46,231	3.13%
16	Iowa	33,214	2.25%
24	Kansas	25,304	1.71%
25	Kentucky	24,966	1.69%
17	Louisiana	32,367	2.19%
37	Maine	9,241	0.62%
22	Maryland	25,977	1.76%
8	Massachusetts	48,276	3.26%
11	Michigan	46,198	3.12%
13	Minnesota	43,298	2.93%
31	Mississippi	14,819	1.00%
12	Missouri	45,745	3.09%
41	Montana	6,297	0.43%
29	Nebraska	17,779	1.20%
47	Nevada	3,043	0.21%
39	New Hampshire	7,523	0.51%
14	New Jersey	40,068	2.71%
42	New Mexico	5,834	0.39%
1	New York	99,372	6.72%
19	North Carolina	28,546	1.93%
40	North Dakota	6,784	0.46%
6	Ohio	77,676	5.25%
21	Oklahoma	27,456	1.86%
32	Oregon	13,392	0.91%
5	Pennsylvania	83,107	5.62%
36	Rhode Island	9,440	0.64%
33	South Carolina	13,089	0.89%
38	South Dakota	8,192	0.55%
18	Tennessee	32,304	2.18%
3	Texas	90,405	6.11%
43	Utah	5,544	0.37%
46	Vermont	3,591	0.24%
23	Virginia	25,775	1.74%
26	Washington	24,525	1.66%
35	West Virginia	9,809	0.66%
9	Wisconsin	46,898	3.17%
49	Wyoming	2,211	0.15%

RANK ORDER

RANK	STATE	POPULATION	% of USA
1	New York	99,372	6.72%
2	California	98,885	6.69%
3	Texas	90,405	6.11%
4	Illinois	87,540	5.92%
5	Pennsylvania	83,107	5.62%
6	Ohio	77,676	5.25%
7	Florida	59,878	4.05%
8	Massachusetts	48,276	3.26%
9	Wisconsin	46,898	3.17%
10	Indiana	46,231	3.13%
11	Michigan	46,198	3.12%
12	Missouri	45,745	3.09%
13	Minnesota	43,298	2.93%
14	New Jersey	40,068	2.71%
15	Georgia	34,728	2.35%
16	Iowa	33,214	2.25%
17	Louisiana	32,367	2.19%
18	Tennessee	32,304	2.18%
19	North Carolina	28,546	1.93%
20	Connecticut	27,921	1.89%
21	Oklahoma	27,456	1.86%
22	Maryland	25,977	1.76%
23	Virginia	25,775	1.74%
24	Kansas	25,304	1.71%
25	Kentucky	24,966	1.69%
26	Washington	24,525	1.66%
27	Alabama	21,675	1.47%
28	Arkansas	20,298	1.37%
29	Nebraska	17,779	1.20%
30	Colorado	15,871	1.07%
31	Mississippi	14,819	1.00%
32	Oregon	13,392	0.91%
33	South Carolina	13,089	0.89%
34	Arizona	12,103	0.82%
35	West Virginia	9,809	0.66%
36	Rhode Island	9,440	0.64%
37	Maine	9,241	0.62%
38	South Dakota	8,192	0.55%
39	New Hampshire	7,523	0.51%
40	North Dakota	6,784	0.46%
41	Montana	6,297	0.43%
42	New Mexico	5,834	0.39%
43	Utah	5,544	0.37%
44	Idaho	4,871	0.33%
45	Delaware	4,308	0.29%
46	Vermont	3,591	0.24%
47	Nevada	3,043	0.21%
48	Hawaii	2,840	0.19%
49	Wyoming	2,211	0.15%
50	Alaska	808	0.05%
	District of Columbia	2,881	0.19%

Source: U.S. Department of Health and Human Services, National Center for Health Statistics "National Health Provider Inventory" (Advance Data, No. 266, September 19, 1995)
A nursing home is facility with three or more beds that is either licensed as a nursing home, certified as a nursing facility under Medicare or Medicaid, identified as a nursing care unit of a retirement center or determined to provide nursing or medical care.

Percent of Nursing Home Population 65 Years Old or Older in 1991

National Percent = 92.3% of Nursing Home Population*

ALPHA ORDER

RANK ORDER

RANK	STATE	PERCENT	RANK	STATE	PERCENT
25	Alabama	92.5	1	Rhode Island	96.5
50	Alaska	78.7	2	South Dakota	95.7
36	Arizona	91.9	3	Maine	95.6
44	Arkansas	90.5	4	North Dakota	95.4
47	California	88.8	5	Iowa	95.2
41	Colorado	90.9	6	New Hampshire	95.1
28	Connecticut	92.3	7	Florida	94.9
28	Delaware	92.3	8	Vermont	94.5
7	Florida	94.9	9	Minnesota	94.3
42	Georgia	90.7	10	West Virginia	94.2
33	Hawaii	92.0	11	New York	94.1
42	Idaho	90.7	12	Pennsylvania	94.0
46	Illinois	89.0	13	Nebraska	93.9
40	Indiana	91.1	14	Wyoming	93.6
5	Iowa	95.2	15	Massachusetts	93.5
22	Kansas	92.7	16	New Jersey	93.4
31	Kentucky	92.1	17	Missouri	93.1
45	Louisiana	89.1	18	Oregon	93.0
3	Maine	95.6	18	Texas	93.0
33	Maryland	92.0	20	Mississippi	92.9
15	Massachusetts	93.5	21	Oklahoma	92.8
39	Michigan	91.5	22	Kansas	92.7
9	Minnesota	94.3	22	Tennessee	92.7
20	Mississippi	92.9	24	South Carolina	92.6
17	Missouri	93.1	25	Alabama	92.5
25	Montana	92.5	25	Montana	92.5
13	Nebraska	93.9	27	Virginia	92.4
48	Nevada	88.0	28	Connecticut	92.3
6	New Hampshire	95.1	28	Delaware	92.3
16	New Jersey	93.4	28	North Carolina	92.3
33	New Mexico	92.0	31	Kentucky	92.1
11	New York	94.1	31	Washington	92.1
28	North Carolina	92.3	33	Hawaii	92.0
4	North Dakota	95.4	33	Maryland	92.0
37	Ohio	91.7	33	New Mexico	92.0
21	Oklahoma	92.8	36	Arizona	91.9
18	Oregon	93.0	37	Ohio	91.7
12	Pennsylvania	94.0	38	Wisconsin	91.6
1	Rhode Island	96.5	39	Michigan	91.5
24	South Carolina	92.6	40	Indiana	91.1
2	South Dakota	95.7	41	Colorado	90.9
22	Tennessee	92.7	42	Georgia	90.7
18	Texas	93.0	42	Idaho	90.7
49	Utah	86.5	44	Arkansas	90.5
8	Vermont	94.5	45	Louisiana	89.1
27	Virginia	92.4	46	Illinois	89.0
31	Washington	92.1	47	California	88.8
10	West Virginia	94.2	48	Nevada	88.0
38	Wisconsin	91.6	49	Utah	86.5
14	Wyoming	93.6	50	Alaska	78.7

| | | | | District of Columbia | 93.3 |

Source: U.S. Department of Health and Human Services, National Center for Health Statistics
"National Health Provider Inventory" (Advance Data, No. 266, September 19, 1995)
*A nursing home is facility with three or more beds that is either licensed as a nursing home, certified as a nursing facility under Medicare or Medicaid, identified as a nursing care unit of a retirement center or determined to provide nursing or medical care.

Percent of Nursing Home Population 85 Years Old or Older in 1991

National Percent = 33.7% of Nursing Home Population*

ALPHA ORDER				RANK ORDER		
RANK	STATE	PERCENT		RANK	STATE	PERCENT
43	Alabama	28.6		1	New Hampshire	49.0
48	Alaska	24.9		2	Hawaii	46.8
20	Arizona	34.8		3	South Dakota	45.5
44	Arkansas	28.5		4	Nebraska	43.8
34	California	31.3		5	Iowa	42.8
15	Colorado	37.3		6	Maine	41.4
37	Connecticut	31.1		7	North Dakota	41.3
15	Delaware	37.3		8	Kansas	40.0
22	Florida	34.6		8	Vermont	40.0
37	Georgia	31.1		10	Rhode Island	39.9
2	Hawaii	46.8		11	Massachusetts	38.5
29	Idaho	32.6		12	Minnesota	38.4
32	Illinois	31.8		13	New York	38.3
31	Indiana	32.1		14	Wisconsin	37.7
5	Iowa	42.8		15	Colorado	37.3
8	Kansas	40.0		15	Delaware	37.3
39	Kentucky	30.8		17	Montana	37.1
50	Louisiana	23.8		18	New Jersey	35.6
6	Maine	41.4		19	Wyoming	35.2
46	Maryland	27.8		20	Arizona	34.8
11	Massachusetts	38.5		20	New Mexico	34.8
26	Michigan	33.4		22	Florida	34.6
12	Minnesota	38.4		23	Missouri	33.9
47	Mississippi	27.5		23	South Carolina	33.9
23	Missouri	33.9		23	Virginia	33.9
17	Montana	37.1		26	Michigan	33.4
4	Nebraska	43.8		27	Oklahoma	33.2
49	Nevada	24.2		28	Pennsylvania	33.0
1	New Hampshire	49.0		29	Idaho	32.6
18	New Jersey	35.6		29	Oregon	32.6
20	New Mexico	34.8		31	Indiana	32.1
13	New York	38.3		32	Illinois	31.8
45	North Carolina	28.4		32	Ohio	31.8
7	North Dakota	41.3		34	California	31.3
32	Ohio	31.8		34	Texas	31.3
27	Oklahoma	33.2		36	Tennessee	31.2
29	Oregon	32.6		37	Connecticut	31.1
28	Pennsylvania	33.0		37	Georgia	31.1
10	Rhode Island	39.9		39	Kentucky	30.8
23	South Carolina	33.9		40	West Virginia	30.5
3	South Dakota	45.5		41	Washington	30.4
36	Tennessee	31.2		42	Utah	29.3
34	Texas	31.3		43	Alabama	28.6
42	Utah	29.3		44	Arkansas	28.5
8	Vermont	40.0		45	North Carolina	28.4
23	Virginia	33.9		46	Maryland	27.8
41	Washington	30.4		47	Mississippi	27.5
40	West Virginia	30.5		48	Alaska	24.9
14	Wisconsin	37.7		49	Nevada	24.2
19	Wyoming	35.2		50	Louisiana	23.8
					District of Columbia	26.5

Source: Morgan Quitno Press using data from U.S. Dept of Health & Human Serv's, Nat'l Center for Health Statistics
"National Health Provider Inventory" (unpublished data)

*A nursing home is facility with three or more beds that is either licensed as a nursing home, certified as a nursing facility under Medicare or Medicaid, identified as a nursing care unit of a retirement center or determined to provide nursing or medical care.

Health Service Establishments in 1996

National Total = 482,617 Establishments*

ALPHA ORDER

RANK	STATE	ESTABLISH'S	% of USA
25	Alabama	6,308	1.3%
48	Alaska	1,026	0.2%
19	Arizona	7,928	1.6%
32	Arkansas	4,167	0.9%
1	California	63,279	13.1%
20	Colorado	7,889	1.6%
23	Connecticut	7,037	1.5%
45	Delaware	1,291	0.3%
4	Florida	32,877	6.8%
10	Georgia	12,259	2.5%
39	Hawaii	2,413	0.5%
41	Idaho	2,112	0.4%
6	Illinois	20,183	4.2%
16	Indiana	9,424	2.0%
30	Iowa	4,712	1.0%
31	Kansas	4,488	0.9%
26	Kentucky	6,303	1.3%
22	Louisiana	7,588	1.6%
40	Maine	2,376	0.5%
15	Maryland	9,933	2.1%
11	Massachusetts	11,285	2.3%
9	Michigan	17,050	3.5%
24	Minnesota	6,948	1.4%
33	Mississippi	3,498	0.7%
17	Missouri	9,094	1.9%
44	Montana	1,804	0.4%
38	Nebraska	2,583	0.5%
37	Nevada	2,763	0.6%
42	New Hampshire	2,036	0.4%
8	New Jersey	17,807	3.7%
36	New Mexico	2,778	0.6%
2	New York	35,502	7.4%
13	North Carolina	10,256	2.1%
49	North Dakota	974	0.2%
7	Ohio	19,757	4.1%
27	Oklahoma	6,096	1.3%
28	Oregon	6,039	1.3%
5	Pennsylvania	23,329	4.8%
43	Rhode Island	1,989	0.4%
29	South Carolina	5,270	1.1%
46	South Dakota	1,226	0.3%
18	Tennessee	8,976	1.9%
3	Texas	33,628	7.0%
34	Utah	3,484	0.7%
47	Vermont	1,109	0.2%
12	Virginia	10,483	2.2%
14	Washington	10,062	2.1%
35	West Virginia	3,026	0.6%
21	Wisconsin	7,878	1.6%
50	Wyoming	887	0.2%

RANK ORDER

RANK	STATE	ESTABLISH'S	% of USA
1	California	63,279	13.1%
2	New York	35,502	7.4%
3	Texas	33,628	7.0%
4	Florida	32,877	6.8%
5	Pennsylvania	23,329	4.8%
6	Illinois	20,183	4.2%
7	Ohio	19,757	4.1%
8	New Jersey	17,807	3.7%
9	Michigan	17,050	3.5%
10	Georgia	12,259	2.5%
11	Massachusetts	11,285	2.3%
12	Virginia	10,483	2.2%
13	North Carolina	10,256	2.1%
14	Washington	10,062	2.1%
15	Maryland	9,933	2.1%
16	Indiana	9,424	2.0%
17	Missouri	9,094	1.9%
18	Tennessee	8,976	1.9%
19	Arizona	7,928	1.6%
20	Colorado	7,889	1.6%
21	Wisconsin	7,878	1.6%
22	Louisiana	7,588	1.6%
23	Connecticut	7,037	1.5%
24	Minnesota	6,948	1.4%
25	Alabama	6,308	1.3%
26	Kentucky	6,303	1.3%
27	Oklahoma	6,096	1.3%
28	Oregon	6,039	1.3%
29	South Carolina	5,270	1.1%
30	Iowa	4,712	1.0%
31	Kansas	4,488	0.9%
32	Arkansas	4,167	0.9%
33	Mississippi	3,498	0.7%
34	Utah	3,484	0.7%
35	West Virginia	3,026	0.6%
36	New Mexico	2,778	0.6%
37	Nevada	2,763	0.6%
38	Nebraska	2,583	0.5%
39	Hawaii	2,413	0.5%
40	Maine	2,376	0.5%
41	Idaho	2,112	0.4%
42	New Hampshire	2,036	0.4%
43	Rhode Island	1,989	0.4%
44	Montana	1,804	0.4%
45	Delaware	1,291	0.3%
46	South Dakota	1,226	0.3%
47	Vermont	1,109	0.2%
48	Alaska	1,026	0.2%
49	North Dakota	974	0.2%
50	Wyoming	887	0.2%
	District of Columbia	1,407	0.3%

Source: U.S. Bureau of the Census
   "1996 County Business Patterns"
*Includes establishments exempt from, as well as subject to, the federal income tax. Includes those establishments within the Standard Industry Classification (SIC) 8000. These include those primarily engaged in furnishing medical, surgical and other health services to persons.

Offices and Clinics of Doctors of Medicine in 1992

National Total = 197,701 Establishments*

ALPHA ORDER

RANK	STATE	ESTABLISH'S	% of USA
23	Alabama	2,611	1.32%
47	Alaska	349	0.18%
20	Arizona	3,150	1.59%
29	Arkansas	1,664	0.84%
1	California	28,494	14.41%
22	Colorado	2,698	1.36%
21	Connecticut	3,039	1.54%
45	Delaware	587	0.30%
3	Florida	14,487	7.33%
10	Georgia	5,214	2.64%
37	Hawaii	1,066	0.54%
43	Idaho	728	0.37%
6	Illinois	8,424	4.26%
16	Indiana	3,744	1.89%
33	Iowa	1,349	0.68%
32	Kansas	1,382	0.70%
24	Kentucky	2,565	1.30%
18	Louisiana	3,293	1.67%
39	Maine	914	0.46%
11	Maryland	4,760	2.41%
13	Massachusetts	4,524	2.29%
9	Michigan	5,935	3.00%
30	Minnesota	1,480	0.75%
31	Mississippi	1,458	0.74%
19	Missouri	3,280	1.66%
44	Montana	599	0.30%
41	Nebraska	886	0.45%
36	Nevada	1,096	0.55%
42	New Hampshire	754	0.38%
8	New Jersey	7,718	3.90%
38	New Mexico	1,033	0.52%
2	New York	16,226	8.21%
15	North Carolina	3,826	1.94%
50	North Dakota	243	0.12%
7	Ohio	8,004	4.05%
28	Oklahoma	2,052	1.04%
26	Oregon	2,263	1.14%
5	Pennsylvania	9,347	4.73%
40	Rhode Island	889	0.45%
27	South Carolina	2,219	1.12%
47	South Dakota	349	0.18%
14	Tennessee	3,840	1.94%
4	Texas	14,367	7.27%
35	Utah	1,261	0.64%
46	Vermont	393	0.20%
12	Virginia	4,724	2.39%
17	Washington	3,464	1.75%
34	West Virginia	1,340	0.68%
25	Wisconsin	2,546	1.29%
49	Wyoming	294	0.15%

RANK ORDER

RANK	STATE	ESTABLISH'S	% of USA
1	California	28,494	14.41%
2	New York	16,226	8.21%
3	Florida	14,487	7.33%
4	Texas	14,367	7.27%
5	Pennsylvania	9,347	4.73%
6	Illinois	8,424	4.26%
7	Ohio	8,004	4.05%
8	New Jersey	7,718	3.90%
9	Michigan	5,935	3.00%
10	Georgia	5,214	2.64%
11	Maryland	4,760	2.41%
12	Virginia	4,724	2.39%
13	Massachusetts	4,524	2.29%
14	Tennessee	3,840	1.94%
15	North Carolina	3,826	1.94%
16	Indiana	3,744	1.89%
17	Washington	3,464	1.75%
18	Louisiana	3,293	1.67%
19	Missouri	3,280	1.66%
20	Arizona	3,150	1.59%
21	Connecticut	3,039	1.54%
22	Colorado	2,698	1.36%
23	Alabama	2,611	1.32%
24	Kentucky	2,565	1.30%
25	Wisconsin	2,546	1.29%
26	Oregon	2,263	1.14%
27	South Carolina	2,219	1.12%
28	Oklahoma	2,052	1.04%
29	Arkansas	1,664	0.84%
30	Minnesota	1,480	0.75%
31	Mississippi	1,458	0.74%
32	Kansas	1,382	0.70%
33	Iowa	1,349	0.68%
34	West Virginia	1,340	0.68%
35	Utah	1,261	0.64%
36	Nevada	1,096	0.55%
37	Hawaii	1,066	0.54%
38	New Mexico	1,033	0.52%
39	Maine	914	0.46%
40	Rhode Island	889	0.45%
41	Nebraska	886	0.45%
42	New Hampshire	754	0.38%
43	Idaho	728	0.37%
44	Montana	599	0.30%
45	Delaware	587	0.30%
46	Vermont	393	0.20%
47	Alaska	349	0.18%
47	South Dakota	349	0.18%
49	Wyoming	294	0.15%
50	North Dakota	243	0.12%
	District of Columbia	773	0.39%

Source: U.S. Bureau of the Census
"1992 Census of Service Industries, Geographic Area Series, United States" (SC92-A-52)
*Includes only establishments subject to the federal income tax.

Offices and Clinics of Dentists in 1992

National Total = 108,804 Establishments*

ALPHA ORDER

ALPHA ORDER

RANK	STATE	ESTABLISH'S	% of USA
27	Alabama	1,331	1.22%
45	Alaska	262	0.24%
25	Arizona	1,522	1.40%
33	Arkansas	822	0.76%
1	California	14,806	13.61%
21	Colorado	1,911	1.76%
22	Connecticut	1,740	1.60%
49	Delaware	215	0.20%
4	Florida	5,374	4.94%
13	Georgia	2,346	2.16%
36	Hawaii	640	0.59%
42	Idaho	455	0.42%
6	Illinois	5,156	4.74%
16	Indiana	2,177	2.00%
30	Iowa	1,149	1.06%
31	Kansas	1,003	0.92%
26	Kentucky	1,462	1.34%
24	Louisiana	1,548	1.42%
41	Maine	458	0.42%
15	Maryland	2,195	2.02%
10	Massachusetts	2,941	2.70%
8	Michigan	4,348	4.00%
19	Minnesota	2,010	1.85%
34	Mississippi	784	0.72%
18	Missouri	2,047	1.88%
44	Montana	397	0.36%
35	Nebraska	747	0.69%
40	Nevada	478	0.44%
39	New Hampshire	514	0.47%
9	New Jersey	4,033	3.71%
38	New Mexico	532	0.49%
2	New York	8,560	7.87%
17	North Carolina	2,162	1.99%
47	North Dakota	250	0.23%
7	Ohio	4,497	4.13%
28	Oklahoma	1,229	1.13%
23	Oregon	1,587	1.46%
5	Pennsylvania	5,316	4.89%
43	Rhode Island	406	0.37%
29	South Carolina	1,153	1.06%
46	South Dakota	260	0.24%
20	Tennessee	1,984	1.82%
3	Texas	6,233	5.73%
32	Utah	974	0.90%
48	Vermont	245	0.23%
12	Virginia	2,524	2.32%
11	Washington	2,674	2.46%
37	West Virginia	563	0.52%
14	Wisconsin	2,235	2.05%
50	Wyoming	202	0.19%

RANK ORDER

RANK	STATE	ESTABLISH'S	% of USA
1	California	14,806	13.61%
2	New York	8,560	7.87%
3	Texas	6,233	5.73%
4	Florida	5,374	4.94%
5	Pennsylvania	5,316	4.89%
6	Illinois	5,156	4.74%
7	Ohio	4,497	4.13%
8	Michigan	4,348	4.00%
9	New Jersey	4,033	3.71%
10	Massachusetts	2,941	2.70%
11	Washington	2,674	2.46%
12	Virginia	2,524	2.32%
13	Georgia	2,346	2.16%
14	Wisconsin	2,235	2.05%
15	Maryland	2,195	2.02%
16	Indiana	2,177	2.00%
17	North Carolina	2,162	1.99%
18	Missouri	2,047	1.88%
19	Minnesota	2,010	1.85%
20	Tennessee	1,984	1.82%
21	Colorado	1,911	1.76%
22	Connecticut	1,740	1.60%
23	Oregon	1,587	1.46%
24	Louisiana	1,548	1.42%
25	Arizona	1,522	1.40%
26	Kentucky	1,462	1.34%
27	Alabama	1,331	1.22%
28	Oklahoma	1,229	1.13%
29	South Carolina	1,153	1.06%
30	Iowa	1,149	1.06%
31	Kansas	1,003	0.92%
32	Utah	974	0.90%
33	Arkansas	822	0.76%
34	Mississippi	784	0.72%
35	Nebraska	747	0.69%
36	Hawaii	640	0.59%
37	West Virginia	563	0.52%
38	New Mexico	532	0.49%
39	New Hampshire	514	0.47%
40	Nevada	478	0.44%
41	Maine	458	0.42%
42	Idaho	455	0.42%
43	Rhode Island	406	0.37%
44	Montana	397	0.36%
45	Alaska	262	0.24%
46	South Dakota	260	0.24%
47	North Dakota	250	0.23%
48	Vermont	245	0.23%
49	Delaware	215	0.20%
50	Wyoming	202	0.19%
	District of Columbia	347	0.32%

Source: U.S. Bureau of the Census
"1992 Census of Service Industries, Geographic Area Series, United States" (SC92-A-52)
*Includes only establishments subject to the federal income tax.

Offices and Clinics of Doctors of Osteopathy in 1992

National Total = 8,708 Establishments*

ALPHA ORDER

RANK	STATE	ESTABLISH'S	% of USA
31	Alabama	32	0.37%
41	Alaska	11	0.13%
10	Arizona	317	3.64%
32	Arkansas	26	0.30%
9	California	322	3.70%
11	Colorado	207	2.38%
38	Connecticut	14	0.16%
26	Delaware	50	0.57%
4	Florida	762	8.75%
17	Georgia	124	1.42%
41	Hawaii	11	0.13%
39	Idaho	13	0.15%
14	Illinois	173	1.99%
16	Indiana	142	1.63%
13	Iowa	193	2.22%
20	Kansas	97	1.11%
30	Kentucky	38	0.44%
47	Louisiana	6	0.07%
18	Maine	120	1.38%
36	Maryland	16	0.18%
28	Massachusetts	40	0.46%
1	Michigan	1,201	13.79%
36	Minnesota	16	0.18%
34	Mississippi	20	0.23%
6	Missouri	446	5.12%
40	Montana	12	0.14%
49	Nebraska	2	0.02%
27	Nevada	41	0.47%
45	New Hampshire	9	0.10%
7	New Jersey	399	4.58%
23	New Mexico	57	0.65%
12	New York	201	2.31%
35	North Carolina	19	0.22%
49	North Dakota	2	0.02%
3	Ohio	821	9.43%
8	Oklahoma	328	3.77%
19	Oregon	112	1.29%
2	Pennsylvania	1,062	12.20%
24	Rhode Island	55	0.63%
33	South Carolina	21	0.24%
45	South Dakota	9	0.10%
25	Tennessee	52	0.60%
5	Texas	707	8.12%
43	Utah	10	0.11%
47	Vermont	6	0.07%
29	Virginia	39	0.45%
15	Washington	149	1.71%
22	West Virginia	90	1.03%
21	Wisconsin	96	1.10%
43	Wyoming	10	0.11%

RANK ORDER

RANK	STATE	ESTABLISH'S	% of USA
1	Michigan	1,201	13.79%
2	Pennsylvania	1,062	12.20%
3	Ohio	821	9.43%
4	Florida	762	8.75%
5	Texas	707	8.12%
6	Missouri	446	5.12%
7	New Jersey	399	4.58%
8	Oklahoma	328	3.77%
9	California	322	3.70%
10	Arizona	317	3.64%
11	Colorado	207	2.38%
12	New York	201	2.31%
13	Iowa	193	2.22%
14	Illinois	173	1.99%
15	Washington	149	1.71%
16	Indiana	142	1.63%
17	Georgia	124	1.42%
18	Maine	120	1.38%
19	Oregon	112	1.29%
20	Kansas	97	1.11%
21	Wisconsin	96	1.10%
22	West Virginia	90	1.03%
23	New Mexico	57	0.65%
24	Rhode Island	55	0.63%
25	Tennessee	52	0.60%
26	Delaware	50	0.57%
27	Nevada	41	0.47%
28	Massachusetts	40	0.46%
29	Virginia	39	0.45%
30	Kentucky	38	0.44%
31	Alabama	32	0.37%
32	Arkansas	26	0.30%
33	South Carolina	21	0.24%
34	Mississippi	20	0.23%
35	North Carolina	19	0.22%
36	Maryland	16	0.18%
36	Minnesota	16	0.18%
38	Connecticut	14	0.16%
39	Idaho	13	0.15%
40	Montana	12	0.14%
41	Alaska	11	0.13%
41	Hawaii	11	0.13%
43	Utah	10	0.11%
43	Wyoming	10	0.11%
45	New Hampshire	9	0.10%
45	South Dakota	9	0.10%
47	Louisiana	6	0.07%
47	Vermont	6	0.07%
49	Nebraska	2	0.02%
49	North Dakota	2	0.02%
	District of Columbia	2	0.02%

Source: U.S. Bureau of the Census
"1992 Census of Service Industries, Geographic Area Series, United States" (SC92-A-52)
Includes only establishments subject to the federal income tax.

Offices and Clinics of Chiropractors in 1992

National Total = 27,329 Establishments*

<u>ALPHA ORDER</u>

RANK	STATE	ESTABLISH'S	% of USA
29	Alabama	282	1.03%
47	Alaska	71	0.26%
14	Arizona	622	2.28%
31	Arkansas	237	0.87%
1	California	4,364	15.97%
16	Colorado	589	2.16%
24	Connecticut	347	1.27%
49	Delaware	50	0.18%
2	Florida	1,847	6.76%
12	Georgia	760	2.78%
39	Hawaii	119	0.44%
37	Idaho	134	0.49%
7	Illinois	1,068	3.91%
20	Indiana	436	1.60%
18	Iowa	446	1.63%
25	Kansas	321	1.17%
30	Kentucky	269	0.98%
28	Louisiana	284	1.04%
38	Maine	126	0.46%
32	Maryland	231	0.85%
17	Massachusetts	575	2.10%
8	Michigan	938	3.43%
10	Minnesota	824	3.02%
42	Mississippi	113	0.41%
15	Missouri	598	2.19%
41	Montana	117	0.43%
35	Nebraska	163	0.60%
34	Nevada	166	0.61%
43	New Hampshire	108	0.40%
6	New Jersey	1,245	4.56%
33	New Mexico	185	0.68%
3	New York	1,741	6.37%
19	North Carolina	439	1.61%
45	North Dakota	90	0.33%
9	Ohio	871	3.19%
27	Oklahoma	316	1.16%
21	Oregon	428	1.57%
5	Pennsylvania	1,310	4.79%
46	Rhode Island	79	0.29%
26	South Carolina	319	1.17%
40	South Dakota	118	0.43%
22	Tennessee	356	1.30%
4	Texas	1,426	5.22%
36	Utah	153	0.56%
48	Vermont	65	0.24%
23	Virginia	355	1.30%
11	Washington	804	2.94%
44	West Virginia	105	0.38%
13	Wisconsin	665	2.43%
50	Wyoming	41	0.15%

<u>RANK ORDER</u>

RANK	STATE	ESTABLISH'S	% of USA
1	California	4,364	15.97%
2	Florida	1,847	6.76%
3	New York	1,741	6.37%
4	Texas	1,426	5.22%
5	Pennsylvania	1,310	4.79%
6	New Jersey	1,245	4.56%
7	Illinois	1,068	3.91%
8	Michigan	938	3.43%
9	Ohio	871	3.19%
10	Minnesota	824	3.02%
11	Washington	804	2.94%
12	Georgia	760	2.78%
13	Wisconsin	665	2.43%
14	Arizona	622	2.28%
15	Missouri	598	2.19%
16	Colorado	589	2.16%
17	Massachusetts	575	2.10%
18	Iowa	446	1.63%
19	North Carolina	439	1.61%
20	Indiana	436	1.60%
21	Oregon	428	1.57%
22	Tennessee	356	1.30%
23	Virginia	355	1.30%
24	Connecticut	347	1.27%
25	Kansas	321	1.17%
26	South Carolina	319	1.17%
27	Oklahoma	316	1.16%
28	Louisiana	284	1.04%
29	Alabama	282	1.03%
30	Kentucky	269	0.98%
31	Arkansas	237	0.87%
32	Maryland	231	0.85%
33	New Mexico	185	0.68%
34	Nevada	166	0.61%
35	Nebraska	163	0.60%
36	Utah	153	0.56%
37	Idaho	134	0.49%
38	Maine	126	0.46%
39	Hawaii	119	0.44%
40	South Dakota	118	0.43%
41	Montana	117	0.43%
42	Mississippi	113	0.41%
43	New Hampshire	108	0.40%
44	West Virginia	105	0.38%
45	North Dakota	90	0.33%
46	Rhode Island	79	0.29%
47	Alaska	71	0.26%
48	Vermont	65	0.24%
49	Delaware	50	0.18%
50	Wyoming	41	0.15%
	District of Columbia	13	0.05%

Source: U.S. Bureau of the Census
"1992 Census of Service Industries, Geographic Area Series, United States" (SC92-A-52)
Includes only establishments subject to the federal income tax.

Offices and Clinics of Optometrists in 1992

National Total = 17,135 Establishments*

ALPHA ORDER					RANK ORDER			

RANK	STATE	ESTABLISH'S	% of USA
26	Alabama	229	1.34%
49	Alaska	44	0.26%
32	Arizona	189	1.10%
29	Arkansas	202	1.18%
1	California	2,382	13.90%
22	Colorado	257	1.50%
27	Connecticut	228	1.33%
50	Delaware	40	0.23%
4	Florida	854	4.98%
13	Georgia	373	2.18%
40	Hawaii	99	0.58%
41	Idaho	94	0.55%
7	Illinois	698	4.07%
11	Indiana	463	2.70%
21	Iowa	270	1.58%
24	Kansas	247	1.44%
23	Kentucky	248	1.45%
31	Louisiana	196	1.14%
35	Maine	123	0.72%
25	Maryland	235	1.37%
14	Massachusetts	370	2.16%
8	Michigan	607	3.54%
20	Minnesota	281	1.64%
34	Mississippi	148	0.86%
19	Missouri	301	1.76%
39	Montana	103	0.60%
36	Nebraska	121	0.71%
37	Nevada	110	0.64%
44	New Hampshire	74	0.43%
9	New Jersey	550	3.21%
38	New Mexico	104	0.61%
6	New York	791	4.62%
10	North Carolina	498	2.91%
46	North Dakota	64	0.37%
5	Ohio	836	4.88%
18	Oklahoma	317	1.85%
28	Oregon	222	1.30%
3	Pennsylvania	869	5.07%
45	Rhode Island	72	0.42%
30	South Carolina	198	1.16%
43	South Dakota	80	0.47%
15	Tennessee	364	2.12%
2	Texas	1,100	6.42%
42	Utah	81	0.47%
48	Vermont	50	0.29%
12	Virginia	436	2.54%
17	Washington	341	1.99%
33	West Virginia	151	0.88%
16	Wisconsin	347	2.03%
47	Wyoming	54	0.32%

RANK	STATE	ESTABLISH'S	% of USA
1	California	2,382	13.90%
2	Texas	1,100	6.42%
3	Pennsylvania	869	5.07%
4	Florida	854	4.98%
5	Ohio	836	4.88%
6	New York	791	4.62%
7	Illinois	698	4.07%
8	Michigan	607	3.54%
9	New Jersey	550	3.21%
10	North Carolina	498	2.91%
11	Indiana	463	2.70%
12	Virginia	436	2.54%
13	Georgia	373	2.18%
14	Massachusetts	370	2.16%
15	Tennessee	364	2.12%
16	Wisconsin	347	2.03%
17	Washington	341	1.99%
18	Oklahoma	317	1.85%
19	Missouri	301	1.76%
20	Minnesota	281	1.64%
21	Iowa	270	1.58%
22	Colorado	257	1.50%
23	Kentucky	248	1.45%
24	Kansas	247	1.44%
25	Maryland	235	1.37%
26	Alabama	229	1.34%
27	Connecticut	228	1.33%
28	Oregon	222	1.30%
29	Arkansas	202	1.18%
30	South Carolina	198	1.16%
31	Louisiana	196	1.14%
32	Arizona	189	1.10%
33	West Virginia	151	0.88%
34	Mississippi	148	0.86%
35	Maine	123	0.72%
36	Nebraska	121	0.71%
37	Nevada	110	0.64%
38	New Mexico	104	0.61%
39	Montana	103	0.60%
40	Hawaii	99	0.58%
41	Idaho	94	0.55%
42	Utah	81	0.47%
43	South Dakota	80	0.47%
44	New Hampshire	74	0.43%
45	Rhode Island	72	0.42%
46	North Dakota	64	0.37%
47	Wyoming	54	0.32%
48	Vermont	50	0.29%
49	Alaska	44	0.26%
50	Delaware	40	0.23%
	District of Columbia	24	0.14%

Source: U.S. Bureau of the Census
   "1992 Census of Service Industries, Geographic Area Series, United States" (SC92-A-52)
*Includes only establishments subject to the federal income tax.

Offices and Clinics of Podiatrists in 1992

National Total = 7,948 Establishments*

ALPHA ORDER					RANK ORDER			
RANK	STATE		ESTABLISH'S	% of USA	RANK	STATE	ESTABLISH'S	% of USA
29	Alabama		49	0.62%	1	New York	938	11.80%
49	Alaska		5	0.06%	2	California	930	11.70%
18	Arizona		121	1.52%	3	Pennsylvania	589	7.41%
41	Arkansas		20	0.25%	4	Florida	564	7.10%
2	California		930	11.70%	5	Ohio	490	6.17%
22	Colorado		88	1.11%	6	New Jersey	449	5.65%
14	Connecticut		152	1.91%	7	Illinois	419	5.27%
39	Delaware		25	0.31%	8	Michigan	400	5.03%
4	Florida		564	7.10%	9	Texas	382	4.81%
17	Georgia		139	1.75%	10	Maryland	211	2.65%
44	Hawaii		16	0.20%	11	Massachusetts	208	2.62%
43	Idaho		17	0.21%	12	Indiana	166	2.09%
7	Illinois		419	5.27%	13	Virginia	164	2.06%
12	Indiana		166	2.09%	14	Connecticut	152	1.91%
23	Iowa		75	0.94%	15	Washington	146	1.84%
26	Kansas		55	0.69%	16	North Carolina	140	1.76%
31	Kentucky		46	0.58%	17	Georgia	139	1.75%
30	Louisiana		48	0.60%	18	Arizona	121	1.52%
34	Maine		36	0.45%	19	Wisconsin	119	1.50%
10	Maryland		211	2.65%	20	Missouri	98	1.23%
11	Massachusetts		208	2.62%	21	Tennessee	90	1.13%
8	Michigan		400	5.03%	22	Colorado	88	1.11%
25	Minnesota		60	0.75%	23	Iowa	75	0.94%
42	Mississippi		18	0.23%	24	Oregon	61	0.77%
20	Missouri		98	1.23%	25	Minnesota	60	0.75%
44	Montana		16	0.20%	26	Kansas	55	0.69%
35	Nebraska		34	0.43%	27	Oklahoma	52	0.65%
37	Nevada		28	0.35%	28	Rhode Island	50	0.63%
40	New Hampshire		24	0.30%	29	Alabama	49	0.62%
6	New Jersey		449	5.65%	30	Louisiana	48	0.60%
36	New Mexico		33	0.42%	31	Kentucky	46	0.58%
1	New York		938	11.80%	32	Utah	44	0.55%
16	North Carolina		140	1.76%	33	South Carolina	40	0.50%
48	North Dakota		7	0.09%	34	Maine	36	0.45%
5	Ohio		490	6.17%	35	Nebraska	34	0.43%
27	Oklahoma		52	0.65%	36	New Mexico	33	0.42%
24	Oregon		61	0.77%	37	Nevada	28	0.35%
3	Pennsylvania		589	7.41%	38	West Virginia	26	0.33%
28	Rhode Island		50	0.63%	39	Delaware	25	0.31%
33	South Carolina		40	0.50%	40	New Hampshire	24	0.30%
46	South Dakota		14	0.18%	41	Arkansas	20	0.25%
21	Tennessee		90	1.13%	42	Mississippi	18	0.23%
9	Texas		382	4.81%	43	Idaho	17	0.21%
32	Utah		44	0.55%	44	Hawaii	16	0.20%
47	Vermont		9	0.11%	44	Montana	16	0.20%
13	Virginia		164	2.06%	46	South Dakota	14	0.18%
15	Washington		146	1.84%	47	Vermont	9	0.11%
38	West Virginia		26	0.33%	48	North Dakota	7	0.09%
19	Wisconsin		119	1.50%	49	Alaska	5	0.06%
49	Wyoming		5	0.06%	49	Wyoming	5	0.06%
						District of Columbia	32	0.40%

Source: U.S. Bureau of the Census
 "1992 Census of Service Industries, Geographic Area Series, United States" (SC92-A-52)
*Includes only establishments subject to the federal income tax.

IV. FINANCE

IV. FINANCE (Continued)

National Health Care Finance Data 1997

Total Health Care Expenditures = $1,092,400,000,000*

The 1993 health care expenditures broken down to the state level and shown in this book were released in the fall of 1995. The Health Care Financing Administration (HCFA) is committed to updating these numbers. Updates were expected in the summer of 1997 but difficulties inherent in allocating more than one trillion dollars in expenditures among the states have delayed the release of any updates a number of times. As we go to press in March of 1999, we are told that updates should be expected later this year.

Given the high level of interest in health care finance data, we have assembled a table showing the most recent national level health care expenditure data. We will continue to monitor HCFA data releases and will include the state expenditure updates in forthcoming editions. The percent change numbers are based on updated 1996 figures.

	EXPENDITURES IN 1997	PERCENT CHANGE: 1996 TO 1997
Total Health Care Expenditures	$1,092,400,000,000	4.8
Per Capita Total Health Care Expenditures	$4,080	3.8
Personal Health Care Expenditures	$969,000,000,000	4.9
Per Capita Personal Health Care Expenditures	$3,619	3.9
Hospital Care Expenditures	$371,100,000,000	2.9
Per Capita Hospital Care Expenditures	$1,386	1.8
Physician Services Expenditures	$217,600,000,000	4.4
Per Capita Physician Services Expenditures	$813	3.4
Dental Services Expenditures	$50,600,000,000	6.5
Per Capita Dental Services Expenditures	$189	5.6
Other Professional Services	$61,900,000,000	7.7
Per Capita Other Professional Services	$231	6.5
Home Health Care Expenditures	$32,300,000,000	3.5
Per Capita Home Health Care Expenditures	$121	2.5
Drugs and Other Medical Nondurables	$108,900,000,000	10.8
Per Capita Drugs and Other Medical Nondurables	$407	9.7
Vision Products and Other Medical Durables	$13,900,000,000	3.7
Per Capita Vision Products and Other Medical Durables	$52	2.0
Nursing Home Care	$82,800,000,000	4.3
Per Capita Nursing Home Care	$309	3.3
Other Personal Care Expenditures	$29,900,000,000	9.1
Per Capita Other Personal Care Expenditures	$112	8.7

Source: U.S. Department of Health and Human Services, Health Care Financing Administration
   "National Health Expenditures Aggregate Amounts and Average Annual Percent Change, by Type of Expenditure"
      (www.hcfa.gov/stats/nhe-oact/tables/t10.htm)
*Per Capita figures calculated by Morgan Quitno Press. For definitions see the corresponding 1993 state tables in this chapter.

Personal Health Care Expenditures in 1993

National Total = $778,510,000,000*

ALPHA ORDER					RANK ORDER			
RANK	STATE	EXPENDITURES	% of USA		RANK	STATE	EXPENDITURES	% of USA
23	Alabama	$12,060,000,000	1.55%		1	California	$94,178,000,000	12.10%
48	Alaska	1,573,000,000	0.20%		2	New York	67,033,000,000	8.61%
24	Arizona	10,635,000,000	1.37%		3	Texas	49,816,000,000	6.40%
33	Arkansas	6,111,000,000	0.78%		4	Florida	44,811,000,000	5.76%
1	California	94,178,000,000	12.10%		5	Pennsylvania	41,521,000,000	5.33%
26	Colorado	10,066,000,000	1.29%		6	Illinois	34,747,000,000	4.46%
22	Connecticut	12,216,000,000	1.57%		7	Ohio	33,456,000,000	4.30%
44	Delaware	2,260,000,000	0.29%		8	Michigan	27,136,000,000	3.49%
4	Florida	44,811,000,000	5.76%		9	New Jersey	25,741,000,000	3.31%
11	Georgia	20,104,000,000	2.58%		10	Massachusetts	23,421,000,000	3.01%
39	Hawaii	3,485,000,000	0.45%		11	Georgia	20,104,000,000	2.58%
43	Idaho	2,277,000,000	0.29%		12	North Carolina	18,241,000,000	2.34%
6	Illinois	34,747,000,000	4.46%		13	Virginia	16,682,000,000	2.14%
14	Indiana	16,401,000,000	2.11%		14	Indiana	16,401,000,000	2.11%
30	Iowa	7,341,000,000	0.94%		15	Tennessee	16,203,000,000	2.08%
31	Kansas	6,903,000,000	0.89%		16	Missouri	15,949,000,000	2.05%
25	Kentucky	10,384,000,000	1.33%		17	Maryland	15,154,000,000	1.95%
21	Louisiana	13,014,000,000	1.67%		18	Washington	15,129,000,000	1.94%
41	Maine	3,433,000,000	0.44%		19	Wisconsin	14,502,000,000	1.86%
17	Maryland	15,154,000,000	1.95%		20	Minnesota	14,194,000,000	1.82%
10	Massachusetts	23,421,000,000	3.01%		21	Louisiana	13,014,000,000	1.67%
8	Michigan	27,136,000,000	3.49%		22	Connecticut	12,216,000,000	1.57%
20	Minnesota	14,194,000,000	1.82%		23	Alabama	12,060,000,000	1.55%
32	Mississippi	6,187,000,000	0.79%		24	Arizona	10,635,000,000	1.37%
16	Missouri	15,949,000,000	2.05%		25	Kentucky	10,384,000,000	1.33%
45	Montana	2,103,000,000	0.27%		26	Colorado	10,066,000,000	1.29%
35	Nebraska	4,400,000,000	0.57%		27	South Carolina	9,029,000,000	1.16%
38	Nevada	3,747,000,000	0.48%		28	Oklahoma	8,041,000,000	1.03%
40	New Hampshire	3,452,000,000	0.44%		29	Oregon	7,999,000,000	1.03%
9	New Jersey	25,741,000,000	3.31%		30	Iowa	7,341,000,000	0.94%
37	New Mexico	3,878,000,000	0.50%		31	Kansas	6,903,000,000	0.89%
2	New York	67,033,000,000	8.61%		32	Mississippi	6,187,000,000	0.79%
12	North Carolina	18,241,000,000	2.34%		33	Arkansas	6,111,000,000	0.78%
46	North Dakota	2,021,000,000	0.26%		34	West Virginia	5,197,000,000	0.67%
7	Ohio	33,456,000,000	4.30%		35	Nebraska	4,400,000,000	0.57%
28	Oklahoma	8,041,000,000	1.03%		36	Utah	4,118,000,000	0.53%
29	Oregon	7,999,000,000	1.03%		37	New Mexico	3,878,000,000	0.50%
5	Pennsylvania	41,521,000,000	5.33%		38	Nevada	3,747,000,000	0.48%
42	Rhode Island	3,428,000,000	0.44%		39	Hawaii	3,485,000,000	0.45%
27	South Carolina	9,029,000,000	1.16%		40	New Hampshire	3,452,000,000	0.44%
47	South Dakota	1,953,000,000	0.25%		41	Maine	3,433,000,000	0.44%
15	Tennessee	16,203,000,000	2.08%		42	Rhode Island	3,428,000,000	0.44%
3	Texas	49,816,000,000	6.40%		43	Idaho	2,277,000,000	0.29%
36	Utah	4,118,000,000	0.53%		44	Delaware	2,260,000,000	0.29%
49	Vermont	1,499,000,000	0.19%		45	Montana	2,103,000,000	0.27%
13	Virginia	16,682,000,000	2.14%		46	North Dakota	2,021,000,000	0.26%
18	Washington	15,129,000,000	1.94%		47	South Dakota	1,953,000,000	0.25%
34	West Virginia	5,197,000,000	0.67%		48	Alaska	1,573,000,000	0.20%
19	Wisconsin	14,502,000,000	1.86%		49	Vermont	1,499,000,000	0.19%
50	Wyoming	998,000,000	0.13%		50	Wyoming	998,000,000	0.13%
						District of Columbia	4,285,000,000	0.55%

Source: U.S. Department of Health and Human Services, Health Care Financing Administration
"State Health Expenditure Accounts" (Health Care Financing Review, Fall 1995, Volume 17, Number 1)
By state of provider. Includes hospital care, physician services, dental services, home health care, drugs, vision products and other personal health care services and products.

Health Care Expenditures as a Percent of Gross State Product in 1993

National Percent = 12.1% of Total Gross State Product*

ALPHA ORDER

RANK	STATE	PERCENT
6	Alabama	14.6
50	Alaska	6.3
19	Arizona	12.6
13	Arkansas	13.1
36	California	11.2
40	Colorado	10.8
33	Connecticut	11.5
48	Delaware	9.3
3	Florida	15.0
30	Georgia	11.8
46	Hawaii	9.6
44	Idaho	10.2
37	Illinois	11.1
16	Indiana	12.9
28	Iowa	11.9
28	Kansas	11.9
16	Kentucky	12.9
8	Louisiana	13.8
9	Maine	13.7
25	Maryland	12.2
10	Massachusetts	13.4
21	Michigan	12.5
22	Minnesota	12.3
10	Mississippi	13.4
10	Missouri	13.4
15	Montana	13.0
33	Nebraska	11.5
47	Nevada	9.5
18	New Hampshire	12.7
43	New Jersey	10.5
35	New Mexico	11.3
22	New York	12.3
40	North Carolina	10.8
2	North Dakota	16.0
13	Ohio	13.1
19	Oklahoma	12.6
32	Oregon	11.6
4	Pennsylvania	14.7
4	Rhode Island	14.7
27	South Carolina	12.0
26	South Dakota	12.1
7	Tennessee	14.0
37	Texas	11.1
40	Utah	10.8
30	Vermont	11.8
45	Virginia	9.8
37	Washington	11.1
1	West Virginia	16.2
22	Wisconsin	12.3
49	Wyoming	6.7

RANK ORDER

RANK	STATE	PERCENT
1	West Virginia	16.2
2	North Dakota	16.0
3	Florida	15.0
4	Pennsylvania	14.7
4	Rhode Island	14.7
6	Alabama	14.6
7	Tennessee	14.0
8	Louisiana	13.8
9	Maine	13.7
10	Massachusetts	13.4
10	Mississippi	13.4
10	Missouri	13.4
13	Arkansas	13.1
13	Ohio	13.1
15	Montana	13.0
16	Indiana	12.9
16	Kentucky	12.9
18	New Hampshire	12.7
19	Arizona	12.6
19	Oklahoma	12.6
21	Michigan	12.5
22	Minnesota	12.3
22	New York	12.3
22	Wisconsin	12.3
25	Maryland	12.2
26	South Dakota	12.1
27	South Carolina	12.0
28	Iowa	11.9
28	Kansas	11.9
30	Georgia	11.8
30	Vermont	11.8
32	Oregon	11.6
33	Connecticut	11.5
33	Nebraska	11.5
35	New Mexico	11.3
36	California	11.2
37	Illinois	11.1
37	Texas	11.1
37	Washington	11.1
40	Colorado	10.8
40	North Carolina	10.8
40	Utah	10.8
43	New Jersey	10.5
44	Idaho	10.2
45	Virginia	9.8
46	Hawaii	9.6
47	Nevada	9.5
48	Delaware	9.3
49	Wyoming	6.7
50	Alaska	6.3

District of Columbia 9.1

Source: Morgan Quitno Press using data from U.S. Dept of Health & Human Services, Health Care Financing Admin. "State Health Expenditure Accounts" (Health Care Financing Review, Fall 1995, Volume 17, Number 1)
*By state of provider. Includes hospital care, physician services, dental services, home health care, drugs, vision products and other personal health care services and products.

Per Capita Personal Health Care Expenditures in 1993

National Per Capita = $3,020*

ALPHA ORDER			RANK ORDER		
RANK	STATE	PER CAPITA	RANK	STATE	PER CAPITA
21	Alabama	$2,884	1	Massachusetts	$3,892
37	Alaska	2,630	2	Connecticut	3,727
35	Arizona	2,697	3	New York	3,693
42	Arkansas	2,520	4	Pennsylvania	3,451
17	California	3,017	5	Rhode Island	3,431
27	Colorado	2,821	6	New Jersey	3,275
2	Connecticut	3,727	7	Florida	3,266
8	Delaware	3,233	8	Delaware	3,233
7	Florida	3,266	9	Tennessee	3,181
20	Georgia	2,913	10	North Dakota	3,173
18	Hawaii	2,989	11	Minnesota	3,137
50	Idaho	2,068	12	New Hampshire	3,074
19	Illinois	2,972	13	Maryland	3,060
24	Indiana	2,874	14	Missouri	3,047
40	Iowa	2,601	15	Louisiana	3,034
31	Kansas	2,726	16	Ohio	3,025
30	Kentucky	2,738	17	California	3,017
15	Louisiana	3,034	18	Hawaii	2,989
28	Maine	2,771	19	Illinois	2,972
13	Maryland	3,060	20	Georgia	2,913
1	Massachusetts	3,892	21	Alabama	2,884
25	Michigan	2,869	22	Washington	2,879
11	Minnesota	3,137	23	Wisconsin	2,875
47	Mississippi	2,344	24	Indiana	2,874
14	Missouri	3,047	25	Michigan	2,869
43	Montana	2,501	26	West Virginia	2,859
31	Nebraska	2,726	27	Colorado	2,821
34	Nevada	2,705	28	Maine	2,771
12	New Hampshire	3,074	29	Texas	2,760
6	New Jersey	3,275	30	Kentucky	2,738
46	New Mexico	2,400	31	Kansas	2,726
3	New York	3,693	31	Nebraska	2,726
38	North Carolina	2,623	33	South Dakota	2,724
10	North Dakota	3,173	34	Nevada	2,705
16	Ohio	3,025	35	Arizona	2,697
45	Oklahoma	2,488	36	Oregon	2,636
36	Oregon	2,636	37	Alaska	2,630
4	Pennsylvania	3,451	38	North Carolina	2,623
5	Rhode Island	3,431	39	Vermont	2,602
44	South Carolina	2,489	40	Iowa	2,601
33	South Dakota	2,724	41	Virginia	2,576
9	Tennessee	3,181	42	Arkansas	2,520
29	Texas	2,760	43	Montana	2,501
48	Utah	2,214	44	South Carolina	2,489
39	Vermont	2,602	45	Oklahoma	2,488
41	Virginia	2,576	46	New Mexico	2,400
22	Washington	2,879	47	Mississippi	2,344
26	West Virginia	2,859	48	Utah	2,214
23	Wisconsin	2,875	49	Wyoming	2,123
49	Wyoming	2,123	50	Idaho	2,068
				District of Columbia	7,413

Source: Morgan Quitno Press using data from U.S. Dept of Health & Human Services, Health Care Financing Admin. "State Health Expenditure Accounts" (Health Care Financing Review, Fall 1995, Volume 17, Number 1)
*By state of provider. Includes hospital care, physician services, dental services, home health care, drugs, vision products and other personal health care services and products.

Percent Change in Personal Health Care Expenditures: 1990 to 1993

National Percent Change = 28.0% Increase*

ALPHA ORDER

RANK	STATE	PERCENT CHANGE
13	Alabama	31.7
32	Alaska	27.0
41	Arizona	25.4
37	Arkansas	26.1
30	California	27.1
20	Colorado	30.3
48	Connecticut	22.5
12	Delaware	32.2
28	Florida	27.6
15	Georgia	31.5
29	Hawaii	27.5
1	Idaho	37.4
34	Illinois	26.7
19	Indiana	30.7
50	Iowa	21.9
43	Kansas	25.3
11	Kentucky	32.7
14	Louisiana	31.6
30	Maine	27.1
27	Maryland	28.0
49	Massachusetts	22.2
46	Michigan	23.5
47	Minnesota	23.3
16	Mississippi	31.2
34	Missouri	26.7
17	Montana	30.9
36	Nebraska	26.5
3	Nevada	35.4
2	New Hampshire	36.9
23	New Jersey	29.0
6	New Mexico	34.0
44	New York	24.8
8	North Carolina	33.1
44	North Dakota	24.8
41	Ohio	25.4
24	Oklahoma	28.1
20	Oregon	30.3
24	Pennsylvania	28.1
40	Rhode Island	25.5
5	South Carolina	34.8
18	South Dakota	30.8
8	Tennessee	33.1
7	Texas	33.7
22	Utah	29.9
33	Vermont	26.8
38	Virginia	25.9
3	Washington	35.4
8	West Virginia	33.1
24	Wisconsin	28.1
39	Wyoming	25.7

RANK ORDER

RANK	STATE	PERCENT CHANGE
1	Idaho	37.4
2	New Hampshire	36.9
3	Nevada	35.4
3	Washington	35.4
5	South Carolina	34.8
6	New Mexico	34.0
7	Texas	33.7
8	North Carolina	33.1
8	Tennessee	33.1
8	West Virginia	33.1
11	Kentucky	32.7
12	Delaware	32.2
13	Alabama	31.7
14	Louisiana	31.6
15	Georgia	31.5
16	Mississippi	31.2
17	Montana	30.9
18	South Dakota	30.8
19	Indiana	30.7
20	Colorado	30.3
20	Oregon	30.3
22	Utah	29.9
23	New Jersey	29.0
24	Oklahoma	28.1
24	Pennsylvania	28.1
24	Wisconsin	28.1
27	Maryland	28.0
28	Florida	27.6
29	Hawaii	27.5
30	California	27.1
30	Maine	27.1
32	Alaska	27.0
33	Vermont	26.8
34	Illinois	26.7
34	Missouri	26.7
36	Nebraska	26.5
37	Arkansas	26.1
38	Virginia	25.9
39	Wyoming	25.7
40	Rhode Island	25.5
41	Arizona	25.4
41	Ohio	25.4
43	Kansas	25.3
44	New York	24.8
44	North Dakota	24.8
46	Michigan	23.5
47	Minnesota	23.3
48	Connecticut	22.5
49	Massachusetts	22.2
50	Iowa	21.9

District of Columbia — 21.2

Source: Morgan Quitno Press using data from U.S. Dept of Health & Human Services, Health Care Financing Admin.
"State Health Expenditure Accounts" (Health Care Financing Review, Fall 1995, Volume 17, Number 1)
*By state of provider. Includes hospital care, physician services, dental services, home health care, drugs, vision products and other personal health care services and products.

Percent Change in Per Capita Expenditures for
Personal Health Care: 1990 to 1993
National Percent Change = 23.5% Increase*

ALPHA ORDER

RANK ORDER

RANK	STATE	PERCENT CHANGE
8	Alabama	27.2
49	Alaska	16.7
50	Arizona	16.6
35	Arkansas	22.2
41	California	21.1
42	Colorado	20.3
33	Connecticut	22.8
16	Delaware	25.9
42	Florida	20.3
31	Georgia	23.4
40	Hawaii	21.2
18	Idaho	25.7
26	Illinois	23.9
11	Indiana	26.9
46	Iowa	20.0
34	Kansas	22.6
5	Kentucky	29.0
3	Louisiana	29.5
14	Maine	26.0
30	Maryland	23.6
36	Massachusetts	22.1
38	Michigan	21.4
47	Minnesota	19.3
6	Mississippi	28.0
27	Missouri	23.8
23	Montana	24.4
28	Nebraska	23.7
48	Nevada	17.5
1	New Hampshire	35.2
11	New Jersey	26.9
19	New Mexico	25.6
28	New York	23.7
9	North Carolina	27.0
21	North Dakota	25.2
32	Ohio	23.0
22	Oklahoma	24.6
36	Oregon	22.1
13	Pennsylvania	26.5
14	Rhode Island	26.0
3	South Carolina	29.5
9	South Dakota	27.0
7	Tennessee	27.4
17	Texas	25.8
42	Utah	20.3
25	Vermont	24.0
42	Virginia	20.3
20	Washington	25.4
2	West Virginia	31.3
24	Wisconsin	24.2
38	Wyoming	21.4

RANK	STATE	PERCENT CHANGE
1	New Hampshire	35.2
2	West Virginia	31.3
3	Louisiana	29.5
3	South Carolina	29.5
5	Kentucky	29.0
6	Mississippi	28.0
7	Tennessee	27.4
8	Alabama	27.2
9	North Carolina	27.0
9	South Dakota	27.0
11	Indiana	26.9
11	New Jersey	26.9
13	Pennsylvania	26.5
14	Maine	26.0
14	Rhode Island	26.0
16	Delaware	25.9
17	Texas	25.8
18	Idaho	25.7
19	New Mexico	25.6
20	Washington	25.4
21	North Dakota	25.2
22	Oklahoma	24.6
23	Montana	24.4
24	Wisconsin	24.2
25	Vermont	24.0
26	Illinois	23.9
27	Missouri	23.8
28	Nebraska	23.7
28	New York	23.7
30	Maryland	23.6
31	Georgia	23.4
32	Ohio	23.0
33	Connecticut	22.8
34	Kansas	22.6
35	Arkansas	22.2
36	Massachusetts	22.1
36	Oregon	22.1
38	Michigan	21.4
38	Wyoming	21.4
40	Hawaii	21.2
41	California	21.1
42	Colorado	20.3
42	Florida	20.3
42	Utah	20.3
42	Virginia	20.3
46	Iowa	20.0
47	Minnesota	19.3
48	Nevada	17.5
49	Alaska	16.7
50	Arizona	16.6

District of Columbia   27.3

*Source: Morgan Quitno Press using data from U.S. Dept of Health & Human Services, Health Care Financing Admin.
"State Health Expenditure Accounts" (Health Care Financing Review, Fall 1995, Volume 17, Number 1)
By state of provider. Includes hospital care, physician services, dental services, home health care, drugs, vision products and other personal health care services and products.

Average Annual Change in Expenditures for Personal Health Care: 1980 to 1993
National Percent = 10.3% Average Annual Growth*

ALPHA ORDER

RANK	STATE	PERCENT
16	Alabama	10.9
27	Alaska	10.2
5	Arizona	11.9
32	Arkansas	10.1
27	California	10.2
23	Colorado	10.5
15	Connecticut	11.0
9	Delaware	11.3
2	Florida	12.4
4	Georgia	12.1
19	Hawaii	10.8
24	Idaho	10.4
47	Illinois	8.7
26	Indiana	10.3
50	Iowa	8.3
45	Kansas	9.0
16	Kentucky	10.9
24	Louisiana	10.4
21	Maine	10.6
21	Maryland	10.6
27	Massachusetts	10.2
49	Michigan	8.5
37	Minnesota	9.7
32	Mississippi	10.1
39	Missouri	9.6
35	Montana	9.8
46	Nebraska	8.9
3	Nevada	12.2
1	New Hampshire	13.0
10	New Jersey	11.2
8	New Mexico	11.7
37	New York	9.7
5	North Carolina	11.9
43	North Dakota	9.4
39	Ohio	9.6
44	Oklahoma	9.1
34	Oregon	9.9
27	Pennsylvania	10.2
27	Rhode Island	10.2
5	South Carolina	11.9
35	South Dakota	9.8
10	Tennessee	11.2
12	Texas	11.1
12	Utah	11.1
19	Vermont	10.8
16	Virginia	10.9
12	Washington	11.1
39	West Virginia	9.6
42	Wisconsin	9.5
47	Wyoming	8.7

RANK ORDER

RANK	STATE	PERCENT
1	New Hampshire	13.0
2	Florida	12.4
3	Nevada	12.2
4	Georgia	12.1
5	Arizona	11.9
5	North Carolina	11.9
5	South Carolina	11.9
8	New Mexico	11.7
9	Delaware	11.3
10	New Jersey	11.2
10	Tennessee	11.2
12	Texas	11.1
12	Utah	11.1
12	Washington	11.1
15	Connecticut	11.0
16	Alabama	10.9
16	Kentucky	10.9
16	Virginia	10.9
19	Hawaii	10.8
19	Vermont	10.8
21	Maine	10.6
21	Maryland	10.6
23	Colorado	10.5
24	Idaho	10.4
24	Louisiana	10.4
26	Indiana	10.3
27	Alaska	10.2
27	California	10.2
27	Massachusetts	10.2
27	Pennsylvania	10.2
27	Rhode Island	10.2
32	Arkansas	10.1
32	Mississippi	10.1
34	Oregon	9.9
35	Montana	9.8
35	South Dakota	9.8
37	Minnesota	9.7
37	New York	9.7
39	Missouri	9.6
39	Ohio	9.6
39	West Virginia	9.6
42	Wisconsin	9.5
43	North Dakota	9.4
44	Oklahoma	9.1
45	Kansas	9.0
46	Nebraska	8.9
47	Illinois	8.7
47	Wyoming	8.7
49	Michigan	8.5
50	Iowa	8.3
	District of Columbia	9.1

Source: U.S. Department of Health and Human Services, Health Care Financing Administration
   "State Health Expenditure Accounts" (Health Care Financing Review, Fall 1995, Volume 17, Number 1)
*By state of provider. Includes hospital care, physician services, dental services, home health care, drugs, vision products and other personal health care services and products.

Average Annual Change in Per Capita Expenditures
For Personal Health Care: 1980 to 1993
National Percent = 9.3% Average Annual Increase*

ALPHA ORDER

RANK	STATE	PERCENT
7	Alabama	10.3
50	Alaska	6.8
38	Arizona	8.8
21	Arkansas	9.6
48	California	7.9
38	Colorado	8.8
5	Connecticut	10.5
13	Delaware	10.0
23	Florida	9.5
11	Georgia	10.1
30	Hawaii	9.2
31	Idaho	9.1
45	Illinois	8.5
13	Indiana	10.0
42	Iowa	8.6
46	Kansas	8.4
3	Kentucky	10.6
7	Louisiana	10.3
16	Maine	9.8
27	Maryland	9.3
16	Massachusetts	9.8
46	Michigan	8.4
37	Minnesota	8.9
19	Mississippi	9.7
31	Missouri	9.1
27	Montana	9.3
42	Nebraska	8.6
49	Nevada	7.6
1	New Hampshire	11.3
2	New Jersey	10.7
15	New Mexico	9.9
25	New York	9.4
5	North Carolina	10.5
21	North Dakota	9.6
25	Ohio	9.4
42	Oklahoma	8.6
40	Oregon	8.7
11	Pennsylvania	10.1
19	Rhode Island	9.7
3	South Carolina	10.6
23	South Dakota	9.5
7	Tennessee	10.3
31	Texas	9.1
35	Utah	9.0
16	Vermont	9.8
27	Virginia	9.3
31	Washington	9.1
10	West Virginia	10.2
35	Wisconsin	9.0
40	Wyoming	8.7

RANK ORDER

RANK	STATE	PERCENT
1	New Hampshire	11.3
2	New Jersey	10.7
3	Kentucky	10.6
3	South Carolina	10.6
5	Connecticut	10.5
5	North Carolina	10.5
7	Alabama	10.3
7	Louisiana	10.3
7	Tennessee	10.3
10	West Virginia	10.2
11	Georgia	10.1
11	Pennsylvania	10.1
13	Delaware	10.0
13	Indiana	10.0
15	New Mexico	9.9
16	Maine	9.8
16	Massachusetts	9.8
16	Vermont	9.8
19	Mississippi	9.7
19	Rhode Island	9.7
21	Arkansas	9.6
21	North Dakota	9.6
23	Florida	9.5
23	South Dakota	9.5
25	New York	9.4
25	Ohio	9.4
27	Maryland	9.3
27	Montana	9.3
27	Virginia	9.3
30	Hawaii	9.2
31	Idaho	9.1
31	Missouri	9.1
31	Texas	9.1
31	Washington	9.1
35	Utah	9.0
35	Wisconsin	9.0
37	Minnesota	8.9
38	Arizona	8.8
38	Colorado	8.8
40	Oregon	8.7
40	Wyoming	8.7
42	Iowa	8.6
42	Nebraska	8.6
42	Oklahoma	8.6
45	Illinois	8.5
46	Kansas	8.4
46	Michigan	8.4
48	California	7.9
49	Nevada	7.6
50	Alaska	6.8

| | District of Columbia | 9.9 |

Source: Morgan Quitno Press using data from U.S. Dept of Health & Human Services, Health Care Financing Admin.
"State Health Expenditure Accounts" (Health Care Financing Review, Fall 1995, Volume 17, Number 1)
*By state of provider. Includes hospital care, physician services, dental services, home health care, drugs, vision products and other personal health care services and products.

Expenditures for Hospital Care in 1993

National Total = $323,919,000,000*

ALPHA ORDER

RANK	STATE	EXPENDITURES	% of USA
21	Alabama	$5,301,000,000	1.64%
48	Alaska	701,000,000	0.22%
26	Arizona	3,999,000,000	1.24%
33	Arkansas	2,723,000,000	0.84%
1	California	34,827,000,000	10.77%
27	Colorado	3,932,000,000	1.22%
24	Connecticut	4,380,000,000	1.35%
43	Delaware	937,000,000	0.29%
5	Florida	17,131,000,000	5.30%
11	Georgia	8,704,000,000	2.69%
38	Hawaii	1,460,000,000	0.45%
46	Idaho	900,000,000	0.28%
6	Illinois	15,621,000,000	4.83%
16	Indiana	6,998,000,000	2.16%
29	Iowa	3,111,000,000	0.96%
32	Kansas	2,868,000,000	0.89%
23	Kentucky	4,515,000,000	1.40%
17	Louisiana	5,956,000,000	1.84%
40	Maine	1,376,000,000	0.43%
18	Maryland	5,926,000,000	1.83%
10	Massachusetts	10,034,000,000	3.10%
8	Michigan	11,711,000,000	3.62%
22	Minnesota	4,796,000,000	1.48%
31	Mississippi	2,897,000,000	0.90%
13	Missouri	7,652,000,000	2.37%
47	Montana	894,000,000	0.28%
35	Nebraska	2,003,000,000	0.62%
41	Nevada	1,362,000,000	0.42%
39	New Hampshire	1,388,000,000	0.43%
9	New Jersey	10,312,000,000	3.19%
36	New Mexico	1,848,000,000	0.57%
2	New York	28,001,000,000	8.66%
12	North Carolina	7,801,000,000	2.41%
45	North Dakota	903,000,000	0.28%
7	Ohio	14,305,000,000	4.42%
28	Oklahoma	3,329,000,000	1.03%
30	Oregon	2,966,000,000	0.92%
4	Pennsylvania	19,540,000,000	6.04%
42	Rhode Island	1,314,000,000	0.41%
25	South Carolina	4,221,000,000	1.30%
44	South Dakota	920,000,000	0.28%
14	Tennessee	7,208,000,000	2.23%
3	Texas	21,592,000,000	6.68%
37	Utah	1,743,000,000	0.54%
49	Vermont	562,000,000	0.17%
15	Virginia	7,031,000,000	2.17%
20	Washington	5,305,000,000	1.64%
34	West Virginia	2,346,000,000	0.73%
19	Wisconsin	5,537,000,000	1.71%
50	Wyoming	417,000,000	0.13%

RANK ORDER

RANK	STATE	EXPENDITURES	% of USA
1	California	$34,827,000,000	10.77%
2	New York	28,001,000,000	8.66%
3	Texas	21,592,000,000	6.68%
4	Pennsylvania	19,540,000,000	6.04%
5	Florida	17,131,000,000	5.30%
6	Illinois	15,621,000,000	4.83%
7	Ohio	14,305,000,000	4.42%
8	Michigan	11,711,000,000	3.62%
9	New Jersey	10,312,000,000	3.19%
10	Massachusetts	10,034,000,000	3.10%
11	Georgia	8,704,000,000	2.69%
12	North Carolina	7,801,000,000	2.41%
13	Missouri	7,652,000,000	2.37%
14	Tennessee	7,208,000,000	2.23%
15	Virginia	7,031,000,000	2.17%
16	Indiana	6,998,000,000	2.16%
17	Louisiana	5,956,000,000	1.84%
18	Maryland	5,926,000,000	1.83%
19	Wisconsin	5,537,000,000	1.71%
20	Washington	5,305,000,000	1.64%
21	Alabama	5,301,000,000	1.64%
22	Minnesota	4,796,000,000	1.48%
23	Kentucky	4,515,000,000	1.40%
24	Connecticut	4,380,000,000	1.35%
25	South Carolina	4,221,000,000	1.30%
26	Arizona	3,999,000,000	1.24%
27	Colorado	3,932,000,000	1.22%
28	Oklahoma	3,329,000,000	1.03%
29	Iowa	3,111,000,000	0.96%
30	Oregon	2,966,000,000	0.92%
31	Mississippi	2,897,000,000	0.90%
32	Kansas	2,868,000,000	0.89%
33	Arkansas	2,723,000,000	0.84%
34	West Virginia	2,346,000,000	0.73%
35	Nebraska	2,003,000,000	0.62%
36	New Mexico	1,848,000,000	0.57%
37	Utah	1,743,000,000	0.54%
38	Hawaii	1,460,000,000	0.45%
39	New Hampshire	1,388,000,000	0.43%
40	Maine	1,376,000,000	0.43%
41	Nevada	1,362,000,000	0.42%
42	Rhode Island	1,314,000,000	0.41%
43	Delaware	937,000,000	0.29%
44	South Dakota	920,000,000	0.28%
45	North Dakota	903,000,000	0.28%
46	Idaho	900,000,000	0.28%
47	Montana	894,000,000	0.28%
48	Alaska	701,000,000	0.22%
49	Vermont	562,000,000	0.17%
50	Wyoming	417,000,000	0.13%
	District of Columbia	2,612,000,000	0.81%

Source: U.S. Department of Health and Human Services, Health Care Financing Administration
"State Health Expenditure Accounts" (Health Care Financing Review, Fall 1995, Volume 17, Number 1)
*By state of provider.

Percent of Total Personal Health Care Expenditures
Spent on Hospital Care in 1993
National Percent = 41.6%*

ALPHA ORDER

RANK	STATE	PERCENT
15	Alabama	44.0
12	Alaska	44.6
43	Arizona	37.6
12	Arkansas	44.6
46	California	37.0
38	Colorado	39.1
48	Connecticut	35.9
31	Delaware	41.5
41	Florida	38.2
17	Georgia	43.3
28	Hawaii	41.9
37	Idaho	39.5
10	Illinois	45.0
23	Indiana	42.7
25	Iowa	42.4
31	Kansas	41.5
16	Kentucky	43.5
7	Louisiana	45.8
35	Maine	40.1
38	Maryland	39.1
20	Massachusetts	42.8
19	Michigan	43.2
50	Minnesota	33.8
5	Mississippi	46.8
1	Missouri	48.0
24	Montana	42.5
8	Nebraska	45.5
47	Nevada	36.3
34	New Hampshire	40.2
35	New Jersey	40.1
2	New Mexico	47.7
29	New York	41.8
20	North Carolina	42.8
11	North Dakota	44.7
20	Ohio	42.8
33	Oklahoma	41.4
45	Oregon	37.1
3	Pennsylvania	47.1
40	Rhode Island	38.3
6	South Carolina	46.7
3	South Dakota	47.1
14	Tennessee	44.5
17	Texas	43.3
26	Utah	42.3
44	Vermont	37.5
27	Virginia	42.1
49	Washington	35.1
9	West Virginia	45.1
41	Wisconsin	38.2
29	Wyoming	41.8

RANK ORDER

RANK	STATE	PERCENT
1	Missouri	48.0
2	New Mexico	47.7
3	Pennsylvania	47.1
3	South Dakota	47.1
5	Mississippi	46.8
6	South Carolina	46.7
7	Louisiana	45.8
8	Nebraska	45.5
9	West Virginia	45.1
10	Illinois	45.0
11	North Dakota	44.7
12	Alaska	44.6
12	Arkansas	44.6
14	Tennessee	44.5
15	Alabama	44.0
16	Kentucky	43.5
17	Georgia	43.3
17	Texas	43.3
19	Michigan	43.2
20	Massachusetts	42.8
20	North Carolina	42.8
20	Ohio	42.8
23	Indiana	42.7
24	Montana	42.5
25	Iowa	42.4
26	Utah	42.3
27	Virginia	42.1
28	Hawaii	41.9
29	New York	41.8
29	Wyoming	41.8
31	Delaware	41.5
31	Kansas	41.5
33	Oklahoma	41.4
34	New Hampshire	40.2
35	Maine	40.1
35	New Jersey	40.1
37	Idaho	39.5
38	Colorado	39.1
38	Maryland	39.1
40	Rhode Island	38.3
41	Florida	38.2
41	Wisconsin	38.2
43	Arizona	37.6
44	Vermont	37.5
45	Oregon	37.1
46	California	37.0
47	Nevada	36.3
48	Connecticut	35.9
49	Washington	35.1
50	Minnesota	33.8

District of Columbia   61.0

Source: Morgan Quitno Press using data from U.S. Dept of Health & Human Services, Health Care Financing Admin.
"State Health Expenditure Accounts" (Health Care Financing Review, Fall 1995, Volume 17, Number 1)
*By state of provider.

Per Capita Expenditures for Hospital Care in 1993

National Per Capita = $1,256*

ALPHA ORDER

ALPHA ORDER

RANK	STATE	PER CAPITA		RANK	STATE	PER CAPITA
16	Alabama	$1,268		1	Massachusetts	$1,667
27	Alaska	1,172		2	Pennsylvania	1,624
43	Arizona	1,014		3	New York	1,542
31	Arkansas	1,123		4	Missouri	1,462
33	California	1,116		5	North Dakota	1,418
35	Colorado	1,102		6	Tennessee	1,415
9	Connecticut	1,336		7	Louisiana	1,389
8	Delaware	1,340		8	Delaware	1,340
19	Florida	1,248		9	Connecticut	1,336
17	Georgia	1,261		9	Illinois	1,336
18	Hawaii	1,252		11	Rhode Island	1,315
50	Idaho	817		12	New Jersey	1,312
9	Illinois	1,336		13	Ohio	1,293
23	Indiana	1,226		14	West Virginia	1,290
35	Iowa	1,102		15	South Dakota	1,283
30	Kansas	1,133		16	Alabama	1,268
26	Kentucky	1,190		17	Georgia	1,261
7	Louisiana	1,389		18	Hawaii	1,252
34	Maine	1,111		19	Florida	1,248
24	Maryland	1,197		20	Nebraska	1,241
1	Massachusetts	1,667		21	Michigan	1,238
21	Michigan	1,238		22	New Hampshire	1,236
41	Minnesota	1,060		23	Indiana	1,226
37	Mississippi	1,098		24	Maryland	1,197
4	Missouri	1,462		25	Texas	1,196
40	Montana	1,063		26	Kentucky	1,190
20	Nebraska	1,241		27	Alaska	1,172
45	Nevada	983		28	South Carolina	1,164
22	New Hampshire	1,236		29	New Mexico	1,144
12	New Jersey	1,312		30	Kansas	1,133
29	New Mexico	1,144		31	Arkansas	1,123
3	New York	1,542		32	North Carolina	1,122
32	North Carolina	1,122		33	California	1,116
5	North Dakota	1,418		34	Maine	1,111
13	Ohio	1,293		35	Colorado	1,102
42	Oklahoma	1,030		35	Iowa	1,102
46	Oregon	977		37	Mississippi	1,098
2	Pennsylvania	1,624		37	Wisconsin	1,098
11	Rhode Island	1,315		39	Virginia	1,086
28	South Carolina	1,164		40	Montana	1,063
15	South Dakota	1,283		41	Minnesota	1,060
6	Tennessee	1,415		42	Oklahoma	1,030
25	Texas	1,196		43	Arizona	1,014
48	Utah	937		44	Washington	1,010
47	Vermont	976		45	Nevada	983
39	Virginia	1,086		46	Oregon	977
44	Washington	1,010		47	Vermont	976
14	West Virginia	1,290		48	Utah	937
37	Wisconsin	1,098		49	Wyoming	887
49	Wyoming	887		50	Idaho	817

District of Columbia** 4,519

Source: Morgan Quitno Press using data from U.S. Dept of Health & Human Services, Health Care Financing Admin.
"State Health Expenditure Accounts" (Health Care Financing Review, Fall 1995, Volume 17, Number 1)
By state of provider.
**The District of Columbia's per capita is greatly affected by residents of Maryland and Virginia receiving services.

Percent Change in Expenditures for Hospital Care: 1990 to 1993

National Percent Change = 27.4% Increase*

ALPHA ORDER

RANK	STATE	PERCENT
12	Alabama	32.0
33	Alaska	25.9
40	Arizona	24.3
22	Arkansas	29.1
38	California	24.6
29	Colorado	26.8
47	Connecticut	19.5
10	Delaware	32.2
26	Florida	27.3
21	Georgia	30.2
28	Hawaii	27.2
4	Idaho	35.3
32	Illinois	26.0
9	Indiana	32.3
48	Iowa	18.1
37	Kansas	24.7
15	Kentucky	31.4
24	Louisiana	28.7
44	Maine	23.0
26	Maryland	27.3
44	Massachusetts	23.0
42	Michigan	23.3
50	Minnesota	17.1
8	Mississippi	32.5
25	Missouri	27.8
13	Montana	31.7
31	Nebraska	26.2
20	Nevada	30.6
15	New Hampshire	31.4
18	New Jersey	31.2
2	New Mexico	35.5
43	New York	23.1
10	North Carolina	32.2
33	North Dakota	25.9
36	Ohio	25.3
39	Oklahoma	24.5
22	Oregon	29.1
15	Pennsylvania	31.4
46	Rhode Island	20.0
1	South Carolina	35.8
7	South Dakota	32.6
19	Tennessee	30.8
2	Texas	35.5
14	Utah	31.5
35	Vermont	25.7
41	Virginia	24.2
5	Washington	33.9
6	West Virginia	33.1
30	Wisconsin	26.5
48	Wyoming	18.1

RANK ORDER

RANK	STATE	PERCENT
1	South Carolina	35.8
2	New Mexico	35.5
2	Texas	35.5
4	Idaho	35.3
5	Washington	33.9
6	West Virginia	33.1
7	South Dakota	32.6
8	Mississippi	32.5
9	Indiana	32.3
10	Delaware	32.2
10	North Carolina	32.2
12	Alabama	32.0
13	Montana	31.7
14	Utah	31.5
15	Kentucky	31.4
15	New Hampshire	31.4
15	Pennsylvania	31.4
18	New Jersey	31.2
19	Tennessee	30.8
20	Nevada	30.6
21	Georgia	30.2
22	Arkansas	29.1
22	Oregon	29.1
24	Louisiana	28.7
25	Missouri	27.8
26	Florida	27.3
26	Maryland	27.3
28	Hawaii	27.2
29	Colorado	26.8
30	Wisconsin	26.5
31	Nebraska	26.2
32	Illinois	26.0
33	Alaska	25.9
33	North Dakota	25.9
35	Vermont	25.7
36	Ohio	25.3
37	Kansas	24.7
38	California	24.6
39	Oklahoma	24.5
40	Arizona	24.3
41	Virginia	24.2
42	Michigan	23.3
43	New York	23.1
44	Maine	23.0
44	Massachusetts	23.0
46	Rhode Island	20.0
47	Connecticut	19.5
48	Iowa	18.1
48	Wyoming	18.1
50	Minnesota	17.1

District of Columbia   22.5

Source: Morgan Quitno Press using data from U.S. Dept of Health & Human Services, Health Care Financing Admin.
"State Health Expenditure Accounts" (Health Care Financing Review, Fall 1995, Volume 17, Number 1)
*By state of provider.

Percent Change in Per Capita Expenditures for Hospital Care: 1990 to 1993

National Percent Change = 22.9% Increase*

ALPHA ORDER				RANK ORDER		
RANK	STATE	PERCENT CHANGE		RANK	STATE	PERCENT CHANGE
10	Alabama	27.6		1	West Virginia	31.2
46	Alaska	15.7		2	South Carolina	30.5
47	Arizona	15.5		3	New Hampshire	29.8
17	Arkansas	25.2		4	Pennsylvania	29.7
42	California	18.8		5	Mississippi	29.3
44	Colorado	17.1		6	New Jersey	29.1
41	Connecticut	19.8		7	South Dakota	28.7
16	Delaware	25.8		8	Indiana	28.5
40	Florida	19.9		9	Kentucky	27.7
30	Georgia	22.2		10	Alabama	27.6
38	Hawaii	20.8		11	Texas	27.5
22	Idaho	23.8		12	New Mexico	27.1
24	Illinois	23.1		13	Louisiana	26.7
8	Indiana	28.5		14	North Dakota	26.4
45	Iowa	16.1		15	North Carolina	26.1
31	Kansas	22.1		16	Delaware	25.8
9	Kentucky	27.7		17	Arkansas	25.2
13	Louisiana	26.7		17	Tennessee	25.2
32	Maine	22.0		19	Montana	25.1
25	Maryland	22.9		20	Missouri	25.0
25	Massachusetts	22.9		21	Washington	24.1
36	Michigan	21.1		22	Idaho	23.8
49	Minnesota	13.2		23	Nebraska	23.4
5	Mississippi	29.3		24	Illinois	23.1
20	Missouri	25.0		25	Maryland	22.9
19	Montana	25.1		25	Massachusetts	22.9
23	Nebraska	23.4		25	Vermont	22.9
49	Nevada	13.2		28	Ohio	22.8
3	New Hampshire	29.8		29	Wisconsin	22.7
6	New Jersey	29.1		30	Georgia	22.2
12	New Mexico	27.1		31	Kansas	22.1
32	New York	22.0		32	Maine	22.0
15	North Carolina	26.1		32	New York	22.0
14	North Dakota	26.4		34	Utah	21.8
28	Ohio	22.8		35	Oklahoma	21.2
35	Oklahoma	21.2		36	Michigan	21.1
37	Oregon	20.9		37	Oregon	20.9
4	Pennsylvania	29.7		38	Hawaii	20.8
39	Rhode Island	20.4		39	Rhode Island	20.4
2	South Carolina	30.5		40	Florida	19.9
7	South Dakota	28.7		41	Connecticut	19.8
17	Tennessee	25.2		42	California	18.8
11	Texas	27.5		43	Virginia	18.7
34	Utah	21.8		44	Colorado	17.1
25	Vermont	22.9		45	Iowa	16.1
43	Virginia	18.7		46	Alaska	15.7
21	Washington	24.1		47	Arizona	15.5
1	West Virginia	31.2		48	Wyoming	14.0
29	Wisconsin	22.7		49	Minnesota	13.2
48	Wyoming	14.0		49	Nevada	13.2
				District of Columbia		28.6

Source: Morgan Quitno Press using data from U.S. Dept of Health & Human Services, Health Care Financing Admin.
"State Health Expenditure Accounts" (Health Care Financing Review, Fall 1995, Volume 17, Number 1)
*By state of provider.

Average Annual Change in Expenditures for Hospital Care: 1980 to 1993

National Percent = 9.4% Average Annual Growth*

ALPHA ORDER				RANK ORDER		
RANK	STATE	PERCENT		RANK	STATE	PERCENT
23	Alabama	9.8		1	New Hampshire	12.2
19	Alaska	10.2		2	South Carolina	12.0
15	Arizona	10.5		3	Hawaii	11.5
13	Arkansas	10.6		3	New Mexico	11.5
33	California	8.8		5	Georgia	11.4
27	Colorado	9.5		6	North Carolina	11.3
31	Connecticut	9.2		7	Florida	11.1
16	Delaware	10.4		7	Texas	11.1
7	Florida	11.1		9	Utah	11.0
5	Georgia	11.4		10	Washington	10.9
3	Hawaii	11.5		11	Idaho	10.7
11	Idaho	10.7		11	New Jersey	10.7
50	Illinois	7.4		13	Arkansas	10.6
26	Indiana	9.7		13	Kentucky	10.6
47	Iowa	7.8		15	Arizona	10.5
47	Kansas	7.8		16	Delaware	10.4
13	Kentucky	10.6		17	Nevada	10.3
20	Louisiana	10.0		17	Tennessee	10.3
33	Maine	8.8		19	Alaska	10.2
37	Maryland	8.6		20	Louisiana	10.0
45	Massachusetts	8.1		21	Montana	9.9
49	Michigan	7.7		21	Virginia	9.9
44	Minnesota	8.2		23	Alabama	9.8
23	Mississippi	9.8		23	Mississippi	9.8
32	Missouri	8.9		23	South Dakota	9.8
21	Montana	9.9		26	Indiana	9.7
33	Nebraska	8.8		27	Colorado	9.5
17	Nevada	10.3		27	Pennsylvania	9.5
1	New Hampshire	12.2		27	Vermont	9.5
11	New Jersey	10.7		30	Oregon	9.4
3	New Mexico	11.5		31	Connecticut	9.2
37	New York	8.6		32	Missouri	8.9
6	North Carolina	11.3		33	California	8.8
39	North Dakota	8.5		33	Maine	8.8
33	Ohio	8.8		33	Nebraska	8.8
39	Oklahoma	8.5		33	Ohio	8.8
30	Oregon	9.4		37	Maryland	8.6
27	Pennsylvania	9.5		37	New York	8.6
45	Rhode Island	8.1		39	North Dakota	8.5
2	South Carolina	12.0		39	Oklahoma	8.5
23	South Dakota	9.8		39	Wyoming	8.5
17	Tennessee	10.3		42	West Virginia	8.4
7	Texas	11.1		42	Wisconsin	8.4
9	Utah	11.0		44	Minnesota	8.2
27	Vermont	9.5		45	Massachusetts	8.1
21	Virginia	9.9		45	Rhode Island	8.1
10	Washington	10.9		47	Iowa	7.8
42	West Virginia	8.4		47	Kansas	7.8
42	Wisconsin	8.4		49	Michigan	7.7
39	Wyoming	8.5		50	Illinois	7.4
					District of Columbia	8.4

Source: U.S. Department of Health and Human Services, Health Care Financing Administration
    "State Health Expenditure Accounts" (Health Care Financing Review, Fall 1995, Volume 17, Number 1)
*By state of provider.

Average Annual Change in Per Capita Expenditures
For Hospital Care: 1980 to 1993
National Percent = 8.3% Average Annual Increase*

ALPHA ORDER

RANK	STATE	PERCENT
18	Alabama	9.1
48	Alaska	6.9
43	Arizona	7.4
5	Arkansas	10.0
49	California	6.5
39	Colorado	7.7
24	Connecticut	8.7
19	Delaware	9.0
32	Florida	8.2
10	Georgia	9.4
6	Hawaii	9.8
14	Idaho	9.3
44	Illinois	7.2
14	Indiana	9.3
35	Iowa	8.0
44	Kansas	7.2
3	Kentucky	10.2
8	Louisiana	9.7
35	Maine	8.0
44	Maryland	7.2
39	Massachusetts	7.7
42	Michigan	7.5
44	Minnesota	7.2
14	Mississippi	9.3
27	Missouri	8.4
14	Montana	9.3
27	Nebraska	8.4
50	Nevada	5.6
2	New Hampshire	10.4
4	New Jersey	10.1
9	New Mexico	9.6
31	New York	8.3
6	North Carolina	9.8
24	North Dakota	8.7
26	Ohio	8.6
37	Oklahoma	7.8
32	Oregon	8.2
10	Pennsylvania	9.4
41	Rhode Island	7.6
1	South Carolina	10.6
10	South Dakota	9.4
10	Tennessee	9.4
19	Texas	9.0
21	Utah	8.9
27	Vermont	8.4
32	Virginia	8.2
23	Washington	8.8
21	West Virginia	8.9
37	Wisconsin	7.8
27	Wyoming	8.4

RANK ORDER

RANK	STATE	PERCENT
1	South Carolina	10.6
2	New Hampshire	10.4
3	Kentucky	10.2
4	New Jersey	10.1
5	Arkansas	10.0
6	Hawaii	9.8
6	North Carolina	9.8
8	Louisiana	9.7
9	New Mexico	9.6
10	Georgia	9.4
10	Pennsylvania	9.4
10	South Dakota	9.4
10	Tennessee	9.4
14	Idaho	9.3
14	Indiana	9.3
14	Mississippi	9.3
14	Montana	9.3
18	Alabama	9.1
19	Delaware	9.0
19	Texas	9.0
21	Utah	8.9
21	West Virginia	8.9
23	Washington	8.8
24	Connecticut	8.7
24	North Dakota	8.7
26	Ohio	8.6
27	Missouri	8.4
27	Nebraska	8.4
27	Vermont	8.4
27	Wyoming	8.4
31	New York	8.3
32	Florida	8.2
32	Oregon	8.2
32	Virginia	8.2
35	Iowa	8.0
35	Maine	8.0
37	Oklahoma	7.8
37	Wisconsin	7.8
39	Colorado	7.7
39	Massachusetts	7.7
41	Rhode Island	7.6
42	Michigan	7.5
43	Arizona	7.4
44	Illinois	7.2
44	Kansas	7.2
44	Maryland	7.2
44	Minnesota	7.2
48	Alaska	6.9
49	California	6.5
50	Nevada	5.6

District of Columbia   9.3

Source: Morgan Quitno Press using data from U.S. Dept of Health & Human Services, Health Care Financing Admin.
"State Health Expenditure Accounts" (Health Care Financing Review, Fall 1995, Volume 17, Number 1)
*By state of provider.

Expenditures for Physician Services in 1993

National Total = $171,226,000,000*

ALPHA ORDER

RANK ORDER

RANK	STATE	EXPENDITURES	% of USA
22	Alabama	$2,631,000,000	1.54%
48	Alaska	301,000,000	0.18%
21	Arizona	2,799,000,000	1.63%
32	Arkansas	1,244,000,000	0.73%
1	California	28,981,000,000	16.93%
25	Colorado	2,452,000,000	1.43%
23	Connecticut	2,587,000,000	1.51%
44	Delaware	466,000,000	0.27%
4	Florida	10,498,000,000	6.13%
10	Georgia	4,543,000,000	2.65%
39	Hawaii	771,000,000	0.45%
43	Idaho	486,000,000	0.28%
7	Illinois	6,970,000,000	4.07%
18	Indiana	3,263,000,000	1.91%
31	Iowa	1,376,000,000	0.80%
30	Kansas	1,425,000,000	0.83%
26	Kentucky	2,038,000,000	1.19%
24	Louisiana	2,537,000,000	1.48%
41	Maine	601,000,000	0.35%
15	Maryland	3,704,000,000	2.16%
11	Massachusetts	4,442,000,000	2.59%
9	Michigan	5,562,000,000	3.25%
16	Minnesota	3,617,000,000	2.11%
33	Mississippi	1,107,000,000	0.65%
20	Missouri	2,958,000,000	1.73%
46	Montana	392,000,000	0.23%
37	Nebraska	825,000,000	0.48%
34	Nevada	1,029,000,000	0.60%
38	New Hampshire	780,000,000	0.46%
8	New Jersey	5,776,000,000	3.37%
40	New Mexico	716,000,000	0.42%
2	New York	12,003,000,000	7.01%
14	North Carolina	3,717,000,000	2.17%
45	North Dakota	445,000,000	0.26%
6	Ohio	7,118,000,000	4.16%
29	Oklahoma	1,640,000,000	0.96%
27	Oregon	1,904,000,000	1.11%
5	Pennsylvania	7,460,000,000	4.36%
42	Rhode Island	575,000,000	0.34%
28	South Carolina	1,685,000,000	0.98%
47	South Dakota	342,000,000	0.20%
19	Tennessee	3,137,000,000	1.83%
3	Texas	10,526,000,000	6.15%
36	Utah	864,000,000	0.50%
49	Vermont	265,000,000	0.15%
12	Virginia	3,769,000,000	2.20%
13	Washington	3,720,000,000	2.17%
35	West Virginia	988,000,000	0.58%
17	Wisconsin	3,362,000,000	1.96%
50	Wyoming	160,000,000	0.09%

RANK	STATE	EXPENDITURES	% of USA
1	California	$28,981,000,000	16.93%
2	New York	12,003,000,000	7.01%
3	Texas	10,526,000,000	6.15%
4	Florida	10,498,000,000	6.13%
5	Pennsylvania	7,460,000,000	4.36%
6	Ohio	7,118,000,000	4.16%
7	Illinois	6,970,000,000	4.07%
8	New Jersey	5,776,000,000	3.37%
9	Michigan	5,562,000,000	3.25%
10	Georgia	4,543,000,000	2.65%
11	Massachusetts	4,442,000,000	2.59%
12	Virginia	3,769,000,000	2.20%
13	Washington	3,720,000,000	2.17%
14	North Carolina	3,717,000,000	2.17%
15	Maryland	3,704,000,000	2.16%
16	Minnesota	3,617,000,000	2.11%
17	Wisconsin	3,362,000,000	1.96%
18	Indiana	3,263,000,000	1.91%
19	Tennessee	3,137,000,000	1.83%
20	Missouri	2,958,000,000	1.73%
21	Arizona	2,799,000,000	1.63%
22	Alabama	2,631,000,000	1.54%
23	Connecticut	2,587,000,000	1.51%
24	Louisiana	2,537,000,000	1.48%
25	Colorado	2,452,000,000	1.43%
26	Kentucky	2,038,000,000	1.19%
27	Oregon	1,904,000,000	1.11%
28	South Carolina	1,685,000,000	0.98%
29	Oklahoma	1,640,000,000	0.96%
30	Kansas	1,425,000,000	0.83%
31	Iowa	1,376,000,000	0.80%
32	Arkansas	1,244,000,000	0.73%
33	Mississippi	1,107,000,000	0.65%
34	Nevada	1,029,000,000	0.60%
35	West Virginia	988,000,000	0.58%
36	Utah	864,000,000	0.50%
37	Nebraska	825,000,000	0.48%
38	New Hampshire	780,000,000	0.46%
39	Hawaii	771,000,000	0.45%
40	New Mexico	716,000,000	0.42%
41	Maine	601,000,000	0.35%
42	Rhode Island	575,000,000	0.34%
43	Idaho	486,000,000	0.28%
44	Delaware	466,000,000	0.27%
45	North Dakota	445,000,000	0.26%
46	Montana	392,000,000	0.23%
47	South Dakota	342,000,000	0.20%
48	Alaska	301,000,000	0.18%
49	Vermont	265,000,000	0.15%
50	Wyoming	160,000,000	0.09%
	District of Columbia	672,000,000	0.39%

Source: U.S. Department of Health and Human Services, Health Care Financing Administration
    "State Health Expenditure Accounts" (Health Care Financing Review, Fall 1995, Volume 17, Number 1)
*By state of provider.

Percent of Total Personal Health Care Expenditures
Spent on Physician Services in 1993
National Percent = 22.0%*

ALPHA ORDER

RANK ORDER

RANK	STATE	PERCENT		RANK	STATE	PERCENT
17	Alabama	21.8		1	California	30.8
34	Alaska	19.1		2	Nevada	27.5
3	Arizona	26.3		3	Arizona	26.3
26	Arkansas	20.4		4	Minnesota	25.5
1	California	30.8		5	Washington	24.6
6	Colorado	24.4		6	Colorado	24.4
20	Connecticut	21.2		6	Maryland	24.4
23	Delaware	20.6		8	Oregon	23.8
9	Florida	23.4		9	Florida	23.4
11	Georgia	22.6		10	Wisconsin	23.2
15	Hawaii	22.1		11	Georgia	22.6
18	Idaho	21.3		11	New Hampshire	22.6
29	Illinois	20.1		11	Virginia	22.6
30	Indiana	19.9		14	New Jersey	22.4
38	Iowa	18.7		15	Hawaii	22.1
23	Kansas	20.6		16	North Dakota	22.0
31	Kentucky	19.6		17	Alabama	21.8
32	Louisiana	19.5		18	Idaho	21.3
47	Maine	17.5		18	Ohio	21.3
6	Maryland	24.4		20	Connecticut	21.2
35	Massachusetts	19.0		21	Texas	21.1
25	Michigan	20.5		22	Utah	21.0
4	Minnesota	25.5		23	Delaware	20.6
44	Mississippi	17.9		23	Kansas	20.6
41	Missouri	18.5		25	Michigan	20.5
40	Montana	18.6		26	Arkansas	20.4
37	Nebraska	18.8		26	North Carolina	20.4
2	Nevada	27.5		26	Oklahoma	20.4
11	New Hampshire	22.6		29	Illinois	20.1
14	New Jersey	22.4		30	Indiana	19.9
41	New Mexico	18.5		31	Kentucky	19.6
44	New York	17.9		32	Louisiana	19.5
26	North Carolina	20.4		33	Tennessee	19.4
16	North Dakota	22.0		34	Alaska	19.1
18	Ohio	21.3		35	Massachusetts	19.0
26	Oklahoma	20.4		35	West Virginia	19.0
8	Oregon	23.8		37	Nebraska	18.8
43	Pennsylvania	18.0		38	Iowa	18.7
49	Rhode Island	16.8		38	South Carolina	18.7
38	South Carolina	18.7		40	Montana	18.6
47	South Dakota	17.5		41	Missouri	18.5
33	Tennessee	19.4		41	New Mexico	18.5
21	Texas	21.1		43	Pennsylvania	18.0
22	Utah	21.0		44	Mississippi	17.9
46	Vermont	17.7		44	New York	17.9
11	Virginia	22.6		46	Vermont	17.7
5	Washington	24.6		47	Maine	17.5
35	West Virginia	19.0		47	South Dakota	17.5
10	Wisconsin	23.2		49	Rhode Island	16.8
50	Wyoming	16.0		50	Wyoming	16.0

District of Columbia 15.7

Source: Morgan Quitno Press using data from U.S. Dept of Health & Human Services, Health Care Financing Admin.
   "State Health Expenditure Accounts" (Health Care Financing Review, Fall 1995, Volume 17, Number 1)
By state of provider.

Per Capita Expenditures for Physician Services in 1993

National Per Capita = $664*

ALPHA ORDER			RANK ORDER		
RANK	STATE	PER CAPITA	RANK	STATE	PER CAPITA
20	Alabama	$629	1	California	$928
39	Alaska	503	2	Minnesota	800
9	Arizona	710	3	Connecticut	789
36	Arkansas	513	4	Florida	765
1	California	928	5	Maryland	748
13	Colorado	687	6	Nevada	743
3	Connecticut	789	7	Massachusetts	738
14	Delaware	667	8	New Jersey	735
4	Florida	765	9	Arizona	710
18	Georgia	658	10	Washington	708
16	Hawaii	661	11	North Dakota	699
48	Idaho	441	12	New Hampshire	695
24	Illinois	596	13	Colorado	687
30	Indiana	572	14	Delaware	667
40	Iowa	488	14	Wisconsin	667
32	Kansas	563	16	Hawaii	661
34	Kentucky	537	16	New York	661
25	Louisiana	592	18	Georgia	658
41	Maine	485	19	Ohio	644
5	Maryland	748	20	Alabama	629
7	Massachusetts	738	21	Oregon	627
26	Michigan	588	22	Pennsylvania	620
2	Minnesota	800	23	Tennessee	616
49	Mississippi	419	24	Illinois	596
31	Missouri	565	25	Louisiana	592
43	Montana	466	26	Michigan	588
37	Nebraska	511	27	Texas	583
6	Nevada	743	28	Virginia	582
12	New Hampshire	695	29	Rhode Island	576
8	New Jersey	735	30	Indiana	572
47	New Mexico	443	31	Missouri	565
16	New York	661	32	Kansas	563
35	North Carolina	535	33	West Virginia	543
11	North Dakota	699	34	Kentucky	537
19	Ohio	644	35	North Carolina	535
38	Oklahoma	507	36	Arkansas	513
21	Oregon	627	37	Nebraska	511
22	Pennsylvania	620	38	Oklahoma	507
29	Rhode Island	576	39	Alaska	503
44	South Carolina	465	40	Iowa	488
42	South Dakota	477	41	Maine	485
23	Tennessee	616	42	South Dakota	477
27	Texas	583	43	Montana	466
44	Utah	465	44	South Carolina	465
46	Vermont	460	44	Utah	465
28	Virginia	582	46	Vermont	460
10	Washington	708	47	New Mexico	443
33	West Virginia	543	48	Idaho	441
14	Wisconsin	667	49	Mississippi	419
50	Wyoming	340	50	Wyoming	340
				District of Columbia**	1,163

Source: Morgan Quitno Press using data from U.S. Dept of Health & Human Services, Health Care Financing Admin.
"State Health Expenditure Accounts" (Health Care Financing Review, Fall 1995, Volume 17, Number 1)
*By state of provider.
**The District of Columbia's per capita is greatly affected by residents of Maryland and Virginia receiving services.

Percent Change in Expenditures for Physician Services: 1990 to 1993

National Percent Change = 21.9% Increase*

ALPHA ORDER				RANK ORDER		
RANK	STATE	PERCENT CHANGE		RANK	STATE	PERCENT CHANGE
42	Alabama	17.1		1	New Hampshire	58.9
44	Alaska	16.7		2	Washington	31.3
46	Arizona	12.0		3	Wisconsin	31.1
49	Arkansas	9.7		4	Idaho	29.9
6	California	29.6		5	Colorado	29.7
5	Colorado	29.7		6	California	29.6
37	Connecticut	18.4		7	New Jersey	27.8
19	Delaware	23.6		8	South Carolina	27.2
48	Florida	11.2		9	Nevada	26.7
15	Georgia	24.6		10	Montana	26.0
20	Hawaii	22.6		11	Maine	25.2
4	Idaho	29.9		12	Maryland	24.8
34	Illinois	18.9		12	South Dakota	24.8
23	Indiana	21.8		14	New Mexico	24.7
25	Iowa	20.5		15	Georgia	24.6
40	Kansas	17.7		16	Kentucky	24.3
16	Kentucky	24.3		17	New York	23.8
30	Louisiana	19.2		18	North Carolina	23.7
11	Maine	25.2		19	Delaware	23.6
12	Maryland	24.8		20	Hawaii	22.6
38	Massachusetts	18.0		21	Minnesota	22.3
30	Michigan	19.2		22	Tennessee	22.1
21	Minnesota	22.3		23	Indiana	21.8
28	Mississippi	19.7		24	North Dakota	20.9
33	Missouri	19.0		25	Iowa	20.5
10	Montana	26.0		26	Nebraska	19.9
26	Nebraska	19.9		26	Vermont	19.9
9	Nevada	26.7		28	Mississippi	19.7
1	New Hampshire	58.9		29	Pennsylvania	19.3
7	New Jersey	27.8		30	Louisiana	19.2
14	New Mexico	24.7		30	Michigan	19.2
17	New York	23.8		30	Oregon	19.2
18	North Carolina	23.7		33	Missouri	19.0
24	North Dakota	20.9		34	Illinois	18.9
40	Ohio	17.7		35	Virginia	18.8
36	Oklahoma	18.7		36	Oklahoma	18.7
30	Oregon	19.2		37	Connecticut	18.4
29	Pennsylvania	19.3		38	Massachusetts	18.0
47	Rhode Island	11.9		38	Texas	18.0
8	South Carolina	27.2		40	Kansas	17.7
12	South Dakota	24.8		40	Ohio	17.7
22	Tennessee	22.1		42	Alabama	17.1
38	Texas	18.0		43	Utah	16.9
43	Utah	16.9		44	Alaska	16.7
26	Vermont	19.9		45	West Virginia	15.4
35	Virginia	18.8		46	Arizona	12.0
2	Washington	31.3		47	Rhode Island	11.9
45	West Virginia	15.4		48	Florida	11.2
3	Wisconsin	31.1		49	Arkansas	9.7
50	Wyoming	9.6		50	Wyoming	9.6
					District of Columbia	2.3

Source: Morgan Quitno Press using data from U.S. Dept of Health & Human Services, Health Care Financing Admin. "State Health Expenditure Accounts" (Health Care Financing Review, Fall 1995, Volume 17, Number 1)
*By state of provider.

Percent Change in Per Capita Expenditures for Physician Services: 1990 to 1993

National Percent Change = 17.5% Increase*

ALPHA ORDER				RANK ORDER		
RANK	STATE	PERCENT CHANGE		RANK	STATE	PERCENT CHANGE
40	Alabama	13.1		1	New Hampshire	56.9
46	Alaska	7.2		2	Wisconsin	27.3
50	Arizona	4.1		3	New Jersey	25.6
47	Arkansas	6.4		4	Maine	24.0
5	California	23.4		5	California	23.4
14	Colorado	19.7		6	New York	22.6
17	Connecticut	18.6		7	South Carolina	22.4
23	Delaware	17.8		8	Washington	21.6
49	Florida	4.8		9	North Dakota	21.4
28	Georgia	16.9		10	South Dakota	21.1
32	Hawaii	16.4		11	Kentucky	20.7
15	Idaho	18.9		12	Maryland	20.5
34	Illinois	16.2		13	Montana	19.8
18	Indiana	18.4		14	Colorado	19.7
16	Iowa	18.7		15	Idaho	18.9
37	Kansas	15.1		16	Iowa	18.7
11	Kentucky	20.7		17	Connecticut	18.6
24	Louisiana	17.2		18	Indiana	18.4
4	Maine	24.0		19	Minnesota	18.3
12	Maryland	20.5		20	North Carolina	18.1
21	Massachusetts	17.9		21	Massachusetts	17.9
26	Michigan	17.1		21	Pennsylvania	17.9
19	Minnesota	18.3		23	Delaware	17.8
31	Mississippi	16.7		24	Louisiana	17.2
33	Missouri	16.3		24	Nebraska	17.2
13	Montana	19.8		26	Michigan	17.1
24	Nebraska	17.2		27	Vermont	17.0
44	Nevada	9.9		28	Georgia	16.9
1	New Hampshire	56.9		28	New Mexico	16.9
3	New Jersey	25.6		28	Tennessee	16.9
28	New Mexico	16.9		31	Mississippi	16.7
6	New York	22.6		32	Hawaii	16.4
20	North Carolina	18.1		33	Missouri	16.3
9	North Dakota	21.4		34	Illinois	16.2
36	Ohio	15.4		35	Oklahoma	15.5
35	Oklahoma	15.5		36	Ohio	15.4
42	Oregon	11.6		37	Kansas	15.1
21	Pennsylvania	17.9		38	West Virginia	13.8
41	Rhode Island	12.5		39	Virginia	13.5
7	South Carolina	22.4		40	Alabama	13.1
10	South Dakota	21.1		41	Rhode Island	12.5
28	Tennessee	16.9		42	Oregon	11.6
43	Texas	11.0		43	Texas	11.0
45	Utah	8.4		44	Nevada	9.9
27	Vermont	17.0		45	Utah	8.4
39	Virginia	13.5		46	Alaska	7.2
8	Washington	21.6		47	Arkansas	6.4
38	West Virginia	13.8		48	Wyoming	5.6
2	Wisconsin	27.3		49	Florida	4.8
48	Wyoming	5.6		50	Arizona	4.1
					District of Columbia	7.5

Source: Morgan Quitno Press using data from U.S. Dept of Health & Human Services, Health Care Financing Admin.
    "State Health Expenditure Accounts" (Health Care Financing Review, Fall 1995, Volume 17, Number 1)
*By state of provider.

Average Annual Change in Expenditures for Physician Services: 1980 to 1993

National Percent = 10.8% Average Annual Increase*

ALPHA ORDER

RANK	STATE	PERCENT CHANGE
14	Alabama	11.6
41	Alaska	9.1
5	Arizona	12.1
36	Arkansas	9.7
14	California	11.6
16	Colorado	11.4
5	Connecticut	12.1
20	Delaware	11.0
11	Florida	11.7
3	Georgia	12.5
41	Hawaii	9.1
29	Idaho	10.1
38	Illinois	9.6
24	Indiana	10.5
48	Iowa	8.3
41	Kansas	9.1
25	Kentucky	10.4
32	Louisiana	9.9
11	Maine	11.7
5	Maryland	12.1
4	Massachusetts	12.3
49	Michigan	8.2
21	Minnesota	10.9
33	Mississippi	9.8
33	Missouri	9.8
47	Montana	8.4
45	Nebraska	8.8
2	Nevada	13.1
1	New Hampshire	14.8
9	New Jersey	11.8
18	New Mexico	11.1
25	New York	10.4
8	North Carolina	11.9
39	North Dakota	9.4
36	Ohio	9.7
44	Oklahoma	9.0
40	Oregon	9.3
21	Pennsylvania	10.9
31	Rhode Island	10.0
11	South Carolina	11.7
33	South Dakota	9.8
23	Tennessee	10.7
29	Texas	10.1
28	Utah	10.2
18	Vermont	11.1
9	Virginia	11.8
16	Washington	11.4
45	West Virginia	8.8
27	Wisconsin	10.3
50	Wyoming	7.3

RANK ORDER

RANK	STATE	PERCENT CHANGE
1	New Hampshire	14.8
2	Nevada	13.1
3	Georgia	12.5
4	Massachusetts	12.3
5	Arizona	12.1
5	Connecticut	12.1
5	Maryland	12.1
8	North Carolina	11.9
9	New Jersey	11.8
9	Virginia	11.8
11	Florida	11.7
11	Maine	11.7
11	South Carolina	11.7
14	Alabama	11.6
14	California	11.6
16	Colorado	11.4
16	Washington	11.4
18	New Mexico	11.1
18	Vermont	11.1
20	Delaware	11.0
21	Minnesota	10.9
21	Pennsylvania	10.9
23	Tennessee	10.7
24	Indiana	10.5
25	Kentucky	10.4
25	New York	10.4
27	Wisconsin	10.3
28	Utah	10.2
29	Idaho	10.1
29	Texas	10.1
31	Rhode Island	10.0
32	Louisiana	9.9
33	Mississippi	9.8
33	Missouri	9.8
33	South Dakota	9.8
36	Arkansas	9.7
36	Ohio	9.7
38	Illinois	9.6
39	North Dakota	9.4
40	Oregon	9.3
41	Alaska	9.1
41	Hawaii	9.1
41	Kansas	9.1
44	Oklahoma	9.0
45	Nebraska	8.8
45	West Virginia	8.8
47	Montana	8.4
48	Iowa	8.3
49	Michigan	8.2
50	Wyoming	7.3
	District of Columbia	8.4

Source: U.S. Department of Health and Human Services, Health Care Financing Administration
   "State Health Expenditure Accounts" (Health Care Financing Review, Fall 1995, Volume 17, Number 1)
*By state of provider.

Average Annual Change in Per Capita Expenditures
For Physician Services: 1980 to 1993
National Percent = 9.7% Average Annual Increase*

ALPHA ORDER

RANK	STATE	PERCENT
5	Alabama	11.0
50	Alaska	5.8
35	Arizona	8.9
33	Arkansas	9.2
33	California	9.2
21	Colorado	9.6
3	Connecticut	11.6
21	Delaware	9.6
36	Florida	8.8
9	Georgia	10.4
48	Hawaii	7.5
36	Idaho	8.8
26	Illinois	9.4
12	Indiana	10.2
38	Iowa	8.6
39	Kansas	8.5
13	Kentucky	10.1
20	Louisiana	9.7
6	Maine	10.9
7	Maryland	10.8
2	Massachusetts	12.0
46	Michigan	8.0
16	Minnesota	10.0
26	Mississippi	9.4
31	Missouri	9.3
47	Montana	7.8
39	Nebraska	8.5
41	Nevada	8.4
1	New Hampshire	13.1
4	New Jersey	11.2
31	New Mexico	9.3
13	New York	10.1
9	North Carolina	10.4
21	North Dakota	9.6
25	Ohio	9.5
41	Oklahoma	8.4
43	Oregon	8.2
7	Pennsylvania	10.8
21	Rhode Island	9.6
9	South Carolina	10.4
26	South Dakota	9.4
18	Tennessee	9.8
45	Texas	8.1
43	Utah	8.2
16	Vermont	10.0
13	Virginia	10.1
26	Washington	9.4
26	West Virginia	9.4
18	Wisconsin	9.8
49	Wyoming	7.3

RANK ORDER

RANK	STATE	PERCENT
1	New Hampshire	13.1
2	Massachusetts	12.0
3	Connecticut	11.6
4	New Jersey	11.2
5	Alabama	11.0
6	Maine	10.9
7	Maryland	10.8
7	Pennsylvania	10.8
9	Georgia	10.4
9	North Carolina	10.4
9	South Carolina	10.4
12	Indiana	10.2
13	Kentucky	10.1
13	New York	10.1
13	Virginia	10.1
16	Minnesota	10.0
16	Vermont	10.0
18	Tennessee	9.8
18	Wisconsin	9.8
20	Louisiana	9.7
21	Colorado	9.6
21	Delaware	9.6
21	North Dakota	9.6
21	Rhode Island	9.6
25	Ohio	9.5
26	Illinois	9.4
26	Mississippi	9.4
26	South Dakota	9.4
26	Washington	9.4
26	West Virginia	9.4
31	Missouri	9.3
31	New Mexico	9.3
33	Arkansas	9.2
33	California	9.2
35	Arizona	8.9
36	Florida	8.8
36	Idaho	8.8
38	Iowa	8.6
39	Kansas	8.5
39	Nebraska	8.5
41	Nevada	8.4
41	Oklahoma	8.4
43	Oregon	8.2
43	Utah	8.2
45	Texas	8.1
46	Michigan	8.0
47	Montana	7.8
48	Hawaii	7.5
49	Wyoming	7.3
50	Alaska	5.8

District of Columbia 9.2

Source: Morgan Quitno Press using data from U.S. Dept of Health & Human Services, Health Care Financing Admin.
"State Health Expenditure Accounts" (Health Care Financing Review, Fall 1995, Volume 17, Number 1)
*By state of provider.

Expenditures for Prescription Drugs in 1993

National Total = $48,840,000,000*

ALPHA ORDER

RANK	STATE	EXPENDITURES	% of USA
18	Alabama	$904,000,000	1.85%
49	Alaska	85,000,000	0.17%
24	Arizona	728,000,000	1.49%
31	Arkansas	484,000,000	0.99%
1	California	5,501,000,000	11.26%
28	Colorado	534,000,000	1.09%
26	Connecticut	650,000,000	1.33%
44	Delaware	129,000,000	0.26%
4	Florida	2,832,000,000	5.80%
10	Georgia	1,397,000,000	2.86%
41	Hawaii	197,000,000	0.40%
43	Idaho	182,000,000	0.37%
6	Illinois	2,206,000,000	4.52%
16	Indiana	1,106,000,000	2.26%
29	Iowa	516,000,000	1.06%
32	Kansas	465,000,000	0.95%
21	Kentucky	846,000,000	1.73%
22	Louisiana	832,000,000	1.70%
39	Maine	213,000,000	0.44%
15	Maryland	1,140,000,000	2.33%
13	Massachusetts	1,337,000,000	2.74%
8	Michigan	2,054,000,000	4.21%
23	Minnesota	739,000,000	1.51%
30	Mississippi	499,000,000	1.02%
17	Missouri	975,000,000	2.00%
45	Montana	120,000,000	0.25%
36	Nebraska	293,000,000	0.60%
38	Nevada	246,000,000	0.50%
41	New Hampshire	197,000,000	0.40%
9	New Jersey	1,601,000,000	3.28%
37	New Mexico	259,000,000	0.53%
2	New York	3,232,000,000	6.62%
11	North Carolina	1,392,000,000	2.85%
48	North Dakota	103,000,000	0.21%
7	Ohio	2,095,000,000	4.29%
27	Oklahoma	569,000,000	1.17%
33	Oregon	431,000,000	0.88%
5	Pennsylvania	2,386,000,000	4.89%
40	Rhode Island	206,000,000	0.42%
25	South Carolina	665,000,000	1.36%
47	South Dakota	104,000,000	0.21%
14	Tennessee	1,153,000,000	2.36%
3	Texas	3,153,000,000	6.46%
35	Utah	302,000,000	0.62%
46	Vermont	108,000,000	0.22%
12	Virginia	1,343,000,000	2.75%
20	Washington	853,000,000	1.75%
34	West Virginia	412,000,000	0.84%
19	Wisconsin	899,000,000	1.84%
50	Wyoming	64,000,000	0.13%

RANK ORDER

RANK	STATE	EXPENDITURES	% of USA
1	California	$5,501,000,000	11.26%
2	New York	3,232,000,000	6.62%
3	Texas	3,153,000,000	6.46%
4	Florida	2,832,000,000	5.80%
5	Pennsylvania	2,386,000,000	4.89%
6	Illinois	2,206,000,000	4.52%
7	Ohio	2,095,000,000	4.29%
8	Michigan	2,054,000,000	4.21%
9	New Jersey	1,601,000,000	3.28%
10	Georgia	1,397,000,000	2.86%
11	North Carolina	1,392,000,000	2.85%
12	Virginia	1,343,000,000	2.75%
13	Massachusetts	1,337,000,000	2.74%
14	Tennessee	1,153,000,000	2.36%
15	Maryland	1,140,000,000	2.33%
16	Indiana	1,106,000,000	2.26%
17	Missouri	975,000,000	2.00%
18	Alabama	904,000,000	1.85%
19	Wisconsin	899,000,000	1.84%
20	Washington	853,000,000	1.75%
21	Kentucky	846,000,000	1.73%
22	Louisiana	832,000,000	1.70%
23	Minnesota	739,000,000	1.51%
24	Arizona	728,000,000	1.49%
25	South Carolina	665,000,000	1.36%
26	Connecticut	650,000,000	1.33%
27	Oklahoma	569,000,000	1.17%
28	Colorado	534,000,000	1.09%
29	Iowa	516,000,000	1.06%
30	Mississippi	499,000,000	1.02%
31	Arkansas	484,000,000	0.99%
32	Kansas	465,000,000	0.95%
33	Oregon	431,000,000	0.88%
34	West Virginia	412,000,000	0.84%
35	Utah	302,000,000	0.62%
36	Nebraska	293,000,000	0.60%
37	New Mexico	259,000,000	0.53%
38	Nevada	246,000,000	0.50%
39	Maine	213,000,000	0.44%
40	Rhode Island	206,000,000	0.42%
41	Hawaii	197,000,000	0.40%
41	New Hampshire	197,000,000	0.40%
43	Idaho	182,000,000	0.37%
44	Delaware	129,000,000	0.26%
45	Montana	120,000,000	0.25%
46	Vermont	108,000,000	0.22%
47	South Dakota	104,000,000	0.21%
48	North Dakota	103,000,000	0.21%
49	Alaska	85,000,000	0.17%
50	Wyoming	64,000,000	0.13%
	District of Columbia	103,000,000	0.21%

Source: U.S. Department of Health and Human Services, Health Care Financing Administration
"State Health Expenditure Accounts" (Health Care Financing Review, Fall 1995, Volume 17, Number 1)
Purchases in retail outlets. By state of outlet. This is a subset of overall "Drug and Other Medical Non-Durable Expenditures" shown elsewhere in this book.

Percent of Total Personal Health Care Expenditures
Spent on Prescription Drugs in 1993
National Percent = 6.3%*

ALPHA ORDER

RANK	STATE	PERCENT
9	Alabama	7.5
43	Alaska	5.4
18	Arizona	6.8
5	Arkansas	7.9
35	California	5.8
45	Colorado	5.3
45	Connecticut	5.3
36	Delaware	5.7
26	Florida	6.3
17	Georgia	6.9
36	Hawaii	5.7
4	Idaho	8.0
26	Illinois	6.3
19	Indiana	6.7
16	Iowa	7.0
19	Kansas	6.7
1	Kentucky	8.1
24	Louisiana	6.4
30	Maine	6.2
9	Maryland	7.5
36	Massachusetts	5.7
7	Michigan	7.6
48	Minnesota	5.2
1	Mississippi	8.1
33	Missouri	6.1
36	Montana	5.7
19	Nebraska	6.7
23	Nevada	6.6
36	New Hampshire	5.7
30	New Jersey	6.2
19	New Mexico	6.7
50	New York	4.8
7	North Carolina	7.6
49	North Dakota	5.1
26	Ohio	6.3
14	Oklahoma	7.1
43	Oregon	5.4
36	Pennsylvania	5.7
34	Rhode Island	6.0
11	South Carolina	7.4
45	South Dakota	5.3
14	Tennessee	7.1
26	Texas	6.3
12	Utah	7.3
13	Vermont	7.2
1	Virginia	8.1
42	Washington	5.6
5	West Virginia	7.9
30	Wisconsin	6.2
24	Wyoming	6.4

RANK ORDER

RANK	STATE	PERCENT
1	Kentucky	8.1
1	Mississippi	8.1
1	Virginia	8.1
4	Idaho	8.0
5	Arkansas	7.9
5	West Virginia	7.9
7	Michigan	7.6
7	North Carolina	7.6
9	Alabama	7.5
9	Maryland	7.5
11	South Carolina	7.4
12	Utah	7.3
13	Vermont	7.2
14	Oklahoma	7.1
14	Tennessee	7.1
16	Iowa	7.0
17	Georgia	6.9
18	Arizona	6.8
19	Indiana	6.7
19	Kansas	6.7
19	Nebraska	6.7
19	New Mexico	6.7
23	Nevada	6.6
24	Louisiana	6.4
24	Wyoming	6.4
26	Florida	6.3
26	Illinois	6.3
26	Ohio	6.3
26	Texas	6.3
30	Maine	6.2
30	New Jersey	6.2
30	Wisconsin	6.2
33	Missouri	6.1
34	Rhode Island	6.0
35	California	5.8
36	Delaware	5.7
36	Hawaii	5.7
36	Massachusetts	5.7
36	Montana	5.7
36	New Hampshire	5.7
36	Pennsylvania	5.7
42	Washington	5.6
43	Alaska	5.4
43	Oregon	5.4
45	Colorado	5.3
45	Connecticut	5.3
45	South Dakota	5.3
48	Minnesota	5.2
49	North Dakota	5.1
50	New York	4.8

District of Columbia 2.4

*Source: Morgan Quitno Press using data from U.S. Dept of Health & Human Services, Health Care Financing Admin.
"State Health Expenditure Accounts" (Health Care Financing Review, Fall 1995, Volume 17, Number 1)
*Purchases in retail outlets. By state of outlet. This is a subset of overall "Drug and Other Medical Non-Durable
Expenditures" shown elsewhere in this book.*

Per Capita Expenditures for Prescription Drugs in 1993

National Per Capita = $189*

ALPHA ORDER

RANK	STATE	PER CAPITA
7	Alabama	$216
48	Alaska	142
24	Arizona	185
13	Arkansas	200
33	California	176
45	Colorado	150
15	Connecticut	198
24	Delaware	185
9	Florida	206
12	Georgia	202
38	Hawaii	169
39	Idaho	165
19	Illinois	189
17	Indiana	194
27	Iowa	183
26	Kansas	184
4	Kentucky	223
17	Louisiana	194
37	Maine	172
1	Maryland	230
5	Massachusetts	222
6	Michigan	217
40	Minnesota	163
19	Mississippi	189
23	Missouri	186
47	Montana	143
29	Nebraska	182
30	Nevada	178
35	New Hampshire	175
11	New Jersey	204
44	New Mexico	160
30	New York	178
13	North Carolina	200
41	North Dakota	162
19	Ohio	189
33	Oklahoma	176
48	Oregon	142
15	Pennsylvania	198
9	Rhode Island	206
27	South Carolina	183
46	South Dakota	145
3	Tennessee	226
35	Texas	175
41	Utah	162
22	Vermont	188
8	Virginia	207
41	Washington	162
2	West Virginia	227
30	Wisconsin	178
50	Wyoming	136

RANK ORDER

RANK	STATE	PER CAPITA
1	Maryland	$230
2	West Virginia	227
3	Tennessee	226
4	Kentucky	223
5	Massachusetts	222
6	Michigan	217
7	Alabama	216
8	Virginia	207
9	Florida	206
9	Rhode Island	206
11	New Jersey	204
12	Georgia	202
13	Arkansas	200
13	North Carolina	200
15	Connecticut	198
15	Pennsylvania	198
17	Indiana	194
17	Louisiana	194
19	Illinois	189
19	Mississippi	189
19	Ohio	189
22	Vermont	188
23	Missouri	186
24	Arizona	185
24	Delaware	185
26	Kansas	184
27	Iowa	183
27	South Carolina	183
29	Nebraska	182
30	Nevada	178
30	New York	178
30	Wisconsin	178
33	California	176
33	Oklahoma	176
35	New Hampshire	175
35	Texas	175
37	Maine	172
38	Hawaii	169
39	Idaho	165
40	Minnesota	163
41	North Dakota	162
41	Utah	162
41	Washington	162
44	New Mexico	160
45	Colorado	150
46	South Dakota	145
47	Montana	143
48	Alaska	142
48	Oregon	142
50	Wyoming	136
	District of Columbia	178

Source: Morgan Quitno Press using data from U.S. Dept of Health & Human Services, Health Care Financing Admin. "State Health Expenditure Accounts" (Health Care Financing Review, Fall 1995, Volume 17, Number 1)
Purchases in retail outlets. By state of outlet. This is a subset of overall "Drug and Other Medical Non-Durable Expenditures" shown elsewhere in this book.

Percent Change in Expenditures for Prescription Drugs: 1990 to 1993

National Percent Change = 27.9% Increase*

ALPHA ORDER

RANK	STATE	PERCENT CHANGE
23	Alabama	27.9
2	Alaska	46.6
6	Arizona	38.4
28	Arkansas	26.7
19	California	30.3
4	Colorado	40.9
49	Connecticut	19.5
15	Delaware	31.6
14	Florida	32.6
10	Georgia	35.0
13	Hawaii	33.1
3	Idaho	41.1
35	Illinois	24.6
29	Indiana	26.5
42	Iowa	23.2
33	Kansas	24.7
26	Kentucky	26.8
35	Louisiana	24.6
45	Maine	22.4
22	Maryland	28.4
47	Massachusetts	20.1
39	Michigan	24.2
24	Minnesota	27.4
32	Mississippi	25.1
37	Missouri	24.5
12	Montana	33.3
33	Nebraska	24.7
1	Nevada	55.7
43	New Hampshire	23.1
41	New Jersey	23.3
8	New Mexico	36.3
46	New York	21.3
16	North Carolina	31.2
48	North Dakota	19.8
38	Ohio	24.4
30	Oklahoma	26.4
9	Oregon	35.5
44	Pennsylvania	22.5
50	Rhode Island	18.4
20	South Carolina	30.1
26	South Dakota	26.8
20	Tennessee	30.1
11	Texas	34.4
5	Utah	38.5
31	Vermont	25.6
17	Virginia	30.9
7	Washington	38.0
40	West Virginia	23.7
25	Wisconsin	27.0
18	Wyoming	30.6

RANK ORDER

RANK	STATE	PERCENT CHANGE
1	Nevada	55.7
2	Alaska	46.6
3	Idaho	41.1
4	Colorado	40.9
5	Utah	38.5
6	Arizona	38.4
7	Washington	38.0
8	New Mexico	36.3
9	Oregon	35.5
10	Georgia	35.0
11	Texas	34.4
12	Montana	33.3
13	Hawaii	33.1
14	Florida	32.6
15	Delaware	31.6
16	North Carolina	31.2
17	Virginia	30.9
18	Wyoming	30.6
19	California	30.3
20	South Carolina	30.1
20	Tennessee	30.1
22	Maryland	28.4
23	Alabama	27.9
24	Minnesota	27.4
25	Wisconsin	27.0
26	Kentucky	26.8
26	South Dakota	26.8
28	Arkansas	26.7
29	Indiana	26.5
30	Oklahoma	26.4
31	Vermont	25.6
32	Mississippi	25.1
33	Kansas	24.7
33	Nebraska	24.7
35	Illinois	24.6
35	Louisiana	24.6
37	Missouri	24.5
38	Ohio	24.4
39	Michigan	24.2
40	West Virginia	23.7
41	New Jersey	23.3
42	Iowa	23.2
43	New Hampshire	23.1
44	Pennsylvania	22.5
45	Maine	22.4
46	New York	21.3
47	Massachusetts	20.1
48	North Dakota	19.8
49	Connecticut	19.5
50	Rhode Island	18.4

| | District of Columbia | 10.8 |

Source: Morgan Quitno Press using data from U.S. Dept of Health & Human Services, Health Care Financing Admin.
"State Health Expenditure Accounts" (Health Care Financing Review, Fall 1995, Volume 17, Number 1)
*Purchases in retail outlets. By state of outlet. This is a subset of overall "Drug and Other Medical Non-Durable Expenditures" shown elsewhere in this book.

Percent Change in Per Capita Expenditures for Prescription Drugs: 1990 to 1993

National Percent Change = 22.7% Increase*

ALPHA ORDER

RANK ORDER

RANK	STATE	PERCENT CHANGE		RANK	STATE	PERCENT CHANGE
24	Alabama	23.4		1	Nevada	35.9
2	Alaska	35.2		2	Alaska	35.2
5	Arizona	28.5		3	Colorado	30.4
23	Arkansas	23.5		4	Idaho	28.9
21	California	23.9		5	Arizona	28.5
3	Colorado	30.4		6	New Mexico	28.0
49	Connecticut	19.3		7	Utah	27.6
14	Delaware	25.9		7	Washington	27.6
17	Florida	24.8		9	Oregon	26.8
12	Georgia	26.3		9	Texas	26.8
13	Hawaii	26.1		11	Montana	26.5
4	Idaho	28.9		12	Georgia	26.3
35	Illinois	21.9		13	Hawaii	26.1
29	Indiana	22.8		14	Delaware	25.9
43	Iowa	21.2		14	Wyoming	25.9
35	Kansas	21.9		16	North Carolina	25.0
25	Kentucky	23.2		17	Florida	24.8
29	Louisiana	22.8		18	Virginia	24.7
44	Maine	21.1		19	South Carolina	24.5
22	Maryland	23.7		20	Tennessee	24.2
47	Massachusetts	20.0		21	California	23.9
35	Michigan	21.9		22	Maryland	23.7
32	Minnesota	22.6		23	Arkansas	23.5
35	Mississippi	21.9		24	Alabama	23.4
40	Missouri	21.6		25	Kentucky	23.2
11	Montana	26.5		26	Oklahoma	23.1
33	Nebraska	22.1		27	South Dakota	22.9
1	Nevada	35.9		27	Vermont	22.9
41	New Hampshire	21.5		29	Indiana	22.8
42	New Jersey	21.4		29	Louisiana	22.8
6	New Mexico	28.0		29	Wisconsin	22.8
46	New York	20.3		32	Minnesota	22.6
16	North Carolina	25.0		33	Nebraska	22.1
47	North Dakota	20.0		34	West Virginia	22.0
35	Ohio	21.9		35	Illinois	21.9
26	Oklahoma	23.1		35	Kansas	21.9
9	Oregon	26.8		35	Michigan	21.9
45	Pennsylvania	20.7		35	Mississippi	21.9
50	Rhode Island	19.1		35	Ohio	21.9
19	South Carolina	24.5		40	Missouri	21.6
27	South Dakota	22.9		41	New Hampshire	21.5
20	Tennessee	24.2		42	New Jersey	21.4
9	Texas	26.8		43	Iowa	21.2
7	Utah	27.6		44	Maine	21.1
27	Vermont	22.9		45	Pennsylvania	20.7
18	Virginia	24.7		46	New York	20.3
7	Washington	27.6		47	Massachusetts	20.0
34	West Virginia	22.0		47	North Dakota	20.0
29	Wisconsin	22.8		49	Connecticut	19.3
14	Wyoming	25.9		50	Rhode Island	19.1

District of Columbia   16.3

Source: Morgan Quitno Press using data from U.S. Dept of Health & Human Services, Health Care Financing Admin. "State Health Expenditure Accounts" (Health Care Financing Review, Fall 1995, Volume 17, Number 1)
*Purchases in retail outlets. By state of outlet. This is a subset of overall "Drug and Other Medical Non-Durable Expenditures" shown elsewhere in this book.

Average Annual Change in Expenditures for Prescription Drugs: 1980 to 1993

National Percent = 11.4% Average Annual Increase*

RANK	STATE	PERCENT
32	Alabama	10.9
4	Alaska	13.7
2	Arizona	14.7
49	Arkansas	9.3
16	California	11.8
18	Colorado	11.7
33	Connecticut	10.7
6	Delaware	13.3
4	Florida	13.7
12	Georgia	12.7
14	Hawaii	12.2
20	Idaho	11.6
26	Illinois	11.1
39	Indiana	10.4
46	Iowa	9.6
37	Kansas	10.5
33	Kentucky	10.7
47	Louisiana	9.5
20	Maine	11.6
6	Maryland	13.3
13	Massachusetts	12.5
28	Michigan	11.0
28	Minnesota	11.0
42	Mississippi	10.1
41	Missouri	10.2
28	Montana	11.0
37	Nebraska	10.5
1	Nevada	15.8
6	New Hampshire	13.3
18	New Jersey	11.7
9	New Mexico	13.2
26	New York	11.1
22	North Carolina	11.5
35	North Dakota	10.6
43	Ohio	10.0
47	Oklahoma	9.5
43	Oregon	10.0
28	Pennsylvania	11.0
16	Rhode Island	11.8
15	South Carolina	11.9
43	South Dakota	10.0
25	Tennessee	11.2
35	Texas	10.6
3	Utah	14.2
10	Vermont	13.0
10	Virginia	13.0
24	Washington	11.3
40	West Virginia	10.3
22	Wisconsin	11.5
50	Wyoming	8.2

RANK	STATE	PERCENT
1	Nevada	15.8
2	Arizona	14.7
3	Utah	14.2
4	Alaska	13.7
4	Florida	13.7
6	Delaware	13.3
6	Maryland	13.3
6	New Hampshire	13.3
9	New Mexico	13.2
10	Vermont	13.0
10	Virginia	13.0
12	Georgia	12.7
13	Massachusetts	12.5
14	Hawaii	12.2
15	South Carolina	11.9
16	California	11.8
16	Rhode Island	11.8
18	Colorado	11.7
18	New Jersey	11.7
20	Idaho	11.6
20	Maine	11.6
22	North Carolina	11.5
22	Wisconsin	11.5
24	Washington	11.3
25	Tennessee	11.2
26	Illinois	11.1
26	New York	11.1
28	Michigan	11.0
28	Minnesota	11.0
28	Montana	11.0
28	Pennsylvania	11.0
32	Alabama	10.9
33	Connecticut	10.7
33	Kentucky	10.7
35	North Dakota	10.6
35	Texas	10.6
37	Kansas	10.5
37	Nebraska	10.5
39	Indiana	10.4
40	West Virginia	10.3
41	Missouri	10.2
42	Mississippi	10.1
43	Ohio	10.0
43	Oregon	10.0
43	South Dakota	10.0
46	Iowa	9.6
47	Louisiana	9.5
47	Oklahoma	9.5
49	Arkansas	9.3
50	Wyoming	8.2
	District of Columbia	9.5

Source: U.S. Department of Health and Human Services, Health Care Financing Administration
"State Health Expenditure Accounts" (Health Care Financing Review, Fall 1995, Volume 17, Number 1)
*Purchases in retail outlets. By state of outlet. This is a subset of overall "Drug and Other Medical Non-Durable Expenditures" shown elsewhere in this book.

Average Annual Change in Per Capita Expenditures
For Prescription Drugs: 1980 to 1993
National Percent = 10.3% Average Annual Increase*

ALPHA ORDER

RANK	STATE	PERCENT
27	Alabama	10.4
30	Alaska	10.2
7	Arizona	11.5
48	Arkansas	8.8
43	California	9.4
36	Colorado	9.9
30	Connecticut	10.2
1	Delaware	12.1
20	Florida	10.7
20	Georgia	10.7
24	Hawaii	10.5
32	Idaho	10.1
14	Illinois	10.9
33	Indiana	10.0
38	Iowa	9.8
36	Kansas	9.9
24	Kentucky	10.5
43	Louisiana	9.4
14	Maine	10.9
5	Maryland	11.8
2	Massachusetts	12.0
17	Michigan	10.8
33	Minnesota	10.0
38	Mississippi	9.8
42	Missouri	9.7
24	Montana	10.5
28	Nebraska	10.3
11	Nevada	11.2
6	New Hampshire	11.6
12	New Jersey	11.1
9	New Mexico	11.3
17	New York	10.8
33	North Carolina	10.0
20	North Dakota	10.7
38	Ohio	9.8
46	Oklahoma	8.9
46	Oregon	8.9
17	Pennsylvania	10.8
9	Rhode Island	11.3
20	South Carolina	10.7
38	South Dakota	9.8
28	Tennessee	10.3
49	Texas	8.6
2	Utah	12.0
2	Vermont	12.0
8	Virginia	11.4
45	Washington	9.3
14	West Virginia	10.9
13	Wisconsin	11.0
50	Wyoming	8.2

RANK ORDER

RANK	STATE	PERCENT
1	Delaware	12.1
2	Massachusetts	12.0
2	Utah	12.0
2	Vermont	12.0
5	Maryland	11.8
6	New Hampshire	11.6
7	Arizona	11.5
8	Virginia	11.4
9	New Mexico	11.3
9	Rhode Island	11.3
11	Nevada	11.2
12	New Jersey	11.1
13	Wisconsin	11.0
14	Illinois	10.9
14	Maine	10.9
14	West Virginia	10.9
17	Michigan	10.8
17	New York	10.8
17	Pennsylvania	10.8
20	Florida	10.7
20	Georgia	10.7
20	North Dakota	10.7
20	South Carolina	10.7
24	Hawaii	10.5
24	Kentucky	10.5
24	Montana	10.5
27	Alabama	10.4
28	Nebraska	10.3
28	Tennessee	10.3
30	Alaska	10.2
30	Connecticut	10.2
32	Idaho	10.1
33	Indiana	10.0
33	Minnesota	10.0
33	North Carolina	10.0
36	Colorado	9.9
36	Kansas	9.9
38	Iowa	9.8
38	Mississippi	9.8
38	Ohio	9.8
38	South Dakota	9.8
42	Missouri	9.7
43	California	9.4
43	Louisiana	9.4
45	Washington	9.3
46	Oklahoma	8.9
46	Oregon	8.9
48	Arkansas	8.8
49	Texas	8.6
50	Wyoming	8.2

District of Columbia	10.3

Source: Morgan Quitno Press using data from U.S. Dept of Health & Human Services, Health Care Financing Admin.
"State Health Expenditure Accounts" (Health Care Financing Review, Fall 1995, Volume 17, Number 1)
*Purchases in retail outlets. By state of outlet. This is a subset of overall "Drug and Other Medical Non-Durable Expenditures" shown elsewhere in this book.

Expenditures for Dental Service in 1993

National Total = $37,383,000,000*

ALPHA ORDER

RANK	STATE	EXPENDITURES	% of USA
25	Alabama	$456,000,000	1.22%
44	Alaska	124,000,000	0.33%
24	Arizona	551,000,000	1.47%
33	Arkansas	242,000,000	0.65%
1	California	5,664,000,000	15.15%
21	Colorado	605,000,000	1.62%
19	Connecticut	685,000,000	1.83%
45	Delaware	104,000,000	0.28%
4	Florida	2,029,000,000	5.43%
12	Georgia	898,000,000	2.40%
34	Hawaii	235,000,000	0.63%
41	Idaho	163,000,000	0.44%
6	Illinois	1,588,000,000	4.25%
18	Indiana	692,000,000	1.85%
30	Iowa	341,000,000	0.91%
31	Kansas	325,000,000	0.87%
28	Kentucky	369,000,000	0.99%
26	Louisiana	432,000,000	1.16%
42	Maine	157,000,000	0.42%
16	Maryland	749,000,000	2.00%
11	Massachusetts	1,022,000,000	2.73%
7	Michigan	1,531,000,000	4.10%
17	Minnesota	741,000,000	1.98%
36	Mississippi	214,000,000	0.57%
22	Missouri	602,000,000	1.61%
46	Montana	103,000,000	0.28%
37	Nebraska	191,000,000	0.51%
35	Nevada	215,000,000	0.58%
39	New Hampshire	177,000,000	0.47%
8	New Jersey	1,460,000,000	3.91%
40	New Mexico	175,000,000	0.47%
2	New York	2,837,000,000	7.59%
14	North Carolina	810,000,000	2.17%
49	North Dakota	78,000,000	0.21%
9	Ohio	1,398,000,000	3.74%
29	Oklahoma	356,000,000	0.95%
23	Oregon	578,000,000	1.55%
5	Pennsylvania	1,634,000,000	4.37%
43	Rhode Island	150,000,000	0.40%
27	South Carolina	387,000,000	1.04%
47	South Dakota	87,000,000	0.23%
20	Tennessee	609,000,000	1.63%
3	Texas	2,081,000,000	5.57%
32	Utah	276,000,000	0.74%
48	Vermont	84,000,000	0.22%
13	Virginia	863,000,000	2.31%
10	Washington	1,189,000,000	3.18%
38	West Virginia	182,000,000	0.49%
15	Wisconsin	765,000,000	2.05%
50	Wyoming	57,000,000	0.15%

RANK ORDER

RANK	STATE	EXPENDITURES	% of USA
1	California	$5,664,000,000	15.15%
2	New York	2,837,000,000	7.59%
3	Texas	2,081,000,000	5.57%
4	Florida	2,029,000,000	5.43%
5	Pennsylvania	1,634,000,000	4.37%
6	Illinois	1,588,000,000	4.25%
7	Michigan	1,531,000,000	4.10%
8	New Jersey	1,460,000,000	3.91%
9	Ohio	1,398,000,000	3.74%
10	Washington	1,189,000,000	3.18%
11	Massachusetts	1,022,000,000	2.73%
12	Georgia	898,000,000	2.40%
13	Virginia	863,000,000	2.31%
14	North Carolina	810,000,000	2.17%
15	Wisconsin	765,000,000	2.05%
16	Maryland	749,000,000	2.00%
17	Minnesota	741,000,000	1.98%
18	Indiana	692,000,000	1.85%
19	Connecticut	685,000,000	1.83%
20	Tennessee	609,000,000	1.63%
21	Colorado	605,000,000	1.62%
22	Missouri	602,000,000	1.61%
23	Oregon	578,000,000	1.55%
24	Arizona	551,000,000	1.47%
25	Alabama	456,000,000	1.22%
26	Louisiana	432,000,000	1.16%
27	South Carolina	387,000,000	1.04%
28	Kentucky	369,000,000	0.99%
29	Oklahoma	356,000,000	0.95%
30	Iowa	341,000,000	0.91%
31	Kansas	325,000,000	0.87%
32	Utah	276,000,000	0.74%
33	Arkansas	242,000,000	0.65%
34	Hawaii	235,000,000	0.63%
35	Nevada	215,000,000	0.58%
36	Mississippi	214,000,000	0.57%
37	Nebraska	191,000,000	0.51%
38	West Virginia	182,000,000	0.49%
39	New Hampshire	177,000,000	0.47%
40	New Mexico	175,000,000	0.47%
41	Idaho	163,000,000	0.44%
42	Maine	157,000,000	0.42%
43	Rhode Island	150,000,000	0.40%
44	Alaska	124,000,000	0.33%
45	Delaware	104,000,000	0.28%
46	Montana	103,000,000	0.28%
47	South Dakota	87,000,000	0.23%
48	Vermont	84,000,000	0.22%
49	North Dakota	78,000,000	0.21%
50	Wyoming	57,000,000	0.15%
	District of Columbia	119,000,000	0.32%

Source: U.S. Department of Health and Human Services, Health Care Financing Administration
   "State Health Expenditure Accounts" (Health Care Financing Review, Fall 1995, Volume 17, Number 1)
*By state of provider.

Percent of Total Personal Health Care Expenditures
Spent on Dental Service in 1993
National Percent = 4.8%*

ALPHA ORDER

RANK	STATE	PERCENT
44	Alabama	3.8
1	Alaska	7.9
16	Arizona	5.2
41	Arkansas	4.0
7	California	6.0
7	Colorado	6.0
12	Connecticut	5.6
23	Delaware	4.6
27	Florida	4.5
27	Georgia	4.5
5	Hawaii	6.7
3	Idaho	7.2
23	Illinois	4.6
37	Indiana	4.2
23	Iowa	4.6
22	Kansas	4.7
47	Kentucky	3.6
50	Louisiana	3.3
23	Maine	4.6
20	Maryland	4.9
31	Massachusetts	4.4
12	Michigan	5.6
16	Minnesota	5.2
48	Mississippi	3.5
44	Missouri	3.8
20	Montana	4.9
35	Nebraska	4.3
9	Nevada	5.7
19	New Hampshire	5.1
9	New Jersey	5.7
27	New Mexico	4.5
37	New York	4.2
31	North Carolina	4.4
42	North Dakota	3.9
37	Ohio	4.2
31	Oklahoma	4.4
3	Oregon	7.2
42	Pennsylvania	3.9
31	Rhode Island	4.4
35	South Carolina	4.3
27	South Dakota	4.5
44	Tennessee	3.8
37	Texas	4.2
5	Utah	6.7
12	Vermont	5.6
16	Virginia	5.2
1	Washington	7.9
48	West Virginia	3.5
15	Wisconsin	5.3
9	Wyoming	5.7

RANK ORDER

RANK	STATE	PERCENT
1	Alaska	7.9
1	Washington	7.9
3	Idaho	7.2
3	Oregon	7.2
5	Hawaii	6.7
5	Utah	6.7
7	California	6.0
7	Colorado	6.0
9	Nevada	5.7
9	New Jersey	5.7
9	Wyoming	5.7
12	Connecticut	5.6
12	Michigan	5.6
12	Vermont	5.6
15	Wisconsin	5.3
16	Arizona	5.2
16	Minnesota	5.2
16	Virginia	5.2
19	New Hampshire	5.1
20	Maryland	4.9
20	Montana	4.9
22	Kansas	4.7
23	Delaware	4.6
23	Illinois	4.6
23	Iowa	4.6
23	Maine	4.6
27	Florida	4.5
27	Georgia	4.5
27	New Mexico	4.5
27	South Dakota	4.5
31	Massachusetts	4.4
31	North Carolina	4.4
31	Oklahoma	4.4
31	Rhode Island	4.4
35	Nebraska	4.3
35	South Carolina	4.3
37	Indiana	4.2
37	New York	4.2
37	Ohio	4.2
37	Texas	4.2
41	Arkansas	4.0
42	North Dakota	3.9
42	Pennsylvania	3.9
44	Alabama	3.8
44	Missouri	3.8
44	Tennessee	3.8
47	Kentucky	3.6
48	Mississippi	3.5
48	West Virginia	3.5
50	Louisiana	3.3
	District of Columbia	2.8

*Source: Morgan Quitno Press using data from U.S. Dept of Health & Human Services, Health Care Financing Admin.
"State Health Expenditure Accounts" (Health Care Financing Review, Fall 1995, Volume 17, Number 1)*
By state of provider.

Per Capita Expenditures for Dental Service in 1993

National Per Capita = $145*

<table>
<tr><td colspan="3">ALPHA ORDER</td><td colspan="3">RANK ORDER</td></tr>
<tr><td>RANK</td><td>STATE</td><td>PER CAPITA</td><td>RANK</td><td>STATE</td><td>PER CAPITA</td></tr>
<tr><td>43</td><td>Alabama</td><td>$109</td><td>1</td><td>Washington</td><td>$226</td></tr>
<tr><td>3</td><td>Alaska</td><td>207</td><td>2</td><td>Connecticut</td><td>209</td></tr>
<tr><td>23</td><td>Arizona</td><td>140</td><td>3</td><td>Alaska</td><td>207</td></tr>
<tr><td>47</td><td>Arkansas</td><td>100</td><td>4</td><td>Hawaii</td><td>202</td></tr>
<tr><td>7</td><td>California</td><td>181</td><td>5</td><td>Oregon</td><td>190</td></tr>
<tr><td>8</td><td>Colorado</td><td>170</td><td>6</td><td>New Jersey</td><td>186</td></tr>
<tr><td>2</td><td>Connecticut</td><td>209</td><td>7</td><td>California</td><td>181</td></tr>
<tr><td>18</td><td>Delaware</td><td>149</td><td>8</td><td>Colorado</td><td>170</td></tr>
<tr><td>19</td><td>Florida</td><td>148</td><td>8</td><td>Massachusetts</td><td>170</td></tr>
<tr><td>27</td><td>Georgia</td><td>130</td><td>10</td><td>Minnesota</td><td>164</td></tr>
<tr><td>4</td><td>Hawaii</td><td>202</td><td>11</td><td>Michigan</td><td>162</td></tr>
<tr><td>19</td><td>Idaho</td><td>148</td><td>12</td><td>New Hampshire</td><td>158</td></tr>
<tr><td>24</td><td>Illinois</td><td>136</td><td>13</td><td>New York</td><td>156</td></tr>
<tr><td>33</td><td>Indiana</td><td>121</td><td>14</td><td>Nevada</td><td>155</td></tr>
<tr><td>33</td><td>Iowa</td><td>121</td><td>15</td><td>Wisconsin</td><td>152</td></tr>
<tr><td>28</td><td>Kansas</td><td>128</td><td>16</td><td>Maryland</td><td>151</td></tr>
<tr><td>49</td><td>Kentucky</td><td>97</td><td>17</td><td>Rhode Island</td><td>150</td></tr>
<tr><td>46</td><td>Louisiana</td><td>101</td><td>18</td><td>Delaware</td><td>149</td></tr>
<tr><td>29</td><td>Maine</td><td>127</td><td>19</td><td>Florida</td><td>148</td></tr>
<tr><td>16</td><td>Maryland</td><td>151</td><td>19</td><td>Idaho</td><td>148</td></tr>
<tr><td>8</td><td>Massachusetts</td><td>170</td><td>19</td><td>Utah</td><td>148</td></tr>
<tr><td>11</td><td>Michigan</td><td>162</td><td>22</td><td>Vermont</td><td>146</td></tr>
<tr><td>10</td><td>Minnesota</td><td>164</td><td>23</td><td>Arizona</td><td>140</td></tr>
<tr><td>50</td><td>Mississippi</td><td>81</td><td>24</td><td>Illinois</td><td>136</td></tr>
<tr><td>40</td><td>Missouri</td><td>115</td><td>24</td><td>Pennsylvania</td><td>136</td></tr>
<tr><td>31</td><td>Montana</td><td>122</td><td>26</td><td>Virginia</td><td>133</td></tr>
<tr><td>38</td><td>Nebraska</td><td>118</td><td>27</td><td>Georgia</td><td>130</td></tr>
<tr><td>14</td><td>Nevada</td><td>155</td><td>28</td><td>Kansas</td><td>128</td></tr>
<tr><td>12</td><td>New Hampshire</td><td>158</td><td>29</td><td>Maine</td><td>127</td></tr>
<tr><td>6</td><td>New Jersey</td><td>186</td><td>30</td><td>Ohio</td><td>126</td></tr>
<tr><td>44</td><td>New Mexico</td><td>108</td><td>31</td><td>Montana</td><td>122</td></tr>
<tr><td>13</td><td>New York</td><td>156</td><td>31</td><td>North Dakota</td><td>122</td></tr>
<tr><td>39</td><td>North Carolina</td><td>116</td><td>33</td><td>Indiana</td><td>121</td></tr>
<tr><td>31</td><td>North Dakota</td><td>122</td><td>33</td><td>Iowa</td><td>121</td></tr>
<tr><td>30</td><td>Ohio</td><td>126</td><td>33</td><td>South Dakota</td><td>121</td></tr>
<tr><td>42</td><td>Oklahoma</td><td>110</td><td>33</td><td>Wyoming</td><td>121</td></tr>
<tr><td>5</td><td>Oregon</td><td>190</td><td>37</td><td>Tennessee</td><td>120</td></tr>
<tr><td>24</td><td>Pennsylvania</td><td>136</td><td>38</td><td>Nebraska</td><td>118</td></tr>
<tr><td>17</td><td>Rhode Island</td><td>150</td><td>39</td><td>North Carolina</td><td>116</td></tr>
<tr><td>45</td><td>South Carolina</td><td>107</td><td>40</td><td>Missouri</td><td>115</td></tr>
<tr><td>33</td><td>South Dakota</td><td>121</td><td>40</td><td>Texas</td><td>115</td></tr>
<tr><td>37</td><td>Tennessee</td><td>120</td><td>42</td><td>Oklahoma</td><td>110</td></tr>
<tr><td>40</td><td>Texas</td><td>115</td><td>43</td><td>Alabama</td><td>109</td></tr>
<tr><td>19</td><td>Utah</td><td>148</td><td>44</td><td>New Mexico</td><td>108</td></tr>
<tr><td>22</td><td>Vermont</td><td>146</td><td>45</td><td>South Carolina</td><td>107</td></tr>
<tr><td>26</td><td>Virginia</td><td>133</td><td>46</td><td>Louisiana</td><td>101</td></tr>
<tr><td>1</td><td>Washington</td><td>226</td><td>47</td><td>Arkansas</td><td>100</td></tr>
<tr><td>47</td><td>West Virginia</td><td>100</td><td>47</td><td>West Virginia</td><td>100</td></tr>
<tr><td>15</td><td>Wisconsin</td><td>152</td><td>49</td><td>Kentucky</td><td>97</td></tr>
<tr><td>33</td><td>Wyoming</td><td>121</td><td>50</td><td>Mississippi</td><td>81</td></tr>
</table>

District of Columbia   206

Source: Morgan Quitno Press using data from U.S. Dept of Health & Human Services, Health Care Financing Admin.
"State Health Expenditure Accounts" (Health Care Financing Review, Fall 1995, Volume 17, Number 1)
*By state of provider.

Expenditures for Other Professional Health Care Services in 1993

National Total = $51,200,000,000*

ALPHA ORDER

RANK	STATE	EXPENDITURES	% of USA
26	Alabama	$641,000,000	1.25%
45	Alaska	127,000,000	0.25%
21	Arizona	821,000,000	1.60%
32	Arkansas	332,000,000	0.65%
1	California	6,859,000,000	13.39%
23	Colorado	751,000,000	1.47%
22	Connecticut	769,000,000	1.50%
44	Delaware	156,000,000	0.30%
4	Florida	3,505,000,000	6.84%
11	Georgia	1,226,000,000	2.39%
40	Hawaii	222,000,000	0.43%
46	Idaho	126,000,000	0.25%
6	Illinois	2,063,000,000	4.03%
16	Indiana	993,000,000	1.94%
31	Iowa	431,000,000	0.84%
30	Kansas	470,000,000	0.92%
25	Kentucky	691,000,000	1.35%
24	Louisiana	736,000,000	1.44%
42	Maine	210,000,000	0.41%
18	Maryland	942,000,000	1.84%
10	Massachusetts	1,524,000,000	2.98%
9	Michigan	1,844,000,000	3.60%
19	Minnesota	933,000,000	1.82%
35	Mississippi	288,000,000	0.56%
15	Missouri	1,013,000,000	1.98%
43	Montana	166,000,000	0.32%
39	Nebraska	225,000,000	0.44%
34	Nevada	307,000,000	0.60%
36	New Hampshire	269,000,000	0.53%
8	New Jersey	1,870,000,000	3.65%
37	New Mexico	254,000,000	0.50%
2	New York	3,717,000,000	7.26%
13	North Carolina	1,102,000,000	2.15%
49	North Dakota	93,000,000	0.18%
7	Ohio	1,969,000,000	3.84%
28	Oklahoma	504,000,000	0.98%
27	Oregon	530,000,000	1.03%
5	Pennsylvania	3,005,000,000	5.87%
38	Rhode Island	239,000,000	0.47%
29	South Carolina	472,000,000	0.92%
48	South Dakota	117,000,000	0.23%
12	Tennessee	1,166,000,000	2.28%
3	Texas	3,591,000,000	7.01%
41	Utah	220,000,000	0.43%
47	Vermont	122,000,000	0.24%
17	Virginia	970,000,000	1.89%
13	Washington	1,102,000,000	2.15%
33	West Virginia	326,000,000	0.64%
20	Wisconsin	875,000,000	1.71%
50	Wyoming	68,000,000	0.13%

RANK ORDER

RANK	STATE	EXPENDITURES	% of USA
1	California	$6,859,000,000	13.39%
2	New York	3,717,000,000	7.26%
3	Texas	3,591,000,000	7.01%
4	Florida	3,505,000,000	6.84%
5	Pennsylvania	3,005,000,000	5.87%
6	Illinois	2,063,000,000	4.03%
7	Ohio	1,969,000,000	3.84%
8	New Jersey	1,870,000,000	3.65%
9	Michigan	1,844,000,000	3.60%
10	Massachusetts	1,524,000,000	2.98%
11	Georgia	1,226,000,000	2.39%
12	Tennessee	1,166,000,000	2.28%
13	North Carolina	1,102,000,000	2.15%
13	Washington	1,102,000,000	2.15%
15	Missouri	1,013,000,000	1.98%
16	Indiana	993,000,000	1.94%
17	Virginia	970,000,000	1.89%
18	Maryland	942,000,000	1.84%
19	Minnesota	933,000,000	1.82%
20	Wisconsin	875,000,000	1.71%
21	Arizona	821,000,000	1.60%
22	Connecticut	769,000,000	1.50%
23	Colorado	751,000,000	1.47%
24	Louisiana	736,000,000	1.44%
25	Kentucky	691,000,000	1.35%
26	Alabama	641,000,000	1.25%
27	Oregon	530,000,000	1.03%
28	Oklahoma	504,000,000	0.98%
29	South Carolina	472,000,000	0.92%
30	Kansas	470,000,000	0.92%
31	Iowa	431,000,000	0.84%
32	Arkansas	332,000,000	0.65%
33	West Virginia	326,000,000	0.64%
34	Nevada	307,000,000	0.60%
35	Mississippi	288,000,000	0.56%
36	New Hampshire	269,000,000	0.53%
37	New Mexico	254,000,000	0.50%
38	Rhode Island	239,000,000	0.47%
39	Nebraska	225,000,000	0.44%
40	Hawaii	222,000,000	0.43%
41	Utah	220,000,000	0.43%
42	Maine	210,000,000	0.41%
43	Montana	166,000,000	0.32%
44	Delaware	156,000,000	0.30%
45	Alaska	127,000,000	0.25%
46	Idaho	126,000,000	0.25%
47	Vermont	122,000,000	0.24%
48	South Dakota	117,000,000	0.23%
49	North Dakota	93,000,000	0.18%
50	Wyoming	68,000,000	0.13%
	District of Columbia	267,000,000	0.52%

Source: U.S. Department of Health and Human Services, Health Care Financing Administration
   "State Health Expenditure Accounts" (Health Care Financing Review, Fall 1995, Volume 17, Number 1)
*By state of provider. Includes services by chiropractors, optometrists and podiatrists. Also includes spending in kidney dialysis clinics, alcohol treatment centers, rehabilitation clinics and other health care establishments not elsewhere classified. Medicare ambulance expenditures are also included.

Percent of Total Personal Health Care Expenditures
Spent on Other Professional Services in 1993
National Percent = 6.6%*

ALPHA ORDER

RANK	STATE	PERCENT
45	Alabama	5.3
2	Alaska	8.1
7	Arizona	7.7
44	Arkansas	5.4
9	California	7.3
8	Colorado	7.5
27	Connecticut	6.3
16	Delaware	6.9
5	Florida	7.8
31	Georgia	6.1
25	Hawaii	6.4
42	Idaho	5.5
37	Illinois	5.9
31	Indiana	6.1
37	Iowa	5.9
17	Kansas	6.8
20	Kentucky	6.7
41	Louisiana	5.7
31	Maine	6.1
30	Maryland	6.2
23	Massachusetts	6.5
17	Michigan	6.8
21	Minnesota	6.6
49	Mississippi	4.7
25	Missouri	6.4
4	Montana	7.9
48	Nebraska	5.1
1	Nevada	8.2
5	New Hampshire	7.8
9	New Jersey	7.3
23	New Mexico	6.5
42	New York	5.5
34	North Carolina	6.0
50	North Dakota	4.6
37	Ohio	5.9
27	Oklahoma	6.3
21	Oregon	6.6
12	Pennsylvania	7.2
15	Rhode Island	7.0
47	South Carolina	5.2
34	South Dakota	6.0
12	Tennessee	7.2
12	Texas	7.2
45	Utah	5.3
2	Vermont	8.1
40	Virginia	5.8
9	Washington	7.3
27	West Virginia	6.3
34	Wisconsin	6.0
17	Wyoming	6.8

RANK ORDER

RANK	STATE	PERCENT
1	Nevada	8.2
2	Alaska	8.1
2	Vermont	8.1
4	Montana	7.9
5	Florida	7.8
5	New Hampshire	7.8
7	Arizona	7.7
8	Colorado	7.5
9	California	7.3
9	New Jersey	7.3
9	Washington	7.3
12	Pennsylvania	7.2
12	Tennessee	7.2
12	Texas	7.2
15	Rhode Island	7.0
16	Delaware	6.9
17	Kansas	6.8
17	Michigan	6.8
17	Wyoming	6.8
20	Kentucky	6.7
21	Minnesota	6.6
21	Oregon	6.6
23	Massachusetts	6.5
23	New Mexico	6.5
25	Hawaii	6.4
25	Missouri	6.4
27	Connecticut	6.3
27	Oklahoma	6.3
27	West Virginia	6.3
30	Maryland	6.2
31	Georgia	6.1
31	Indiana	6.1
31	Maine	6.1
34	North Carolina	6.0
34	South Dakota	6.0
34	Wisconsin	6.0
37	Illinois	5.9
37	Iowa	5.9
37	Ohio	5.9
40	Virginia	5.8
41	Louisiana	5.7
42	Idaho	5.5
42	New York	5.5
44	Arkansas	5.4
45	Alabama	5.3
45	Utah	5.3
47	South Carolina	5.2
48	Nebraska	5.1
49	Mississippi	4.7
50	North Dakota	4.6

District of Columbia 6.2

Source: Morgan Quitno Press using data from U.S. Dept of Health & Human Services, Health Care Financing Admin. "State Health Expenditure Accounts" (Health Care Financing Review, Fall 1995, Volume 17, Number 1)
*By state of provider. Includes services by chiropractors, optometrists and podiatrists. Also includes spending in kidney dialysis clinics, alcohol treatment centers, rehabilitation clinics and other health care establishments not elsewhere classified. Medicare ambulance expenditures are also included.

Per Capita Expenditures for Other Professional Health Care Services in 1993

National Per Capita = $199*

ALPHA ORDER

RANK	STATE	PER CAPITA
40	Alabama	$153
12	Alaska	212
16	Arizona	208
46	Arkansas	137
11	California	220
14	Colorado	210
7	Connecticut	235
9	Delaware	223
1	Florida	255
28	Georgia	178
23	Hawaii	190
49	Idaho	114
30	Illinois	176
32	Indiana	174
40	Iowa	153
25	Kansas	186
26	Kentucky	182
34	Louisiana	172
35	Maine	169
23	Maryland	190
2	Massachusetts	253
21	Michigan	195
17	Minnesota	206
50	Mississippi	109
22	Missouri	194
20	Montana	197
45	Nebraska	139
10	Nevada	222
4	New Hampshire	240
6	New Jersey	238
38	New Mexico	157
18	New York	205
37	North Carolina	158
43	North Dakota	146
28	Ohio	178
39	Oklahoma	156
31	Oregon	175
3	Pennsylvania	250
5	Rhode Island	239
47	South Carolina	130
36	South Dakota	163
8	Tennessee	229
19	Texas	199
48	Utah	118
12	Vermont	212
42	Virginia	150
14	Washington	210
27	West Virginia	179
33	Wisconsin	173
44	Wyoming	145

RANK ORDER

RANK	STATE	PER CAPITA
1	Florida	$255
2	Massachusetts	253
3	Pennsylvania	250
4	New Hampshire	240
5	Rhode Island	239
6	New Jersey	238
7	Connecticut	235
8	Tennessee	229
9	Delaware	223
10	Nevada	222
11	California	220
12	Alaska	212
12	Vermont	212
14	Colorado	210
14	Washington	210
16	Arizona	208
17	Minnesota	206
18	New York	205
19	Texas	199
20	Montana	197
21	Michigan	195
22	Missouri	194
23	Hawaii	190
23	Maryland	190
25	Kansas	186
26	Kentucky	182
27	West Virginia	179
28	Georgia	178
28	Ohio	178
30	Illinois	176
31	Oregon	175
32	Indiana	174
33	Wisconsin	173
34	Louisiana	172
35	Maine	169
36	South Dakota	163
37	North Carolina	158
38	New Mexico	157
39	Oklahoma	156
40	Alabama	153
40	Iowa	153
42	Virginia	150
43	North Dakota	146
44	Wyoming	145
45	Nebraska	139
46	Arkansas	137
47	South Carolina	130
48	Utah	118
49	Idaho	114
50	Mississippi	109

District of Columbia   462

Source: Morgan Quitno Press using data from U.S. Dept of Health & Human Services, Health Care Financing Admin. "State Health Expenditure Accounts" (Health Care Financing Review, Fall 1995, Volume 17, Number 1)
*By state of provider. Includes services by chiropractors, optometrists and podiatrists. Also includes spending in kidney dialysis clinics, alcohol treatment centers, rehabilitation clinics and other health care establishments not elsewhere classified. Medicare ambulance expenditures are also included.

Expenditures for Home Health Care in 1993

National Total = $22,982,000,000*

ALPHA ORDER

RANK	STATE	EXPENDITURES	% of USA
13	Alabama	$602,000,000	2.62%
50	Alaska	5,000,000	0.02%
22	Arizona	317,000,000	1.38%
32	Arkansas	145,000,000	0.63%
3	California	1,640,000,000	7.14%
29	Colorado	195,000,000	0.85%
17	Connecticut	391,000,000	1.70%
43	Delaware	51,000,000	0.22%
2	Florida	2,323,000,000	10.11%
9	Georgia	729,000,000	3.17%
46	Hawaii	32,000,000	0.14%
45	Idaho	49,000,000	0.21%
6	Illinois	853,000,000	3.71%
24	Indiana	308,000,000	1.34%
33	Iowa	137,000,000	0.60%
30	Kansas	152,000,000	0.66%
20	Kentucky	357,000,000	1.55%
16	Louisiana	410,000,000	1.78%
36	Maine	104,000,000	0.45%
23	Maryland	314,000,000	1.37%
7	Massachusetts	835,000,000	3.63%
11	Michigan	714,000,000	3.11%
15	Minnesota	414,000,000	1.80%
25	Mississippi	300,000,000	1.31%
21	Missouri	347,000,000	1.51%
44	Montana	50,000,000	0.22%
39	Nebraska	74,000,000	0.32%
35	Nevada	120,000,000	0.52%
40	New Hampshire	71,000,000	0.31%
10	New Jersey	718,000,000	3.12%
41	New Mexico	62,000,000	0.27%
1	New York	3,562,000,000	15.50%
14	North Carolina	541,000,000	2.35%
48	North Dakota	16,000,000	0.07%
12	Ohio	649,000,000	2.82%
26	Oklahoma	273,000,000	1.19%
34	Oregon	122,000,000	0.53%
8	Pennsylvania	796,000,000	3.46%
37	Rhode Island	103,000,000	0.45%
28	South Carolina	216,000,000	0.94%
48	South Dakota	16,000,000	0.07%
5	Tennessee	899,000,000	3.91%
4	Texas	1,583,000,000	6.89%
38	Utah	100,000,000	0.44%
42	Vermont	52,000,000	0.23%
19	Virginia	368,000,000	1.60%
18	Washington	380,000,000	1.65%
31	West Virginia	150,000,000	0.65%
27	Wisconsin	265,000,000	1.15%
47	Wyoming	29,000,000	0.13%

RANK ORDER

RANK	STATE	EXPENDITURES	% of USA
1	New York	$3,562,000,000	15.50%
2	Florida	2,323,000,000	10.11%
3	California	1,640,000,000	7.14%
4	Texas	1,583,000,000	6.89%
5	Tennessee	899,000,000	3.91%
6	Illinois	853,000,000	3.71%
7	Massachusetts	835,000,000	3.63%
8	Pennsylvania	796,000,000	3.46%
9	Georgia	729,000,000	3.17%
10	New Jersey	718,000,000	3.12%
11	Michigan	714,000,000	3.11%
12	Ohio	649,000,000	2.82%
13	Alabama	602,000,000	2.62%
14	North Carolina	541,000,000	2.35%
15	Minnesota	414,000,000	1.80%
16	Louisiana	410,000,000	1.78%
17	Connecticut	391,000,000	1.70%
18	Washington	380,000,000	1.65%
19	Virginia	368,000,000	1.60%
20	Kentucky	357,000,000	1.55%
21	Missouri	347,000,000	1.51%
22	Arizona	317,000,000	1.38%
23	Maryland	314,000,000	1.37%
24	Indiana	308,000,000	1.34%
25	Mississippi	300,000,000	1.31%
26	Oklahoma	273,000,000	1.19%
27	Wisconsin	265,000,000	1.15%
28	South Carolina	216,000,000	0.94%
29	Colorado	195,000,000	0.85%
30	Kansas	152,000,000	0.66%
31	West Virginia	150,000,000	0.65%
32	Arkansas	145,000,000	0.63%
33	Iowa	137,000,000	0.60%
34	Oregon	122,000,000	0.53%
35	Nevada	120,000,000	0.52%
36	Maine	104,000,000	0.45%
37	Rhode Island	103,000,000	0.45%
38	Utah	100,000,000	0.44%
39	Nebraska	74,000,000	0.32%
40	New Hampshire	71,000,000	0.31%
41	New Mexico	62,000,000	0.27%
42	Vermont	52,000,000	0.23%
43	Delaware	51,000,000	0.22%
44	Montana	50,000,000	0.22%
45	Idaho	49,000,000	0.21%
46	Hawaii	32,000,000	0.14%
47	Wyoming	29,000,000	0.13%
48	North Dakota	16,000,000	0.07%
48	South Dakota	16,000,000	0.07%
50	Alaska	5,000,000	0.02%
	District of Columbia	45,000,000	0.20%

Source: U.S. Department of Health and Human Services, Health Care Financing Administration
   "State Health Expenditure Accounts" (Health Care Financing Review, Fall 1995, Volume 17, Number 1)
*By state of provider. Includes spending for services and products by public and private freestanding home health agencies. Excludes home health care services provided by hospital-based agencies which are included in hospital expenditures.

Percent of Total Personal Health Care Expenditures
Spent on Home Health Care in 1993
National Percent = 3.0%*

ALPHA ORDER

RANK	STATE	PERCENT
4	Alabama	5.0
50	Alaska	0.3
15	Arizona	3.0
26	Arkansas	2.4
43	California	1.7
37	Colorado	1.9
11	Connecticut	3.2
30	Delaware	2.3
3	Florida	5.2
6	Georgia	3.6
47	Hawaii	0.9
31	Idaho	2.2
24	Illinois	2.5
37	Indiana	1.9
37	Iowa	1.9
31	Kansas	2.2
9	Kentucky	3.4
11	Louisiana	3.2
15	Maine	3.0
35	Maryland	2.1
6	Massachusetts	3.6
23	Michigan	2.6
19	Minnesota	2.9
5	Mississippi	4.8
31	Missouri	2.2
26	Montana	2.4
43	Nebraska	1.7
11	Nevada	3.2
35	New Hampshire	2.1
22	New Jersey	2.8
45	New Mexico	1.6
2	New York	5.3
15	North Carolina	3.0
48	North Dakota	0.8
37	Ohio	1.9
9	Oklahoma	3.4
46	Oregon	1.5
37	Pennsylvania	1.9
15	Rhode Island	3.0
26	South Carolina	2.4
48	South Dakota	0.8
1	Tennessee	5.5
11	Texas	3.2
26	Utah	2.4
8	Vermont	3.5
31	Virginia	2.2
24	Washington	2.5
19	West Virginia	2.9
42	Wisconsin	1.8
19	Wyoming	2.9

RANK ORDER

RANK	STATE	PERCENT
1	Tennessee	5.5
2	New York	5.3
3	Florida	5.2
4	Alabama	5.0
5	Mississippi	4.8
6	Georgia	3.6
6	Massachusetts	3.6
8	Vermont	3.5
9	Kentucky	3.4
9	Oklahoma	3.4
11	Connecticut	3.2
11	Louisiana	3.2
11	Nevada	3.2
11	Texas	3.2
15	Arizona	3.0
15	Maine	3.0
15	North Carolina	3.0
15	Rhode Island	3.0
19	Minnesota	2.9
19	West Virginia	2.9
19	Wyoming	2.9
22	New Jersey	2.8
23	Michigan	2.6
24	Illinois	2.5
24	Washington	2.5
26	Arkansas	2.4
26	Montana	2.4
26	South Carolina	2.4
26	Utah	2.4
30	Delaware	2.3
31	Idaho	2.2
31	Kansas	2.2
31	Missouri	2.2
31	Virginia	2.2
35	Maryland	2.1
35	New Hampshire	2.1
37	Colorado	1.9
37	Indiana	1.9
37	Iowa	1.9
37	Ohio	1.9
37	Pennsylvania	1.9
42	Wisconsin	1.8
43	California	1.7
43	Nebraska	1.7
45	New Mexico	1.6
46	Oregon	1.5
47	Hawaii	0.9
48	North Dakota	0.8
48	South Dakota	0.8
50	Alaska	0.3
	District of Columbia	1.1

Source: Morgan Quitno Press using data from U.S. Dept of Health & Human Services, Health Care Financing Admin.
"State Health Expenditure Accounts" (Health Care Financing Review, Fall 1995, Volume 17, Number 1)
*By state of provider. Includes spending for services and products by public and private freestanding home health agencies. Excludes home health care services provided by hospital-based agencies which are included in hospital expenditures.

Per Capita Expenditures for Home Health Care in 1993

National Per Capita = $89*

<table>
<tr><td colspan="3"><u>ALPHA ORDER</u></td><td colspan="3"><u>RANK ORDER</u></td></tr>
<tr><th>RANK</th><th>STATE</th><th>PER CAPITA</th><th>RANK</th><th>STATE</th><th>PER CAPITA</th></tr>
<tr><td>4</td><td>Alabama</td><td>$144</td><td>1</td><td>New York</td><td>$196</td></tr>
<tr><td>50</td><td>Alaska</td><td>8</td><td>2</td><td>Tennessee</td><td>177</td></tr>
<tr><td>20</td><td>Arizona</td><td>80</td><td>3</td><td>Florida</td><td>169</td></tr>
<tr><td>31</td><td>Arkansas</td><td>60</td><td>4</td><td>Alabama</td><td>144</td></tr>
<tr><td>40</td><td>California</td><td>53</td><td>5</td><td>Massachusetts</td><td>139</td></tr>
<tr><td>37</td><td>Colorado</td><td>55</td><td>6</td><td>Connecticut</td><td>119</td></tr>
<tr><td>6</td><td>Connecticut</td><td>119</td><td>7</td><td>Mississippi</td><td>114</td></tr>
<tr><td>23</td><td>Delaware</td><td>73</td><td>8</td><td>Georgia</td><td>106</td></tr>
<tr><td>3</td><td>Florida</td><td>169</td><td>9</td><td>Rhode Island</td><td>103</td></tr>
<tr><td>8</td><td>Georgia</td><td>106</td><td>10</td><td>Louisiana</td><td>96</td></tr>
<tr><td>47</td><td>Hawaii</td><td>27</td><td>11</td><td>Kentucky</td><td>94</td></tr>
<tr><td>44</td><td>Idaho</td><td>45</td><td>12</td><td>Minnesota</td><td>92</td></tr>
<tr><td>23</td><td>Illinois</td><td>73</td><td>13</td><td>New Jersey</td><td>91</td></tr>
<tr><td>38</td><td>Indiana</td><td>54</td><td>14</td><td>Vermont</td><td>90</td></tr>
<tr><td>42</td><td>Iowa</td><td>49</td><td>15</td><td>Texas</td><td>88</td></tr>
<tr><td>31</td><td>Kansas</td><td>60</td><td>16</td><td>Nevada</td><td>87</td></tr>
<tr><td>11</td><td>Kentucky</td><td>94</td><td>17</td><td>Maine</td><td>84</td></tr>
<tr><td>10</td><td>Louisiana</td><td>96</td><td>17</td><td>Oklahoma</td><td>84</td></tr>
<tr><td>17</td><td>Maine</td><td>84</td><td>19</td><td>West Virginia</td><td>83</td></tr>
<tr><td>28</td><td>Maryland</td><td>63</td><td>20</td><td>Arizona</td><td>80</td></tr>
<tr><td>5</td><td>Massachusetts</td><td>139</td><td>21</td><td>North Carolina</td><td>78</td></tr>
<tr><td>22</td><td>Michigan</td><td>75</td><td>22</td><td>Michigan</td><td>75</td></tr>
<tr><td>12</td><td>Minnesota</td><td>92</td><td>23</td><td>Delaware</td><td>73</td></tr>
<tr><td>7</td><td>Mississippi</td><td>114</td><td>23</td><td>Illinois</td><td>73</td></tr>
<tr><td>26</td><td>Missouri</td><td>66</td><td>25</td><td>Washington</td><td>72</td></tr>
<tr><td>34</td><td>Montana</td><td>59</td><td>26</td><td>Missouri</td><td>66</td></tr>
<tr><td>43</td><td>Nebraska</td><td>46</td><td>26</td><td>Pennsylvania</td><td>66</td></tr>
<tr><td>16</td><td>Nevada</td><td>87</td><td>28</td><td>Maryland</td><td>63</td></tr>
<tr><td>28</td><td>New Hampshire</td><td>63</td><td>28</td><td>New Hampshire</td><td>63</td></tr>
<tr><td>13</td><td>New Jersey</td><td>91</td><td>30</td><td>Wyoming</td><td>62</td></tr>
<tr><td>46</td><td>New Mexico</td><td>38</td><td>31</td><td>Arkansas</td><td>60</td></tr>
<tr><td>1</td><td>New York</td><td>196</td><td>31</td><td>Kansas</td><td>60</td></tr>
<tr><td>21</td><td>North Carolina</td><td>78</td><td>31</td><td>South Carolina</td><td>60</td></tr>
<tr><td>48</td><td>North Dakota</td><td>25</td><td>34</td><td>Montana</td><td>59</td></tr>
<tr><td>34</td><td>Ohio</td><td>59</td><td>34</td><td>Ohio</td><td>59</td></tr>
<tr><td>17</td><td>Oklahoma</td><td>84</td><td>36</td><td>Virginia</td><td>57</td></tr>
<tr><td>45</td><td>Oregon</td><td>40</td><td>37</td><td>Colorado</td><td>55</td></tr>
<tr><td>26</td><td>Pennsylvania</td><td>66</td><td>38</td><td>Indiana</td><td>54</td></tr>
<tr><td>9</td><td>Rhode Island</td><td>103</td><td>38</td><td>Utah</td><td>54</td></tr>
<tr><td>31</td><td>South Carolina</td><td>60</td><td>40</td><td>California</td><td>53</td></tr>
<tr><td>49</td><td>South Dakota</td><td>22</td><td>40</td><td>Wisconsin</td><td>53</td></tr>
<tr><td>2</td><td>Tennessee</td><td>177</td><td>42</td><td>Iowa</td><td>49</td></tr>
<tr><td>15</td><td>Texas</td><td>88</td><td>43</td><td>Nebraska</td><td>46</td></tr>
<tr><td>38</td><td>Utah</td><td>54</td><td>44</td><td>Idaho</td><td>45</td></tr>
<tr><td>14</td><td>Vermont</td><td>90</td><td>45</td><td>Oregon</td><td>40</td></tr>
<tr><td>36</td><td>Virginia</td><td>57</td><td>46</td><td>New Mexico</td><td>38</td></tr>
<tr><td>25</td><td>Washington</td><td>72</td><td>47</td><td>Hawaii</td><td>27</td></tr>
<tr><td>19</td><td>West Virginia</td><td>83</td><td>48</td><td>North Dakota</td><td>25</td></tr>
<tr><td>40</td><td>Wisconsin</td><td>53</td><td>49</td><td>South Dakota</td><td>22</td></tr>
<tr><td>30</td><td>Wyoming</td><td>62</td><td>50</td><td>Alaska</td><td>8</td></tr>
<tr><td></td><td></td><td></td><td></td><td>District of Columbia</td><td>78</td></tr>
</table>

Source: Morgan Quitno Press using data from U.S. Dept of Health & Human Services, Health Care Financing Admin.
"State Health Expenditure Accounts" (Health Care Financing Review, Fall 1995, Volume 17, Number 1)
*By state of provider. Includes spending for services and products by public and private freestanding home health agencies. Excludes home health care services provided by hospital-based agencies which are included in hospital expenditures.

Expenditures for Drugs and Other Medical Non-Durables in 1993

National Total = $74,956,000,000*

ALPHA ORDER

RANK	STATE	EXPENDITURES	% of USA
21	Alabama	$1,247,000,000	1.66%
46	Alaska	165,000,000	0.22%
24	Arizona	1,124,000,000	1.50%
33	Arkansas	684,000,000	0.91%
1	California	9,017,000,000	12.03%
27	Colorado	919,000,000	1.23%
25	Connecticut	996,000,000	1.33%
44	Delaware	214,000,000	0.29%
4	Florida	4,450,000,000	5.94%
10	Georgia	2,117,000,000	2.82%
37	Hawaii	416,000,000	0.55%
43	Idaho	265,000,000	0.35%
6	Illinois	3,263,000,000	4.35%
16	Indiana	1,594,000,000	2.13%
30	Iowa	743,000,000	0.99%
32	Kansas	695,000,000	0.93%
22	Kentucky	1,196,000,000	1.60%
20	Louisiana	1,269,000,000	1.69%
40	Maine	333,000,000	0.44%
14	Maryland	1,749,000,000	2.33%
13	Massachusetts	1,961,000,000	2.62%
8	Michigan	2,937,000,000	3.92%
23	Minnesota	1,146,000,000	1.53%
31	Mississippi	720,000,000	0.96%
18	Missouri	1,420,000,000	1.89%
45	Montana	209,000,000	0.28%
36	Nebraska	421,000,000	0.56%
39	Nevada	408,000,000	0.54%
41	New Hampshire	319,000,000	0.43%
9	New Jersey	2,452,000,000	3.27%
38	New Mexico	409,000,000	0.55%
3	New York	5,081,000,000	6.78%
11	North Carolina	2,027,000,000	2.70%
49	North Dakota	160,000,000	0.21%
7	Ohio	3,218,000,000	4.29%
28	Oklahoma	874,000,000	1.17%
29	Oregon	762,000,000	1.02%
5	Pennsylvania	3,519,000,000	4.69%
42	Rhode Island	310,000,000	0.41%
26	South Carolina	978,000,000	1.30%
47	South Dakota	163,000,000	0.22%
15	Tennessee	1,635,000,000	2.18%
2	Texas	5,131,000,000	6.85%
35	Utah	439,000,000	0.59%
48	Vermont	161,000,000	0.21%
12	Virginia	2,015,000,000	2.69%
17	Washington	1,474,000,000	1.97%
34	West Virginia	574,000,000	0.77%
19	Wisconsin	1,290,000,000	1.72%
50	Wyoming	113,000,000	0.15%

RANK ORDER

RANK	STATE	EXPENDITURES	% of USA
1	California	$9,017,000,000	12.03%
2	Texas	5,131,000,000	6.85%
3	New York	5,081,000,000	6.78%
4	Florida	4,450,000,000	5.94%
5	Pennsylvania	3,519,000,000	4.69%
6	Illinois	3,263,000,000	4.35%
7	Ohio	3,218,000,000	4.29%
8	Michigan	2,937,000,000	3.92%
9	New Jersey	2,452,000,000	3.27%
10	Georgia	2,117,000,000	2.82%
11	North Carolina	2,027,000,000	2.70%
12	Virginia	2,015,000,000	2.69%
13	Massachusetts	1,961,000,000	2.62%
14	Maryland	1,749,000,000	2.33%
15	Tennessee	1,635,000,000	2.18%
16	Indiana	1,594,000,000	2.13%
17	Washington	1,474,000,000	1.97%
18	Missouri	1,420,000,000	1.89%
19	Wisconsin	1,290,000,000	1.72%
20	Louisiana	1,269,000,000	1.69%
21	Alabama	1,247,000,000	1.66%
22	Kentucky	1,196,000,000	1.60%
23	Minnesota	1,146,000,000	1.53%
24	Arizona	1,124,000,000	1.50%
25	Connecticut	996,000,000	1.33%
26	South Carolina	978,000,000	1.30%
27	Colorado	919,000,000	1.23%
28	Oklahoma	874,000,000	1.17%
29	Oregon	762,000,000	1.02%
30	Iowa	743,000,000	0.99%
31	Mississippi	720,000,000	0.96%
32	Kansas	695,000,000	0.93%
33	Arkansas	684,000,000	0.91%
34	West Virginia	574,000,000	0.77%
35	Utah	439,000,000	0.59%
36	Nebraska	421,000,000	0.56%
37	Hawaii	416,000,000	0.55%
38	New Mexico	409,000,000	0.55%
39	Nevada	408,000,000	0.54%
40	Maine	333,000,000	0.44%
41	New Hampshire	319,000,000	0.43%
42	Rhode Island	310,000,000	0.41%
43	Idaho	265,000,000	0.35%
44	Delaware	214,000,000	0.29%
45	Montana	209,000,000	0.28%
46	Alaska	165,000,000	0.22%
47	South Dakota	163,000,000	0.22%
48	Vermont	161,000,000	0.21%
49	North Dakota	160,000,000	0.21%
50	Wyoming	113,000,000	0.15%
	District of Columbia	175,000,000	0.23%

Source: U.S. Department of Health and Human Services, Health Care Financing Administration
"State Health Expenditure Accounts" (Health Care Financing Review, Fall 1995, Volume 17, Number 1)
*By state of provider. Includes prescription and over-the-counter drugs and sundries. Limited to spending that occurs in retail outlets such as food stores, drug stores, HMO pharmacies or through mail-order pharmacies.

Percent of Total Personal Health Care Expenditures
Spent on Drugs and Other Medical Non-Durables in 1993
National Percent = 9.6%*

ALPHA ORDER

RANK	STATE	PERCENT
21	Alabama	10.3
18	Alaska	10.5
17	Arizona	10.6
8	Arkansas	11.2
32	California	9.6
40	Colorado	9.1
47	Connecticut	8.2
35	Delaware	9.5
26	Florida	9.9
18	Georgia	10.5
2	Hawaii	11.9
3	Idaho	11.6
38	Illinois	9.4
29	Indiana	9.7
23	Iowa	10.1
23	Kansas	10.1
5	Kentucky	11.5
28	Louisiana	9.8
29	Maine	9.7
5	Maryland	11.5
45	Massachusetts	8.4
13	Michigan	10.8
48	Minnesota	8.1
3	Mississippi	11.6
42	Missouri	8.9
26	Montana	9.9
32	Nebraska	9.6
11	Nevada	10.9
39	New Hampshire	9.2
35	New Jersey	9.5
18	New Mexico	10.5
50	New York	7.6
9	North Carolina	11.1
49	North Dakota	7.9
32	Ohio	9.6
11	Oklahoma	10.9
35	Oregon	9.5
44	Pennsylvania	8.5
41	Rhode Island	9.0
13	South Carolina	10.8
46	South Dakota	8.3
23	Tennessee	10.1
21	Texas	10.3
15	Utah	10.7
15	Vermont	10.7
1	Virginia	12.1
29	Washington	9.7
10	West Virginia	11.0
42	Wisconsin	8.9
7	Wyoming	11.3

RANK ORDER

RANK	STATE	PERCENT
1	Virginia	12.1
2	Hawaii	11.9
3	Idaho	11.6
3	Mississippi	11.6
5	Kentucky	11.5
5	Maryland	11.5
7	Wyoming	11.3
8	Arkansas	11.2
9	North Carolina	11.1
10	West Virginia	11.0
11	Nevada	10.9
11	Oklahoma	10.9
13	Michigan	10.8
13	South Carolina	10.8
15	Utah	10.7
15	Vermont	10.7
17	Arizona	10.6
18	Alaska	10.5
18	Georgia	10.5
18	New Mexico	10.5
21	Alabama	10.3
21	Texas	10.3
23	Iowa	10.1
23	Kansas	10.1
23	Tennessee	10.1
26	Florida	9.9
26	Montana	9.9
28	Louisiana	9.8
29	Indiana	9.7
29	Maine	9.7
29	Washington	9.7
32	California	9.6
32	Nebraska	9.6
32	Ohio	9.6
35	Delaware	9.5
35	New Jersey	9.5
35	Oregon	9.5
38	Illinois	9.4
39	New Hampshire	9.2
40	Colorado	9.1
41	Rhode Island	9.0
42	Missouri	8.9
42	Wisconsin	8.9
44	Pennsylvania	8.5
45	Massachusetts	8.4
46	South Dakota	8.3
47	Connecticut	8.2
48	Minnesota	8.1
49	North Dakota	7.9
50	New York	7.6

District of Columbia 4.1

Source: Morgan Quitno Press using data from U.S. Dept of Health & Human Services, Health Care Financing Admin.
"State Health Expenditure Accounts" (Health Care Financing Review, Fall 1995, Volume 17, Number 1)
By state of provider. Includes prescription and over-the-counter drugs and sundries. Limited to spending that
occurs in retail outlets such as food stores, drug stores, HMO pharmacies or through mail-order pharmacies.

Expenditures for Other Professional Health Care Services in 1993

National Total = $51,200,000,000*

ALPHA ORDER

RANK	STATE	EXPENDITURES	% of USA
26	Alabama	$641,000,000	1.25%
45	Alaska	127,000,000	0.25%
21	Arizona	821,000,000	1.60%
32	Arkansas	332,000,000	0.65%
1	California	6,859,000,000	13.39%
23	Colorado	751,000,000	1.47%
22	Connecticut	769,000,000	1.50%
44	Delaware	156,000,000	0.30%
4	Florida	3,505,000,000	6.84%
11	Georgia	1,226,000,000	2.39%
40	Hawaii	222,000,000	0.43%
46	Idaho	126,000,000	0.25%
6	Illinois	2,063,000,000	4.03%
16	Indiana	993,000,000	1.94%
31	Iowa	431,000,000	0.84%
30	Kansas	470,000,000	0.92%
25	Kentucky	691,000,000	1.35%
24	Louisiana	736,000,000	1.44%
42	Maine	210,000,000	0.41%
18	Maryland	942,000,000	1.84%
10	Massachusetts	1,524,000,000	2.98%
9	Michigan	1,844,000,000	3.60%
19	Minnesota	933,000,000	1.82%
35	Mississippi	288,000,000	0.56%
15	Missouri	1,013,000,000	1.98%
43	Montana	166,000,000	0.32%
39	Nebraska	225,000,000	0.44%
34	Nevada	307,000,000	0.60%
36	New Hampshire	269,000,000	0.53%
8	New Jersey	1,870,000,000	3.65%
37	New Mexico	254,000,000	0.50%
2	New York	3,717,000,000	7.26%
13	North Carolina	1,102,000,000	2.15%
49	North Dakota	93,000,000	0.18%
7	Ohio	1,969,000,000	3.84%
28	Oklahoma	504,000,000	0.98%
27	Oregon	530,000,000	1.03%
5	Pennsylvania	3,005,000,000	5.87%
38	Rhode Island	239,000,000	0.47%
29	South Carolina	472,000,000	0.92%
48	South Dakota	117,000,000	0.23%
12	Tennessee	1,166,000,000	2.28%
3	Texas	3,591,000,000	7.01%
41	Utah	220,000,000	0.43%
47	Vermont	122,000,000	0.24%
17	Virginia	970,000,000	1.89%
13	Washington	1,102,000,000	2.15%
33	West Virginia	326,000,000	0.64%
20	Wisconsin	875,000,000	1.71%
50	Wyoming	68,000,000	0.13%

RANK ORDER

RANK	STATE	EXPENDITURES	% of USA
1	California	$6,859,000,000	13.39%
2	New York	3,717,000,000	7.26%
3	Texas	3,591,000,000	7.01%
4	Florida	3,505,000,000	6.84%
5	Pennsylvania	3,005,000,000	5.87%
6	Illinois	2,063,000,000	4.03%
7	Ohio	1,969,000,000	3.84%
8	New Jersey	1,870,000,000	3.65%
9	Michigan	1,844,000,000	3.60%
10	Massachusetts	1,524,000,000	2.98%
11	Georgia	1,226,000,000	2.39%
12	Tennessee	1,166,000,000	2.28%
13	North Carolina	1,102,000,000	2.15%
13	Washington	1,102,000,000	2.15%
15	Missouri	1,013,000,000	1.98%
16	Indiana	993,000,000	1.94%
17	Virginia	970,000,000	1.89%
18	Maryland	942,000,000	1.84%
19	Minnesota	933,000,000	1.82%
20	Wisconsin	875,000,000	1.71%
21	Arizona	821,000,000	1.60%
22	Connecticut	769,000,000	1.50%
23	Colorado	751,000,000	1.47%
24	Louisiana	736,000,000	1.44%
25	Kentucky	691,000,000	1.35%
26	Alabama	641,000,000	1.25%
27	Oregon	530,000,000	1.03%
28	Oklahoma	504,000,000	0.98%
29	South Carolina	472,000,000	0.92%
30	Kansas	470,000,000	0.92%
31	Iowa	431,000,000	0.84%
32	Arkansas	332,000,000	0.65%
33	West Virginia	326,000,000	0.64%
34	Nevada	307,000,000	0.60%
35	Mississippi	288,000,000	0.56%
36	New Hampshire	269,000,000	0.53%
37	New Mexico	254,000,000	0.50%
38	Rhode Island	239,000,000	0.47%
39	Nebraska	225,000,000	0.44%
40	Hawaii	222,000,000	0.43%
41	Utah	220,000,000	0.43%
42	Maine	210,000,000	0.41%
43	Montana	166,000,000	0.32%
44	Delaware	156,000,000	0.30%
45	Alaska	127,000,000	0.25%
46	Idaho	126,000,000	0.25%
47	Vermont	122,000,000	0.24%
48	South Dakota	117,000,000	0.23%
49	North Dakota	93,000,000	0.18%
50	Wyoming	68,000,000	0.13%
	District of Columbia	267,000,000	0.52%

Source: U.S. Department of Health and Human Services, Health Care Financing Administration
"State Health Expenditure Accounts" (Health Care Financing Review, Fall 1995, Volume 17, Number 1)
By state of provider. Includes services by chiropractors, optometrists and podiatrists. Also includes spending in kidney dialysis clinics, alcohol treatment centers, rehabilitation clinics and other health care establishments not elsewhere classified. Medicare ambulance expenditures are also included.

Expenditures for Vision Products and Other Medical Durables in 1993

National Total = $12,636,000,000*

RANK	STATE	EXPENDITURES	% of USA
	ALPHA ORDER		
25	Alabama	$155,000,000	1.23%
48	Alaska	26,000,000	0.21%
21	Arizona	227,000,000	1.80%
39	Arkansas	56,000,000	0.44%
1	California	1,522,000,000	12.04%
22	Colorado	226,000,000	1.79%
23	Connecticut	192,000,000	1.52%
43	Delaware	35,000,000	0.28%
4	Florida	872,000,000	6.90%
10	Georgia	331,000,000	2.62%
37	Hawaii	64,000,000	0.51%
43	Idaho	35,000,000	0.28%
6	Illinois	604,000,000	4.78%
14	Indiana	270,000,000	2.14%
26	Iowa	148,000,000	1.17%
31	Kansas	107,000,000	0.85%
27	Kentucky	141,000,000	1.12%
24	Louisiana	160,000,000	1.27%
40	Maine	46,000,000	0.36%
13	Maryland	272,000,000	2.15%
15	Massachusetts	269,000,000	2.13%
8	Michigan	457,000,000	3.62%
12	Minnesota	277,000,000	2.19%
38	Mississippi	60,000,000	0.47%
17	Missouri	244,000,000	1.93%
42	Montana	36,000,000	0.28%
33	Nebraska	80,000,000	0.63%
34	Nevada	76,000,000	0.60%
41	New Hampshire	43,000,000	0.34%
8	New Jersey	457,000,000	3.62%
36	New Mexico	69,000,000	0.55%
2	New York	1,090,000,000	8.63%
16	North Carolina	268,000,000	2.12%
47	North Dakota	28,000,000	0.22%
7	Ohio	531,000,000	4.20%
28	Oklahoma	121,000,000	0.96%
32	Oregon	91,000,000	0.72%
5	Pennsylvania	617,000,000	4.88%
45	Rhode Island	33,000,000	0.26%
30	South Carolina	115,000,000	0.91%
46	South Dakota	30,000,000	0.24%
20	Tennessee	228,000,000	1.80%
3	Texas	883,000,000	6.99%
29	Utah	117,000,000	0.93%
49	Vermont	24,000,000	0.19%
11	Virginia	295,000,000	2.33%
18	Washington	242,000,000	1.92%
35	West Virginia	74,000,000	0.59%
19	Wisconsin	240,000,000	1.90%
50	Wyoming	17,000,000	0.13%

RANK	STATE	EXPENDITURES	% of USA
	RANK ORDER		
1	California	$1,522,000,000	12.04%
2	New York	1,090,000,000	8.63%
3	Texas	883,000,000	6.99%
4	Florida	872,000,000	6.90%
5	Pennsylvania	617,000,000	4.88%
6	Illinois	604,000,000	4.78%
7	Ohio	531,000,000	4.20%
8	Michigan	457,000,000	3.62%
8	New Jersey	457,000,000	3.62%
10	Georgia	331,000,000	2.62%
11	Virginia	295,000,000	2.33%
12	Minnesota	277,000,000	2.19%
13	Maryland	272,000,000	2.15%
14	Indiana	270,000,000	2.14%
15	Massachusetts	269,000,000	2.13%
16	North Carolina	268,000,000	2.12%
17	Missouri	244,000,000	1.93%
18	Washington	242,000,000	1.92%
19	Wisconsin	240,000,000	1.90%
20	Tennessee	228,000,000	1.80%
21	Arizona	227,000,000	1.80%
22	Colorado	226,000,000	1.79%
23	Connecticut	192,000,000	1.52%
24	Louisiana	160,000,000	1.27%
25	Alabama	155,000,000	1.23%
26	Iowa	148,000,000	1.17%
27	Kentucky	141,000,000	1.12%
28	Oklahoma	121,000,000	0.96%
29	Utah	117,000,000	0.93%
30	South Carolina	115,000,000	0.91%
31	Kansas	107,000,000	0.85%
32	Oregon	91,000,000	0.72%
33	Nebraska	80,000,000	0.63%
34	Nevada	76,000,000	0.60%
35	West Virginia	74,000,000	0.59%
36	New Mexico	69,000,000	0.55%
37	Hawaii	64,000,000	0.51%
38	Mississippi	60,000,000	0.47%
39	Arkansas	56,000,000	0.44%
40	Maine	46,000,000	0.36%
41	New Hampshire	43,000,000	0.34%
42	Montana	36,000,000	0.28%
43	Delaware	35,000,000	0.28%
43	Idaho	35,000,000	0.28%
45	Rhode Island	33,000,000	0.26%
46	South Dakota	30,000,000	0.24%
47	North Dakota	28,000,000	0.22%
48	Alaska	26,000,000	0.21%
49	Vermont	24,000,000	0.19%
50	Wyoming	17,000,000	0.13%
	District of Columbia	34,000,000	0.27%

Source: U.S. Department of Health and Human Services, Health Care Financing Administration
"State Health Expenditure Accounts" (Health Care Financing Review, Fall 1995, Volume 17, Number 1)
*By state of provider. Includes eyeglasses, hearing aids, surgical appliances and supplies, bulk and cylinder oxygen and medical equipment rentals.

Percent of Total Personal Health Care Expenditures
Spent on Vision Products and Other Medical Durables in 1993
National Percent = 1.6%*

ALPHA ORDER

RANK	STATE	PERCENT
41	Alabama	1.3
15	Alaska	1.7
3	Arizona	2.1
50	Arkansas	0.9
21	California	1.6
2	Colorado	2.2
21	Connecticut	1.6
30	Delaware	1.5
7	Florida	1.9
21	Georgia	1.6
8	Hawaii	1.8
30	Idaho	1.5
15	Illinois	1.7
21	Indiana	1.6
4	Iowa	2.0
21	Kansas	1.6
37	Kentucky	1.4
44	Louisiana	1.2
41	Maine	1.3
8	Maryland	1.8
46	Massachusetts	1.1
15	Michigan	1.7
4	Minnesota	2.0
48	Mississippi	1.0
30	Missouri	1.5
15	Montana	1.7
8	Nebraska	1.8
4	Nevada	2.0
44	New Hampshire	1.2
8	New Jersey	1.8
8	New Mexico	1.8
21	New York	1.6
30	North Carolina	1.5
37	North Dakota	1.4
21	Ohio	1.6
30	Oklahoma	1.5
46	Oregon	1.1
30	Pennsylvania	1.5
48	Rhode Island	1.0
41	South Carolina	1.3
30	South Dakota	1.5
37	Tennessee	1.4
8	Texas	1.8
1	Utah	2.8
21	Vermont	1.6
8	Virginia	1.8
21	Washington	1.6
37	West Virginia	1.4
15	Wisconsin	1.7
15	Wyoming	1.7

RANK ORDER

RANK	STATE	PERCENT
1	Utah	2.8
2	Colorado	2.2
3	Arizona	2.1
4	Iowa	2.0
4	Minnesota	2.0
4	Nevada	2.0
7	Florida	1.9
8	Hawaii	1.8
8	Maryland	1.8
8	Nebraska	1.8
8	New Jersey	1.8
8	New Mexico	1.8
8	Texas	1.8
8	Virginia	1.8
15	Alaska	1.7
15	Illinois	1.7
15	Michigan	1.7
15	Montana	1.7
15	Wisconsin	1.7
15	Wyoming	1.7
21	California	1.6
21	Connecticut	1.6
21	Georgia	1.6
21	Indiana	1.6
21	Kansas	1.6
21	New York	1.6
21	Ohio	1.6
21	Vermont	1.6
21	Washington	1.6
30	Delaware	1.5
30	Idaho	1.5
30	Missouri	1.5
30	North Carolina	1.5
30	Oklahoma	1.5
30	Pennsylvania	1.5
30	South Dakota	1.5
37	Kentucky	1.4
37	North Dakota	1.4
37	Tennessee	1.4
37	West Virginia	1.4
41	Alabama	1.3
41	Maine	1.3
41	South Carolina	1.3
44	Louisiana	1.2
44	New Hampshire	1.2
46	Massachusetts	1.1
46	Oregon	1.1
48	Mississippi	1.0
48	Rhode Island	1.0
50	Arkansas	0.9

District of Columbia   0.8

Source: Morgan Quitno Press using data from U.S. Dept of Health & Human Services, Health Care Financing Admin. "State Health Expenditure Accounts" (Health Care Financing Review, Fall 1995, Volume 17, Number 1)
By state of provider. Includes eyeglasses, hearing aids, surgical appliances and supplies, bulk and cylinder oxygen and medical equipment rentals.

Per Capita Expenditures for Vision Products and Other Medical Durables in 1993

National Per Capita = $49*

ALPHA ORDER

RANK ORDER

RANK	STATE	PER CAPITA	RANK	STATE	PER CAPITA
39	Alabama	$37	1	Florida	$64
30	Alaska	43	2	Colorado	63
7	Arizona	58	2	Utah	63
49	Arkansas	23	4	Minnesota	61
17	California	49	5	New York	60
2	Colorado	63	6	Connecticut	59
6	Connecticut	59	7	Arizona	58
15	Delaware	50	7	New Jersey	58
1	Florida	64	9	Hawaii	55
19	Georgia	48	9	Maryland	55
9	Hawaii	55	9	Nevada	55
46	Idaho	32	12	Illinois	52
12	Illinois	52	12	Iowa	52
23	Indiana	47	14	Pennsylvania	51
12	Iowa	52	15	Delaware	50
33	Kansas	42	15	Nebraska	50
39	Kentucky	37	17	California	49
39	Louisiana	37	17	Texas	49
39	Maine	37	19	Georgia	48
9	Maryland	55	19	Michigan	48
27	Massachusetts	45	19	Ohio	48
19	Michigan	48	19	Wisconsin	48
4	Minnesota	61	23	Indiana	47
49	Mississippi	23	23	Missouri	47
23	Missouri	47	25	Virginia	46
30	Montana	43	25	Washington	46
15	Nebraska	50	27	Massachusetts	45
9	Nevada	55	27	Tennessee	45
38	New Hampshire	38	29	North Dakota	44
7	New Jersey	58	30	Alaska	43
30	New Mexico	43	30	Montana	43
5	New York	60	30	New Mexico	43
37	North Carolina	39	33	Kansas	42
29	North Dakota	44	33	South Dakota	42
19	Ohio	48	33	Vermont	42
39	Oklahoma	37	36	West Virginia	41
48	Oregon	30	37	North Carolina	39
14	Pennsylvania	51	38	New Hampshire	38
45	Rhode Island	33	39	Alabama	37
46	South Carolina	32	39	Kentucky	37
33	South Dakota	42	39	Louisiana	37
27	Tennessee	45	39	Maine	37
17	Texas	49	39	Oklahoma	37
2	Utah	63	44	Wyoming	36
33	Vermont	42	45	Rhode Island	33
25	Virginia	46	46	Idaho	32
25	Washington	46	46	South Carolina	32
36	West Virginia	41	48	Oregon	30
19	Wisconsin	48	49	Arkansas	23
44	Wyoming	36	49	Mississippi	23
				District of Columbia	59

Source: Morgan Quitno Press using data from U.S. Dept of Health & Human Services, Health Care Financing Admin.
"State Health Expenditure Accounts" (Health Care Financing Review, Fall 1995, Volume 17, Number 1)
*By state of provider. Includes eyeglasses, hearing aids, surgical appliances and supplies, bulk and cylinder oxygen and medical equipment rentals.

Expenditures for Nursing Home Care in 1993

National Total = $66,201,000,000*

ALPHA ORDER

RANK ORDER

RANK	STATE	EXPENDITURES	% of USA
27	Alabama	$703,000,000	1.06%
50	Alaska	56,000,000	0.08%
31	Arizona	567,000,000	0.86%
32	Arkansas	558,000,000	0.84%
3	California	4,103,000,000	6.20%
28	Colorado	661,000,000	1.00%
14	Connecticut	1,749,000,000	2.64%
41	Delaware	217,000,000	0.33%
7	Florida	3,089,000,000	4.67%
21	Georgia	1,038,000,000	1.57%
45	Hawaii	181,000,000	0.27%
44	Idaho	197,000,000	0.30%
5	Illinois	3,148,000,000	4.76%
10	Indiana	2,018,000,000	3.05%
23	Iowa	927,000,000	1.40%
26	Kansas	721,000,000	1.09%
24	Kentucky	850,000,000	1.28%
18	Louisiana	1,186,000,000	1.79%
36	Maine	453,000,000	0.68%
19	Maryland	1,185,000,000	1.79%
8	Massachusetts	2,737,000,000	4.13%
12	Michigan	1,849,000,000	2.79%
11	Minnesota	1,884,000,000	2.85%
35	Mississippi	460,000,000	0.69%
16	Missouri	1,368,000,000	2.07%
46	Montana	178,000,000	0.27%
34	Nebraska	482,000,000	0.73%
47	Nevada	164,000,000	0.25%
38	New Hampshire	268,000,000	0.40%
9	New Jersey	2,128,000,000	3.21%
43	New Mexico	215,000,000	0.32%
1	New York	9,106,000,000	13.76%
15	North Carolina	1,562,000,000	2.36%
40	North Dakota	246,000,000	0.37%
4	Ohio	3,758,000,000	5.68%
25	Oklahoma	748,000,000	1.13%
29	Oregon	656,000,000	0.99%
2	Pennsylvania	4,153,000,000	6.27%
33	Rhode Island	485,000,000	0.73%
30	South Carolina	638,000,000	0.96%
42	South Dakota	216,000,000	0.33%
20	Tennessee	1,085,000,000	1.64%
6	Texas	3,104,000,000	4.69%
39	Utah	260,000,000	0.39%
48	Vermont	148,000,000	0.22%
22	Virginia	976,000,000	1.47%
17	Washington	1,291,000,000	1.95%
37	West Virginia	365,000,000	0.55%
13	Wisconsin	1,752,000,000	2.65%
49	Wyoming	83,000,000	0.13%

RANK	STATE	EXPENDITURES	% of USA
1	New York	$9,106,000,000	13.76%
2	Pennsylvania	4,153,000,000	6.27%
3	California	4,103,000,000	6.20%
4	Ohio	3,758,000,000	5.68%
5	Illinois	3,148,000,000	4.76%
6	Texas	3,104,000,000	4.69%
7	Florida	3,089,000,000	4.67%
8	Massachusetts	2,737,000,000	4.13%
9	New Jersey	2,128,000,000	3.21%
10	Indiana	2,018,000,000	3.05%
11	Minnesota	1,884,000,000	2.85%
12	Michigan	1,849,000,000	2.79%
13	Wisconsin	1,752,000,000	2.65%
14	Connecticut	1,749,000,000	2.64%
15	North Carolina	1,562,000,000	2.36%
16	Missouri	1,368,000,000	2.07%
17	Washington	1,291,000,000	1.95%
18	Louisiana	1,186,000,000	1.79%
19	Maryland	1,185,000,000	1.79%
20	Tennessee	1,085,000,000	1.64%
21	Georgia	1,038,000,000	1.57%
22	Virginia	976,000,000	1.47%
23	Iowa	927,000,000	1.40%
24	Kentucky	850,000,000	1.28%
25	Oklahoma	748,000,000	1.13%
26	Kansas	721,000,000	1.09%
27	Alabama	703,000,000	1.06%
28	Colorado	661,000,000	1.00%
29	Oregon	656,000,000	0.99%
30	South Carolina	638,000,000	0.96%
31	Arizona	567,000,000	0.86%
32	Arkansas	558,000,000	0.84%
33	Rhode Island	485,000,000	0.73%
34	Nebraska	482,000,000	0.73%
35	Mississippi	460,000,000	0.69%
36	Maine	453,000,000	0.68%
37	West Virginia	365,000,000	0.55%
38	New Hampshire	268,000,000	0.40%
39	Utah	260,000,000	0.39%
40	North Dakota	246,000,000	0.37%
41	Delaware	217,000,000	0.33%
42	South Dakota	216,000,000	0.33%
43	New Mexico	215,000,000	0.32%
44	Idaho	197,000,000	0.30%
45	Hawaii	181,000,000	0.27%
46	Montana	178,000,000	0.27%
47	Nevada	164,000,000	0.25%
48	Vermont	148,000,000	0.22%
49	Wyoming	83,000,000	0.13%
50	Alaska	56,000,000	0.08%
	District of Columbia	231,000,000	0.35%

Source: U.S. Department of Health and Human Services, Health Care Financing Administration
   "State Health Expenditure Accounts" (Health Care Financing Review, Fall 1995, Volume 17, Number 1)
By state of provider. Includes freestanding nursing and personal-care facilities. Includes Medicare- and Medicaid-certified skilled nursing and intermediate care facilities as well as facilities that are not certified. Excludes hospital-based facilities as they are counted in hospital care expenditures.

Percent of Total Personal Health Care Expenditures
Spent on Nursing Home Care in 1993
National Percent = 8.5%*

ALPHA ORDER

RANK	STATE	PERCENT
43	Alabama	5.8
50	Alaska	3.6
45	Arizona	5.3
19	Arkansas	9.1
48	California	4.4
39	Colorado	6.6
1	Connecticut	14.3
17	Delaware	9.6
36	Florida	6.9
46	Georgia	5.2
46	Hawaii	5.2
22	Idaho	8.7
19	Illinois	9.1
7	Indiana	12.3
6	Iowa	12.6
14	Kansas	10.4
29	Kentucky	8.2
19	Louisiana	9.1
5	Maine	13.2
31	Maryland	7.8
10	Massachusetts	11.7
37	Michigan	6.8
4	Minnesota	13.3
33	Mississippi	7.4
23	Missouri	8.6
25	Montana	8.5
13	Nebraska	11.0
48	Nevada	4.4
31	New Hampshire	7.8
27	New Jersey	8.3
44	New Mexico	5.5
3	New York	13.6
23	North Carolina	8.6
8	North Dakota	12.2
11	Ohio	11.2
18	Oklahoma	9.3
29	Oregon	8.2
15	Pennsylvania	10.0
2	Rhode Island	14.1
34	South Carolina	7.1
12	South Dakota	11.1
38	Tennessee	6.7
41	Texas	6.2
40	Utah	6.3
16	Vermont	9.9
42	Virginia	5.9
25	Washington	8.5
35	West Virginia	7.0
9	Wisconsin	12.1
27	Wyoming	8.3

RANK ORDER

RANK	STATE	PERCENT
1	Connecticut	14.3
2	Rhode Island	14.1
3	New York	13.6
4	Minnesota	13.3
5	Maine	13.2
6	Iowa	12.6
7	Indiana	12.3
8	North Dakota	12.2
9	Wisconsin	12.1
10	Massachusetts	11.7
11	Ohio	11.2
12	South Dakota	11.1
13	Nebraska	11.0
14	Kansas	10.4
15	Pennsylvania	10.0
16	Vermont	9.9
17	Delaware	9.6
18	Oklahoma	9.3
19	Arkansas	9.1
19	Illinois	9.1
19	Louisiana	9.1
22	Idaho	8.7
23	Missouri	8.6
23	North Carolina	8.6
25	Montana	8.5
25	Washington	8.5
27	New Jersey	8.3
27	Wyoming	8.3
29	Kentucky	8.2
29	Oregon	8.2
31	Maryland	7.8
31	New Hampshire	7.8
33	Mississippi	7.4
34	South Carolina	7.1
35	West Virginia	7.0
36	Florida	6.9
37	Michigan	6.8
38	Tennessee	6.7
39	Colorado	6.6
40	Utah	6.3
41	Texas	6.2
42	Virginia	5.9
43	Alabama	5.8
44	New Mexico	5.5
45	Arizona	5.3
46	Georgia	5.2
46	Hawaii	5.2
48	California	4.4
48	Nevada	4.4
50	Alaska	3.6

| | District of Columbia | 5.4 |

*Source: Morgan Quitno Press using data from U.S. Dept of Health & Human Services, Health Care Financing Admin.
"State Health Expenditure Accounts" (Health Care Financing Review, Fall 1995, Volume 17, Number 1)
*By state of provider. Includes freestanding nursing and personal-care facilities. Includes Medicare- and
Medicaid-certified skilled nursing and intermediate care facilities as well as facilities that are not certified.
Excludes hospital-based facilities as they are counted in hospital care expenditures.*

Per Capita Expenditures for Nursing Home Care in 1993

National Per Capita = $257*

<table>
<tr><td colspan="3">ALPHA ORDER</td><td colspan="3">RANK ORDER</td></tr>
<tr><td>RANK</td><td>STATE</td><td>PER CAPITA</td><td>RANK</td><td>STATE</td><td>PER CAPITA</td></tr>
<tr><td>41</td><td>Alabama</td><td>$168</td><td>1</td><td>Connecticut</td><td>$534</td></tr>
<tr><td>50</td><td>Alaska</td><td>94</td><td>2</td><td>New York</td><td>502</td></tr>
<tr><td>45</td><td>Arizona</td><td>144</td><td>3</td><td>Rhode Island</td><td>485</td></tr>
<tr><td>26</td><td>Arkansas</td><td>230</td><td>4</td><td>Massachusetts</td><td>455</td></tr>
<tr><td>48</td><td>California</td><td>131</td><td>5</td><td>Minnesota</td><td>416</td></tr>
<tr><td>35</td><td>Colorado</td><td>185</td><td>6</td><td>North Dakota</td><td>386</td></tr>
<tr><td>1</td><td>Connecticut</td><td>534</td><td>7</td><td>Maine</td><td>366</td></tr>
<tr><td>13</td><td>Delaware</td><td>310</td><td>8</td><td>Indiana</td><td>354</td></tr>
<tr><td>27</td><td>Florida</td><td>225</td><td>9</td><td>Wisconsin</td><td>347</td></tr>
<tr><td>44</td><td>Georgia</td><td>150</td><td>10</td><td>Pennsylvania</td><td>345</td></tr>
<tr><td>42</td><td>Hawaii</td><td>155</td><td>11</td><td>Ohio</td><td>340</td></tr>
<tr><td>36</td><td>Idaho</td><td>179</td><td>12</td><td>Iowa</td><td>328</td></tr>
<tr><td>19</td><td>Illinois</td><td>269</td><td>13</td><td>Delaware</td><td>310</td></tr>
<tr><td>8</td><td>Indiana</td><td>354</td><td>14</td><td>South Dakota</td><td>301</td></tr>
<tr><td>12</td><td>Iowa</td><td>328</td><td>15</td><td>Nebraska</td><td>299</td></tr>
<tr><td>16</td><td>Kansas</td><td>285</td><td>16</td><td>Kansas</td><td>285</td></tr>
<tr><td>29</td><td>Kentucky</td><td>224</td><td>17</td><td>Louisiana</td><td>277</td></tr>
<tr><td>17</td><td>Louisiana</td><td>277</td><td>18</td><td>New Jersey</td><td>271</td></tr>
<tr><td>7</td><td>Maine</td><td>366</td><td>19</td><td>Illinois</td><td>269</td></tr>
<tr><td>23</td><td>Maryland</td><td>239</td><td>20</td><td>Missouri</td><td>261</td></tr>
<tr><td>4</td><td>Massachusetts</td><td>455</td><td>21</td><td>Vermont</td><td>257</td></tr>
<tr><td>34</td><td>Michigan</td><td>196</td><td>22</td><td>Washington</td><td>246</td></tr>
<tr><td>5</td><td>Minnesota</td><td>416</td><td>23</td><td>Maryland</td><td>239</td></tr>
<tr><td>39</td><td>Mississippi</td><td>174</td><td>23</td><td>New Hampshire</td><td>239</td></tr>
<tr><td>20</td><td>Missouri</td><td>261</td><td>25</td><td>Oklahoma</td><td>231</td></tr>
<tr><td>32</td><td>Montana</td><td>212</td><td>26</td><td>Arkansas</td><td>230</td></tr>
<tr><td>15</td><td>Nebraska</td><td>299</td><td>27</td><td>Florida</td><td>225</td></tr>
<tr><td>49</td><td>Nevada</td><td>118</td><td>27</td><td>North Carolina</td><td>225</td></tr>
<tr><td>23</td><td>New Hampshire</td><td>239</td><td>29</td><td>Kentucky</td><td>224</td></tr>
<tr><td>18</td><td>New Jersey</td><td>271</td><td>30</td><td>Oregon</td><td>216</td></tr>
<tr><td>47</td><td>New Mexico</td><td>133</td><td>31</td><td>Tennessee</td><td>213</td></tr>
<tr><td>2</td><td>New York</td><td>502</td><td>32</td><td>Montana</td><td>212</td></tr>
<tr><td>27</td><td>North Carolina</td><td>225</td><td>33</td><td>West Virginia</td><td>201</td></tr>
<tr><td>6</td><td>North Dakota</td><td>386</td><td>34</td><td>Michigan</td><td>196</td></tr>
<tr><td>11</td><td>Ohio</td><td>340</td><td>35</td><td>Colorado</td><td>185</td></tr>
<tr><td>25</td><td>Oklahoma</td><td>231</td><td>36</td><td>Idaho</td><td>179</td></tr>
<tr><td>30</td><td>Oregon</td><td>216</td><td>37</td><td>Wyoming</td><td>177</td></tr>
<tr><td>10</td><td>Pennsylvania</td><td>345</td><td>38</td><td>South Carolina</td><td>176</td></tr>
<tr><td>3</td><td>Rhode Island</td><td>485</td><td>39</td><td>Mississippi</td><td>174</td></tr>
<tr><td>38</td><td>South Carolina</td><td>176</td><td>40</td><td>Texas</td><td>172</td></tr>
<tr><td>14</td><td>South Dakota</td><td>301</td><td>41</td><td>Alabama</td><td>168</td></tr>
<tr><td>31</td><td>Tennessee</td><td>213</td><td>42</td><td>Hawaii</td><td>155</td></tr>
<tr><td>40</td><td>Texas</td><td>172</td><td>43</td><td>Virginia</td><td>151</td></tr>
<tr><td>46</td><td>Utah</td><td>140</td><td>44</td><td>Georgia</td><td>150</td></tr>
<tr><td>21</td><td>Vermont</td><td>257</td><td>45</td><td>Arizona</td><td>144</td></tr>
<tr><td>43</td><td>Virginia</td><td>151</td><td>46</td><td>Utah</td><td>140</td></tr>
<tr><td>22</td><td>Washington</td><td>246</td><td>47</td><td>New Mexico</td><td>133</td></tr>
<tr><td>33</td><td>West Virginia</td><td>201</td><td>48</td><td>California</td><td>131</td></tr>
<tr><td>9</td><td>Wisconsin</td><td>347</td><td>49</td><td>Nevada</td><td>118</td></tr>
<tr><td>37</td><td>Wyoming</td><td>177</td><td>50</td><td>Alaska</td><td>94</td></tr>
<tr><td></td><td></td><td></td><td></td><td>District of Columbia</td><td>400</td></tr>
</table>

Source: Morgan Quitno Press using data from U.S. Dept of Health & Human Services, Health Care Financing Admin. "State Health Expenditure Accounts" (Health Care Financing Review, Fall 1995, Volume 17, Number 1)
*By state of provider. Includes freestanding nursing and personal-care facilities. Includes Medicare- and Medicaid-certified skilled nursing and intermediate care facilities as well as facilities that are not certified. Excludes hospital-based facilities as they are counted in hospital care expenditures.

Persons Not Covered by Health Insurance in 1997

National Total = 43,448,000 Uninsured

ALPHA ORDER

RANK	STATE	UNINSURED	% of USA
20	Alabama	659,000	1.5%
43	Alaska	116,000	0.3%
10	Arizona	1,141,000	2.6%
23	Arkansas	639,000	1.5%
1	California	7,095,000	16.3%
25	Colorado	592,000	1.4%
32	Connecticut	395,000	0.9%
44	Delaware	98,000	0.2%
4	Florida	2,817,000	6.5%
6	Georgia	1,344,000	3.1%
47	Hawaii	89,000	0.2%
38	Idaho	223,000	0.5%
5	Illinois	1,506,000	3.5%
18	Indiana	669,000	1.5%
33	Iowa	340,000	0.8%
34	Kansas	304,000	0.7%
26	Kentucky	587,000	1.4%
14	Louisiana	827,000	1.9%
39	Maine	182,000	0.4%
17	Maryland	677,000	1.6%
16	Massachusetts	755,000	1.7%
12	Michigan	1,133,000	2.6%
29	Minnesota	438,000	1.0%
27	Mississippi	550,000	1.3%
18	Missouri	669,000	1.5%
41	Montana	174,000	0.4%
40	Nebraska	180,000	0.4%
35	Nevada	301,000	0.7%
42	New Hampshire	141,000	0.3%
7	New Jersey	1,320,000	3.0%
30	New Mexico	413,000	1.0%
3	New York	3,174,000	7.3%
10	North Carolina	1,141,000	2.6%
45	North Dakota	97,000	0.2%
8	Ohio	1,297,000	3.0%
24	Oklahoma	593,000	1.4%
28	Oregon	440,000	1.0%
9	Pennsylvania	1,209,000	2.8%
46	Rhode Island	96,000	0.2%
22	South Carolina	640,000	1.5%
48	South Dakota	84,000	0.2%
15	Tennessee	756,000	1.7%
2	Texas	4,836,000	11.1%
37	Utah	280,000	0.6%
50	Vermont	55,000	0.1%
13	Virginia	854,000	2.0%
21	Washington	655,000	1.5%
36	West Virginia	300,000	0.7%
31	Wisconsin	409,000	0.9%
49	Wyoming	76,000	0.2%

RANK ORDER

RANK	STATE	UNINSURED	% of USA
1	California	7,095,000	16.3%
2	Texas	4,836,000	11.1%
3	New York	3,174,000	7.3%
4	Florida	2,817,000	6.5%
5	Illinois	1,506,000	3.5%
6	Georgia	1,344,000	3.1%
7	New Jersey	1,320,000	3.0%
8	Ohio	1,297,000	3.0%
9	Pennsylvania	1,209,000	2.8%
10	Arizona	1,141,000	2.6%
10	North Carolina	1,141,000	2.6%
12	Michigan	1,133,000	2.6%
13	Virginia	854,000	2.0%
14	Louisiana	827,000	1.9%
15	Tennessee	756,000	1.7%
16	Massachusetts	755,000	1.7%
17	Maryland	677,000	1.6%
18	Indiana	669,000	1.5%
18	Missouri	669,000	1.5%
20	Alabama	659,000	1.5%
21	Washington	655,000	1.5%
22	South Carolina	640,000	1.5%
23	Arkansas	639,000	1.5%
24	Oklahoma	593,000	1.4%
25	Colorado	592,000	1.4%
26	Kentucky	587,000	1.4%
27	Mississippi	550,000	1.3%
28	Oregon	440,000	1.0%
29	Minnesota	438,000	1.0%
30	New Mexico	413,000	1.0%
31	Wisconsin	409,000	0.9%
32	Connecticut	395,000	0.9%
33	Iowa	340,000	0.8%
34	Kansas	304,000	0.7%
35	Nevada	301,000	0.7%
36	West Virginia	300,000	0.7%
37	Utah	280,000	0.6%
38	Idaho	223,000	0.5%
39	Maine	182,000	0.4%
40	Nebraska	180,000	0.4%
41	Montana	174,000	0.4%
42	New Hampshire	141,000	0.3%
43	Alaska	116,000	0.3%
44	Delaware	98,000	0.2%
45	North Dakota	97,000	0.2%
46	Rhode Island	96,000	0.2%
47	Hawaii	89,000	0.2%
48	South Dakota	84,000	0.2%
49	Wyoming	76,000	0.2%
50	Vermont	55,000	0.1%
	District of Columbia	84,000	0.2%

Source: U.S. Bureau of the Census
"Health Insurance Coverage: 1997" (http://www.census.gov/hhes/hlthins/hlthin97.html)

Percent of Population Not Covered by Health Insurance in 1997

National Percent = 16.1% Not Covered by Health Insurance

ALPHA ORDER

RANK	STATE	PERCENT
18	Alabama	15.5
9	Alaska	18.1
1	Arizona	24.5
3	Arkansas	24.4
5	California	21.5
22	Colorado	15.1
35	Connecticut	12.0
30	Delaware	13.1
7	Florida	19.6
12	Georgia	17.6
50	Hawaii	7.5
11	Idaho	17.7
34	Illinois	12.4
42	Indiana	11.4
35	Iowa	12.0
39	Kansas	11.7
23	Kentucky	15.0
24	Louisiana	14.9
24	Maine	14.9
27	Maryland	13.4
31	Massachusetts	12.6
40	Michigan	11.6
48	Minnesota	9.2
6	Mississippi	20.1
31	Missouri	12.6
8	Montana	19.5
44	Nebraska	10.8
13	Nevada	17.5
37	New Hampshire	11.8
17	New Jersey	16.5
4	New Mexico	22.6
13	New York	17.5
18	North Carolina	15.5
21	North Dakota	15.2
41	Ohio	11.5
10	Oklahoma	17.8
29	Oregon	13.3
46	Pennsylvania	10.1
45	Rhode Island	10.2
16	South Carolina	16.8
37	South Dakota	11.8
26	Tennessee	13.6
1	Texas	24.5
27	Utah	13.4
47	Vermont	9.5
31	Virginia	12.6
42	Washington	11.4
15	West Virginia	17.2
49	Wisconsin	8.0
18	Wyoming	15.5

RANK ORDER

RANK	STATE	PERCENT
1	Arizona	24.5
1	Texas	24.5
3	Arkansas	24.4
4	New Mexico	22.6
5	California	21.5
6	Mississippi	20.1
7	Florida	19.6
8	Montana	19.5
9	Alaska	18.1
10	Oklahoma	17.8
11	Idaho	17.7
12	Georgia	17.6
13	Nevada	17.5
13	New York	17.5
15	West Virginia	17.2
16	South Carolina	16.8
17	New Jersey	16.5
18	Alabama	15.5
18	North Carolina	15.5
18	Wyoming	15.5
21	North Dakota	15.2
22	Colorado	15.1
23	Kentucky	15.0
24	Louisiana	14.9
24	Maine	14.9
26	Tennessee	13.6
27	Maryland	13.4
27	Utah	13.4
29	Oregon	13.3
30	Delaware	13.1
31	Massachusetts	12.6
31	Missouri	12.6
31	Virginia	12.6
34	Illinois	12.4
35	Connecticut	12.0
35	Iowa	12.0
37	New Hampshire	11.8
37	South Dakota	11.8
39	Kansas	11.7
40	Michigan	11.6
41	Ohio	11.5
42	Indiana	11.4
42	Washington	11.4
44	Nebraska	10.8
45	Rhode Island	10.2
46	Pennsylvania	10.1
47	Vermont	9.5
48	Minnesota	9.2
49	Wisconsin	8.0
50	Hawaii	7.5
	District of Columbia	16.2

Source: U.S. Bureau of the Census
   "Health Insurance Coverage: 1997" (http://www.census.gov/hhes/hlthins/hlthin97.html)

Persons Covered by Health Insurance in 1997

National Total = 225,646,000 Insured

ALPHA ORDER

RANK ORDER

RANK	STATE	INSURED	% of USA
21	Alabama	3,588,000	1.6%
49	Alaska	525,000	0.2%
22	Arizona	3,514,000	1.6%
33	Arkansas	1,983,000	0.9%
1	California	25,892,000	11.5%
24	Colorado	3,337,000	1.5%
27	Connecticut	2,904,000	1.3%
45	Delaware	652,000	0.3%
4	Florida	11,582,000	5.1%
10	Georgia	6,303,000	2.8%
39	Hawaii	1,094,000	0.5%
42	Idaho	1,034,000	0.5%
6	Illinois	10,592,000	4.7%
14	Indiana	5,196,000	2.3%
30	Iowa	2,490,000	1.1%
31	Kansas	2,286,000	1.0%
25	Kentucky	3,335,000	1.5%
23	Louisiana	3,423,000	1.5%
41	Maine	1,043,000	0.5%
19	Maryland	4,380,000	1.9%
13	Massachusetts	5,249,000	2.3%
8	Michigan	8,661,000	3.8%
20	Minnesota	4,329,000	1.9%
32	Mississippi	2,187,000	1.0%
18	Missouri	4,653,000	2.1%
44	Montana	720,000	0.3%
35	Nebraska	1,482,000	0.7%
37	Nevada	1,423,000	0.6%
40	New Hampshire	1,059,000	0.5%
9	New Jersey	6,657,000	3.0%
38	New Mexico	1,414,000	0.6%
2	New York	14,969,000	6.6%
11	North Carolina	6,211,000	2.8%
47	North Dakota	542,000	0.2%
7	Ohio	9,934,000	4.4%
29	Oklahoma	2,745,000	1.2%
28	Oregon	2,858,000	1.3%
5	Pennsylvania	10,713,000	4.7%
43	Rhode Island	848,000	0.4%
26	South Carolina	3,175,000	1.4%
46	South Dakota	628,000	0.3%
16	Tennessee	4,786,000	2.1%
3	Texas	14,915,000	6.6%
34	Utah	1,805,000	0.8%
48	Vermont	526,000	0.2%
12	Virginia	5,898,000	2.6%
15	Washington	5,093,000	2.3%
36	West Virginia	1,447,000	0.6%
17	Wisconsin	4,717,000	2.1%
50	Wyoming	415,000	0.2%

RANK	STATE	INSURED	% of USA
1	California	25,892,000	11.5%
2	New York	14,969,000	6.6%
3	Texas	14,915,000	6.6%
4	Florida	11,582,000	5.1%
5	Pennsylvania	10,713,000	4.7%
6	Illinois	10,592,000	4.7%
7	Ohio	9,934,000	4.4%
8	Michigan	8,661,000	3.8%
9	New Jersey	6,657,000	3.0%
10	Georgia	6,303,000	2.8%
11	North Carolina	6,211,000	2.8%
12	Virginia	5,898,000	2.6%
13	Massachusetts	5,249,000	2.3%
14	Indiana	5,196,000	2.3%
15	Washington	5,093,000	2.3%
16	Tennessee	4,786,000	2.1%
17	Wisconsin	4,717,000	2.1%
18	Missouri	4,653,000	2.1%
19	Maryland	4,380,000	1.9%
20	Minnesota	4,329,000	1.9%
21	Alabama	3,588,000	1.6%
22	Arizona	3,514,000	1.6%
23	Louisiana	3,423,000	1.5%
24	Colorado	3,337,000	1.5%
25	Kentucky	3,335,000	1.5%
26	South Carolina	3,175,000	1.4%
27	Connecticut	2,904,000	1.3%
28	Oregon	2,858,000	1.3%
29	Oklahoma	2,745,000	1.2%
30	Iowa	2,490,000	1.1%
31	Kansas	2,286,000	1.0%
32	Mississippi	2,187,000	1.0%
33	Arkansas	1,983,000	0.9%
34	Utah	1,805,000	0.8%
35	Nebraska	1,482,000	0.7%
36	West Virginia	1,447,000	0.6%
37	Nevada	1,423,000	0.6%
38	New Mexico	1,414,000	0.6%
39	Hawaii	1,094,000	0.5%
40	New Hampshire	1,059,000	0.5%
41	Maine	1,043,000	0.5%
42	Idaho	1,034,000	0.5%
43	Rhode Island	848,000	0.4%
44	Montana	720,000	0.3%
45	Delaware	652,000	0.3%
46	South Dakota	628,000	0.3%
47	North Dakota	542,000	0.2%
48	Vermont	526,000	0.2%
49	Alaska	525,000	0.2%
50	Wyoming	415,000	0.2%
	District of Columbia	434,000	0.2%

Source: U.S. Bureau of the Census
"Health Insurance Coverage: 1997" (http://www.census.gov/hhes/hlthins/hlthin97.html)

Percent of Population Covered by Health Insurance in 1997

National Percent = 83.9% of Population Covered by Health Insurance

ALPHA ORDER

RANK	STATE	PERCENT
31	Alabama	84.5
42	Alaska	81.9
49	Arizona	75.5
48	Arkansas	75.6
46	California	78.5
29	Colorado	84.9
15	Connecticut	88.0
21	Delaware	86.9
44	Florida	80.4
39	Georgia	82.4
1	Hawaii	92.5
40	Idaho	82.3
17	Illinois	87.6
8	Indiana	88.6
15	Iowa	88.0
12	Kansas	88.3
28	Kentucky	85.0
26	Louisiana	85.1
26	Maine	85.1
23	Maryland	86.6
18	Massachusetts	87.4
11	Michigan	88.4
3	Minnesota	90.8
45	Mississippi	79.9
18	Missouri	87.4
43	Montana	80.5
7	Nebraska	89.2
37	Nevada	82.5
13	New Hampshire	88.2
34	New Jersey	83.5
47	New Mexico	77.4
37	New York	82.5
31	North Carolina	84.5
30	North Dakota	84.8
10	Ohio	88.5
41	Oklahoma	82.2
22	Oregon	86.7
5	Pennsylvania	89.9
6	Rhode Island	89.8
35	South Carolina	83.2
13	South Dakota	88.2
25	Tennessee	86.4
49	Texas	75.5
23	Utah	86.6
4	Vermont	90.5
18	Virginia	87.4
8	Washington	88.6
36	West Virginia	82.8
2	Wisconsin	92.0
31	Wyoming	84.5

RANK ORDER

RANK	STATE	PERCENT
1	Hawaii	92.5
2	Wisconsin	92.0
3	Minnesota	90.8
4	Vermont	90.5
5	Pennsylvania	89.9
6	Rhode Island	89.8
7	Nebraska	89.2
8	Indiana	88.6
8	Washington	88.6
10	Ohio	88.5
11	Michigan	88.4
12	Kansas	88.3
13	New Hampshire	88.2
13	South Dakota	88.2
15	Connecticut	88.0
15	Iowa	88.0
17	Illinois	87.6
18	Massachusetts	87.4
18	Missouri	87.4
18	Virginia	87.4
21	Delaware	86.9
22	Oregon	86.7
23	Maryland	86.6
23	Utah	86.6
25	Tennessee	86.4
26	Louisiana	85.1
26	Maine	85.1
28	Kentucky	85.0
29	Colorado	84.9
30	North Dakota	84.8
31	Alabama	84.5
31	North Carolina	84.5
31	Wyoming	84.5
34	New Jersey	83.5
35	South Carolina	83.2
36	West Virginia	82.8
37	Nevada	82.5
37	New York	82.5
39	Georgia	82.4
40	Idaho	82.3
41	Oklahoma	82.2
42	Alaska	81.9
43	Montana	80.5
44	Florida	80.4
45	Mississippi	79.9
46	California	78.5
47	New Mexico	77.4
48	Arkansas	75.6
49	Arizona	75.5
49	Texas	75.5
	District of Columbia	83.8

Source: Morgan Quitno Press using data from U.S. Bureau of the Census
"Health Insurance Coverage: 1997" (http://www.census.gov/hhes/hlthins/hlthin97.html)

Persons Not Covered by Health Insurance in 1992

National Total = 38,641,000 Uninsured

ALPHA ORDER

RANK	STATE	UNINSURED	% of USA
16	Alabama	710,000	1.8%
43	Alaska	96,000	0.2%
21	Arizona	596,000	1.5%
26	Arkansas	491,000	1.3%
1	California	6,344,000	16.4%
28	Colorado	441,000	1.1%
36	Connecticut	270,000	0.7%
46	Delaware	79,000	0.2%
3	Florida	2,719,000	7.0%
6	Georgia	1,279,000	3.3%
47	Hawaii	72,000	0.2%
38	Idaho	181,000	0.5%
5	Illinois	1,570,000	4.1%
20	Indiana	618,000	1.6%
33	Iowa	294,000	0.8%
35	Kansas	274,000	0.7%
23	Kentucky	544,000	1.4%
10	Louisiana	950,000	2.5%
41	Maine	138,000	0.4%
22	Maryland	559,000	1.4%
19	Massachusetts	622,000	1.6%
12	Michigan	934,000	2.4%
30	Minnesota	350,000	0.9%
25	Mississippi	529,000	1.4%
14	Missouri	728,000	1.9%
45	Montana	81,000	0.2%
39	Nebraska	151,000	0.4%
32	Nevada	312,000	0.8%
40	New Hampshire	141,000	0.4%
9	New Jersey	1,035,000	2.7%
31	New Mexico	320,000	0.8%
4	New York	2,500,000	6.5%
11	North Carolina	949,000	2.5%
50	North Dakota	51,000	0.1%
7	Ohio	1,235,000	3.2%
15	Oklahoma	721,000	1.9%
29	Oregon	412,000	1.1%
8	Pennsylvania	1,042,000	2.7%
44	Rhode Island	91,000	0.2%
18	South Carolina	632,000	1.6%
42	South Dakota	108,000	0.3%
17	Tennessee	687,000	1.8%
2	Texas	4,144,000	10.7%
37	Utah	217,000	0.6%
48	Vermont	55,000	0.1%
13	Virginia	912,000	2.4%
24	Washington	533,000	1.4%
34	West Virginia	277,000	0.7%
27	Wisconsin	465,000	1.2%
48	Wyoming	55,000	0.1%

RANK ORDER

RANK	STATE	UNINSURED	% of USA
1	California	6,344,000	16.4%
2	Texas	4,144,000	10.7%
3	Florida	2,719,000	7.0%
4	New York	2,500,000	6.5%
5	Illinois	1,570,000	4.1%
6	Georgia	1,279,000	3.3%
7	Ohio	1,235,000	3.2%
8	Pennsylvania	1,042,000	2.7%
9	New Jersey	1,035,000	2.7%
10	Louisiana	950,000	2.5%
11	North Carolina	949,000	2.5%
12	Michigan	934,000	2.4%
13	Virginia	912,000	2.4%
14	Missouri	728,000	1.9%
15	Oklahoma	721,000	1.9%
16	Alabama	710,000	1.8%
17	Tennessee	687,000	1.8%
18	South Carolina	632,000	1.6%
19	Massachusetts	622,000	1.6%
20	Indiana	618,000	1.6%
21	Arizona	596,000	1.5%
22	Maryland	559,000	1.4%
23	Kentucky	544,000	1.4%
24	Washington	533,000	1.4%
25	Mississippi	529,000	1.4%
26	Arkansas	491,000	1.3%
27	Wisconsin	465,000	1.2%
28	Colorado	441,000	1.1%
29	Oregon	412,000	1.1%
30	Minnesota	350,000	0.9%
31	New Mexico	320,000	0.8%
32	Nevada	312,000	0.8%
33	Iowa	294,000	0.8%
34	West Virginia	277,000	0.7%
35	Kansas	274,000	0.7%
36	Connecticut	270,000	0.7%
37	Utah	217,000	0.6%
38	Idaho	181,000	0.5%
39	Nebraska	151,000	0.4%
40	New Hampshire	141,000	0.4%
41	Maine	138,000	0.4%
42	South Dakota	108,000	0.3%
43	Alaska	96,000	0.2%
44	Rhode Island	91,000	0.2%
45	Montana	81,000	0.2%
46	Delaware	79,000	0.2%
47	Hawaii	72,000	0.2%
48	Vermont	55,000	0.1%
48	Wyoming	55,000	0.1%
50	North Dakota	51,000	0.1%
	District of Columbia	128,000	0.3%

Source: U.S. Bureau of the Census
Table HI-4. "Health Insurance Coverage Status and Type of Coverage by State - 1987 to 1997"

Percent of Persons Not Covered by Health Insurance in 1992

National Percent = 15.0% Not Covered by Health Insurance

ALPHA ORDER				RANK ORDER		
RANK	STATE	PERCENT		RANK	STATE	PERCENT
12	Alabama	16.8		1	Texas	23.1
12	Alaska	16.8		2	Nevada	23.0
15	Arizona	15.5		3	Louisiana	22.3
6	Arkansas	19.9		4	Oklahoma	22.0
5	California	20.0		5	California	20.0
27	Colorado	12.7		6	Arkansas	19.9
47	Connecticut	8.2		7	Florida	19.8
32	Delaware	11.2		7	New Mexico	19.8
7	Florida	19.8		9	Mississippi	19.4
10	Georgia	19.1		10	Georgia	19.1
50	Hawaii	6.1		11	South Carolina	17.2
14	Idaho	16.5		12	Alabama	16.8
26	Illinois	13.2		12	Alaska	16.8
34	Indiana	11.0		14	Idaho	16.5
39	Iowa	10.3		15	Arizona	15.5
36	Kansas	10.9		16	West Virginia	15.4
18	Kentucky	14.6		17	South Dakota	15.1
3	Louisiana	22.3		18	Kentucky	14.6
33	Maine	11.1		18	Virginia	14.6
31	Maryland	11.3		20	Missouri	14.4
37	Massachusetts	10.6		21	New York	13.9
40	Michigan	10.0		21	North Carolina	13.9
49	Minnesota	8.1		23	Oregon	13.6
9	Mississippi	19.4		23	Tennessee	13.6
20	Missouri	14.4		25	New Jersey	13.3
43	Montana	9.4		26	Illinois	13.2
43	Nebraska	9.4		27	Colorado	12.7
2	Nevada	23.0		28	New Hampshire	12.6
28	New Hampshire	12.6		29	Utah	11.8
25	New Jersey	13.3		30	Wyoming	11.7
7	New Mexico	19.8		31	Maryland	11.3
21	New York	13.9		32	Delaware	11.2
21	North Carolina	13.9		33	Maine	11.1
47	North Dakota	8.2		34	Indiana	11.0
34	Ohio	11.0		34	Ohio	11.0
4	Oklahoma	22.0		36	Kansas	10.9
23	Oregon	13.6		37	Massachusetts	10.6
46	Pennsylvania	8.7		38	Washington	10.4
41	Rhode Island	9.5		39	Iowa	10.3
11	South Carolina	17.2		40	Michigan	10.0
17	South Dakota	15.1		41	Rhode Island	9.5
23	Tennessee	13.6		41	Vermont	9.5
1	Texas	23.1		43	Montana	9.4
29	Utah	11.8		43	Nebraska	9.4
41	Vermont	9.5		45	Wisconsin	9.1
18	Virginia	14.6		46	Pennsylvania	8.7
38	Washington	10.4		47	Connecticut	8.2
16	West Virginia	15.4		47	North Dakota	8.2
45	Wisconsin	9.1		49	Minnesota	8.1
30	Wyoming	11.7		50	Hawaii	6.1
				District of Columbia		21.7

Source: U.S. Bureau of the Census
Table HI-4: "Health Insurance Coverage Status and Type of Coverage by State - 1987 to 1997"

Change in Number of Persons Uninsured: 1992 to 1997

National Change = 4,807,000 Increase

ALPHA ORDER

RANK	STATE	CHANGE
44	Alabama	(51,000)
35	Alaska	20,000
4	Arizona	545,000
10	Arkansas	148,000
1	California	751,000
9	Colorado	151,000
12	Connecticut	125,000
36	Delaware	19,000
15	Florida	98,000
20	Georgia	65,000
37	Hawaii	17,000
28	Idaho	42,000
48	Illinois	(64,000)
23	Indiana	51,000
24	Iowa	46,000
29	Kansas	30,000
27	Kentucky	43,000
49	Louisiana	(123,000)
26	Maine	44,000
14	Maryland	118,000
11	Massachusetts	133,000
6	Michigan	199,000
18	Minnesota	88,000
33	Mississippi	21,000
47	Missouri	(59,000)
16	Montana	93,000
30	Nebraska	29,000
42	Nevada	(11,000)
40	New Hampshire	0
5	New Jersey	285,000
16	New Mexico	93,000
3	New York	674,000
7	North Carolina	192,000
24	North Dakota	46,000
22	Ohio	62,000
50	Oklahoma	(128,000)
31	Oregon	28,000
8	Pennsylvania	167,000
39	Rhode Island	5,000
38	South Carolina	8,000
43	South Dakota	(24,000)
19	Tennessee	69,000
2	Texas	692,000
21	Utah	63,000
40	Vermont	0
46	Virginia	(58,000)
13	Washington	122,000
32	West Virginia	23,000
45	Wisconsin	(56,000)
33	Wyoming	21,000

RANK ORDER

RANK	STATE	CHANGE
1	California	751,000
2	Texas	692,000
3	New York	674,000
4	Arizona	545,000
5	New Jersey	285,000
6	Michigan	199,000
7	North Carolina	192,000
8	Pennsylvania	167,000
9	Colorado	151,000
10	Arkansas	148,000
11	Massachusetts	133,000
12	Connecticut	125,000
13	Washington	122,000
14	Maryland	118,000
15	Florida	98,000
16	Montana	93,000
16	New Mexico	93,000
18	Minnesota	88,000
19	Tennessee	69,000
20	Georgia	65,000
21	Utah	63,000
22	Ohio	62,000
23	Indiana	51,000
24	Iowa	46,000
24	North Dakota	46,000
26	Maine	44,000
27	Kentucky	43,000
28	Idaho	42,000
29	Kansas	30,000
30	Nebraska	29,000
31	Oregon	28,000
32	West Virginia	23,000
33	Mississippi	21,000
33	Wyoming	21,000
35	Alaska	20,000
36	Delaware	19,000
37	Hawaii	17,000
38	South Carolina	8,000
39	Rhode Island	5,000
40	New Hampshire	0
40	Vermont	0
42	Nevada	(11,000)
43	South Dakota	(24,000)
44	Alabama	(51,000)
45	Wisconsin	(56,000)
46	Virginia	(58,000)
47	Missouri	(59,000)
48	Illinois	(64,000)
49	Louisiana	(123,000)
50	Oklahoma	(128,000)

District of Columbia (44,000)

Source: Morgan Quitno Press using data from U.S. Bureau of the Census
"Health Insurance Coverage: 1997" (http://www.census.gov/hhes/hlthins/hlthin97.html)
Table HI-4: "Health Insurance Coverage Status and Type of Coverage by State - 1987 to 1997"

Percent Change in Number of Uninsured: 1992 to 1997

National Percent Change = 12.4% Increase

<table>
<tr><td colspan="3">ALPHA ORDER</td><td colspan="3">RANK ORDER</td></tr>
<tr><td>RANK</td><td>STATE</td><td>PERCENT CHANGE</td><td>RANK</td><td>STATE</td><td>PERCENT CHANGE</td></tr>
<tr><td>45</td><td>Alabama</td><td>(7.2)</td><td>1</td><td>Montana</td><td>114.8</td></tr>
<tr><td>21</td><td>Alaska</td><td>20.8</td><td>2</td><td>Arizona</td><td>91.4</td></tr>
<tr><td>2</td><td>Arizona</td><td>91.4</td><td>3</td><td>North Dakota</td><td>90.2</td></tr>
<tr><td>8</td><td>Arkansas</td><td>30.1</td><td>4</td><td>Connecticut</td><td>46.3</td></tr>
<tr><td>27</td><td>California</td><td>11.8</td><td>5</td><td>Wyoming</td><td>38.2</td></tr>
<tr><td>6</td><td>Colorado</td><td>34.2</td><td>6</td><td>Colorado</td><td>34.2</td></tr>
<tr><td>4</td><td>Connecticut</td><td>46.3</td><td>7</td><td>Maine</td><td>31.9</td></tr>
<tr><td>14</td><td>Delaware</td><td>24.1</td><td>8</td><td>Arkansas</td><td>30.1</td></tr>
<tr><td>38</td><td>Florida</td><td>3.6</td><td>9</td><td>New Mexico</td><td>29.1</td></tr>
<tr><td>35</td><td>Georgia</td><td>5.1</td><td>10</td><td>Utah</td><td>29.0</td></tr>
<tr><td>15</td><td>Hawaii</td><td>23.6</td><td>11</td><td>New Jersey</td><td>27.5</td></tr>
<tr><td>16</td><td>Idaho</td><td>23.2</td><td>12</td><td>New York</td><td>27.0</td></tr>
<tr><td>43</td><td>Illinois</td><td>(4.1)</td><td>13</td><td>Minnesota</td><td>25.1</td></tr>
<tr><td>30</td><td>Indiana</td><td>8.3</td><td>14</td><td>Delaware</td><td>24.1</td></tr>
<tr><td>26</td><td>Iowa</td><td>15.6</td><td>15</td><td>Hawaii</td><td>23.6</td></tr>
<tr><td>28</td><td>Kansas</td><td>10.9</td><td>16</td><td>Idaho</td><td>23.2</td></tr>
<tr><td>32</td><td>Kentucky</td><td>7.9</td><td>17</td><td>Washington</td><td>22.9</td></tr>
<tr><td>48</td><td>Louisiana</td><td>(12.9)</td><td>18</td><td>Massachusetts</td><td>21.4</td></tr>
<tr><td>7</td><td>Maine</td><td>31.9</td><td>19</td><td>Michigan</td><td>21.3</td></tr>
<tr><td>20</td><td>Maryland</td><td>21.1</td><td>20</td><td>Maryland</td><td>21.1</td></tr>
<tr><td>18</td><td>Massachusetts</td><td>21.4</td><td>21</td><td>Alaska</td><td>20.8</td></tr>
<tr><td>19</td><td>Michigan</td><td>21.3</td><td>22</td><td>North Carolina</td><td>20.2</td></tr>
<tr><td>13</td><td>Minnesota</td><td>25.1</td><td>23</td><td>Nebraska</td><td>19.2</td></tr>
<tr><td>37</td><td>Mississippi</td><td>4.0</td><td>24</td><td>Texas</td><td>16.7</td></tr>
<tr><td>46</td><td>Missouri</td><td>(8.1)</td><td>25</td><td>Pennsylvania</td><td>16.0</td></tr>
<tr><td>1</td><td>Montana</td><td>114.8</td><td>26</td><td>Iowa</td><td>15.6</td></tr>
<tr><td>23</td><td>Nebraska</td><td>19.2</td><td>27</td><td>California</td><td>11.8</td></tr>
<tr><td>42</td><td>Nevada</td><td>(3.5)</td><td>28</td><td>Kansas</td><td>10.9</td></tr>
<tr><td>40</td><td>New Hampshire</td><td>0.0</td><td>29</td><td>Tennessee</td><td>10.0</td></tr>
<tr><td>11</td><td>New Jersey</td><td>27.5</td><td>30</td><td>Indiana</td><td>8.3</td></tr>
<tr><td>9</td><td>New Mexico</td><td>29.1</td><td>30</td><td>West Virginia</td><td>8.3</td></tr>
<tr><td>12</td><td>New York</td><td>27.0</td><td>32</td><td>Kentucky</td><td>7.9</td></tr>
<tr><td>22</td><td>North Carolina</td><td>20.2</td><td>33</td><td>Oregon</td><td>6.8</td></tr>
<tr><td>3</td><td>North Dakota</td><td>90.2</td><td>34</td><td>Rhode Island</td><td>5.5</td></tr>
<tr><td>36</td><td>Ohio</td><td>5.0</td><td>35</td><td>Georgia</td><td>5.1</td></tr>
<tr><td>49</td><td>Oklahoma</td><td>(17.8)</td><td>36</td><td>Ohio</td><td>5.0</td></tr>
<tr><td>33</td><td>Oregon</td><td>6.8</td><td>37</td><td>Mississippi</td><td>4.0</td></tr>
<tr><td>25</td><td>Pennsylvania</td><td>16.0</td><td>38</td><td>Florida</td><td>3.6</td></tr>
<tr><td>34</td><td>Rhode Island</td><td>5.5</td><td>39</td><td>South Carolina</td><td>1.3</td></tr>
<tr><td>39</td><td>South Carolina</td><td>1.3</td><td>40</td><td>New Hampshire</td><td>0.0</td></tr>
<tr><td>50</td><td>South Dakota</td><td>(22.2)</td><td>40</td><td>Vermont</td><td>0.0</td></tr>
<tr><td>29</td><td>Tennessee</td><td>10.0</td><td>42</td><td>Nevada</td><td>(3.5)</td></tr>
<tr><td>24</td><td>Texas</td><td>16.7</td><td>43</td><td>Illinois</td><td>(4.1)</td></tr>
<tr><td>10</td><td>Utah</td><td>29.0</td><td>44</td><td>Virginia</td><td>(6.4)</td></tr>
<tr><td>40</td><td>Vermont</td><td>0.0</td><td>45</td><td>Alabama</td><td>(7.2)</td></tr>
<tr><td>44</td><td>Virginia</td><td>(6.4)</td><td>46</td><td>Missouri</td><td>(8.1)</td></tr>
<tr><td>17</td><td>Washington</td><td>22.9</td><td>47</td><td>Wisconsin</td><td>(12.0)</td></tr>
<tr><td>30</td><td>West Virginia</td><td>8.3</td><td>48</td><td>Louisiana</td><td>(12.9)</td></tr>
<tr><td>47</td><td>Wisconsin</td><td>(12.0)</td><td>49</td><td>Oklahoma</td><td>(17.8)</td></tr>
<tr><td>5</td><td>Wyoming</td><td>38.2</td><td>50</td><td>South Dakota</td><td>(22.2)</td></tr>
<tr><td></td><td></td><td></td><td></td><td>District of Columbia</td><td>(34.4)</td></tr>
</table>

Source: Morgan Quitno Press using data from U.S. Bureau of the Census
"Health Insurance Coverage: 1997" (http://www.census.gov/hhes/hlthins/hlthin97.html)
Table HI-4: "Health Insurance Coverage Status and Type of Coverage by State - 1987 to 1997"

Change in Percent of Population Uninsured: 1992 to 1997

National Percent Change = 7.3% Increase

RANK	STATE	PERCENT CHANGE
42	Alabama	(7.7)
25	Alaska	7.7
3	Arizona	58.1
10	Arkansas	22.6
26	California	7.5
11	Colorado	18.9
4	Connecticut	46.3
14	Delaware	17.0
37	Florida	(1.0)
43	Georgia	(7.9)
9	Hawaii	23.0
28	Idaho	7.3
40	Illinois	(6.1)
32	Indiana	3.6
15	Iowa	16.5
28	Kansas	7.3
34	Kentucky	2.7
50	Louisiana	(33.2)
5	Maine	34.2
13	Maryland	18.6
11	Massachusetts	18.9
17	Michigan	16.0
20	Minnesota	13.6
32	Mississippi	3.6
45	Missouri	(12.5)
1	Montana	107.4
18	Nebraska	14.9
49	Nevada	(23.9)
41	New Hampshire	(6.3)
8	New Jersey	24.1
19	New Mexico	14.1
7	New York	25.9
23	North Carolina	11.5
2	North Dakota	85.4
31	Ohio	4.5
47	Oklahoma	(19.1)
38	Oregon	(2.2)
16	Pennsylvania	16.1
27	Rhode Island	7.4
39	South Carolina	(2.3)
48	South Dakota	(21.9)
35	Tennessee	0.0
30	Texas	6.1
20	Utah	13.6
35	Vermont	0.0
46	Virginia	(13.7)
24	Washington	9.6
22	West Virginia	11.7
44	Wisconsin	(12.1)
6	Wyoming	32.5

RANK	STATE	PERCENT CHANGE
1	Montana	107.4
2	North Dakota	85.4
3	Arizona	58.1
4	Connecticut	46.3
5	Maine	34.2
6	Wyoming	32.5
7	New York	25.9
8	New Jersey	24.1
9	Hawaii	23.0
10	Arkansas	22.6
11	Colorado	18.9
11	Massachusetts	18.9
13	Maryland	18.6
14	Delaware	17.0
15	Iowa	16.5
16	Pennsylvania	16.1
17	Michigan	16.0
18	Nebraska	14.9
19	New Mexico	14.1
20	Minnesota	13.6
20	Utah	13.6
22	West Virginia	11.7
23	North Carolina	11.5
24	Washington	9.6
25	Alaska	7.7
26	California	7.5
27	Rhode Island	7.4
28	Idaho	7.3
28	Kansas	7.3
30	Texas	6.1
31	Ohio	4.5
32	Indiana	3.6
32	Mississippi	3.6
34	Kentucky	2.7
35	Tennessee	0.0
35	Vermont	0.0
37	Florida	(1.0)
38	Oregon	(2.2)
39	South Carolina	(2.3)
40	Illinois	(6.1)
41	New Hampshire	(6.3)
42	Alabama	(7.7)
43	Georgia	(7.9)
44	Wisconsin	(12.1)
45	Missouri	(12.5)
46	Virginia	(13.7)
47	Oklahoma	(19.1)
48	South Dakota	(21.9)
49	Nevada	(23.9)
50	Louisiana	(33.2)

| | District of Columbia | (25.3) |

Source: Morgan Quitno Press using data from U.S. Bureau of the Census
"Health Insurance Coverage: 1997" (http://www.census.gov/hhes/hlthins/hlthin97.html)
Table HI-4: "Health Insurance Coverage Status and Type of Coverage by State - 1987 to 1997"

Preferred Provider Organizations (PPOs) in 1995

National Total = 1,023 PPOs*

ALPHA ORDER

RANK	STATE	PPOs	% of USA
15	Alabama	25	2.44%
45	Alaska	3	0.29%
11	Arizona	27	2.64%
36	Arkansas	8	0.78%
1	California	72	7.04%
10	Colorado	28	2.74%
31	Connecticut	11	1.08%
40	Delaware	5	0.49%
1	Florida	72	7.04%
7	Georgia	37	3.62%
40	Hawaii	5	0.49%
47	Idaho	1	0.10%
5	Illinois	46	4.50%
9	Indiana	30	2.93%
30	Iowa	13	1.27%
26	Kansas	17	1.66%
28	Kentucky	16	1.56%
13	Louisiana	26	2.54%
37	Maine	7	0.68%
23	Maryland	18	1.76%
21	Massachusetts	19	1.86%
11	Michigan	27	2.64%
28	Minnesota	16	1.56%
37	Mississippi	7	0.68%
15	Missouri	25	2.44%
49	Montana	0	0.00%
31	Nebraska	11	1.08%
17	Nevada	24	2.35%
42	New Hampshire	4	0.39%
21	New Jersey	19	1.86%
34	New Mexico	9	0.88%
19	New York	22	2.15%
18	North Carolina	23	2.25%
47	North Dakota	1	0.10%
6	Ohio	44	4.30%
23	Oklahoma	18	1.76%
33	Oregon	10	0.98%
4	Pennsylvania	54	5.28%
42	Rhode Island	4	0.39%
26	South Carolina	17	1.66%
42	South Dakota	4	0.39%
7	Tennessee	37	3.62%
3	Texas	71	6.94%
34	Utah	9	0.88%
46	Vermont	2	0.20%
23	Virginia	18	1.76%
20	Washington	21	2.05%
39	West Virginia	6	0.59%
13	Wisconsin	26	2.54%
49	Wyoming	0	0.00%

RANK ORDER

RANK	STATE	PPOs	% of USA
1	California	72	7.04%
1	Florida	72	7.04%
3	Texas	71	6.94%
4	Pennsylvania	54	5.28%
5	Illinois	46	4.50%
6	Ohio	44	4.30%
7	Georgia	37	3.62%
7	Tennessee	37	3.62%
9	Indiana	30	2.93%
10	Colorado	28	2.74%
11	Arizona	27	2.64%
11	Michigan	27	2.64%
13	Louisiana	26	2.54%
13	Wisconsin	26	2.54%
15	Alabama	25	2.44%
15	Missouri	25	2.44%
17	Nevada	24	2.35%
18	North Carolina	23	2.25%
19	New York	22	2.15%
20	Washington	21	2.05%
21	Massachusetts	19	1.86%
21	New Jersey	19	1.86%
23	Maryland	18	1.76%
23	Oklahoma	18	1.76%
23	Virginia	18	1.76%
26	Kansas	17	1.66%
26	South Carolina	17	1.66%
28	Kentucky	16	1.56%
28	Minnesota	16	1.56%
30	Iowa	13	1.27%
31	Connecticut	11	1.08%
31	Nebraska	11	1.08%
33	Oregon	10	0.98%
34	New Mexico	9	0.88%
34	Utah	9	0.88%
36	Arkansas	8	0.78%
37	Maine	7	0.68%
37	Mississippi	7	0.68%
39	West Virginia	6	0.59%
40	Delaware	5	0.49%
40	Hawaii	5	0.49%
42	New Hampshire	4	0.39%
42	Rhode Island	4	0.39%
42	South Dakota	4	0.39%
45	Alaska	3	0.29%
46	Vermont	2	0.20%
47	Idaho	1	0.10%
47	North Dakota	1	0.10%
49	Montana	0	0.00%
49	Wyoming	0	0.00%
	District of Columbia	6	0.59%

Source: American Association of Health Plans (formerly American Managed Care and Review Association)
   "1995-1996 Managed Health Care Overview"

As of October 1995. Total does not include two PPOs in Puerto Rico. Health plans are allocated to states based upon their primary service areas. This means each plan is counted once. However, many plans serve more than one state.

Health Maintenance Organizations (HMOs) in 1998

National Total = 648 HMOs*

ALPHA ORDER

RANK	STATE	HMOs	% of USA
22	Alabama	10	1.5%
49	Alaska	0	0.0%
22	Arizona	10	1.5%
38	Arkansas	5	0.8%
4	California	37	5.7%
12	Colorado	17	2.6%
17	Connecticut	14	2.2%
35	Delaware	6	0.9%
2	Florida	41	6.3%
16	Georgia	15	2.3%
31	Hawaii	8	1.2%
41	Idaho	3	0.5%
6	Illinois	29	4.5%
12	Indiana	17	2.6%
41	Iowa	3	0.5%
22	Kansas	10	1.5%
20	Kentucky	11	1.7%
17	Louisiana	14	2.2%
41	Maine	3	0.5%
27	Maryland	9	1.4%
20	Massachusetts	11	1.7%
7	Michigan	24	3.7%
27	Minnesota	9	1.4%
27	Mississippi	9	1.4%
8	Missouri	21	3.2%
41	Montana	3	0.5%
35	Nebraska	6	0.9%
27	Nevada	9	1.4%
40	New Hampshire	4	0.6%
12	New Jersey	17	2.6%
35	New Mexico	6	0.9%
5	New York	35	5.4%
11	North Carolina	20	3.1%
46	North Dakota	2	0.3%
3	Ohio	40	6.2%
22	Oklahoma	10	1.5%
31	Oregon	8	1.2%
8	Pennsylvania	21	3.2%
46	Rhode Island	2	0.3%
34	South Carolina	7	1.1%
41	South Dakota	3	0.5%
12	Tennessee	17	2.6%
1	Texas	42	6.5%
31	Utah	8	1.2%
49	Vermont	0	0.0%
19	Virginia	13	2.0%
22	Washington	10	1.5%
38	West Virginia	5	0.8%
8	Wisconsin	21	3.2%
48	Wyoming	1	0.2%

RANK ORDER

RANK	STATE	HMOs	% of USA
1	Texas	42	6.5%
2	Florida	41	6.3%
3	Ohio	40	6.2%
4	California	37	5.7%
5	New York	35	5.4%
6	Illinois	29	4.5%
7	Michigan	24	3.7%
8	Missouri	21	3.2%
8	Pennsylvania	21	3.2%
8	Wisconsin	21	3.2%
11	North Carolina	20	3.1%
12	Colorado	17	2.6%
12	Indiana	17	2.6%
12	New Jersey	17	2.6%
12	Tennessee	17	2.6%
16	Georgia	15	2.3%
17	Connecticut	14	2.2%
17	Louisiana	14	2.2%
19	Virginia	13	2.0%
20	Kentucky	11	1.7%
20	Massachusetts	11	1.7%
22	Alabama	10	1.5%
22	Arizona	10	1.5%
22	Kansas	10	1.5%
22	Oklahoma	10	1.5%
22	Washington	10	1.5%
27	Maryland	9	1.4%
27	Minnesota	9	1.4%
27	Mississippi	9	1.4%
27	Nevada	9	1.4%
31	Hawaii	8	1.2%
31	Oregon	8	1.2%
31	Utah	8	1.2%
34	South Carolina	7	1.1%
35	Delaware	6	0.9%
35	Nebraska	6	0.9%
35	New Mexico	6	0.9%
38	Arkansas	5	0.8%
38	West Virginia	5	0.8%
40	New Hampshire	4	0.6%
41	Idaho	3	0.5%
41	Iowa	3	0.5%
41	Maine	3	0.5%
41	Montana	3	0.5%
41	South Dakota	3	0.5%
46	North Dakota	2	0.3%
46	Rhode Island	2	0.3%
48	Wyoming	1	0.2%
49	Alaska	0	0.0%
49	Vermont	0	0.0%
	District of Columbia	2	0.3%

Source: InterStudy Publications (Minneapolis, MN)
     "The Competitive Edge Industry Report 8.2" (Press Release, November 3, 1998)
*As of January 1, 1998. Total does not include two HMOs in Guam and one in Puerto Rico. Health plans are allocated to states based upon their primary service areas. This means each plan is counted once. However, many plans serve more than one state. Total does not include three HMOs in U.S. territories.

Enrollees in Health Maintenance Organizations (HMOs) in 1998

National Total = 76,158,995 Enrollees*

ALPHA ORDER

RANK	STATE	ENROLLEES	% of USA
29	Alabama	468,534	0.6%
49	Alaska	0	0.0%
19	Arizona	1,378,468	1.8%
39	Arkansas	270,855	0.4%
1	California	15,184,126	19.9%
17	Colorado	1,418,757	1.9%
18	Connecticut	1,403,610	1.8%
36	Delaware	351,989	0.5%
3	Florida	4,614,895	6.1%
22	Georgia	1,160,645	1.5%
33	Hawaii	388,915	0.5%
44	Idaho	68,838	0.1%
9	Illinois	2,473,647	3.2%
25	Indiana	820,998	1.1%
42	Iowa	139,291	0.2%
34	Kansas	374,446	0.5%
24	Kentucky	1,087,203	1.4%
27	Louisiana	723,280	0.9%
40	Maine	236,675	0.3%
11	Maryland	2,220,329	2.9%
6	Massachusetts	3,313,951	4.4%
10	Michigan	2,470,436	3.2%
14	Minnesota	1,520,377	2.0%
43	Mississippi	98,877	0.1%
12	Missouri	1,822,532	2.4%
46	Montana	33,997	0.0%
38	Nebraska	280,320	0.4%
31	Nevada	449,858	0.6%
32	New Hampshire	396,395	0.5%
8	New Jersey	2,522,029	3.3%
28	New Mexico	558,008	0.7%
2	New York	6,859,973	9.0%
21	North Carolina	1,268,684	1.7%
47	North Dakota	14,360	0.0%
7	Ohio	2,619,944	3.4%
30	Oklahoma	457,559	0.6%
16	Oregon	1,468,925	1.9%
4	Pennsylvania	4,457,387	5.9%
37	Rhode Island	294,136	0.4%
35	South Carolina	371,575	0.5%
45	South Dakota	37,353	0.0%
20	Tennessee	1,292,729	1.7%
5	Texas	3,460,565	4.5%
26	Utah	732,092	1.0%
49	Vermont	0	0.0%
23	Virginia**	1,137,333	1.5%
15	Washington	1,474,979	1.9%
41	West Virginia	193,894	0.3%
13	Wisconsin	1,590,064	2.1%
48	Wyoming	3,515	0.0%

RANK ORDER

RANK	STATE	ENROLLEES	% of USA
1	California	15,184,126	19.9%
2	New York	6,859,973	9.0%
3	Florida	4,614,895	6.1%
4	Pennsylvania	4,457,387	5.9%
5	Texas	3,460,565	4.5%
6	Massachusetts	3,313,951	4.4%
7	Ohio	2,619,944	3.4%
8	New Jersey	2,522,029	3.3%
9	Illinois	2,473,647	3.2%
10	Michigan	2,470,436	3.2%
11	Maryland	2,220,329	2.9%
12	Missouri	1,822,532	2.4%
13	Wisconsin	1,590,064	2.1%
14	Minnesota	1,520,377	2.0%
15	Washington	1,474,979	1.9%
16	Oregon	1,468,925	1.9%
17	Colorado	1,418,757	1.9%
18	Connecticut	1,403,610	1.8%
19	Arizona	1,378,468	1.8%
20	Tennessee	1,292,729	1.7%
21	North Carolina	1,268,684	1.7%
22	Georgia	1,160,645	1.5%
23	Virginia**	1,137,333	1.5%
24	Kentucky	1,087,203	1.4%
25	Indiana	820,998	1.1%
26	Utah	732,092	1.0%
27	Louisiana	723,280	0.9%
28	New Mexico	558,008	0.7%
29	Alabama	468,534	0.6%
30	Oklahoma	457,559	0.6%
31	Nevada	449,858	0.6%
32	New Hampshire	396,395	0.5%
33	Hawaii	388,915	0.5%
34	Kansas	374,446	0.5%
35	South Carolina	371,575	0.5%
36	Delaware	351,989	0.5%
37	Rhode Island	294,136	0.4%
38	Nebraska	280,320	0.4%
39	Arkansas	270,855	0.4%
40	Maine	236,675	0.3%
41	West Virginia	193,894	0.3%
42	Iowa	139,291	0.2%
43	Mississippi	98,877	0.1%
44	Idaho	68,838	0.1%
45	South Dakota	37,353	0.0%
46	Montana	33,997	0.0%
47	North Dakota	14,360	0.0%
48	Wyoming	3,515	0.0%
49	Alaska	0	0.0%
49	Vermont	0	0.0%
	District of Columbia	171,647	0.2%

Source: InterStudy Publications (Minneapolis, MN)
   "The Competitive Edge Industry Report 8.2" (Press Release, November 3, 1998)
*As of January 1, 1998. Total does not include 475,273 enrollees in U.S. territories.
**Virginia includes enrollment from two HMOs serving the Washington, DC metropolitan area.

Percent Change in Enrollees in Health Maintenance Organizations (HMOs): 1997 to 1998
National Percent Change = 14.7% Increase*

ALPHA ORDER

ALPHA ORDER

RANK	STATE	PERCENT CHANGE
34	Alabama	11.8
NA	Alaska**	NA
39	Arizona	8.1
21	Arkansas	23.6
38	California	8.7
26	Colorado	19.3
22	Connecticut	23.4
17	Delaware	25.3
36	Florida	10.5
18	Georgia	24.2
13	Hawaii	31.3
10	Idaho	34.1
24	Illinois	21.9
30	Indiana	17.8
40	Iowa	6.5
15	Kansas	27.0
43	Kentucky	2.0
32	Louisiana	12.9
25	Maine	19.6
9	Maryland	34.2
23	Massachusetts	22.0
46	Michigan	(3.2)
44	Minnesota	(0.3)
5	Mississippi	52.9
33	Missouri	12.6
16	Montana	26.6
36	Nebraska	10.5
8	Nevada	34.9
7	New Hampshire	42.9
31	New Jersey	15.0
4	New Mexico	54.9
42	New York	5.8
28	North Carolina	18.5
12	North Dakota	31.9
11	Ohio	33.3
35	Oklahoma	11.5
45	Oregon	(2.8)
19	Pennsylvania	23.8
1	Rhode Island	152.8
27	South Carolina	19.1
6	South Dakota	44.0
3	Tennessee	55.4
29	Texas	18.1
47	Utah	(10.0)
NA	Vermont**	NA
14	Virginia	27.8
41	Washington	6.4
48	West Virginia	(26.6)
19	Wisconsin	23.8
2	Wyoming	76.6

RANK ORDER

RANK	STATE	PERCENT CHANGE
1	Rhode Island	152.8
2	Wyoming	76.6
3	Tennessee	55.4
4	New Mexico	54.9
5	Mississippi	52.9
6	South Dakota	44.0
7	New Hampshire	42.9
8	Nevada	34.9
9	Maryland	34.2
10	Idaho	34.1
11	Ohio	33.3
12	North Dakota	31.9
13	Hawaii	31.3
14	Virginia	27.8
15	Kansas	27.0
16	Montana	26.6
17	Delaware	25.3
18	Georgia	24.2
19	Pennsylvania	23.8
19	Wisconsin	23.8
21	Arkansas	23.6
22	Connecticut	23.4
23	Massachusetts	22.0
24	Illinois	21.9
25	Maine	19.6
26	Colorado	19.3
27	South Carolina	19.1
28	North Carolina	18.5
29	Texas	18.1
30	Indiana	17.8
31	New Jersey	15.0
32	Louisiana	12.9
33	Missouri	12.6
34	Alabama	11.8
35	Oklahoma	11.5
36	Florida	10.5
36	Nebraska	10.5
38	California	8.7
39	Arizona	8.1
40	Iowa	6.5
41	Washington	6.4
42	New York	5.8
43	Kentucky	2.0
44	Minnesota	(0.3)
45	Oregon	(2.8)
46	Michigan	(3.2)
47	Utah	(10.0)
48	West Virginia	(26.6)
NA	Alaska**	NA
NA	Vermont**	NA
	District of Columbia	(23.5)

Source: InterStudy Publications (Minneapolis, MN)
   "The Competitive Edge Industry Report 8.2" (Press Release, November 3, 1998)
*As of January 1, 1998. National rate includes enrollees in U.S. territories.
**Not applicable.

Percent of Population Enrolled in Health Maintenance Organizations (HMOs) in 1998
National Percent = 28.6% Enrolled in HMOs*

ALPHA ORDER

RANK	STATE	PERCENT
38	Alabama	10.8
49	Alaska	0.0
20	Arizona	30.3
39	Arkansas	10.7
3	California	47.1
9	Colorado	36.4
6	Connecticut	42.9
2	Delaware	48.1
17	Florida	31.5
34	Georgia	15.5
14	Hawaii	32.8
42	Idaho	5.7
27	Illinois	20.8
36	Indiana	14.0
44	Iowa	4.9
35	Kansas	14.4
11	Kentucky	35.1
33	Louisiana	16.6
28	Maine	19.1
5	Maryland	43.6
1	Massachusetts	54.2
24	Michigan	25.3
15	Minnesota	32.4
46	Mississippi	3.6
13	Missouri	33.7
45	Montana	3.9
31	Nebraska	16.9
22	Nevada	26.8
12	New Hampshire	33.8
18	New Jersey	31.3
16	New Mexico	32.3
7	New York	37.8
30	North Carolina	17.1
47	North Dakota	2.2
26	Ohio	23.4
37	Oklahoma	13.8
4	Oregon	45.3
8	Pennsylvania	37.1
21	Rhode Island	29.8
41	South Carolina	9.9
43	South Dakota	5.1
25	Tennessee	24.1
29	Texas	17.8
10	Utah	35.5
49	Vermont	0.0
31	Virginia	16.9
23	Washington	26.3
39	West Virginia	10.7
19	Wisconsin	30.8
48	Wyoming	0.7

RANK ORDER

RANK	STATE	PERCENT
1	Massachusetts	54.2
2	Delaware	48.1
3	California	47.1
4	Oregon	45.3
5	Maryland	43.6
6	Connecticut	42.9
7	New York	37.8
8	Pennsylvania	37.1
9	Colorado	36.4
10	Utah	35.5
11	Kentucky	35.1
12	New Hampshire	33.8
13	Missouri	33.7
14	Hawaii	32.8
15	Minnesota	32.4
16	New Mexico	32.3
17	Florida	31.5
18	New Jersey	31.3
19	Wisconsin	30.8
20	Arizona	30.3
21	Rhode Island	29.8
22	Nevada	26.8
23	Washington	26.3
24	Michigan	25.3
25	Tennessee	24.1
26	Ohio	23.4
27	Illinois	20.8
28	Maine	19.1
29	Texas	17.8
30	North Carolina	17.1
31	Nebraska	16.9
31	Virginia	16.9
33	Louisiana	16.6
34	Georgia	15.5
35	Kansas	14.4
36	Indiana	14.0
37	Oklahoma	13.8
38	Alabama	10.8
39	Arkansas	10.7
39	West Virginia	10.7
41	South Carolina	9.9
42	Idaho	5.7
43	South Dakota	5.1
44	Iowa	4.9
45	Montana	3.9
46	Mississippi	3.6
47	North Dakota	2.2
48	Wyoming	0.7
49	Alaska	0.0
49	Vermont	0.0
	District of Columbia	33.0

Source: InterStudy Publications (Minneapolis, MN)
"The Competitive Edge Industry Report 8.2" (Press Release, November 3, 1998)
*As of January 1, 1998.

Percent of Insured Population
Enrolled in Health Maintenance Organizations (HMOs) in 1998
National Percent = 33.3% of Insured are Enrolled in HMOs*

ALPHA ORDER

RANK ORDER

RANK	STATE	PERCENT		RANK	STATE	PERCENT
40	Alabama	13.1		1	Massachusetts	63.1
49	Alaska	0.0		2	California	58.6
13	Arizona	39.2		3	Delaware	54.0
38	Arkansas	13.7		4	Oregon	51.4
2	California	58.6		5	Maryland	50.7
8	Colorado	42.5		6	Connecticut	48.3
6	Connecticut	48.3		7	New York	45.8
3	Delaware	54.0		8	Colorado	42.5
11	Florida	39.8		9	Pennsylvania	41.6
34	Georgia	18.4		10	Utah	40.6
17	Hawaii	35.5		11	Florida	39.8
42	Idaho	6.7		12	New Mexico	39.5
27	Illinois	23.4		13	Arizona	39.2
37	Indiana	15.8		13	Missouri	39.2
44	Iowa	5.6		15	New Jersey	37.9
36	Kansas	16.4		16	New Hampshire	37.4
21	Kentucky	32.6		17	Hawaii	35.5
30	Louisiana	21.1		18	Minnesota	35.1
29	Maine	22.7		19	Rhode Island	34.7
5	Maryland	50.7		20	Wisconsin	33.7
1	Massachusetts	63.1		21	Kentucky	32.6
24	Michigan	28.5		22	Nevada	31.6
18	Minnesota	35.1		23	Washington	29.0
46	Mississippi	4.5		24	Michigan	28.5
13	Missouri	39.2		25	Tennessee	27.0
45	Montana	4.7		26	Ohio	26.4
33	Nebraska	18.9		27	Illinois	23.4
22	Nevada	31.6		28	Texas	23.2
16	New Hampshire	37.4		29	Maine	22.7
15	New Jersey	37.9		30	Louisiana	21.1
12	New Mexico	39.5		31	North Carolina	20.4
7	New York	45.8		32	Virginia	19.3
31	North Carolina	20.4		33	Nebraska	18.9
47	North Dakota	2.6		34	Georgia	18.4
26	Ohio	26.4		35	Oklahoma	16.7
35	Oklahoma	16.7		36	Kansas	16.4
4	Oregon	51.4		37	Indiana	15.8
9	Pennsylvania	41.6		38	Arkansas	13.7
19	Rhode Island	34.7		39	West Virginia	13.4
41	South Carolina	11.7		40	Alabama	13.1
43	South Dakota	5.9		41	South Carolina	11.7
25	Tennessee	27.0		42	Idaho	6.7
28	Texas	23.2		43	South Dakota	5.9
10	Utah	40.6		44	Iowa	5.6
49	Vermont	0.0		45	Montana	4.7
32	Virginia	19.3		46	Mississippi	4.5
23	Washington	29.0		47	North Dakota	2.6
39	West Virginia	13.4		48	Wyoming	0.8
20	Wisconsin	33.7		49	Alaska	0.0
48	Wyoming	0.8		49	Vermont	0.0

District of Columbia		39.6

Source: Morgan Quitno Press using data from InterStudy Publications (Minneapolis, MN)
"The Competitive Edge Industry Report 8.2" (Press Release, November 3, 1998)
*As of January 1, 1998. Calculated using estimated number of insured as of 1997 from Census.

Persons Eligible for the Civilian Health and Medical Program
Of the Uniformed Services (CHAMPUS) in 1998
National Total = 5,025,087 Eligible to Enroll*

<u>ALPHA ORDER</u>

RANK	STATE	ELIGIBLE	% of USA
11	Alabama	123,647	2.5%
29	Alaska	47,670	0.9%
12	Arizona	115,955	2.3%
27	Arkansas	50,891	1.0%
1	California	545,555	10.9%
10	Colorado	131,320	2.6%
37	Connecticut	27,373	0.5%
43	Delaware	18,454	0.4%
4	Florida	419,298	8.3%
5	Georgia	256,638	5.1%
15	Hawaii	91,272	1.8%
39	Idaho	27,054	0.5%
17	Illinois	80,510	1.6%
32	Indiana	40,746	0.8%
44	Iowa	17,580	0.3%
23	Kansas	68,481	1.4%
22	Kentucky	74,250	1.5%
19	Louisiana	79,902	1.6%
36	Maine	27,763	0.6%
8	Maryland	141,958	2.8%
33	Massachusetts	34,092	0.7%
30	Michigan	47,590	0.9%
40	Minnesota	24,135	0.5%
24	Mississippi	66,164	1.3%
20	Missouri	78,962	1.6%
42	Montana	19,315	0.4%
31	Nebraska	42,114	0.8%
26	Nevada	56,553	1.1%
47	New Hampshire	15,234	0.3%
28	New Jersey	48,725	1.0%
25	New Mexico	61,137	1.2%
18	New York	80,101	1.6%
6	North Carolina	245,271	4.9%
41	North Dakota	21,923	0.4%
16	Ohio	89,871	1.8%
14	Oklahoma	98,707	2.0%
34	Oregon	34,051	0.7%
21	Pennsylvania	76,542	1.5%
49	Rhode Island	12,976	0.3%
9	South Carolina	139,945	2.8%
46	South Dakota	17,120	0.3%
13	Tennessee	103,339	2.1%
2	Texas	465,702	9.3%
35	Utah	32,727	0.7%
50	Vermont	4,995	0.1%
3	Virginia	444,022	8.8%
7	Washington	214,907	4.3%
45	West Virginia	17,481	0.3%
38	Wisconsin	27,084	0.5%
48	Wyoming	13,295	0.3%

<u>RANK ORDER</u>

RANK	STATE	ELIGIBLE	% of USA
1	California	545,555	10.9%
2	Texas	465,702	9.3%
3	Virginia	444,022	8.8%
4	Florida	419,298	8.3%
5	Georgia	256,638	5.1%
6	North Carolina	245,271	4.9%
7	Washington	214,907	4.3%
8	Maryland	141,958	2.8%
9	South Carolina	139,945	2.8%
10	Colorado	131,320	2.6%
11	Alabama	123,647	2.5%
12	Arizona	115,955	2.3%
13	Tennessee	103,339	2.1%
14	Oklahoma	98,707	2.0%
15	Hawaii	91,272	1.8%
16	Ohio	89,871	1.8%
17	Illinois	80,510	1.6%
18	New York	80,101	1.6%
19	Louisiana	79,902	1.6%
20	Missouri	78,962	1.6%
21	Pennsylvania	76,542	1.5%
22	Kentucky	74,250	1.5%
23	Kansas	68,481	1.4%
24	Mississippi	66,164	1.3%
25	New Mexico	61,137	1.2%
26	Nevada	56,553	1.1%
27	Arkansas	50,891	1.0%
28	New Jersey	48,725	1.0%
29	Alaska	47,670	0.9%
30	Michigan	47,590	0.9%
31	Nebraska	42,114	0.8%
32	Indiana	40,746	0.8%
33	Massachusetts	34,092	0.7%
34	Oregon	34,051	0.7%
35	Utah	32,727	0.7%
36	Maine	27,763	0.6%
37	Connecticut	27,373	0.5%
38	Wisconsin	27,084	0.5%
39	Idaho	27,054	0.5%
40	Minnesota	24,135	0.5%
41	North Dakota	21,923	0.4%
42	Montana	19,315	0.4%
43	Delaware	18,454	0.4%
44	Iowa	17,580	0.3%
45	West Virginia	17,481	0.3%
46	South Dakota	17,120	0.3%
47	New Hampshire	15,234	0.3%
48	Wyoming	13,295	0.3%
49	Rhode Island	12,976	0.3%
50	Vermont	4,995	0.1%
	District of Columbia	4,690	0.1%

Source: U.S. Department of Defense, Office of CHAMPUS
    "Defense Enrollment Eligibility Reporting System (DEERS) Report" (August 10, 1998)
*As of July 31, 1998. National total does not include 28,982 eligible in U.S. territories and possessions.
CHAMPUS provides health care coverage for current or former U.S. military personnel and their dependents.

Percent of Population Eligible for CHAMPUS in 1998

National Percent = 1.9% of Population Eligible*

ALPHA ORDER				RANK ORDER		
RANK	STATE	PERCENT		RANK	STATE	PERCENT
13	Alabama	2.8		1	Alaska	7.8
1	Alaska	7.8		2	Hawaii	7.7
18	Arizona	2.5		3	Virginia	6.5
27	Arkansas	2.0		4	Washington	3.8
31	California	1.7		5	South Carolina	3.6
9	Colorado	3.3		6	New Mexico	3.5
38	Connecticut	0.8		7	Georgia	3.4
18	Delaware	2.5		7	North Dakota	3.4
13	Florida	2.8		9	Colorado	3.3
7	Georgia	3.4		9	North Carolina	3.3
2	Hawaii	7.7		11	Nevada	3.2
24	Idaho	2.2		12	Oklahoma	2.9
41	Illinois	0.7		13	Alabama	2.8
41	Indiana	0.7		13	Florida	2.8
43	Iowa	0.6		13	Maryland	2.8
17	Kansas	2.6		13	Wyoming	2.8
28	Kentucky	1.9		17	Kansas	2.6
30	Louisiana	1.8		18	Arizona	2.5
24	Maine	2.2		18	Delaware	2.5
13	Maryland	2.8		18	Nebraska	2.5
43	Massachusetts	0.6		21	Mississippi	2.4
47	Michigan	0.5		21	Texas	2.4
47	Minnesota	0.5		23	South Dakota	2.3
21	Mississippi	2.4		24	Idaho	2.2
33	Missouri	1.5		24	Maine	2.2
24	Montana	2.2		24	Montana	2.2
18	Nebraska	2.5		27	Arkansas	2.0
11	Nevada	3.2		28	Kentucky	1.9
34	New Hampshire	1.3		28	Tennessee	1.9
43	New Jersey	0.6		30	Louisiana	1.8
6	New Mexico	3.5		31	California	1.7
50	New York	0.4		32	Utah	1.6
9	North Carolina	3.3		33	Missouri	1.5
7	North Dakota	3.4		34	New Hampshire	1.3
38	Ohio	0.8		34	Rhode Island	1.3
12	Oklahoma	2.9		36	Oregon	1.0
36	Oregon	1.0		36	West Virginia	1.0
43	Pennsylvania	0.6		38	Connecticut	0.8
34	Rhode Island	1.3		38	Ohio	0.8
5	South Carolina	3.6		38	Vermont	0.8
23	South Dakota	2.3		41	Illinois	0.7
28	Tennessee	1.9		41	Indiana	0.7
21	Texas	2.4		43	Iowa	0.6
32	Utah	1.6		43	Massachusetts	0.6
38	Vermont	0.8		43	New Jersey	0.6
3	Virginia	6.5		43	Pennsylvania	0.6
4	Washington	3.8		47	Michigan	0.5
36	West Virginia	1.0		47	Minnesota	0.5
47	Wisconsin	0.5		47	Wisconsin	0.5
13	Wyoming	2.8		50	New York	0.4
					District of Columbia	0.9

Source: Morgan Quitno Press using data from U.S. Department of Defense, Office of CHAMPUS
"Defense Enrollment Eligibility Reporting System (DEERS) Report" (August 10, 1998)
*As of July 31, 1998. National total does not include 28,982 eligible in U.S. territories and possessions.
CHAMPUS provides health care coverage for current or former U.S. military personnel and their dependents.

Medicare Benefit Payments in 1998

National Total = $210,101,815,777*

ALPHA ORDER

RANK	STATE	BENEFITS	% of USA
19	Alabama	$3,560,717,508	1.7%
50	Alaska	159,758,199	0.1%
22	Arizona	2,985,530,968	1.4%
30	Arkansas	1,928,749,334	0.9%
1	California	22,557,637,106	10.7%
28	Colorado	2,278,634,923	1.1%
21	Connecticut	3,128,330,518	1.5%
47	Delaware	405,179,514	0.2%
2	Florida	17,902,925,272	8.5%
15	Georgia	4,287,055,620	2.0%
42	Hawaii	638,739,135	0.3%
43	Idaho	600,569,407	0.3%
7	Illinois	8,490,218,565	4.0%
16	Indiana	4,263,103,328	2.0%
32	Iowa	1,809,851,994	0.9%
33	Kansas	1,808,698,803	0.9%
23	Kentucky	2,897,036,258	1.4%
14	Louisiana	4,293,485,495	2.0%
40	Maine	793,293,556	0.4%
18	Maryland	3,641,544,943	1.7%
10	Massachusetts	5,806,660,558	2.8%
8	Michigan	7,710,609,123	3.7%
25	Minnesota	2,798,007,301	1.3%
29	Mississippi	2,216,407,663	1.1%
13	Missouri	4,695,447,829	2.2%
44	Montana	534,258,341	0.3%
36	Nebraska	1,079,689,239	0.5%
35	Nevada	1,105,343,755	0.5%
41	New Hampshire	647,514,836	0.3%
9	New Jersey	6,907,721,916	3.3%
39	New Mexico	829,432,056	0.4%
3	New York	17,065,062,152	8.1%
11	North Carolina	5,295,680,613	2.5%
46	North Dakota	480,392,514	0.2%
6	Ohio	8,834,503,816	4.2%
27	Oklahoma	2,372,547,734	1.1%
31	Oregon	1,831,805,057	0.9%
5	Pennsylvania	13,183,135,104	6.3%
37	Rhode Island	1,022,126,351	0.5%
26	South Carolina	2,563,287,620	1.2%
45	South Dakota	503,514,478	0.2%
12	Tennessee	4,728,188,173	2.3%
4	Texas	14,666,114,703	7.0%
38	Utah	888,315,472	0.4%
48	Vermont	289,235,157	0.1%
17	Virginia	3,657,019,701	1.7%
24	Washington	2,883,183,663	1.4%
34	West Virginia	1,528,209,589	0.7%
20	Wisconsin	3,267,431,972	1.6%
49	Wyoming	218,451,250	0.1%

RANK ORDER

RANK	STATE	BENEFITS	% of USA
1	California	$22,557,637,106	10.7%
2	Florida	17,902,925,272	8.5%
3	New York	17,065,062,152	8.1%
4	Texas	14,666,114,703	7.0%
5	Pennsylvania	13,183,135,104	6.3%
6	Ohio	8,834,503,816	4.2%
7	Illinois	8,490,218,565	4.0%
8	Michigan	7,710,609,123	3.7%
9	New Jersey	6,907,721,916	3.3%
10	Massachusetts	5,806,660,558	2.8%
11	North Carolina	5,295,680,613	2.5%
12	Tennessee	4,728,188,173	2.3%
13	Missouri	4,695,447,829	2.2%
14	Louisiana	4,293,485,495	2.0%
15	Georgia	4,287,055,620	2.0%
16	Indiana	4,263,103,328	2.0%
17	Virginia	3,657,019,701	1.7%
18	Maryland	3,641,544,943	1.7%
19	Alabama	3,560,717,508	1.7%
20	Wisconsin	3,267,431,972	1.6%
21	Connecticut	3,128,330,518	1.5%
22	Arizona	2,985,530,968	1.4%
23	Kentucky	2,897,036,258	1.4%
24	Washington	2,883,183,663	1.4%
25	Minnesota	2,798,007,301	1.3%
26	South Carolina	2,563,287,620	1.2%
27	Oklahoma	2,372,547,734	1.1%
28	Colorado	2,278,634,923	1.1%
29	Mississippi	2,216,407,663	1.1%
30	Arkansas	1,928,749,334	0.9%
31	Oregon	1,831,805,057	0.9%
32	Iowa	1,809,851,994	0.9%
33	Kansas	1,808,698,803	0.9%
34	West Virginia	1,528,209,589	0.7%
35	Nevada	1,105,343,755	0.5%
36	Nebraska	1,079,689,239	0.5%
37	Rhode Island	1,022,126,351	0.5%
38	Utah	888,315,472	0.4%
39	New Mexico	829,432,056	0.4%
40	Maine	793,293,556	0.4%
41	New Hampshire	647,514,836	0.3%
42	Hawaii	638,739,135	0.3%
43	Idaho	600,569,407	0.3%
44	Montana	534,258,341	0.3%
45	South Dakota	503,514,478	0.2%
46	North Dakota	480,392,514	0.2%
47	Delaware	405,179,514	0.2%
48	Vermont	289,235,157	0.1%
49	Wyoming	218,451,250	0.1%
50	Alaska	159,758,199	0.1%
	District of Columbia	922,292,162	0.4%

Source: U.S. Department of Health and Human Services, Health Care Financing Administration
unpublished data

*For fiscal year 1998. Includes payments to aged and disabled enrollees. Total includes $1,085,621,690 in payments to enrollees in Puerto Rico and $53,543,743 to enrollees in "other outlying areas."

Medicare Enrollees in 1998

National Total = 38,444,739 Enrollees*

ALPHA ORDER

RANK	STATE	ENROLLEES	% of USA
19	Alabama	662,299	1.7%
50	Alaska	36,522	0.1%
21	Arizona	636,450	1.7%
31	Arkansas	431,020	1.1%
1	California	3,738,081	9.7%
30	Colorado	442,452	1.2%
26	Connecticut	507,927	1.3%
46	Delaware	105,693	0.3%
2	Florida	2,727,545	7.1%
12	Georgia	869,443	2.3%
42	Hawaii	156,103	0.4%
43	Idaho	155,810	0.4%
7	Illinois	1,622,181	4.2%
15	Indiana	835,183	2.2%
29	Iowa	475,786	1.2%
33	Kansas	387,589	1.0%
23	Kentucky	602,570	1.6%
24	Louisiana	592,543	1.5%
38	Maine	207,784	0.5%
22	Maryland	619,700	1.6%
11	Massachusetts	946,879	2.5%
8	Michigan	1,369,629	3.6%
20	Minnesota	639,293	1.7%
32	Mississippi	407,440	1.1%
14	Missouri	844,920	2.2%
44	Montana	133,089	0.3%
35	Nebraska	251,029	0.7%
37	Nevada	213,742	0.6%
41	New Hampshire	161,759	0.4%
9	New Jersey	1,182,204	3.1%
36	New Mexico	221,061	0.6%
3	New York	2,651,677	6.9%
10	North Carolina	1,073,564	2.8%
47	North Dakota	102,764	0.3%
6	Ohio	1,683,167	4.4%
27	Oklahoma	497,066	1.3%
28	Oregon	477,022	1.2%
5	Pennsylvania	2,084,565	5.4%
40	Rhode Island	169,359	0.4%
25	South Carolina	534,827	1.4%
45	South Dakota	117,931	0.3%
16	Tennessee	796,692	2.1%
4	Texas	2,162,917	5.6%
39	Utah	195,326	0.5%
48	Vermont	85,562	0.2%
13	Virginia	849,493	2.2%
18	Washington	708,607	1.8%
34	West Virginia	333,217	0.9%
17	Wisconsin	770,405	2.0%
49	Wyoming	62,654	0.2%

RANK ORDER

RANK	STATE	ENROLLEES	% of USA
1	California	3,738,081	9.7%
2	Florida	2,727,545	7.1%
3	New York	2,651,677	6.9%
4	Texas	2,162,917	5.6%
5	Pennsylvania	2,084,565	5.4%
6	Ohio	1,683,167	4.4%
7	Illinois	1,622,181	4.2%
8	Michigan	1,369,629	3.6%
9	New Jersey	1,182,204	3.1%
10	North Carolina	1,073,564	2.8%
11	Massachusetts	946,879	2.5%
12	Georgia	869,443	2.3%
13	Virginia	849,493	2.2%
14	Missouri	844,920	2.2%
15	Indiana	835,183	2.2%
16	Tennessee	796,692	2.1%
17	Wisconsin	770,405	2.0%
18	Washington	708,607	1.8%
19	Alabama	662,299	1.7%
20	Minnesota	639,293	1.7%
21	Arizona	636,450	1.7%
22	Maryland	619,700	1.6%
23	Kentucky	602,570	1.6%
24	Louisiana	592,543	1.5%
25	South Carolina	534,827	1.4%
26	Connecticut	507,927	1.3%
27	Oklahoma	497,066	1.3%
28	Oregon	477,022	1.2%
29	Iowa	475,786	1.2%
30	Colorado	442,452	1.2%
31	Arkansas	431,020	1.1%
32	Mississippi	407,440	1.1%
33	Kansas	387,589	1.0%
34	West Virginia	333,217	0.9%
35	Nebraska	251,029	0.7%
36	New Mexico	221,061	0.6%
37	Nevada	213,742	0.6%
38	Maine	207,784	0.5%
39	Utah	195,326	0.5%
40	Rhode Island	169,359	0.4%
41	New Hampshire	161,759	0.4%
42	Hawaii	156,103	0.4%
43	Idaho	155,810	0.4%
44	Montana	133,089	0.3%
45	South Dakota	117,931	0.3%
46	Delaware	105,693	0.3%
47	North Dakota	102,764	0.3%
48	Vermont	85,562	0.2%
49	Wyoming	62,654	0.2%
50	Alaska	36,522	0.1%
	District of Columbia	78,151	0.2%

Source: U.S. Department of Health and Human Services, Health Care Financing Administration
 unpublished data

*For fiscal year 1998. Includes aged and disabled enrollees. Total includes 502,780 enrollees in Puerto Rico and 323,287 enrollees in "other outlying areas."

Medicare Payments per Enrollee in 1998

National Rate = $5,465*

ALPHA ORDER

RANK	STATE	PER ENROLLEE
16	Alabama	$5,376
34	Alaska	4,374
27	Arizona	4,691
32	Arkansas	4,475
8	California	6,035
20	Colorado	5,150
6	Connecticut	6,159
45	Delaware	3,834
3	Florida	6,564
23	Georgia	4,931
39	Hawaii	4,092
43	Idaho	3,854
18	Illinois	5,234
21	Indiana	5,104
47	Iowa	3,804
29	Kansas	4,667
24	Kentucky	4,808
1	Louisiana	7,246
46	Maine	3,818
11	Maryland	5,876
7	Massachusetts	6,132
13	Michigan	5,630
33	Minnesota	4,377
15	Mississippi	5,440
14	Missouri	5,557
41	Montana	4,014
36	Nebraska	4,301
19	Nevada	5,171
42	New Hampshire	4,003
12	New Jersey	5,843
48	New Mexico	3,752
4	New York	6,436
22	North Carolina	4,933
28	North Dakota	4,675
17	Ohio	5,249
26	Oklahoma	4,773
44	Oregon	3,840
5	Pennsylvania	6,324
8	Rhode Island	6,035
25	South Carolina	4,793
37	South Dakota	4,270
10	Tennessee	5,935
2	Texas	6,781
31	Utah	4,548
50	Vermont	3,380
35	Virginia	4,305
40	Washington	4,069
30	West Virginia	4,586
38	Wisconsin	4,241
49	Wyoming	3,487

RANK ORDER

RANK	STATE	PER ENROLLEE
1	Louisiana	$7,246
2	Texas	6,781
3	Florida	6,564
4	New York	6,436
5	Pennsylvania	6,324
6	Connecticut	6,159
7	Massachusetts	6,132
8	California	6,035
8	Rhode Island	6,035
10	Tennessee	5,935
11	Maryland	5,876
12	New Jersey	5,843
13	Michigan	5,630
14	Missouri	5,557
15	Mississippi	5,440
16	Alabama	5,376
17	Ohio	5,249
18	Illinois	5,234
19	Nevada	5,171
20	Colorado	5,150
21	Indiana	5,104
22	North Carolina	4,933
23	Georgia	4,931
24	Kentucky	4,808
25	South Carolina	4,793
26	Oklahoma	4,773
27	Arizona	4,691
28	North Dakota	4,675
29	Kansas	4,667
30	West Virginia	4,586
31	Utah	4,548
32	Arkansas	4,475
33	Minnesota	4,377
34	Alaska	4,374
35	Virginia	4,305
36	Nebraska	4,301
37	South Dakota	4,270
38	Wisconsin	4,241
39	Hawaii	4,092
40	Washington	4,069
41	Montana	4,014
42	New Hampshire	4,003
43	Idaho	3,854
44	Oregon	3,840
45	Delaware	3,834
46	Maine	3,818
47	Iowa	3,804
48	New Mexico	3,752
49	Wyoming	3,487
50	Vermont	3,380

District of Columbia	11,801

Source: U.S. Department of Health and Human Services, Health Care Financing Administration unpublished data

*For fiscal year 1998. Includes aged and disabled enrollees. National rate includes payments to enrollees in Puerto Rico and in "other outlying areas."

Percent of Population Enrolled in Medicare in 1998

National Percent = 13.9% of Population*

ALPHA ORDER

RANK	STATE	RATE
14	Alabama	15.2
50	Alaska	5.9
32	Arizona	13.6
5	Arkansas	17.0
45	California	11.4
47	Colorado	11.1
10	Connecticut	15.5
27	Delaware	14.2
2	Florida	18.3
45	Georgia	11.4
37	Hawaii	13.1
39	Idaho	12.7
35	Illinois	13.5
27	Indiana	14.2
7	Iowa	16.6
20	Kansas	14.7
13	Kentucky	15.3
32	Louisiana	13.6
6	Maine	16.7
44	Maryland	12.1
12	Massachusetts	15.4
30	Michigan	14.0
35	Minnesota	13.5
19	Mississippi	14.8
10	Missouri	15.5
15	Montana	15.1
15	Nebraska	15.1
43	Nevada	12.2
32	New Hampshire	13.6
23	New Jersey	14.6
39	New Mexico	12.7
23	New York	14.6
27	North Carolina	14.2
8	North Dakota	16.1
17	Ohio	15.0
18	Oklahoma	14.9
25	Oregon	14.5
3	Pennsylvania	17.4
4	Rhode Island	17.1
31	South Carolina	13.9
9	South Dakota	16.0
20	Tennessee	14.7
48	Texas	10.9
49	Utah	9.3
25	Vermont	14.5
41	Virginia	12.5
41	Washington	12.5
1	West Virginia	18.4
20	Wisconsin	14.7
38	Wyoming	13.0

RANK ORDER

RANK	STATE	RATE
1	West Virginia	18.4
2	Florida	18.3
3	Pennsylvania	17.4
4	Rhode Island	17.1
5	Arkansas	17.0
6	Maine	16.7
7	Iowa	16.6
8	North Dakota	16.1
9	South Dakota	16.0
10	Connecticut	15.5
10	Missouri	15.5
12	Massachusetts	15.4
13	Kentucky	15.3
14	Alabama	15.2
15	Montana	15.1
15	Nebraska	15.1
17	Ohio	15.0
18	Oklahoma	14.9
19	Mississippi	14.8
20	Kansas	14.7
20	Tennessee	14.7
20	Wisconsin	14.7
23	New Jersey	14.6
23	New York	14.6
25	Oregon	14.5
25	Vermont	14.5
27	Delaware	14.2
27	Indiana	14.2
27	North Carolina	14.2
30	Michigan	14.0
31	South Carolina	13.9
32	Arizona	13.6
32	Louisiana	13.6
32	New Hampshire	13.6
35	Illinois	13.5
35	Minnesota	13.5
37	Hawaii	13.1
38	Wyoming	13.0
39	Idaho	12.7
39	New Mexico	12.7
41	Virginia	12.5
41	Washington	12.5
43	Nevada	12.2
44	Maryland	12.1
45	California	11.4
45	Georgia	11.4
47	Colorado	11.1
48	Texas	10.9
49	Utah	9.3
50	Alaska	5.9
	District of Columbia	14.9

Source: Morgan Quitno Press using data from U.S. Dept. of Health and Human Services, Health Care Financing Admn
    unpublished data
*For fiscal year 1998. Includes aged and disabled enrollees. National rate includes only residents of the 50 states
and the District of Columbia.

Medicare Health Maintenance Organizations (HMOs) in 1998

National Total = 282 Medicare HMOs*

ALPHA ORDER

RANK	STATE	HMOs	% of USA
32	Alabama	2	0.7%
46	Alaska	0	0.0%
8	Arizona	10	3.5%
27	Arkansas	3	1.1%
2	California	23	8.2%
11	Colorado	9	3.2%
12	Connecticut	7	2.5%
32	Delaware	2	0.7%
1	Florida	24	8.5%
23	Georgia	4	1.4%
40	Hawaii	1	0.4%
40	Idaho	1	0.4%
8	Illinois	10	3.5%
15	Indiana	6	2.1%
32	Iowa	2	0.7%
23	Kansas	4	1.4%
32	Kentucky	2	0.7%
15	Louisiana	6	2.1%
46	Maine	0	0.0%
18	Maryland	5	1.8%
12	Massachusetts	7	2.5%
6	Michigan	12	4.3%
18	Minnesota	5	1.8%
40	Mississippi	1	0.4%
18	Missouri	5	1.8%
40	Montana	1	0.4%
32	Nebraska	2	0.7%
27	Nevada	3	1.1%
27	New Hampshire	3	1.1%
8	New Jersey	10	3.5%
23	New Mexico	4	1.4%
3	New York	21	7.4%
18	North Carolina	5	1.8%
40	North Dakota	1	0.4%
5	Ohio	16	5.7%
23	Oklahoma	4	1.4%
15	Oregon	6	2.1%
7	Pennsylvania	11	3.9%
32	Rhode Island	2	0.7%
32	South Carolina	2	0.7%
46	South Dakota	0	0.0%
27	Tennessee	3	1.1%
4	Texas	18	6.4%
32	Utah	2	0.7%
46	Vermont	0	0.0%
27	Virginia	3	1.1%
12	Washington	7	2.5%
40	West Virginia	1	0.4%
18	Wisconsin	5	1.8%
46	Wyoming	0	0.0%

RANK ORDER

RANK	STATE	HMOs	% of USA
1	Florida	24	8.5%
2	California	23	8.2%
3	New York	21	7.4%
4	Texas	18	6.4%
5	Ohio	16	5.7%
6	Michigan	12	4.3%
7	Pennsylvania	11	3.9%
8	Arizona	10	3.5%
8	Illinois	10	3.5%
8	New Jersey	10	3.5%
11	Colorado	9	3.2%
12	Connecticut	7	2.5%
12	Massachusetts	7	2.5%
12	Washington	7	2.5%
15	Indiana	6	2.1%
15	Louisiana	6	2.1%
15	Oregon	6	2.1%
18	Maryland	5	1.8%
18	Minnesota	5	1.8%
18	Missouri	5	1.8%
18	North Carolina	5	1.8%
18	Wisconsin	5	1.8%
23	Georgia	4	1.4%
23	Kansas	4	1.4%
23	New Mexico	4	1.4%
23	Oklahoma	4	1.4%
27	Arkansas	3	1.1%
27	Nevada	3	1.1%
27	New Hampshire	3	1.1%
27	Tennessee	3	1.1%
27	Virginia	3	1.1%
32	Alabama	2	0.7%
32	Delaware	2	0.7%
32	Iowa	2	0.7%
32	Kentucky	2	0.7%
32	Nebraska	2	0.7%
32	Rhode Island	2	0.7%
32	South Carolina	2	0.7%
32	Utah	2	0.7%
40	Hawaii	1	0.4%
40	Idaho	1	0.4%
40	Mississippi	1	0.4%
40	Montana	1	0.4%
40	North Dakota	1	0.4%
40	West Virginia	1	0.4%
46	Alaska	0	0.0%
46	Maine	0	0.0%
46	South Dakota	0	0.0%
46	Vermont	0	0.0%
46	Wyoming	0	0.0%
	District of Columbia	1	0.4%

Source: InterStudy Publications (Minneapolis, MN)
   "The Competitive Edge Industry Report 8.2" (Press Release, November 3, 1998)
*As of January 1, 1998. Health plans are allocated to states based upon their primary service areas. This means each plan is counted once. However, many plans serve more than one state.

Medicare Managed Care Enrollees in 1998

National Total = 6,759,542 Enrollees*

ALPHA ORDER

RANK ORDER

RANK	STATE	ENROLLEES	% of USA		RANK	STATE	ENROLLEES	% of USA
25	Alabama	46,149	0.7%		1	California	1,556,130	23.0%
47	Alaska	0	0.0%		2	Florida	786,025	11.6%
6	Arizona	254,917	3.8%		3	Pennsylvania	549,502	8.1%
34	Arkansas	14,351	0.2%		4	New York	517,517	7.7%
1	California	1,556,130	23.0%		5	Texas	353,235	5.2%
12	Colorado	156,219	2.3%		6	Arizona	254,917	3.8%
16	Connecticut	107,842	1.6%		7	Ohio	234,008	3.5%
47	Delaware	0	0.0%		8	Massachusetts	218,946	3.2%
2	Florida	786,025	11.6%		9	Oregon	192,749	2.9%
22	Georgia	56,616	0.8%		10	Washington	182,544	2.7%
24	Hawaii	55,032	0.8%		11	Illinois	180,964	2.7%
37	Idaho	8,929	0.1%		12	Colorado	156,219	2.3%
11	Illinois	180,964	2.7%		13	New Jersey	153,576	2.3%
20	Indiana	78,278	1.2%		14	Missouri	142,694	2.1%
38	Iowa	7,907	0.1%		15	Maryland	110,718	1.6%
40	Kansas	6,784	0.1%		16	Connecticut	107,842	1.6%
36	Kentucky	13,153	0.2%		17	Louisiana	107,811	1.6%
17	Louisiana	107,811	1.6%		18	Minnesota	106,240	1.6%
46	Maine	482	0.0%		19	Nevada	78,495	1.2%
15	Maryland	110,718	1.6%		20	Indiana	78,278	1.2%
8	Massachusetts	218,946	3.2%		21	Rhode Island	66,902	1.0%
23	Michigan	56,125	0.8%		22	Georgia	56,616	0.8%
18	Minnesota	106,240	1.6%		23	Michigan	56,125	0.8%
43	Mississippi	1,101	0.0%		24	Hawaii	55,032	0.8%
14	Missouri	142,694	2.1%		25	Alabama	46,149	0.7%
41	Montana	1,965	0.0%		26	New Mexico	44,707	0.7%
35	Nebraska	14,074	0.2%		27	Oklahoma	43,933	0.6%
19	Nevada	78,495	1.2%		28	Wisconsin	40,676	0.6%
33	New Hampshire	14,952	0.2%		29	Utah	35,952	0.5%
13	New Jersey	153,576	2.3%		30	North Carolina	35,261	0.5%
26	New Mexico	44,707	0.7%		31	Tennessee	23,985	0.4%
4	New York	517,517	7.7%		32	Virginia	21,496	0.3%
30	North Carolina	35,261	0.5%		33	New Hampshire	14,952	0.2%
45	North Dakota	866	0.0%		34	Arkansas	14,351	0.2%
7	Ohio	234,008	3.5%		35	Nebraska	14,074	0.2%
27	Oklahoma	43,933	0.6%		36	Kentucky	13,153	0.2%
9	Oregon	192,749	2.9%		37	Idaho	8,929	0.1%
3	Pennsylvania	549,502	8.1%		38	Iowa	7,907	0.1%
21	Rhode Island	66,902	1.0%		39	West Virginia	7,408	0.1%
44	South Carolina	1,094	0.0%		40	Kansas	6,784	0.1%
47	South Dakota	0	0.0%		41	Montana	1,965	0.0%
31	Tennessee	23,985	0.4%		42	Vermont	1,646	0.0%
5	Texas	353,235	5.2%		43	Mississippi	1,101	0.0%
29	Utah	35,952	0.5%		44	South Carolina	1,094	0.0%
42	Vermont	1,646	0.0%		45	North Dakota	866	0.0%
32	Virginia	21,496	0.3%		46	Maine	482	0.0%
10	Washington	182,544	2.7%		47	Alaska	0	0.0%
39	West Virginia	7,408	0.1%		47	Delaware	0	0.0%
28	Wisconsin	40,676	0.6%		47	South Dakota	0	0.0%
47	Wyoming	0	0.0%		47	Wyoming	0	0.0%
						District of Columbia	0	0.0%

Source: U.S. Department of Health and Human Services, Health Care Financing Administration
    "Medicare Managed Care Contract Report" (December 1, 1998, http://www.hcfa.gov/stats/mmcc1298.txt)
*As of December 1st. Includes TEFRA, Cost, and Health Care Prepayment Plans (HCPP). National total includes
163,908 enrollees in "Other Demonstration" plans. National total includes 69,586 enrollees in the United Mine
Workers' plan not shown separately by state.

Percent of Medicare Enrollees in Managed Care Programs in 1998

National Percent = 18.0% of Medicare Enrollees*

ALPHA ORDER

RANK	STATE	PERCENT
27	Alabama	7.0
47	Alaska	0.0
3	Arizona	40.1
33	Arkansas	3.3
1	California	41.6
6	Colorado	35.3
12	Connecticut	21.2
47	Delaware	0.0
8	Florida	28.8
28	Georgia	6.5
6	Hawaii	35.3
29	Idaho	5.7
23	Illinois	11.2
24	Indiana	9.4
41	Iowa	1.7
40	Kansas	1.8
37	Kentucky	2.2
16	Louisiana	18.2
45	Maine	0.2
17	Maryland	17.9
11	Massachusetts	23.1
32	Michigan	4.1
19	Minnesota	16.6
44	Mississippi	0.3
18	Missouri	16.9
42	Montana	1.5
30	Nebraska	5.6
5	Nevada	36.7
25	New Hampshire	9.2
22	New Jersey	13.0
13	New Mexico	20.2
14	New York	19.5
33	North Carolina	3.3
43	North Dakota	0.8
21	Ohio	13.9
26	Oklahoma	8.8
2	Oregon	40.4
9	Pennsylvania	26.4
4	Rhode Island	39.5
45	South Carolina	0.2
47	South Dakota	0.0
35	Tennessee	3.0
20	Texas	16.3
15	Utah	18.4
39	Vermont	1.9
36	Virginia	2.5
10	Washington	25.8
37	West Virginia	2.2
31	Wisconsin	5.3
47	Wyoming	0.0

RANK ORDER

RANK	STATE	PERCENT
1	California	41.6
2	Oregon	40.4
3	Arizona	40.1
4	Rhode Island	39.5
5	Nevada	36.7
6	Colorado	35.3
6	Hawaii	35.3
8	Florida	28.8
9	Pennsylvania	26.4
10	Washington	25.8
11	Massachusetts	23.1
12	Connecticut	21.2
13	New Mexico	20.2
14	New York	19.5
15	Utah	18.4
16	Louisiana	18.2
17	Maryland	17.9
18	Missouri	16.9
19	Minnesota	16.6
20	Texas	16.3
21	Ohio	13.9
22	New Jersey	13.0
23	Illinois	11.2
24	Indiana	9.4
25	New Hampshire	9.2
26	Oklahoma	8.8
27	Alabama	7.0
28	Georgia	6.5
29	Idaho	5.7
30	Nebraska	5.6
31	Wisconsin	5.3
32	Michigan	4.1
33	Arkansas	3.3
33	North Carolina	3.3
35	Tennessee	3.0
36	Virginia	2.5
37	Kentucky	2.2
37	West Virginia	2.2
39	Vermont	1.9
40	Kansas	1.8
41	Iowa	1.7
42	Montana	1.5
43	North Dakota	0.8
44	Mississippi	0.3
45	Maine	0.2
45	South Carolina	0.2
47	Alaska	0.0
47	Delaware	0.0
47	South Dakota	0.0
47	Wyoming	0.0
	District of Columbia	0.0

Source: Morgan Quitno Press using data from U.S. Dept. of Health and Human Services, Health Care Financing Admin.
"Medicare Managed Care Contract Report" (December 1, 1998, http://www.hcfa.gov/stats/mmcc1298.txt)
*As of December 1st. Includes aged and disabled enrollees. National percent does not include enrollees in Puerto Rico and other outlying areas."

Medicare Physicians in 1998

National Total = 807,674 Physicians*

ALPHA ORDER

RANK ORDER

RANK	STATE	PHYSICIANS	% of USA		RANK	STATE	PHYSICIANS	% of USA
25	Alabama	9,685	1.2%		1	California	96,634	12.0%
49	Alaska	1,412	0.2%		2	New York	73,813	9.1%
24	Arizona	11,127	1.4%		3	Pennsylvania	50,141	6.2%
31	Arkansas	6,866	0.9%		4	Texas	48,958	6.1%
1	California	96,634	12.0%		5	Florida	41,483	5.1%
22	Colorado	12,619	1.6%		6	Ohio	31,875	3.9%
23	Connecticut	11,878	1.5%		7	Illinois	31,869	3.9%
45	Delaware	2,294	0.3%		8	Michigan	28,234	3.5%
5	Florida	41,483	5.1%		9	Massachusetts	27,476	3.4%
12	Georgia	18,489	2.3%		10	New Jersey	27,448	3.4%
40	Hawaii**	3,871	0.5%		11	Maryland	18,572	2.3%
44	Idaho	2,451	0.3%		12	Georgia	18,489	2.3%
7	Illinois	31,869	3.9%		13	North Carolina	17,615	2.2%
19	Indiana	15,293	1.9%		14	Virginia	16,829	2.1%
28	Iowa	8,492	1.1%		15	Washington	16,407	2.0%
32	Kansas	6,793	0.8%		16	Missouri	16,301	2.0%
27	Kentucky	9,092	1.1%		17	Wisconsin	16,074	2.0%
21	Louisiana	13,156	1.6%		18	Minnesota	15,367	1.9%
36	Maine	4,425	0.5%		19	Indiana	15,293	1.9%
11	Maryland	18,572	2.3%		20	Tennessee	14,773	1.8%
9	Massachusetts	27,476	3.4%		21	Louisiana	13,156	1.6%
8	Michigan	28,234	3.5%		22	Colorado	12,619	1.6%
18	Minnesota	15,367	1.9%		23	Connecticut	11,878	1.5%
33	Mississippi	5,274	0.7%		24	Arizona	11,127	1.4%
16	Missouri	16,301	2.0%		25	Alabama	9,685	1.2%
43	Montana	2,571	0.3%		26	Oregon	9,447	1.2%
37	Nebraska	4,226	0.5%		27	Kentucky	9,092	1.1%
41	Nevada	3,383	0.4%		28	Iowa	8,492	1.1%
38	New Hampshire	4,200	0.5%		29	South Carolina	8,444	1.0%
10	New Jersey	27,448	3.4%		30	Oklahoma	7,332	0.9%
39	New Mexico	4,012	0.5%		31	Arkansas	6,866	0.9%
2	New York	73,813	9.1%		32	Kansas	6,793	0.8%
13	North Carolina	17,615	2.2%		33	Mississippi	5,274	0.7%
46	North Dakota	2,244	0.3%		34	Utah	4,879	0.6%
6	Ohio	31,875	3.9%		35	West Virginia	4,708	0.6%
30	Oklahoma	7,332	0.9%		36	Maine	4,425	0.5%
26	Oregon	9,447	1.2%		37	Nebraska	4,226	0.5%
3	Pennsylvania	50,141	6.2%		38	New Hampshire	4,200	0.5%
42	Rhode Island	3,340	0.4%		39	New Mexico	4,012	0.5%
29	South Carolina	8,444	1.0%		40	Hawaii**	3,871	0.5%
47	South Dakota	2,173	0.3%		41	Nevada	3,383	0.4%
20	Tennessee	14,773	1.8%		42	Rhode Island	3,340	0.4%
4	Texas	48,958	6.1%		43	Montana	2,571	0.3%
34	Utah	4,879	0.6%		44	Idaho	2,451	0.3%
48	Vermont	2,116	0.3%		45	Delaware	2,294	0.3%
14	Virginia	16,829	2.1%		46	North Dakota	2,244	0.3%
15	Washington	16,407	2.0%		47	South Dakota	2,173	0.3%
35	West Virginia	4,708	0.6%		48	Vermont	2,116	0.3%
17	Wisconsin	16,074	2.0%		49	Alaska	1,412	0.2%
50	Wyoming	1,238	0.2%		50	Wyoming	1,238	0.2%
						District of Columbia	4,235	0.5%

Source: U.S. Department of Health and Human Services, Health Care Financing Administration
   "Medicare Physician Registry" (August 1998)
*Medicare Part B. "Physicians" include MD, DO, DDM, DDS, DPM, OD and CH. National total includes 6,265
physicians in Puerto Rico and the Virgin Islands.
**Physicians for Guam are included in Hawaii's total.

Percent of Physicians Participating in Medicare in 1997

National Percent = 80.2% of Physicians Participate in Medicare*

ALPHA ORDER			RANK ORDER		
RANK	STATE	PERCENT	RANK	STATE	PERCENT
1	Alabama	93.5	1	Alabama	93.5
36	Alaska	79.0	2	North Dakota	93.2
17	Arizona	86.6	3	Ohio	92.7
37	Arkansas	78.9	4	Nevada	92.2
31	California	80.9	5	Kansas	91.8
30	Colorado	81.4	6	West Virginia	90.8
18	Connecticut	86.4	7	Utah	90.2
43	Delaware	74.4	8	Washington	89.9
44	Florida	73.9	9	Maryland	89.6
11	Georgia	88.6	10	Kentucky	88.7
23	Hawaii	84.0	11	Georgia	88.6
48	Idaho	67.6	12	Iowa	88.5
25	Illinois	83.3	13	Missouri	88.1
42	Indiana	76.8	14	Oregon	87.6
12	Iowa	88.5	15	Tennessee	87.5
5	Kansas	91.8	16	Nebraska	87.2
10	Kentucky	88.7	17	Arizona	86.6
49	Louisiana	64.6	18	Connecticut	86.4
32	Maine	79.9	19	Virginia	85.7
9	Maryland	89.6	20	South Carolina	85.5
41	Massachusetts	77.2	21	Wisconsin	85.2
27	Michigan	82.6	22	North Carolina	84.6
40	Minnesota	77.3	23	Hawaii	84.0
34	Mississippi	79.3	23	Oklahoma	84.0
13	Missouri	88.1	25	Illinois	83.3
38	Montana	78.7	25	Wyoming	83.3
16	Nebraska	87.2	27	Michigan	82.6
4	Nevada	92.2	28	Texas	82.1
33	New Hampshire	79.7	29	New Mexico	81.7
50	New Jersey	62.8	30	Colorado	81.4
29	New Mexico	81.7	31	California	80.9
46	New York	70.0	32	Maine	79.9
22	North Carolina	84.6	33	New Hampshire	79.7
2	North Dakota	93.2	34	Mississippi	79.3
3	Ohio	92.7	34	South Dakota	79.3
23	Oklahoma	84.0	36	Alaska	79.0
14	Oregon	87.6	37	Arkansas	78.9
45	Pennsylvania	72.0	38	Montana	78.7
47	Rhode Island	68.4	39	Vermont	78.6
20	South Carolina	85.5	40	Minnesota	77.3
34	South Dakota	79.3	41	Massachusetts	77.2
15	Tennessee	87.5	42	Indiana	76.8
28	Texas	82.1	43	Delaware	74.4
7	Utah	90.2	44	Florida	73.9
39	Vermont	78.6	45	Pennsylvania	72.0
19	Virginia	85.7	46	New York	70.0
8	Washington	89.9	47	Rhode Island	68.4
6	West Virginia	90.8	48	Idaho	67.6
21	Wisconsin	85.2	49	Louisiana	64.6
25	Wyoming	83.3	50	New Jersey	62.8
				District of Columbia	68.6

Source: U.S. Department of Health and Human Services, Health Care Financing Administration
    "Practitioner Enrollment in Medicare Program Increases for 1997" (Press Release, May 6, 1997)
*Medicare Part B. Physicians include MD's, DO's, limited license practitioners and non-physician practitioners.

Medicaid Expenditures in 1997

National Total = $123,552,098,563*

ALPHA ORDER

RANK	STATE	EXPENDITURES	% of USA
24	Alabama	$1,571,203,728	1.3%
43	Alaska	320,829,650	0.3%
48	Arizona	245,821,514	0.2%
28	Arkansas	1,301,593,755	1.1%
2	California	11,433,311,901	9.3%
30	Colorado	1,123,843,562	0.9%
20	Connecticut	2,003,015,959	1.6%
47	Delaware	274,826,560	0.2%
6	Florida	4,884,588,899	4.0%
12	Georgia	3,090,016,213	2.5%
50	Hawaii	0	0.0%
39	Idaho	432,361,263	0.3%
5	Illinois	5,782,847,483	4.7%
14	Indiana	2,381,860,140	1.9%
31	Iowa	1,084,248,482	0.9%
33	Kansas	919,272,243	0.7%
17	Kentucky	2,268,938,421	1.8%
16	Louisiana	2,336,007,497	1.9%
35	Maine	779,569,232	0.6%
18	Maryland	2,200,668,586	1.8%
8	Massachusetts	3,855,391,508	3.1%
10	Michigan	3,591,221,336	2.9%
15	Minnesota	2,358,826,359	1.9%
26	Mississippi	1,424,219,167	1.2%
19	Missouri	2,097,275,522	1.7%
45	Montana	317,733,011	0.3%
37	Nebraska	696,226,804	0.6%
41	Nevada	372,877,260	0.3%
38	New Hampshire	553,935,895	0.4%
11	New Jersey	3,569,003,878	2.9%
34	New Mexico	822,360,613	0.7%
1	New York	21,339,566,488	17.3%
9	North Carolina	3,788,456,205	3.1%
42	North Dakota	328,362,994	0.3%
4	Ohio	5,847,639,671	4.7%
32	Oklahoma	1,038,028,999	0.8%
25	Oregon	1,474,863,025	1.2%
7	Pennsylvania	4,689,468,962	3.8%
36	Rhode Island	737,994,298	0.6%
23	South Carolina	1,607,427,848	1.3%
44	South Dakota	318,474,724	0.3%
13	Tennessee	2,936,393,617	2.4%
3	Texas	7,345,173,561	5.9%
40	Utah	423,724,395	0.3%
46	Vermont	308,611,188	0.2%
22	Virginia	1,857,931,916	1.5%
27	Washington	1,392,671,086	1.1%
29	West Virginia	1,256,997,370	1.0%
21	Wisconsin	1,878,572,907	1.5%
49	Wyoming	184,256,251	0.1%

RANK ORDER

RANK	STATE	EXPENDITURES	% of USA
1	New York	$21,339,566,488	17.3%
2	California	11,433,311,901	9.3%
3	Texas	7,345,173,561	5.9%
4	Ohio	5,847,639,671	4.7%
5	Illinois	5,782,847,483	4.7%
6	Florida	4,884,588,899	4.0%
7	Pennsylvania	4,689,468,962	3.8%
8	Massachusetts	3,855,391,508	3.1%
9	North Carolina	3,788,456,205	3.1%
10	Michigan	3,591,221,336	2.9%
11	New Jersey	3,569,003,878	2.9%
12	Georgia	3,090,016,213	2.5%
13	Tennessee	2,936,393,617	2.4%
14	Indiana	2,381,860,140	1.9%
15	Minnesota	2,358,826,359	1.9%
16	Louisiana	2,336,007,497	1.9%
17	Kentucky	2,268,938,421	1.8%
18	Maryland	2,200,668,586	1.8%
19	Missouri	2,097,275,522	1.7%
20	Connecticut	2,003,015,959	1.6%
21	Wisconsin	1,878,572,907	1.5%
22	Virginia	1,857,931,916	1.5%
23	South Carolina	1,607,427,848	1.3%
24	Alabama	1,571,203,728	1.3%
25	Oregon	1,474,863,025	1.2%
26	Mississippi	1,424,219,167	1.2%
27	Washington	1,392,671,086	1.1%
28	Arkansas	1,301,593,755	1.1%
29	West Virginia	1,256,997,370	1.0%
30	Colorado	1,123,843,562	0.9%
31	Iowa	1,084,248,482	0.9%
32	Oklahoma	1,038,028,999	0.8%
33	Kansas	919,272,243	0.7%
34	New Mexico	822,360,613	0.7%
35	Maine	779,569,232	0.6%
36	Rhode Island	737,994,298	0.6%
37	Nebraska	696,226,804	0.6%
38	New Hampshire	553,935,895	0.4%
39	Idaho	432,361,263	0.3%
40	Utah	423,724,395	0.3%
41	Nevada	372,877,260	0.3%
42	North Dakota	328,362,994	0.3%
43	Alaska	320,829,650	0.3%
44	South Dakota	318,474,724	0.3%
45	Montana	317,733,011	0.3%
46	Vermont	308,611,188	0.2%
47	Delaware	274,826,560	0.2%
48	Arizona	245,821,514	0.2%
49	Wyoming	184,256,251	0.1%
50	Hawaii	0	0.0%
	District of Columbia	696,209,244	0.6%

Source: U.S. Department of Health and Human Services, Health Care Financing Administration
"Medicaid Medical Vendor Payments by Type of Service, Region and State: FY 1997" (HCFA-2082)
*For fiscal year ending September 30, 1997. National total includes $7,377,373 for the Virgin Islands.

Percent Change in Medicaid Expenditures: 1990 to 1997

National Percent Change = 90.5% Increase*

ALPHA ORDER			RANK ORDER		
RANK	STATE	PERCENT CHANGE	RANK	STATE	PERCENT CHANGE
8	Alabama	157.9	1	West Virginia	248.1
15	Alaska	130.6	2	Wyoming	212.7
NA	Arizona**	NA	3	New Mexico	198.8
20	Arkansas	117.2	4	Oregon	184.3
34	California	75.7	5	Idaho	166.6
19	Colorado	117.9	6	North Carolina	165.7
40	Connecticut	66.2	7	Texas	164.1
18	Delaware	123.1	8	Alabama	157.9
22	Florida	106.9	9	Tennessee	152.5
46	Georgia	48.8	10	Nevada	150.9
NA	Hawaii**	NA	11	Mississippi	143.0
5	Idaho	166.6	12	Illinois	138.6
12	Illinois	138.6	13	Missouri	133.7
33	Indiana	77.4	14	Kentucky	132.3
35	Iowa	74.8	15	Alaska	130.6
27	Kansas	87.4	16	New Hampshire	127.9
14	Kentucky	132.3	17	Nebraska	125.1
32	Louisiana	77.7	18	Delaware	123.1
30	Maine	80.5	19	Colorado	117.9
23	Maryland	101.8	20	Arkansas	117.2
48	Massachusetts	41.2	21	South Carolina	116.3
41	Michigan	63.6	22	Florida	106.9
38	Minnesota	67.2	23	Maryland	101.8
11	Mississippi	143.0	23	Vermont	101.8
13	Missouri	133.7	25	South Dakota	91.8
29	Montana	86.3	26	Virginia	88.6
17	Nebraska	125.1	27	Kansas	87.4
10	Nevada	150.9	28	Ohio	86.7
16	New Hampshire	127.9	29	Montana	86.3
43	New Jersey	55.3	30	Maine	80.5
3	New Mexico	198.8	31	New York	79.7
31	New York	79.7	32	Louisiana	77.7
6	North Carolina	165.7	33	Indiana	77.4
37	North Dakota	69.4	34	California	75.7
28	Ohio	86.7	35	Iowa	74.8
44	Oklahoma	51.0	36	Utah	71.8
4	Oregon	184.3	37	North Dakota	69.4
42	Pennsylvania	62.7	38	Minnesota	67.2
39	Rhode Island	66.9	39	Rhode Island	66.9
21	South Carolina	116.3	40	Connecticut	66.2
25	South Dakota	91.8	41	Michigan	63.6
9	Tennessee	152.5	42	Pennsylvania	62.7
7	Texas	164.1	43	New Jersey	55.3
36	Utah	71.8	44	Oklahoma	51.0
23	Vermont	101.8	45	Wisconsin	50.5
26	Virginia	88.6	46	Georgia	48.8
47	Washington	46.2	47	Washington	46.2
1	West Virginia	248.1	48	Massachusetts	41.2
45	Wisconsin	50.5	NA	Arizona**	NA
2	Wyoming	212.7	NA	Hawaii**	NA

District of Columbia   183.3

Source: Morgan Quitno Press using data from U.S. Dept. of Health & Human Services, Health Care Financing Admin.
     "Medicaid Recipients, Vendor Payments and Average Cost per Recipient by State: FY 1997" (HCFA-2082)
*For fiscal year ending September 30, 1997.
**Not available.

Medicaid Recipients in 1997

National Total = 33,579,168 Recipients*

<u>ALPHA ORDER</u>

RANK	STATE	RECIPIENTS	% of USA
17	Alabama	546,152	1.6%
47	Alaska	73,050	0.2%
18	Arizona	540,785	1.6%
28	Arkansas	370,386	1.1%
1	California	4,854,546	14.5%
33	Colorado	251,423	0.7%
36	Connecticut	201,779	0.6%
45	Delaware	83,956	0.3%
4	Florida	1,597,461	4.8%
8	Georgia	1,208,445	3.6%
50	Hawaii	0	0.0%
40	Idaho	115,087	0.3%
6	Illinois	1,399,960	4.2%
23	Indiana	514,683	1.5%
32	Iowa	293,784	0.9%
34	Kansas	232,888	0.7%
14	Kentucky	664,454	2.0%
12	Louisiana	746,461	2.2%
37	Maine	167,221	0.5%
25	Maryland	402,002	1.2%
13	Massachusetts	723,472	2.2%
9	Michigan	1,132,783	3.4%
27	Minnesota	371,483	1.1%
24	Mississippi	504,017	1.5%
19	Missouri	540,487	1.6%
43	Montana	95,562	0.3%
35	Nebraska	203,340	0.6%
42	Nevada	105,588	0.3%
44	New Hampshire	95,215	0.3%
20	New Jersey	537,890	1.6%
30	New Mexico	320,223	1.0%
2	New York	3,151,837	9.4%
10	North Carolina	1,112,931	3.3%
48	North Dakota	61,117	0.2%
7	Ohio	1,395,540	4.2%
31	Oklahoma	315,801	0.9%
21	Oregon	531,242	1.6%
11	Pennsylvania	1,024,993	3.1%
39	Rhode Island	116,766	0.3%
22	South Carolina	519,875	1.5%
46	South Dakota	75,444	0.2%
5	Tennessee	1,415,612	4.2%
3	Texas	2,538,655	7.6%
38	Utah	144,749	0.4%
41	Vermont	109,283	0.3%
16	Virginia	595,234	1.8%
15	Washington	630,165	1.9%
29	West Virginia	359,091	1.1%
26	Wisconsin	392,223	1.2%
49	Wyoming	48,865	0.1%

<u>RANK ORDER</u>

RANK	STATE	RECIPIENTS	% of USA
1	California	4,854,546	14.5%
2	New York	3,151,837	9.4%
3	Texas	2,538,655	7.6%
4	Florida	1,597,461	4.8%
5	Tennessee	1,415,612	4.2%
6	Illinois	1,399,960	4.2%
7	Ohio	1,395,540	4.2%
8	Georgia	1,208,445	3.6%
9	Michigan	1,132,783	3.4%
10	North Carolina	1,112,931	3.3%
11	Pennsylvania	1,024,993	3.1%
12	Louisiana	746,461	2.2%
13	Massachusetts	723,472	2.2%
14	Kentucky	664,454	2.0%
15	Washington	630,165	1.9%
16	Virginia	595,234	1.8%
17	Alabama	546,152	1.6%
18	Arizona	540,785	1.6%
19	Missouri	540,487	1.6%
20	New Jersey	537,890	1.6%
21	Oregon	531,242	1.6%
22	South Carolina	519,875	1.5%
23	Indiana	514,683	1.5%
24	Mississippi	504,017	1.5%
25	Maryland	402,002	1.2%
26	Wisconsin	392,223	1.2%
27	Minnesota	371,483	1.1%
28	Arkansas	370,386	1.1%
29	West Virginia	359,091	1.1%
30	New Mexico	320,223	1.0%
31	Oklahoma	315,801	0.9%
32	Iowa	293,784	0.9%
33	Colorado	251,423	0.7%
34	Kansas	232,888	0.7%
35	Nebraska	203,340	0.6%
36	Connecticut	201,779	0.6%
37	Maine	167,221	0.5%
38	Utah	144,749	0.4%
39	Rhode Island	116,766	0.3%
40	Idaho	115,087	0.3%
41	Vermont	109,283	0.3%
42	Nevada	105,588	0.3%
43	Montana	95,562	0.3%
44	New Hampshire	95,215	0.3%
45	Delaware	83,956	0.3%
46	South Dakota	75,444	0.2%
47	Alaska	73,050	0.2%
48	North Dakota	61,117	0.2%
49	Wyoming	48,865	0.1%
50	Hawaii	0	0.0%
	District of Columbia	128,008	0.4%

Source: U.S. Department of Health and Human Services, Health Care Financing Administration
    "Medicaid Recipients by Basis of Eligibility and by State: FY 1997" (HCFA-2082)
*For fiscal year ending September 30, 1997. National total includes 17,154 recipients in the Virgin Islands.

Percent Change in Number of Medicaid Recipients: 1990 to 1997

National Percent Change = 33.0% Increase*

ALPHA ORDER				RANK ORDER		
RANK	STATE	PERCENT CHANGE		RANK	STATE	PERCENT CHANGE
18	Alabama	55.2		1	New Mexico	146.6
9	Alaska	87.1		2	Oregon	133.8
NA	Arizona**	NA		3	Tennessee	130.8
25	Arkansas	40.1		4	Nevada	124.6
27	California	33.9		5	New Hampshire	112.4
29	Colorado	31.9		6	Idaho	111.0
48	Connecticut	(19.2)		7	Delaware	104.7
7	Delaware	104.7		8	North Carolina	97.6
19	Florida	53.8		9	Alaska	87.1
10	Georgia	85.7		10	Georgia	85.7
NA	Hawaii**	NA		11	Vermont	80.9
6	Idaho	111.0		12	Texas	76.0
30	Illinois	31.1		13	Nebraska	70.6
21	Indiana	48.0		14	Wyoming	68.8
34	Iowa	22.6		15	South Carolina	63.9
38	Kansas	19.8		16	Virginia	56.9
23	Kentucky	42.1		17	Montana	56.5
31	Louisiana	27.6		18	Alabama	55.2
32	Maine	25.7		19	Florida	53.8
36	Maryland	21.7		20	South Dakota	53.0
35	Massachusetts	22.5		21	Indiana	48.0
42	Michigan	8.1		22	West Virginia	43.5
45	Minnesota	(2.3)		23	Kentucky	42.1
39	Mississippi	16.4		24	Washington	40.8
37	Missouri	20.6		25	Arkansas	40.1
17	Montana	56.5		26	New York	35.3
13	Nebraska	70.6		27	California	33.9
4	Nevada	124.6		28	Utah	33.7
5	New Hampshire	112.4		29	Colorado	31.9
46	New Jersey	(5.1)		30	Illinois	31.1
1	New Mexico	146.6		31	Louisiana	27.6
26	New York	35.3		32	Maine	25.7
8	North Carolina	97.6		33	North Dakota	24.7
33	North Dakota	24.7		34	Iowa	22.6
41	Ohio	14.3		35	Massachusetts	22.5
40	Oklahoma	15.6		36	Maryland	21.7
2	Oregon	133.8		37	Missouri	20.6
47	Pennsylvania	(12.9)		38	Kansas	19.8
44	Rhode Island	(0.2)		39	Mississippi	16.4
15	South Carolina	63.9		40	Oklahoma	15.6
20	South Dakota	53.0		41	Ohio	14.3
3	Tennessee	130.8		42	Michigan	8.1
12	Texas	76.0		43	Wisconsin	(0.1)
28	Utah	33.7		44	Rhode Island	(0.2)
11	Vermont	80.9		45	Minnesota	(2.3)
16	Virginia	56.9		46	New Jersey	(5.1)
24	Washington	40.8		47	Pennsylvania	(12.9)
22	West Virginia	43.5		48	Connecticut	(19.2)
43	Wisconsin	(0.1)		NA	Arizona**	NA
14	Wyoming	68.8		NA	Hawaii**	NA
					District of Columbia	36.9

Source: Morgan Quitno Press using data from U.S. Dept. of Health & Human Services, Health Care Financing Admin.
   "HCFA-2082 Report" (FY97 and FY90)
*For fiscal year ending September 30, 1997. National rate includes recipients Puerto Rico and the Virgin Islands.
**Not available.

Medicaid Cost per Recipient in 1997

National Rate = $3,679 per Recipient*

ALPHA ORDER

RANK	STATE	PER CAPITA
40	Alabama	$2,877
15	Alaska	4,392
49	Arizona	455
25	Arkansas	3,514
46	California	2,355
14	Colorado	4,470
1	Connecticut	9,927
32	Delaware	3,273
37	Florida	3,058
45	Georgia	2,557
NA	Hawaii**	NA
22	Idaho	3,757
18	Illinois	4,131
12	Indiana	4,628
23	Iowa	3,691
19	Kansas	3,947
28	Kentucky	3,415
34	Louisiana	3,129
11	Maine	4,662
7	Maryland	5,474
9	Massachusetts	5,329
33	Michigan	3,170
4	Minnesota	6,350
41	Mississippi	2,826
20	Missouri	3,880
30	Montana	3,325
27	Nebraska	3,424
24	Nevada	3,531
6	New Hampshire	5,818
3	New Jersey	6,635
44	New Mexico	2,568
2	New York	6,771
29	North Carolina	3,404
8	North Dakota	5,373
17	Ohio	4,190
31	Oklahoma	3,287
43	Oregon	2,776
13	Pennsylvania	4,575
5	Rhode Island	6,320
36	South Carolina	3,092
16	South Dakota	4,221
48	Tennessee	2,074
39	Texas	2,893
38	Utah	2,927
42	Vermont	2,824
35	Virginia	3,121
47	Washington	2,210
26	West Virginia	3,500
10	Wisconsin	4,790
21	Wyoming	3,771

RANK ORDER

RANK	STATE	PER CAPITA
1	Connecticut	$9,927
2	New York	6,771
3	New Jersey	6,635
4	Minnesota	6,350
5	Rhode Island	6,320
6	New Hampshire	5,818
7	Maryland	5,474
8	North Dakota	5,373
9	Massachusetts	5,329
10	Wisconsin	4,790
11	Maine	4,662
12	Indiana	4,628
13	Pennsylvania	4,575
14	Colorado	4,470
15	Alaska	4,392
16	South Dakota	4,221
17	Ohio	4,190
18	Illinois	4,131
19	Kansas	3,947
20	Missouri	3,880
21	Wyoming	3,771
22	Idaho	3,757
23	Iowa	3,691
24	Nevada	3,531
25	Arkansas	3,514
26	West Virginia	3,500
27	Nebraska	3,424
28	Kentucky	3,415
29	North Carolina	3,404
30	Montana	3,325
31	Oklahoma	3,287
32	Delaware	3,273
33	Michigan	3,170
34	Louisiana	3,129
35	Virginia	3,121
36	South Carolina	3,092
37	Florida	3,058
38	Utah	2,927
39	Texas	2,893
40	Alabama	2,877
41	Mississippi	2,826
42	Vermont	2,824
43	Oregon	2,776
44	New Mexico	2,568
45	Georgia	2,557
46	California	2,355
47	Washington	2,210
48	Tennessee	2,074
49	Arizona	455
NA	Hawaii**	NA

District of Columbia 5,439

Source: Morgan Quitno Press using data from U.S. Dept. of Health & Human Services, Health Care Financing Admin. "HCFA-2082 Report: FY97" (www.hcfa.gov/medicaid/mstats.htm)

For fiscal year ending September 30, 1997.

**Not available.*

Percent Change in Cost per Medicaid Recipient: 1990 to 1997

National Percent Change = 43.3% Increase*

ALPHA ORDER

RANK	STATE	PERCENT CHANGE
10	Alabama	66.2
35	Alaska	23.3
NA	Arizona**	NA
17	Arkansas	55.0
30	California	31.2
12	Colorado	65.2
3	Connecticut	105.6
45	Delaware	9.0
25	Florida	34.5
48	Georgia	(19.8)
NA	Hawaii**	NA
33	Idaho	26.4
7	Illinois	81.9
39	Indiana	19.9
22	Iowa	42.6
16	Kansas	56.4
14	Kentucky	63.5
23	Louisiana	39.3
21	Maine	43.5
11	Maryland	65.9
41	Massachusetts	15.3
18	Michigan	51.4
8	Minnesota	71.2
2	Mississippi	108.7
4	Missouri	93.8
40	Montana	19.0
29	Nebraska	31.9
42	Nevada	11.7
46	New Hampshire	7.3
13	New Jersey	63.7
37	New Mexico	21.1
27	New York	32.8
25	North Carolina	34.5
24	North Dakota	35.9
15	Ohio	63.3
31	Oklahoma	30.6
36	Oregon	21.6
5	Pennsylvania	86.8
9	Rhode Island	67.3
28	South Carolina	32.0
34	South Dakota	25.3
44	Tennessee	9.4
20	Texas	50.1
32	Utah	28.4
43	Vermont	11.6
38	Virginia	20.2
47	Washington	3.9
1	West Virginia	142.6
19	Wisconsin	50.7
6	Wyoming	85.2

RANK ORDER

RANK	STATE	PERCENT CHANGE
1	West Virginia	142.6
2	Mississippi	108.7
3	Connecticut	105.6
4	Missouri	93.8
5	Pennsylvania	86.8
6	Wyoming	85.2
7	Illinois	81.9
8	Minnesota	71.2
9	Rhode Island	67.3
10	Alabama	66.2
11	Maryland	65.9
12	Colorado	65.2
13	New Jersey	63.7
14	Kentucky	63.5
15	Ohio	63.3
16	Kansas	56.4
17	Arkansas	55.0
18	Michigan	51.4
19	Wisconsin	50.7
20	Texas	50.1
21	Maine	43.5
22	Iowa	42.6
23	Louisiana	39.3
24	North Dakota	35.9
25	Florida	34.5
25	North Carolina	34.5
27	New York	32.8
28	South Carolina	32.0
29	Nebraska	31.9
30	California	31.2
31	Oklahoma	30.6
32	Utah	28.4
33	Idaho	26.4
34	South Dakota	25.3
35	Alaska	23.3
36	Oregon	21.6
37	New Mexico	21.1
38	Virginia	20.2
39	Indiana	19.9
40	Montana	19.0
41	Massachusetts	15.3
42	Nevada	11.7
43	Vermont	11.6
44	Tennessee	9.4
45	Delaware	9.0
46	New Hampshire	7.3
47	Washington	3.9
48	Georgia	(19.8)
NA	Arizona**	NA
NA	Hawaii**	NA

District of Columbia 106.9

Source: Morgan Quitno Press using data from U.S. Dept. of Health & Human Services, Health Care Financing Admin.
    "Medicaid Recipients, Vendor Payments and Average Cost per Recipient by State: FY 1997" (HCFA-2082)
*For fiscal year ending September 30, 1997.
**Not available.

Federal Medicaid Matching Fund Rate for 1999

National Average = 72.47% of States' Funds Matched by Federal Government*

ALPHA ORDER

RANK	STATE	RATE
13	Alabama	78.49
29	Alaska	71.86
16	Arizona	75.85
4	Arkansas	81.07
38	California	66.09
40	Colorado	65.42
41	Connecticut	65.00
41	Delaware	65.00
32	Florida	69.07
26	Georgia	72.33
41	Hawaii	65.00
11	Idaho	78.89
41	Illinois	65.00
24	Indiana	72.71
18	Iowa	74.32
28	Kansas	72.03
8	Kentucky	79.37
9	Louisiana	79.26
15	Maine	76.48
41	Maryland	65.00
41	Massachusetts	65.00
35	Michigan	66.91
39	Minnesota	66.05
1	Mississippi	83.75
27	Missouri	72.17
6	Montana	80.21
23	Nebraska	73.02
41	Nevada	65.00
41	New Hampshire	65.00
41	New Jersey	65.00
3	New Mexico	81.09
41	New York	65.00
20	North Carolina	74.15
10	North Dakota	78.96
31	Ohio	70.78
7	Oklahoma	79.59
25	Oregon	72.38
34	Pennsylvania	67.64
33	Rhode Island	67.83
11	South Carolina	78.89
14	South Dakota	77.71
19	Tennessee	74.16
21	Texas	73.72
5	Utah	80.25
22	Vermont	73.38
37	Virginia	66.12
36	Washington	66.75
2	West Virginia	82.13
30	Wisconsin	71.20
17	Wyoming	74.86

RANK ORDER

RANK	STATE	RATE
1	Mississippi	83.75
2	West Virginia	82.13
3	New Mexico	81.09
4	Arkansas	81.07
5	Utah	80.25
6	Montana	80.21
7	Oklahoma	79.59
8	Kentucky	79.37
9	Louisiana	79.26
10	North Dakota	78.96
11	Idaho	78.89
11	South Carolina	78.89
13	Alabama	78.49
14	South Dakota	77.71
15	Maine	76.48
16	Arizona	75.85
17	Wyoming	74.86
18	Iowa	74.32
19	Tennessee	74.16
20	North Carolina	74.15
21	Texas	73.72
22	Vermont	73.38
23	Nebraska	73.02
24	Indiana	72.71
25	Oregon	72.38
26	Georgia	72.33
27	Missouri	72.17
28	Kansas	72.03
29	Alaska	71.86
30	Wisconsin	71.20
31	Ohio	70.78
32	Florida	69.07
33	Rhode Island	67.83
34	Pennsylvania	67.64
35	Michigan	66.91
36	Washington	66.75
37	Virginia	66.12
38	California	66.09
39	Minnesota	66.05
40	Colorado	65.42
41	Connecticut	65.00
41	Delaware	65.00
41	Hawaii	65.00
41	Illinois	65.00
41	Maryland	65.00
41	Massachusetts	65.00
41	Nevada	65.00
41	New Hampshire	65.00
41	New Jersey	65.00
41	New York	65.00
	District of Columbia	79.00

*Source: U.S. Department of Health and Human Services, Health Care Financing Administration
"Enhanced Federal Medical Assistance Percentages" (Federal Register, 11/24/97)*
*For fiscal year 1999. These are "enhanced" matching rates established by the Children's Health Insurance
Program, signed into law in August 1997. Sixty-five percent is the minimum. National average is a simple average of
the 51 individual rates and is not weighted for population or funds.*

Percent of Population Receiving Medicaid in 1997

National Percent = 12.5% of Population*

RANK	STATE (ALPHA ORDER)	PERCENT		RANK	STATE (RANK ORDER)	PERCENT
17	Alabama	12.6		1	Tennessee	26.4
20	Alaska	12.0		2	West Virginia	19.8
21	Arizona	11.9		3	New Mexico	18.6
13	Arkansas	14.7		3	Vermont	18.6
11	California	15.1		5	Mississippi	18.5
47	Colorado	6.5		6	New York	17.4
49	Connecticut	6.2		7	Louisiana	17.1
26	Delaware	11.4		8	Kentucky	17.0
28	Florida	10.9		9	Oregon	16.4
10	Georgia	16.1		10	Georgia	16.1
50	Hawaii	0.0		11	California	15.1
34	Idaho	9.5		12	North Carolina	15.0
24	Illinois	11.7		13	Arkansas	14.7
38	Indiana	8.8		14	South Carolina	13.7
30	Iowa	10.3		15	Maine	13.5
37	Kansas	9.0		16	Texas	13.1
8	Kentucky	17.0		17	Alabama	12.6
7	Louisiana	17.1		18	Ohio	12.5
15	Maine	13.5		19	Nebraska	12.3
42	Maryland	7.9		20	Alaska	12.0
22	Massachusetts	11.8		21	Arizona	11.9
25	Michigan	11.6		22	Massachusetts	11.8
42	Minnesota	7.9		22	Rhode Island	11.8
5	Mississippi	18.5		24	Illinois	11.7
33	Missouri	10.0		25	Michigan	11.6
28	Montana	10.9		26	Delaware	11.4
19	Nebraska	12.3		27	Washington	11.2
48	Nevada	6.3		28	Florida	10.9
41	New Hampshire	8.1		28	Montana	10.9
46	New Jersey	6.7		30	Iowa	10.3
3	New Mexico	18.6		31	South Dakota	10.2
6	New York	17.4		31	Wyoming	10.2
12	North Carolina	15.0		33	Missouri	10.0
34	North Dakota	9.5		34	Idaho	9.5
18	Ohio	12.5		34	North Dakota	9.5
34	Oklahoma	9.5		34	Oklahoma	9.5
9	Oregon	16.4		37	Kansas	9.0
40	Pennsylvania	8.5		38	Indiana	8.8
22	Rhode Island	11.8		38	Virginia	8.8
14	South Carolina	13.7		40	Pennsylvania	8.5
31	South Dakota	10.2		41	New Hampshire	8.1
1	Tennessee	26.4		42	Maryland	7.9
16	Texas	13.1		42	Minnesota	7.9
45	Utah	7.0		44	Wisconsin	7.5
3	Vermont	18.6		45	Utah	7.0
38	Virginia	8.8		46	New Jersey	6.7
27	Washington	11.2		47	Colorado	6.5
2	West Virginia	19.8		48	Nevada	6.3
44	Wisconsin	7.5		49	Connecticut	6.2
31	Wyoming	10.2		50	Hawaii	0.0

District of Columbia   24.2

Source: Morgan Quitno Press using data from US Dept. of Health & Human Services, Health Care Financing Admin.
"Medicaid Recipients by Basis of Eligibility and by State: FY 1997" (HCFA-2082)
*For fiscal year ending September 30, 1997. National percent does not include recipients in the Virgin Islands.

Medicaid Managed Care Enrollment in 1997

National Total = 15,345,502 Medicaid Enrollees*

ALPHA ORDER

RANK	STATE	ENROLLEES	% of USA
10	Alabama	407,643	2.66%
NA	Alaska**	NA	NA
14	Arizona	349,142	2.28%
28	Arkansas	159,458	1.04%
1	California	1,854,294	12.08%
26	Colorado	184,000	1.20%
21	Connecticut	231,966	1.51%
38	Delaware	65,061	0.42%
3	Florida	896,559	5.84%
8	Georgia	560,771	3.65%
30	Hawaii	135,200	0.88%
42	Idaho	32,428	0.21%
25	Illinois	187,048	1.22%
23	Indiana	220,000	1.43%
35	Iowa	88,282	0.58%
32	Kansas	94,430	0.62%
19	Kentucky	268,205	1.75%
41	Louisiana	40,469	0.26%
47	Maine	12,511	0.08%
15	Maryland	347,640	2.27%
9	Massachusetts	461,989	3.01%
5	Michigan	865,434	5.64%
27	Minnesota	169,329	1.10%
36	Mississippi	81,255	0.53%
20	Missouri	264,496	1.72%
39	Montana	62,004	0.40%
34	Nebraska	93,085	0.61%
43	Nevada	26,376	0.17%
48	New Hampshire	9,102	0.06%
11	New Jersey	384,644	2.51%
29	New Mexico	139,337	0.91%
7	New York	660,725	4.31%
13	North Carolina	351,043	2.29%
44	North Dakota	24,295	0.16%
12	Ohio	352,833	2.30%
22	Oklahoma	222,818	1.45%
16	Oregon	312,345	2.04%
4	Pennsylvania	870,365	5.67%
37	Rhode Island	70,944	0.46%
46	South Carolina	14,311	0.09%
40	South Dakota	41,542	0.27%
2	Tennessee	1,188,570	7.75%
18	Texas	275,951	1.80%
33	Utah	93,785	0.61%
45	Vermont	22,946	0.15%
17	Virginia	306,804	2.00%
6	Washington	730,052	4.76%
31	West Virginia	125,521	0.82%
24	Wisconsin	205,523	1.34%
NA	Wyoming**	NA	NA

RANK ORDER

RANK	STATE	ENROLLEES	% of USA
1	California	1,854,294	12.08%
2	Tennessee	1,188,570	7.75%
3	Florida	896,559	5.84%
4	Pennsylvania	870,365	5.67%
5	Michigan	865,434	5.64%
6	Washington	730,052	4.76%
7	New York	660,725	4.31%
8	Georgia	560,771	3.65%
9	Massachusetts	461,989	3.01%
10	Alabama	407,643	2.66%
11	New Jersey	384,644	2.51%
12	Ohio	352,833	2.30%
13	North Carolina	351,043	2.29%
14	Arizona	349,142	2.28%
15	Maryland	347,640	2.27%
16	Oregon	312,345	2.04%
17	Virginia	306,804	2.00%
18	Texas	275,951	1.80%
19	Kentucky	268,205	1.75%
20	Missouri	264,496	1.72%
21	Connecticut	231,966	1.51%
22	Oklahoma	222,818	1.45%
23	Indiana	220,000	1.43%
24	Wisconsin	205,523	1.34%
25	Illinois	187,048	1.22%
26	Colorado	184,000	1.20%
27	Minnesota	169,329	1.10%
28	Arkansas	159,458	1.04%
29	New Mexico	139,337	0.91%
30	Hawaii	135,200	0.88%
31	West Virginia	125,521	0.82%
32	Kansas	94,430	0.62%
33	Utah	93,785	0.61%
34	Nebraska	93,085	0.61%
35	Iowa	88,282	0.58%
36	Mississippi	81,255	0.53%
37	Rhode Island	70,944	0.46%
38	Delaware	65,061	0.42%
39	Montana	62,004	0.40%
40	South Dakota	41,542	0.27%
41	Louisiana	40,469	0.26%
42	Idaho	32,428	0.21%
43	Nevada	26,376	0.17%
44	North Dakota	24,295	0.16%
45	Vermont	22,946	0.15%
46	South Carolina	14,311	0.09%
47	Maine	12,511	0.08%
48	New Hampshire	9,102	0.06%
NA	Alaska**	NA	NA
NA	Wyoming**	NA	NA
	District of Columbia	80,721	0.53%

Source: U.S. Department of Health and Human Services, Health Care Financing Administration
"Medicaid Managed Care State Enrollment" (http://www.hcfa.gov/medicaid/plantyp7.htm)
As of June 30, 1997. Enrollment in state health care reform programs that expand eligibility beyond traditional Medicaid standards. National total includes 702,250 Medicaid enrollees in Puerto Rico.
***None or not available.*

Medicaid Health Maintenance Organizations (HMOs) in 1998

National Total = 284 Medicaid HMOs*

ALPHA ORDER

RANK	STATE	HMOs	% of USA
36	Alabama	2	0.7%
NA	Alaska**	NA	NA
27	Arizona	3	1.1%
40	Arkansas	1	0.4%
1	California	22	7.7%
12	Colorado	7	2.5%
21	Connecticut	4	1.4%
21	Delaware	4	1.4%
5	Florida	15	5.3%
27	Georgia	3	1.1%
21	Hawaii	4	1.4%
40	Idaho	1	0.4%
9	Illinois	10	3.5%
36	Indiana	2	0.7%
40	Iowa	1	0.4%
27	Kansas	3	1.1%
27	Kentucky	3	1.1%
46	Louisiana	0	0.0%
40	Maine	1	0.4%
21	Maryland	4	1.4%
16	Massachusetts	5	1.8%
3	Michigan	19	6.7%
12	Minnesota	7	2.5%
16	Mississippi	5	1.8%
9	Missouri	10	3.5%
40	Montana	1	0.4%
27	Nebraska	3	1.1%
21	Nevada	4	1.4%
27	New Hampshire	3	1.1%
7	New Jersey	13	4.6%
27	New Mexico	3	1.1%
2	New York	21	7.4%
16	North Carolina	5	1.8%
40	North Dakota	1	0.4%
5	Ohio	15	5.3%
27	Oklahoma	3	1.1%
21	Oregon	4	1.4%
9	Pennsylvania	10	3.5%
36	Rhode Island	2	0.7%
27	South Carolina	3	1.1%
46	South Dakota	0	0.0%
12	Tennessee	7	2.5%
8	Texas	12	4.2%
15	Utah	6	2.1%
46	Vermont	0	0.0%
16	Virginia	5	1.8%
16	Washington	5	1.8%
36	West Virginia	2	0.7%
4	Wisconsin	18	6.3%
46	Wyoming	0	0.0%

RANK ORDER

RANK	STATE	HMOs	% of USA
1	California	22	7.7%
2	New York	21	7.4%
3	Michigan	19	6.7%
4	Wisconsin	18	6.3%
5	Florida	15	5.3%
5	Ohio	15	5.3%
7	New Jersey	13	4.6%
8	Texas	12	4.2%
9	Illinois	10	3.5%
9	Missouri	10	3.5%
9	Pennsylvania	10	3.5%
12	Colorado	7	2.5%
12	Minnesota	7	2.5%
12	Tennessee	7	2.5%
15	Utah	6	2.1%
16	Massachusetts	5	1.8%
16	Mississippi	5	1.8%
16	North Carolina	5	1.8%
16	Virginia	5	1.8%
16	Washington	5	1.8%
21	Connecticut	4	1.4%
21	Delaware	4	1.4%
21	Hawaii	4	1.4%
21	Maryland	4	1.4%
21	Nevada	4	1.4%
21	Oregon	4	1.4%
27	Arizona	3	1.1%
27	Georgia	3	1.1%
27	Kansas	3	1.1%
27	Kentucky	3	1.1%
27	Nebraska	3	1.1%
27	New Hampshire	3	1.1%
27	New Mexico	3	1.1%
27	Oklahoma	3	1.1%
27	South Carolina	3	1.1%
36	Alabama	2	0.7%
36	Indiana	2	0.7%
36	Rhode Island	2	0.7%
36	West Virginia	2	0.7%
40	Arkansas	1	0.4%
40	Idaho	1	0.4%
40	Iowa	1	0.4%
40	Maine	1	0.4%
40	Montana	1	0.4%
40	North Dakota	1	0.4%
46	Louisiana	0	0.0%
46	South Dakota	0	0.0%
46	Vermont	0	0.0%
46	Wyoming	0	0.0%
NA	Alaska**	NA	NA
	District of Columbia	1	0.4%

Source: InterStudy Publications (Minneapolis, MN)
   "The Competitive Edge Industry Report 8.2" (Press Release, November 3, 1998)
As of January 1, 1998. Health plans are allocated to states based upon their primary service areas. This means each plan is counted once. However, many plans serve more than one state. National total includes one HMO in Puerto Rico.

Medicaid Health Maintenance Organization (HMOs) Enrollment in 1998

National Total = 7,834,419 Enrollees*

ALPHA ORDER

RANK	STATE	ENROLLEES	% of USA
29	Alabama	35,189	0.4%
NA	Alaska**	NA	NA
34	Arizona	21,082	0.3%
45	Arkansas	0	0.0%
1	California	1,386,134	17.7%
23	Colorado	72,125	0.9%
16	Connecticut	148,826	1.9%
22	Delaware	75,799	1.0%
6	Florida	372,820	4.8%
28	Georgia	36,377	0.5%
25	Hawaii	61,150	0.8%
41	Idaho	3,171	0.0%
13	Illinois	203,607	2.6%
24	Indiana	67,812	0.9%
42	Iowa	1,074	0.0%
35	Kansas	19,018	0.2%
32	Kentucky	26,992	0.3%
45	Louisiana	0	0.0%
39	Maine	4,729	0.1%
9	Maryland	242,151	3.1%
18	Massachusetts	144,795	1.8%
4	Michigan	455,183	5.8%
12	Minnesota	205,598	2.6%
37	Mississippi	10,074	0.1%
10	Missouri	221,080	2.8%
44	Montana	540	0.0%
36	Nebraska	18,709	0.2%
31	Nevada	28,574	0.4%
38	New Hampshire	8,037	0.1%
7	New Jersey	348,690	4.5%
17	New Mexico	147,724	1.9%
5	New York	412,449	5.3%
33	North Carolina	25,957	0.3%
43	North Dakota	846	0.0%
8	Ohio	347,056	4.4%
26	Oklahoma	50,220	0.6%
19	Oregon	139,159	1.8%
2	Pennsylvania	715,330	9.1%
27	Rhode Island	42,362	0.5%
40	South Carolina	3,261	0.0%
45	South Dakota	0	0.0%
3	Tennessee	533,538	6.8%
14	Texas	197,500	2.5%
20	Utah	103,031	1.3%
45	Vermont	0	0.0%
21	Virginia	88,690	1.1%
15	Washington	178,245	2.3%
30	West Virginia	31,741	0.4%
11	Wisconsin	206,148	2.6%
45	Wyoming	0	0.0%

RANK ORDER

RANK	STATE	ENROLLEES	% of USA
1	California	1,386,134	17.7%
2	Pennsylvania	715,330	9.1%
3	Tennessee	533,538	6.8%
4	Michigan	455,183	5.8%
5	New York	412,449	5.3%
6	Florida	372,820	4.8%
7	New Jersey	348,690	4.5%
8	Ohio	347,056	4.4%
9	Maryland	242,151	3.1%
10	Missouri	221,080	2.8%
11	Wisconsin	206,148	2.6%
12	Minnesota	205,598	2.6%
13	Illinois	203,607	2.6%
14	Texas	197,500	2.5%
15	Washington	178,245	2.3%
16	Connecticut	148,826	1.9%
17	New Mexico	147,724	1.9%
18	Massachusetts	144,795	1.8%
19	Oregon	139,159	1.8%
20	Utah	103,031	1.3%
21	Virginia	88,690	1.1%
22	Delaware	75,799	1.0%
23	Colorado	72,125	0.9%
24	Indiana	67,812	0.9%
25	Hawaii	61,150	0.8%
26	Oklahoma	50,220	0.6%
27	Rhode Island	42,362	0.5%
28	Georgia	36,377	0.5%
29	Alabama	35,189	0.4%
30	West Virginia	31,741	0.4%
31	Nevada	28,574	0.4%
32	Kentucky	26,992	0.3%
33	North Carolina	25,957	0.3%
34	Arizona	21,082	0.3%
35	Kansas	19,018	0.2%
36	Nebraska	18,709	0.2%
37	Mississippi	10,074	0.1%
38	New Hampshire	8,037	0.1%
39	Maine	4,729	0.1%
40	South Carolina	3,261	0.0%
41	Idaho	3,171	0.0%
42	Iowa	1,074	0.0%
43	North Dakota	846	0.0%
44	Montana	540	0.0%
45	Arkansas	0	0.0%
45	Louisiana	0	0.0%
45	South Dakota	0	0.0%
45	Vermont	0	0.0%
45	Wyoming	0	0.0%
NA	Alaska**	NA	NA
	District of Columbia	2,196	0.0%

Source: InterStudy Publications (Minneapolis, MN)
   "The Competitive Edge Industry Report 8.2" (Press Release, November 3, 1998)
*As of January 1, 1998. Health plans are allocated to states based upon their primary service areas. This means each plan is counted once. However, many plans serve more than one state. National total includes 389,630 enrollees in Puerto Rico.

Medicaid Costs Related to Smoking in 1993

National Total = $12,893,507,000

ALPHA ORDER

RANK	STATE	COSTS	% of USA
29	Alabama	$107,304,000	0.8%
46	Alaska	23,617,000	0.2%
26	Arizona	121,846,000	0.9%
36	Arkansas	78,456,000	0.6%
2	California	1,732,749,000	13.4%
24	Colorado	151,500,000	1.2%
22	Connecticut	181,755,000	1.4%
47	Delaware	22,845,000	0.2%
9	Florida	516,980,000	4.0%
14	Georgia	251,936,000	2.0%
40	Hawaii	44,059,000	0.3%
45	Idaho	25,343,000	0.2%
6	Illinois	560,629,000	4.3%
13	Indiana	254,892,000	2.0%
35	Iowa	79,384,000	0.6%
37	Kansas	72,300,000	0.6%
19	Kentucky	200,740,000	1.6%
10	Louisiana	417,026,000	3.2%
31	Maine	95,862,000	0.7%
16	Maryland	212,304,000	1.6%
11	Massachusetts	405,943,000	3.1%
8	Michigan	532,580,000	4.1%
21	Minnesota	186,846,000	1.4%
28	Mississippi	111,130,000	0.9%
17	Missouri	206,923,000	1.6%
44	Montana	28,065,000	0.2%
41	Nebraska	43,434,000	0.3%
38	Nevada	50,137,000	0.4%
32	New Hampshire	94,531,000	0.7%
7	New Jersey	544,708,000	4.2%
39	New Mexico	48,314,000	0.4%
1	New York	1,850,692,000	14.4%
18	North Carolina	205,600,000	1.6%
49	North Dakota	19,056,000	0.1%
5	Ohio	597,217,000	4.6%
34	Oklahoma	80,105,000	0.6%
33	Oregon	89,231,000	0.7%
4	Pennsylvania	605,516,000	4.7%
30	Rhode Island	96,884,000	0.8%
25	South Carolina	142,044,000	1.1%
48	South Dakota	20,740,000	0.2%
12	Tennessee	299,880,000	2.3%
3	Texas	654,003,000	5.1%
42	Utah	34,211,000	0.3%
43	Vermont	29,025,000	0.2%
23	Virginia	162,564,000	1.3%
15	Washington	237,159,000	1.8%
27	West Virginia	119,235,000	0.9%
20	Wisconsin	197,927,000	1.5%
50	Wyoming	11,449,000	0.1%

RANK ORDER

RANK	STATE	COSTS	% of USA
1	New York	$1,850,692,000	14.4%
2	California	1,732,749,000	13.4%
3	Texas	654,003,000	5.1%
4	Pennsylvania	605,516,000	4.7%
5	Ohio	597,217,000	4.6%
6	Illinois	560,629,000	4.3%
7	New Jersey	544,708,000	4.2%
8	Michigan	532,580,000	4.1%
9	Florida	516,980,000	4.0%
10	Louisiana	417,026,000	3.2%
11	Massachusetts	405,943,000	3.1%
12	Tennessee	299,880,000	2.3%
13	Indiana	254,892,000	2.0%
14	Georgia	251,936,000	2.0%
15	Washington	237,159,000	1.8%
16	Maryland	212,304,000	1.6%
17	Missouri	206,923,000	1.6%
18	North Carolina	205,600,000	1.6%
19	Kentucky	200,740,000	1.6%
20	Wisconsin	197,927,000	1.5%
21	Minnesota	186,846,000	1.4%
22	Connecticut	181,755,000	1.4%
23	Virginia	162,564,000	1.3%
24	Colorado	151,500,000	1.2%
25	South Carolina	142,044,000	1.1%
26	Arizona	121,846,000	0.9%
27	West Virginia	119,235,000	0.9%
28	Mississippi	111,130,000	0.9%
29	Alabama	107,304,000	0.8%
30	Rhode Island	96,884,000	0.8%
31	Maine	95,862,000	0.7%
32	New Hampshire	94,531,000	0.7%
33	Oregon	89,231,000	0.7%
34	Oklahoma	80,105,000	0.6%
35	Iowa	79,384,000	0.6%
36	Arkansas	78,456,000	0.6%
37	Kansas	72,300,000	0.6%
38	Nevada	50,137,000	0.4%
39	New Mexico	48,314,000	0.4%
40	Hawaii	44,059,000	0.3%
41	Nebraska	43,434,000	0.3%
42	Utah	34,211,000	0.3%
43	Vermont	29,025,000	0.2%
44	Montana	28,065,000	0.2%
45	Idaho	25,343,000	0.2%
46	Alaska	23,617,000	0.2%
47	Delaware	22,845,000	0.2%
48	South Dakota	20,740,000	0.2%
49	North Dakota	19,056,000	0.1%
50	Wyoming	11,449,000	0.1%
	District of Columbia	35,830,000	0.3%

Source: Centers for Disease Control and Prevention, Office on Smoking and Health
"State and National Tobacco Control Highlights" (http://www.cdc.gov/nccdphp/osh/statehi/statehi.htm)

Estimated State Funds from the Tobacco Settlement Through 2025

National Total = $195,918,675,920*

ALPHA ORDER

RANK	STATE	FUNDS	% of USA
21	Alabama	$3,166,302,119	1.6%
45	Alaska	668,903,057	0.3%
22	Arizona	2,887,614,909	1.5%
30	Arkansas	1,622,336,126	0.8%
1	California	25,006,972,511	12.8%
23	Colorado	2,685,773,549	1.4%
19	Connecticut	3,637,303,382	1.9%
41	Delaware	774,798,677	0.4%
NA	Florida**	NA	NA
9	Georgia	4,808,740,669	2.5%
35	Hawaii	1,179,165,923	0.6%
43	Idaho	711,700,479	0.4%
5	Illinois	9,118,539,559	4.7%
18	Indiana	3,996,355,551	2.0%
28	Iowa	1,703,839,986	0.9%
29	Kansas	1,633,317,646	0.8%
20	Kentucky	3,450,438,586	1.8%
14	Louisiana	4,418,657,915	2.3%
31	Maine	1,507,301,276	0.8%
13	Maryland	4,428,657,384	2.3%
7	Massachusetts	7,913,114,213	4.0%
6	Michigan	8,526,278,034	4.4%
NA	Minnesota**	NA	NA
NA	Mississippi**	NA	NA
12	Missouri	4,456,368,286	2.3%
39	Montana	832,182,431	0.4%
37	Nebraska	1,165,683,457	0.6%
34	Nevada	1,194,976,855	0.6%
33	New Hampshire	1,304,689,150	0.7%
8	New Jersey	7,576,167,918	3.9%
36	New Mexico	1,168,438,809	0.6%
2	New York	25,003,202,243	12.8%
11	North Carolina	4,569,381,898	2.3%
42	North Dakota	717,089,369	0.4%
4	Ohio	9,869,422,449	5.0%
26	Oklahoma	2,029,985,862	1.0%
25	Oregon	2,248,476,833	1.1%
3	Pennsylvania	11,259,169,603	5.7%
32	Rhode Island	1,408,469,747	0.7%
24	South Carolina	2,304,693,120	1.2%
44	South Dakota	683,650,009	0.3%
10	Tennessee	4,782,168,127	2.4%
NA	Texas**	NA	NA
38	Utah	871,616,513	0.4%
40	Vermont	805,588,329	0.4%
17	Virginia	4,006,037,550	2.0%
16	Washington	4,022,716,267	2.1%
27	West Virginia	1,736,741,427	0.9%
15	Wisconsin	4,059,511,421	2.1%
46	Wyoming	486,553,976	0.2%

RANK ORDER

RANK	STATE	FUNDS	% of USA
1	California	$25,006,972,511	12.8%
2	New York	25,003,202,243	12.8%
3	Pennsylvania	11,259,169,603	5.7%
4	Ohio	9,869,422,449	5.0%
5	Illinois	9,118,539,559	4.7%
6	Michigan	8,526,278,034	4.4%
7	Massachusetts	7,913,114,213	4.0%
8	New Jersey	7,576,167,918	3.9%
9	Georgia	4,808,740,669	2.5%
10	Tennessee	4,782,168,127	2.4%
11	North Carolina	4,569,381,898	2.3%
12	Missouri	4,456,368,286	2.3%
13	Maryland	4,428,657,384	2.3%
14	Louisiana	4,418,657,915	2.3%
15	Wisconsin	4,059,511,421	2.1%
16	Washington	4,022,716,267	2.1%
17	Virginia	4,006,037,550	2.0%
18	Indiana	3,996,355,551	2.0%
19	Connecticut	3,637,303,382	1.9%
20	Kentucky	3,450,438,586	1.8%
21	Alabama	3,166,302,119	1.6%
22	Arizona	2,887,614,909	1.5%
23	Colorado	2,685,773,549	1.4%
24	South Carolina	2,304,693,120	1.2%
25	Oregon	2,248,476,833	1.1%
26	Oklahoma	2,029,985,862	1.0%
27	West Virginia	1,736,741,427	0.9%
28	Iowa	1,703,839,986	0.9%
29	Kansas	1,633,317,646	0.8%
30	Arkansas	1,622,336,126	0.8%
31	Maine	1,507,301,276	0.8%
32	Rhode Island	1,408,469,747	0.7%
33	New Hampshire	1,304,689,150	0.7%
34	Nevada	1,194,976,855	0.6%
35	Hawaii	1,179,165,923	0.6%
36	New Mexico	1,168,438,809	0.6%
37	Nebraska	1,165,683,457	0.6%
38	Utah	871,616,513	0.4%
39	Montana	832,182,431	0.4%
40	Vermont	805,588,329	0.4%
41	Delaware	774,798,677	0.4%
42	North Dakota	717,089,369	0.4%
43	Idaho	711,700,479	0.4%
44	South Dakota	683,650,009	0.3%
45	Alaska	668,903,057	0.3%
46	Wyoming	486,553,976	0.2%
NA	Florida**	NA	NA
NA	Minnesota**	NA	NA
NA	Mississippi**	NA	NA
NA	Texas**	NA	NA
	District of Columbia	1,189,458,106	0.6%

Source: National Association of Attorneys General
"Attorneys General Announce Tobacco Settlement Proposal" (News release, http://www.naag.org/tob2.htm)
*This settlement was reached in November 1998. National total includes $4,640,249,229 for U.S. territories.
**Total does not include $40 billion in previous settlements with Florida, Minnesota, Mississippi and Texas.

331

State Government Expenditures for Health Programs in 1997

National Total = $33,879,585,000*

<table>
<tr><td colspan="4">ALPHA ORDER</td><td colspan="4">RANK ORDER</td></tr>
<tr><th>RANK</th><th>STATE</th><th>EXPENDITURES</th><th>% of USA</th><th>RANK</th><th>STATE</th><th>EXPENDITURES</th><th>% of USA</th></tr>
<tr><td>18</td><td>Alabama</td><td>$566,651,000</td><td>1.7%</td><td>1</td><td>California</td><td>$6,083,766,000</td><td>18.0%</td></tr>
<tr><td>42</td><td>Alaska</td><td>159,454,000</td><td>0.5%</td><td>2</td><td>New York</td><td>2,147,669,000</td><td>6.3%</td></tr>
<tr><td>19</td><td>Arizona</td><td>558,780,000</td><td>1.6%</td><td>3</td><td>Michigan</td><td>2,046,674,000</td><td>6.0%</td></tr>
<tr><td>32</td><td>Arkansas</td><td>261,311,000</td><td>0.8%</td><td>4</td><td>Florida</td><td>1,850,393,000</td><td>5.5%</td></tr>
<tr><td>1</td><td>California</td><td>6,083,766,000</td><td>18.0%</td><td>5</td><td>Illinois</td><td>1,702,964,000</td><td>5.0%</td></tr>
<tr><td>35</td><td>Colorado</td><td>247,006,000</td><td>0.7%</td><td>6</td><td>Pennsylvania</td><td>1,379,050,000</td><td>4.1%</td></tr>
<tr><td>24</td><td>Connecticut</td><td>402,219,000</td><td>1.2%</td><td>7</td><td>Ohio</td><td>1,352,057,000</td><td>4.0%</td></tr>
<tr><td>40</td><td>Delaware</td><td>166,892,000</td><td>0.5%</td><td>8</td><td>Texas</td><td>1,331,742,000</td><td>3.9%</td></tr>
<tr><td>4</td><td>Florida</td><td>1,850,393,000</td><td>5.5%</td><td>9</td><td>Massachusetts</td><td>1,325,680,000</td><td>3.9%</td></tr>
<tr><td>15</td><td>Georgia</td><td>691,605,000</td><td>2.0%</td><td>10</td><td>Washington</td><td>1,009,328,000</td><td>3.0%</td></tr>
<tr><td>30</td><td>Hawaii</td><td>276,988,000</td><td>0.8%</td><td>11</td><td>North Carolina</td><td>899,998,000</td><td>2.7%</td></tr>
<tr><td>45</td><td>Idaho</td><td>92,562,000</td><td>0.3%</td><td>12</td><td>Maryland</td><td>779,238,000</td><td>2.3%</td></tr>
<tr><td>5</td><td>Illinois</td><td>1,702,964,000</td><td>5.0%</td><td>13</td><td>New Jersey</td><td>754,228,000</td><td>2.2%</td></tr>
<tr><td>23</td><td>Indiana</td><td>406,647,000</td><td>1.2%</td><td>14</td><td>South Carolina</td><td>703,186,000</td><td>2.1%</td></tr>
<tr><td>38</td><td>Iowa</td><td>185,579,000</td><td>0.5%</td><td>15</td><td>Georgia</td><td>691,605,000</td><td>2.0%</td></tr>
<tr><td>29</td><td>Kansas</td><td>301,760,000</td><td>0.9%</td><td>16</td><td>Tennessee</td><td>572,837,000</td><td>1.7%</td></tr>
<tr><td>28</td><td>Kentucky</td><td>302,747,000</td><td>0.9%</td><td>17</td><td>Missouri</td><td>569,282,000</td><td>1.7%</td></tr>
<tr><td>25</td><td>Louisiana</td><td>395,194,000</td><td>1.2%</td><td>18</td><td>Alabama</td><td>566,651,000</td><td>1.7%</td></tr>
<tr><td>37</td><td>Maine</td><td>207,689,000</td><td>0.6%</td><td>19</td><td>Arizona</td><td>558,780,000</td><td>1.6%</td></tr>
<tr><td>12</td><td>Maryland</td><td>779,238,000</td><td>2.3%</td><td>20</td><td>Virginia</td><td>540,595,000</td><td>1.6%</td></tr>
<tr><td>9</td><td>Massachusetts</td><td>1,325,680,000</td><td>3.9%</td><td>21</td><td>Minnesota</td><td>501,351,000</td><td>1.5%</td></tr>
<tr><td>3</td><td>Michigan</td><td>2,046,674,000</td><td>6.0%</td><td>22</td><td>Wisconsin</td><td>497,319,000</td><td>1.5%</td></tr>
<tr><td>21</td><td>Minnesota</td><td>501,351,000</td><td>1.5%</td><td>23</td><td>Indiana</td><td>406,647,000</td><td>1.2%</td></tr>
<tr><td>34</td><td>Mississippi</td><td>247,910,000</td><td>0.7%</td><td>24</td><td>Connecticut</td><td>402,219,000</td><td>1.2%</td></tr>
<tr><td>17</td><td>Missouri</td><td>569,282,000</td><td>1.7%</td><td>25</td><td>Louisiana</td><td>395,194,000</td><td>1.2%</td></tr>
<tr><td>41</td><td>Montana</td><td>162,858,000</td><td>0.5%</td><td>26</td><td>Oregon</td><td>366,493,000</td><td>1.1%</td></tr>
<tr><td>36</td><td>Nebraska</td><td>215,305,000</td><td>0.6%</td><td>27</td><td>Oklahoma</td><td>324,915,000</td><td>1.0%</td></tr>
<tr><td>46</td><td>Nevada</td><td>89,068,000</td><td>0.3%</td><td>28</td><td>Kentucky</td><td>302,747,000</td><td>0.9%</td></tr>
<tr><td>43</td><td>New Hampshire</td><td>138,275,000</td><td>0.4%</td><td>29</td><td>Kansas</td><td>301,760,000</td><td>0.9%</td></tr>
<tr><td>13</td><td>New Jersey</td><td>754,228,000</td><td>2.2%</td><td>30</td><td>Hawaii</td><td>276,988,000</td><td>0.8%</td></tr>
<tr><td>31</td><td>New Mexico</td><td>269,931,000</td><td>0.8%</td><td>31</td><td>New Mexico</td><td>269,931,000</td><td>0.8%</td></tr>
<tr><td>2</td><td>New York</td><td>2,147,669,000</td><td>6.3%</td><td>32</td><td>Arkansas</td><td>261,311,000</td><td>0.8%</td></tr>
<tr><td>11</td><td>North Carolina</td><td>899,998,000</td><td>2.7%</td><td>33</td><td>Rhode Island</td><td>248,079,000</td><td>0.7%</td></tr>
<tr><td>49</td><td>North Dakota</td><td>56,870,000</td><td>0.2%</td><td>34</td><td>Mississippi</td><td>247,910,000</td><td>0.7%</td></tr>
<tr><td>7</td><td>Ohio</td><td>1,352,057,000</td><td>4.0%</td><td>35</td><td>Colorado</td><td>247,006,000</td><td>0.7%</td></tr>
<tr><td>27</td><td>Oklahoma</td><td>324,915,000</td><td>1.0%</td><td>36</td><td>Nebraska</td><td>215,305,000</td><td>0.6%</td></tr>
<tr><td>26</td><td>Oregon</td><td>366,493,000</td><td>1.1%</td><td>37</td><td>Maine</td><td>207,689,000</td><td>0.6%</td></tr>
<tr><td>6</td><td>Pennsylvania</td><td>1,379,050,000</td><td>4.1%</td><td>38</td><td>Iowa</td><td>185,579,000</td><td>0.5%</td></tr>
<tr><td>33</td><td>Rhode Island</td><td>248,079,000</td><td>0.7%</td><td>39</td><td>Utah</td><td>172,481,000</td><td>0.5%</td></tr>
<tr><td>14</td><td>South Carolina</td><td>703,186,000</td><td>2.1%</td><td>40</td><td>Delaware</td><td>166,892,000</td><td>0.5%</td></tr>
<tr><td>48</td><td>South Dakota</td><td>58,861,000</td><td>0.2%</td><td>41</td><td>Montana</td><td>162,858,000</td><td>0.5%</td></tr>
<tr><td>16</td><td>Tennessee</td><td>572,837,000</td><td>1.7%</td><td>42</td><td>Alaska</td><td>159,454,000</td><td>0.5%</td></tr>
<tr><td>8</td><td>Texas</td><td>1,331,742,000</td><td>3.9%</td><td>43</td><td>New Hampshire</td><td>138,275,000</td><td>0.4%</td></tr>
<tr><td>39</td><td>Utah</td><td>172,481,000</td><td>0.5%</td><td>44</td><td>West Virginia</td><td>134,349,000</td><td>0.4%</td></tr>
<tr><td>50</td><td>Vermont</td><td>49,852,000</td><td>0.1%</td><td>45</td><td>Idaho</td><td>92,562,000</td><td>0.3%</td></tr>
<tr><td>20</td><td>Virginia</td><td>540,595,000</td><td>1.6%</td><td>46</td><td>Nevada</td><td>89,068,000</td><td>0.3%</td></tr>
<tr><td>10</td><td>Washington</td><td>1,009,328,000</td><td>3.0%</td><td>47</td><td>Wyoming</td><td>73,897,000</td><td>0.2%</td></tr>
<tr><td>44</td><td>West Virginia</td><td>134,349,000</td><td>0.4%</td><td>48</td><td>South Dakota</td><td>58,861,000</td><td>0.2%</td></tr>
<tr><td>22</td><td>Wisconsin</td><td>497,319,000</td><td>1.5%</td><td>49</td><td>North Dakota</td><td>56,870,000</td><td>0.2%</td></tr>
<tr><td>47</td><td>Wyoming</td><td>73,897,000</td><td>0.2%</td><td>50</td><td>Vermont</td><td>49,852,000</td><td>0.1%</td></tr>
<tr><td></td><td></td><td></td><td></td><td colspan="2">District of Columbia**</td><td>NA</td><td>NA</td></tr>
</table>

Source: U.S. Bureau of the Census, Governments Division
   "1997 State Government Finance Data" (http://www.census.gov/govs/www/st97.html)
*Includes outpatient health services other than hospital care, research and education, categorical health programs, treatment and immunization clinics, nursing and environmental health activities. Includes capital expenditures.
**Not applicable.

Per Capita State Government Expenditures for Health Programs in 1997

National Per Capita = $127*

ALPHA ORDER

RANK	STATE	PER CAPITA
16	Alabama	$131
1	Alaska	262
19	Arizona	123
31	Arkansas	104
7	California	189
49	Colorado	63
19	Connecticut	123
4	Delaware	227
18	Florida	126
35	Georgia	92
3	Hawaii	232
43	Idaho	77
15	Illinois	142
46	Indiana	69
48	Iowa	65
25	Kansas	116
43	Kentucky	77
36	Louisiana	91
11	Maine	167
14	Maryland	153
5	Massachusetts	217
6	Michigan	209
28	Minnesota	107
36	Mississippi	91
30	Missouri	105
9	Montana	185
17	Nebraska	130
50	Nevada	53
23	New Hampshire	118
34	New Jersey	94
12	New Mexico	157
23	New York	118
21	North Carolina	121
38	North Dakota	89
21	Ohio	121
32	Oklahoma	98
27	Oregon	113
26	Pennsylvania	115
2	Rhode Island	251
8	South Carolina	186
41	South Dakota	80
28	Tennessee	107
46	Texas	69
40	Utah	84
39	Vermont	85
41	Virginia	80
10	Washington	180
45	West Virginia	74
33	Wisconsin	96
13	Wyoming	154

RANK ORDER

RANK	STATE	PER CAPITA
1	Alaska	$262
2	Rhode Island	251
3	Hawaii	232
4	Delaware	227
5	Massachusetts	217
6	Michigan	209
7	California	189
8	South Carolina	186
9	Montana	185
10	Washington	180
11	Maine	167
12	New Mexico	157
13	Wyoming	154
14	Maryland	153
15	Illinois	142
16	Alabama	131
17	Nebraska	130
18	Florida	126
19	Arizona	123
19	Connecticut	123
21	North Carolina	121
21	Ohio	121
23	New Hampshire	118
23	New York	118
25	Kansas	116
26	Pennsylvania	115
27	Oregon	113
28	Minnesota	107
28	Tennessee	107
30	Missouri	105
31	Arkansas	104
32	Oklahoma	98
33	Wisconsin	96
34	New Jersey	94
35	Georgia	92
36	Louisiana	91
36	Mississippi	91
38	North Dakota	89
39	Vermont	85
40	Utah	84
41	South Dakota	80
41	Virginia	80
43	Idaho	77
43	Kentucky	77
45	West Virginia	74
46	Indiana	69
46	Texas	69
48	Iowa	65
49	Colorado	63
50	Nevada	53

District of Columbia**   NA

Source: Morgan Quitno Press using data from U.S. Bureau of the Census, Governments Division
"1997 State Government Finance Data" (http://www.census.gov/govs/www/st97.html)
*Includes outpatient health services other than hospital care, research and education, categorical health programs, treatment and immunization clinics, nursing and environmental health activities. Includes capital expenditures.
**Not applicable.

State Government Expenditures for Hospitals in 1997

National Total = $29,313,344,000*

ALPHA ORDER

RANK	STATE	EXPENDITURES	% of USA
11	Alabama	$882,613,000	3.0%
49	Alaska	28,220,000	0.1%
41	Arizona	54,907,000	0.2%
27	Arkansas	362,721,000	1.2%
2	California	2,917,670,000	10.0%
36	Colorado	145,875,000	0.5%
8	Connecticut	977,504,000	3.3%
40	Delaware	60,422,000	0.2%
18	Florida	551,166,000	1.9%
15	Georgia	652,117,000	2.2%
34	Hawaii	237,641,000	0.8%
46	Idaho	37,764,000	0.1%
13	Illinois	846,042,000	2.9%
35	Indiana	227,424,000	0.8%
20	Iowa	493,587,000	1.7%
32	Kansas	303,263,000	1.0%
21	Kentucky	447,971,000	1.5%
7	Louisiana	1,063,310,000	3.6%
42	Maine	53,917,000	0.2%
31	Maryland	319,502,000	1.1%
10	Massachusetts	886,275,000	3.0%
5	Michigan	1,420,141,000	4.8%
25	Minnesota	428,811,000	1.5%
26	Mississippi	422,071,000	1.4%
23	Missouri	441,048,000	1.5%
47	Montana	28,715,000	0.1%
28	Nebraska	328,258,000	1.1%
39	Nevada	67,089,000	0.2%
44	New Hampshire	41,250,000	0.1%
9	New Jersey	974,484,000	3.3%
29	New Mexico	320,578,000	1.1%
1	New York	3,311,633,000	11.3%
14	North Carolina	781,710,000	2.7%
43	North Dakota	44,984,000	0.2%
12	Ohio	875,478,000	3.0%
33	Oklahoma	290,809,000	1.0%
24	Oregon	438,214,000	1.5%
4	Pennsylvania	1,697,003,000	5.8%
38	Rhode Island	79,877,000	0.3%
16	South Carolina	611,090,000	2.1%
45	South Dakota	39,703,000	0.1%
19	Tennessee	544,800,000	1.9%
3	Texas	1,961,616,000	6.7%
30	Utah	319,921,000	1.1%
50	Vermont	8,714,000	0.0%
6	Virginia	1,163,248,000	4.0%
17	Washington	564,674,000	1.9%
37	West Virginia	82,939,000	0.3%
22	Wisconsin	446,159,000	1.5%
48	Wyoming	28,416,000	0.1%

RANK ORDER

RANK	STATE	EXPENDITURES	% of USA
1	New York	$3,311,633,000	11.3%
2	California	2,917,670,000	10.0%
3	Texas	1,961,616,000	6.7%
4	Pennsylvania	1,697,003,000	5.8%
5	Michigan	1,420,141,000	4.8%
6	Virginia	1,163,248,000	4.0%
7	Louisiana	1,063,310,000	3.6%
8	Connecticut	977,504,000	3.3%
9	New Jersey	974,484,000	3.3%
10	Massachusetts	886,275,000	3.0%
11	Alabama	882,613,000	3.0%
12	Ohio	875,478,000	3.0%
13	Illinois	846,042,000	2.9%
14	North Carolina	781,710,000	2.7%
15	Georgia	652,117,000	2.2%
16	South Carolina	611,090,000	2.1%
17	Washington	564,674,000	1.9%
18	Florida	551,166,000	1.9%
19	Tennessee	544,800,000	1.9%
20	Iowa	493,587,000	1.7%
21	Kentucky	447,971,000	1.5%
22	Wisconsin	446,159,000	1.5%
23	Missouri	441,048,000	1.5%
24	Oregon	438,214,000	1.5%
25	Minnesota	428,811,000	1.5%
26	Mississippi	422,071,000	1.4%
27	Arkansas	362,721,000	1.2%
28	Nebraska	328,258,000	1.1%
29	New Mexico	320,578,000	1.1%
30	Utah	319,921,000	1.1%
31	Maryland	319,502,000	1.1%
32	Kansas	303,263,000	1.0%
33	Oklahoma	290,809,000	1.0%
34	Hawaii	237,641,000	0.8%
35	Indiana	227,424,000	0.8%
36	Colorado	145,875,000	0.5%
37	West Virginia	82,939,000	0.3%
38	Rhode Island	79,877,000	0.3%
39	Nevada	67,089,000	0.2%
40	Delaware	60,422,000	0.2%
41	Arizona	54,907,000	0.2%
42	Maine	53,917,000	0.2%
43	North Dakota	44,984,000	0.2%
44	New Hampshire	41,250,000	0.1%
45	South Dakota	39,703,000	0.1%
46	Idaho	37,764,000	0.1%
47	Montana	28,715,000	0.1%
48	Wyoming	28,416,000	0.1%
49	Alaska	28,220,000	0.1%
50	Vermont	8,714,000	0.0%
	District of Columbia**	NA	NA

Source: U.S. Bureau of the Census, Governments Division
"1997 State Government Finance Data" (http://www.census.gov/govs/www/st97.html)
*Financing, construction, acquisition, maintenance or operation of hospital facilities, provision of hospital care and support of public or private hospitals.
**Not applicable.

Per Capita State Government Expenditures for Hospitals in 1997

National Per Capita = $109*

ALPHA ORDER

RANK	STATE	PER CAPITA
3	Alabama	$204
39	Alaska	46
50	Arizona	12
15	Arkansas	144
25	California	91
45	Colorado	37
1	Connecticut	299
30	Delaware	82
44	Florida	38
28	Georgia	87
4	Hawaii	199
48	Idaho	31
34	Illinois	71
43	Indiana	39
8	Iowa	173
19	Kansas	117
20	Kentucky	115
2	Louisiana	244
41	Maine	43
36	Maryland	63
13	Massachusetts	145
13	Michigan	145
25	Minnesota	91
11	Mississippi	155
30	Missouri	82
47	Montana	33
5	Nebraska	198
42	Nevada	40
46	New Hampshire	35
18	New Jersey	121
6	New Mexico	186
7	New York	182
21	North Carolina	105
35	North Dakota	70
33	Ohio	78
27	Oklahoma	88
17	Oregon	135
16	Pennsylvania	141
32	Rhode Island	81
10	South Carolina	161
38	South Dakota	54
22	Tennessee	101
22	Texas	101
11	Utah	155
49	Vermont	15
8	Virginia	173
22	Washington	101
39	West Virginia	46
29	Wisconsin	86
37	Wyoming	59

RANK ORDER

RANK	STATE	PER CAPITA
1	Connecticut	$299
2	Louisiana	244
3	Alabama	204
4	Hawaii	199
5	Nebraska	198
6	New Mexico	186
7	New York	182
8	Iowa	173
8	Virginia	173
10	South Carolina	161
11	Mississippi	155
11	Utah	155
13	Massachusetts	145
13	Michigan	145
15	Arkansas	144
16	Pennsylvania	141
17	Oregon	135
18	New Jersey	121
19	Kansas	117
20	Kentucky	115
21	North Carolina	105
22	Tennessee	101
22	Texas	101
22	Washington	101
25	California	91
25	Minnesota	91
27	Oklahoma	88
28	Georgia	87
29	Wisconsin	86
30	Delaware	82
30	Missouri	82
32	Rhode Island	81
33	Ohio	78
34	Illinois	71
35	North Dakota	70
36	Maryland	63
37	Wyoming	59
38	South Dakota	54
39	Alaska	46
39	West Virginia	46
41	Maine	43
42	Nevada	40
43	Indiana	39
44	Florida	38
45	Colorado	37
46	New Hampshire	35
47	Montana	33
48	Idaho	31
49	Vermont	15
50	Arizona	12

District of Columbia**	NA

Source: Morgan Quitno Press using data from U.S. Bureau of the Census, Governments Division
"1997 State Government Finance Data" (http://www.census.gov/govs/www/st97.html)
*Financing, construction, acquisition, maintenance or operation of hospital facilities, provision of hospital care and support of public or private hospitals.
**Not applicable.

Payroll of Health Service Establishments in 1996

National Total = $328,578,123,000

ALPHA ORDER

RANK	STATE	PAYROLL	% of USA
23	Alabama	$5,119,562,000	1.6%
48	Alaska	741,991,000	0.2%
24	Arizona	4,549,936,000	1.4%
33	Arkansas	2,617,240,000	0.8%
1	California	33,758,246,000	10.3%
26	Colorado	4,227,556,000	1.3%
21	Connecticut	5,689,623,000	1.7%
44	Delaware	1,017,855,000	0.3%
4	Florida	18,811,953,000	5.7%
11	Georgia	8,552,487,000	2.6%
42	Hawaii	1,369,000,000	0.4%
43	Idaho	1,030,264,000	0.3%
7	Illinois	14,510,905,000	4.4%
14	Indiana	6,816,043,000	2.1%
29	Iowa	3,376,346,000	1.0%
31	Kansas	3,175,416,000	1.0%
25	Kentucky	4,292,538,000	1.3%
22	Louisiana	5,337,798,000	1.6%
39	Maine	1,559,043,000	0.5%
19	Maryland	6,508,781,000	2.0%
10	Massachusetts	10,936,545,000	3.3%
8	Michigan	12,135,176,000	3.7%
16	Minnesota	6,762,620,000	2.1%
32	Mississippi	2,644,280,000	0.8%
15	Missouri	6,814,324,000	2.1%
47	Montana	840,140,000	0.3%
35	Nebraska	1,874,633,000	0.6%
37	Nevada	1,583,651,000	0.5%
41	New Hampshire	1,416,167,000	0.4%
9	New Jersey	11,472,176,000	3.5%
38	New Mexico	1,572,454,000	0.5%
2	New York	29,686,442,000	9.0%
12	North Carolina	8,299,603,000	2.5%
46	North Dakota	890,862,000	0.3%
6	Ohio	14,656,575,000	4.5%
28	Oklahoma	3,508,386,000	1.1%
30	Oregon	3,316,622,000	1.0%
5	Pennsylvania	17,552,425,000	5.3%
40	Rhode Island	1,483,679,000	0.5%
27	South Carolina	3,689,833,000	1.1%
45	South Dakota	939,810,000	0.3%
13	Tennessee	7,069,956,000	2.2%
3	Texas	20,499,773,000	6.2%
36	Utah	1,734,398,000	0.5%
49	Vermont	540,879,000	0.2%
17	Virginia	6,728,133,000	2.0%
20	Washington	6,079,507,000	1.9%
34	West Virginia	2,008,203,000	0.6%
18	Wisconsin	6,568,410,000	2.0%
50	Wyoming	435,342,000	0.1%

RANK ORDER

RANK	STATE	PAYROLL	% of USA
1	California	$33,758,246,000	10.3%
2	New York	29,686,442,000	9.0%
3	Texas	20,499,773,000	6.2%
4	Florida	18,811,953,000	5.7%
5	Pennsylvania	17,552,425,000	5.3%
6	Ohio	14,656,575,000	4.5%
7	Illinois	14,510,905,000	4.4%
8	Michigan	12,135,176,000	3.7%
9	New Jersey	11,472,176,000	3.5%
10	Massachusetts	10,936,545,000	3.3%
11	Georgia	8,552,487,000	2.6%
12	North Carolina	8,299,603,000	2.5%
13	Tennessee	7,069,956,000	2.2%
14	Indiana	6,816,043,000	2.1%
15	Missouri	6,814,324,000	2.1%
16	Minnesota	6,762,620,000	2.1%
17	Virginia	6,728,133,000	2.0%
18	Wisconsin	6,568,410,000	2.0%
19	Maryland	6,508,781,000	2.0%
20	Washington	6,079,507,000	1.9%
21	Connecticut	5,689,623,000	1.7%
22	Louisiana	5,337,798,000	1.6%
23	Alabama	5,119,562,000	1.6%
24	Arizona	4,549,936,000	1.4%
25	Kentucky	4,292,538,000	1.3%
26	Colorado	4,227,556,000	1.3%
27	South Carolina	3,689,833,000	1.1%
28	Oklahoma	3,508,386,000	1.1%
29	Iowa	3,376,346,000	1.0%
30	Oregon	3,316,622,000	1.0%
31	Kansas	3,175,416,000	1.0%
32	Mississippi	2,644,280,000	0.8%
33	Arkansas	2,617,240,000	0.8%
34	West Virginia	2,008,203,000	0.6%
35	Nebraska	1,874,633,000	0.6%
36	Utah	1,734,398,000	0.5%
37	Nevada	1,583,651,000	0.5%
38	New Mexico	1,572,454,000	0.5%
39	Maine	1,559,043,000	0.5%
40	Rhode Island	1,483,679,000	0.5%
41	New Hampshire	1,416,167,000	0.4%
42	Hawaii	1,369,000,000	0.4%
43	Idaho	1,030,264,000	0.3%
44	Delaware	1,017,855,000	0.3%
45	South Dakota	939,810,000	0.3%
46	North Dakota	890,862,000	0.3%
47	Montana	840,140,000	0.3%
48	Alaska	741,991,000	0.2%
49	Vermont	540,879,000	0.2%
50	Wyoming	435,342,000	0.1%
	District of Columbia	1,774,536,000	0.5%

Source: U.S. Bureau of the Census
"1996 County Business Patterns"

Includes establishments exempt from as well as subject to the federal income tax. Includes those establishments within the Standard Industry Classification (SIC) 8000. These include those primarily engaged in furnishing medical, surgical and other health services to persons. See Facilities Chapter for establishments.

Average Pay per Health Service Establishment Employee in 1996

National Average = $29,897 per Employee*

ALPHA ORDER

RANK	STATE	AVERAGE PAY
25	Alabama	$28,822
1	Alaska	40,358
9	Arizona	31,792
40	Arkansas	25,856
6	California	33,173
16	Colorado	30,230
5	Connecticut	33,240
7	Delaware	32,646
13	Florida	30,572
12	Georgia	30,661
2	Hawaii	36,226
34	Idaho	26,514
20	Illinois	30,061
32	Indiana	27,015
50	Iowa	24,700
43	Kansas	25,577
35	Kentucky	26,439
44	Louisiana	25,557
37	Maine	26,309
10	Maryland	31,613
14	Massachusetts	30,373
11	Michigan	30,948
26	Minnesota	28,710
38	Mississippi	26,260
31	Missouri	27,016
48	Montana	25,015
42	Nebraska	25,609
3	Nevada	34,599
24	New Hampshire	28,944
4	New Jersey	33,859
33	New Mexico	26,939
8	New York	32,079
23	North Carolina	29,638
45	North Dakota	25,457
29	Ohio	28,417
46	Oklahoma	25,413
15	Oregon	30,327
19	Pennsylvania	30,064
27	Rhode Island	28,695
21	South Carolina	29,938
49	South Dakota	25,007
18	Tennessee	30,158
30	Texas	28,125
41	Utah	25,642
47	Vermont	25,082
22	Virginia	29,801
17	Washington	30,211
36	West Virginia	26,403
28	Wisconsin	28,578
39	Wyoming	26,019

RANK ORDER

RANK	STATE	AVERAGE PAY
1	Alaska	$40,358
2	Hawaii	36,226
3	Nevada	34,599
4	New Jersey	33,859
5	Connecticut	33,240
6	California	33,173
7	Delaware	32,646
8	New York	32,079
9	Arizona	31,792
10	Maryland	31,613
11	Michigan	30,948
12	Georgia	30,661
13	Florida	30,572
14	Massachusetts	30,373
15	Oregon	30,327
16	Colorado	30,230
17	Washington	30,211
18	Tennessee	30,158
19	Pennsylvania	30,064
20	Illinois	30,061
21	South Carolina	29,938
22	Virginia	29,801
23	North Carolina	29,638
24	New Hampshire	28,944
25	Alabama	28,822
26	Minnesota	28,710
27	Rhode Island	28,695
28	Wisconsin	28,578
29	Ohio	28,417
30	Texas	28,125
31	Missouri	27,016
32	Indiana	27,015
33	New Mexico	26,939
34	Idaho	26,514
35	Kentucky	26,439
36	West Virginia	26,403
37	Maine	26,309
38	Mississippi	26,260
39	Wyoming	26,019
40	Arkansas	25,856
41	Utah	25,642
42	Nebraska	25,609
43	Kansas	25,577
44	Louisiana	25,557
45	North Dakota	25,457
46	Oklahoma	25,413
47	Vermont	25,082
48	Montana	25,015
49	South Dakota	25,007
50	Iowa	24,700
	District of Columbia	39,090

Source: Morgan Quitno Press using data from U.S. Bureau of the Census
 "1996 County Business Patterns"
Includes establishments exempt from as well as subject to the federal income tax. Includes those establishments within the Standard Industry Classification (SIC) 8000. These include those primarily engaged in furnishing medical, surgical and other health services to persons. See Facilities Chapter for establishments.

Receipts of Health Services Establishments in 1992

National Total = $623,480,434,000*

ALPHA ORDER

RANK	STATE	RECEIPTS	% of USA
23	Alabama	$9,400,816,000	1.51%
48	Alaska	1,225,327,000	0.20%
24	Arizona	8,624,782,000	1.38%
32	Arkansas	4,791,668,000	0.77%
1	California	79,130,980,000	12.69%
25	Colorado	8,000,876,000	1.28%
22	Connecticut	9,932,092,000	1.59%
43	Delaware	1,780,075,000	0.29%
4	Florida	36,667,132,000	5.88%
11	Georgia	15,774,705,000	2.53%
39	Hawaii	2,757,575,000	0.44%
44	Idaho	1,775,447,000	0.28%
6	Illinois	27,961,997,000	4.48%
14	Indiana	13,010,617,000	2.09%
30	Iowa	5,852,492,000	0.94%
31	Kansas	5,763,990,000	0.92%
26	Kentucky	7,923,070,000	1.27%
21	Louisiana	10,204,980,000	1.64%
40	Maine	2,666,876,000	0.43%
18	Maryland	11,824,018,000	1.90%
10	Massachusetts	19,296,743,000	3.10%
8	Michigan	21,891,285,000	3.51%
20	Minnesota	11,199,561,000	1.80%
33	Mississippi	4,605,036,000	0.74%
15	Missouri	12,918,009,000	2.07%
46	Montana	1,589,295,000	0.25%
35	Nebraska	3,483,096,000	0.56%
37	Nevada	3,016,118,000	0.48%
41	New Hampshire	2,642,095,000	0.42%
9	New Jersey	21,102,821,000	3.38%
38	New Mexico	2,881,524,000	0.46%
2	New York	53,091,018,000	8.52%
12	North Carolina	14,227,452,000	2.28%
45	North Dakota	1,651,634,000	0.26%
7	Ohio	27,492,361,000	4.41%
28	Oklahoma	6,268,749,000	1.01%
29	Oregon	6,137,525,000	0.98%
5	Pennsylvania	33,155,698,000	5.32%
42	Rhode Island	2,617,386,000	0.42%
27	South Carolina	6,612,570,000	1.06%
47	South Dakota	1,543,627,000	0.25%
16	Tennessee	12,807,220,000	2.05%
3	Texas	38,769,630,000	6.22%
36	Utah	3,216,121,000	0.52%
49	Vermont	1,121,735,000	0.18%
13	Virginia	13,140,339,000	2.11%
17	Washington	12,022,436,000	1.93%
34	West Virginia	4,040,621,000	0.65%
19	Wisconsin	11,288,091,000	1.81%
50	Wyoming	708,286,000	0.11%

RANK ORDER

RANK	STATE	RECEIPTS	% of USA
1	California	$79,130,980,000	12.69%
2	New York	53,091,018,000	8.52%
3	Texas	38,769,630,000	6.22%
4	Florida	36,667,132,000	5.88%
5	Pennsylvania	33,155,698,000	5.32%
6	Illinois	27,961,997,000	4.48%
7	Ohio	27,492,361,000	4.41%
8	Michigan	21,891,285,000	3.51%
9	New Jersey	21,102,821,000	3.38%
10	Massachusetts	19,296,743,000	3.10%
11	Georgia	15,774,705,000	2.53%
12	North Carolina	14,227,452,000	2.28%
13	Virginia	13,140,339,000	2.11%
14	Indiana	13,010,617,000	2.09%
15	Missouri	12,918,009,000	2.07%
16	Tennessee	12,807,220,000	2.05%
17	Washington	12,022,436,000	1.93%
18	Maryland	11,824,018,000	1.90%
19	Wisconsin	11,288,091,000	1.81%
20	Minnesota	11,199,561,000	1.80%
21	Louisiana	10,204,980,000	1.64%
22	Connecticut	9,932,092,000	1.59%
23	Alabama	9,400,816,000	1.51%
24	Arizona	8,624,782,000	1.38%
25	Colorado	8,000,876,000	1.28%
26	Kentucky	7,923,070,000	1.27%
27	South Carolina	6,612,570,000	1.06%
28	Oklahoma	6,268,749,000	1.01%
29	Oregon	6,137,525,000	0.98%
30	Iowa	5,852,492,000	0.94%
31	Kansas	5,763,990,000	0.92%
32	Arkansas	4,791,668,000	0.77%
33	Mississippi	4,605,036,000	0.74%
34	West Virginia	4,040,621,000	0.65%
35	Nebraska	3,483,096,000	0.56%
36	Utah	3,216,121,000	0.52%
37	Nevada	3,016,118,000	0.48%
38	New Mexico	2,881,524,000	0.46%
39	Hawaii	2,757,575,000	0.44%
40	Maine	2,666,876,000	0.43%
41	New Hampshire	2,642,095,000	0.42%
42	Rhode Island	2,617,386,000	0.42%
43	Delaware	1,780,075,000	0.29%
44	Idaho	1,775,447,000	0.28%
45	North Dakota	1,651,634,000	0.26%
46	Montana	1,589,295,000	0.25%
47	South Dakota	1,543,627,000	0.25%
48	Alaska	1,225,327,000	0.20%
49	Vermont	1,121,735,000	0.18%
50	Wyoming	708,286,000	0.11%
	District of Columbia	3,872,837,000	0.62%

Source: Morgan Quitno Press using data from U.S. Bureau of the Census
    "1992 Census of Service Industries, Geographic Area Series, United States" (SC92-A-52)
*Includes establishments exempt from as well as subject to the federal income tax. Includes those establishments within the Standard Industry Classification (SIC) 8000. These include those primarily engaged in furnishing medical, surgical and other health services to persons. See Facilities Chapter for establishments.

Receipts per Health Service Establishment in 1992

National Rate = $1,339,792 per Establishment*

ALPHA ORDER

RANK ORDER

RANK	STATE	PER ESTABLISHMENT
4	Alabama	$1,606,428
27	Alaska	1,304,928
40	Arizona	1,155,517
31	Arkansas	1,261,297
33	California	1,251,696
44	Colorado	1,081,199
10	Connecticut	1,430,931
13	Delaware	1,419,518
38	Florida	1,201,768
19	Georgia	1,375,541
39	Hawaii	1,183,509
48	Idaho	966,493
14	Illinois	1,415,296
15	Indiana	1,392,701
32	Iowa	1,252,942
20	Kansas	1,360,073
24	Kentucky	1,322,495
11	Louisiana	1,430,872
42	Maine	1,114,449
35	Maryland	1,244,110
2	Massachusetts	1,700,753
26	Michigan	1,307,333
3	Minnesota	1,676,581
16	Mississippi	1,391,670
8	Missouri	1,452,768
49	Montana	944,323
22	Nebraska	1,348,469
29	Nevada	1,274,237
25	New Hampshire	1,312,516
36	New Jersey	1,239,884
43	New Mexico	1,109,132
5	New York	1,549,922
6	North Carolina	1,520,839
1	North Dakota	1,736,734
17	Ohio	1,388,854
41	Oklahoma	1,116,032
45	Oregon	1,041,317
12	Pennsylvania	1,420,492
30	Rhode Island	1,265,661
21	South Carolina	1,357,817
23	South Dakota	1,348,146
7	Tennessee	1,478,040
34	Texas	1,249,666
47	Utah	1,021,964
46	Vermont	1,040,571
28	Virginia	1,298,581
37	Washington	1,237,003
18	West Virginia	1,378,111
9	Wisconsin	1,438,340
50	Wyoming	897,701

RANK	STATE	PER ESTABLISHMENT
1	North Dakota	$1,736,734
2	Massachusetts	1,700,753
3	Minnesota	1,676,581
4	Alabama	1,606,428
5	New York	1,549,922
6	North Carolina	1,520,839
7	Tennessee	1,478,040
8	Missouri	1,452,768
9	Wisconsin	1,438,340
10	Connecticut	1,430,931
11	Louisiana	1,430,872
12	Pennsylvania	1,420,492
13	Delaware	1,419,518
14	Illinois	1,415,296
15	Indiana	1,392,701
16	Mississippi	1,391,670
17	Ohio	1,388,854
18	West Virginia	1,378,111
19	Georgia	1,375,541
20	Kansas	1,360,073
21	South Carolina	1,357,817
22	Nebraska	1,348,469
23	South Dakota	1,348,146
24	Kentucky	1,322,495
25	New Hampshire	1,312,516
26	Michigan	1,307,333
27	Alaska	1,304,928
28	Virginia	1,298,581
29	Nevada	1,274,237
30	Rhode Island	1,265,661
31	Arkansas	1,261,297
32	Iowa	1,252,942
33	California	1,251,696
34	Texas	1,249,666
35	Maryland	1,244,110
36	New Jersey	1,239,884
37	Washington	1,237,003
38	Florida	1,201,768
39	Hawaii	1,183,509
40	Arizona	1,155,517
41	Oklahoma	1,116,032
42	Maine	1,114,449
43	New Mexico	1,109,132
44	Colorado	1,081,199
45	Oregon	1,041,317
46	Vermont	1,040,571
47	Utah	1,021,964
48	Idaho	966,493
49	Montana	944,323
50	Wyoming	897,701
	District of Columbia	2,639,971

Source: Morgan Quitno Press using data from U.S. Bureau of the Census
   "1992 Census of Service Industries, Geographic Area Series, United States" (SC92-A-52)
*Includes establishments exempt from as well as subject to the federal income tax. Includes those establishments
within the Standard Industry Classification (SIC) 8000. These include those primarily engaged in furnishing medical,
surgical and other health services to persons. See Facilities Chapter for establishments.

Receipts of Offices and Clinics of Doctors of Medicine in 1992

National Total = $141,429,109,000*

ALPHA ORDER

RANK	STATE	RECEIPTS	% of USA
23	Alabama	$2,194,200,000	1.55%
48	Alaska	257,847,000	0.18%
21	Arizona	2,358,063,000	1.67%
31	Arkansas	1,184,434,000	0.84%
1	California	21,969,551,000	15.53%
26	Colorado	1,823,874,000	1.29%
22	Connecticut	2,264,576,000	1.60%
45	Delaware	402,076,000	0.28%
2	Florida	10,360,884,000	7.33%
9	Georgia	4,096,050,000	2.90%
38	Hawaii	621,177,000	0.44%
43	Idaho	435,493,000	0.31%
5	Illinois	6,252,042,000	4.42%
16	Indiana	2,829,577,000	2.00%
32	Iowa	1,169,464,000	0.83%
30	Kansas	1,269,708,000	0.90%
25	Kentucky	1,867,177,000	1.32%
20	Louisiana	2,411,609,000	1.71%
41	Maine	493,897,000	0.35%
14	Maryland	3,054,253,000	2.16%
13	Massachusetts	3,103,826,000	2.19%
10	Michigan	3,899,622,000	2.76%
24	Minnesota	1,964,322,000	1.39%
33	Mississippi	968,510,000	0.68%
17	Missouri	2,562,807,000	1.81%
46	Montana	336,865,000	0.24%
37	Nebraska	750,417,000	0.53%
34	Nevada	947,372,000	0.67%
40	New Hampshire	495,024,000	0.35%
8	New Jersey	5,079,647,000	3.59%
39	New Mexico	620,805,000	0.44%
3	New York	9,895,040,000	7.00%
12	North Carolina	3,170,587,000	2.24%
44	North Dakota	422,058,000	0.30%
7	Ohio	5,703,695,000	4.03%
29	Oklahoma	1,366,055,000	0.97%
27	Oregon	1,491,857,000	1.05%
6	Pennsylvania	6,183,845,000	4.37%
42	Rhode Island	458,399,000	0.32%
28	South Carolina	1,491,246,000	1.05%
47	South Dakota	305,158,000	0.22%
15	Tennessee	2,927,905,000	2.07%
4	Texas	9,488,688,000	6.71%
36	Utah	816,997,000	0.58%
49	Vermont	187,557,000	0.13%
11	Virginia	3,207,044,000	2.27%
19	Washington	2,415,635,000	1.71%
35	West Virginia	848,606,000	0.60%
18	Wisconsin	2,415,679,000	1.71%
50	Wyoming	148,221,000	0.10%

RANK ORDER

RANK	STATE	RECEIPTS	% of USA
1	California	$21,969,551,000	15.53%
2	Florida	10,360,884,000	7.33%
3	New York	9,895,040,000	7.00%
4	Texas	9,488,688,000	6.71%
5	Illinois	6,252,042,000	4.42%
6	Pennsylvania	6,183,845,000	4.37%
7	Ohio	5,703,695,000	4.03%
8	New Jersey	5,079,647,000	3.59%
9	Georgia	4,096,050,000	2.90%
10	Michigan	3,899,622,000	2.76%
11	Virginia	3,207,044,000	2.27%
12	North Carolina	3,170,587,000	2.24%
13	Massachusetts	3,103,826,000	2.19%
14	Maryland	3,054,253,000	2.16%
15	Tennessee	2,927,905,000	2.07%
16	Indiana	2,829,577,000	2.00%
17	Missouri	2,562,807,000	1.81%
18	Wisconsin	2,415,679,000	1.71%
19	Washington	2,415,635,000	1.71%
20	Louisiana	2,411,609,000	1.71%
21	Arizona	2,358,063,000	1.67%
22	Connecticut	2,264,576,000	1.60%
23	Alabama	2,194,200,000	1.55%
24	Minnesota	1,964,322,000	1.39%
25	Kentucky	1,867,177,000	1.32%
26	Colorado	1,823,874,000	1.29%
27	Oregon	1,491,857,000	1.05%
28	South Carolina	1,491,246,000	1.05%
29	Oklahoma	1,366,055,000	0.97%
30	Kansas	1,269,708,000	0.90%
31	Arkansas	1,184,434,000	0.84%
32	Iowa	1,169,464,000	0.83%
33	Mississippi	968,510,000	0.68%
34	Nevada	947,372,000	0.67%
35	West Virginia	848,606,000	0.60%
36	Utah	816,997,000	0.58%
37	Nebraska	750,417,000	0.53%
38	Hawaii	621,177,000	0.44%
39	New Mexico	620,805,000	0.44%
40	New Hampshire	495,024,000	0.35%
41	Maine	493,897,000	0.35%
42	Rhode Island	458,399,000	0.32%
43	Idaho	435,493,000	0.31%
44	North Dakota	422,058,000	0.30%
45	Delaware	402,076,000	0.28%
46	Montana	336,865,000	0.24%
47	South Dakota	305,158,000	0.22%
48	Alaska	257,847,000	0.18%
49	Vermont	187,557,000	0.13%
50	Wyoming	148,221,000	0.10%
	District of Columbia	439,668,000	0.31%

Source: U.S. Bureau of the Census
   "1992 Census of Service Industries, Geographic Area Series, United States" (SC92-A-52)
*Includes only establishments subject to the federal income tax. See Facilities Chapter for establishments.

Receipts per Office or Clinic of Doctors of Medicine in 1992

National Rate = $715,369 per Establishment*

ALPHA ORDER

RANK	STATE	PER ESTABLISHMENT
9	Alabama	$840,368
19	Alaska	738,817
16	Arizona	748,591
24	Arkansas	711,799
13	California	771,024
29	Colorado	676,010
17	Connecticut	745,171
27	Delaware	684,968
22	Florida	715,185
11	Georgia	785,587
45	Hawaii	582,718
44	Idaho	598,205
18	Illinois	742,170
15	Indiana	755,763
6	Iowa	866,912
4	Kansas	918,747
21	Kentucky	727,944
20	Louisiana	732,344
47	Maine	540,369
40	Maryland	641,650
26	Massachusetts	686,080
37	Michigan	657,055
2	Minnesota	1,327,245
32	Mississippi	664,273
12	Missouri	781,344
46	Montana	562,379
8	Nebraska	846,972
7	Nevada	864,391
38	New Hampshire	656,531
36	New Jersey	658,156
43	New Mexico	600,973
42	New York	609,826
10	North Carolina	828,695
1	North Dakota	1,736,864
23	Ohio	712,606
31	Oklahoma	665,719
35	Oregon	659,239
33	Pennsylvania	661,586
48	Rhode Island	515,634
30	South Carolina	672,035
5	South Dakota	874,378
14	Tennessee	762,475
34	Texas	660,450
39	Utah	647,896
50	Vermont	477,244
28	Virginia	678,883
25	Washington	697,354
41	West Virginia	633,288
3	Wisconsin	948,813
49	Wyoming	504,153

RANK ORDER

RANK	STATE	PER ESTABLISHMENT
1	North Dakota	$1,736,864
2	Minnesota	1,327,245
3	Wisconsin	948,813
4	Kansas	918,747
5	South Dakota	874,378
6	Iowa	866,912
7	Nevada	864,391
8	Nebraska	846,972
9	Alabama	840,368
10	North Carolina	828,695
11	Georgia	785,587
12	Missouri	781,344
13	California	771,024
14	Tennessee	762,475
15	Indiana	755,763
16	Arizona	748,591
17	Connecticut	745,171
18	Illinois	742,170
19	Alaska	738,817
20	Louisiana	732,344
21	Kentucky	727,944
22	Florida	715,185
23	Ohio	712,606
24	Arkansas	711,799
25	Washington	697,354
26	Massachusetts	686,080
27	Delaware	684,968
28	Virginia	678,883
29	Colorado	676,010
30	South Carolina	672,035
31	Oklahoma	665,719
32	Mississippi	664,273
33	Pennsylvania	661,586
34	Texas	660,450
35	Oregon	659,239
36	New Jersey	658,156
37	Michigan	657,055
38	New Hampshire	656,531
39	Utah	647,896
40	Maryland	641,650
41	West Virginia	633,288
42	New York	609,826
43	New Mexico	600,973
44	Idaho	598,205
45	Hawaii	582,718
46	Montana	562,379
47	Maine	540,369
48	Rhode Island	515,634
49	Wyoming	504,153
50	Vermont	477,244
	District of Columbia	568,781

Source: Morgan Quitno Press using data from U.S. Bureau of the Census
"1992 Census of Service Industries, Geographic Area Series, United States" (SC92-A-52)
*Includes only establishments subject to the federal income tax. See Facilities Chapter for establishments.

Receipts of Offices and Clinics of Dentists in 1992

National Total = $35,522,953,000*

ALPHA ORDER

RANK	STATE	RECEIPTS	% of USA
25	Alabama	$423,367,000	1.30%
44	Alaska	114,760,000	0.35%
24	Arizona	506,268,000	1.56%
33	Arkansas	226,609,000	0.70%
1	California	5,523,663,000	16.98%
22	Colorado	555,652,000	1.71%
18	Connecticut	669,243,000	2.06%
45	Delaware	102,416,000	0.31%
4	Florida	1,893,179,000	5.82%
19	Georgia	644,777,000	1.98%
34	Hawaii	219,683,000	0.68%
42	Idaho	150,221,000	0.46%
6	Illinois	1,510,700,000	4.65%
12	Indiana	840,283,000	2.58%
30	Iowa	320,371,000	0.99%
31	Kansas	306,171,000	0.94%
28	Kentucky	338,975,000	1.04%
26	Louisiana	409,110,000	1.26%
41	Maine	150,904,000	0.46%
16	Maryland	713,076,000	2.19%
11	Massachusetts	992,382,000	3.05%
7	Michigan	1,475,023,000	4.54%
17	Minnesota	686,914,000	2.11%
36	Mississippi	198,070,000	0.61%
21	Missouri	569,399,000	1.75%
46	Montana	96,335,000	0.30%
37	Nebraska	185,366,000	0.57%
35	Nevada	204,068,000	0.63%
39	New Hampshire	167,595,000	0.52%
8	New Jersey	1,415,884,000	4.35%
40	New Mexico	160,064,000	0.49%
2	New York	2,770,069,000	8.52%
14	North Carolina	760,910,000	2.34%
49	North Dakota	70,632,000	0.22%
9	Ohio	1,337,215,000	4.11%
29	Oklahoma	338,025,000	1.04%
23	Oregon	526,242,000	1.62%
5	Pennsylvania	1,571,424,000	4.83%
43	Rhode Island	148,838,000	0.46%
27	South Carolina	364,380,000	1.12%
47	South Dakota	79,410,000	0.24%
20	Tennessee	572,138,000	1.76%
3	Texas	1,919,816,000	5.90%
32	Utah	257,633,000	0.79%
48	Vermont	78,673,000	0.24%
13	Virginia	811,992,000	2.50%
10	Washington	1,088,396,000	3.35%
38	West Virginia	174,028,000	0.54%
15	Wisconsin	718,189,000	2.21%
50	Wyoming	52,712,000	0.16%

RANK ORDER

RANK	STATE	RECEIPTS	% of USA
1	California	$5,523,663,000	16.98%
2	New York	2,770,069,000	8.52%
3	Texas	1,919,816,000	5.90%
4	Florida	1,893,179,000	5.82%
5	Pennsylvania	1,571,424,000	4.83%
6	Illinois	1,510,700,000	4.65%
7	Michigan	1,475,023,000	4.54%
8	New Jersey	1,415,884,000	4.35%
9	Ohio	1,337,215,000	4.11%
10	Washington	1,088,396,000	3.35%
11	Massachusetts	992,382,000	3.05%
12	Indiana	840,283,000	2.58%
13	Virginia	811,992,000	2.50%
14	North Carolina	760,910,000	2.34%
15	Wisconsin	718,189,000	2.21%
16	Maryland	713,076,000	2.19%
17	Minnesota	686,914,000	2.11%
18	Connecticut	669,243,000	2.06%
19	Georgia	644,777,000	1.98%
20	Tennessee	572,138,000	1.76%
21	Missouri	569,399,000	1.75%
22	Colorado	555,652,000	1.71%
23	Oregon	526,242,000	1.62%
24	Arizona	506,268,000	1.56%
25	Alabama	423,367,000	1.30%
26	Louisiana	409,110,000	1.26%
27	South Carolina	364,380,000	1.12%
28	Kentucky	338,975,000	1.04%
29	Oklahoma	338,025,000	1.04%
30	Iowa	320,371,000	0.99%
31	Kansas	306,171,000	0.94%
32	Utah	257,633,000	0.79%
33	Arkansas	226,609,000	0.70%
34	Hawaii	219,683,000	0.68%
35	Nevada	204,068,000	0.63%
36	Mississippi	198,070,000	0.61%
37	Nebraska	185,366,000	0.57%
38	West Virginia	174,028,000	0.54%
39	New Hampshire	167,595,000	0.52%
40	New Mexico	160,064,000	0.49%
41	Maine	150,904,000	0.46%
42	Idaho	150,221,000	0.46%
43	Rhode Island	148,838,000	0.46%
44	Alaska	114,760,000	0.35%
45	Delaware	102,416,000	0.31%
46	Montana	96,335,000	0.30%
47	South Dakota	79,410,000	0.24%
48	Vermont	78,673,000	0.24%
49	North Dakota	70,632,000	0.22%
50	Wyoming	52,712,000	0.16%
	District of Columbia	111,703,000	0.34%

Source: U.S. Bureau of the Census
    "1992 Census of Service Industries, Geographic Area Series, United States" (SC92-A-52)
*Includes only establishments subject to the federal income tax. See Facilities Chapter for establishments.

Receipts per Office or Clinic of Dentists in 1992

National Rate = $326,486 per Establishment*

RANK	STATE	PER ESTABLISHMENT
26	Alabama	$318,082
2	Alaska	438,015
16	Arizona	332,633
41	Arkansas	275,680
7	California	373,069
36	Colorado	290,765
6	Connecticut	384,622
1	Delaware	476,353
9	Florida	352,285
43	Georgia	274,841
12	Hawaii	343,255
18	Idaho	330,156
35	Illinois	292,998
5	Indiana	385,982
39	Iowa	278,826
31	Kansas	305,255
50	Kentucky	231,857
45	Louisiana	264,283
19	Maine	329,485
21	Maryland	324,864
15	Massachusetts	337,430
14	Michigan	339,242
13	Minnesota	341,748
47	Mississippi	252,640
40	Missouri	278,163
49	Montana	242,657
48	Nebraska	248,147
3	Nevada	426,921
20	New Hampshire	326,060
11	New Jersey	351,075
32	New Mexico	300,872
22	New York	323,606
10	North Carolina	351,947
38	North Dakota	282,528
33	Ohio	297,357
42	Oklahoma	275,041
17	Oregon	331,595
34	Pennsylvania	295,603
8	Rhode Island	366,596
27	South Carolina	316,028
30	South Dakota	305,423
37	Tennessee	288,376
29	Texas	308,008
44	Utah	264,510
25	Vermont	321,114
23	Virginia	321,708
4	Washington	407,029
28	West Virginia	309,108
24	Wisconsin	321,337
46	Wyoming	260,950

RANK	STATE	PER ESTABLISHMENT
1	Delaware	$476,353
2	Alaska	438,015
3	Nevada	426,921
4	Washington	407,029
5	Indiana	385,982
6	Connecticut	384,622
7	California	373,069
8	Rhode Island	366,596
9	Florida	352,285
10	North Carolina	351,947
11	New Jersey	351,075
12	Hawaii	343,255
13	Minnesota	341,748
14	Michigan	339,242
15	Massachusetts	337,430
16	Arizona	332,633
17	Oregon	331,595
18	Idaho	330,156
19	Maine	329,485
20	New Hampshire	326,060
21	Maryland	324,864
22	New York	323,606
23	Virginia	321,708
24	Wisconsin	321,337
25	Vermont	321,114
26	Alabama	318,082
27	South Carolina	316,028
28	West Virginia	309,108
29	Texas	308,008
30	South Dakota	305,423
31	Kansas	305,255
32	New Mexico	300,872
33	Ohio	297,357
34	Pennsylvania	295,603
35	Illinois	292,998
36	Colorado	290,765
37	Tennessee	288,376
38	North Dakota	282,528
39	Iowa	278,826
40	Missouri	278,163
41	Arkansas	275,680
42	Oklahoma	275,041
43	Georgia	274,841
44	Utah	264,510
45	Louisiana	264,283
46	Wyoming	260,950
47	Mississippi	252,640
48	Nebraska	248,147
49	Montana	242,657
50	Kentucky	231,857
	District of Columbia	321,911

Source: Morgan Quitno Press using data from U.S. Bureau of the Census
    "1992 Census of Service Industries, Geographic Area Series, United States" (SC92-A-52)
*Includes only establishments subject to the federal income tax. See Facilities Chapter for establishments.

Receipts of Offices and Clinics of Doctors of Osteopathy in 1992

National Total = $3,638,144,000*

ALPHA ORDER

RANK	STATE	RECEIPTS	% of USA
31	Alabama	$10,073,000	0.28%
36	Alaska	5,757,000	0.16%
8	Arizona	141,382,000	3.89%
33	Arkansas	7,486,000	0.21%
9	California	128,791,000	3.54%
13	Colorado	68,206,000	1.87%
NA	Connecticut**	NA	NA
23	Delaware	23,457,000	0.64%
4	Florida	325,522,000	8.95%
17	Georgia	42,184,000	1.16%
NA	Hawaii**	NA	NA
37	Idaho	4,797,000	0.13%
14	Illinois	62,781,000	1.73%
15	Indiana	54,594,000	1.50%
11	Iowa	77,485,000	2.13%
18	Kansas	39,828,000	1.09%
30	Kentucky	10,275,000	0.28%
44	Louisiana	1,804,000	0.05%
20	Maine	36,670,000	1.01%
38	Maryland	4,765,000	0.13%
29	Massachusetts	10,746,000	0.30%
1	Michigan	593,339,000	16.31%
NA	Minnesota**	NA	NA
32	Mississippi	8,865,000	0.24%
7	Missouri	160,312,000	4.41%
41	Montana	3,003,000	0.08%
NA	Nebraska**	NA	NA
27	Nevada	16,329,000	0.45%
42	New Hampshire	2,867,000	0.08%
6	New Jersey	213,199,000	5.86%
25	New Mexico	18,596,000	0.51%
12	New York	74,955,000	2.06%
35	North Carolina	6,445,000	0.18%
NA	North Dakota**	NA	NA
3	Ohio	386,003,000	10.61%
10	Oklahoma	127,260,000	3.50%
22	Oregon	32,862,000	0.90%
2	Pennsylvania	447,326,000	12.30%
26	Rhode Island	16,940,000	0.47%
34	South Carolina	6,489,000	0.18%
39	South Dakota	3,914,000	0.11%
24	Tennessee	22,588,000	0.62%
5	Texas	286,680,000	7.88%
40	Utah	3,446,000	0.09%
45	Vermont	1,074,000	0.03%
28	Virginia	13,366,000	0.37%
16	Washington	46,322,000	1.27%
19	West Virginia	37,666,000	1.04%
21	Wisconsin	36,056,000	0.99%
43	Wyoming	2,617,000	0.07%

RANK ORDER

RANK	STATE	RECEIPTS	% of USA
1	Michigan	$593,339,000	16.31%
2	Pennsylvania	447,326,000	12.30%
3	Ohio	386,003,000	10.61%
4	Florida	325,522,000	8.95%
5	Texas	286,680,000	7.88%
6	New Jersey	213,199,000	5.86%
7	Missouri	160,312,000	4.41%
8	Arizona	141,382,000	3.89%
9	California	128,791,000	3.54%
10	Oklahoma	127,260,000	3.50%
11	Iowa	77,485,000	2.13%
12	New York	74,955,000	2.06%
13	Colorado	68,206,000	1.87%
14	Illinois	62,781,000	1.73%
15	Indiana	54,594,000	1.50%
16	Washington	46,322,000	1.27%
17	Georgia	42,184,000	1.16%
18	Kansas	39,828,000	1.09%
19	West Virginia	37,666,000	1.04%
20	Maine	36,670,000	1.01%
21	Wisconsin	36,056,000	0.99%
22	Oregon	32,862,000	0.90%
23	Delaware	23,457,000	0.64%
24	Tennessee	22,588,000	0.62%
25	New Mexico	18,596,000	0.51%
26	Rhode Island	16,940,000	0.47%
27	Nevada	16,329,000	0.45%
28	Virginia	13,366,000	0.37%
29	Massachusetts	10,746,000	0.30%
30	Kentucky	10,275,000	0.28%
31	Alabama	10,073,000	0.28%
32	Mississippi	8,865,000	0.24%
33	Arkansas	7,486,000	0.21%
34	South Carolina	6,489,000	0.18%
35	North Carolina	6,445,000	0.18%
36	Alaska	5,757,000	0.16%
37	Idaho	4,797,000	0.13%
38	Maryland	4,765,000	0.13%
39	South Dakota	3,914,000	0.11%
40	Utah	3,446,000	0.09%
41	Montana	3,003,000	0.08%
42	New Hampshire	2,867,000	0.08%
43	Wyoming	2,617,000	0.07%
44	Louisiana	1,804,000	0.05%
45	Vermont	1,074,000	0.03%
NA	Connecticut**	NA	NA
NA	Hawaii**	NA	NA
NA	Minnesota**	NA	NA
NA	Nebraska**	NA	NA
NA	North Dakota**	NA	NA
	District of Columbia**	NA	NA

Source: U.S. Bureau of the Census
   "1992 Census of Service Industries, Geographic Area Series, United States" (SC92-A-52)
*Includes only establishments subject to the federal income tax. See Facilities Chapter for establishments.
**Not available.

Receipts per Office or Clinic of Doctors of Osteopathy in 1992

National Rate = $417,793 per Establishment*

ALPHA ORDER

ALPHA ORDER

RANK	STATE	PER ESTABLISHMENT	RANK	STATE	PER ESTABLISHMENT
32	Alabama	$314,781	1	New Jersey	$534,333
2	Alaska	523,364	2	Alaska	523,364
6	Arizona	446,000	3	Michigan	494,037
40	Arkansas	287,923	4	Ohio	470,162
16	California	399,972	5	Delaware	469,140
29	Colorado	329,498	6	Arizona	446,000
NA	Connecticut**	NA	7	Mississippi	443,250
5	Delaware	469,140	8	South Dakota	434,889
10	Florida	427,194	9	Tennessee	434,385
27	Georgia	340,194	10	Florida	427,194
NA	Hawaii**	NA	11	Pennsylvania	421,211
22	Idaho	369,000	12	West Virginia	418,511
23	Illinois	362,896	13	Kansas	410,598
19	Indiana	384,465	14	Texas	405,488
15	Iowa	401,477	15	Iowa	401,477
13	Kansas	410,598	16	California	399,972
41	Kentucky	270,395	17	Nevada	398,268
37	Louisiana	300,667	18	Oklahoma	387,988
36	Maine	305,583	19	Indiana	384,465
38	Maryland	297,813	20	Wisconsin	375,583
42	Massachusetts	268,650	21	New York	372,910
3	Michigan	494,037	22	Idaho	369,000
NA	Minnesota**	NA	23	Illinois	362,896
7	Mississippi	443,250	24	Missouri	359,444
24	Missouri	359,444	25	Utah	344,600
44	Montana	250,250	26	Virginia	342,718
NA	Nebraska**	NA	27	Georgia	340,194
17	Nevada	398,268	28	North Carolina	339,211
31	New Hampshire	318,556	29	Colorado	329,498
1	New Jersey	534,333	30	New Mexico	326,246
30	New Mexico	326,246	31	New Hampshire	318,556
21	New York	372,910	32	Alabama	314,781
28	North Carolina	339,211	33	Washington	310,886
NA	North Dakota**	NA	34	South Carolina	309,000
4	Ohio	470,162	35	Rhode Island	308,000
18	Oklahoma	387,988	36	Maine	305,583
39	Oregon	293,411	37	Louisiana	300,667
11	Pennsylvania	421,211	38	Maryland	297,813
35	Rhode Island	308,000	39	Oregon	293,411
34	South Carolina	309,000	40	Arkansas	287,923
8	South Dakota	434,889	41	Kentucky	270,395
9	Tennessee	434,385	42	Massachusetts	268,650
14	Texas	405,488	43	Wyoming	261,700
25	Utah	344,600	44	Montana	250,250
45	Vermont	179,000	45	Vermont	179,000
26	Virginia	342,718	NA	Connecticut**	NA
33	Washington	310,886	NA	Hawaii**	NA
12	West Virginia	418,511	NA	Minnesota**	NA
20	Wisconsin	375,583	NA	Nebraska**	NA
43	Wyoming	261,700	NA	North Dakota**	NA
				District of Columbia**	NA

Source: Morgan Quitno Press using data from U.S. Bureau of the Census
"1992 Census of Service Industries, Geographic Area Series, United States" (SC92-A-52)
*Includes only establishments subject to the federal income tax. See Facilities Chapter for establishments.
**Not available.

Receipts of Offices and Clinics of Chiropractors in 1992

National Total = $5,917,909,000*

RANK	STATE	RECEIPTS	% of USA
31	Alabama	$50,995,000	0.86%
41	Alaska	21,901,000	0.37%
15	Arizona	123,169,000	2.08%
33	Arkansas	39,365,000	0.67%
1	California	972,152,000	16.43%
17	Colorado	100,648,000	1.70%
16	Connecticut	101,975,000	1.72%
48	Delaware	13,666,000	0.23%
2	Florida	444,248,000	7.51%
12	Georgia	154,081,000	2.60%
34	Hawaii	38,828,000	0.66%
40	Idaho	22,470,000	0.38%
8	Illinois	216,560,000	3.66%
19	Indiana	98,161,000	1.66%
24	Iowa	68,192,000	1.15%
28	Kansas	58,992,000	1.00%
30	Kentucky	51,115,000	0.86%
29	Louisiana	58,506,000	0.99%
38	Maine	26,779,000	0.45%
22	Maryland	76,300,000	1.29%
9	Massachusetts	163,870,000	2.77%
11	Michigan	155,693,000	2.63%
10	Minnesota	160,994,000	2.72%
44	Mississippi	19,203,000	0.32%
20	Missouri	89,333,000	1.51%
46	Montana	16,310,000	0.28%
36	Nebraska	30,074,000	0.51%
32	Nevada	47,657,000	0.81%
42	New Hampshire	21,688,000	0.37%
5	New Jersey	326,710,000	5.52%
35	New Mexico	34,298,000	0.58%
3	New York	388,348,000	6.56%
18	North Carolina	99,116,000	1.67%
47	North Dakota	14,992,000	0.25%
7	Ohio	237,979,000	4.02%
25	Oklahoma	66,456,000	1.12%
27	Oregon	60,225,000	1.02%
6	Pennsylvania	293,051,000	4.95%
45	Rhode Island	17,967,000	0.30%
26	South Carolina	60,285,000	1.02%
43	South Dakota	20,907,000	0.35%
23	Tennessee	74,113,000	1.25%
4	Texas	331,418,000	5.60%
37	Utah	27,714,000	0.47%
49	Vermont	10,566,000	0.18%
21	Virginia	85,384,000	1.44%
13	Washington	147,177,000	2.49%
39	West Virginia	24,442,000	0.41%
14	Wisconsin	142,761,000	2.41%
50	Wyoming	6,966,000	0.12%

RANK	STATE	RECEIPTS	% of USA
1	California	$972,152,000	16.43%
2	Florida	444,248,000	7.51%
3	New York	388,348,000	6.56%
4	Texas	331,418,000	5.60%
5	New Jersey	326,710,000	5.52%
6	Pennsylvania	293,051,000	4.95%
7	Ohio	237,979,000	4.02%
8	Illinois	216,560,000	3.66%
9	Massachusetts	163,870,000	2.77%
10	Minnesota	160,994,000	2.72%
11	Michigan	155,693,000	2.63%
12	Georgia	154,081,000	2.60%
13	Washington	147,177,000	2.49%
14	Wisconsin	142,761,000	2.41%
15	Arizona	123,169,000	2.08%
16	Connecticut	101,975,000	1.72%
17	Colorado	100,648,000	1.70%
18	North Carolina	99,116,000	1.67%
19	Indiana	98,161,000	1.66%
20	Missouri	89,333,000	1.51%
21	Virginia	85,384,000	1.44%
22	Maryland	76,300,000	1.29%
23	Tennessee	74,113,000	1.25%
24	Iowa	68,192,000	1.15%
25	Oklahoma	66,456,000	1.12%
26	South Carolina	60,285,000	1.02%
27	Oregon	60,225,000	1.02%
28	Kansas	58,992,000	1.00%
29	Louisiana	58,506,000	0.99%
30	Kentucky	51,115,000	0.86%
31	Alabama	50,995,000	0.86%
32	Nevada	47,657,000	0.81%
33	Arkansas	39,365,000	0.67%
34	Hawaii	38,828,000	0.66%
35	New Mexico	34,298,000	0.58%
36	Nebraska	30,074,000	0.51%
37	Utah	27,714,000	0.47%
38	Maine	26,779,000	0.45%
39	West Virginia	24,442,000	0.41%
40	Idaho	22,470,000	0.38%
41	Alaska	21,901,000	0.37%
42	New Hampshire	21,688,000	0.37%
43	South Dakota	20,907,000	0.35%
44	Mississippi	19,203,000	0.32%
45	Rhode Island	17,967,000	0.30%
46	Montana	16,310,000	0.28%
47	North Dakota	14,992,000	0.25%
48	Delaware	13,666,000	0.23%
49	Vermont	10,566,000	0.18%
50	Wyoming	6,966,000	0.12%
	District of Columbia	4,109,000	0.07%

Source: U.S. Bureau of the Census
"1992 Census of Service Industries, Geographic Area Series, United States" (SC92-A-52)
*Includes only establishments subject to the federal income tax. See Facilities Chapter for establishments.

Receipts per Office or Clinic of Chiropractors in 1992

National Rate = $216,543 per Establishment*

ALPHA ORDER			RANK ORDER		
RANK	STATE	PER ESTABLISHMENT	RANK	STATE	PER ESTABLISHMENT
37	Alabama	$180,833	1	Maryland	$330,303
3	Alaska	308,465	2	Hawaii	326,286
28	Arizona	198,021	3	Alaska	308,465
44	Arkansas	166,097	4	Connecticut	293,876
19	California	222,766	5	Nevada	287,090
39	Colorado	170,879	6	Massachusetts	284,991
4	Connecticut	293,876	7	Delaware	273,320
7	Delaware	273,320	8	Ohio	273,225
10	Florida	240,524	9	New Jersey	262,418
26	Georgia	202,738	10	Florida	240,524
2	Hawaii	326,286	11	Virginia	240,518
42	Idaho	167,687	12	West Virginia	232,781
25	Illinois	202,772	13	Texas	232,411
16	Indiana	225,140	14	Rhode Island	227,430
47	Iowa	152,897	15	North Carolina	225,777
34	Kansas	183,776	16	Indiana	225,140
30	Kentucky	190,019	17	Pennsylvania	223,703
24	Louisiana	206,007	18	New York	223,060
21	Maine	212,532	19	California	222,766
1	Maryland	330,303	20	Wisconsin	214,678
6	Massachusetts	284,991	21	Maine	212,532
45	Michigan	165,984	22	Oklahoma	210,304
29	Minnesota	195,381	23	Tennessee	208,183
40	Mississippi	169,938	24	Louisiana	206,007
48	Missouri	149,386	25	Illinois	202,772
50	Montana	139,402	26	Georgia	202,738
33	Nebraska	184,503	27	New Hampshire	200,815
5	Nevada	287,090	28	Arizona	198,021
27	New Hampshire	200,815	29	Minnesota	195,381
9	New Jersey	262,418	30	Kentucky	190,019
32	New Mexico	185,395	31	South Carolina	188,981
18	New York	223,060	32	New Mexico	185,395
15	North Carolina	225,777	33	Nebraska	184,503
43	North Dakota	166,578	34	Kansas	183,776
8	Ohio	273,225	35	Washington	183,056
22	Oklahoma	210,304	36	Utah	181,137
49	Oregon	140,713	37	Alabama	180,833
17	Pennsylvania	223,703	38	South Dakota	177,178
14	Rhode Island	227,430	39	Colorado	170,879
31	South Carolina	188,981	40	Mississippi	169,938
38	South Dakota	177,178	41	Wyoming	169,902
23	Tennessee	208,183	42	Idaho	167,687
13	Texas	232,411	43	North Dakota	166,578
36	Utah	181,137	44	Arkansas	166,097
46	Vermont	162,554	45	Michigan	165,984
11	Virginia	240,518	46	Vermont	162,554
35	Washington	183,056	47	Iowa	152,897
12	West Virginia	232,781	48	Missouri	149,386
20	Wisconsin	214,678	49	Oregon	140,713
41	Wyoming	169,902	50	Montana	139,402
				District of Columbia	316,077

Source: Morgan Quitno Press using data from U.S. Bureau of the Census
"1992 Census of Service Industries, Geographic Area Series, United States" (SC92-A-52)
*Includes only establishments subject to the federal income tax. See Facilities Chapter for establishments.

Receipts of Offices and Clinics of Optometrists in 1992

National Total = $4,939,521,000*

<table>
<tr><td colspan="4">ALPHA ORDER</td><td colspan="4">RANK ORDER</td></tr>
<tr><th>RANK</th><th>STATE</th><th>RECEIPTS</th><th>% of USA</th><th>RANK</th><th>STATE</th><th>RECEIPTS</th><th>% of USA</th></tr>
<tr><td>27</td><td>Alabama</td><td>$65,608,000</td><td>1.33%</td><td>1</td><td>California</td><td>$754,317,000</td><td>15.27%</td></tr>
<tr><td>47</td><td>Alaska</td><td>17,112,000</td><td>0.35%</td><td>2</td><td>Texas</td><td>329,294,000</td><td>6.67%</td></tr>
<tr><td>31</td><td>Arizona</td><td>49,165,000</td><td>1.00%</td><td>3</td><td>Pennsylvania</td><td>246,226,000</td><td>4.98%</td></tr>
<tr><td>29</td><td>Arkansas</td><td>56,672,000</td><td>1.15%</td><td>4</td><td>New York</td><td>226,940,000</td><td>4.59%</td></tr>
<tr><td>1</td><td>California</td><td>754,317,000</td><td>15.27%</td><td>5</td><td>Florida</td><td>221,280,000</td><td>4.48%</td></tr>
<tr><td>24</td><td>Colorado</td><td>73,235,000</td><td>1.48%</td><td>6</td><td>Ohio</td><td>218,608,000</td><td>4.43%</td></tr>
<tr><td>23</td><td>Connecticut</td><td>73,960,000</td><td>1.50%</td><td>7</td><td>Illinois</td><td>213,734,000</td><td>4.33%</td></tr>
<tr><td>49</td><td>Delaware</td><td>12,873,000</td><td>0.26%</td><td>8</td><td>Michigan</td><td>203,832,000</td><td>4.13%</td></tr>
<tr><td>5</td><td>Florida</td><td>221,280,000</td><td>4.48%</td><td>9</td><td>New Jersey</td><td>147,976,000</td><td>3.00%</td></tr>
<tr><td>13</td><td>Georgia</td><td>102,345,000</td><td>2.07%</td><td>10</td><td>North Carolina</td><td>146,551,000</td><td>2.97%</td></tr>
<tr><td>39</td><td>Hawaii</td><td>27,647,000</td><td>0.56%</td><td>11</td><td>Indiana</td><td>133,059,000</td><td>2.69%</td></tr>
<tr><td>40</td><td>Idaho</td><td>24,607,000</td><td>0.50%</td><td>12</td><td>Virginia</td><td>115,755,000</td><td>2.34%</td></tr>
<tr><td>7</td><td>Illinois</td><td>213,734,000</td><td>4.33%</td><td>13</td><td>Georgia</td><td>102,345,000</td><td>2.07%</td></tr>
<tr><td>11</td><td>Indiana</td><td>133,059,000</td><td>2.69%</td><td>14</td><td>Tennessee</td><td>101,398,000</td><td>2.05%</td></tr>
<tr><td>19</td><td>Iowa</td><td>79,034,000</td><td>1.60%</td><td>15</td><td>Massachusetts</td><td>97,781,000</td><td>1.98%</td></tr>
<tr><td>20</td><td>Kansas</td><td>78,371,000</td><td>1.59%</td><td>16</td><td>Washington</td><td>95,398,000</td><td>1.93%</td></tr>
<tr><td>25</td><td>Kentucky</td><td>72,650,000</td><td>1.47%</td><td>17</td><td>Wisconsin</td><td>94,432,000</td><td>1.91%</td></tr>
<tr><td>32</td><td>Louisiana</td><td>48,393,000</td><td>0.98%</td><td>18</td><td>Missouri</td><td>88,489,000</td><td>1.79%</td></tr>
<tr><td>37</td><td>Maine</td><td>35,347,000</td><td>0.72%</td><td>19</td><td>Iowa</td><td>79,034,000</td><td>1.60%</td></tr>
<tr><td>21</td><td>Maryland</td><td>78,104,000</td><td>1.58%</td><td>20</td><td>Kansas</td><td>78,371,000</td><td>1.59%</td></tr>
<tr><td>15</td><td>Massachusetts</td><td>97,781,000</td><td>1.98%</td><td>21</td><td>Maryland</td><td>78,104,000</td><td>1.58%</td></tr>
<tr><td>8</td><td>Michigan</td><td>203,832,000</td><td>4.13%</td><td>22</td><td>Oklahoma</td><td>76,308,000</td><td>1.54%</td></tr>
<tr><td>26</td><td>Minnesota</td><td>71,690,000</td><td>1.45%</td><td>23</td><td>Connecticut</td><td>73,960,000</td><td>1.50%</td></tr>
<tr><td>35</td><td>Mississippi</td><td>37,655,000</td><td>0.76%</td><td>24</td><td>Colorado</td><td>73,235,000</td><td>1.48%</td></tr>
<tr><td>18</td><td>Missouri</td><td>88,489,000</td><td>1.79%</td><td>25</td><td>Kentucky</td><td>72,650,000</td><td>1.47%</td></tr>
<tr><td>41</td><td>Montana</td><td>24,435,000</td><td>0.49%</td><td>26</td><td>Minnesota</td><td>71,690,000</td><td>1.45%</td></tr>
<tr><td>34</td><td>Nebraska</td><td>38,725,000</td><td>0.78%</td><td>27</td><td>Alabama</td><td>65,608,000</td><td>1.33%</td></tr>
<tr><td>36</td><td>Nevada</td><td>36,924,000</td><td>0.75%</td><td>28</td><td>South Carolina</td><td>58,093,000</td><td>1.18%</td></tr>
<tr><td>45</td><td>New Hampshire</td><td>20,073,000</td><td>0.41%</td><td>29</td><td>Arkansas</td><td>56,672,000</td><td>1.15%</td></tr>
<tr><td>9</td><td>New Jersey</td><td>147,976,000</td><td>3.00%</td><td>30</td><td>Oregon</td><td>51,605,000</td><td>1.04%</td></tr>
<tr><td>38</td><td>New Mexico</td><td>30,091,000</td><td>0.61%</td><td>31</td><td>Arizona</td><td>49,165,000</td><td>1.00%</td></tr>
<tr><td>4</td><td>New York</td><td>226,940,000</td><td>4.59%</td><td>32</td><td>Louisiana</td><td>48,393,000</td><td>0.98%</td></tr>
<tr><td>10</td><td>North Carolina</td><td>146,551,000</td><td>2.97%</td><td>33</td><td>West Virginia</td><td>43,184,000</td><td>0.87%</td></tr>
<tr><td>43</td><td>North Dakota</td><td>21,635,000</td><td>0.44%</td><td>34</td><td>Nebraska</td><td>38,725,000</td><td>0.78%</td></tr>
<tr><td>6</td><td>Ohio</td><td>218,608,000</td><td>4.43%</td><td>35</td><td>Mississippi</td><td>37,655,000</td><td>0.76%</td></tr>
<tr><td>22</td><td>Oklahoma</td><td>76,308,000</td><td>1.54%</td><td>36</td><td>Nevada</td><td>36,924,000</td><td>0.75%</td></tr>
<tr><td>30</td><td>Oregon</td><td>51,605,000</td><td>1.04%</td><td>37</td><td>Maine</td><td>35,347,000</td><td>0.72%</td></tr>
<tr><td>3</td><td>Pennsylvania</td><td>246,226,000</td><td>4.98%</td><td>38</td><td>New Mexico</td><td>30,091,000</td><td>0.61%</td></tr>
<tr><td>44</td><td>Rhode Island</td><td>21,103,000</td><td>0.43%</td><td>39</td><td>Hawaii</td><td>27,647,000</td><td>0.56%</td></tr>
<tr><td>28</td><td>South Carolina</td><td>58,093,000</td><td>1.18%</td><td>40</td><td>Idaho</td><td>24,607,000</td><td>0.50%</td></tr>
<tr><td>46</td><td>South Dakota</td><td>19,165,000</td><td>0.39%</td><td>41</td><td>Montana</td><td>24,435,000</td><td>0.49%</td></tr>
<tr><td>14</td><td>Tennessee</td><td>101,398,000</td><td>2.05%</td><td>42</td><td>Utah</td><td>21,944,000</td><td>0.44%</td></tr>
<tr><td>2</td><td>Texas</td><td>329,294,000</td><td>6.67%</td><td>43</td><td>North Dakota</td><td>21,635,000</td><td>0.44%</td></tr>
<tr><td>42</td><td>Utah</td><td>21,944,000</td><td>0.44%</td><td>44</td><td>Rhode Island</td><td>21,103,000</td><td>0.43%</td></tr>
<tr><td>50</td><td>Vermont</td><td>11,768,000</td><td>0.24%</td><td>45</td><td>New Hampshire</td><td>20,073,000</td><td>0.41%</td></tr>
<tr><td>12</td><td>Virginia</td><td>115,755,000</td><td>2.34%</td><td>46</td><td>South Dakota</td><td>19,165,000</td><td>0.39%</td></tr>
<tr><td>16</td><td>Washington</td><td>95,398,000</td><td>1.93%</td><td>47</td><td>Alaska</td><td>17,112,000</td><td>0.35%</td></tr>
<tr><td>33</td><td>West Virginia</td><td>43,184,000</td><td>0.87%</td><td>48</td><td>Wyoming</td><td>15,714,000</td><td>0.32%</td></tr>
<tr><td>17</td><td>Wisconsin</td><td>94,432,000</td><td>1.91%</td><td>49</td><td>Delaware</td><td>12,873,000</td><td>0.26%</td></tr>
<tr><td>48</td><td>Wyoming</td><td>15,714,000</td><td>0.32%</td><td>50</td><td>Vermont</td><td>11,768,000</td><td>0.24%</td></tr>
<tr><td></td><td></td><td></td><td></td><td></td><td>District of Columbia</td><td>9,216,000</td><td>0.19%</td></tr>
</table>

Source: U.S. Bureau of the Census
  "1992 Census of Service Industries, Geographic Area Series, United States" (SC92-A-52)
*Includes only establishments subject to the federal income tax. See Facilities Chapter for establishments.

Receipts per Office or Clinic of Optometrists in 1992

National Rate = $288,271 per Establishment*

ALPHA ORDER

RANK ORDER

RANK	STATE	PER ESTABLISHMENT
24	Alabama	$286,498
1	Alaska	388,909
41	Arizona	260,132
28	Arkansas	280,554
10	California	316,674
26	Colorado	284,961
6	Connecticut	324,386
7	Delaware	321,825
42	Florida	259,110
32	Georgia	274,383
30	Hawaii	279,263
39	Idaho	261,777
11	Illinois	306,209
21	Indiana	287,384
18	Iowa	292,719
9	Kansas	317,291
17	Kentucky	292,944
45	Louisiana	246,903
22	Maine	287,374
5	Maryland	332,357
38	Massachusetts	264,273
3	Michigan	335,802
43	Minnesota	255,125
44	Mississippi	254,426
14	Missouri	293,983
48	Montana	237,233
8	Nebraska	320,041
4	Nevada	335,673
34	New Hampshire	271,257
36	New Jersey	269,047
20	New Mexico	289,337
23	New York	286,903
13	North Carolina	294,279
2	North Dakota	338,047
40	Ohio	261,493
46	Oklahoma	240,719
50	Oregon	232,455
27	Pennsylvania	283,344
16	Rhode Island	293,097
15	South Carolina	293,399
47	South Dakota	239,563
31	Tennessee	278,566
12	Texas	299,358
35	Utah	270,914
49	Vermont	235,360
37	Virginia	265,493
29	Washington	279,760
25	West Virginia	285,987
33	Wisconsin	272,138
19	Wyoming	291,000

RANK	STATE	PER ESTABLISHMENT
1	Alaska	$388,909
2	North Dakota	338,047
3	Michigan	335,802
4	Nevada	335,673
5	Maryland	332,357
6	Connecticut	324,386
7	Delaware	321,825
8	Nebraska	320,041
9	Kansas	317,291
10	California	316,674
11	Illinois	306,209
12	Texas	299,358
13	North Carolina	294,279
14	Missouri	293,983
15	South Carolina	293,399
16	Rhode Island	293,097
17	Kentucky	292,944
18	Iowa	292,719
19	Wyoming	291,000
20	New Mexico	289,337
21	Indiana	287,384
22	Maine	287,374
23	New York	286,903
24	Alabama	286,498
25	West Virginia	285,987
26	Colorado	284,961
27	Pennsylvania	283,344
28	Arkansas	280,554
29	Washington	279,760
30	Hawaii	279,263
31	Tennessee	278,566
32	Georgia	274,383
33	Wisconsin	272,138
34	New Hampshire	271,257
35	Utah	270,914
36	New Jersey	269,047
37	Virginia	265,493
38	Massachusetts	264,273
39	Idaho	261,777
40	Ohio	261,493
41	Arizona	260,132
42	Florida	259,110
43	Minnesota	255,125
44	Mississippi	254,426
45	Louisiana	246,903
46	Oklahoma	240,719
47	South Dakota	239,563
48	Montana	237,233
49	Vermont	235,360
50	Oregon	232,455
	District of Columbia	384,000

Source: Morgan Quitno Press using data from U.S. Bureau of the Census
  "1992 Census of Service Industries, Geographic Area Series, United States" (SC92-A-52)
*Includes only establishments subject to the federal income tax. See Facilities Chapter for establishments.

Receipts of Offices and Clinics of Podiatrists in 1992

National Total = $1,920,076,000*

ALPHA ORDER

RANK	STATE	RECEIPTS	% of USA
23	Alabama	$15,910,000	0.83%
46	Alaska	2,222,000	0.12%
18	Arizona	27,962,000	1.46%
42	Arkansas	5,017,000	0.26%
1	California	217,602,000	11.33%
22	Colorado	18,980,000	0.99%
11	Connecticut	48,830,000	2.54%
37	Delaware	6,801,000	0.35%
3	Florida	147,168,000	7.66%
12	Georgia	47,600,000	2.48%
43	Hawaii	3,871,000	0.20%
40	Idaho	5,283,000	0.28%
7	Illinois	105,745,000	5.51%
14	Indiana	41,792,000	2.18%
24	Iowa	14,998,000	0.78%
29	Kansas	12,107,000	0.63%
31	Kentucky	10,299,000	0.54%
26	Louisiana	13,876,000	0.72%
38	Maine	6,464,000	0.34%
10	Maryland	56,379,000	2.94%
13	Massachusetts	43,366,000	2.26%
5	Michigan	112,871,000	5.88%
28	Minnesota	12,440,000	0.65%
44	Mississippi	3,801,000	0.20%
20	Missouri	24,462,000	1.27%
45	Montana	3,441,000	0.18%
36	Nebraska	7,020,000	0.37%
35	Nevada	7,995,000	0.42%
41	New Hampshire	5,180,000	0.27%
9	New Jersey	103,924,000	5.41%
34	New Mexico	8,215,000	0.43%
2	New York	209,057,000	10.89%
16	North Carolina	35,032,000	1.82%
48	North Dakota	1,382,000	0.07%
6	Ohio	109,704,000	5.71%
25	Oklahoma	14,850,000	0.77%
27	Oregon	13,796,000	0.72%
4	Pennsylvania	118,882,000	6.19%
30	Rhode Island	11,842,000	0.62%
32	South Carolina	9,906,000	0.52%
47	South Dakota	1,774,000	0.09%
21	Tennessee	23,034,000	1.20%
8	Texas	104,569,000	5.45%
33	Utah	9,326,000	0.49%
49	Vermont	1,157,000	0.06%
15	Virginia	40,402,000	2.10%
17	Washington	31,204,000	1.63%
39	West Virginia	5,602,000	0.29%
19	Wisconsin	27,720,000	1.44%
50	Wyoming	1,035,000	0.05%

RANK ORDER

RANK	STATE	RECEIPTS	% of USA
1	California	$217,602,000	11.33%
2	New York	209,057,000	10.89%
3	Florida	147,168,000	7.66%
4	Pennsylvania	118,882,000	6.19%
5	Michigan	112,871,000	5.88%
6	Ohio	109,704,000	5.71%
7	Illinois	105,745,000	5.51%
8	Texas	104,569,000	5.45%
9	New Jersey	103,924,000	5.41%
10	Maryland	56,379,000	2.94%
11	Connecticut	48,830,000	2.54%
12	Georgia	47,600,000	2.48%
13	Massachusetts	43,366,000	2.26%
14	Indiana	41,792,000	2.18%
15	Virginia	40,402,000	2.10%
16	North Carolina	35,032,000	1.82%
17	Washington	31,204,000	1.63%
18	Arizona	27,962,000	1.46%
19	Wisconsin	27,720,000	1.44%
20	Missouri	24,462,000	1.27%
21	Tennessee	23,034,000	1.20%
22	Colorado	18,980,000	0.99%
23	Alabama	15,910,000	0.83%
24	Iowa	14,998,000	0.78%
25	Oklahoma	14,850,000	0.77%
26	Louisiana	13,876,000	0.72%
27	Oregon	13,796,000	0.72%
28	Minnesota	12,440,000	0.65%
29	Kansas	12,107,000	0.63%
30	Rhode Island	11,842,000	0.62%
31	Kentucky	10,299,000	0.54%
32	South Carolina	9,906,000	0.52%
33	Utah	9,326,000	0.49%
34	New Mexico	8,215,000	0.43%
35	Nevada	7,995,000	0.42%
36	Nebraska	7,020,000	0.37%
37	Delaware	6,801,000	0.35%
38	Maine	6,464,000	0.34%
39	West Virginia	5,602,000	0.29%
40	Idaho	5,283,000	0.28%
41	New Hampshire	5,180,000	0.27%
42	Arkansas	5,017,000	0.26%
43	Hawaii	3,871,000	0.20%
44	Mississippi	3,801,000	0.20%
45	Montana	3,441,000	0.18%
46	Alaska	2,222,000	0.12%
47	South Dakota	1,774,000	0.09%
48	North Dakota	1,382,000	0.07%
49	Vermont	1,157,000	0.06%
50	Wyoming	1,035,000	0.05%
	District of Columbia	8,181,000	0.43%

Source: U.S. Bureau of the Census
  "1992 Census of Service Industries, Geographic Area Series, United States" (SC92-A-52)
Includes only establishments subject to the federal income tax. See Facilities Chapter for establishments.

Receipts per Office or Clinic of Podiatrists in 1992

National Rate = $241,580 per Establishment*

ALPHA ORDER				RANK ORDER		
RANK	STATE	PER ESTABLISHMENT		RANK	STATE	PER ESTABLISHMENT
3	Alabama	$324,694		1	Alaska	$444,400
1	Alaska	444,400		2	Georgia	342,446
28	Arizona	231,091		3	Alabama	324,694
17	Arkansas	250,850		4	Connecticut	321,250
25	California	233,981		5	Idaho	310,765
35	Colorado	215,682		6	Louisiana	289,083
4	Connecticut	321,250		7	Oklahoma	285,577
11	Delaware	272,040		8	Nevada	285,536
13	Florida	260,936		9	Michigan	282,178
2	Georgia	342,446		10	Texas	273,741
23	Hawaii	241,938		11	Delaware	272,040
5	Idaho	310,765		12	Maryland	267,199
15	Illinois	252,375		13	Florida	260,936
16	Indiana	251,759		14	Tennessee	255,933
46	Iowa	199,973		15	Illinois	252,375
33	Kansas	220,127		16	Indiana	251,759
30	Kentucky	223,891		17	Arkansas	250,850
6	Louisiana	289,083		18	North Carolina	250,229
48	Maine	179,556		19	Missouri	249,612
12	Maryland	267,199		20	New Mexico	248,939
41	Massachusetts	208,490		21	South Carolina	247,650
9	Michigan	282,178		22	Virginia	246,354
42	Minnesota	207,333		23	Hawaii	241,938
40	Mississippi	211,167		24	Rhode Island	236,840
19	Missouri	249,612		25	California	233,981
37	Montana	215,063		26	Wisconsin	232,941
44	Nebraska	206,471		27	New Jersey	231,457
8	Nevada	285,536		28	Arizona	231,091
34	New Hampshire	215,833		29	Oregon	226,164
27	New Jersey	231,457		30	Kentucky	223,891
20	New Mexico	248,939		31	Ohio	223,886
32	New York	222,875		32	New York	222,875
18	North Carolina	250,229		33	Kansas	220,127
47	North Dakota	197,429		34	New Hampshire	215,833
31	Ohio	223,886		35	Colorado	215,682
7	Oklahoma	285,577		36	West Virginia	215,462
29	Oregon	226,164		37	Montana	215,063
45	Pennsylvania	201,837		38	Washington	213,726
24	Rhode Island	236,840		39	Utah	211,955
21	South Carolina	247,650		40	Mississippi	211,167
50	South Dakota	126,714		41	Massachusetts	208,490
14	Tennessee	255,933		42	Minnesota	207,333
10	Texas	273,741		43	Wyoming	207,000
39	Utah	211,955		44	Nebraska	206,471
49	Vermont	128,556		45	Pennsylvania	201,837
22	Virginia	246,354		46	Iowa	199,973
38	Washington	213,726		47	North Dakota	197,429
36	West Virginia	215,462		48	Maine	179,556
26	Wisconsin	232,941		49	Vermont	128,556
43	Wyoming	207,000		50	South Dakota	126,714
					District of Columbia	255,656

Source: Morgan Quitno Press using data from U.S. Bureau of the Census
"1992 Census of Service Industries, Geographic Area Series, United States" (SC92-A-52)
*Includes only establishments subject to the federal income tax. See Facilities Chapter for establishments.

Receipts of Hospitals in 1992

National Total = $310,818,211,000*

ALPHA ORDER

RANK	STATE	RECEIPTS	% of USA
21	Alabama	$5,114,698,000	1.65%
NA	Alaska**	NA	NA
23	Arizona	4,064,528,000	1.31%
30	Arkansas	2,601,895,000	0.84%
1	California	34,552,067,000	11.12%
24	Colorado	3,876,008,000	1.25%
NA	Connecticut**	NA	NA
37	Delaware	903,055,000	0.29%
5	Florida	16,528,209,000	5.32%
11	Georgia	8,079,353,000	2.60%
NA	Hawaii**	NA	NA
38	Idaho	880,530,000	0.28%
6	Illinois	14,715,279,000	4.73%
16	Indiana	6,590,871,000	2.12%
NA	Iowa**	NA	NA
27	Kansas	2,856,257,000	0.92%
22	Kentucky	4,185,657,000	1.35%
17	Louisiana	5,658,657,000	1.82%
NA	Maine**	NA	NA
18	Maryland	5,440,457,000	1.75%
10	Massachusetts	9,714,787,000	3.13%
8	Michigan	11,444,321,000	3.68%
NA	Minnesota**	NA	NA
29	Mississippi	2,627,692,000	0.85%
13	Missouri	7,217,462,000	2.32%
39	Montana	864,812,000	0.28%
NA	Nebraska**	NA	NA
34	Nevada	1,296,942,000	0.42%
36	New Hampshire	1,250,889,000	0.40%
9	New Jersey	9,842,808,000	3.17%
33	New Mexico	1,558,035,000	0.50%
2	New York	27,722,480,000	8.92%
12	North Carolina	7,408,964,000	2.38%
NA	North Dakota**	NA	NA
7	Ohio	13,998,840,000	4.50%
26	Oklahoma	3,232,112,000	1.04%
28	Oregon	2,835,585,000	0.91%
4	Pennsylvania	18,019,449,000	5.80%
35	Rhode Island	1,257,773,000	0.40%
25	South Carolina	3,833,754,000	1.23%
NA	South Dakota**	NA	NA
15	Tennessee	6,770,631,000	2.18%
3	Texas	20,081,248,000	6.46%
32	Utah	1,626,872,000	0.52%
40	Vermont	545,676,000	0.18%
14	Virginia	6,793,601,000	2.19%
20	Washington	5,193,838,000	1.67%
31	West Virginia	2,243,147,000	0.72%
19	Wisconsin	5,262,803,000	1.69%
NA	Wyoming**	NA	NA

RANK ORDER

RANK	STATE	RECEIPTS	% of USA
1	California	$34,552,067,000	11.12%
2	New York	27,722,480,000	8.92%
3	Texas	20,081,248,000	6.46%
4	Pennsylvania	18,019,449,000	5.80%
5	Florida	16,528,209,000	5.32%
6	Illinois	14,715,279,000	4.73%
7	Ohio	13,998,840,000	4.50%
8	Michigan	11,444,321,000	3.68%
9	New Jersey	9,842,808,000	3.17%
10	Massachusetts	9,714,787,000	3.13%
11	Georgia	8,079,353,000	2.60%
12	North Carolina	7,408,964,000	2.38%
13	Missouri	7,217,462,000	2.32%
14	Virginia	6,793,601,000	2.19%
15	Tennessee	6,770,631,000	2.18%
16	Indiana	6,590,871,000	2.12%
17	Louisiana	5,658,657,000	1.82%
18	Maryland	5,440,457,000	1.75%
19	Wisconsin	5,262,803,000	1.69%
20	Washington	5,193,838,000	1.67%
21	Alabama	5,114,698,000	1.65%
22	Kentucky	4,185,657,000	1.35%
23	Arizona	4,064,528,000	1.31%
24	Colorado	3,876,008,000	1.25%
25	South Carolina	3,833,754,000	1.23%
26	Oklahoma	3,232,112,000	1.04%
27	Kansas	2,856,257,000	0.92%
28	Oregon	2,835,585,000	0.91%
29	Mississippi	2,627,692,000	0.85%
30	Arkansas	2,601,895,000	0.84%
31	West Virginia	2,243,147,000	0.72%
32	Utah	1,626,872,000	0.52%
33	New Mexico	1,558,035,000	0.50%
34	Nevada	1,296,942,000	0.42%
35	Rhode Island	1,257,773,000	0.40%
36	New Hampshire	1,250,889,000	0.40%
37	Delaware	903,055,000	0.29%
38	Idaho	880,530,000	0.28%
39	Montana	864,812,000	0.28%
40	Vermont	545,676,000	0.18%
NA	Alaska**	NA	NA
NA	Connecticut**	NA	NA
NA	Hawaii**	NA	NA
NA	Iowa**	NA	NA
NA	Maine**	NA	NA
NA	Minnesota**	NA	NA
NA	Nebraska**	NA	NA
NA	North Dakota**	NA	NA
NA	South Dakota**	NA	NA
NA	Wyoming**	NA	NA
	District of Columbia**	NA	NA

Source: Morgan Quitno Press using data from U.S. Bureau of the Census
"1992 Census of Service Industries, Geographic Area Series, United States" (SC92-A-52)
*Includes establishments exempt from as well as subject to the federal income tax. Includes general medical and surgical hospitals, psychiatric hospitals and other specialty hospitals. Includes government owned hospitals.
**Not available.

Receipts per Hospital in 1992

National Rate = $43,654,243 per Hospital*

ALPHA ORDER

RANK	STATE	PER HOSPITAL
24	Alabama	$36,533,557
NA	Alaska**	NA
18	Arizona	40,645,280
34	Arkansas	25,508,775
9	California	57,205,409
21	Colorado	38,760,080
NA	Connecticut**	NA
10	Delaware	56,440,938
12	Florida	50,237,717
23	Georgia	38,473,110
NA	Hawaii**	NA
39	Idaho	16,306,111
8	Illinois	57,257,895
20	Indiana	40,434,791
NA	Iowa**	NA
38	Kansas	17,631,216
28	Kentucky	32,700,445
31	Louisiana	30,422,887
NA	Maine**	NA
3	Maryland	64,005,376
4	Massachusetts	60,717,419
11	Michigan	52,257,174
NA	Minnesota**	NA
36	Mississippi	22,268,576
16	Missouri	41,242,640
40	Montana	13,304,800
NA	Nebraska**	NA
19	Nevada	40,529,438
30	New Hampshire	30,509,488
2	New Jersey	72,909,689
35	New Mexico	23,254,254
1	New York	85,038,282
15	North Carolina	42,580,253
NA	North Dakota**	NA
6	Ohio	57,608,395
37	Oklahoma	21,547,413
25	Oregon	35,893,481
7	Pennsylvania	57,386,780
5	Rhode Island	59,893,952
17	South Carolina	41,223,161
NA	South Dakota**	NA
22	Tennessee	38,689,320
26	Texas	34,326,920
33	Utah	29,051,286
32	Vermont	30,315,333
13	Virginia	48,525,721
14	Washington	43,645,697
29	West Virginia	31,154,819
27	Wisconsin	33,521,038
NA	Wyoming**	NA

RANK ORDER

RANK	STATE	PER HOSPITAL
1	New York	$85,038,282
2	New Jersey	72,909,689
3	Maryland	64,005,376
4	Massachusetts	60,717,419
5	Rhode Island	59,893,952
6	Ohio	57,608,395
7	Pennsylvania	57,386,780
8	Illinois	57,257,895
9	California	57,205,409
10	Delaware	56,440,938
11	Michigan	52,257,174
12	Florida	50,237,717
13	Virginia	48,525,721
14	Washington	43,645,697
15	North Carolina	42,580,253
16	Missouri	41,242,640
17	South Carolina	41,223,161
18	Arizona	40,645,280
19	Nevada	40,529,438
20	Indiana	40,434,791
21	Colorado	38,760,080
22	Tennessee	38,689,320
23	Georgia	38,473,110
24	Alabama	36,533,557
25	Oregon	35,893,481
26	Texas	34,326,920
27	Wisconsin	33,521,038
28	Kentucky	32,700,445
29	West Virginia	31,154,819
30	New Hampshire	30,509,488
31	Louisiana	30,422,887
32	Vermont	30,315,333
33	Utah	29,051,286
34	Arkansas	25,508,775
35	New Mexico	23,254,254
36	Mississippi	22,268,576
37	Oklahoma	21,547,413
38	Kansas	17,631,216
39	Idaho	16,306,111
40	Montana	13,304,800
NA	Alaska**	NA
NA	Connecticut**	NA
NA	Hawaii**	NA
NA	Iowa**	NA
NA	Maine**	NA
NA	Minnesota**	NA
NA	Nebraska**	NA
NA	North Dakota**	NA
NA	South Dakota**	NA
NA	Wyoming**	NA
	District of Columbia**	NA

Source: Morgan Quitno Press using data from U.S. Bureau of the Census
  "1992 Census of Service Industries, Geographic Area Series, United States" (SC92-A-52)
*Calculated using Census Bureau count of 7,120 hospitals. Includes establishments exempt from as well as subject to the federal income tax. Includes general medical and surgical hospitals, psychiatric hospitals and other specialty hospitals. Includes government owned hospitals.
**Not available.

V. INCIDENCE OF DISEASE

V. INCIDENCE OF DISEASE (Continued)

Estimated New Cancer Cases in 1999

National Estimated Total = 1,221,800 New Cases*

ALPHA ORDER

RANK	STATE	CASES	% of USA
20	Alabama	21,100	1.7%
50	Alaska	1,400	0.1%
23	Arizona	20,000	1.6%
30	Arkansas	13,800	1.1%
1	California	112,300	9.2%
31	Colorado	13,300	1.1%
28	Connecticut	15,100	1.2%
45	Delaware	3,800	0.3%
2	Florida	88,000	7.2%
12	Georgia	29,100	2.4%
43	Hawaii	4,300	0.4%
42	Idaho	4,600	0.4%
6	Illinois	56,800	4.6%
14	Indiana	27,900	2.3%
29	Iowa	14,300	1.2%
33	Kansas	12,000	1.0%
21	Kentucky	20,500	1.7%
22	Louisiana	20,300	1.7%
37	Maine	7,000	0.6%
19	Maryland	22,600	1.8%
11	Massachusetts	30,700	2.5%
8	Michigan	44,200	3.6%
24	Minnesota	19,400	1.6%
32	Mississippi	13,000	1.1%
14	Missouri	27,900	2.3%
44	Montana	4,100	0.3%
36	Nebraska	7,400	0.6%
35	Nevada	8,100	0.7%
39	New Hampshire	5,400	0.4%
9	New Jersey	40,000	3.3%
38	New Mexico	6,500	0.5%
3	New York	83,100	6.8%
10	North Carolina	35,500	2.9%
47	North Dakota	3,100	0.3%
7	Ohio	56,500	4.6%
27	Oklahoma	15,800	1.3%
26	Oregon	15,900	1.3%
5	Pennsylvania	66,600	5.5%
40	Rhode Island	5,200	0.4%
25	South Carolina	17,900	1.5%
46	South Dakota	3,400	0.3%
16	Tennessee	26,800	2.2%
4	Texas	77,400	6.3%
40	Utah	5,200	0.4%
48	Vermont	2,600	0.2%
13	Virginia	29,000	2.4%
17	Washington	23,800	1.9%
34	West Virginia	10,600	0.9%
18	Wisconsin	23,700	1.9%
49	Wyoming	2,000	0.2%

RANK ORDER

RANK	STATE	CASES	% of USA
1	California	112,300	9.2%
2	Florida	88,000	7.2%
3	New York	83,100	6.8%
4	Texas	77,400	6.3%
5	Pennsylvania	66,600	5.5%
6	Illinois	56,800	4.6%
7	Ohio	56,500	4.6%
8	Michigan	44,200	3.6%
9	New Jersey	40,000	3.3%
10	North Carolina	35,500	2.9%
11	Massachusetts	30,700	2.5%
12	Georgia	29,100	2.4%
13	Virginia	29,000	2.4%
14	Indiana	27,900	2.3%
14	Missouri	27,900	2.3%
16	Tennessee	26,800	2.2%
17	Washington	23,800	1.9%
18	Wisconsin	23,700	1.9%
19	Maryland	22,600	1.8%
20	Alabama	21,100	1.7%
21	Kentucky	20,500	1.7%
22	Louisiana	20,300	1.7%
23	Arizona	20,000	1.6%
24	Minnesota	19,400	1.6%
25	South Carolina	17,900	1.5%
26	Oregon	15,900	1.3%
27	Oklahoma	15,800	1.3%
28	Connecticut	15,100	1.2%
29	Iowa	14,300	1.2%
30	Arkansas	13,800	1.1%
31	Colorado	13,300	1.1%
32	Mississippi	13,000	1.1%
33	Kansas	12,000	1.0%
34	West Virginia	10,600	0.9%
35	Nevada	8,100	0.7%
36	Nebraska	7,400	0.6%
37	Maine	7,000	0.6%
38	New Mexico	6,500	0.5%
39	New Hampshire	5,400	0.4%
40	Rhode Island	5,200	0.4%
40	Utah	5,200	0.4%
42	Idaho	4,600	0.4%
43	Hawaii	4,300	0.4%
44	Montana	4,100	0.3%
45	Delaware	3,800	0.3%
46	South Dakota	3,400	0.3%
47	North Dakota	3,100	0.3%
48	Vermont	2,600	0.2%
49	Wyoming	2,000	0.2%
50	Alaska	1,400	0.1%
	District of Columbia	3,000	0.2%

Source: American Cancer Society

"1999 Facts & Figures" (Copyright 1999, Reprinted with permission from the American Cancer Society)
These estimates are offered as a rough guide and should not be regarded as definitive. They are calculated according to the distribution of estimated 1999 cancer deaths by state. Totals do not include basal and squamous cell skin cancers or in situ carcinomas except urinary bladder.

Estimated Rate of New Cancer Cases in 1999

National Estimated Rate = 452.0 New Cases per 100,000 Population*

ALPHA ORDER

RANK	STATE	RATE
16	Alabama	484.8
50	Alaska	228.0
37	Arizona	428.4
5	Arkansas	543.7
47	California	343.8
48	Colorado	334.9
27	Connecticut	461.2
9	Delaware	511.0
1	Florida	590.0
43	Georgia	380.8
46	Hawaii	360.4
44	Idaho	374.4
21	Illinois	471.6
18	Indiana	472.9
11	Iowa	499.6
30	Kansas	456.4
7	Kentucky	520.8
25	Louisiana	464.6
3	Maine	562.6
35	Maryland	440.1
12	Massachusetts	499.4
33	Michigan	450.2
41	Minnesota	410.5
19	Mississippi	472.4
8	Missouri	513.0
24	Montana	465.7
34	Nebraska	445.1
26	Nevada	463.7
31	New Hampshire	455.7
14	New Jersey	492.9
45	New Mexico	374.2
29	New York	457.2
22	North Carolina	470.4
15	North Dakota	485.7
10	Ohio	504.0
20	Oklahoma	472.1
17	Oregon	484.5
4	Pennsylvania	554.9
6	Rhode Island	526.1
23	South Carolina	466.6
28	South Dakota	460.6
13	Tennessee	493.5
42	Texas	391.7
49	Utah	247.6
36	Vermont	440.0
38	Virginia	427.0
39	Washington	418.3
2	West Virginia	585.3
32	Wisconsin	453.7
40	Wyoming	415.9

RANK ORDER

RANK	STATE	RATE
1	Florida	590.0
2	West Virginia	585.3
3	Maine	562.6
4	Pennsylvania	554.9
5	Arkansas	543.7
6	Rhode Island	526.1
7	Kentucky	520.8
8	Missouri	513.0
9	Delaware	511.0
10	Ohio	504.0
11	Iowa	499.6
12	Massachusetts	499.4
13	Tennessee	493.5
14	New Jersey	492.9
15	North Dakota	485.7
16	Alabama	484.8
17	Oregon	484.5
18	Indiana	472.9
19	Mississippi	472.4
20	Oklahoma	472.1
21	Illinois	471.6
22	North Carolina	470.4
23	South Carolina	466.6
24	Montana	465.7
25	Louisiana	464.6
26	Nevada	463.7
27	Connecticut	461.2
28	South Dakota	460.6
29	New York	457.2
30	Kansas	456.4
31	New Hampshire	455.7
32	Wisconsin	453.7
33	Michigan	450.2
34	Nebraska	445.1
35	Maryland	440.1
36	Vermont	440.0
37	Arizona	428.4
38	Virginia	427.0
39	Washington	418.3
40	Wyoming	415.9
41	Minnesota	410.5
42	Texas	391.7
43	Georgia	380.8
44	Idaho	374.4
45	New Mexico	374.2
46	Hawaii	360.4
47	California	343.8
48	Colorado	334.9
49	Utah	247.6
50	Alaska	228.0
	District of Columbia	573.5

Source: Morgan Quitno Press using data from American Cancer Society
"1999 Facts & Figures" (Copyright 1999, Reprinted with permission from the American Cancer Society)
*These estimates are offered as a rough guide and should not be regarded as definitive. They are calculated according to the distribution of estimated 1999 cancer deaths by state. Totals do not include basal and squamous cell skin cancers or in situ carcinomas except urinary bladder. Rates calculated using 1998 Census resident population estimates.

Estimated New Cases of Bladder Cancer in 1999

National Estimated Total = 54,200 New Cases*

ALPHA ORDER

RANK	STATE	CASES	% of USA
20	Alabama	800	1.5%
NA	Alaska**	NA	NA
20	Arizona	800	1.5%
31	Arkansas	500	0.9%
1	California	5,200	9.6%
30	Colorado	600	1.1%
20	Connecticut	800	1.5%
35	Delaware	300	0.6%
2	Florida	4,300	7.9%
19	Georgia	900	1.7%
47	Hawaii	100	0.2%
35	Idaho	300	0.6%
7	Illinois	2,500	4.6%
12	Indiana	1,200	2.2%
25	Iowa	700	1.3%
31	Kansas	500	0.9%
25	Kentucky	700	1.3%
25	Louisiana	700	1.3%
35	Maine	300	0.6%
17	Maryland	1,000	1.8%
10	Massachusetts	1,700	3.1%
8	Michigan	2,100	3.9%
20	Minnesota	800	1.5%
34	Mississippi	400	0.7%
15	Missouri	1,100	2.0%
41	Montana	200	0.4%
35	Nebraska	300	0.6%
35	Nevada	300	0.6%
41	New Hampshire	200	0.4%
8	New Jersey	2,100	3.9%
41	New Mexico	200	0.4%
3	New York	4,200	7.7%
11	North Carolina	1,400	2.6%
41	North Dakota	200	0.4%
6	Ohio	2,700	5.0%
25	Oklahoma	700	1.3%
25	Oregon	700	1.3%
4	Pennsylvania	3,100	5.7%
35	Rhode Island	300	0.6%
20	South Carolina	800	1.5%
41	South Dakota	200	0.4%
17	Tennessee	1,000	1.8%
5	Texas	2,800	5.2%
41	Utah	200	0.4%
47	Vermont	100	0.2%
15	Virginia	1,100	2.0%
12	Washington	1,200	2.2%
31	West Virginia	500	0.9%
12	Wisconsin	1,200	2.2%
47	Wyoming	100	0.2%

RANK ORDER

RANK	STATE	CASES	% of USA
1	California	5,200	9.6%
2	Florida	4,300	7.9%
3	New York	4,200	7.7%
4	Pennsylvania	3,100	5.7%
5	Texas	2,800	5.2%
6	Ohio	2,700	5.0%
7	Illinois	2,500	4.6%
8	Michigan	2,100	3.9%
8	New Jersey	2,100	3.9%
10	Massachusetts	1,700	3.1%
11	North Carolina	1,400	2.6%
12	Indiana	1,200	2.2%
12	Washington	1,200	2.2%
12	Wisconsin	1,200	2.2%
15	Missouri	1,100	2.0%
15	Virginia	1,100	2.0%
17	Maryland	1,000	1.8%
17	Tennessee	1,000	1.8%
19	Georgia	900	1.7%
20	Alabama	800	1.5%
20	Arizona	800	1.5%
20	Connecticut	800	1.5%
20	Minnesota	800	1.5%
20	South Carolina	800	1.5%
25	Iowa	700	1.3%
25	Kentucky	700	1.3%
25	Louisiana	700	1.3%
25	Oklahoma	700	1.3%
25	Oregon	700	1.3%
30	Colorado	600	1.1%
31	Arkansas	500	0.9%
31	Kansas	500	0.9%
31	West Virginia	500	0.9%
34	Mississippi	400	0.7%
35	Delaware	300	0.6%
35	Idaho	300	0.6%
35	Maine	300	0.6%
35	Nebraska	300	0.6%
35	Nevada	300	0.6%
35	Rhode Island	300	0.6%
41	Montana	200	0.4%
41	New Hampshire	200	0.4%
41	New Mexico	200	0.4%
41	North Dakota	200	0.4%
41	South Dakota	200	0.4%
41	Utah	200	0.4%
47	Hawaii	100	0.2%
47	Vermont	100	0.2%
47	Wyoming	100	0.2%
NA	Alaska**	NA	NA
	District of Columbia	100	0.2%

Source: American Cancer Society
    "1999 Facts & Figures" (Copyright 1999, Reprinted with permission from the American Cancer Society)
*These estimates are offered as a rough guide and should be interpreted with caution. They are calculated according to the distribution of estimated 1999 cancer deaths by state.
**Fewer than 50 cases.

Estimated Rate of New Cases of Bladder Cancer in 1999

National Estimated Rate = 20.1 New Cases per 100,000 Population*

ALPHA ORDER				RANK ORDER		
RANK	STATE	RATE		RANK	STATE	RATE
31	Alabama	18.4		1	Delaware	40.3
NA	Alaska**	NA		2	North Dakota	31.3
36	Arizona	17.1		3	Rhode Island	30.3
27	Arkansas	19.7		4	Florida	28.8
42	California	15.9		5	Massachusetts	27.7
43	Colorado	15.1		6	West Virginia	27.6
11	Connecticut	24.4		7	South Dakota	27.1
1	Delaware	40.3		8	New Jersey	25.9
4	Florida	28.8		9	Pennsylvania	25.8
46	Georgia	11.8		10	Iowa	24.5
49	Hawaii	8.4		11	Connecticut	24.4
11	Idaho	24.4		11	Idaho	24.4
23	Illinois	20.8		13	Maine	24.1
25	Indiana	20.3		13	Ohio	24.1
10	Iowa	24.5		15	New York	23.1
29	Kansas	19.0		16	Wisconsin	23.0
34	Kentucky	17.8		17	Montana	22.7
41	Louisiana	16.0		18	Michigan	21.4
13	Maine	24.1		19	Oregon	21.3
28	Maryland	19.5		20	Washington	21.1
5	Massachusetts	27.7		21	Oklahoma	20.9
18	Michigan	21.4		21	South Carolina	20.9
37	Minnesota	16.9		23	Illinois	20.8
44	Mississippi	14.5		23	Wyoming	20.8
26	Missouri	20.2		25	Indiana	20.3
17	Montana	22.7		26	Missouri	20.2
33	Nebraska	18.0		27	Arkansas	19.7
35	Nevada	17.2		28	Maryland	19.5
37	New Hampshire	16.9		29	Kansas	19.0
8	New Jersey	25.9		30	North Carolina	18.6
47	New Mexico	11.5		31	Alabama	18.4
15	New York	23.1		31	Tennessee	18.4
30	North Carolina	18.6		33	Nebraska	18.0
2	North Dakota	31.3		34	Kentucky	17.8
13	Ohio	24.1		35	Nevada	17.2
21	Oklahoma	20.9		36	Arizona	17.1
19	Oregon	21.3		37	Minnesota	16.9
9	Pennsylvania	25.8		37	New Hampshire	16.9
3	Rhode Island	30.3		37	Vermont	16.9
21	South Carolina	20.9		40	Virginia	16.2
7	South Dakota	27.1		41	Louisiana	16.0
31	Tennessee	18.4		42	California	15.9
45	Texas	14.2		43	Colorado	15.1
48	Utah	9.5		44	Mississippi	14.5
37	Vermont	16.9		45	Texas	14.2
40	Virginia	16.2		46	Georgia	11.8
20	Washington	21.1		47	New Mexico	11.5
6	West Virginia	27.6		48	Utah	9.5
16	Wisconsin	23.0		49	Hawaii	8.4
23	Wyoming	20.8		NA	Alaska**	NA
					District of Columbia	19.1

Source: Morgan Quitno Press using data from American Cancer Society
"1999 Facts & Figures" (Copyright 1999, Reprinted with permission from the American Cancer Society)
*These estimates are offered as a rough guide and should be interpreted with caution. They are calculated according to the distribution of estimated 1999 cancer deaths by state. Rates calculated using 1998 Census resident population estimates.
**Fewer than 50 cases.

Estimated New Female Breast Cancer Cases in 1999

National Estimated Total = 175,000 New Cases*

ALPHA ORDER

RANK	STATE	CASES	% of USA
25	Alabama	2,500	1.4%
50	Alaska	200	0.1%
23	Arizona	2,600	1.5%
31	Arkansas	1,700	1.0%
1	California	16,900	9.7%
30	Colorado	2,000	1.1%
27	Connecticut	2,100	1.2%
44	Delaware	500	0.3%
3	Florida	11,900	6.8%
13	Georgia	4,000	2.3%
44	Hawaii	500	0.3%
40	Idaho	700	0.4%
6	Illinois	8,500	4.9%
14	Indiana	3,900	2.2%
27	Iowa	2,100	1.2%
31	Kansas	1,700	1.0%
22	Kentucky	2,700	1.5%
20	Louisiana	3,100	1.8%
35	Maine	1,000	0.6%
17	Maryland	3,500	2.0%
11	Massachusetts	4,400	2.5%
8	Michigan	6,500	3.7%
21	Minnesota	2,800	1.6%
31	Mississippi	1,700	1.0%
16	Missouri	3,600	2.1%
43	Montana	600	0.3%
35	Nebraska	1,000	0.6%
35	Nevada	1,000	0.6%
40	New Hampshire	700	0.4%
9	New Jersey	5,900	3.4%
35	New Mexico	1,000	0.6%
2	New York	13,000	7.4%
10	North Carolina	4,700	2.7%
47	North Dakota	400	0.2%
7	Ohio	8,400	4.8%
26	Oklahoma	2,300	1.3%
27	Oregon	2,100	1.2%
5	Pennsylvania	10,000	5.7%
40	Rhode Island	700	0.4%
23	South Carolina	2,600	1.5%
44	South Dakota	500	0.3%
14	Tennessee	3,900	2.2%
4	Texas	11,300	6.5%
39	Utah	800	0.5%
48	Vermont	300	0.2%
12	Virginia	4,200	2.4%
19	Washington	3,300	1.9%
34	West Virginia	1,200	0.7%
18	Wisconsin	3,400	1.9%
48	Wyoming	300	0.2%

RANK ORDER

RANK	STATE	CASES	% of USA
1	California	16,900	9.7%
2	New York	13,000	7.4%
3	Florida	11,900	6.8%
4	Texas	11,300	6.5%
5	Pennsylvania	10,000	5.7%
6	Illinois	8,500	4.9%
7	Ohio	8,400	4.8%
8	Michigan	6,500	3.7%
9	New Jersey	5,900	3.4%
10	North Carolina	4,700	2.7%
11	Massachusetts	4,400	2.5%
12	Virginia	4,200	2.4%
13	Georgia	4,000	2.3%
14	Indiana	3,900	2.2%
14	Tennessee	3,900	2.2%
16	Missouri	3,600	2.1%
17	Maryland	3,500	2.0%
18	Wisconsin	3,400	1.9%
19	Washington	3,300	1.9%
20	Louisiana	3,100	1.8%
21	Minnesota	2,800	1.6%
22	Kentucky	2,700	1.5%
23	Arizona	2,600	1.5%
23	South Carolina	2,600	1.5%
25	Alabama	2,500	1.4%
26	Oklahoma	2,300	1.3%
27	Connecticut	2,100	1.2%
27	Iowa	2,100	1.2%
27	Oregon	2,100	1.2%
30	Colorado	2,000	1.1%
31	Arkansas	1,700	1.0%
31	Kansas	1,700	1.0%
31	Mississippi	1,700	1.0%
34	West Virginia	1,200	0.7%
35	Maine	1,000	0.6%
35	Nebraska	1,000	0.6%
35	Nevada	1,000	0.6%
35	New Mexico	1,000	0.6%
39	Utah	800	0.5%
40	Idaho	700	0.4%
40	New Hampshire	700	0.4%
40	Rhode Island	700	0.4%
43	Montana	600	0.3%
44	Delaware	500	0.3%
44	Hawaii	500	0.3%
44	South Dakota	500	0.3%
47	North Dakota	400	0.2%
48	Vermont	300	0.2%
48	Wyoming	300	0.2%
50	Alaska	200	0.1%
	District of Columbia	500	0.3%

Source: American Cancer Society
    "1999 Facts & Figures" (Copyright 1999, Reprinted with permission from the American Cancer Society)
*These estimates are offered as a rough guide and should be interpreted with caution. They are calculated according to the distribution of estimated 1999 cancer deaths by state.

Estimated Rate of New Female Breast Cancer Cases in 1999

National Estimated Rate = 128.1 New Cases per 100,000 Female Population*

ALPHA ORDER

RANK	STATE	RATE
43	Alabama	111.5
50	Alaska	69.2
42	Arizona	113.2
20	Arkansas	130.6
44	California	104.9
46	Colorado	102.0
29	Connecticut	125.0
19	Delaware	133.3
2	Florida	158.0
45	Georgia	104.3
48	Hawaii	84.8
39	Idaho	115.7
8	Illinois	139.7
21	Indiana	129.8
5	Iowa	143.8
25	Kansas	129.1
15	Kentucky	134.4
11	Louisiana	137.5
3	Maine	157.5
16	Maryland	133.9
9	Massachusetts	139.1
21	Michigan	129.8
36	Minnesota	118.0
34	Mississippi	119.8
23	Missouri	129.5
13	Montana	136.1
35	Nebraska	118.4
33	Nevada	121.7
37	New Hampshire	117.7
6	New Jersey	142.3
41	New Mexico	114.0
10	New York	138.4
31	North Carolina	123.2
30	North Dakota	124.5
4	Ohio	145.6
14	Oklahoma	135.8
26	Oregon	128.1
1	Pennsylvania	160.5
12	Rhode Island	136.7
17	South Carolina	133.8
18	South Dakota	133.6
7	Tennessee	140.7
40	Texas	115.0
49	Utah	77.4
47	Vermont	100.4
32	Virginia	122.2
38	Washington	117.3
27	West Virginia	127.8
23	Wisconsin	129.5
28	Wyoming	126.0

RANK ORDER

RANK	STATE	RATE
1	Pennsylvania	160.5
2	Florida	158.0
3	Maine	157.5
4	Ohio	145.6
5	Iowa	143.8
6	New Jersey	142.3
7	Tennessee	140.7
8	Illinois	139.7
9	Massachusetts	139.1
10	New York	138.4
11	Louisiana	137.5
12	Rhode Island	136.7
13	Montana	136.1
14	Oklahoma	135.8
15	Kentucky	134.4
16	Maryland	133.9
17	South Carolina	133.8
18	South Dakota	133.6
19	Delaware	133.3
20	Arkansas	130.6
21	Indiana	129.8
21	Michigan	129.8
23	Missouri	129.5
23	Wisconsin	129.5
25	Kansas	129.1
26	Oregon	128.1
27	West Virginia	127.8
28	Wyoming	126.0
29	Connecticut	125.0
30	North Dakota	124.5
31	North Carolina	123.2
32	Virginia	122.2
33	Nevada	121.7
34	Mississippi	119.8
35	Nebraska	118.4
36	Minnesota	118.0
37	New Hampshire	117.7
38	Washington	117.3
39	Idaho	115.7
40	Texas	115.0
41	New Mexico	114.0
42	Arizona	113.2
43	Alabama	111.5
44	California	104.9
45	Georgia	104.3
46	Colorado	102.0
47	Vermont	100.4
48	Hawaii	84.8
49	Utah	77.4
50	Alaska	69.2
	District of Columbia	178.1

Source: Morgan Quitno Press using data from American Cancer Society
"1999 Facts & Figures" (Copyright 1999, Reprinted with permission from the American Cancer Society)
These estimates are offered as a rough guide and should be interpreted with caution. They are calculated according to the distribution of estimated 1999 cancer deaths by state. Rates calculated using 1997 Census female resident population estimates.

Percent of Women Age 50 and Older
Who Had a Breast Exam Within the Past Two Years: 1997
National Median = 77.0% of Women 50 Years and Older

ALPHA ORDER

RANK	STATE	PERCENT
34	Alabama	74.0
15	Alaska	79.7
29	Arizona	75.6
50	Arkansas	63.4
25	California	77.2
18	Colorado	78.5
26	Connecticut	76.4
11	Delaware	81.3
21	Florida	78.2
7	Georgia	82.8
12	Hawaii	80.9
43	Idaho	71.7
41	Illinois	72.4
48	Indiana	69.4
35	Iowa	73.7
26	Kansas	76.4
36	Kentucky	73.3
49	Louisiana	64.8
5	Maine	83.0
3	Maryland	84.5
4	Massachusetts	83.8
23	Michigan	77.6
17	Minnesota	78.7
36	Mississippi	73.3
33	Missouri	74.5
20	Montana	78.4
44	Nebraska	71.1
47	Nevada	69.8
2	New Hampshire	85.3
38	New Jersey	73.2
40	New Mexico	72.5
1	New York	86.4
8	North Carolina	82.4
29	North Dakota	75.6
9	Ohio	81.7
9	Oklahoma	81.7
13	Oregon	80.1
46	Pennsylvania	70.3
15	Rhode Island	79.7
5	South Carolina	83.0
28	South Dakota	75.9
14	Tennessee	79.8
42	Texas	71.9
24	Utah	77.3
31	Vermont	75.5
18	Virginia	78.5
22	Washington	77.7
39	West Virginia	72.7
32	Wisconsin	75.3
45	Wyoming	70.8

RANK ORDER

RANK	STATE	PERCENT
1	New York	86.4
2	New Hampshire	85.3
3	Maryland	84.5
4	Massachusetts	83.8
5	Maine	83.0
5	South Carolina	83.0
7	Georgia	82.8
8	North Carolina	82.4
9	Ohio	81.7
9	Oklahoma	81.7
11	Delaware	81.3
12	Hawaii	80.9
13	Oregon	80.1
14	Tennessee	79.8
15	Alaska	79.7
15	Rhode Island	79.7
17	Minnesota	78.7
18	Colorado	78.5
18	Virginia	78.5
20	Montana	78.4
21	Florida	78.2
22	Washington	77.7
23	Michigan	77.6
24	Utah	77.3
25	California	77.2
26	Connecticut	76.4
26	Kansas	76.4
28	South Dakota	75.9
29	Arizona	75.6
29	North Dakota	75.6
31	Vermont	75.5
32	Wisconsin	75.3
33	Missouri	74.5
34	Alabama	74.0
35	Iowa	73.7
36	Kentucky	73.3
36	Mississippi	73.3
38	New Jersey	73.2
39	West Virginia	72.7
40	New Mexico	72.5
41	Illinois	72.4
42	Texas	71.9
43	Idaho	71.7
44	Nebraska	71.1
45	Wyoming	70.8
46	Pennsylvania	70.3
47	Nevada	69.8
48	Indiana	69.4
49	Louisiana	64.8
50	Arkansas	63.4

| | District of Columbia | 83.3 |

Source: U.S. Department of Health and Human Services, Centers for Disease Control and Prevention
"1997 Behavioral Risk Factor Surveillance Summary Prevalence Report" (August 17, 1998)

Estimated New Colon and Rectum Cancer Cases in 1999

National Estimated Total = 129,400 New Cases*

ALPHA ORDER

RANK	STATE	CASES	% of USA
26	Alabama	1,600	1.2%
49	Alaska	200	0.2%
22	Arizona	2,000	1.5%
30	Arkansas	1,400	1.1%
1	California	11,200	8.7%
31	Colorado	1,300	1.0%
28	Connecticut	1,500	1.2%
42	Delaware	400	0.3%
3	Florida	8,900	6.9%
16	Georgia	2,700	2.1%
42	Hawaii	400	0.3%
42	Idaho	400	0.3%
6	Illinois	6,200	4.8%
12	Indiana	3,000	2.3%
25	Iowa	1,700	1.3%
33	Kansas	1,200	0.9%
20	Kentucky	2,200	1.7%
20	Louisiana	2,200	1.7%
37	Maine	700	0.5%
17	Maryland	2,600	2.0%
11	Massachusetts	3,600	2.8%
8	Michigan	4,800	3.7%
22	Minnesota	2,000	1.5%
31	Mississippi	1,300	1.0%
12	Missouri	3,000	2.3%
42	Montana	400	0.3%
35	Nebraska	1,000	0.8%
36	Nevada	800	0.6%
38	New Hampshire	600	0.5%
9	New Jersey	4,700	3.6%
38	New Mexico	600	0.5%
2	New York	9,400	7.3%
10	North Carolina	3,900	3.0%
42	North Dakota	400	0.3%
7	Ohio	6,100	4.7%
26	Oklahoma	1,600	1.2%
28	Oregon	1,500	1.2%
5	Pennsylvania	7,700	6.0%
38	Rhode Island	600	0.5%
24	South Carolina	1,900	1.5%
47	South Dakota	300	0.2%
15	Tennessee	2,800	2.2%
4	Texas	8,400	6.5%
38	Utah	600	0.5%
47	Vermont	300	0.2%
12	Virginia	3,000	2.3%
19	Washington	2,300	1.8%
34	West Virginia	1,100	0.9%
18	Wisconsin	2,500	1.9%
49	Wyoming	200	0.2%

RANK ORDER

RANK	STATE	CASES	% of USA
1	California	11,200	8.7%
2	New York	9,400	7.3%
3	Florida	8,900	6.9%
4	Texas	8,400	6.5%
5	Pennsylvania	7,700	6.0%
6	Illinois	6,200	4.8%
7	Ohio	6,100	4.7%
8	Michigan	4,800	3.7%
9	New Jersey	4,700	3.6%
10	North Carolina	3,900	3.0%
11	Massachusetts	3,600	2.8%
12	Indiana	3,000	2.3%
12	Missouri	3,000	2.3%
12	Virginia	3,000	2.3%
15	Tennessee	2,800	2.2%
16	Georgia	2,700	2.1%
17	Maryland	2,600	2.0%
18	Wisconsin	2,500	1.9%
19	Washington	2,300	1.8%
20	Kentucky	2,200	1.7%
20	Louisiana	2,200	1.7%
22	Arizona	2,000	1.5%
22	Minnesota	2,000	1.5%
24	South Carolina	1,900	1.5%
25	Iowa	1,700	1.3%
26	Alabama	1,600	1.2%
26	Oklahoma	1,600	1.2%
28	Connecticut	1,500	1.2%
28	Oregon	1,500	1.2%
30	Arkansas	1,400	1.1%
31	Colorado	1,300	1.0%
31	Mississippi	1,300	1.0%
33	Kansas	1,200	0.9%
34	West Virginia	1,100	0.9%
35	Nebraska	1,000	0.8%
36	Nevada	800	0.6%
37	Maine	700	0.5%
38	New Hampshire	600	0.5%
38	New Mexico	600	0.5%
38	Rhode Island	600	0.5%
38	Utah	600	0.5%
42	Delaware	400	0.3%
42	Hawaii	400	0.3%
42	Idaho	400	0.3%
42	Montana	400	0.3%
42	North Dakota	400	0.3%
47	South Dakota	300	0.2%
47	Vermont	300	0.2%
49	Alaska	200	0.2%
49	Wyoming	200	0.2%
	District of Columbia	300	0.2%

Source: American Cancer Society
"1999 Facts & Figures" (Copyright 1999, Reprinted with permission from the American Cancer Society)
These estimates are offered as a rough guide and should be interpreted with caution. They are calculated according to the distribution of estimated 1999 cancer deaths by state.

Estimated Rate of New Colon and Rectum Cancer Cases in 1999

National Estimated Rate = 47.9 New Cases per 100,000 Population*

ALPHA ORDER				RANK ORDER		
RANK	STATE	RATE		RANK	STATE	RATE
42	Alabama	36.8		1	Pennsylvania	64.2
48	Alaska	32.6		2	North Dakota	62.7
36	Arizona	42.8		3	Rhode Island	60.7
12	Arkansas	55.2		3	West Virginia	60.7
45	California	34.3		5	Nebraska	60.1
47	Colorado	32.7		6	Florida	59.7
30	Connecticut	45.8		7	Iowa	59.4
15	Delaware	53.8		8	Massachusetts	58.6
6	Florida	59.7		9	New Jersey	57.9
43	Georgia	35.3		10	Maine	56.3
46	Hawaii	33.5		11	Kentucky	55.9
48	Idaho	32.6		12	Arkansas	55.2
19	Illinois	51.5		12	Missouri	55.2
20	Indiana	50.9		14	Ohio	54.4
7	Iowa	59.4		15	Delaware	53.8
33	Kansas	45.6		16	New York	51.7
11	Kentucky	55.9		16	North Carolina	51.7
24	Louisiana	50.4		18	Tennessee	51.6
10	Maine	56.3		19	Illinois	51.5
22	Maryland	50.6		20	Indiana	50.9
8	Massachusetts	58.6		21	Vermont	50.8
26	Michigan	48.9		22	Maryland	50.6
38	Minnesota	42.3		22	New Hampshire	50.6
29	Mississippi	47.2		24	Louisiana	50.4
12	Missouri	55.2		25	South Carolina	49.5
34	Montana	45.4		26	Michigan	48.9
5	Nebraska	60.1		27	Wisconsin	47.9
30	Nevada	45.8		28	Oklahoma	47.8
22	New Hampshire	50.6		29	Mississippi	47.2
9	New Jersey	57.9		30	Connecticut	45.8
44	New Mexico	34.5		30	Nevada	45.8
16	New York	51.7		32	Oregon	45.7
16	North Carolina	51.7		33	Kansas	45.6
2	North Dakota	62.7		34	Montana	45.4
14	Ohio	54.4		35	Virginia	44.2
28	Oklahoma	47.8		36	Arizona	42.8
32	Oregon	45.7		37	Texas	42.5
1	Pennsylvania	64.2		38	Minnesota	42.3
3	Rhode Island	60.7		39	Wyoming	41.6
25	South Carolina	49.5		40	South Dakota	40.6
40	South Dakota	40.6		41	Washington	40.4
18	Tennessee	51.6		42	Alabama	36.8
37	Texas	42.5		43	Georgia	35.3
50	Utah	28.6		44	New Mexico	34.5
21	Vermont	50.8		45	California	34.3
35	Virginia	44.2		46	Hawaii	33.5
41	Washington	40.4		47	Colorado	32.7
3	West Virginia	60.7		48	Alaska	32.6
27	Wisconsin	47.9		48	Idaho	32.6
39	Wyoming	41.6		50	Utah	28.6
					District of Columbia	57.3

Source: Morgan Quitno Press using data from American Cancer Society
    "1999 Facts & Figures" (Copyright 1999, Reprinted with permission from the American Cancer Society)
*These estimates are offered as a rough guide and should be interpreted with caution. They are calculated
according to the distribution of estimated 1999 cancer deaths by state. Rates calculated using 1998 Census
resident population estimates.

Estimated New Lung Cancer Cases in 1999

National Estimated Total = 171,600 New Cases*

ALPHA ORDER

RANK	STATE	CASES	% of USA
21	Alabama	2,900	1.7%
50	Alaska	200	0.1%
22	Arizona	2,800	1.6%
27	Arkansas	2,300	1.3%
1	California	14,600	8.5%
33	Colorado	1,600	0.9%
29	Connecticut	2,000	1.2%
41	Delaware	600	0.3%
2	Florida	13,000	7.6%
11	Georgia	4,400	2.6%
41	Hawaii	600	0.3%
41	Idaho	600	0.3%
7	Illinois	7,800	4.5%
13	Indiana	4,300	2.5%
29	Iowa	2,000	1.2%
33	Kansas	1,600	0.9%
17	Kentucky	3,500	2.0%
20	Louisiana	3,000	1.7%
36	Maine	1,100	0.6%
19	Maryland	3,200	1.9%
15	Massachusetts	4,100	2.4%
8	Michigan	6,400	3.7%
26	Minnesota	2,400	1.4%
31	Mississippi	1,800	1.0%
11	Missouri	4,400	2.6%
41	Montana	600	0.3%
37	Nebraska	1,000	0.6%
35	Nevada	1,200	0.7%
38	New Hampshire	800	0.5%
10	New Jersey	4,900	2.9%
38	New Mexico	800	0.5%
4	New York	10,700	6.2%
9	North Carolina	5,300	3.1%
45	North Dakota	400	0.2%
6	Ohio	8,300	4.8%
24	Oklahoma	2,500	1.5%
28	Oregon	2,200	1.3%
5	Pennsylvania	9,000	5.2%
38	Rhode Island	800	0.5%
24	South Carolina	2,500	1.5%
45	South Dakota	400	0.2%
13	Tennessee	4,300	2.5%
3	Texas	11,500	6.7%
45	Utah	400	0.2%
45	Vermont	400	0.2%
15	Virginia	4,100	2.4%
18	Washington	3,400	2.0%
32	West Virginia	1,700	1.0%
22	Wisconsin	2,800	1.6%
49	Wyoming	300	0.2%

RANK ORDER

RANK	STATE	CASES	% of USA
1	California	14,600	8.5%
2	Florida	13,000	7.6%
3	Texas	11,500	6.7%
4	New York	10,700	6.2%
5	Pennsylvania	9,000	5.2%
6	Ohio	8,300	4.8%
7	Illinois	7,800	4.5%
8	Michigan	6,400	3.7%
9	North Carolina	5,300	3.1%
10	New Jersey	4,900	2.9%
11	Georgia	4,400	2.6%
11	Missouri	4,400	2.6%
13	Indiana	4,300	2.5%
13	Tennessee	4,300	2.5%
15	Massachusetts	4,100	2.4%
15	Virginia	4,100	2.4%
17	Kentucky	3,500	2.0%
18	Washington	3,400	2.0%
19	Maryland	3,200	1.9%
20	Louisiana	3,000	1.7%
21	Alabama	2,900	1.7%
22	Arizona	2,800	1.6%
22	Wisconsin	2,800	1.6%
24	Oklahoma	2,500	1.5%
24	South Carolina	2,500	1.5%
26	Minnesota	2,400	1.4%
27	Arkansas	2,300	1.3%
28	Oregon	2,200	1.3%
29	Connecticut	2,000	1.2%
29	Iowa	2,000	1.2%
31	Mississippi	1,800	1.0%
32	West Virginia	1,700	1.0%
33	Colorado	1,600	0.9%
33	Kansas	1,600	0.9%
35	Nevada	1,200	0.7%
36	Maine	1,100	0.6%
37	Nebraska	1,000	0.6%
38	New Hampshire	800	0.5%
38	New Mexico	800	0.5%
38	Rhode Island	800	0.5%
41	Delaware	600	0.3%
41	Hawaii	600	0.3%
41	Idaho	600	0.3%
41	Montana	600	0.3%
45	North Dakota	400	0.2%
45	South Dakota	400	0.2%
45	Utah	400	0.2%
45	Vermont	400	0.2%
49	Wyoming	300	0.2%
50	Alaska	200	0.1%
	District of Columbia	400	0.2%

Source: American Cancer Society
"1999 Facts & Figures" (Copyright 1999, Reprinted with permission from the American Cancer Society)
These estimates are offered as a rough guide and should be interpreted with caution. They are calculated according to the distribution of estimated 1999 cancer deaths by state.

Estimated Rate of New Lung Cancer Cases in 1999

National Estimated Rate = 63.5 New Cases per 100,000 Population*

ALPHA ORDER			RANK ORDER		
RANK	STATE	RATE	RANK	STATE	RATE
23	Alabama	66.6	1	West Virginia	93.9
49	Alaska	32.6	2	Arkansas	90.6
36	Arizona	60.0	3	Kentucky	88.9
2	Arkansas	90.6	4	Maine	88.4
47	California	44.7	5	Florida	87.2
48	Colorado	40.3	6	Missouri	80.9
31	Connecticut	61.1	6	Rhode Island	80.9
8	Delaware	80.7	8	Delaware	80.7
5	Florida	87.2	9	Tennessee	79.2
40	Georgia	57.6	10	Pennsylvania	75.0
44	Hawaii	50.3	11	Oklahoma	74.7
45	Idaho	48.8	12	Ohio	74.0
27	Illinois	64.8	13	Indiana	72.9
13	Indiana	72.9	14	North Carolina	70.2
15	Iowa	69.9	15	Iowa	69.9
32	Kansas	60.9	16	Louisiana	68.7
3	Kentucky	88.9	16	Nevada	68.7
16	Louisiana	68.7	18	Montana	68.1
4	Maine	88.4	19	Vermont	67.7
30	Maryland	62.3	20	New Hampshire	67.5
22	Massachusetts	66.7	21	Oregon	67.0
25	Michigan	65.2	22	Massachusetts	66.7
43	Minnesota	50.8	23	Alabama	66.6
24	Mississippi	65.4	24	Mississippi	65.4
6	Missouri	80.9	25	Michigan	65.2
18	Montana	68.1	25	South Carolina	65.2
35	Nebraska	60.1	27	Illinois	64.8
16	Nevada	68.7	28	North Dakota	62.7
20	New Hampshire	67.5	29	Wyoming	62.4
33	New Jersey	60.4	30	Maryland	62.3
46	New Mexico	46.1	31	Connecticut	61.1
38	New York	58.9	32	Kansas	60.9
14	North Carolina	70.2	33	New Jersey	60.4
28	North Dakota	62.7	33	Virginia	60.4
12	Ohio	74.0	35	Nebraska	60.1
11	Oklahoma	74.7	36	Arizona	60.0
21	Oregon	67.0	37	Washington	59.8
10	Pennsylvania	75.0	38	New York	58.9
6	Rhode Island	80.9	39	Texas	58.2
25	South Carolina	65.2	40	Georgia	57.6
41	South Dakota	54.2	41	South Dakota	54.2
9	Tennessee	79.2	42	Wisconsin	53.6
39	Texas	58.2	43	Minnesota	50.8
50	Utah	19.0	44	Hawaii	50.3
19	Vermont	67.7	45	Idaho	48.8
33	Virginia	60.4	46	New Mexico	46.1
37	Washington	59.8	47	California	44.7
1	West Virginia	93.9	48	Colorado	40.3
42	Wisconsin	53.6	49	Alaska	32.6
29	Wyoming	62.4	50	Utah	19.0
				District of Columbia	76.5

Source: Morgan Quitno Press using data from American Cancer Society
"1999 Facts & Figures" (Copyright 1999, Reprinted with permission from the American Cancer Society)
These estimates are offered as a rough guide and should be interpreted with caution. They are calculated according to the distribution of estimated 1999 cancer deaths by state. Rates calculated using 1998 Census resident population estimates.

Estimated New Non-Hodgkin's Lymphoma Cases in 1999

National Estimated Total = 56,800 New Cases*

ALPHA ORDER

RANK	STATE	CASES	% of USA
20	Alabama	900	1.6%
NA	Alaska**	NA	NA
20	Arizona	900	1.6%
30	Arkansas	600	1.1%
1	California	5,000	8.8%
29	Colorado	700	1.2%
23	Connecticut	800	1.4%
42	Delaware	200	0.4%
3	Florida	4,000	7.0%
19	Georgia	1,000	1.8%
42	Hawaii	200	0.4%
42	Idaho	200	0.4%
7	Illinois	2,700	4.8%
12	Indiana	1,300	2.3%
23	Iowa	800	1.4%
30	Kansas	600	1.1%
23	Kentucky	800	1.4%
23	Louisiana	800	1.4%
36	Maine	300	0.5%
20	Maryland	900	1.6%
10	Massachusetts	1,500	2.6%
8	Michigan	2,100	3.7%
14	Minnesota	1,200	2.1%
33	Mississippi	500	0.9%
14	Missouri	1,200	2.1%
42	Montana	200	0.4%
36	Nebraska	300	0.5%
36	Nevada	300	0.5%
36	New Hampshire	300	0.5%
9	New Jersey	2,000	3.5%
36	New Mexico	300	0.5%
2	New York	4,100	7.2%
11	North Carolina	1,400	2.5%
42	North Dakota	200	0.4%
6	Ohio	2,800	4.9%
23	Oklahoma	800	1.4%
23	Oregon	800	1.4%
5	Pennsylvania	3,200	5.6%
36	Rhode Island	300	0.5%
30	South Carolina	600	1.1%
42	South Dakota	200	0.4%
14	Tennessee	1,200	2.1%
4	Texas	3,900	6.9%
34	Utah	400	0.7%
48	Vermont	100	0.2%
14	Virginia	1,200	2.1%
18	Washington	1,100	1.9%
34	West Virginia	400	0.7%
12	Wisconsin	1,300	2.3%
48	Wyoming	100	0.2%

RANK ORDER

RANK	STATE	CASES	% of USA
1	California	5,000	8.8%
2	New York	4,100	7.2%
3	Florida	4,000	7.0%
4	Texas	3,900	6.9%
5	Pennsylvania	3,200	5.6%
6	Ohio	2,800	4.9%
7	Illinois	2,700	4.8%
8	Michigan	2,100	3.7%
9	New Jersey	2,000	3.5%
10	Massachusetts	1,500	2.6%
11	North Carolina	1,400	2.5%
12	Indiana	1,300	2.3%
12	Wisconsin	1,300	2.3%
14	Minnesota	1,200	2.1%
14	Missouri	1,200	2.1%
14	Tennessee	1,200	2.1%
14	Virginia	1,200	2.1%
18	Washington	1,100	1.9%
19	Georgia	1,000	1.8%
20	Alabama	900	1.6%
20	Arizona	900	1.6%
20	Maryland	900	1.6%
23	Connecticut	800	1.4%
23	Iowa	800	1.4%
23	Kentucky	800	1.4%
23	Louisiana	800	1.4%
23	Oklahoma	800	1.4%
23	Oregon	800	1.4%
29	Colorado	700	1.2%
30	Arkansas	600	1.1%
30	Kansas	600	1.1%
30	South Carolina	600	1.1%
33	Mississippi	500	0.9%
34	Utah	400	0.7%
34	West Virginia	400	0.7%
36	Maine	300	0.5%
36	Nebraska	300	0.5%
36	Nevada	300	0.5%
36	New Hampshire	300	0.5%
36	New Mexico	300	0.5%
36	Rhode Island	300	0.5%
42	Delaware	200	0.4%
42	Hawaii	200	0.4%
42	Idaho	200	0.4%
42	Montana	200	0.4%
42	North Dakota	200	0.4%
42	South Dakota	200	0.4%
48	Vermont	100	0.2%
48	Wyoming	100	0.2%
NA	Alaska**	NA	NA
	District of Columbia	100	0.2%

Source: American Cancer Society
   "1999 Facts & Figures" (Copyright 1999, Reprinted with permission from the American Cancer Society)
*These estimates are offered as a rough guide and should be interpreted with caution. They are calculated according to the distribution of estimated 1999 cancer deaths by state.
**Fewer than 50 cases.

Estimated Rate of New Non-Hodgkin's Lymphoma Cases in 1999

National Estimated Rate = 21.0 New Cases per 100,000 Population*

ALPHA ORDER

RANK	STATE	RATE
29	Alabama	20.7
NA	Alaska**	NA
32	Arizona	19.3
18	Arkansas	23.6
48	California	15.3
40	Colorado	17.6
13	Connecticut	24.4
5	Delaware	26.9
6	Florida	26.8
49	Georgia	13.1
45	Hawaii	16.8
46	Idaho	16.3
22	Illinois	22.4
26	Indiana	22.0
3	Iowa	27.9
19	Kansas	22.8
30	Kentucky	20.3
36	Louisiana	18.3
16	Maine	24.1
41	Maryland	17.5
13	Massachusetts	24.4
27	Michigan	21.4
8	Minnesota	25.4
37	Mississippi	18.2
23	Missouri	22.1
20	Montana	22.7
38	Nebraska	18.0
43	Nevada	17.2
9	New Hampshire	25.3
12	New Jersey	24.6
42	New Mexico	17.3
21	New York	22.6
35	North Carolina	18.6
1	North Dakota	31.3
10	Ohio	25.0
17	Oklahoma	23.9
13	Oregon	24.4
7	Pennsylvania	26.7
2	Rhode Island	30.3
47	South Carolina	15.6
4	South Dakota	27.1
23	Tennessee	22.1
31	Texas	19.7
34	Utah	19.0
44	Vermont	16.9
39	Virginia	17.7
32	Washington	19.3
23	West Virginia	22.1
11	Wisconsin	24.9
28	Wyoming	20.8

RANK ORDER

RANK	STATE	RATE
1	North Dakota	31.3
2	Rhode Island	30.3
3	Iowa	27.9
4	South Dakota	27.1
5	Delaware	26.9
6	Florida	26.8
7	Pennsylvania	26.7
8	Minnesota	25.4
9	New Hampshire	25.3
10	Ohio	25.0
11	Wisconsin	24.9
12	New Jersey	24.6
13	Connecticut	24.4
13	Massachusetts	24.4
13	Oregon	24.4
16	Maine	24.1
17	Oklahoma	23.9
18	Arkansas	23.6
19	Kansas	22.8
20	Montana	22.7
21	New York	22.6
22	Illinois	22.4
23	Missouri	22.1
23	Tennessee	22.1
23	West Virginia	22.1
26	Indiana	22.0
27	Michigan	21.4
28	Wyoming	20.8
29	Alabama	20.7
30	Kentucky	20.3
31	Texas	19.7
32	Arizona	19.3
32	Washington	19.3
34	Utah	19.0
35	North Carolina	18.6
36	Louisiana	18.3
37	Mississippi	18.2
38	Nebraska	18.0
39	Virginia	17.7
40	Colorado	17.6
41	Maryland	17.5
42	New Mexico	17.3
43	Nevada	17.2
44	Vermont	16.9
45	Hawaii	16.8
46	Idaho	16.3
47	South Carolina	15.6
48	California	15.3
49	Georgia	13.1
NA	Alaska**	NA
	District of Columbia	19.1

Source: Morgan Quitno Press using data from American Cancer Society
   "1999 Facts & Figures" (Copyright 1999, Reprinted with permission from the American Cancer Society)
*These estimates are offered as a rough guide and should be interpreted with caution. They are calculated according to the distribution of estimated 1999 cancer deaths by state. Rates calculated using 1998 Census resident population estimates.

Estimated New Ovarian Cancer Cases in 1999

National Estimated Total = 25,200 New Cases*

ALPHA ORDER

RANK	STATE	CASES	% of USA
20	Alabama	400	1.6%
NA	Alaska**	NA	NA
17	Arizona	500	2.0%
26	Arkansas	300	1.2%
1	California	2,600	10.3%
32	Colorado	200	0.8%
26	Connecticut	300	1.2%
35	Delaware	100	0.4%
2	Florida	1,800	7.1%
11	Georgia	600	2.4%
35	Hawaii	100	0.4%
35	Idaho	100	0.4%
6	Illinois	1,100	4.4%
11	Indiana	600	2.4%
26	Iowa	300	1.2%
26	Kansas	300	1.2%
20	Kentucky	400	1.6%
26	Louisiana	300	1.2%
35	Maine	100	0.4%
20	Maryland	400	1.6%
17	Massachusetts	500	2.0%
9	Michigan	800	3.2%
20	Minnesota	400	1.6%
32	Mississippi	200	0.8%
11	Missouri	600	2.4%
35	Montana	100	0.4%
35	Nebraska	100	0.4%
35	Nevada	100	0.4%
35	New Hampshire	100	0.4%
8	New Jersey	900	3.6%
35	New Mexico	100	0.4%
2	New York	1,800	7.1%
10	North Carolina	700	2.8%
35	North Dakota	100	0.4%
7	Ohio	1,000	4.0%
26	Oklahoma	300	1.2%
20	Oregon	400	1.6%
5	Pennsylvania	1,400	5.6%
35	Rhode Island	100	0.4%
20	South Carolina	400	1.6%
35	South Dakota	100	0.4%
11	Tennessee	600	2.4%
4	Texas	1,500	6.0%
35	Utah	100	0.4%
35	Vermont	100	0.4%
17	Virginia	500	2.0%
11	Washington	600	2.4%
32	West Virginia	200	0.8%
11	Wisconsin	600	2.4%
NA	Wyoming**	NA	NA

RANK ORDER

RANK	STATE	CASES	% of USA
1	California	2,600	10.3%
2	Florida	1,800	7.1%
2	New York	1,800	7.1%
4	Texas	1,500	6.0%
5	Pennsylvania	1,400	5.6%
6	Illinois	1,100	4.4%
7	Ohio	1,000	4.0%
8	New Jersey	900	3.6%
9	Michigan	800	3.2%
10	North Carolina	700	2.8%
11	Georgia	600	2.4%
11	Indiana	600	2.4%
11	Missouri	600	2.4%
11	Tennessee	600	2.4%
11	Washington	600	2.4%
11	Wisconsin	600	2.4%
17	Arizona	500	2.0%
17	Massachusetts	500	2.0%
17	Virginia	500	2.0%
20	Alabama	400	1.6%
20	Kentucky	400	1.6%
20	Maryland	400	1.6%
20	Minnesota	400	1.6%
20	Oregon	400	1.6%
20	South Carolina	400	1.6%
26	Arkansas	300	1.2%
26	Connecticut	300	1.2%
26	Iowa	300	1.2%
26	Kansas	300	1.2%
26	Louisiana	300	1.2%
26	Oklahoma	300	1.2%
32	Colorado	200	0.8%
32	Mississippi	200	0.8%
32	West Virginia	200	0.8%
35	Delaware	100	0.4%
35	Hawaii	100	0.4%
35	Idaho	100	0.4%
35	Maine	100	0.4%
35	Montana	100	0.4%
35	Nebraska	100	0.4%
35	Nevada	100	0.4%
35	New Hampshire	100	0.4%
35	New Mexico	100	0.4%
35	North Dakota	100	0.4%
35	Rhode Island	100	0.4%
35	South Dakota	100	0.4%
35	Utah	100	0.4%
35	Vermont	100	0.4%
NA	Alaska**	NA	NA
NA	Wyoming**	NA	NA
	District of Columbia	100	0.4%

Source: American Cancer Society
"1999 Facts & Figures" (Copyright 1999, Reprinted with permission from the American Cancer Society)
*These estimates are offered as a rough guide and should be interpreted with caution. They are calculated according to the distribution of estimated 1999 cancer deaths by state.
**Fewer than 50 cases.

Estimated Rate of New Ovarian Cancer Cases in 1999

National Estimated Rate = 18.4 New Cases per 100,000 Female Population*

<table>
<tr><td colspan="3">ALPHA ORDER</td><td colspan="3">RANK ORDER</td></tr>
<tr><td>RANK</td><td>STATE</td><td>RATE</td><td>RANK</td><td>STATE</td><td>RATE</td></tr>
<tr><td>27</td><td>Alabama</td><td>17.8</td><td>1</td><td>Vermont</td><td>33.5</td></tr>
<tr><td>NA</td><td>Alaska**</td><td>NA</td><td>2</td><td>North Dakota</td><td>31.1</td></tr>
<tr><td>12</td><td>Arizona</td><td>21.8</td><td>3</td><td>Delaware</td><td>26.7</td></tr>
<tr><td>7</td><td>Arkansas</td><td>23.1</td><td>3</td><td>South Dakota</td><td>26.7</td></tr>
<tr><td>34</td><td>California</td><td>16.1</td><td>5</td><td>Oregon</td><td>24.4</td></tr>
<tr><td>47</td><td>Colorado</td><td>10.2</td><td>6</td><td>Florida</td><td>23.9</td></tr>
<tr><td>26</td><td>Connecticut</td><td>17.9</td><td>7</td><td>Arkansas</td><td>23.1</td></tr>
<tr><td>3</td><td>Delaware</td><td>26.7</td><td>8</td><td>Wisconsin</td><td>22.9</td></tr>
<tr><td>6</td><td>Florida</td><td>23.9</td><td>9</td><td>Kansas</td><td>22.8</td></tr>
<tr><td>38</td><td>Georgia</td><td>15.6</td><td>10</td><td>Montana</td><td>22.7</td></tr>
<tr><td>30</td><td>Hawaii</td><td>17.0</td><td>11</td><td>Pennsylvania</td><td>22.5</td></tr>
<tr><td>33</td><td>Idaho</td><td>16.5</td><td>12</td><td>Arizona</td><td>21.8</td></tr>
<tr><td>25</td><td>Illinois</td><td>18.1</td><td>13</td><td>New Jersey</td><td>21.7</td></tr>
<tr><td>20</td><td>Indiana</td><td>20.0</td><td>14</td><td>Missouri</td><td>21.6</td></tr>
<tr><td>19</td><td>Iowa</td><td>20.5</td><td>14</td><td>Tennessee</td><td>21.6</td></tr>
<tr><td>9</td><td>Kansas</td><td>22.8</td><td>16</td><td>Washington</td><td>21.3</td></tr>
<tr><td>21</td><td>Kentucky</td><td>19.9</td><td>16</td><td>West Virginia</td><td>21.3</td></tr>
<tr><td>43</td><td>Louisiana</td><td>13.3</td><td>18</td><td>South Carolina</td><td>20.6</td></tr>
<tr><td>37</td><td>Maine</td><td>15.7</td><td>19</td><td>Iowa</td><td>20.5</td></tr>
<tr><td>39</td><td>Maryland</td><td>15.3</td><td>20</td><td>Indiana</td><td>20.0</td></tr>
<tr><td>36</td><td>Massachusetts</td><td>15.8</td><td>21</td><td>Kentucky</td><td>19.9</td></tr>
<tr><td>35</td><td>Michigan</td><td>16.0</td><td>22</td><td>Rhode Island</td><td>19.5</td></tr>
<tr><td>31</td><td>Minnesota</td><td>16.9</td><td>23</td><td>New York</td><td>19.2</td></tr>
<tr><td>42</td><td>Mississippi</td><td>14.1</td><td>24</td><td>North Carolina</td><td>18.4</td></tr>
<tr><td>14</td><td>Missouri</td><td>21.6</td><td>25</td><td>Illinois</td><td>18.1</td></tr>
<tr><td>10</td><td>Montana</td><td>22.7</td><td>26</td><td>Connecticut</td><td>17.9</td></tr>
<tr><td>45</td><td>Nebraska</td><td>11.8</td><td>27</td><td>Alabama</td><td>17.8</td></tr>
<tr><td>44</td><td>Nevada</td><td>12.2</td><td>28</td><td>Oklahoma</td><td>17.7</td></tr>
<tr><td>32</td><td>New Hampshire</td><td>16.8</td><td>29</td><td>Ohio</td><td>17.3</td></tr>
<tr><td>13</td><td>New Jersey</td><td>21.7</td><td>30</td><td>Hawaii</td><td>17.0</td></tr>
<tr><td>46</td><td>New Mexico</td><td>11.4</td><td>31</td><td>Minnesota</td><td>16.9</td></tr>
<tr><td>23</td><td>New York</td><td>19.2</td><td>32</td><td>New Hampshire</td><td>16.8</td></tr>
<tr><td>24</td><td>North Carolina</td><td>18.4</td><td>33</td><td>Idaho</td><td>16.5</td></tr>
<tr><td>2</td><td>North Dakota</td><td>31.1</td><td>34</td><td>California</td><td>16.1</td></tr>
<tr><td>29</td><td>Ohio</td><td>17.3</td><td>35</td><td>Michigan</td><td>16.0</td></tr>
<tr><td>28</td><td>Oklahoma</td><td>17.7</td><td>36</td><td>Massachusetts</td><td>15.8</td></tr>
<tr><td>5</td><td>Oregon</td><td>24.4</td><td>37</td><td>Maine</td><td>15.7</td></tr>
<tr><td>11</td><td>Pennsylvania</td><td>22.5</td><td>38</td><td>Georgia</td><td>15.6</td></tr>
<tr><td>22</td><td>Rhode Island</td><td>19.5</td><td>39</td><td>Maryland</td><td>15.3</td></tr>
<tr><td>18</td><td>South Carolina</td><td>20.6</td><td>39</td><td>Texas</td><td>15.3</td></tr>
<tr><td>3</td><td>South Dakota</td><td>26.7</td><td>41</td><td>Virginia</td><td>14.6</td></tr>
<tr><td>14</td><td>Tennessee</td><td>21.6</td><td>42</td><td>Mississippi</td><td>14.1</td></tr>
<tr><td>39</td><td>Texas</td><td>15.3</td><td>43</td><td>Louisiana</td><td>13.3</td></tr>
<tr><td>48</td><td>Utah</td><td>9.7</td><td>44</td><td>Nevada</td><td>12.2</td></tr>
<tr><td>1</td><td>Vermont</td><td>33.5</td><td>45</td><td>Nebraska</td><td>11.8</td></tr>
<tr><td>41</td><td>Virginia</td><td>14.6</td><td>46</td><td>New Mexico</td><td>11.4</td></tr>
<tr><td>16</td><td>Washington</td><td>21.3</td><td>47</td><td>Colorado</td><td>10.2</td></tr>
<tr><td>16</td><td>West Virginia</td><td>21.3</td><td>48</td><td>Utah</td><td>9.7</td></tr>
<tr><td>8</td><td>Wisconsin</td><td>22.9</td><td>NA</td><td>Alaska**</td><td>NA</td></tr>
<tr><td>NA</td><td>Wyoming**</td><td>NA</td><td>NA</td><td>Wyoming**</td><td>NA</td></tr>
<tr><td></td><td></td><td></td><td></td><td>District of Columbia</td><td>35.6</td></tr>
</table>

Source: Morgan Quitno Press using data from American Cancer Society
"1999 Facts & Figures" (Copyright 1999, Reprinted with permission from the American Cancer Society)
*These estimates are offered as a rough guide and should be interpreted with caution. They are calculated according to the distribution of estimated 1999 cancer deaths by state. Rates calculated using 1997 Census female resident population estimates.
**Fewer than 50 cases.

Estimated New Prostate Cancer Cases in 1999

National Estimated Total = 179,300 New Cases*

ALPHA ORDER

RANK	STATE	CASES	% of USA
22	Alabama	3,100	1.7%
50	Alaska	200	0.1%
18	Arizona	3,300	1.8%
26	Arkansas	2,400	1.3%
1	California	16,300	9.1%
31	Colorado	2,000	1.1%
29	Connecticut	2,200	1.2%
47	Delaware	500	0.3%
2	Florida	13,600	7.6%
11	Georgia	4,300	2.4%
41	Hawaii	700	0.4%
40	Idaho	900	0.5%
7	Illinois	7,700	4.3%
16	Indiana	3,700	2.1%
30	Iowa	2,100	1.2%
33	Kansas	1,900	1.1%
25	Kentucky	2,600	1.5%
23	Louisiana	3,000	1.7%
38	Maine	1,000	0.6%
19	Maryland	3,200	1.8%
14	Massachusetts	4,000	2.2%
8	Michigan	6,400	3.6%
19	Minnesota	3,200	1.8%
28	Mississippi	2,300	1.3%
15	Missouri	3,900	2.2%
44	Montana	600	0.3%
35	Nebraska	1,100	0.6%
35	Nevada	1,100	0.6%
41	New Hampshire	700	0.4%
9	New Jersey	5,600	3.1%
38	New Mexico	1,000	0.6%
4	New York	11,500	6.4%
10	North Carolina	5,400	3.0%
44	North Dakota	600	0.3%
6	Ohio	7,900	4.4%
31	Oklahoma	2,000	1.1%
26	Oregon	2,400	1.3%
5	Pennsylvania	9,900	5.5%
44	Rhode Island	600	0.3%
24	South Carolina	2,900	1.6%
41	South Dakota	700	0.4%
17	Tennessee	3,400	1.9%
3	Texas	11,600	6.5%
35	Utah	1,100	0.6%
48	Vermont	300	0.2%
11	Virginia	4,300	2.4%
19	Washington	3,200	1.8%
34	West Virginia	1,500	0.8%
13	Wisconsin	4,100	2.3%
48	Wyoming	300	0.2%

RANK ORDER

RANK	STATE	CASES	% of USA
1	California	16,300	9.1%
2	Florida	13,600	7.6%
3	Texas	11,600	6.5%
4	New York	11,500	6.4%
5	Pennsylvania	9,900	5.5%
6	Ohio	7,900	4.4%
7	Illinois	7,700	4.3%
8	Michigan	6,400	3.6%
9	New Jersey	5,600	3.1%
10	North Carolina	5,400	3.0%
11	Georgia	4,300	2.4%
11	Virginia	4,300	2.4%
13	Wisconsin	4,100	2.3%
14	Massachusetts	4,000	2.2%
15	Missouri	3,900	2.2%
16	Indiana	3,700	2.1%
17	Tennessee	3,400	1.9%
18	Arizona	3,300	1.8%
19	Maryland	3,200	1.8%
19	Minnesota	3,200	1.8%
19	Washington	3,200	1.8%
22	Alabama	3,100	1.7%
23	Louisiana	3,000	1.7%
24	South Carolina	2,900	1.6%
25	Kentucky	2,600	1.5%
26	Arkansas	2,400	1.3%
26	Oregon	2,400	1.3%
28	Mississippi	2,300	1.3%
29	Connecticut	2,200	1.2%
30	Iowa	2,100	1.2%
31	Colorado	2,000	1.1%
31	Oklahoma	2,000	1.1%
33	Kansas	1,900	1.1%
34	West Virginia	1,500	0.8%
35	Nebraska	1,100	0.6%
35	Nevada	1,100	0.6%
35	Utah	1,100	0.6%
38	Maine	1,000	0.6%
38	New Mexico	1,000	0.6%
40	Idaho	900	0.5%
41	Hawaii	700	0.4%
41	New Hampshire	700	0.4%
41	South Dakota	700	0.4%
44	Montana	600	0.3%
44	North Dakota	600	0.3%
44	Rhode Island	600	0.3%
47	Delaware	500	0.3%
48	Vermont	300	0.2%
48	Wyoming	300	0.2%
50	Alaska	200	0.1%
	District of Columbia	600	0.3%

Source: American Cancer Society
   "1999 Facts & Figures" (Copyright 1999, Reprinted with permission from the American Cancer Society)
*These estimates are offered as a rough guide and should be interpreted with caution. They are calculated according to the distribution of estimated 1999 cancer deaths by state.

Estimated Rate of New Prostate Cancer Cases in 1999

National Estimated Rate = 136.9 News Cases per 100,000 Male Population*

ALPHA ORDER

RANK ORDER

RANK	STATE	RATE	RANK	STATE	RATE
14	Alabama	149.3	1	Arkansas	196.5
50	Alaska	62.5	2	South Dakota	192.4
18	Arizona	146.1	3	Florida	190.9
1	Arkansas	196.5	4	North Dakota	187.7
49	California	100.9	5	Mississippi	175.3
47	Colorado	103.6	6	West Virginia	171.1
23	Connecticut	138.4	7	Pennsylvania	171.0
22	Delaware	140.2	8	Maine	164.8
3	Florida	190.9	9	Wisconsin	161.1
42	Georgia	117.8	10	South Carolina	159.6
43	Hawaii	117.3	11	Iowa	150.9
16	Idaho	148.7	12	Oregon	149.6
30	Illinois	132.5	13	North Carolina	149.5
34	Indiana	129.4	14	Alabama	149.3
11	Iowa	150.9	15	Missouri	148.8
16	Kansas	148.7	16	Idaho	148.7
26	Kentucky	136.9	16	Kansas	148.7
21	Louisiana	143.0	18	Arizona	146.1
8	Maine	164.8	19	Ohio	145.8
35	Maryland	129.0	20	New Jersey	143.3
27	Massachusetts	135.4	21	Louisiana	143.0
29	Michigan	134.3	22	Delaware	140.2
23	Minnesota	138.4	23	Connecticut	138.4
5	Mississippi	175.3	23	Minnesota	138.4
15	Missouri	148.8	25	Montana	137.0
25	Montana	137.0	26	Kentucky	136.9
27	Nebraska	135.4	27	Massachusetts	135.4
36	Nevada	128.6	27	Nebraska	135.4
40	New Hampshire	121.1	29	Michigan	134.3
20	New Jersey	143.3	30	Illinois	132.5
44	New Mexico	117.2	31	New York	131.5
31	New York	131.5	32	Tennessee	131.0
13	North Carolina	149.5	33	Virginia	130.4
4	North Dakota	187.7	34	Indiana	129.4
19	Ohio	145.8	35	Maryland	129.0
39	Oklahoma	123.2	36	Nevada	128.6
12	Oregon	149.6	37	Rhode Island	126.2
7	Pennsylvania	171.0	38	Wyoming	124.2
37	Rhode Island	126.2	39	Oklahoma	123.2
10	South Carolina	159.6	40	New Hampshire	121.1
2	South Dakota	192.4	41	Texas	120.7
32	Tennessee	131.0	42	Georgia	117.8
41	Texas	120.7	43	Hawaii	117.3
46	Utah	107.3	44	New Mexico	117.2
48	Vermont	103.4	45	Washington	114.4
33	Virginia	130.4	46	Utah	107.3
45	Washington	114.4	47	Colorado	103.6
6	West Virginia	171.1	48	Vermont	103.4
9	Wisconsin	161.1	49	California	100.9
38	Wyoming	124.2	50	Alaska	62.5
				District of Columbia	241.7

Source: Morgan Quitno Press using data from American Cancer Society
   "1999 Facts & Figures" (Copyright 1999, Reprinted with permission from the American Cancer Society)
*These estimates are offered as a rough guide and should be interpreted with caution. They are calculated according to the distribution of estimated 1999 cancer deaths by state. Rates calculated using 1997 Census male resident population estimates.

Estimated New Skin Melanoma Cases in 1999

National Estimated Total = 44,200 New Cases*

ALPHA ORDER

RANK	STATE	CASES	% of USA
21	Alabama	700	1.6%
NA	Alaska**	NA	NA
15	Arizona	1,000	2.3%
32	Arkansas	400	0.9%
1	California	4,800	10.9%
26	Colorado	600	1.4%
26	Connecticut	600	1.4%
45	Delaware	100	0.2%
2	Florida	3,000	6.8%
15	Georgia	1,000	2.3%
45	Hawaii	100	0.2%
38	Idaho	200	0.5%
6	Illinois	1,900	4.3%
13	Indiana	1,100	2.5%
31	Iowa	500	1.1%
26	Kansas	600	1.4%
19	Kentucky	800	1.8%
21	Louisiana	700	1.6%
38	Maine	200	0.5%
21	Maryland	700	1.6%
10	Massachusetts	1,200	2.7%
9	Michigan	1,300	2.9%
26	Minnesota	600	1.4%
36	Mississippi	300	0.7%
15	Missouri	1,000	2.3%
45	Montana	100	0.2%
38	Nebraska	200	0.5%
32	Nevada	400	0.9%
38	New Hampshire	200	0.5%
8	New Jersey	1,500	3.4%
36	New Mexico	300	0.7%
4	New York	2,400	5.4%
10	North Carolina	1,200	2.7%
45	North Dakota	100	0.2%
7	Ohio	1,600	3.6%
26	Oklahoma	600	1.4%
21	Oregon	700	1.6%
5	Pennsylvania	2,300	5.2%
38	Rhode Island	200	0.5%
21	South Carolina	700	1.6%
38	South Dakota	200	0.5%
10	Tennessee	1,200	2.7%
3	Texas	2,900	6.6%
32	Utah	400	0.9%
38	Vermont	200	0.5%
13	Virginia	1,100	2.5%
19	Washington	800	1.8%
32	West Virginia	400	0.9%
18	Wisconsin	900	2.0%
45	Wyoming	100	0.2%

RANK ORDER

RANK	STATE	CASES	% of USA
1	California	4,800	10.9%
2	Florida	3,000	6.8%
3	Texas	2,900	6.6%
4	New York	2,400	5.4%
5	Pennsylvania	2,300	5.2%
6	Illinois	1,900	4.3%
7	Ohio	1,600	3.6%
8	New Jersey	1,500	3.4%
9	Michigan	1,300	2.9%
10	Massachusetts	1,200	2.7%
10	North Carolina	1,200	2.7%
10	Tennessee	1,200	2.7%
13	Indiana	1,100	2.5%
13	Virginia	1,100	2.5%
15	Arizona	1,000	2.3%
15	Georgia	1,000	2.3%
15	Missouri	1,000	2.3%
18	Wisconsin	900	2.0%
19	Kentucky	800	1.8%
19	Washington	800	1.8%
21	Alabama	700	1.6%
21	Louisiana	700	1.6%
21	Maryland	700	1.6%
21	Oregon	700	1.6%
21	South Carolina	700	1.6%
26	Colorado	600	1.4%
26	Connecticut	600	1.4%
26	Kansas	600	1.4%
26	Minnesota	600	1.4%
26	Oklahoma	600	1.4%
31	Iowa	500	1.1%
32	Arkansas	400	0.9%
32	Nevada	400	0.9%
32	Utah	400	0.9%
32	West Virginia	400	0.9%
36	Mississippi	300	0.7%
36	New Mexico	300	0.7%
38	Idaho	200	0.5%
38	Maine	200	0.5%
38	Nebraska	200	0.5%
38	New Hampshire	200	0.5%
38	Rhode Island	200	0.5%
38	South Dakota	200	0.5%
38	Vermont	200	0.5%
45	Delaware	100	0.2%
45	Hawaii	100	0.2%
45	Montana	100	0.2%
45	North Dakota	100	0.2%
45	Wyoming	100	0.2%
NA	Alaska**	NA	NA
	District of Columbia**	NA	NA

Source: American Cancer Society
   "1999 Facts & Figures" (Copyright 1999, Reprinted with permission from the American Cancer Society)
*These estimates are offered as a rough guide and should be interpreted with caution. They are calculated according to the distribution of estimated 1999 cancer deaths by state.
**Fewer than 50 cases.

Estimated Rate of New Skin Melanoma Cases in 1999

National Estimated Rate = 16.4 New Cases per 100,000 Population*

ALPHA ORDER				RANK ORDER		
RANK	STATE	RATE		RANK	STATE	RATE
28	Alabama	16.1		1	Vermont	33.8
NA	Alaska**	NA		2	South Dakota	27.1
7	Arizona	21.4		3	Nevada	22.9
32	Arkansas	15.8		4	Kansas	22.8
36	California	14.7		5	Tennessee	22.1
35	Colorado	15.1		5	West Virginia	22.1
19	Connecticut	18.3		7	Arizona	21.4
41	Delaware	13.4		8	Oregon	21.3
12	Florida	20.1		9	Wyoming	20.8
44	Georgia	13.1		10	Kentucky	20.3
49	Hawaii	8.4		11	Rhode Island	20.2
26	Idaho	16.3		12	Florida	20.1
32	Illinois	15.8		13	Massachusetts	19.5
16	Indiana	18.6		14	Pennsylvania	19.2
22	Iowa	17.5		15	Utah	19.0
4	Kansas	22.8		16	Indiana	18.6
10	Kentucky	20.3		17	New Jersey	18.5
30	Louisiana	16.0		18	Missouri	18.4
28	Maine	16.1		19	Connecticut	18.3
40	Maryland	13.6		20	South Carolina	18.2
13	Massachusetts	19.5		21	Oklahoma	17.9
42	Michigan	13.2		22	Iowa	17.5
45	Minnesota	12.7		23	New Mexico	17.3
48	Mississippi	10.9		24	Wisconsin	17.2
18	Missouri	18.4		25	New Hampshire	16.9
47	Montana	11.4		26	Idaho	16.3
46	Nebraska	12.0		27	Virginia	16.2
3	Nevada	22.9		28	Alabama	16.1
25	New Hampshire	16.9		28	Maine	16.1
17	New Jersey	18.5		30	Louisiana	16.0
23	New Mexico	17.3		31	North Carolina	15.9
42	New York	13.2		32	Arkansas	15.8
31	North Carolina	15.9		32	Illinois	15.8
34	North Dakota	15.7		34	North Dakota	15.7
38	Ohio	14.3		35	Colorado	15.1
21	Oklahoma	17.9		36	California	14.7
8	Oregon	21.3		36	Texas	14.7
14	Pennsylvania	19.2		38	Ohio	14.3
11	Rhode Island	20.2		39	Washington	14.1
20	South Carolina	18.2		40	Maryland	13.6
2	South Dakota	27.1		41	Delaware	13.4
5	Tennessee	22.1		42	Michigan	13.2
36	Texas	14.7		42	New York	13.2
15	Utah	19.0		44	Georgia	13.1
1	Vermont	33.8		45	Minnesota	12.7
27	Virginia	16.2		46	Nebraska	12.0
39	Washington	14.1		47	Montana	11.4
5	West Virginia	22.1		48	Mississippi	10.9
24	Wisconsin	17.2		49	Hawaii	8.4
9	Wyoming	20.8		NA	Alaska**	NA
					District of Columbia**	NA

Source: Morgan Quitno Press using data from American Cancer Society
    "1999 Facts & Figures" (Copyright 1999, Reprinted with permission from the American Cancer Society)
*These estimates are offered as a rough guide and should be interpreted with caution. They are calculated
according to the distribution of estimated 1999 cancer deaths by state. Rates calculated using 1998 Census
resident population estimates.
**Fewer than 50 cases.

Estimated New Cancer of the Uterus (Cervix) Cases in 1999

National Estimated Total = 12,800 New Cases*

ALPHA ORDER

RANK	STATE	CASES	% of USA
18	Alabama	200	1.6%
NA	Alaska**	NA	NA
18	Arizona	200	1.6%
18	Arkansas	200	1.6%
1	California	1,300	10.2%
18	Colorado	200	1.6%
29	Connecticut	100	0.8%
29	Delaware	100	0.8%
4	Florida	800	6.3%
11	Georgia	300	2.3%
NA	Hawaii**	NA	NA
NA	Idaho**	NA	NA
5	Illinois	600	4.7%
11	Indiana	300	2.3%
29	Iowa	100	0.8%
29	Kansas	100	0.8%
11	Kentucky	300	2.3%
18	Louisiana	200	1.6%
29	Maine	100	0.8%
11	Maryland	300	2.3%
18	Massachusetts	200	1.6%
8	Michigan	500	3.9%
29	Minnesota	100	0.8%
18	Mississippi	200	1.6%
11	Missouri	300	2.3%
NA	Montana**	NA	NA
29	Nebraska	100	0.8%
29	Nevada	100	0.8%
29	New Hampshire	100	0.8%
9	New Jersey	400	3.1%
29	New Mexico	100	0.8%
3	New York	900	7.0%
11	North Carolina	300	2.3%
NA	North Dakota**	NA	NA
5	Ohio	600	4.7%
18	Oklahoma	200	1.6%
29	Oregon	100	0.8%
5	Pennsylvania	600	4.7%
29	Rhode Island	100	0.8%
18	South Carolina	200	1.6%
NA	South Dakota**	NA	NA
9	Tennessee	400	3.1%
2	Texas	1,100	8.6%
29	Utah	100	0.8%
29	Vermont	100	0.8%
11	Virginia	300	2.3%
18	Washington	200	1.6%
29	West Virginia	·100	0.8%
18	Wisconsin	200	1.6%
NA	Wyoming**	NA	NA

RANK ORDER

RANK	STATE	CASES	% of USA
1	California	1,300	10.2%
2	Texas	1,100	8.6%
3	New York	900	7.0%
4	Florida	800	6.3%
5	Illinois	600	4.7%
5	Ohio	600	4.7%
5	Pennsylvania	600	4.7%
8	Michigan	500	3.9%
9	New Jersey	400	3.1%
9	Tennessee	400	3.1%
11	Georgia	300	2.3%
11	Indiana	300	2.3%
11	Kentucky	300	2.3%
11	Maryland	300	2.3%
11	Missouri	300	2.3%
11	North Carolina	300	2.3%
11	Virginia	300	2.3%
18	Alabama	200	1.6%
18	Arizona	200	1.6%
18	Arkansas	200	1.6%
18	Colorado	200	1.6%
18	Louisiana	200	1.6%
18	Massachusetts	200	1.6%
18	Mississippi	200	1.6%
18	Oklahoma	200	1.6%
18	South Carolina	200	1.6%
18	Washington	200	1.6%
18	Wisconsin	200	1.6%
29	Connecticut	100	0.8%
29	Delaware	100	0.8%
29	Iowa	100	0.8%
29	Kansas	100	0.8%
29	Maine	100	0.8%
29	Minnesota	100	0.8%
29	Nebraska	100	0.8%
29	Nevada	100	0.8%
29	New Hampshire	100	0.8%
29	New Mexico	100	0.8%
29	Oregon	100	0.8%
29	Rhode Island	100	0.8%
29	Utah	100	0.8%
29	Vermont	100	0.8%
29	West Virginia	100	0.8%
NA	Alaska**	NA	NA
NA	Hawaii**	NA	NA
NA	Idaho**	NA	NA
NA	Montana**	NA	NA
NA	North Dakota**	NA	NA
NA	South Dakota**	NA	NA
NA	Wyoming**	NA	NA
	District of Columbia**	NA	NA

Source: American Cancer Society
"1999 Facts & Figures" (Copyright 1999, Reprinted with permission from the American Cancer Society)
*These estimates are offered as a rough guide and should be interpreted with caution. They are calculated according to the distribution of estimated 1999 cancer deaths by state.
**Fewer than 50 cases.

Estimated Rate of New Cancer of the Uterus (Cervix) Cases in 1999

National Estimated Rate = 9.4 New Cases per 100,000 Female Population*

ALPHA ORDER

RANK	STATE	RATE
29	Alabama	8.9
NA	Alaska**	NA
31	Arizona	8.7
6	Arkansas	15.4
33	California	8.1
21	Colorado	10.2
42	Connecticut	6.0
2	Delaware	26.7
17	Florida	10.6
35	Georgia	7.8
NA	Hawaii**	NA
NA	Idaho**	NA
24	Illinois	9.9
22	Indiana	10.0
39	Iowa	6.8
36	Kansas	7.6
7	Kentucky	14.9
29	Louisiana	8.9
5	Maine	15.7
13	Maryland	11.5
40	Massachusetts	6.3
22	Michigan	10.0
43	Minnesota	4.2
9	Mississippi	14.1
16	Missouri	10.8
NA	Montana**	NA
11	Nebraska	11.8
10	Nevada	12.2
4	New Hampshire	16.8
25	New Jersey	9.7
14	New Mexico	11.4
27	New York	9.6
34	North Carolina	7.9
NA	North Dakota**	NA
19	Ohio	10.4
11	Oklahoma	11.8
41	Oregon	6.1
27	Pennsylvania	9.6
3	Rhode Island	19.5
20	South Carolina	10.3
NA	South Dakota**	NA
8	Tennessee	14.4
15	Texas	11.2
25	Utah	9.7
1	Vermont	33.5
31	Virginia	8.7
38	Washington	7.1
17	West Virginia	10.6
36	Wisconsin	7.6
NA	Wyoming**	NA

RANK ORDER

RANK	STATE	RATE
1	Vermont	33.5
2	Delaware	26.7
3	Rhode Island	19.5
4	New Hampshire	16.8
5	Maine	15.7
6	Arkansas	15.4
7	Kentucky	14.9
8	Tennessee	14.4
9	Mississippi	14.1
10	Nevada	12.2
11	Nebraska	11.8
11	Oklahoma	11.8
13	Maryland	11.5
14	New Mexico	11.4
15	Texas	11.2
16	Missouri	10.8
17	Florida	10.6
17	West Virginia	10.6
19	Ohio	10.4
20	South Carolina	10.3
21	Colorado	10.2
22	Indiana	10.0
22	Michigan	10.0
24	Illinois	9.9
25	New Jersey	9.7
25	Utah	9.7
27	New York	9.6
27	Pennsylvania	9.6
29	Alabama	8.9
29	Louisiana	8.9
31	Arizona	8.7
31	Virginia	8.7
33	California	8.1
34	North Carolina	7.9
35	Georgia	7.8
36	Kansas	7.6
36	Wisconsin	7.6
38	Washington	7.1
39	Iowa	6.8
40	Massachusetts	6.3
41	Oregon	6.1
42	Connecticut	6.0
43	Minnesota	4.2
NA	Alaska**	NA
NA	Hawaii**	NA
NA	Idaho**	NA
NA	Montana**	NA
NA	North Dakota**	NA
NA	South Dakota**	NA
NA	Wyoming**	NA
	District of Columbia**	NA

Source: Morgan Quitno Press using data from American Cancer Society
"1999 Facts & Figures" (Copyright 1999, Reprinted with permission from the American Cancer Society)
*These estimates are offered as a rough guide and should be interpreted with caution. They are calculated according to the distribution of estimated 1999 cancer deaths by state. Rates calculated using 1997 Census female resident population estimates.
**Fewer than 50 cases.

Percent of Women 18 Years and Older
Who Had a Pap Smear Within the Past Three Years: 1997
National Median = 84.7% of Women 18 Years and Older*

ALPHA ORDER

RANK	STATE	PERCENT
19	Alabama	86.0
2	Alaska	90.3
46	Arizona	79.3
49	Arkansas	78.2
NA	California**	NA
10	Colorado	87.6
36	Connecticut	83.0
3	Delaware	89.8
25	Florida	84.7
1	Georgia	92.3
17	Hawaii	86.9
41	Idaho	81.6
37	Illinois	82.7
27	Indiana	84.5
45	Iowa	80.5
21	Kansas	85.9
40	Kentucky	81.7
32	Louisiana	83.8
7	Maine	88.1
5	Maryland	88.7
6	Massachusetts	88.4
18	Michigan	86.3
35	Minnesota	83.4
21	Mississippi	85.9
31	Missouri	83.9
26	Montana	84.6
29	Nebraska	84.1
23	Nevada	85.6
14	New Hampshire	87.0
42	New Jersey	81.3
44	New Mexico	80.6
14	New York	87.0
11	North Carolina	87.4
38	North Dakota	82.4
13	Ohio	87.3
28	Oklahoma	84.4
19	Oregon	86.0
39	Pennsylvania	82.3
11	Rhode Island	87.4
4	South Carolina	89.7
24	South Dakota	85.0
9	Tennessee	87.8
43	Texas	80.9
48	Utah	78.5
29	Vermont	84.1
8	Virginia	87.9
14	Washington	87.0
47	West Virginia	78.9
32	Wisconsin	83.8
34	Wyoming	83.7

RANK ORDER

RANK	STATE	PERCENT
1	Georgia	92.3
2	Alaska	90.3
3	Delaware	89.8
4	South Carolina	89.7
5	Maryland	88.7
6	Massachusetts	88.4
7	Maine	88.1
8	Virginia	87.9
9	Tennessee	87.8
10	Colorado	87.6
11	North Carolina	87.4
11	Rhode Island	87.4
13	Ohio	87.3
14	New Hampshire	87.0
14	New York	87.0
14	Washington	87.0
17	Hawaii	86.9
18	Michigan	86.3
19	Alabama	86.0
19	Oregon	86.0
21	Kansas	85.9
21	Mississippi	85.9
23	Nevada	85.6
24	South Dakota	85.0
25	Florida	84.7
26	Montana	84.6
27	Indiana	84.5
28	Oklahoma	84.4
29	Nebraska	84.1
29	Vermont	84.1
31	Missouri	83.9
32	Louisiana	83.8
32	Wisconsin	83.8
34	Wyoming	83.7
35	Minnesota	83.4
36	Connecticut	83.0
37	Illinois	82.7
38	North Dakota	82.4
39	Pennsylvania	82.3
40	Kentucky	81.7
41	Idaho	81.6
42	New Jersey	81.3
43	Texas	80.9
44	New Mexico	80.6
45	Iowa	80.5
46	Arizona	79.3
47	West Virginia	78.9
48	Utah	78.5
49	Arkansas	78.2
NA	California**	NA

District of Columbia 92.1

Source: U.S. Department of Health and Human Services, Centers for Disease Control and Prevention
"1997 Behavioral Risk Factor Surveillance Summary Prevalence Report" (August 17, 1998)
*A test for cancer, especially of the female genital tract. Named after George Papanicolaou (1883-1962), American anatomist.
**Not available.

375

AIDS Cases Reported in 1998

National Total = 52,215 New AIDS Cases*

ALPHA ORDER

RANK	STATE	CASES	% of USA
19	Alabama	603	1.2%
43	Alaska	41	0.1%
20	Arizona	548	1.0%
30	Arkansas	225	0.4%
2	California	6,336	12.1%
26	Colorado	317	0.6%
12	Connecticut	894	1.7%
34	Delaware	161	0.3%
3	Florida	5,489	10.5%
9	Georgia	1,362	2.6%
39	Hawaii	128	0.2%
45	Idaho	39	0.1%
7	Illinois	1,782	3.4%
23	Indiana	487	0.9%
40	Iowa	97	0.2%
36	Kansas	147	0.3%
27	Kentucky	312	0.6%
10	Louisiana	1,064	2.0%
43	Maine	41	0.1%
8	Maryland	1,629	3.1%
16	Massachusetts	784	1.5%
14	Michigan	804	1.5%
33	Minnesota	177	0.3%
25	Mississippi	359	0.7%
21	Missouri	543	1.0%
46	Montana	34	0.1%
41	Nebraska	77	0.1%
24	Nevada	484	0.9%
42	New Hampshire	60	0.1%
5	New Jersey	2,507	4.8%
32	New Mexico	220	0.4%
1	New York	11,329	21.7%
13	North Carolina	812	1.6%
49	North Dakota	10	0.0%
15	Ohio	785	1.5%
28	Oklahoma	298	0.6%
29	Oregon	234	0.4%
6	Pennsylvania	1,897	3.6%
37	Rhode Island	141	0.3%
17	South Carolina	777	1.5%
48	South Dakota	17	0.0%
18	Tennessee	694	1.3%
4	Texas	4,472	8.6%
35	Utah	150	0.3%
47	Vermont	21	0.0%
11	Virginia	999	1.9%
22	Washington	528	1.0%
38	West Virginia	130	0.2%
31	Wisconsin	222	0.4%
50	Wyoming	5	0.0%

RANK ORDER

RANK	STATE	CASES	% of USA
1	New York	11,329	21.7%
2	California	6,336	12.1%
3	Florida	5,489	10.5%
4	Texas	4,472	8.6%
5	New Jersey	2,507	4.8%
6	Pennsylvania	1,897	3.6%
7	Illinois	1,782	3.4%
8	Maryland	1,629	3.1%
9	Georgia	1,362	2.6%
10	Louisiana	1,064	2.0%
11	Virginia	999	1.9%
12	Connecticut	894	1.7%
13	North Carolina	812	1.6%
14	Michigan	804	1.5%
15	Ohio	785	1.5%
16	Massachusetts	784	1.5%
17	South Carolina	777	1.5%
18	Tennessee	694	1.3%
19	Alabama	603	1.2%
20	Arizona	548	1.0%
21	Missouri	543	1.0%
22	Washington	528	1.0%
23	Indiana	487	0.9%
24	Nevada	484	0.9%
25	Mississippi	359	0.7%
26	Colorado	317	0.6%
27	Kentucky	312	0.6%
28	Oklahoma	298	0.6%
29	Oregon	234	0.4%
30	Arkansas	225	0.4%
31	Wisconsin	222	0.4%
32	New Mexico	220	0.4%
33	Minnesota	177	0.3%
34	Delaware	161	0.3%
35	Utah	150	0.3%
36	Kansas	147	0.3%
37	Rhode Island	141	0.3%
38	West Virginia	130	0.2%
39	Hawaii	128	0.2%
40	Iowa	97	0.2%
41	Nebraska	77	0.1%
42	New Hampshire	60	0.1%
43	Alaska	41	0.1%
43	Maine	41	0.1%
45	Idaho	39	0.1%
46	Montana	34	0.1%
47	Vermont	21	0.0%
48	South Dakota	17	0.0%
49	North Dakota	10	0.0%
50	Wyoming	5	0.0%
	District of Columbia	943	1.8%

Source: U.S. Department of Health and Human Services, Centers for Disease Control and Prevention
   "HIV/AIDS Surveillance Report, 1998" (Mid-year Edition, Vol. 10, No. 1)
*July 1997-June 1998. AIDS is Acquired Immunodeficiency Syndrome. It is a specific group of diseases or conditions which are indicative of severe immunosuppression related to infection with the Human Immunodeficiency Virus (HIV). National total does not include 2,020 cases in Puerto Rico or 64 cases in the Virgin Islands.

AIDS Rate in 1998

National Rate = 19.5 New AIDS Cases Reported per 100,000 Population*

ALPHA ORDER				RANK ORDER		
RANK	STATE	RATE		RANK	STATE	RATE
17	Alabama	14.0		1	New York	62.5
37	Alaska	6.7		2	Florida	37.5
22	Arizona	12.0		3	Maryland	32.0
28	Arkansas	8.9		4	New Jersey	31.1
11	California	19.6		5	Nevada	28.9
31	Colorado	8.1		6	Connecticut	27.3
6	Connecticut	27.3		7	Louisiana	24.4
9	Delaware	22.0		8	Texas	23.0
2	Florida	37.5		9	Delaware	22.0
12	Georgia	18.2		10	South Carolina	20.7
24	Hawaii	10.8		11	California	19.6
47	Idaho	3.2		12	Georgia	18.2
14	Illinois	15.0		13	Pennsylvania	15.8
29	Indiana	8.3		14	Illinois	15.0
45	Iowa	3.4		15	Virginia	14.8
38	Kansas	5.7		16	Rhode Island	14.3
32	Kentucky	8.0		17	Alabama	14.0
7	Louisiana	24.4		18	Mississippi	13.1
46	Maine	3.3		19	Tennessee	12.9
3	Maryland	32.0		20	Massachusetts	12.8
20	Massachusetts	12.8		21	New Mexico	12.7
30	Michigan	8.2		22	Arizona	12.0
43	Minnesota	3.8		23	North Carolina	10.9
18	Mississippi	13.1		24	Hawaii	10.8
25	Missouri	10.1		25	Missouri	10.1
42	Montana	3.9		26	Washington	9.4
40	Nebraska	4.6		27	Oklahoma	9.0
5	Nevada	28.9		28	Arkansas	8.9
39	New Hampshire	5.1		29	Indiana	8.3
4	New Jersey	31.1		30	Michigan	8.2
21	New Mexico	12.7		31	Colorado	8.1
1	New York	62.5		32	Kentucky	8.0
23	North Carolina	10.9		33	Utah	7.3
49	North Dakota	1.6		34	Oregon	7.2
36	Ohio	7.0		34	West Virginia	7.2
27	Oklahoma	9.0		36	Ohio	7.0
34	Oregon	7.2		37	Alaska	6.7
13	Pennsylvania	15.8		38	Kansas	5.7
16	Rhode Island	14.3		39	New Hampshire	5.1
10	South Carolina	20.7		40	Nebraska	4.6
48	South Dakota	2.3		41	Wisconsin	4.3
19	Tennessee	12.9		42	Montana	3.9
8	Texas	23.0		43	Minnesota	3.8
33	Utah	7.3		44	Vermont	3.6
44	Vermont	3.6		45	Iowa	3.4
15	Virginia	14.8		46	Maine	3.3
26	Washington	9.4		47	Idaho	3.2
34	West Virginia	7.2		48	South Dakota	2.3
41	Wisconsin	4.3		49	North Dakota	1.6
50	Wyoming	1.0		50	Wyoming	1.0
					District of Columbia	178.3

Source: U.S. Department of Health and Human Services, Centers for Disease Control and Prevention
"HIV/AIDS Surveillance Report, 1998" (Mid-year Edition, Vol. 10, No. 1)
*July 1997-June 1998. AIDS is Acquired Immunodeficiency Syndrome. It is a specific group of diseases or conditions which are indicative of severe immunosuppression related to infection with the Human Immunodeficiency Virus (HIV). National rate does not include cases in U.S. territories.

AIDS Cases Reported Through June 1998

National Total = 642,911 Reported AIDS Cases*

ALPHA ORDER

RANK	STATE	CASES	% of USA
24	Alabama	5,108	0.8%
45	Alaska	423	0.1%
22	Arizona	5,786	0.9%
32	Arkansas	2,492	0.4%
2	California	107,468	16.7%
21	Colorado	6,277	1.0%
13	Connecticut	10,061	1.6%
34	Delaware	2,082	0.3%
3	Florida	67,612	10.5%
8	Georgia	19,324	3.0%
33	Hawaii	2,156	0.3%
44	Idaho	432	0.1%
6	Illinois	21,086	3.3%
23	Indiana	5,263	0.8%
39	Iowa	1,121	0.2%
35	Kansas	2,050	0.3%
31	Kentucky	2,707	0.4%
11	Louisiana	10,708	1.7%
42	Maine	824	0.1%
9	Maryland	17,790	2.8%
10	Massachusetts	13,295	2.1%
15	Michigan	9,559	1.5%
28	Minnesota	3,269	0.5%
27	Mississippi	3,404	0.5%
18	Missouri	8,019	1.2%
47	Montana	283	0.0%
41	Nebraska	918	0.1%
26	Nevada	3,773	0.6%
43	New Hampshire	789	0.1%
5	New Jersey	37,342	5.8%
37	New Mexico	1,742	0.3%
1	New York	124,793	19.4%
16	North Carolina	8,553	1.3%
50	North Dakota	94	0.0%
14	Ohio	9,899	1.5%
29	Oklahoma	3,185	0.5%
25	Oregon	4,254	0.7%
7	Pennsylvania	20,266	3.2%
36	Rhode Island	1,801	0.3%
19	South Carolina	7,402	1.2%
49	South Dakota	138	0.0%
20	Tennessee	6,633	1.0%
4	Texas	46,542	7.2%
38	Utah	1,599	0.2%
46	Vermont	338	0.1%
12	Virginia	10,694	1.7%
17	Washington	8,448	1.3%
40	West Virginia	930	0.1%
30	Wisconsin	3,133	0.5%
48	Wyoming	159	0.0%

RANK ORDER

RANK	STATE	CASES	% of USA
1	New York	124,793	19.4%
2	California	107,468	16.7%
3	Florida	67,612	10.5%
4	Texas	46,542	7.2%
5	New Jersey	37,342	5.8%
6	Illinois	21,086	3.3%
7	Pennsylvania	20,266	3.2%
8	Georgia	19,324	3.0%
9	Maryland	17,790	2.8%
10	Massachusetts	13,295	2.1%
11	Louisiana	10,708	1.7%
12	Virginia	10,694	1.7%
13	Connecticut	10,061	1.6%
14	Ohio	9,899	1.5%
15	Michigan	9,559	1.5%
16	North Carolina	8,553	1.3%
17	Washington	8,448	1.3%
18	Missouri	8,019	1.2%
19	South Carolina	7,402	1.2%
20	Tennessee	6,633	1.0%
21	Colorado	6,277	1.0%
22	Arizona	5,786	0.9%
23	Indiana	5,263	0.8%
24	Alabama	5,108	0.8%
25	Oregon	4,254	0.7%
26	Nevada	3,773	0.6%
27	Mississippi	3,404	0.5%
28	Minnesota	3,269	0.5%
29	Oklahoma	3,185	0.5%
30	Wisconsin	3,133	0.5%
31	Kentucky	2,707	0.4%
32	Arkansas	2,492	0.4%
33	Hawaii	2,156	0.3%
34	Delaware	2,082	0.3%
35	Kansas	2,050	0.3%
36	Rhode Island	1,801	0.3%
37	New Mexico	1,742	0.3%
38	Utah	1,599	0.2%
39	Iowa	1,121	0.2%
40	West Virginia	930	0.1%
41	Nebraska	918	0.1%
42	Maine	824	0.1%
43	New Hampshire	789	0.1%
44	Idaho	432	0.1%
45	Alaska	423	0.1%
46	Vermont	338	0.1%
47	Montana	283	0.0%
48	Wyoming	159	0.0%
49	South Dakota	138	0.0%
50	North Dakota	94	0.0%
	District of Columbia	10,887	1.7%

Source: U.S. Department of Health and Human Services, Centers for Disease Control and Prevention
"HIV/AIDS Surveillance Report, 1998" (Mid-year Edition, Vol. 10, No. 1)
Cumulative through June 1998. AIDS is Acquired Immunodeficiency Syndrome. It is a specific group of diseases or conditions which are indicative of severe immunosuppression related to infection with the Human Immunodeficiency Virus (HIV). National total does not include 21,593 cases in Puerto Rico, 393 cases in the Virgin Islands and 23 cases in other U.S. territories.

AIDS Cases in Children 12 Years and Younger Through June 1998

National Total = 7,890 Juvenile AIDS Cases*

ALPHA ORDER

RANK	STATE	CASES	% of USA
18	Alabama	65	0.8%
44	Alaska	5	0.1%
29	Arizona	21	0.3%
23	Arkansas	35	0.4%
4	California	568	7.2%
25	Colorado	27	0.3%
11	Connecticut	174	2.2%
34	Delaware	17	0.2%
2	Florida	1,305	16.5%
10	Georgia	182	2.3%
36	Hawaii	14	0.2%
48	Idaho	2	0.0%
8	Illinois	238	3.0%
22	Indiana	36	0.5%
38	Iowa	9	0.1%
37	Kansas	11	0.1%
29	Kentucky	21	0.3%
14	Louisiana	112	1.4%
38	Maine	9	0.1%
6	Maryland	283	3.6%
9	Massachusetts	199	2.5%
16	Michigan	100	1.3%
29	Minnesota	21	0.3%
20	Mississippi	53	0.7%
19	Missouri	55	0.7%
47	Montana	3	0.0%
38	Nebraska	9	0.1%
26	Nevada	26	0.3%
41	New Hampshire	8	0.1%
3	New Jersey	704	8.9%
41	New Mexico	8	0.1%
1	New York	2,127	27.0%
15	North Carolina	109	1.4%
50	North Dakota	0	0.0%
13	Ohio	116	1.5%
26	Oklahoma	26	0.3%
35	Oregon	16	0.2%
7	Pennsylvania	278	3.5%
33	Rhode Island	19	0.2%
17	South Carolina	74	0.9%
45	South Dakota	4	0.1%
21	Tennessee	47	0.6%
5	Texas	350	4.4%
29	Utah	21	0.3%
45	Vermont	4	0.1%
12	Virginia	157	2.0%
24	Washington	32	0.4%
41	West Virginia	8	0.1%
28	Wisconsin	25	0.3%
48	Wyoming	2	0.0%

RANK ORDER

RANK	STATE	CASES	% of USA
1	New York	2,127	27.0%
2	Florida	1,305	16.5%
3	New Jersey	704	8.9%
4	California	568	7.2%
5	Texas	350	4.4%
6	Maryland	283	3.6%
7	Pennsylvania	278	3.5%
8	Illinois	238	3.0%
9	Massachusetts	199	2.5%
10	Georgia	182	2.3%
11	Connecticut	174	2.2%
12	Virginia	157	2.0%
13	Ohio	116	1.5%
14	Louisiana	112	1.4%
15	North Carolina	109	1.4%
16	Michigan	100	1.3%
17	South Carolina	74	0.9%
18	Alabama	65	0.8%
19	Missouri	55	0.7%
20	Mississippi	53	0.7%
21	Tennessee	47	0.6%
22	Indiana	36	0.5%
23	Arkansas	35	0.4%
24	Washington	32	0.4%
25	Colorado	27	0.3%
26	Nevada	26	0.3%
26	Oklahoma	26	0.3%
28	Wisconsin	25	0.3%
29	Arizona	21	0.3%
29	Kentucky	21	0.3%
29	Minnesota	21	0.3%
29	Utah	21	0.3%
33	Rhode Island	19	0.2%
34	Delaware	17	0.2%
35	Oregon	16	0.2%
36	Hawaii	14	0.2%
37	Kansas	11	0.1%
38	Iowa	9	0.1%
38	Maine	9	0.1%
38	Nebraska	9	0.1%
41	New Hampshire	8	0.1%
41	New Mexico	8	0.1%
41	West Virginia	8	0.1%
44	Alaska	5	0.1%
45	South Dakota	4	0.1%
45	Vermont	4	0.1%
47	Montana	3	0.0%
48	Idaho	2	0.0%
48	Wyoming	2	0.0%
50	North Dakota	0	0.0%
	District of Columbia	155	2.0%

Source: U.S. Department of Health and Human Services, Centers for Disease Control and Prevention
"HIV/AIDS Surveillance Report, 1998" (Mid-year Edition, Vol. 10, No. 1)

*Cumulative through June 1998. AIDS is Acquired Immunodeficiency Syndrome. It is a specific group of diseases or conditions which are indicative of severe immunosuppression related to infection with the Human Immunodeficiency Virus (HIV). National total does not include 373 cases in Puerto Rico and 14 cases in the Virgin Islands.

E-Coli Cases Reported in 1998

National Total = 3,097 Cases*

ALPHA ORDER

RANK	STATE	CASES	% of USA
34	Alabama	25	0.8%
47	Alaska	7	0.2%
36	Arizona	21	0.7%
45	Arkansas	11	0.4%
1	California	268	8.7%
12	Colorado	91	2.9%
17	Connecticut	67	2.2%
50	Delaware*	2	0.1%
21	Florida	57	1.8%
16	Georgia	78	2.5%
41	Hawaii*	16	0.5%
26	Idaho	42	1.4%
8	Illinois	112	3.6%
9	Indiana	105	3.4%
11	Iowa	92	3.0%
31	Kansas	34	1.1%
32	Kentucky	33	1.1%
49	Louisiana	5	0.2%
29	Maine	37	1.2%
28	Maryland	40	1.3%
4	Massachusetts	154	5.0%
7	Michigan	114	3.7%
3	Minnesota	207	6.7%
48	Mississippi	6	0.2%
22	Missouri	56	1.8%
39	Montana	17	0.5%
19	Nebraska	61	2.0%
35	Nevada	22	0.7%
25	New Hampshire	46	1.5%
18	New Jersey	62	2.0%
38	New Mexico	19	0.6%
2	New York	229	7.4%
20	North Carolina	58	1.9%
44	North Dakota	12	0.4%
5	Ohio	128	4.1%
33	Oklahoma	26	0.8%
10	Oregon	104	3.4%
46	Pennsylvania*	10	0.3%
42	Rhode Island	13	0.4%
39	South Carolina	17	0.5%
29	South Dakota	37	1.2%
23	Tennessee	54	1.7%
14	Texas	82	2.6%
15	Utah	79	2.6%
36	Vermont	21	0.7%
26	Virginia*	42	1.4%
6	Washington	123	4.0%
42	West Virginia	13	0.4%
13	Wisconsin*	88	2.8%
24	Wyoming	53	1.7%

RANK ORDER

RANK	STATE	CASES	% of USA
1	California	268	8.7%
2	New York	229	7.4%
3	Minnesota	207	6.7%
4	Massachusetts	154	5.0%
5	Ohio	128	4.1%
6	Washington	123	4.0%
7	Michigan	114	3.7%
8	Illinois	112	3.6%
9	Indiana	105	3.4%
10	Oregon	104	3.4%
11	Iowa	92	3.0%
12	Colorado	91	2.9%
13	Wisconsin*	88	2.8%
14	Texas	82	2.6%
15	Utah	79	2.6%
16	Georgia	78	2.5%
17	Connecticut	67	2.2%
18	New Jersey	62	2.0%
19	Nebraska	61	2.0%
20	North Carolina	58	1.9%
21	Florida	57	1.8%
22	Missouri	56	1.8%
23	Tennessee	54	1.7%
24	Wyoming	53	1.7%
25	New Hampshire	46	1.5%
26	Idaho	42	1.4%
26	Virginia*	42	1.4%
28	Maryland	40	1.3%
29	Maine	37	1.2%
29	South Dakota	37	1.2%
31	Kansas	34	1.1%
32	Kentucky	33	1.1%
33	Oklahoma	26	0.8%
34	Alabama	25	0.8%
35	Nevada	22	0.7%
36	Arizona	21	0.7%
36	Vermont	21	0.7%
38	New Mexico	19	0.6%
39	Montana	17	0.5%
39	South Carolina	17	0.5%
41	Hawaii*	16	0.5%
42	Rhode Island	13	0.4%
42	West Virginia	13	0.4%
44	North Dakota	12	0.4%
45	Arkansas	11	0.4%
46	Pennsylvania*	10	0.3%
47	Alaska	7	0.2%
48	Mississippi	6	0.2%
49	Louisiana	5	0.2%
50	Delaware*	2	0.1%
	District of Columbia	1	0.0%

Source: U.S. Department of Health and Human Services, National Center for Health Statistics
    "Morbidity and Mortality Weekly Report" (January 8, 1999, Vol. 47, No. 51)
*Totals for Delaware, Hawaii, Pennsylvania, Virginia and Wisconsin are from the Public Health Laboratory Information System. All other states' data are from National Electronic Telecommunications System for Surveillance. Escherichia Coli is a common bacterium that normally inhabits the intestinal tracts of humans and animals but can cause infection in other parts of the body, especially the urinary tract. One strain, sometimes transmitted in hamburger meat, can cause serious infection resulting in sickness and death.

E-Coli Rate in 1998

National Rate = 1.1 Cases per 100,000 Population*

<u>ALPHA ORDER</u>

RANK	STATE	RATE
40	Alabama	0.6
26	Alaska	1.1
42	Arizona	0.4
42	Arkansas	0.4
33	California	0.8
13	Colorado	2.3
15	Connecticut	2.0
47	Delaware*	0.3
42	Florida	0.4
29	Georgia	1.0
20	Hawaii*	1.3
8	Idaho	3.4
32	Illinois	0.9
18	Indiana	1.8
9	Iowa	3.2
20	Kansas	1.3
33	Kentucky	0.8
49	Louisiana	0.1
11	Maine	3.0
33	Maryland	0.8
12	Massachusetts	2.5
25	Michigan	1.2
3	Minnesota	4.4
48	Mississippi	0.2
29	Missouri	1.0
16	Montana	1.9
6	Nebraska	3.7
20	Nevada	1.3
4	New Hampshire	3.9
33	New Jersey	0.8
26	New Mexico	1.1
20	New York	1.3
33	North Carolina	0.8
16	North Dakota	1.9
26	Ohio	1.1
33	Oklahoma	0.8
9	Oregon	3.2
49	Pennsylvania*	0.1
20	Rhode Island	1.3
42	South Carolina	0.4
2	South Dakota	5.0
29	Tennessee	1.0
42	Texas	0.4
5	Utah	3.8
7	Vermont	3.6
40	Virginia*	0.6
14	Washington	2.2
39	West Virginia	0.7
19	Wisconsin*	1.7
1	Wyoming	11.0

<u>RANK ORDER</u>

RANK	STATE	RATE
1	Wyoming	11.0
2	South Dakota	5.0
3	Minnesota	4.4
4	New Hampshire	3.9
5	Utah	3.8
6	Nebraska	3.7
7	Vermont	3.6
8	Idaho	3.4
9	Iowa	3.2
9	Oregon	3.2
11	Maine	3.0
12	Massachusetts	2.5
13	Colorado	2.3
14	Washington	2.2
15	Connecticut	2.0
16	Montana	1.9
16	North Dakota	1.9
18	Indiana	1.8
19	Wisconsin*	1.7
20	Hawaii*	1.3
20	Kansas	1.3
20	Nevada	1.3
20	New York	1.3
20	Rhode Island	1.3
25	Michigan	1.2
26	Alaska	1.1
26	New Mexico	1.1
26	Ohio	1.1
29	Georgia	1.0
29	Missouri	1.0
29	Tennessee	1.0
32	Illinois	0.9
33	California	0.8
33	Kentucky	0.8
33	Maryland	0.8
33	New Jersey	0.8
33	North Carolina	0.8
33	Oklahoma	0.8
39	West Virginia	0.7
40	Alabama	0.6
40	Virginia*	0.6
42	Arizona	0.4
42	Arkansas	0.4
42	Florida	0.4
42	South Carolina	0.4
42	Texas	0.4
47	Delaware*	0.3
48	Mississippi	0.2
49	Louisiana	0.1
49	Pennsylvania*	0.1
	District of Columbia	0.2

Source: Morgan Quitno Press using data from U.S. Dept. of Health & Human Serv's, National Center for Health Statistics "Morbidity and Mortality Weekly Report" (January 8, 1999, Vol. 47, No. 51)

*Totals for Delaware, Hawaii, Pennsylvania, Virginia and Wisconsin are from the Public Health Laboratory Information System. All other states' data are from National Electronic Telecommunications System for Surveillance. Escherichia Coli is a common bacterium that normally inhabits the intestinal tracts of humans and animals but can cause infection in other parts of the body, especially the urinary tract. One strain, sometimes transmitted in hamburger meat, can cause serious infection resulting in sickness and death.

German Measles (Rubella) Cases Reported in 1998

National Total = 345 Cases*

ALPHA ORDER

RANK	STATE	CASES	% of USA
22	Alabama	0	0.0%
22	Alaska	0	0.0%
16	Arizona	1	0.3%
22	Arkansas	0	0.0%
10	California	3	0.9%
22	Colorado	0	0.0%
4	Connecticut	29	8.4%
22	Delaware	0	0.0%
9	Florida	4	1.2%
22	Georgia	0	0.0%
12	Hawaii	2	0.6%
22	Idaho	0	0.0%
22	Illinois	0	0.0%
22	Indiana	0	0.0%
22	Iowa	0	0.0%
3	Kansas	31	9.0%
22	Kentucky	0	0.0%
22	Louisiana	0	0.0%
22	Maine	0	0.0%
16	Maryland	1	0.3%
8	Massachusetts	8	2.3%
22	Michigan	0	0.0%
22	Minnesota	0	0.0%
22	Mississippi	0	0.0%
10	Missouri	3	0.9%
22	Montana	0	0.0%
22	Nebraska	0	0.0%
16	Nevada	1	0.3%
22	New Hampshire	0	0.0%
5	New Jersey	13	3.8%
16	New Mexico	1	0.3%
1	New York	129	37.4%
5	North Carolina	13	3.8%
22	North Dakota	0	0.0%
22	Ohio	0	0.0%
22	Oklahoma	0	0.0%
22	Oregon	0	0.0%
12	Pennsylvania	2	0.6%
16	Rhode Island	1	0.3%
22	South Carolina	0	0.0%
22	South Dakota	0	0.0%
12	Tennessee	2	0.6%
2	Texas	89	25.8%
12	Utah	2	0.6%
22	Vermont	0	0.0%
16	Virginia	1	0.3%
7	Washington	9	2.6%
22	West Virginia	0	0.0%
22	Wisconsin	0	0.0%
22	Wyoming	0	0.0%

RANK ORDER

RANK	STATE	CASES	% of USA
1	New York	129	37.4%
2	Texas	89	25.8%
3	Kansas	31	9.0%
4	Connecticut	29	8.4%
5	New Jersey	13	3.8%
5	North Carolina	13	3.8%
7	Washington	9	2.6%
8	Massachusetts	8	2.3%
9	Florida	4	1.2%
10	California	3	0.9%
10	Missouri	3	0.9%
12	Hawaii	2	0.6%
12	Pennsylvania	2	0.6%
12	Tennessee	2	0.6%
12	Utah	2	0.6%
16	Arizona	1	0.3%
16	Maryland	1	0.3%
16	Nevada	1	0.3%
16	New Mexico	1	0.3%
16	Rhode Island	1	0.3%
16	Virginia	1	0.3%
22	Alabama	0	0.0%
22	Alaska	0	0.0%
22	Arkansas	0	0.0%
22	Colorado	0	0.0%
22	Delaware	0	0.0%
22	Georgia	0	0.0%
22	Idaho	0	0.0%
22	Illinois	0	0.0%
22	Indiana	0	0.0%
22	Iowa	0	0.0%
22	Kentucky	0	0.0%
22	Louisiana	0	0.0%
22	Maine	0	0.0%
22	Michigan	0	0.0%
22	Minnesota	0	0.0%
22	Mississippi	0	0.0%
22	Montana	0	0.0%
22	Nebraska	0	0.0%
22	New Hampshire	0	0.0%
22	North Dakota	0	0.0%
22	Ohio	0	0.0%
22	Oklahoma	0	0.0%
22	Oregon	0	0.0%
22	South Carolina	0	0.0%
22	South Dakota	0	0.0%
22	Vermont	0	0.0%
22	West Virginia	0	0.0%
22	Wisconsin	0	0.0%
22	Wyoming	0	0.0%
	District of Columbia	0	0.0%

Source: U.S. Department of Health and Human Services, National Center for Health Statistics
    "Morbidity and Mortality Weekly Report" (January 8, 1999, Vol. 47, No. 51)
*Provisional data. A mild, contagious, eruptive disease caused by a virus and capable of producing congenital
defects in infants born to mothers infected during the first three months of pregnancy.

German Measles (Rubella) Rate in 1998

National Rate = 0.13 Cases per 100,000 Population*

ALPHA ORDER

RANK	STATE	RATE
22	Alabama	0.00
22	Alaska	0.00
17	Arizona	0.02
22	Arkansas	0.00
20	California	0.01
22	Colorado	0.00
2	Connecticut	0.89
22	Delaware	0.00
16	Florida	0.03
22	Georgia	0.00
5	Hawaii	0.17
22	Idaho	0.00
22	Illinois	0.00
22	Indiana	0.00
22	Iowa	0.00
1	Kansas	1.18
22	Kentucky	0.00
22	Louisiana	0.00
22	Maine	0.00
17	Maryland	0.02
9	Massachusetts	0.13
22	Michigan	0.00
22	Minnesota	0.00
22	Mississippi	0.00
12	Missouri	0.06
22	Montana	0.00
22	Nebraska	0.00
12	Nevada	0.06
22	New Hampshire	0.00
7	New Jersey	0.16
12	New Mexico	0.06
3	New York	0.71
5	North Carolina	0.17
22	North Dakota	0.00
22	Ohio	0.00
22	Oklahoma	0.00
22	Oregon	0.00
17	Pennsylvania	0.02
10	Rhode Island	0.10
22	South Carolina	0.00
22	South Dakota	0.00
15	Tennessee	0.04
4	Texas	0.45
10	Utah	0.10
22	Vermont	0.00
20	Virginia	0.01
7	Washington	0.16
22	West Virginia	0.00
22	Wisconsin	0.00
22	Wyoming	0.00

RANK ORDER

RANK	STATE	RATE
1	Kansas	1.18
2	Connecticut	0.89
3	New York	0.71
4	Texas	0.45
5	Hawaii	0.17
5	North Carolina	0.17
7	New Jersey	0.16
7	Washington	0.16
9	Massachusetts	0.13
10	Rhode Island	0.10
10	Utah	0.10
12	Missouri	0.06
12	Nevada	0.06
12	New Mexico	0.06
15	Tennessee	0.04
16	Florida	0.03
17	Arizona	0.02
17	Maryland	0.02
17	Pennsylvania	0.02
20	California	0.01
20	Virginia	0.01
22	Alabama	0.00
22	Alaska	0.00
22	Arkansas	0.00
22	Colorado	0.00
22	Delaware	0.00
22	Georgia	0.00
22	Idaho	0.00
22	Illinois	0.00
22	Indiana	0.00
22	Iowa	0.00
22	Kentucky	0.00
22	Louisiana	0.00
22	Maine	0.00
22	Michigan	0.00
22	Minnesota	0.00
22	Mississippi	0.00
22	Montana	0.00
22	Nebraska	0.00
22	New Hampshire	0.00
22	North Dakota	0.00
22	Ohio	0.00
22	Oklahoma	0.00
22	Oregon	0.00
22	South Carolina	0.00
22	South Dakota	0.00
22	Vermont	0.00
22	West Virginia	0.00
22	Wisconsin	0.00
22	Wyoming	0.00
	District of Columbia	0.00

Source: Morgan Quitno Press using data from U.S. Dept. of Health & Human Serv's, National Center for Health Statistics
"Morbidity and Mortality Weekly Report" (January 8, 1999, Vol. 47, No. 51)
*Provisional data. A mild, contagious, eruptive disease caused by a virus and capable of producing congenital
defects in infants born to mothers infected during the first three months of pregnancy.

Hepatitis (Viral) Cases Reported in 1998

National Total = 30,679 Cases*

ALPHA ORDER

RANK	STATE	CASES	% of USA
32	Alabama	161	0.5%
45	Alaska	29	0.1%
4	Arizona	2,096	6.8%
29	Arkansas	187	0.6%
1	California	5,584	18.2%
20	Colorado	459	1.5%
34	Connecticut	126	0.4%
49	Delaware	10	0.0%
8	Florida	1,003	3.3%
10	Georgia	873	2.8%
40	Hawaii	49	0.2%
26	Idaho	284	0.9%
9	Illinois	905	2.9%
6	Indiana	1,113	3.6%
21	Iowa	456	1.5%
33	Kansas	133	0.4%
38	Kentucky	72	0.2%
23	Louisiana	327	1.1%
46	Maine	25	0.1%
15	Maryland	508	1.7%
31	Massachusetts	166	0.5%
3	Michigan	2,624	8.6%
30	Minnesota	180	0.6%
41	Mississippi	45	0.1%
11	Missouri	852	2.8%
36	Montana	100	0.3%
39	Nebraska	64	0.2%
25	Nevada	296	1.0%
44	New Hampshire	35	0.1%
14	New Jersey	525	1.7%
19	New Mexico	469	1.5%
5	New York	1,288	4.2%
22	North Carolina	372	1.2%
50	North Dakota	8	0.0%
18	Ohio	475	1.5%
12	Oklahoma	764	2.5%
17	Oregon	497	1.6%
13	Pennsylvania	725	2.4%
37	Rhode Island	85	0.3%
35	South Carolina	101	0.3%
43	South Dakota	43	0.1%
16	Tennessee	498	1.6%
2	Texas	4,015	13.1%
27	Utah	262	0.9%
47	Vermont	22	0.1%
24	Virginia	320	1.0%
7	Washington	1,076	3.5%
48	West Virginia	18	0.1%
28	Wisconsin	227	0.7%
42	Wyoming	44	0.1%

RANK ORDER

RANK	STATE	CASES	% of USA
1	California	5,584	18.2%
2	Texas	4,015	13.1%
3	Michigan	2,624	8.6%
4	Arizona	2,096	6.8%
5	New York	1,288	4.2%
6	Indiana	1,113	3.6%
7	Washington	1,076	3.5%
8	Florida	1,003	3.3%
9	Illinois	905	2.9%
10	Georgia	873	2.8%
11	Missouri	852	2.8%
12	Oklahoma	764	2.5%
13	Pennsylvania	725	2.4%
14	New Jersey	525	1.7%
15	Maryland	508	1.7%
16	Tennessee	498	1.6%
17	Oregon	497	1.6%
18	Ohio	475	1.5%
19	New Mexico	469	1.5%
20	Colorado	459	1.5%
21	Iowa	456	1.5%
22	North Carolina	372	1.2%
23	Louisiana	327	1.1%
24	Virginia	320	1.0%
25	Nevada	296	1.0%
26	Idaho	284	0.9%
27	Utah	262	0.9%
28	Wisconsin	227	0.7%
29	Arkansas	187	0.6%
30	Minnesota	180	0.6%
31	Massachusetts	166	0.5%
32	Alabama	161	0.5%
33	Kansas	133	0.4%
34	Connecticut	126	0.4%
35	South Carolina	101	0.3%
36	Montana	100	0.3%
37	Rhode Island	85	0.3%
38	Kentucky	72	0.2%
39	Nebraska	64	0.2%
40	Hawaii	49	0.2%
41	Mississippi	45	0.1%
42	Wyoming	44	0.1%
43	South Dakota	43	0.1%
44	New Hampshire	35	0.1%
45	Alaska	29	0.1%
46	Maine	25	0.1%
47	Vermont	22	0.1%
48	West Virginia	18	0.1%
49	Delaware	10	0.0%
50	North Dakota	8	0.0%
	District of Columbia	83	0.3%

Source: U.S. Department of Health and Human Services, National Center for Health Statistics
   "Morbidity and Mortality Weekly Report" (January 8, 1999, Vol. 47, No. 51)
*Provisional data. An inflammation of the liver. Includes types A and B.

Hepatitis (Viral) Rate in 1998

National Rate = 11.4 Cases per 100,000 Population*

ALPHA ORDER

RANK	STATE	RATE
40	Alabama	3.7
32	Alaska	4.7
1	Arizona	44.9
24	Arkansas	7.4
9	California	17.1
15	Colorado	11.6
37	Connecticut	3.8
48	Delaware	1.3
26	Florida	6.7
16	Georgia	11.4
36	Hawaii	4.1
4	Idaho	23.1
22	Illinois	7.5
7	Indiana	18.9
11	Iowa	15.9
30	Kansas	5.1
46	Kentucky	1.8
22	Louisiana	7.5
45	Maine	2.0
18	Maryland	9.9
43	Massachusetts	2.7
3	Michigan	26.7
37	Minnesota	3.8
47	Mississippi	1.6
12	Missouri	15.7
16	Montana	11.4
37	Nebraska	3.8
10	Nevada	16.9
42	New Hampshire	3.0
27	New Jersey	6.5
2	New Mexico	27.0
25	New York	7.1
31	North Carolina	4.9
48	North Dakota	1.3
35	Ohio	4.2
5	Oklahoma	22.8
13	Oregon	15.1
28	Pennsylvania	6.0
21	Rhode Island	8.6
44	South Carolina	2.6
29	South Dakota	5.8
19	Tennessee	9.2
6	Texas	20.3
14	Utah	12.5
40	Vermont	3.7
32	Virginia	4.7
7	Washington	18.9
50	West Virginia	1.0
34	Wisconsin	4.3
20	Wyoming	9.1

RANK ORDER

RANK	STATE	RATE
1	Arizona	44.9
2	New Mexico	27.0
3	Michigan	26.7
4	Idaho	23.1
5	Oklahoma	22.8
6	Texas	20.3
7	Indiana	18.9
7	Washington	18.9
9	California	17.1
10	Nevada	16.9
11	Iowa	15.9
12	Missouri	15.7
13	Oregon	15.1
14	Utah	12.5
15	Colorado	11.6
16	Georgia	11.4
16	Montana	11.4
18	Maryland	9.9
19	Tennessee	9.2
20	Wyoming	9.1
21	Rhode Island	8.6
22	Illinois	7.5
22	Louisiana	7.5
24	Arkansas	7.4
25	New York	7.1
26	Florida	6.7
27	New Jersey	6.5
28	Pennsylvania	6.0
29	South Dakota	5.8
30	Kansas	5.1
31	North Carolina	4.9
32	Alaska	4.7
32	Virginia	4.7
34	Wisconsin	4.3
35	Ohio	4.2
36	Hawaii	4.1
37	Connecticut	3.8
37	Minnesota	3.8
37	Nebraska	3.8
40	Alabama	3.7
40	Vermont	3.7
42	New Hampshire	3.0
43	Massachusetts	2.7
44	South Carolina	2.6
45	Maine	2.0
46	Kentucky	1.8
47	Mississippi	1.6
48	Delaware	1.3
48	North Dakota	1.3
50	West Virginia	1.0

District of Columbia 15.9

Source: Morgan Quitno Press using data from U.S. Dept. of Health & Human Serv's, National Center for Health Statistics "Morbidity and Mortality Weekly Report" (January 8, 1999, Vol. 47, No. 51)

*Provisional data. An inflammation of the liver. Includes types A and B.

Legionellosis Cases Reported in 1998

National Total = 1,327 Cases*

ALPHA ORDER

RANK	STATE	CASES	% of USA
30	Alabama	9	0.7%
43	Alaska	1	0.1%
20	Arizona	20	1.5%
48	Arkansas	0	0.0%
7	California	55	4.1%
19	Colorado	21	1.6%
23	Connecticut	15	1.1%
26	Delaware	13	1.0%
8	Florida	41	3.1%
31	Georgia	8	0.6%
43	Hawaii	1	0.1%
40	Idaho	3	0.2%
8	Illinois	41	3.1%
4	Indiana	128	9.6%
24	Iowa	14	1.1%
31	Kansas	8	0.6%
12	Kentucky	30	2.3%
38	Louisiana	4	0.3%
43	Maine	1	0.1%
10	Maryland	33	2.5%
11	Massachusetts	32	2.4%
5	Michigan	80	6.0%
31	Minnesota	8	0.6%
35	Mississippi	7	0.5%
14	Missouri	24	1.8%
41	Montana	2	0.2%
20	Nebraska	20	1.5%
31	Nevada	8	0.6%
35	New Hampshire	7	0.5%
22	New Jersey	17	1.3%
41	New Mexico	2	0.2%
3	New York	130	9.8%
24	North Carolina	14	1.1%
48	North Dakota	0	0.0%
2	Ohio	136	10.2%
27	Oklahoma	12	0.9%
43	Oregon	1	0.1%
1	Pennsylvania	155	11.7%
16	Rhode Island	22	1.7%
29	South Carolina	11	0.8%
38	South Dakota	4	0.3%
14	Tennessee	24	1.8%
12	Texas	30	2.3%
16	Utah	22	1.7%
35	Vermont	7	0.5%
16	Virginia	22	1.7%
27	Washington	12	0.9%
NA	West Virginia**	NA	NA
6	Wisconsin	61	4.6%
43	Wyoming	1	0.1%

RANK ORDER

RANK	STATE	CASES	% of USA
1	Pennsylvania	155	11.7%
2	Ohio	136	10.2%
3	New York	130	9.8%
4	Indiana	128	9.6%
5	Michigan	80	6.0%
6	Wisconsin	61	4.6%
7	California	55	4.1%
8	Florida	41	3.1%
8	Illinois	41	3.1%
10	Maryland	33	2.5%
11	Massachusetts	32	2.4%
12	Kentucky	30	2.3%
12	Texas	30	2.3%
14	Missouri	24	1.8%
14	Tennessee	24	1.8%
16	Rhode Island	22	1.7%
16	Utah	22	1.7%
16	Virginia	22	1.7%
19	Colorado	21	1.6%
20	Arizona	20	1.5%
20	Nebraska	20	1.5%
22	New Jersey	17	1.3%
23	Connecticut	15	1.1%
24	Iowa	14	1.1%
24	North Carolina	14	1.1%
26	Delaware	13	1.0%
27	Oklahoma	12	0.9%
27	Washington	12	0.9%
29	South Carolina	11	0.8%
30	Alabama	9	0.7%
31	Georgia	8	0.6%
31	Kansas	8	0.6%
31	Minnesota	8	0.6%
31	Nevada	8	0.6%
35	Mississippi	7	0.5%
35	New Hampshire	7	0.5%
35	Vermont	7	0.5%
38	Louisiana	4	0.3%
38	South Dakota	4	0.3%
40	Idaho	3	0.2%
41	Montana	2	0.2%
41	New Mexico	2	0.2%
43	Alaska	1	0.1%
43	Hawaii	1	0.1%
43	Maine	1	0.1%
43	Oregon	1	0.1%
43	Wyoming	1	0.1%
48	Arkansas	0	0.0%
48	North Dakota	0	0.0%
NA	West Virginia**	NA	NA
	District of Columbia	8	0.6%

Source: U.S. Department of Health and Human Services, National Center for Health Statistics
"Morbidity and Mortality Weekly Report" (January 8, 1999, Vol. 47, No. 51)
Provisional data. A pneumonia-like disease (Legionnaire's Disease).
**Not notifiable.

Legionellosis Rate in 1998

National Rate = 0.5 Cases per 100,000 Population*

ALPHA ORDER

ALPHA ORDER

RANK	STATE	RATE
31	Alabama	0.2
31	Alaska	0.2
21	Arizona	0.4
47	Arkansas	0.0
31	California	0.2
15	Colorado	0.5
15	Connecticut	0.5
3	Delaware	1.7
25	Florida	0.3
42	Georgia	0.1
42	Hawaii	0.1
31	Idaho	0.2
25	Illinois	0.3
1	Indiana	2.2
15	Iowa	0.5
25	Kansas	0.3
10	Kentucky	0.8
42	Louisiana	0.1
42	Maine	0.1
13	Maryland	0.6
15	Massachusetts	0.5
10	Michigan	0.8
31	Minnesota	0.2
25	Mississippi	0.3
21	Missouri	0.4
31	Montana	0.2
5	Nebraska	1.2
15	Nevada	0.5
13	New Hampshire	0.6
31	New Jersey	0.2
42	New Mexico	0.1
12	New York	0.7
31	North Carolina	0.2
47	North Dakota	0.0
5	Ohio	1.2
21	Oklahoma	0.4
47	Oregon	0.0
4	Pennsylvania	1.3
1	Rhode Island	2.2
25	South Carolina	0.3
15	South Dakota	0.5
21	Tennessee	0.4
31	Texas	0.2
9	Utah	1.0
5	Vermont	1.2
25	Virginia	0.3
31	Washington	0.2
NA	West Virginia**	NA
5	Wisconsin	1.2
31	Wyoming	0.2

RANK ORDER

RANK	STATE	RATE
1	Indiana	2.2
1	Rhode Island	2.2
3	Delaware	1.7
4	Pennsylvania	1.3
5	Nebraska	1.2
5	Ohio	1.2
5	Vermont	1.2
5	Wisconsin	1.2
9	Utah	1.0
10	Kentucky	0.8
10	Michigan	0.8
12	New York	0.7
13	Maryland	0.6
13	New Hampshire	0.6
15	Colorado	0.5
15	Connecticut	0.5
15	Iowa	0.5
15	Massachusetts	0.5
15	Nevada	0.5
15	South Dakota	0.5
21	Arizona	0.4
21	Missouri	0.4
21	Oklahoma	0.4
21	Tennessee	0.4
25	Florida	0.3
25	Illinois	0.3
25	Kansas	0.3
25	Mississippi	0.3
25	South Carolina	0.3
25	Virginia	0.3
31	Alabama	0.2
31	Alaska	0.2
31	California	0.2
31	Idaho	0.2
31	Minnesota	0.2
31	Montana	0.2
31	New Jersey	0.2
31	North Carolina	0.2
31	Texas	0.2
31	Washington	0.2
31	Wyoming	0.2
42	Georgia	0.1
42	Hawaii	0.1
42	Louisiana	0.1
42	Maine	0.1
42	New Mexico	0.1
47	Arkansas	0.0
47	North Dakota	0.0
47	Oregon	0.0
NA	West Virginia**	NA

District of Columbia 1.5

Source: Morgan Quitno Press using data from U.S. Dept. of Health & Human Serv's, National Center for Health Statistics "Morbidity and Mortality Weekly Report" (January 8, 1999, Vol. 47, No. 51)
Provisional data. A pneumonia-like disease (Legionnaire's Disease).
Not notifiable.

Lyme Disease Cases in 1998

National Total = 14,646 Cases*

RANK	STATE	CASES	% of USA
20	Alabama	24	0.2%
42	Alaska	1	0.0%
42	Arizona	1	0.0%
30	Arkansas	7	0.0%
9	California	142	1.0%
35	Colorado	6	0.0%
2	Connecticut	2,969	20.3%
15	Delaware	45	0.3%
10	Florida	68	0.5%
37	Georgia	5	0.0%
45	Hawaii	0	0.0%
30	Idaho	7	0.0%
29	Illinois	9	0.1%
12	Indiana	65	0.4%
18	Iowa	26	0.2%
26	Kansas	11	0.1%
19	Kentucky	25	0.2%
30	Louisiana	7	0.0%
24	Maine	12	0.1%
7	Maryland	653	4.5%
5	Massachusetts	782	5.3%
24	Michigan	12	0.1%
8	Minnesota	174	1.2%
39	Mississippi	4	0.0%
41	Missouri	2	0.0%
45	Montana	0	0.0%
37	Nebraska	5	0.0%
35	Nevada	6	0.0%
15	New Hampshire	45	0.3%
4	New Jersey	1,729	11.8%
39	New Mexico	4	0.0%
1	New York	4,251	29.0%
13	North Carolina	63	0.4%
45	North Dakota	0	0.0%
14	Ohio	59	0.4%
28	Oklahoma	10	0.1%
21	Oregon	21	0.1%
3	Pennsylvania	2,524	17.2%
6	Rhode Island	692	4.7%
30	South Carolina	7	0.0%
45	South Dakota	0	0.0%
15	Tennessee	45	0.3%
22	Texas	20	0.1%
45	Utah	0	0.0%
26	Vermont	11	0.1%
10	Virginia	68	0.5%
30	Washington	7	0.0%
23	West Virginia	13	0.1%
NA	Wisconsin**	NA	NA
42	Wyoming	1	0.0%

RANK	STATE	CASES	% of USA
1	New York	4,251	29.0%
2	Connecticut	2,969	20.3%
3	Pennsylvania	2,524	17.2%
4	New Jersey	1,729	11.8%
5	Massachusetts	782	5.3%
6	Rhode Island	692	4.7%
7	Maryland	653	4.5%
8	Minnesota	174	1.2%
9	California	142	1.0%
10	Florida	68	0.5%
10	Virginia	68	0.5%
12	Indiana	65	0.4%
13	North Carolina	63	0.4%
14	Ohio	59	0.4%
15	Delaware	45	0.3%
15	New Hampshire	45	0.3%
15	Tennessee	45	0.3%
18	Iowa	26	0.2%
19	Kentucky	25	0.2%
20	Alabama	24	0.2%
21	Oregon	21	0.1%
22	Texas	20	0.1%
23	West Virginia	13	0.1%
24	Maine	12	0.1%
24	Michigan	12	0.1%
26	Kansas	11	0.1%
26	Vermont	11	0.1%
28	Oklahoma	10	0.1%
29	Illinois	9	0.1%
30	Arkansas	7	0.0%
30	Idaho	7	0.0%
30	Louisiana	7	0.0%
30	South Carolina	7	0.0%
30	Washington	7	0.0%
35	Colorado	6	0.0%
35	Nevada	6	0.0%
37	Georgia	5	0.0%
37	Nebraska	5	0.0%
39	Mississippi	4	0.0%
39	New Mexico	4	0.0%
41	Missouri	2	0.0%
42	Alaska	1	0.0%
42	Arizona	1	0.0%
42	Wyoming	1	0.0%
45	Hawaii	0	0.0%
45	Montana	0	0.0%
45	North Dakota	0	0.0%
45	South Dakota	0	0.0%
45	Utah	0	0.0%
NA	Wisconsin**	NA	NA
	District of Columbia	8	0.1%

*Source: U.S. Department of Health and Human Services, National Center for Health Statistics
"Morbidity and Mortality Weekly Report" (January 8, 1999, Vol. 47, No. 51)*
**Provisional data. Caused by ticks-lesions, followed by arthritis of large joints, myalgia, malaise and neurologic
and cardiac manifestations. Named after Old Lyme, CT, where the disease was first reported.*
**Not available.

Lyme Disease Rate in 1998

National Rate = 5.4 Cases per 100,000 Population*

ALPHA ORDER

RANK	STATE	RATE
19	Alabama	0.6
31	Alaska	0.2
43	Arizona	0.0
27	Arkansas	0.3
25	California	0.4
31	Colorado	0.2
1	Connecticut	90.7
8	Delaware	6.1
23	Florida	0.5
37	Georgia	0.1
43	Hawaii	0.0
19	Idaho	0.6
37	Illinois	0.1
12	Indiana	1.1
15	Iowa	0.9
25	Kansas	0.4
19	Kentucky	0.6
31	Louisiana	0.2
13	Maine	1.0
6	Maryland	12.7
6	Massachusetts	12.7
37	Michigan	0.1
10	Minnesota	3.7
37	Mississippi	0.1
43	Missouri	0.0
43	Montana	0.0
27	Nebraska	0.3
27	Nevada	0.3
9	New Hampshire	3.8
4	New Jersey	21.3
31	New Mexico	0.2
3	New York	23.4
16	North Carolina	0.8
43	North Dakota	0.0
23	Ohio	0.5
27	Oklahoma	0.3
19	Oregon	0.6
5	Pennsylvania	21.0
2	Rhode Island	70.0
31	South Carolina	0.2
43	South Dakota	0.0
16	Tennessee	0.8
37	Texas	0.1
43	Utah	0.0
11	Vermont	1.9
13	Virginia	1.0
37	Washington	0.1
18	West Virginia	0.7
NA	Wisconsin**	NA
31	Wyoming	0.2

RANK ORDER

RANK	STATE	RATE
1	Connecticut	90.7
2	Rhode Island	70.0
3	New York	23.4
4	New Jersey	21.3
5	Pennsylvania	21.0
6	Maryland	12.7
6	Massachusetts	12.7
8	Delaware	6.1
9	New Hampshire	3.8
10	Minnesota	3.7
11	Vermont	1.9
12	Indiana	1.1
13	Maine	1.0
13	Virginia	1.0
15	Iowa	0.9
16	North Carolina	0.8
16	Tennessee	0.8
18	West Virginia	0.7
19	Alabama	0.6
19	Idaho	0.6
19	Kentucky	0.6
19	Oregon	0.6
23	Florida	0.5
23	Ohio	0.5
25	California	0.4
25	Kansas	0.4
27	Arkansas	0.3
27	Nebraska	0.3
27	Nevada	0.3
27	Oklahoma	0.3
31	Alaska	0.2
31	Colorado	0.2
31	Louisiana	0.2
31	New Mexico	0.2
31	South Carolina	0.2
31	Wyoming	0.2
37	Georgia	0.1
37	Illinois	0.1
37	Michigan	0.1
37	Mississippi	0.1
37	Texas	0.1
37	Washington	0.1
43	Arizona	0.0
43	Hawaii	0.0
43	Missouri	0.0
43	Montana	0.0
43	North Dakota	0.0
43	South Dakota	0.0
43	Utah	0.0
NA	Wisconsin**	NA

District of Columbia 1.5

Source: Morgan Quitno Press using data from U.S. Dept. of Health & Human Serv's, National Center for Health Statistics "Morbidity and Mortality Weekly Report" (January 8, 1999, Vol. 47, No. 51)
*Provisional data. Caused by ticks-lesions, followed by arthritis of large joints, myalgia, malaise and neurologic and cardiac manifestations. Named after Old Lyme, CT, where the disease was first reported.
**Not available.

Malaria Cases Reported in 1998

National Total = 1,381 Cases*

RANK	STATE	CASES	% of USA
34	Alabama	6	0.4%
38	Alaska	4	0.3%
28	Arizona	9	0.7%
47	Arkansas	1	0.1%
2	California	217	15.7%
15	Colorado	19	1.4%
16	Connecticut	18	1.3%
40	Delaware	3	0.2%
4	Florida	83	6.0%
11	Georgia	40	2.9%
31	Hawaii	7	0.5%
30	Idaho	8	0.6%
10	Illinois	44	3.2%
26	Indiana	11	0.8%
31	Iowa	7	0.5%
27	Kansas	10	0.7%
31	Kentucky	7	0.5%
19	Louisiana	16	1.2%
36	Maine	5	0.4%
3	Maryland	89	6.4%
19	Massachusetts	16	1.2%
8	Michigan	49	3.5%
5	Minnesota	63	4.6%
42	Mississippi	2	0.1%
21	Missouri	15	1.1%
47	Montana	1	0.1%
42	Nebraska	2	0.1%
24	Nevada	12	0.9%
36	New Hampshire	5	0.4%
7	New Jersey	54	3.9%
24	New Mexico	12	0.9%
1	New York	244	17.7%
13	North Carolina	30	2.2%
40	North Dakota	3	0.2%
21	Ohio	15	1.1%
38	Oklahoma	4	0.3%
17	Oregon	17	1.2%
12	Pennsylvania	34	2.5%
23	Rhode Island	14	1.0%
34	South Carolina	6	0.4%
47	South Dakota	1	0.1%
17	Tennessee	17	1.2%
9	Texas	45	3.3%
42	Utah	2	0.1%
42	Vermont	2	0.1%
6	Virginia	58	4.2%
14	Washington	24	1.7%
42	West Virginia	2	0.1%
28	Wisconsin	9	0.7%
50	Wyoming	0	0.0%

RANK	STATE	CASES	% of USA
1	New York	244	17.7%
2	California	217	15.7%
3	Maryland	89	6.4%
4	Florida	83	6.0%
5	Minnesota	63	4.6%
6	Virginia	58	4.2%
7	New Jersey	54	3.9%
8	Michigan	49	3.5%
9	Texas	45	3.3%
10	Illinois	44	3.2%
11	Georgia	40	2.9%
12	Pennsylvania	34	2.5%
13	North Carolina	30	2.2%
14	Washington	24	1.7%
15	Colorado	19	1.4%
16	Connecticut	18	1.3%
17	Oregon	17	1.2%
17	Tennessee	17	1.2%
19	Louisiana	16	1.2%
19	Massachusetts	16	1.2%
21	Missouri	15	1.1%
21	Ohio	15	1.1%
23	Rhode Island	14	1.0%
24	Nevada	12	0.9%
24	New Mexico	12	0.9%
26	Indiana	11	0.8%
27	Kansas	10	0.7%
28	Arizona	9	0.7%
28	Wisconsin	9	0.7%
30	Idaho	8	0.6%
31	Hawaii	7	0.5%
31	Iowa	7	0.5%
31	Kentucky	7	0.5%
34	Alabama	6	0.4%
34	South Carolina	6	0.4%
36	Maine	5	0.4%
36	New Hampshire	5	0.4%
38	Alaska	4	0.3%
38	Oklahoma	4	0.3%
40	Delaware	3	0.2%
40	North Dakota	3	0.2%
42	Mississippi	2	0.1%
42	Nebraska	2	0.1%
42	Utah	2	0.1%
42	Vermont	2	0.1%
42	West Virginia	2	0.1%
47	Arkansas	1	0.1%
47	Montana	1	0.1%
47	South Dakota	1	0.1%
50	Wyoming	0	0.0%
	District of Columbia	19	1.4%

Source: U.S. Department of Health and Human Services, National Center for Health Statistics
   "Morbidity and Mortality Weekly Report" (January 8, 1999, Vol. 47, No. 51)
*Provisional data. Infectious disease usually transmitted by bites of infected mosquitoes. Symptoms include high fever, shaking chills, sweating and anemia.

Malaria Rate in 1998

National Rate = 0.5 Cases per 100,000 Population*

ALPHA ORDER

RANK	STATE	RATE
40	Alabama	0.1
6	Alaska	0.7
33	Arizona	0.2
49	Arkansas	0.0
6	California	0.7
14	Colorado	0.5
14	Connecticut	0.5
20	Delaware	0.4
12	Florida	0.6
14	Georgia	0.5
12	Hawaii	0.6
6	Idaho	0.7
20	Illinois	0.4
33	Indiana	0.2
33	Iowa	0.2
20	Kansas	0.4
33	Kentucky	0.2
20	Louisiana	0.4
20	Maine	0.4
1	Maryland	1.7
28	Massachusetts	0.3
14	Michigan	0.5
3	Minnesota	1.3
40	Mississippi	0.1
28	Missouri	0.3
40	Montana	0.1
40	Nebraska	0.1
6	Nevada	0.7
20	New Hampshire	0.4
6	New Jersey	0.7
6	New Mexico	0.7
3	New York	1.3
20	North Carolina	0.4
14	North Dakota	0.5
40	Ohio	0.1
40	Oklahoma	0.1
14	Oregon	0.5
28	Pennsylvania	0.3
2	Rhode Island	1.4
33	South Carolina	0.2
40	South Dakota	0.1
28	Tennessee	0.3
33	Texas	0.2
40	Utah	0.1
28	Vermont	0.3
5	Virginia	0.9
20	Washington	0.4
40	West Virginia	0.1
33	Wisconsin	0.2
49	Wyoming	0.0

RANK ORDER

RANK	STATE	RATE
1	Maryland	1.7
2	Rhode Island	1.4
3	Minnesota	1.3
3	New York	1.3
5	Virginia	0.9
6	Alaska	0.7
6	California	0.7
6	Idaho	0.7
6	Nevada	0.7
6	New Jersey	0.7
6	New Mexico	0.7
12	Florida	0.6
12	Hawaii	0.6
14	Colorado	0.5
14	Connecticut	0.5
14	Georgia	0.5
14	Michigan	0.5
14	North Dakota	0.5
14	Oregon	0.5
20	Delaware	0.4
20	Illinois	0.4
20	Kansas	0.4
20	Louisiana	0.4
20	Maine	0.4
20	New Hampshire	0.4
20	North Carolina	0.4
20	Washington	0.4
28	Massachusetts	0.3
28	Missouri	0.3
28	Pennsylvania	0.3
28	Tennessee	0.3
28	Vermont	0.3
33	Arizona	0.2
33	Indiana	0.2
33	Iowa	0.2
33	Kentucky	0.2
33	South Carolina	0.2
33	Texas	0.2
33	Wisconsin	0.2
40	Alabama	0.1
40	Mississippi	0.1
40	Montana	0.1
40	Nebraska	0.1
40	Ohio	0.1
40	Oklahoma	0.1
40	South Dakota	0.1
40	Utah	0.1
40	West Virginia	0.1
49	Arkansas	0.0
49	Wyoming	0.0

District of Columbia   3.6

Source: Morgan Quitno Press using data from U.S. Dept. of Health & Human Serv's, National Center for Health Statistics
"Morbidity and Mortality Weekly Report" (January 8, 1999, Vol. 47, No. 51)
*Provisional data. Infectious disease usually transmitted by bites of infected mosquitoes. Symptoms include high fever, shaking chills, sweating and anemia.

Measles (Rubeola) Cases Reported in 1998

National Total = 89 Cases*

ALPHA ORDER				RANK ORDER			
RANK	STATE	CASES	% of USA	RANK	STATE	CASES	% of USA
13	Alabama	1	1.1%	1	Alaska	29	32.6%
1	Alaska	29	32.6%	2	Michigan	10	11.2%
5	Arizona	5	5.6%	3	California	8	9.0%
24	Arkansas	0	0.0%	3	New Jersey	8	9.0%
3	California	8	9.0%	5	Arizona	5	5.6%
24	Colorado	0	0.0%	6	Pennsylvania	4	4.5%
24	Connecticut	0	0.0%	7	Indiana	3	3.4%
13	Delaware	1	1.1%	7	New York	3	3.4%
9	Florida	2	2.2%	9	Florida	2	2.2%
9	Georgia	2	2.2%	9	Georgia	2	2.2%
24	Hawaii	0	0.0%	9	Massachusetts	2	2.2%
24	Idaho	0	0.0%	9	Virginia	2	2.2%
13	Illinois	1	1.1%	13	Alabama	1	1.1%
7	Indiana	3	3.4%	13	Delaware	1	1.1%
13	Iowa	1	1.1%	13	Illinois	1	1.1%
24	Kansas	0	0.0%	13	Iowa	1	1.1%
24	Kentucky	0	0.0%	13	Louisiana	1	1.1%
13	Louisiana	1	1.1%	13	Maryland	1	1.1%
24	Maine	0	0.0%	13	Ohio	1	1.1%
13	Maryland	1	1.1%	13	Tennessee	1	1.1%
9	Massachusetts	2	2.2%	13	Vermont	1	1.1%
2	Michigan	10	11.2%	13	Washington	1	1.1%
24	Minnesota	0	0.0%	13	Wisconsin	1	1.1%
24	Mississippi	0	0.0%	24	Arkansas	0	0.0%
24	Missouri	0	0.0%	24	Colorado	0	0.0%
24	Montana	0	0.0%	24	Connecticut	0	0.0%
24	Nebraska	0	0.0%	24	Hawaii	0	0.0%
24	Nevada	0	0.0%	24	Idaho	0	0.0%
24	New Hampshire	0	0.0%	24	Kansas	0	0.0%
3	New Jersey	8	9.0%	24	Kentucky	0	0.0%
24	New Mexico	0	0.0%	24	Maine	0	0.0%
7	New York	3	3.4%	24	Minnesota	0	0.0%
24	North Carolina	0	0.0%	24	Mississippi	0	0.0%
24	North Dakota	0	0.0%	24	Missouri	0	0.0%
13	Ohio	1	1.1%	24	Montana	0	0.0%
24	Oklahoma	0	0.0%	24	Nebraska	0	0.0%
24	Oregon	0	0.0%	24	Nevada	0	0.0%
6	Pennsylvania	4	4.5%	24	New Hampshire	0	0.0%
24	Rhode Island	0	0.0%	24	New Mexico	0	0.0%
24	South Carolina	0	0.0%	24	North Carolina	0	0.0%
24	South Dakota	0	0.0%	24	North Dakota	0	0.0%
13	Tennessee	1	1.1%	24	Oklahoma	0	0.0%
24	Texas	0	0.0%	24	Oregon	0	0.0%
24	Utah	0	0.0%	24	Rhode Island	0	0.0%
13	Vermont	1	1.1%	24	South Carolina	0	0.0%
9	Virginia	2	2.2%	24	South Dakota	0	0.0%
13	Washington	1	1.1%	24	Texas	0	0.0%
24	West Virginia	0	0.0%	24	Utah	0	0.0%
13	Wisconsin	1	1.1%	24	West Virginia	0	0.0%
24	Wyoming	0	0.0%	24	Wyoming	0	0.0%
					District of Columbia	0	0.0%

Source: U.S. Department of Health and Human Services, National Center for Health Statistics
   "Morbidity and Mortality Weekly Report" (January 8, 1999, Vol. 47, No. 51)
*Provisional data. Includes indigenous and imported cases.

Measles (Rubeola) Rate in 1998

National Rate = 0.03 Cases per 100,000 Population*

ALPHA ORDER

RANK	STATE	RATE
13	Alabama	0.02
1	Alaska	4.72
4	Arizona	0.11
24	Arkansas	0.00
13	California	0.02
24	Colorado	0.00
24	Connecticut	0.00
3	Delaware	0.13
21	Florida	0.01
8	Georgia	0.03
24	Hawaii	0.00
24	Idaho	0.00
21	Illinois	0.01
7	Indiana	0.05
8	Iowa	0.03
24	Kansas	0.00
24	Kentucky	0.00
13	Louisiana	0.02
24	Maine	0.00
13	Maryland	0.02
8	Massachusetts	0.03
5	Michigan	0.10
24	Minnesota	0.00
24	Mississippi	0.00
24	Missouri	0.00
24	Montana	0.00
24	Nebraska	0.00
24	Nevada	0.00
24	New Hampshire	0.00
5	New Jersey	0.10
24	New Mexico	0.00
13	New York	0.02
24	North Carolina	0.00
24	North Dakota	0.00
21	Ohio	0.01
24	Oklahoma	0.00
24	Oregon	0.00
8	Pennsylvania	0.03
24	Rhode Island	0.00
24	South Carolina	0.00
24	South Dakota	0.00
13	Tennessee	0.02
24	Texas	0.00
24	Utah	0.00
2	Vermont	0.17
8	Virginia	0.03
13	Washington	0.02
24	West Virginia	0.00
13	Wisconsin	0.02
24	Wyoming	0.00

RANK ORDER

RANK	STATE	RATE
1	Alaska	4.72
2	Vermont	0.17
3	Delaware	0.13
4	Arizona	0.11
5	Michigan	0.10
5	New Jersey	0.10
7	Indiana	0.05
8	Georgia	0.03
8	Iowa	0.03
8	Massachusetts	0.03
8	Pennsylvania	0.03
8	Virginia	0.03
13	Alabama	0.02
13	California	0.02
13	Louisiana	0.02
13	Maryland	0.02
13	New York	0.02
13	Tennessee	0.02
13	Washington	0.02
13	Wisconsin	0.02
21	Florida	0.01
21	Illinois	0.01
21	Ohio	0.01
24	Arkansas	0.00
24	Colorado	0.00
24	Connecticut	0.00
24	Hawaii	0.00
24	Idaho	0.00
24	Kansas	0.00
24	Kentucky	0.00
24	Maine	0.00
24	Minnesota	0.00
24	Mississippi	0.00
24	Missouri	0.00
24	Montana	0.00
24	Nebraska	0.00
24	Nevada	0.00
24	New Hampshire	0.00
24	New Mexico	0.00
24	North Carolina	0.00
24	North Dakota	0.00
24	Oklahoma	0.00
24	Oregon	0.00
24	Rhode Island	0.00
24	South Carolina	0.00
24	South Dakota	0.00
24	Texas	0.00
24	Utah	0.00
24	West Virginia	0.00
24	Wyoming	0.00

District of Columbia	0.00

Source: Morgan Quitno Press using data from U.S. Dept. of Health & Human Serv's, National Center for Health Statistics "Morbidity and Mortality Weekly Report" (January 8, 1999, Vol. 47, No. 51)
*Provisional data. Includes indigenous and imported cases.

Meningococcal Infections Reported in 1998

National Total = 2,633 Cases*

ALPHA ORDER

ALPHA ORDER

RANK	STATE	CASES	% of USA
5	Alabama	110	4.2%
49	Alaska	3	0.1%
22	Arizona	47	1.8%
31	Arkansas	31	1.2%
1	California	311	11.8%
32	Colorado	30	1.1%
32	Connecticut	30	1.1%
50	Delaware	2	0.1%
4	Florida	139	5.3%
6	Georgia	98	3.7%
44	Hawaii	5	0.2%
37	Idaho	14	0.5%
9	Illinois	97	3.7%
13	Indiana	71	2.7%
20	Iowa	49	1.9%
30	Kansas	32	1.2%
26	Kentucky	38	1.4%
14	Louisiana	66	2.5%
41	Maine	8	0.3%
28	Maryland	34	1.3%
16	Massachusetts	60	2.3%
24	Michigan	42	1.6%
27	Minnesota	36	1.4%
25	Mississippi	39	1.5%
11	Missouri	83	3.2%
44	Montana	5	0.2%
36	Nebraska	15	0.6%
39	Nevada	10	0.4%
48	New Hampshire	4	0.2%
17	New Jersey	59	2.2%
34	New Mexico	26	1.0%
6	New York	98	3.7%
17	North Carolina	59	2.2%
44	North Dakota	5	0.2%
3	Ohio	143	5.4%
23	Oklahoma	43	1.6%
10	Oregon	91	3.5%
6	Pennsylvania	98	3.7%
41	Rhode Island	8	0.3%
19	South Carolina	57	2.2%
40	South Dakota	9	0.3%
12	Tennessee	72	2.7%
2	Texas	162	6.2%
37	Utah	14	0.5%
44	Vermont	5	0.2%
21	Virginia	48	1.8%
15	Washington	65	2.5%
35	West Virginia	17	0.6%
28	Wisconsin	34	1.3%
43	Wyoming	7	0.3%

RANK ORDER

RANK	STATE	CASES	% of USA
1	California	311	11.8%
2	Texas	162	6.2%
3	Ohio	143	5.4%
4	Florida	139	5.3%
5	Alabama	110	4.2%
6	Georgia	98	3.7%
6	New York	98	3.7%
6	Pennsylvania	98	3.7%
9	Illinois	97	3.7%
10	Oregon	91	3.5%
11	Missouri	83	3.2%
12	Tennessee	72	2.7%
13	Indiana	71	2.7%
14	Louisiana	66	2.5%
15	Washington	65	2.5%
16	Massachusetts	60	2.3%
17	New Jersey	59	2.2%
17	North Carolina	59	2.2%
19	South Carolina	57	2.2%
20	Iowa	49	1.9%
21	Virginia	48	1.8%
22	Arizona	47	1.8%
23	Oklahoma	43	1.6%
24	Michigan	42	1.6%
25	Mississippi	39	1.5%
26	Kentucky	38	1.4%
27	Minnesota	36	1.4%
28	Maryland	34	1.3%
28	Wisconsin	34	1.3%
30	Kansas	32	1.2%
31	Arkansas	31	1.2%
32	Colorado	30	1.1%
32	Connecticut	30	1.1%
34	New Mexico	26	1.0%
35	West Virginia	17	0.6%
36	Nebraska	15	0.6%
37	Idaho	14	0.5%
37	Utah	14	0.5%
39	Nevada	10	0.4%
40	South Dakota	9	0.3%
41	Maine	8	0.3%
41	Rhode Island	8	0.3%
43	Wyoming	7	0.3%
44	Hawaii	5	0.2%
44	Montana	5	0.2%
44	North Dakota	5	0.2%
44	Vermont	5	0.2%
48	New Hampshire	4	0.2%
49	Alaska	3	0.1%
50	Delaware	2	0.1%
	District of Columbia	4	0.2%

Source: U.S. Department of Health and Human Services, National Center for Health Statistics "Morbidity and Mortality Weekly Report" (January 8, 1999, Vol. 47, No. 51)
*Provisional data. A bacterium (Neisseria meningitidis) that causes cerebrospinal meningitis.

Meningococcal Infection Rate in 1998

National Rate = 1.0 Cases per 100,000 Population*

RANK	STATE	RATE
2	Alabama	2.5
45	Alaska	0.5
20	Arizona	1.0
14	Arkansas	1.2
20	California	1.0
28	Colorado	0.8
24	Connecticut	0.9
49	Delaware	0.3
24	Florida	0.9
10	Georgia	1.3
47	Hawaii	0.4
18	Idaho	1.1
28	Illinois	0.8
14	Indiana	1.2
3	Iowa	1.7
14	Kansas	1.2
20	Kentucky	1.0
4	Louisiana	1.5
42	Maine	0.6
37	Maryland	0.7
20	Massachusetts	1.0
47	Michigan	0.4
28	Minnesota	0.8
9	Mississippi	1.4
4	Missouri	1.5
42	Montana	0.6
24	Nebraska	0.9
42	Nevada	0.6
49	New Hampshire	0.3
37	New Jersey	0.7
4	New Mexico	1.5
45	New York	0.5
28	North Carolina	0.8
28	North Dakota	0.8
10	Ohio	1.3
10	Oklahoma	1.3
1	Oregon	2.8
28	Pennsylvania	0.8
28	Rhode Island	0.8
4	South Carolina	1.5
14	South Dakota	1.2
10	Tennessee	1.3
28	Texas	0.8
37	Utah	0.7
28	Vermont	0.8
37	Virginia	0.7
18	Washington	1.1
24	West Virginia	0.9
37	Wisconsin	0.7
4	Wyoming	1.5

RANK	STATE	RATE
1	Oregon	2.8
2	Alabama	2.5
3	Iowa	1.7
4	Louisiana	1.5
4	Missouri	1.5
4	New Mexico	1.5
4	South Carolina	1.5
4	Wyoming	1.5
9	Mississippi	1.4
10	Georgia	1.3
10	Ohio	1.3
10	Oklahoma	1.3
10	Tennessee	1.3
14	Arkansas	1.2
14	Indiana	1.2
14	Kansas	1.2
14	South Dakota	1.2
18	Idaho	1.1
18	Washington	1.1
20	Arizona	1.0
20	California	1.0
20	Kentucky	1.0
20	Massachusetts	1.0
24	Connecticut	0.9
24	Florida	0.9
24	Nebraska	0.9
24	West Virginia	0.9
28	Colorado	0.8
28	Illinois	0.8
28	Minnesota	0.8
28	North Carolina	0.8
28	North Dakota	0.8
28	Pennsylvania	0.8
28	Rhode Island	0.8
28	Texas	0.8
28	Vermont	0.8
37	Maryland	0.7
37	New Jersey	0.7
37	Utah	0.7
37	Virginia	0.7
37	Wisconsin	0.7
42	Maine	0.6
42	Montana	0.6
42	Nevada	0.6
45	Alaska	0.5
45	New York	0.5
47	Hawaii	0.4
47	Michigan	0.4
49	Delaware	0.3
49	New Hampshire	0.3

| | District of Columbia | 0.8 |

Source: Morgan Quitno Press using data from U.S. Dept. of Health & Human Serv's, National Center for Health Statistics "Morbidity and Mortality Weekly Report" (January 8, 1999, Vol. 47, No. 51)

Provisional data. A bacterium (Neisseria meningitidis) that causes cerebrospinal meningitis.

Mumps Cases Reported in 1998

National Total = 606 Cases*

ALPHA ORDER				RANK ORDER			
RANK	STATE	CASES	% of USA	RANK	STATE	CASES	% of USA
18	Alabama	9	1.5%	1	New York	152	25.1%
30	Alaska	2	0.3%	2	California	108	17.8%
22	Arizona	6	1.0%	3	Texas	39	6.4%
11	Arkansas	12	2.0%	4	Michigan	31	5.1%
2	California	108	17.8%	5	Ohio	29	4.8%
19	Colorado	7	1.2%	6	Hawaii	24	4.0%
28	Connecticut	3	0.5%	7	Florida	22	3.6%
38	Delaware	0	0.0%	8	Pennsylvania	19	3.1%
7	Florida	22	3.6%	9	Nevada	14	2.3%
30	Georgia	2	0.3%	10	Minnesota	13	2.1%
6	Hawaii	24	4.0%	11	Arkansas	12	2.0%
19	Idaho	7	1.2%	12	Illinois	11	1.8%
12	Illinois	11	1.8%	12	Iowa	11	1.8%
22	Indiana	6	1.0%	12	North Carolina	11	1.8%
12	Iowa	11	1.8%	12	Washington	11	1.8%
34	Kansas	1	0.2%	16	Louisiana	10	1.7%
34	Kentucky	1	0.2%	16	Virginia	10	1.7%
16	Louisiana	10	1.7%	18	Alabama	9	1.5%
38	Maine	0	0.0%	19	Colorado	7	1.2%
38	Maryland	0	0.0%	19	Idaho	7	1.2%
26	Massachusetts	4	0.7%	19	South Carolina	7	1.2%
4	Michigan	31	5.1%	22	Arizona	6	1.0%
10	Minnesota	13	2.1%	22	Indiana	6	1.0%
22	Mississippi	6	1.0%	22	Mississippi	6	1.0%
26	Missouri	4	0.7%	25	Utah	5	0.8%
38	Montana	0	0.0%	26	Massachusetts	4	0.7%
38	Nebraska	0	0.0%	26	Missouri	4	0.7%
9	Nevada	14	2.3%	28	Connecticut	3	0.5%
38	New Hampshire	0	0.0%	28	New Jersey	3	0.5%
28	New Jersey	3	0.5%	30	Alaska	2	0.3%
NA	New Mexico**	NA	NA	30	Georgia	2	0.3%
1	New York	152	25.1%	30	North Dakota	2	0.3%
12	North Carolina	11	1.8%	30	Tennessee	2	0.3%
30	North Dakota	2	0.3%	34	Kansas	1	0.2%
5	Ohio	29	4.8%	34	Kentucky	1	0.2%
38	Oklahoma	0	0.0%	34	Rhode Island	1	0.2%
NA	Oregon**	NA	NA	34	Wyoming	1	0.2%
8	Pennsylvania	19	3.1%	38	Delaware	0	0.0%
34	Rhode Island	1	0.2%	38	Maine	0	0.0%
19	South Carolina	7	1.2%	38	Maryland	0	0.0%
38	South Dakota	0	0.0%	38	Montana	0	0.0%
30	Tennessee	2	0.3%	38	Nebraska	0	0.0%
3	Texas	39	6.4%	38	New Hampshire	0	0.0%
25	Utah	5	0.8%	38	Oklahoma	0	0.0%
38	Vermont	0	0.0%	38	South Dakota	0	0.0%
16	Virginia	10	1.7%	38	Vermont	0	0.0%
12	Washington	11	1.8%	38	West Virginia	0	0.0%
38	West Virginia	0	0.0%	38	Wisconsin	0	0.0%
38	Wisconsin	0	0.0%	NA	New Mexico**	NA	NA
34	Wyoming	1	0.2%	NA	Oregon**	NA	NA
					District of Columbia	0	0.0%

Source: U.S. Department of Health and Human Services, National Center for Health Statistics
  "Morbidity and Mortality Weekly Report" (January 8, 1999, Vol. 47, No. 51)
*Provisional data. An acute, inflammatory, contagious disease caused by a paramyxovirus and characterized by swelling of the salivary glands, especially the parotids, and sometimes of the pancreas, ovaries, or testes. This disease, mainly affecting children, can be prevented by vaccination.
**Mumps is not a notifiable disease in New Mexico or Oregon.

Mumps Rate in 1998

National Rate = 0.22 Cases per 100,000 Population*

ALPHA ORDER

RANK	STATE	RATE
16	Alabama	0.21
7	Alaska	0.33
26	Arizona	0.13
5	Arkansas	0.47
7	California	0.33
20	Colorado	0.18
29	Connecticut	0.09
38	Delaware	0.00
23	Florida	0.15
36	Georgia	0.03
1	Hawaii	2.01
4	Idaho	0.57
29	Illinois	0.09
27	Indiana	0.10
6	Iowa	0.38
33	Kansas	0.04
36	Kentucky	0.03
14	Louisiana	0.23
38	Maine	0.00
38	Maryland	0.00
31	Massachusetts	0.07
9	Michigan	0.32
11	Minnesota	0.28
15	Mississippi	0.22
31	Missouri	0.07
38	Montana	0.00
38	Nebraska	0.00
3	Nevada	0.80
38	New Hampshire	0.00
33	New Jersey	0.04
NA	New Mexico**	NA
2	New York	0.84
23	North Carolina	0.15
10	North Dakota	0.31
12	Ohio	0.26
38	Oklahoma	0.00
NA	Oregon**	NA
22	Pennsylvania	0.16
27	Rhode Island	0.10
20	South Carolina	0.18
38	South Dakota	0.00
33	Tennessee	0.04
18	Texas	0.20
13	Utah	0.24
38	Vermont	0.00
23	Virginia	0.15
19	Washington	0.19
38	West Virginia	0.00
38	Wisconsin	0.00
16	Wyoming	0.21

RANK ORDER

RANK	STATE	RATE
1	Hawaii	2.01
2	New York	0.84
3	Nevada	0.80
4	Idaho	0.57
5	Arkansas	0.47
6	Iowa	0.38
7	Alaska	0.33
7	California	0.33
9	Michigan	0.32
10	North Dakota	0.31
11	Minnesota	0.28
12	Ohio	0.26
13	Utah	0.24
14	Louisiana	0.23
15	Mississippi	0.22
16	Alabama	0.21
16	Wyoming	0.21
18	Texas	0.20
19	Washington	0.19
20	Colorado	0.18
20	South Carolina	0.18
22	Pennsylvania	0.16
23	Florida	0.15
23	North Carolina	0.15
23	Virginia	0.15
26	Arizona	0.13
27	Indiana	0.10
27	Rhode Island	0.10
29	Connecticut	0.09
29	Illinois	0.09
31	Massachusetts	0.07
31	Missouri	0.07
33	Kansas	0.04
33	New Jersey	0.04
33	Tennessee	0.04
36	Georgia	0.03
36	Kentucky	0.03
38	Delaware	0.00
38	Maine	0.00
38	Maryland	0.00
38	Montana	0.00
38	Nebraska	0.00
38	New Hampshire	0.00
38	Oklahoma	0.00
38	South Dakota	0.00
38	Vermont	0.00
38	West Virginia	0.00
38	Wisconsin	0.00
NA	New Mexico**	NA
NA	Oregon**	NA

District of Columbia   0.00

Source: Morgan Quitno Press using data from U.S. Dept. of Health & Human Serv's, National Center for Health Statistics
"Morbidity and Mortality Weekly Report" (January 8, 1999, Vol. 47, No. 51)
*Provisional data. An acute, inflammatory, contagious disease caused by a paramyxovirus and characterized by swelling of the salivary glands, especially the parotids, and sometimes of the pancreas, ovaries, or testes. This disease, mainly affecting children, can be prevented by vaccination.
**Mumps is not a notifiable disease in New Mexico or Oregon.

Rabies (Animal) Cases Reported in 1997

National Total = 8,105 Cases*

RANK	STATE	CASES	% of USA
24	Alabama	88	1.1%
35	Alaska	29	0.4%
28	Arizona	53	0.7%
27	Arkansas	56	0.7%
6	California	327	4.0%
32	Colorado	34	0.4%
5	Connecticut	544	6.7%
26	Delaware	67	0.8%
9	Florida	278	3.4%
7	Georgia	324	4.0%
48	Hawaii	0	0.0%
48	Idaho	0	0.0%
39	Illinois	20	0.2%
41	Indiana	13	0.2%
15	Iowa	160	2.0%
22	Kansas	89	1.1%
35	Kentucky	29	0.4%
44	Louisiana	7	0.1%
12	Maine	227	2.8%
4	Maryland	603	7.4%
8	Massachusetts	282	3.5%
37	Michigan	28	0.3%
25	Minnesota	70	0.9%
46	Mississippi	5	0.1%
33	Missouri	31	0.4%
29	Montana	52	0.6%
47	Nebraska	2	0.0%
43	Nevada	8	0.1%
30	New Hampshire	49	0.6%
13	New Jersey	190	2.3%
41	New Mexico	13	0.2%
1	New York	1,264	15.6%
2	North Carolina	879	10.8%
21	North Dakota	91	1.1%
17	Ohio	116	1.4%
18	Oklahoma	113	1.4%
40	Oregon	14	0.2%
10	Pennsylvania	268	3.3%
31	Rhode Island	42	0.5%
14	South Carolina	186	2.3%
20	South Dakota	94	1.2%
16	Tennessee	149	1.8%
11	Texas	263	3.2%
45	Utah	6	0.1%
18	Vermont	113	1.4%
3	Virginia	678	8.4%
48	Washington	0	0.0%
22	West Virginia	89	1.1%
38	Wisconsin	26	0.3%
33	Wyoming	31	0.4%

RANK	STATE	CASES	% of USA
1	New York	1,264	15.6%
2	North Carolina	879	10.8%
3	Virginia	678	8.4%
4	Maryland	603	7.4%
5	Connecticut	544	6.7%
6	California	327	4.0%
7	Georgia	324	4.0%
8	Massachusetts	282	3.5%
9	Florida	278	3.4%
10	Pennsylvania	268	3.3%
11	Texas	263	3.2%
12	Maine	227	2.8%
13	New Jersey	190	2.3%
14	South Carolina	186	2.3%
15	Iowa	160	2.0%
16	Tennessee	149	1.8%
17	Ohio	116	1.4%
18	Oklahoma	113	1.4%
18	Vermont	113	1.4%
20	South Dakota	94	1.2%
21	North Dakota	91	1.1%
22	Kansas	89	1.1%
22	West Virginia	89	1.1%
24	Alabama	88	1.1%
25	Minnesota	70	0.9%
26	Delaware	67	0.8%
27	Arkansas	56	0.7%
28	Arizona	53	0.7%
29	Montana	52	0.6%
30	New Hampshire	49	0.6%
31	Rhode Island	42	0.5%
32	Colorado	34	0.4%
33	Missouri	31	0.4%
33	Wyoming	31	0.4%
35	Alaska	29	0.4%
35	Kentucky	29	0.4%
37	Michigan	28	0.3%
38	Wisconsin	26	0.3%
39	Illinois	20	0.2%
40	Oregon	14	0.2%
41	Indiana	13	0.2%
41	New Mexico	13	0.2%
43	Nevada	8	0.1%
44	Louisiana	7	0.1%
45	Utah	6	0.1%
46	Mississippi	5	0.1%
47	Nebraska	2	0.0%
48	Hawaii	0	0.0%
48	Idaho	0	0.0%
48	Washington	0	0.0%
	District of Columbia	5	0.1%

Source: U.S. Department of Health and Human Services, National Center for Health Statistics "Summary of Notifiable Diseases" (MMWR, November 20, 1998, Vol. 46, No. 54)
*Updated data. An acute, infectious, often fatal viral disease of most warm-blooded animals, especially wolves, cats, and dogs, that attacks the central nervous system and is transmitted by the bite of infected animals.

Rabies (Animal) Rate in 1997

National Rate = 3.0 Cases per 100,000 Human Population*

ALPHA ORDER				RANK ORDER		
RANK	STATE	RATE		RANK	STATE	RATE
27	Alabama	2.0		1	Vermont	19.2
16	Alaska	4.8		2	Maine	18.3
31	Arizona	1.2		3	Connecticut	16.7
25	Arkansas	2.2		4	North Dakota	14.2
32	California	1.0		5	South Dakota	12.7
34	Colorado	0.9		6	Maryland	11.8
3	Connecticut	16.7		6	North Carolina	11.8
9	Delaware	9.1		8	Virginia	10.1
28	Florida	1.9		9	Delaware	9.1
18	Georgia	4.3		10	New York	7.0
48	Hawaii	0.0		11	Wyoming	6.5
48	Idaho	0.0		12	Montana	5.9
43	Illinois	0.2		13	Iowa	5.6
43	Indiana	0.2		14	South Carolina	4.9
13	Iowa	5.6		14	West Virginia	4.9
21	Kansas	3.4		16	Alaska	4.8
36	Kentucky	0.7		17	Massachusetts	4.6
43	Louisiana	0.2		18	Georgia	4.3
2	Maine	18.3		18	Rhode Island	4.3
6	Maryland	11.8		20	New Hampshire	4.2
17	Massachusetts	4.6		21	Kansas	3.4
41	Michigan	0.3		21	Oklahoma	3.4
29	Minnesota	1.5		23	Tennessee	2.8
43	Mississippi	0.2		24	New Jersey	2.4
37	Missouri	0.6		25	Arkansas	2.2
12	Montana	5.9		25	Pennsylvania	2.2
47	Nebraska	0.1		27	Alabama	2.0
38	Nevada	0.5		28	Florida	1.9
20	New Hampshire	4.2		29	Minnesota	1.5
24	New Jersey	2.4		30	Texas	1.4
35	New Mexico	0.8		31	Arizona	1.2
10	New York	7.0		32	California	1.0
6	North Carolina	11.8		32	Ohio	1.0
4	North Dakota	14.2		34	Colorado	0.9
32	Ohio	1.0		35	New Mexico	0.8
21	Oklahoma	3.4		36	Kentucky	0.7
40	Oregon	0.4		37	Missouri	0.6
25	Pennsylvania	2.2		38	Nevada	0.5
18	Rhode Island	4.3		38	Wisconsin	0.5
14	South Carolina	4.9		40	Oregon	0.4
5	South Dakota	12.7		41	Michigan	0.3
23	Tennessee	2.8		41	Utah	0.3
30	Texas	1.4		43	Illinois	0.2
41	Utah	0.3		43	Indiana	0.2
1	Vermont	19.2		43	Louisiana	0.2
8	Virginia	10.1		43	Mississippi	0.2
48	Washington	0.0		47	Nebraska	0.1
14	West Virginia	4.9		48	Hawaii	0.0
38	Wisconsin	0.5		48	Idaho	0.0
11	Wyoming	6.5		48	Washington	0.0
					District of Columbia	0.9

Source: Morgan Quitno Press using data from U.S. Dept. of Health & Human Serv's, National Center for Health Statistics "Summary of Notifiable Diseases" (MMWR, November 20, 1998, Vol. 46, No. 54)
Updated data. An acute, infectious, often fatal viral disease of most warm-blooded animals, especially wolves, cats, and dogs, that attacks the central nervous system and is transmitted by the bite of infected animals.

Salmonellosis Cases Reported in 1997

National Total = 41,901 Cases*

ALPHA ORDER				RANK ORDER			
RANK	STATE	CASES	% of USA	RANK	STATE	CASES	% of USA
26	Alabama	470	1.1%	1	California	5,993	14.3%
49	Alaska	50	0.1%	2	New York	3,445	8.2%
16	Arizona	853	2.0%	3	Texas	2,793	6.7%
28	Arkansas	445	1.1%	4	Florida	2,590	6.2%
1	California	5,993	14.3%	5	Illinois	1,935	4.6%
20	Colorado	608	1.5%	6	Pennsylvania	1,559	3.7%
24	Connecticut	546	1.3%	7	Ohio	1,545	3.7%
44	Delaware	101	0.2%	8	New Jersey	1,501	3.6%
4	Florida	2,590	6.2%	9	Georgia	1,356	3.2%
9	Georgia	1,356	3.2%	10	Massachusetts	1,259	3.0%
31	Hawaii	384	0.9%	11	Maryland	1,231	2.9%
41	Idaho	141	0.3%	11	Wisconsin	1,231	2.9%
5	Illinois	1,935	4.6%	13	North Carolina	1,226	2.9%
22	Indiana	590	1.4%	14	Virginia	1,120	2.7%
35	Iowa	297	0.7%	15	Michigan	906	2.2%
27	Kansas	446	1.1%	16	Arizona	853	2.0%
32	Kentucky	373	0.9%	17	Washington	680	1.6%
19	Louisiana	617	1.5%	18	Minnesota	632	1.5%
42	Maine	137	0.3%	19	Louisiana	617	1.5%
11	Maryland	1,231	2.9%	20	Colorado	608	1.5%
10	Massachusetts	1,259	3.0%	21	South Carolina	603	1.4%
15	Michigan	906	2.2%	22	Indiana	590	1.4%
18	Minnesota	632	1.5%	23	Missouri	568	1.4%
25	Mississippi	485	1.2%	24	Connecticut	546	1.3%
23	Missouri	568	1.4%	25	Mississippi	485	1.2%
48	Montana	63	0.2%	26	Alabama	470	1.1%
38	Nebraska	185	0.4%	27	Kansas	446	1.1%
36	Nevada	291	0.7%	28	Arkansas	445	1.1%
40	New Hampshire	151	0.4%	29	Tennessee	443	1.1%
8	New Jersey	1,501	3.6%	30	Oklahoma	391	0.9%
34	New Mexico	311	0.7%	31	Hawaii	384	0.9%
2	New York	3,445	8.2%	32	Kentucky	373	0.9%
13	North Carolina	1,226	2.9%	33	Oregon	368	0.9%
47	North Dakota	69	0.2%	34	New Mexico	311	0.7%
7	Ohio	1,545	3.7%	35	Iowa	297	0.7%
30	Oklahoma	391	0.9%	36	Nevada	291	0.7%
33	Oregon	368	0.9%	37	Utah	271	0.6%
6	Pennsylvania	1,559	3.7%	38	Nebraska	185	0.4%
39	Rhode Island	167	0.4%	39	Rhode Island	167	0.4%
21	South Carolina	603	1.4%	40	New Hampshire	151	0.4%
45	South Dakota	90	0.2%	41	Idaho	141	0.3%
29	Tennessee	443	1.1%	42	Maine	137	0.3%
3	Texas	2,793	6.7%	43	West Virginia	133	0.3%
37	Utah	271	0.6%	44	Delaware	101	0.2%
46	Vermont	88	0.2%	45	South Dakota	90	0.2%
14	Virginia	1,120	2.7%	46	Vermont	88	0.2%
17	Washington	680	1.6%	47	North Dakota	69	0.2%
43	West Virginia	133	0.3%	48	Montana	63	0.2%
11	Wisconsin	1,231	2.9%	49	Alaska	50	0.1%
50	Wyoming	49	0.1%	50	Wyoming	49	0.1%
					District of Columbia	115	0.3%

Source: U.S. Department of Health and Human Services, National Center for Health Statistics
"Summary of Notifiable Diseases" (MMWR, November 20, 1998, Vol. 46, No. 54)
*Final data. Any disease caused by a salmonella infection, which may be manifested as food poisoning with acute gastroenteritis, vomiting and diarrhea.

Salmonellosis Rate in 1997

National Rate = 15.6 Cases per 100,000 Population*

ALPHA ORDER

ALPHA ORDER

RANK	STATE	RATE
39	Alabama	10.9
47	Alaska	8.2
6	Arizona	18.7
12	Arkansas	17.6
7	California	18.6
22	Colorado	15.6
17	Connecticut	16.7
27	Delaware	13.7
12	Florida	17.6
9	Georgia	18.1
1	Hawaii	32.2
35	Idaho	11.7
20	Illinois	16.1
44	Indiana	10.1
42	Iowa	10.4
15	Kansas	17.1
45	Kentucky	9.5
25	Louisiana	14.2
38	Maine	11.0
2	Maryland	24.2
4	Massachusetts	20.6
46	Michigan	9.3
28	Minnesota	13.5
11	Mississippi	17.8
41	Missouri	10.5
50	Montana	7.2
37	Nebraska	11.2
14	Nevada	17.3
31	New Hampshire	12.9
7	New Jersey	18.6
10	New Mexico	18.0
5	New York	19.0
19	North Carolina	16.5
40	North Dakota	10.8
26	Ohio	13.8
34	Oklahoma	11.8
36	Oregon	11.3
30	Pennsylvania	13.0
16	Rhode Island	16.9
21	South Carolina	15.9
32	South Dakota	12.2
47	Tennessee	8.2
24	Texas	14.4
29	Utah	13.1
23	Vermont	14.9
18	Virginia	16.6
33	Washington	12.1
49	West Virginia	7.3
3	Wisconsin	23.7
43	Wyoming	10.2

RANK ORDER

RANK	STATE	RATE
1	Hawaii	32.2
2	Maryland	24.2
3	Wisconsin	23.7
4	Massachusetts	20.6
5	New York	19.0
6	Arizona	18.7
7	California	18.6
7	New Jersey	18.6
9	Georgia	18.1
10	New Mexico	18.0
11	Mississippi	17.8
12	Arkansas	17.6
12	Florida	17.6
14	Nevada	17.3
15	Kansas	17.1
16	Rhode Island	16.9
17	Connecticut	16.7
18	Virginia	16.6
19	North Carolina	16.5
20	Illinois	16.1
21	South Carolina	15.9
22	Colorado	15.6
23	Vermont	14.9
24	Texas	14.4
25	Louisiana	14.2
26	Ohio	13.8
27	Delaware	13.7
28	Minnesota	13.5
29	Utah	13.1
30	Pennsylvania	13.0
31	New Hampshire	12.9
32	South Dakota	12.2
33	Washington	12.1
34	Oklahoma	11.8
35	Idaho	11.7
36	Oregon	11.3
37	Nebraska	11.2
38	Maine	11.0
39	Alabama	10.9
40	North Dakota	10.8
41	Missouri	10.5
42	Iowa	10.4
43	Wyoming	10.2
44	Indiana	10.1
45	Kentucky	9.5
46	Michigan	9.3
47	Alaska	8.2
47	Tennessee	8.2
49	West Virginia	7.3
50	Montana	7.2

District of Columbia   21.7

Source: Morgan Quitno Press using data from U.S. Dept. of Health & Human Serv's, National Center for Health Statistics "Summary of Notifiable Diseases" (MMWR, November 20, 1998, Vol. 46, No. 54)
*Final data. Any disease caused by a salmonella infection, which may be manifested as food poisoning with acute gastroenteritis, vomiting and diarrhea.

Shigellosis Cases Reported in 1997

National Total = 23,117 Cases*

ALPHA ORDER

RANK	STATE	CASES	% of USA
23	Alabama	272	1.2%
49	Alaska	6	0.0%
7	Arizona	1,076	4.7%
22	Arkansas	273	1.2%
1	California	3,528	15.3%
24	Colorado	258	1.1%
32	Connecticut	101	0.4%
42	Delaware	35	0.2%
3	Florida	1,946	8.4%
6	Georgia	1,131	4.9%
39	Hawaii	65	0.3%
38	Idaho	79	0.3%
5	Illinois	1,163	5.0%
36	Indiana	88	0.4%
35	Iowa	90	0.4%
29	Kansas	133	0.6%
11	Kentucky	449	1.9%
27	Louisiana	182	0.8%
45	Maine	15	0.1%
12	Maryland	423	1.8%
18	Massachusetts	316	1.4%
15	Michigan	346	1.5%
28	Minnesota	138	0.6%
31	Mississippi	115	0.5%
25	Missouri	222	1.0%
46	Montana	11	0.0%
21	Nebraska	284	1.2%
41	Nevada	52	0.2%
40	New Hampshire	54	0.2%
10	New Jersey	625	2.7%
16	New Mexico	331	1.4%
4	New York	1,757	7.6%
14	North Carolina	387	1.7%
48	North Dakota	10	0.0%
8	Ohio	835	3.6%
19	Oklahoma	293	1.3%
26	Oregon	189	0.8%
9	Pennsylvania	786	3.4%
34	Rhode Island	95	0.4%
37	South Carolina	87	0.4%
43	South Dakota	31	0.1%
20	Tennessee	291	1.3%
2	Texas	3,504	15.2%
32	Utah	101	0.4%
46	Vermont	11	0.0%
13	Virginia	416	1.8%
17	Washington	318	1.4%
44	West Virginia	27	0.1%
30	Wisconsin	120	0.5%
50	Wyoming	5	0.0%

RANK ORDER

RANK	STATE	CASES	% of USA
1	California	3,528	15.3%
2	Texas	3,504	15.2%
3	Florida	1,946	8.4%
4	New York	1,757	7.6%
5	Illinois	1,163	5.0%
6	Georgia	1,131	4.9%
7	Arizona	1,076	4.7%
8	Ohio	835	3.6%
9	Pennsylvania	786	3.4%
10	New Jersey	625	2.7%
11	Kentucky	449	1.9%
12	Maryland	423	1.8%
13	Virginia	416	1.8%
14	North Carolina	387	1.7%
15	Michigan	346	1.5%
16	New Mexico	331	1.4%
17	Washington	318	1.4%
18	Massachusetts	316	1.4%
19	Oklahoma	293	1.3%
20	Tennessee	291	1.3%
21	Nebraska	284	1.2%
22	Arkansas	273	1.2%
23	Alabama	272	1.2%
24	Colorado	258	1.1%
25	Missouri	222	1.0%
26	Oregon	189	0.8%
27	Louisiana	182	0.8%
28	Minnesota	138	0.6%
29	Kansas	133	0.6%
30	Wisconsin	120	0.5%
31	Mississippi	115	0.5%
32	Connecticut	101	0.4%
32	Utah	101	0.4%
34	Rhode Island	95	0.4%
35	Iowa	90	0.4%
36	Indiana	88	0.4%
37	South Carolina	87	0.4%
38	Idaho	79	0.3%
39	Hawaii	65	0.3%
40	New Hampshire	54	0.2%
41	Nevada	52	0.2%
42	Delaware	35	0.2%
43	South Dakota	31	0.1%
44	West Virginia	27	0.1%
45	Maine	15	0.1%
46	Montana	11	0.0%
46	Vermont	11	0.0%
48	North Dakota	10	0.0%
49	Alaska	6	0.0%
50	Wyoming	5	0.0%
	District of Columbia	47	0.2%

Source: U.S. Department of Health and Human Services, National Center for Health Statistics
  "Summary of Notifiable Diseases" (MMWR, November 20, 1998, Vol. 46, No. 54)
*Final data. Dysentery caused by any of various species of shigellae, occurring most frequently in areas where poor sanitation and malnutrition are prevalent and commonly affecting children and infants.

Shigellosis Rate in 1997

National Rate = 8.6 Cases per 100,000 Population*

ALPHA ORDER

RANK	STATE	RATE
20	Alabama	6.3
49	Alaska	1.0
1	Arizona	23.6
9	Arkansas	10.8
8	California	11.0
17	Colorado	6.6
38	Connecticut	3.1
30	Delaware	4.8
6	Florida	13.3
5	Georgia	15.1
24	Hawaii	5.5
18	Idaho	6.5
10	Illinois	9.7
45	Indiana	1.5
37	Iowa	3.2
28	Kansas	5.1
7	Kentucky	11.5
32	Louisiana	4.2
48	Maine	1.2
14	Maryland	8.3
26	Massachusetts	5.2
36	Michigan	3.5
40	Minnesota	2.9
32	Mississippi	4.2
35	Missouri	4.1
47	Montana	1.3
4	Nebraska	17.1
38	Nevada	3.1
31	New Hampshire	4.6
15	New Jersey	7.8
2	New Mexico	19.2
10	New York	9.7
26	North Carolina	5.2
44	North Dakota	1.6
16	Ohio	7.5
13	Oklahoma	8.8
22	Oregon	5.8
18	Pennsylvania	6.5
12	Rhode Island	9.6
41	South Carolina	2.3
32	South Dakota	4.2
25	Tennessee	5.4
3	Texas	18.1
29	Utah	4.9
43	Vermont	1.9
21	Virginia	6.2
23	Washington	5.7
45	West Virginia	1.5
41	Wisconsin	2.3
49	Wyoming	1.0

RANK ORDER

RANK	STATE	RATE
1	Arizona	23.6
2	New Mexico	19.2
3	Texas	18.1
4	Nebraska	17.1
5	Georgia	15.1
6	Florida	13.3
7	Kentucky	11.5
8	California	11.0
9	Arkansas	10.8
10	Illinois	9.7
10	New York	9.7
12	Rhode Island	9.6
13	Oklahoma	8.8
14	Maryland	8.3
15	New Jersey	7.8
16	Ohio	7.5
17	Colorado	6.6
18	Idaho	6.5
18	Pennsylvania	6.5
20	Alabama	6.3
21	Virginia	6.2
22	Oregon	5.8
23	Washington	5.7
24	Hawaii	5.5
25	Tennessee	5.4
26	Massachusetts	5.2
26	North Carolina	5.2
28	Kansas	5.1
29	Utah	4.9
30	Delaware	4.8
31	New Hampshire	4.6
32	Louisiana	4.2
32	Mississippi	4.2
32	South Dakota	4.2
35	Missouri	4.1
36	Michigan	3.5
37	Iowa	3.2
38	Connecticut	3.1
38	Nevada	3.1
40	Minnesota	2.9
41	South Carolina	2.3
41	Wisconsin	2.3
43	Vermont	1.9
44	North Dakota	1.6
45	Indiana	1.5
45	West Virginia	1.5
47	Montana	1.3
48	Maine	1.2
49	Alaska	1.0
49	Wyoming	1.0
	District of Columbia	8.9

Source: Morgan Quitno Press using data from U.S. Dept. of Health & Human Serv's, National Center for Health Statistics "Summary of Notifiable Diseases" (MMWR, November 20, 1998, Vol. 46, No. 54)
*Final data. Dysentery caused by any of various species of shigellae, occurring most frequently in areas where poor sanitation and malnutrition are prevalent and commonly affecting children and infants.

Tuberculosis Cases Reported in 1998

National Total = 14,756 Cases*

RANK	STATE	CASES	% of USA
11	Alabama	316	2.1%
34	Alaska	54	0.4%
18	Arizona	206	1.4%
24	Arkansas	152	1.0%
1	California	3,256	22.1%
NA	Colorado**	NA	NA
27	Connecticut	106	0.7%
43	Delaware	18	0.1%
31	Florida	70	0.5%
7	Georgia	517	3.5%
20	Hawaii	169	1.1%
45	Idaho	13	0.1%
4	Illinois	655	4.4%
23	Indiana	157	1.1%
36	Iowa	51	0.3%
38	Kansas	44	0.3%
22	Kentucky	158	1.1%
13	Louisiana	274	1.9%
46	Maine	11	0.1%
13	Maryland	274	1.9%
15	Massachusetts	270	1.8%
10	Michigan	360	2.4%
25	Minnesota	149	1.0%
19	Mississippi	186	1.3%
28	Missouri	95	0.6%
42	Montana	19	0.1%
40	Nebraska	31	0.2%
30	Nevada	85	0.6%
44	New Hampshire	14	0.1%
5	New Jersey	631	4.3%
32	New Mexico	65	0.4%
2	New York	1,840	12.5%
8	North Carolina	498	3.4%
47	North Dakota	10	0.1%
29	Ohio	90	0.6%
21	Oklahoma	161	1.1%
26	Oregon	146	1.0%
6	Pennsylvania	532	3.6%
33	Rhode Island	64	0.4%
16	South Carolina	234	1.6%
41	South Dakota	23	0.2%
9	Tennessee	458	3.1%
3	Texas	1,536	10.4%
35	Utah	52	0.4%
48	Vermont	4	0.0%
12	Virginia	280	1.9%
17	Washington	210	1.4%
39	West Virginia	42	0.3%
37	Wisconsin	46	0.3%
48	Wyoming	4	0.0%

RANK	STATE	CASES	% of USA
1	California	3,256	22.1%
2	New York	1,840	12.5%
3	Texas	1,536	10.4%
4	Illinois	655	4.4%
5	New Jersey	631	4.3%
6	Pennsylvania	532	3.6%
7	Georgia	517	3.5%
8	North Carolina	498	3.4%
9	Tennessee	458	3.1%
10	Michigan	360	2.4%
11	Alabama	316	2.1%
12	Virginia	280	1.9%
13	Louisiana	274	1.9%
13	Maryland	274	1.9%
15	Massachusetts	270	1.8%
16	South Carolina	234	1.6%
17	Washington	210	1.4%
18	Arizona	206	1.4%
19	Mississippi	186	1.3%
20	Hawaii	169	1.1%
21	Oklahoma	161	1.1%
22	Kentucky	158	1.1%
23	Indiana	157	1.1%
24	Arkansas	152	1.0%
25	Minnesota	149	1.0%
26	Oregon	146	1.0%
27	Connecticut	106	0.7%
28	Missouri	95	0.6%
29	Ohio	90	0.6%
30	Nevada	85	0.6%
31	Florida	70	0.5%
32	New Mexico	65	0.4%
33	Rhode Island	64	0.4%
34	Alaska	54	0.4%
35	Utah	52	0.4%
36	Iowa	51	0.3%
37	Wisconsin	46	0.3%
38	Kansas	44	0.3%
39	West Virginia	42	0.3%
40	Nebraska	31	0.2%
41	South Dakota	23	0.2%
42	Montana	19	0.1%
43	Delaware	18	0.1%
44	New Hampshire	14	0.1%
45	Idaho	13	0.1%
46	Maine	11	0.1%
47	North Dakota	10	0.1%
48	Vermont	4	0.0%
48	Wyoming	4	0.0%
NA	Colorado**	NA	NA
	District of Columbia	101	0.7%

Source: U.S. Department of Health and Human Services, National Center for Health Statistics
"Morbidity and Mortality Weekly Report" (January 8, 1999, Vol. 47, No. 51)
*Provisional data. An infectious disease caused by the tubercle bacillus and causing the formation of tubercles on the lungs and other tissues of the body, often developing long after the initial infection. Characterized by the coughing up of mucus and sputum, fever, weight loss, and chest pain.
**Not available.

Tuberculosis Rate in 1998

National Rate = 5.5 Cases per 100,000 Population*

ALPHA ORDER

RANK	STATE	RATE
8	Alabama	7.3
4	Alaska	8.8
20	Arizona	4.4
15	Arkansas	6.0
3	California	10.0
NA	Colorado**	NA
29	Connecticut	3.2
34	Delaware	2.4
49	Florida	0.5
9	Georgia	6.8
1	Hawaii	14.2
43	Idaho	1.1
16	Illinois	5.4
32	Indiana	2.7
38	Iowa	1.8
39	Kansas	1.7
25	Kentucky	4.0
13	Louisiana	6.3
44	Maine	0.9
17	Maryland	5.3
20	Massachusetts	4.4
26	Michigan	3.7
29	Minnesota	3.2
9	Mississippi	6.8
39	Missouri	1.7
36	Montana	2.2
37	Nebraska	1.9
18	Nevada	4.9
42	New Hampshire	1.2
6	New Jersey	7.8
26	New Mexico	3.7
2	New York	10.1
11	North Carolina	6.6
41	North Dakota	1.6
46	Ohio	0.8
19	Oklahoma	4.8
20	Oregon	4.4
20	Pennsylvania	4.4
12	Rhode Island	6.5
14	South Carolina	6.1
31	South Dakota	3.1
5	Tennessee	8.4
6	Texas	7.8
33	Utah	2.5
48	Vermont	0.7
24	Virginia	4.1
26	Washington	3.7
35	West Virginia	2.3
44	Wisconsin	0.9
46	Wyoming	0.8

RANK ORDER

RANK	STATE	RATE
1	Hawaii	14.2
2	New York	10.1
3	California	10.0
4	Alaska	8.8
5	Tennessee	8.4
6	New Jersey	7.8
6	Texas	7.8
8	Alabama	7.3
9	Georgia	6.8
9	Mississippi	6.8
11	North Carolina	6.6
12	Rhode Island	6.5
13	Louisiana	6.3
14	South Carolina	6.1
15	Arkansas	6.0
16	Illinois	5.4
17	Maryland	5.3
18	Nevada	4.9
19	Oklahoma	4.8
20	Arizona	4.4
20	Massachusetts	4.4
20	Oregon	4.4
20	Pennsylvania	4.4
24	Virginia	4.1
25	Kentucky	4.0
26	Michigan	3.7
26	New Mexico	3.7
26	Washington	3.7
29	Connecticut	3.2
29	Minnesota	3.2
31	South Dakota	3.1
32	Indiana	2.7
33	Utah	2.5
34	Delaware	2.4
35	West Virginia	2.3
36	Montana	2.2
37	Nebraska	1.9
38	Iowa	1.8
39	Kansas	1.7
39	Missouri	1.7
41	North Dakota	1.6
42	New Hampshire	1.2
43	Idaho	1.1
44	Maine	0.9
44	Wisconsin	0.9
46	Ohio	0.8
46	Wyoming	0.8
48	Vermont	0.7
49	Florida	0.5
NA	Colorado**	NA

District of Columbia 19.3

Source: Morgan Quitno Press using data from U.S. Dept. of Health & Human Serv's, National Center for Health Statistics "Morbidity and Mortality Weekly Report" (January 8, 1999, Vol. 47, No. 51)
Provisional data. An infectious disease caused by the tubercle bacillus and causing the formation of tubercles on the lungs and other tissues of the body, often developing long after the initial infection. Characterized by the coughing up of mucus and sputum, fever, weight loss, and chest pain.
**Not available.*

Whooping Cough (Pertussis) Cases Reported in 1998

National Total = 6,279 Cases*

ALPHA ORDER

RANK	STATE	CASES	% of USA
34	Alabama	32	0.5%
41	Alaska	15	0.2%
12	Arizona	224	3.6%
18	Arkansas	96	1.5%
1	California	958	15.3%
8	Colorado	257	4.1%
29	Connecticut	46	0.7%
47	Delaware	5	0.1%
24	Florida	62	1.0%
36	Georgia	28	0.4%
38	Hawaii	20	0.3%
9	Idaho	246	3.9%
14	Illinois	129	2.1%
13	Indiana	151	2.4%
21	Iowa	73	1.2%
23	Kansas	66	1.1%
27	Kentucky	50	0.8%
44	Louisiana	9	0.1%
47	Maine	5	0.1%
25	Maryland	59	0.9%
2	Massachusetts	686	10.9%
22	Michigan	71	1.1%
4	Minnesota	353	5.6%
50	Mississippi	3	0.0%
27	Missouri	50	0.8%
42	Montana	13	0.2%
38	Nebraska	20	0.3%
31	Nevada	41	0.7%
15	New Hampshire	127	2.0%
43	New Jersey	12	0.2%
17	New Mexico	100	1.6%
3	New York	364	5.8%
16	North Carolina	110	1.8%
30	North Dakota	45	0.7%
6	Ohio	298	4.7%
35	Oklahoma	31	0.5%
19	Oregon	90	1.4%
11	Pennsylvania	229	3.6%
40	Rhode Island	16	0.3%
37	South Carolina	27	0.4%
45	South Dakota	8	0.1%
33	Tennessee	37	0.6%
10	Texas	237	3.8%
7	Utah	266	4.2%
20	Vermont	77	1.2%
26	Virginia	51	0.8%
5	Washington	335	5.3%
49	West Virginia	4	0.1%
32	Wisconsin	38	0.6%
45	Wyoming	8	0.1%

RANK ORDER

RANK	STATE	CASES	% of USA
1	California	958	15.3%
2	Massachusetts	686	10.9%
3	New York	364	5.8%
4	Minnesota	353	5.6%
5	Washington	335	5.3%
6	Ohio	298	4.7%
7	Utah	266	4.2%
8	Colorado	257	4.1%
9	Idaho	246	3.9%
10	Texas	237	3.8%
11	Pennsylvania	229	3.6%
12	Arizona	224	3.6%
13	Indiana	151	2.4%
14	Illinois	129	2.1%
15	New Hampshire	127	2.0%
16	North Carolina	110	1.8%
17	New Mexico	100	1.6%
18	Arkansas	96	1.5%
19	Oregon	90	1.4%
20	Vermont	77	1.2%
21	Iowa	73	1.2%
22	Michigan	71	1.1%
23	Kansas	66	1.1%
24	Florida	62	1.0%
25	Maryland	59	0.9%
26	Virginia	51	0.8%
27	Kentucky	50	0.8%
27	Missouri	50	0.8%
29	Connecticut	46	0.7%
30	North Dakota	45	0.7%
31	Nevada	41	0.7%
32	Wisconsin	38	0.6%
33	Tennessee	37	0.6%
34	Alabama	32	0.5%
35	Oklahoma	31	0.5%
36	Georgia	28	0.4%
37	South Carolina	27	0.4%
38	Hawaii	20	0.3%
38	Nebraska	20	0.3%
40	Rhode Island	16	0.3%
41	Alaska	15	0.2%
42	Montana	13	0.2%
43	New Jersey	12	0.2%
44	Louisiana	9	0.1%
45	South Dakota	8	0.1%
45	Wyoming	8	0.1%
47	Delaware	5	0.1%
47	Maine	5	0.1%
49	West Virginia	4	0.1%
50	Mississippi	3	0.0%
	District of Columbia	1	0.0%

Source: U.S. Department of Health and Human Services, National Center for Health Statistics
"Morbidity and Mortality Weekly Report" (January 8, 1999, Vol. 47, No. 51)
Provisional data. Acute, highly contagious infection of respiratory tract.

Whooping Cough (Pertussis) Rate in 1998

National Rate = 2.3 Cases per 100,000 Population*

ALPHA ORDER

RANK	STATE	RATE
38	Alabama	0.7
19	Alaska	2.4
11	Arizona	4.8
12	Arkansas	3.8
13	California	2.9
8	Colorado	6.5
28	Connecticut	1.4
38	Delaware	0.7
44	Florida	0.4
44	Georgia	0.4
23	Hawaii	1.7
1	Idaho	20.0
32	Illinois	1.1
16	Indiana	2.6
16	Iowa	2.6
18	Kansas	2.5
29	Kentucky	1.3
47	Louisiana	0.2
44	Maine	0.4
32	Maryland	1.1
4	Massachusetts	11.2
38	Michigan	0.7
6	Minnesota	7.5
49	Mississippi	0.1
35	Missouri	0.9
26	Montana	1.5
30	Nebraska	1.2
20	Nevada	2.3
5	New Hampshire	10.7
49	New Jersey	0.1
10	New Mexico	5.8
21	New York	2.0
26	North Carolina	1.5
7	North Dakota	7.1
14	Ohio	2.7
35	Oklahoma	0.9
14	Oregon	2.7
22	Pennsylvania	1.9
25	Rhode Island	1.6
38	South Carolina	0.7
32	South Dakota	1.1
38	Tennessee	0.7
30	Texas	1.2
3	Utah	12.7
2	Vermont	13.0
37	Virginia	0.8
9	Washington	5.9
47	West Virginia	0.2
38	Wisconsin	0.7
23	Wyoming	1.7

RANK ORDER

RANK	STATE	RATE
1	Idaho	20.0
2	Vermont	13.0
3	Utah	12.7
4	Massachusetts	11.2
5	New Hampshire	10.7
6	Minnesota	7.5
7	North Dakota	7.1
8	Colorado	6.5
9	Washington	5.9
10	New Mexico	5.8
11	Arizona	4.8
12	Arkansas	3.8
13	California	2.9
14	Ohio	2.7
14	Oregon	2.7
16	Indiana	2.6
16	Iowa	2.6
18	Kansas	2.5
19	Alaska	2.4
20	Nevada	2.3
21	New York	2.0
22	Pennsylvania	1.9
23	Hawaii	1.7
23	Wyoming	1.7
25	Rhode Island	1.6
26	Montana	1.5
26	North Carolina	1.5
28	Connecticut	1.4
29	Kentucky	1.3
30	Nebraska	1.2
30	Texas	1.2
32	Illinois	1.1
32	Maryland	1.1
32	South Dakota	1.1
35	Missouri	0.9
35	Oklahoma	0.9
37	Virginia	0.8
38	Alabama	0.7
38	Delaware	0.7
38	Michigan	0.7
38	South Carolina	0.7
38	Tennessee	0.7
38	Wisconsin	0.7
44	Florida	0.4
44	Georgia	0.4
44	Maine	0.4
47	Louisiana	0.2
47	West Virginia	0.2
49	Mississippi	0.1
49	New Jersey	0.1
	District of Columbia	0.2

Source: Morgan Quitno Press using data from U.S. Dept. of Health & Human Serv's, National Center for Health Statistics
"Morbidity and Mortality Weekly Report" (January 8, 1999, Vol. 47, No. 51)
*Provisional data. Acute, highly contagious infection of respiratory tract.

Percent of Children Aged 19 to 35 Months Fully Immunized in 1997

National Percent = 76%*

ALPHA ORDER			RANK ORDER		
RANK	STATE	PERCENT	RANK	STATE	PERCENT
21	Alabama	78	1	Connecticut	88
42	Alaska	72	2	Massachusetts	86
47	Arizona	69	3	Maine	85
31	Arkansas	75	4	Vermont	84
31	California	75	5	Minnesota	83
39	Colorado	73	6	Louisiana	82
1	Connecticut	88	6	New Hampshire	82
19	Delaware	79	6	Pennsylvania	82
26	Florida	77	6	South Carolina	82
13	Georgia	80	10	Mississippi	81
13	Hawaii	80	10	Rhode Island	81
50	Idaho	67	10	Washington	81
30	Illinois	76	13	Georgia	80
45	Indiana	71	13	Hawaii	80
13	Iowa	80	13	Iowa	80
26	Kansas	77	13	North Carolina	80
26	Kentucky	77	13	North Dakota	80
6	Louisiana	82	13	West Virginia	80
3	Maine	85	19	Delaware	79
21	Maryland	78	19	Wisconsin	79
2	Massachusetts	86	21	Alabama	78
39	Michigan	73	21	Maryland	78
5	Minnesota	83	21	Montana	78
10	Mississippi	81	21	Nebraska	78
36	Missouri	74	21	Tennessee	78
21	Montana	78	26	Florida	77
21	Nebraska	78	26	Kansas	77
46	Nevada	70	26	Kentucky	77
6	New Hampshire	82	26	South Dakota	77
39	New Jersey	73	30	Illinois	76
31	New Mexico	75	31	Arkansas	75
36	New York	74	31	California	75
13	North Carolina	80	31	New Mexico	75
13	North Dakota	80	31	Ohio	75
31	Ohio	75	31	Virginia	75
47	Oklahoma	69	36	Missouri	74
42	Oregon	72	36	New York	74
6	Pennsylvania	82	36	Wyoming	74
10	Rhode Island	81	39	Colorado	73
6	South Carolina	82	39	Michigan	73
26	South Dakota	77	39	New Jersey	73
21	Tennessee	78	42	Alaska	72
42	Texas	72	42	Oregon	72
49	Utah	68	42	Texas	72
4	Vermont	84	45	Indiana	71
31	Virginia	75	46	Nevada	70
10	Washington	81	47	Arizona	69
13	West Virginia	80	47	Oklahoma	69
19	Wisconsin	79	49	Utah	68
36	Wyoming	74	50	Idaho	67
				District of Columbia**	NA

Source: U.S. Department of Health and Human Services, Centers for Disease Control and Prevention
"State Vaccination Coverage Levels" (Morbidity and Mortality Weekly Report, Vol. 47, No. 6, 02/20/98)
*As of June 1997. Fully immunized children received four doses of DTP/DT (Diphtheria, Tetanus, Pertussis (Whooping Cough)), three doses of OPV (Poliovirus), one dose of MCV (Measles Containing Vaccine) and three doses of Hib (Haemophilus influenzae type b).
**Not available.

Sexually Transmitted Diseases in 1997

National Total = 860,347 Cases*

ALPHA ORDER

RANK	STATE	CASES	% of USA
15	Alabama	21,147	2.5%
42	Alaska	2,008	0.2%
21	Arizona	14,717	1.7%
30	Arkansas	7,059	0.8%
1	California	86,993	10.1%
27	Colorado	9,531	1.1%
28	Connecticut	9,153	1.1%
37	Delaware	3,908	0.5%
4	Florida	46,166	5.4%
8	Georgia	34,898	4.1%
40	Hawaii	2,316	0.3%
43	Idaho	1,868	0.2%
5	Illinois	41,887	4.9%
20	Indiana	15,906	1.8%
31	Iowa	6,225	0.7%
33	Kansas	5,772	0.7%
25	Kentucky	10,494	1.2%
14	Louisiana	22,694	2.6%
46	Maine	1,134	0.1%
11	Maryland	26,223	3.0%
26	Massachusetts	10,291	1.2%
7	Michigan	37,288	4.3%
29	Minnesota	9,064	1.1%
19	Mississippi	16,616	1.9%
17	Missouri	20,363	2.4%
45	Montana	1,212	0.1%
36	Nebraska	3,982	0.5%
38	Nevada	2,511	0.3%
48	New Hampshire	912	0.1%
18	New Jersey	18,085	2.1%
34	New Mexico	4,887	0.6%
3	New York	51,118	5.9%
9	North Carolina	34,726	4.0%
47	North Dakota	970	0.1%
6	Ohio	38,009	4.4%
23	Oklahoma	12,289	1.4%
32	Oregon	6,054	0.7%
10	Pennsylvania	29,928	3.5%
39	Rhode Island	2,493	0.3%
12	South Carolina	24,391	2.8%
44	South Dakota	1,624	0.2%
13	Tennessee	24,273	2.8%
2	Texas	78,016	9.1%
41	Utah	2,057	0.2%
50	Vermont	487	0.1%
16	Virginia	20,583	2.4%
24	Washington	11,561	1.3%
35	West Virginia	4,066	0.5%
22	Wisconsin	13,959	1.6%
49	Wyoming	690	0.1%

RANK ORDER

RANK	STATE	CASES	% of USA
1	California	86,993	10.1%
2	Texas	78,016	9.1%
3	New York	51,118	5.9%
4	Florida	46,166	5.4%
5	Illinois	41,887	4.9%
6	Ohio	38,009	4.4%
7	Michigan	37,288	4.3%
8	Georgia	34,898	4.1%
9	North Carolina	34,726	4.0%
10	Pennsylvania	29,928	3.5%
11	Maryland	26,223	3.0%
12	South Carolina	24,391	2.8%
13	Tennessee	24,273	2.8%
14	Louisiana	22,694	2.6%
15	Alabama	21,147	2.5%
16	Virginia	20,583	2.4%
17	Missouri	20,363	2.4%
18	New Jersey	18,085	2.1%
19	Mississippi	16,616	1.9%
20	Indiana	15,906	1.8%
21	Arizona	14,717	1.7%
22	Wisconsin	13,959	1.6%
23	Oklahoma	12,289	1.4%
24	Washington	11,561	1.3%
25	Kentucky	10,494	1.2%
26	Massachusetts	10,291	1.2%
27	Colorado	9,531	1.1%
28	Connecticut	9,153	1.1%
29	Minnesota	9,064	1.1%
30	Arkansas	7,059	0.8%
31	Iowa	6,225	0.7%
32	Oregon	6,054	0.7%
33	Kansas	5,772	0.7%
34	New Mexico	4,887	0.6%
35	West Virginia	4,066	0.5%
36	Nebraska	3,982	0.5%
37	Delaware	3,908	0.5%
38	Nevada	2,511	0.3%
39	Rhode Island	2,493	0.3%
40	Hawaii	2,316	0.3%
41	Utah	2,057	0.2%
42	Alaska	2,008	0.2%
43	Idaho	1,868	0.2%
44	South Dakota	1,624	0.2%
45	Montana	1,212	0.1%
46	Maine	1,134	0.1%
47	North Dakota	970	0.1%
48	New Hampshire	912	0.1%
49	Wyoming	690	0.1%
50	Vermont	487	0.1%
	District of Columbia	7,743	0.9%

Source: Morgan Quitno Press using data from U.S. Dept. of Health and Human Services, Nat'l Center for Health Statistics "Sexually Transmitted Disease Surveillance 1997" (http://www.cdc.gov/nchstp/dstd/)
Includes chancroid, chlamydia, gonorrhea and primary and secondary syphilis.

Sexually Transmitted Disease Rate in 1997

National Rate = 332.8 Cases per 100,000 Population*

RANK	STATE	RATE	RANK	STATE	RATE
7	Alabama	494.9	1	South Carolina	659.4
18	Alaska	330.9	2	Mississippi	611.8
17	Arizona	332.4	3	Delaware	539.1
22	Arkansas	281.2	4	Louisiana	521.7
24	California	272.9	5	Maryland	517.1
29	Colorado	251.6	6	New York	510.3
23	Connecticut	279.5	7	Alabama	494.9
3	Delaware	539.1	8	Georgia	474.6
19	Florida	320.6	9	North Carolina	474.1
8	Georgia	474.6	10	Tennessee	456.2
38	Hawaii	195.7	11	Texas	407.8
42	Idaho	157.1	12	Michigan	388.6
15	Illinois	353.6	13	Missouri	380.0
25	Indiana	272.4	14	Oklahoma	372.3
36	Iowa	218.3	15	Illinois	353.6
33	Kansas	224.3	16	Ohio	340.2
27	Kentucky	270.2	17	Arizona	332.4
4	Louisiana	521.7	18	Alaska	330.9
48	Maine	91.2	19	Florida	320.6
5	Maryland	517.1	20	Virginia	308.3
41	Massachusetts	168.9	21	New Mexico	285.2
12	Michigan	388.6	22	Arkansas	281.2
39	Minnesota	194.6	23	Connecticut	279.5
2	Mississippi	611.8	24	California	272.9
13	Missouri	380.0	25	Indiana	272.4
46	Montana	137.8	26	Wisconsin	270.5
31	Nebraska	241.0	27	Kentucky	270.2
43	Nevada	156.6	28	Rhode Island	251.7
50	New Hampshire	78.5	29	Colorado	251.6
32	New Jersey	226.4	30	Pennsylvania	248.2
21	New Mexico	285.2	31	Nebraska	241.0
6	New York	510.3	32	New Jersey	226.4
9	North Carolina	474.1	33	Kansas	224.3
44	North Dakota	150.8	34	West Virginia	222.7
16	Ohio	340.2	35	South Dakota	221.7
14	Oklahoma	372.3	36	Iowa	218.3
40	Oregon	188.9	37	Washington	208.9
30	Pennsylvania	248.2	38	Hawaii	195.7
28	Rhode Island	251.7	39	Minnesota	194.6
1	South Carolina	659.4	40	Oregon	188.9
35	South Dakota	221.7	41	Massachusetts	168.9
10	Tennessee	456.2	42	Idaho	157.1
11	Texas	407.8	43	Nevada	156.6
47	Utah	102.8	44	North Dakota	150.8
49	Vermont	82.7	45	Wyoming	143.3
20	Virginia	308.3	46	Montana	137.8
37	Washington	208.9	47	Utah	102.8
34	West Virginia	222.7	48	Maine	91.2
26	Wisconsin	270.5	49	Vermont	82.7
45	Wyoming	143.3	50	New Hampshire	78.5

District of Columbia   1,461.3

Source: Morgan Quitno Press using data from U.S. Dept. of Health and Human Services, Nat'l Center for Health Statistics "Sexually Transmitted Disease Surveillance 1997" (http://www.cdc.gov/nchstp/dstd/)
Includes chancroid, chlamydia, gonorrhea and primary and secondary syphilis.

Chancroid Cases Reported in 1997

National Total = 243 Cases*

ALPHA ORDER

RANK	STATE	CASES	% of USA
12	Alabama	1	0.4%
20	Alaska	0	0.0%
20	Arizona	0	0.0%
12	Arkansas	1	0.4%
3	California	19	7.8%
20	Colorado	0	0.0%
20	Connecticut	0	0.0%
20	Delaware	0	0.0%
8	Florida	3	1.2%
12	Georgia	1	0.4%
20	Hawaii	0	0.0%
20	Idaho	0	0.0%
6	Illinois	5	2.1%
20	Indiana	0	0.0%
20	Iowa	0	0.0%
20	Kansas	0	0.0%
20	Kentucky	0	0.0%
8	Louisiana	3	1.2%
20	Maine	0	0.0%
12	Maryland	1	0.4%
7	Massachusetts	4	1.6%
20	Michigan	0	0.0%
20	Minnesota	0	0.0%
20	Mississippi	0	0.0%
20	Missouri	0	0.0%
20	Montana	0	0.0%
20	Nebraska	0	0.0%
20	Nevada	0	0.0%
20	New Hampshire	0	0.0%
20	New Jersey	0	0.0%
20	New Mexico	0	0.0%
1	New York	119	49.0%
5	North Carolina	9	3.7%
20	North Dakota	0	0.0%
8	Ohio	3	1.2%
20	Oklahoma	0	0.0%
12	Oregon	1	0.4%
20	Pennsylvania	0	0.0%
20	Rhode Island	0	0.0%
4	South Carolina	15	6.2%
20	South Dakota	0	0.0%
12	Tennessee	1	0.4%
2	Texas	53	21.8%
20	Utah	0	0.0%
20	Vermont	0	0.0%
12	Virginia	1	0.4%
11	Washington	2	0.8%
20	West Virginia	0	0.0%
20	Wisconsin	0	0.0%
12	Wyoming	1	0.4%

RANK ORDER

RANK	STATE	CASES	% of USA
1	New York	119	49.0%
2	Texas	53	21.8%
3	California	19	7.8%
4	South Carolina	15	6.2%
5	North Carolina	9	3.7%
6	Illinois	5	2.1%
7	Massachusetts	4	1.6%
8	Florida	3	1.2%
8	Louisiana	3	1.2%
8	Ohio	3	1.2%
11	Washington	2	0.8%
12	Alabama	1	0.4%
12	Arkansas	1	0.4%
12	Georgia	1	0.4%
12	Maryland	1	0.4%
12	Oregon	1	0.4%
12	Tennessee	1	0.4%
12	Virginia	1	0.4%
12	Wyoming	1	0.4%
20	Alaska	0	0.0%
20	Arizona	0	0.0%
20	Colorado	0	0.0%
20	Connecticut	0	0.0%
20	Delaware	0	0.0%
20	Hawaii	0	0.0%
20	Idaho	0	0.0%
20	Indiana	0	0.0%
20	Iowa	0	0.0%
20	Kansas	0	0.0%
20	Kentucky	0	0.0%
20	Maine	0	0.0%
20	Michigan	0	0.0%
20	Minnesota	0	0.0%
20	Mississippi	0	0.0%
20	Missouri	0	0.0%
20	Montana	0	0.0%
20	Nebraska	0	0.0%
20	Nevada	0	0.0%
20	New Hampshire	0	0.0%
20	New Jersey	0	0.0%
20	New Mexico	0	0.0%
20	North Dakota	0	0.0%
20	Oklahoma	0	0.0%
20	Pennsylvania	0	0.0%
20	Rhode Island	0	0.0%
20	South Dakota	0	0.0%
20	Utah	0	0.0%
20	Vermont	0	0.0%
20	West Virginia	0	0.0%
20	Wisconsin	0	0.0%
	District of Columbia	0	0.0%

Source: U.S. Department of Health and Human Services, National Center for Health Statistics
  "Sexually Transmitted Disease Surveillance 1997" (http://www.cdc.gov/nchstp/dstd/)
*A soft, highly infectious, nonsyphilitic venereal ulcer of the genital region, caused by the bacillus Hemophilus ducreyi. Also called soft chancre.

Chancroid Rate in 1997

National Rate = 0.1 Cases per 100,000 Population*

ALPHA ORDER

RANK	STATE	RATE
9	Alabama	0.0
9	Alaska	0.0
9	Arizona	0.0
9	Arkansas	0.0
5	California	0.1
9	Colorado	0.0
9	Connecticut	0.0
9	Delaware	0.0
9	Florida	0.0
9	Georgia	0.0
9	Hawaii	0.0
9	Idaho	0.0
9	Illinois	0.0
9	Indiana	0.0
9	Iowa	0.0
9	Kansas	0.0
9	Kentucky	0.0
5	Louisiana	0.1
9	Maine	0.0
9	Maryland	0.0
5	Massachusetts	0.1
9	Michigan	0.0
9	Minnesota	0.0
9	Mississippi	0.0
9	Missouri	0.0
9	Montana	0.0
9	Nebraska	0.0
9	Nevada	0.0
9	New Hampshire	0.0
9	New Jersey	0.0
9	New Mexico	0.0
1	New York	0.7
5	North Carolina	0.1
9	North Dakota	0.0
9	Ohio	0.0
9	Oklahoma	0.0
9	Oregon	0.0
9	Pennsylvania	0.0
9	Rhode Island	0.0
2	South Carolina	0.4
9	South Dakota	0.0
9	Tennessee	0.0
3	Texas	0.3
9	Utah	0.0
9	Vermont	0.0
9	Virginia	0.0
9	Washington	0.0
9	West Virginia	0.0
9	Wisconsin	0.0
4	Wyoming	0.2

RANK ORDER

RANK	STATE	RATE
1	New York	0.7
2	South Carolina	0.4
3	Texas	0.3
4	Wyoming	0.2
5	California	0.1
5	Louisiana	0.1
5	Massachusetts	0.1
5	North Carolina	0.1
9	Alabama	0.0
9	Alaska	0.0
9	Arizona	0.0
9	Arkansas	0.0
9	Colorado	0.0
9	Connecticut	0.0
9	Delaware	0.0
9	Florida	0.0
9	Georgia	0.0
9	Hawaii	0.0
9	Idaho	0.0
9	Illinois	0.0
9	Indiana	0.0
9	Iowa	0.0
9	Kansas	0.0
9	Kentucky	0.0
9	Maine	0.0
9	Maryland	0.0
9	Michigan	0.0
9	Minnesota	0.0
9	Mississippi	0.0
9	Missouri	0.0
9	Montana	0.0
9	Nebraska	0.0
9	Nevada	0.0
9	New Hampshire	0.0
9	New Jersey	0.0
9	New Mexico	0.0
9	North Dakota	0.0
9	Ohio	0.0
9	Oklahoma	0.0
9	Oregon	0.0
9	Pennsylvania	0.0
9	Rhode Island	0.0
9	South Dakota	0.0
9	Tennessee	0.0
9	Utah	0.0
9	Vermont	0.0
9	Virginia	0.0
9	Washington	0.0
9	West Virginia	0.0
9	Wisconsin	0.0
	District of Columbia	0.0

Source: U.S. Department of Health and Human Services, National Center for Health Statistics
   "Sexually Transmitted Disease Surveillance 1997" (http://www.cdc.gov/nchstp/dstd/)
A soft, highly infectious, nonsyphilitic venereal ulcer of the genital region, caused by the bacillus Hemophilus ducreyi. Also called soft chancre.

Chlamydia Cases Reported in 1997

National Total = 526,653 Cases*

ALPHA ORDER

RANK	STATE	CASES	% of USA
22	Alabama	8,704	1.7%
43	Alaska	1,615	0.3%
17	Arizona	10,783	2.0%
37	Arkansas	2,503	0.5%
1	California	68,647	13.0%
26	Colorado	7,196	1.4%
29	Connecticut	6,064	1.2%
36	Delaware	2,613	0.5%
4	Florida	26,788	5.1%
10	Georgia	15,911	3.0%
40	Hawaii	1,811	0.3%
42	Idaho	1,709	0.3%
5	Illinois	23,024	4.4%
19	Indiana	9,600	1.8%
31	Iowa	4,907	0.9%
33	Kansas	4,003	0.8%
28	Kentucky	6,332	1.2%
16	Louisiana	11,545	2.2%
46	Maine	1,066	0.2%
11	Maryland	13,763	2.6%
23	Massachusetts	7,984	1.5%
7	Michigan	21,399	4.1%
27	Minnesota	6,631	1.3%
24	Mississippi	7,899	1.5%
14	Missouri	12,308	2.3%
45	Montana	1,146	0.2%
35	Nebraska	2,767	0.5%
39	Nevada	1,952	0.4%
48	New Hampshire	816	0.2%
18	New Jersey	10,347	2.0%
32	New Mexico	4,021	0.8%
3	New York	28,468	5.4%
9	North Carolina	17,108	3.2%
47	North Dakota	902	0.2%
6	Ohio	22,827	4.3%
25	Oklahoma	7,416	1.4%
30	Oregon	5,270	1.0%
8	Pennsylvania	19,838	3.8%
38	Rhode Island	2,069	0.4%
12	South Carolina	12,511	2.4%
44	South Dakota	1,450	0.3%
13	Tennessee	12,502	2.4%
2	Texas	50,675	9.6%
41	Utah	1,774	0.3%
50	Vermont	434	0.1%
15	Virginia	11,615	2.2%
20	Washington	9,574	1.8%
34	West Virginia	3,108	0.6%
21	Wisconsin	9,554	1.8%
49	Wyoming	635	0.1%

RANK ORDER

RANK	STATE	CASES	% of USA
1	California	68,647	13.0%
2	Texas	50,675	9.6%
3	New York	28,468	5.4%
4	Florida	26,788	5.1%
5	Illinois	23,024	4.4%
6	Ohio	22,827	4.3%
7	Michigan	21,399	4.1%
8	Pennsylvania	19,838	3.8%
9	North Carolina	17,108	3.2%
10	Georgia	15,911	3.0%
11	Maryland	13,763	2.6%
12	South Carolina	12,511	2.4%
13	Tennessee	12,502	2.4%
14	Missouri	12,308	2.3%
15	Virginia	11,615	2.2%
16	Louisiana	11,545	2.2%
17	Arizona	10,783	2.0%
18	New Jersey	10,347	2.0%
19	Indiana	9,600	1.8%
20	Washington	9,574	1.8%
21	Wisconsin	9,554	1.8%
22	Alabama	8,704	1.7%
23	Massachusetts	7,984	1.5%
24	Mississippi	7,899	1.5%
25	Oklahoma	7,416	1.4%
26	Colorado	7,196	1.4%
27	Minnesota	6,631	1.3%
28	Kentucky	6,332	1.2%
29	Connecticut	6,064	1.2%
30	Oregon	5,270	1.0%
31	Iowa	4,907	0.9%
32	New Mexico	4,021	0.8%
33	Kansas	4,003	0.8%
34	West Virginia	3,108	0.6%
35	Nebraska	2,767	0.5%
36	Delaware	2,613	0.5%
37	Arkansas	2,503	0.5%
38	Rhode Island	2,069	0.4%
39	Nevada	1,952	0.4%
40	Hawaii	1,811	0.3%
41	Utah	1,774	0.3%
42	Idaho	1,709	0.3%
43	Alaska	1,615	0.3%
44	South Dakota	1,450	0.3%
45	Montana	1,146	0.2%
46	Maine	1,066	0.2%
47	North Dakota	902	0.2%
48	New Hampshire	816	0.2%
49	Wyoming	635	0.1%
50	Vermont	434	0.1%
	District of Columbia	3,069	0.6%

Source: U.S. Department of Health and Human Services, National Center for Health Statistics
   "Sexually Transmitted Disease Surveillance 1997" (http://www.cdc.gov/nchstp/dstd/)
*Any of several common, often asymptomatic, sexually transmitted diseases caused by the microorganism Chlamydia trachomatis, including nonspecific urethritis in men.

Chlamydia Rate in 1997

National Rate = 207.0 Cases per 100,000 Population*

ALPHA ORDER

RANK	STATE	RATE
20	Alabama	203.7
6	Alaska	266.1
9	Arizona	243.5
46	Arkansas	99.7
17	California	215.3
23	Colorado	190.5
25	Connecticut	185.2
2	Delaware	360.5
24	Florida	186.0
16	Georgia	216.4
37	Hawaii	153.0
38	Idaho	143.7
22	Illinois	194.4
34	Indiana	164.4
29	Iowa	172.1
36	Kansas	155.6
35	Kentucky	163.0
7	Louisiana	265.4
48	Maine	85.7
5	Maryland	271.4
42	Massachusetts	131.0
15	Michigan	223.0
39	Minnesota	142.4
4	Mississippi	290.8
13	Missouri	229.7
43	Montana	130.3
31	Nebraska	167.5
45	Nevada	121.8
50	New Hampshire	70.2
44	New Jersey	129.5
11	New Mexico	234.7
1	New York	385.7
12	North Carolina	233.6
40	North Dakota	140.2
19	Ohio	204.3
14	Oklahoma	224.7
32	Oregon	164.5
32	Pennsylvania	164.5
18	Rhode Island	208.9
3	South Carolina	338.2
21	South Dakota	198.0
10	Tennessee	235.0
8	Texas	264.9
47	Utah	88.7
49	Vermont	73.7
27	Virginia	174.0
28	Washington	173.0
30	West Virginia	170.2
25	Wisconsin	185.2
41	Wyoming	131.9

RANK ORDER

RANK	STATE	RATE
1	New York	385.7
2	Delaware	360.5
3	South Carolina	338.2
4	Mississippi	290.8
5	Maryland	271.4
6	Alaska	266.1
7	Louisiana	265.4
8	Texas	264.9
9	Arizona	243.5
10	Tennessee	235.0
11	New Mexico	234.7
12	North Carolina	233.6
13	Missouri	229.7
14	Oklahoma	224.7
15	Michigan	223.0
16	Georgia	216.4
17	California	215.3
18	Rhode Island	208.9
19	Ohio	204.3
20	Alabama	203.7
21	South Dakota	198.0
22	Illinois	194.4
23	Colorado	190.5
24	Florida	186.0
25	Connecticut	185.2
25	Wisconsin	185.2
27	Virginia	174.0
28	Washington	173.0
29	Iowa	172.1
30	West Virginia	170.2
31	Nebraska	167.5
32	Oregon	164.5
32	Pennsylvania	164.5
34	Indiana	164.4
35	Kentucky	163.0
36	Kansas	155.6
37	Hawaii	153.0
38	Idaho	143.7
39	Minnesota	142.4
40	North Dakota	140.2
41	Wyoming	131.9
42	Massachusetts	131.0
43	Montana	130.3
44	New Jersey	129.5
45	Nevada	121.8
46	Arkansas	99.7
47	Utah	88.7
48	Maine	85.7
49	Vermont	73.7
50	New Hampshire	70.2
	District of Columbia	579.2

Source: U.S. Department of Health and Human Services, National Center for Health Statistics
"Sexually Transmitted Disease Surveillance 1997" (http://www.cdc.gov/nchstp/dstd/)
*Any of several common, often asymptomatic, sexually transmitted diseases caused by the microorganism Chlamydia trachomatis, including nonspecific urethritis in men.

Gonorrhea Cases Reported in 1997

National Total = 324,901 Cases*

ALPHA ORDER

RANK	STATE	CASES	% of USA
10	Alabama	12,032	3.7%
41	Alaska	392	0.1%
25	Arizona	3,802	1.2%
22	Arkansas	4,382	1.3%
6	California	17,941	5.5%
28	Colorado	2,320	0.7%
26	Connecticut	3,027	0.9%
33	Delaware	1,273	0.4%
3	Florida	19,079	5.9%
4	Georgia	18,471	5.7%
39	Hawaii	504	0.2%
44	Idaho	158	0.0%
5	Illinois	18,423	5.7%
20	Indiana	6,155	1.9%
32	Iowa	1,311	0.4%
31	Kansas	1,740	0.5%
24	Kentucky	4,027	1.2%
14	Louisiana	10,782	3.3%
47	Maine	66	0.0%
11	Maryland	11,568	3.6%
29	Massachusetts	2,225	0.7%
8	Michigan	15,736	4.8%
27	Minnesota	2,417	0.7%
17	Mississippi	8,327	2.6%
18	Missouri	7,941	2.4%
47	Montana	66	0.0%
34	Nebraska	1,210	0.4%
38	Nevada	549	0.2%
45	New Hampshire	96	0.0%
19	New Jersey	7,587	2.3%
36	New Mexico	857	0.3%
2	New York	22,393	6.9%
7	North Carolina	16,888	5.2%
46	North Dakota	68	0.0%
9	Ohio	14,961	4.6%
21	Oklahoma	4,756	1.5%
37	Oregon	773	0.2%
15	Pennsylvania	9,967	3.1%
40	Rhode Island	422	0.1%
12	South Carolina	11,487	3.5%
43	South Dakota	173	0.1%
13	Tennessee	11,023	3.4%
1	Texas	26,612	8.2%
42	Utah	278	0.1%
50	Vermont	53	0.0%
16	Virginia	8,731	2.7%
30	Washington	1,968	0.6%
35	West Virginia	957	0.3%
23	Wisconsin	4,316	1.3%
49	Wyoming	54	0.0%

RANK ORDER

RANK	STATE	CASES	% of USA
1	Texas	26,612	8.2%
2	New York	22,393	6.9%
3	Florida	19,079	5.9%
4	Georgia	18,471	5.7%
5	Illinois	18,423	5.7%
6	California	17,941	5.5%
7	North Carolina	16,888	5.2%
8	Michigan	15,736	4.8%
9	Ohio	14,961	4.6%
10	Alabama	12,032	3.7%
11	Maryland	11,568	3.6%
12	South Carolina	11,487	3.5%
13	Tennessee	11,023	3.4%
14	Louisiana	10,782	3.3%
15	Pennsylvania	9,967	3.1%
16	Virginia	8,731	2.7%
17	Mississippi	8,327	2.6%
18	Missouri	7,941	2.4%
19	New Jersey	7,587	2.3%
20	Indiana	6,155	1.9%
21	Oklahoma	4,756	1.5%
22	Arkansas	4,382	1.3%
23	Wisconsin	4,316	1.3%
24	Kentucky	4,027	1.2%
25	Arizona	3,802	1.2%
26	Connecticut	3,027	0.9%
27	Minnesota	2,417	0.7%
28	Colorado	2,320	0.7%
29	Massachusetts	2,225	0.7%
30	Washington	1,968	0.6%
31	Kansas	1,740	0.5%
32	Iowa	1,311	0.4%
33	Delaware	1,273	0.4%
34	Nebraska	1,210	0.4%
35	West Virginia	957	0.3%
36	New Mexico	857	0.3%
37	Oregon	773	0.2%
38	Nevada	549	0.2%
39	Hawaii	504	0.2%
40	Rhode Island	422	0.1%
41	Alaska	392	0.1%
42	Utah	278	0.1%
43	South Dakota	173	0.1%
44	Idaho	158	0.0%
45	New Hampshire	96	0.0%
46	North Dakota	68	0.0%
47	Maine	66	0.0%
47	Montana	66	0.0%
49	Wyoming	54	0.0%
50	Vermont	53	0.0%
	District of Columbia	4,557	1.4%

Source: U.S. Department of Health and Human Services, National Center for Health Statistics
"Sexually Transmitted Disease Surveillance 1997" (http://www.cdc.gov/nchstp/dstd/)
*Gonorrhea is a sexually transmitted disease caused by gonococcal bacteria that affects the mucous membrane chiefly of the genital and urinary tracts and is characterized by an acute purulent discharge and painful or difficult urination, though women often have no symptoms.

Gonorrhea Rate in 1997

National Rate = 122.5 Cases per 100,000 Population*

RANK	STATE (ALPHA ORDER)	RATE		RANK	STATE (RANK ORDER)	RATE
3	Alabama	281.6		1	South Carolina	310.6
29	Alaska	64.6		2	Mississippi	306.6
24	Arizona	85.9		3	Alabama	281.6
10	Arkansas	174.6		4	Georgia	251.2
31	California	56.3		5	Louisiana	247.8
30	Colorado	60.7		6	North Carolina	230.6
23	Connecticut	92.4		7	Maryland	228.1
9	Delaware	175.6		8	Tennessee	207.2
17	Florida	132.5		9	Delaware	175.6
4	Georgia	251.2		10	Arkansas	174.6
36	Hawaii	42.6		11	Michigan	164.0
44	Idaho	13.3		12	Illinois	155.5
12	Illinois	155.5		13	Missouri	148.2
20	Indiana	105.4		14	Oklahoma	144.1
35	Iowa	46.0		15	Texas	139.1
28	Kansas	67.6		16	Ohio	133.9
21	Kentucky	103.7		17	Florida	132.5
5	Louisiana	247.8		18	Virginia	130.8
50	Maine	5.3		19	New York	123.1
7	Maryland	228.1		20	Indiana	105.4
38	Massachusetts	36.5		21	Kentucky	103.7
11	Michigan	164.0		22	New Jersey	95.0
33	Minnesota	51.9		23	Connecticut	92.4
2	Mississippi	306.6		24	Arizona	85.9
13	Missouri	148.2		25	Wisconsin	83.6
49	Montana	7.5		26	Pennsylvania	82.7
27	Nebraska	73.2		27	Nebraska	73.2
40	Nevada	34.2		28	Kansas	67.6
48	New Hampshire	8.3		29	Alaska	64.6
22	New Jersey	95.0		30	Colorado	60.7
34	New Mexico	50.0		31	California	56.3
19	New York	123.1		32	West Virginia	52.4
6	North Carolina	230.6		33	Minnesota	51.9
46	North Dakota	10.6		34	New Mexico	50.0
16	Ohio	133.9		35	Iowa	46.0
14	Oklahoma	144.1		36	Hawaii	42.6
41	Oregon	24.1		36	Rhode Island	42.6
26	Pennsylvania	82.7		38	Massachusetts	36.5
36	Rhode Island	42.6		39	Washington	35.6
1	South Carolina	310.6		40	Nevada	34.2
42	South Dakota	23.6		41	Oregon	24.1
8	Tennessee	207.2		42	South Dakota	23.6
15	Texas	139.1		43	Utah	13.9
43	Utah	13.9		44	Idaho	13.3
47	Vermont	9.0		45	Wyoming	11.2
18	Virginia	130.8		46	North Dakota	10.6
39	Washington	35.6		47	Vermont	9.0
32	West Virginia	52.4		48	New Hampshire	8.3
25	Wisconsin	83.6		49	Montana	7.5
45	Wyoming	11.2		50	Maine	5.3
					District of Columbia	860.0

Source: U.S. Department of Health and Human Services, National Center for Health Statistics
   "Sexually Transmitted Disease Surveillance 1997" (http://www.cdc.gov/nchstp/dstd/)
*Gonorrhea is a sexually transmitted disease caused by gonococcal bacteria that affects the mucous membrane chiefly of the genital and urinary tracts and is characterized by an acute purulent discharge and painful or difficult urination, though women often have no symptoms.

Syphilis Cases Reported in 1997

National Total = 8,550 Cases*

ALPHA ORDER

RANK ORDER

RANK	STATE	CASES	% of USA
7	Alabama	410	4.8%
41	Alaska	1	0.0%
21	Arizona	132	1.5%
15	Arkansas	173	2.0%
9	California	386	4.5%
32	Colorado	15	0.2%
27	Connecticut	62	0.7%
29	Delaware	22	0.3%
12	Florida	296	3.5%
5	Georgia	515	6.0%
41	Hawaii	1	0.0%
41	Idaho	1	0.0%
6	Illinois	435	5.1%
17	Indiana	151	1.8%
36	Iowa	7	0.1%
28	Kansas	29	0.3%
20	Kentucky	135	1.6%
11	Louisiana	364	4.3%
39	Maine	2	0.0%
1	Maryland	891	10.4%
26	Massachusetts	78	0.9%
16	Michigan	153	1.8%
31	Minnesota	16	0.2%
8	Mississippi	390	4.6%
24	Missouri	114	1.3%
46	Montana	0	0.0%
37	Nebraska	5	0.1%
33	Nevada	10	0.1%
46	New Hampshire	0	0.0%
17	New Jersey	151	1.8%
35	New Mexico	9	0.1%
19	New York	138	1.6%
3	North Carolina	721	8.4%
46	North Dakota	0	0.0%
14	Ohio	218	2.5%
23	Oklahoma	117	1.4%
33	Oregon	10	0.1%
22	Pennsylvania	123	1.4%
39	Rhode Island	2	0.0%
10	South Carolina	378	4.4%
41	South Dakota	1	0.0%
2	Tennessee	747	8.7%
4	Texas	676	7.9%
37	Utah	5	0.1%
46	Vermont	0	0.0%
13	Virginia	236	2.8%
30	Washington	17	0.2%
41	West Virginia	1	0.0%
25	Wisconsin	89	1.0%
46	Wyoming	0	0.0%

RANK	STATE	CASES	% of USA
1	Maryland	891	10.4%
2	Tennessee	747	8.7%
3	North Carolina	721	8.4%
4	Texas	676	7.9%
5	Georgia	515	6.0%
6	Illinois	435	5.1%
7	Alabama	410	4.8%
8	Mississippi	390	4.6%
9	California	386	4.5%
10	South Carolina	378	4.4%
11	Louisiana	364	4.3%
12	Florida	296	3.5%
13	Virginia	236	2.8%
14	Ohio	218	2.5%
15	Arkansas	173	2.0%
16	Michigan	153	1.8%
17	Indiana	151	1.8%
17	New Jersey	151	1.8%
19	New York	138	1.6%
20	Kentucky	135	1.6%
21	Arizona	132	1.5%
22	Pennsylvania	123	1.4%
23	Oklahoma	117	1.4%
24	Missouri	114	1.3%
25	Wisconsin	89	1.0%
26	Massachusetts	78	0.9%
27	Connecticut	62	0.7%
28	Kansas	29	0.3%
29	Delaware	22	0.3%
30	Washington	17	0.2%
31	Minnesota	16	0.2%
32	Colorado	15	0.2%
33	Nevada	10	0.1%
33	Oregon	10	0.1%
35	New Mexico	9	0.1%
36	Iowa	7	0.1%
37	Nebraska	5	0.1%
37	Utah	5	0.1%
39	Maine	2	0.0%
39	Rhode Island	2	0.0%
41	Alaska	1	0.0%
41	Hawaii	1	0.0%
41	Idaho	1	0.0%
41	South Dakota	1	0.0%
41	West Virginia	1	0.0%
46	Montana	0	0.0%
46	New Hampshire	0	0.0%
46	North Dakota	0	0.0%
46	Vermont	0	0.0%
46	Wyoming	0	0.0%

District of Columbia — 117 — 1.4%

Source: U.S. Department of Health and Human Services, National Center for Health Statistics
"Sexually Transmitted Disease Surveillance 1997" (http://www.cdc.gov/nchstp/dstd/)
*Includes only primary and secondary cases. Does not include 37,987 cases in other stages. A chronic infectious disease caused by a spirochete (Treponema pallidum), either transmitted by direct contact, usually in sexual intercourse, or passed from mother to child in utero, and progressing through three stages characterized respectively by local formation of chancres, ulcerous skin eruptions, and systemic infection leading to general paresis.

Syphilis Rate in 1997

National Rate = 3.2 Cases per 100,000 Population*

ALPHA ORDER

RANK	STATE	RATE
6	Alabama	9.6
37	Alaska	0.2
15	Arizona	3.0
9	Arkansas	6.9
26	California	1.2
32	Colorado	0.4
21	Connecticut	1.9
15	Delaware	3.0
18	Florida	2.1
8	Georgia	7.0
42	Hawaii	0.1
42	Idaho	0.1
10	Illinois	3.7
17	Indiana	2.6
37	Iowa	0.2
27	Kansas	1.1
11	Kentucky	3.5
7	Louisiana	8.4
37	Maine	0.2
1	Maryland	17.6
25	Massachusetts	1.3
24	Michigan	1.6
33	Minnesota	0.3
2	Mississippi	14.4
18	Missouri	2.1
46	Montana	0.0
33	Nebraska	0.3
30	Nevada	0.6
46	New Hampshire	0.0
21	New Jersey	1.9
31	New Mexico	0.5
29	New York	0.8
5	North Carolina	9.8
46	North Dakota	0.0
20	Ohio	2.0
11	Oklahoma	3.5
33	Oregon	0.3
28	Pennsylvania	1.0
37	Rhode Island	0.2
4	South Carolina	10.2
42	South Dakota	0.1
3	Tennessee	14.0
11	Texas	3.5
37	Utah	0.2
46	Vermont	0.0
11	Virginia	3.5
33	Washington	0.3
42	West Virginia	0.1
23	Wisconsin	1.7
46	Wyoming	0.0

RANK ORDER

RANK	STATE	RATE
1	Maryland	17.6
2	Mississippi	14.4
3	Tennessee	14.0
4	South Carolina	10.2
5	North Carolina	9.8
6	Alabama	9.6
7	Louisiana	8.4
8	Georgia	7.0
9	Arkansas	6.9
10	Illinois	3.7
11	Kentucky	3.5
11	Oklahoma	3.5
11	Texas	3.5
11	Virginia	3.5
15	Arizona	3.0
15	Delaware	3.0
17	Indiana	2.6
18	Florida	2.1
18	Missouri	2.1
20	Ohio	2.0
21	Connecticut	1.9
21	New Jersey	1.9
23	Wisconsin	1.7
24	Michigan	1.6
25	Massachusetts	1.3
26	California	1.2
27	Kansas	1.1
28	Pennsylvania	1.0
29	New York	0.8
30	Nevada	0.6
31	New Mexico	0.5
32	Colorado	0.4
33	Minnesota	0.3
33	Nebraska	0.3
33	Oregon	0.3
33	Washington	0.3
37	Alaska	0.2
37	Iowa	0.2
37	Maine	0.2
37	Rhode Island	0.2
37	Utah	0.2
42	Hawaii	0.1
42	Idaho	0.1
42	South Dakota	0.1
42	West Virginia	0.1
46	Montana	0.0
46	New Hampshire	0.0
46	North Dakota	0.0
46	Vermont	0.0
46	Wyoming	0.0

	District of Columbia	22.1

Source: U.S. Department of Health and Human Services, National Center for Health Statistics
   "Sexually Transmitted Disease Surveillance 1997" (http://www.cdc.gov/nchstp/dstd/)
*Includes only primary and secondary cases. Does not include 37,987 cases in other stages. A chronic infectious disease caused by a spirochete (Treponema pallidum), either transmitted by direct contact, usually in sexual intercourse, or passed from mother to child in utero, and progressing through three stages characterized respectively by local formation of chancres, ulcerous skin eruptions, and systemic infection leading to general paresis.

VI. PROVIDERS

VI. PROVIDERS (continued)

Physicians in 1997

National Total = 744,934 Physicians*

ALPHA ORDER

RANK	STATE	PHYSICIANS	% of USA
25	Alabama	9,327	1.3%
49	Alaska	1,199	0.2%
23	Arizona	11,124	1.5%
32	Arkansas	5,287	0.7%
1	California	91,287	12.3%
24	Colorado	10,508	1.4%
20	Connecticut	12,531	1.7%
46	Delaware	1,916	0.3%
4	Florida	41,855	5.6%
14	Georgia	17,465	2.3%
38	Hawaii	3,718	0.5%
43	Idaho	2,147	0.3%
6	Illinois	33,359	4.5%
21	Indiana	12,510	1.7%
31	Iowa	5,636	0.8%
30	Kansas	6,103	0.8%
26	Kentucky	8,849	1.2%
22	Louisiana	11,417	1.5%
41	Maine	3,142	0.4%
11	Maryland	22,185	3.0%
8	Massachusetts	26,889	3.6%
10	Michigan	23,619	3.2%
18	Minnesota	13,073	1.8%
33	Mississippi	4,949	0.7%
17	Missouri	13,338	1.8%
45	Montana	1,981	0.3%
37	Nebraska	3,956	0.5%
40	Nevada	3,258	0.4%
42	New Hampshire	3,141	0.4%
9	New Jersey	25,329	3.4%
36	New Mexico	4,258	0.6%
2	New York	73,844	9.9%
12	North Carolina	19,015	2.6%
47	North Dakota	1,570	0.2%
7	Ohio	28,649	3.8%
29	Oklahoma	6,250	0.8%
28	Oregon	8,495	1.1%
5	Pennsylvania	37,528	5.0%
39	Rhode Island	3,552	0.5%
27	South Carolina	8,636	1.2%
48	South Dakota	1,542	0.2%
16	Tennessee	14,351	1.9%
3	Texas	43,130	5.8%
34	Utah	4,596	0.6%
44	Vermont	1,999	0.3%
13	Virginia	18,447	2.5%
15	Washington	15,423	2.1%
35	West Virginia	4,264	0.6%
19	Wisconsin	13,050	1.8%
50	Wyoming	957	0.1%

RANK ORDER

RANK	STATE	PHYSICIANS	% of USA
1	California	91,287	12.3%
2	New York	73,844	9.9%
3	Texas	43,130	5.8%
4	Florida	41,855	5.6%
5	Pennsylvania	37,528	5.0%
6	Illinois	33,359	4.5%
7	Ohio	28,649	3.8%
8	Massachusetts	26,889	3.6%
9	New Jersey	25,329	3.4%
10	Michigan	23,619	3.2%
11	Maryland	22,185	3.0%
12	North Carolina	19,015	2.6%
13	Virginia	18,447	2.5%
14	Georgia	17,465	2.3%
15	Washington	15,423	2.1%
16	Tennessee	14,351	1.9%
17	Missouri	13,338	1.8%
18	Minnesota	13,073	1.8%
19	Wisconsin	13,050	1.8%
20	Connecticut	12,531	1.7%
21	Indiana	12,510	1.7%
22	Louisiana	11,417	1.5%
23	Arizona	11,124	1.5%
24	Colorado	10,508	1.4%
25	Alabama	9,327	1.3%
26	Kentucky	8,849	1.2%
27	South Carolina	8,636	1.2%
28	Oregon	8,495	1.1%
29	Oklahoma	6,250	0.8%
30	Kansas	6,103	0.8%
31	Iowa	5,636	0.8%
32	Arkansas	5,287	0.7%
33	Mississippi	4,949	0.7%
34	Utah	4,596	0.6%
35	West Virginia	4,264	0.6%
36	New Mexico	4,258	0.6%
37	Nebraska	3,956	0.5%
38	Hawaii	3,718	0.5%
39	Rhode Island	3,552	0.5%
40	Nevada	3,258	0.4%
41	Maine	3,142	0.4%
42	New Hampshire	3,141	0.4%
43	Idaho	2,147	0.3%
44	Vermont	1,999	0.3%
45	Montana	1,981	0.3%
46	Delaware	1,916	0.3%
47	North Dakota	1,570	0.2%
48	South Dakota	1,542	0.2%
49	Alaska	1,199	0.2%
50	Wyoming	957	0.1%
	District of Columbia	4,280	0.6%

Source: American Medical Association (Chicago, Illinois)
    "Physician Characteristics and Distribution in the U.S." (1999 Edition)
*As of December 31, 1997. Comprised of federal and nonfederal physicians. Total does not include 11,776 physicians in the U.S. territories and possessions, at APO's and FPO's and whose addresses are unknown.

Male Physicians in 1997

National Total = 581,200 Physicians*

ALPHA ORDER					RANK ORDER			

RANK	STATE	PHYSICIANS	% of USA
25	Alabama	7,751	1.3%
49	Alaska	927	0.2%
23	Arizona	8,925	1.5%
32	Arkansas	4,411	0.8%
1	California	71,294	12.3%
24	Colorado	8,149	1.4%
21	Connecticut	9,641	1.7%
46	Delaware	1,465	0.3%
3	Florida	35,098	6.0%
14	Georgia	13,962	2.4%
38	Hawaii	2,928	0.5%
43	Idaho	1,881	0.3%
6	Illinois	24,649	4.2%
19	Indiana	10,152	1.7%
31	Iowa	4,646	0.8%
30	Kansas	4,866	0.8%
26	Kentucky	7,149	1.2%
22	Louisiana	9,204	1.6%
42	Maine	2,496	0.4%
11	Maryland	16,386	2.8%
8	Massachusetts	19,518	3.4%
10	Michigan	18,105	3.1%
20	Minnesota	10,125	1.7%
33	Mississippi	4,181	0.7%
17	Missouri	10,558	1.8%
44	Montana	1,696	0.3%
36	Nebraska	3,224	0.6%
39	Nevada	2,752	0.5%
41	New Hampshire	2,534	0.4%
9	New Jersey	18,902	3.3%
37	New Mexico	3,142	0.5%
2	New York	54,587	9.4%
12	North Carolina	15,112	2.6%
47	North Dakota	1,337	0.2%
7	Ohio	22,193	3.8%
29	Oklahoma	5,155	0.9%
28	Oregon	6,750	1.2%
5	Pennsylvania	28,885	5.0%
40	Rhode Island	2,674	0.5%
27	South Carolina	7,098	1.2%
48	South Dakota	1,305	0.2%
16	Tennessee	11,725	2.0%
4	Texas	34,254	5.9%
34	Utah	3,893	0.7%
45	Vermont	1,526	0.3%
13	Virginia	14,276	2.5%
15	Washington	12,066	2.1%
35	West Virginia	3,447	0.6%
18	Wisconsin	10,336	1.8%
50	Wyoming	822	0.1%

RANK	STATE	PHYSICIANS	% of USA
1	California	71,294	12.3%
2	New York	54,587	9.4%
3	Florida	35,098	6.0%
4	Texas	34,254	5.9%
5	Pennsylvania	28,885	5.0%
6	Illinois	24,649	4.2%
7	Ohio	22,193	3.8%
8	Massachusetts	19,518	3.4%
9	New Jersey	18,902	3.3%
10	Michigan	18,105	3.1%
11	Maryland	16,386	2.8%
12	North Carolina	15,112	2.6%
13	Virginia	14,276	2.5%
14	Georgia	13,962	2.4%
15	Washington	12,066	2.1%
16	Tennessee	11,725	2.0%
17	Missouri	10,558	1.8%
18	Wisconsin	10,336	1.8%
19	Indiana	10,152	1.7%
20	Minnesota	10,125	1.7%
21	Connecticut	9,641	1.7%
22	Louisiana	9,204	1.6%
23	Arizona	8,925	1.5%
24	Colorado	8,149	1.4%
25	Alabama	7,751	1.3%
26	Kentucky	7,149	1.2%
27	South Carolina	7,098	1.2%
28	Oregon	6,750	1.2%
29	Oklahoma	5,155	0.9%
30	Kansas	4,866	0.8%
31	Iowa	4,646	0.8%
32	Arkansas	4,411	0.8%
33	Mississippi	4,181	0.7%
34	Utah	3,893	0.7%
35	West Virginia	3,447	0.6%
36	Nebraska	3,224	0.6%
37	New Mexico	3,142	0.5%
38	Hawaii	2,928	0.5%
39	Nevada	2,752	0.5%
40	Rhode Island	2,674	0.5%
41	New Hampshire	2,534	0.4%
42	Maine	2,496	0.4%
43	Idaho	1,881	0.3%
44	Montana	1,696	0.3%
45	Vermont	1,526	0.3%
46	Delaware	1,465	0.3%
47	North Dakota	1,337	0.2%
48	South Dakota	1,305	0.2%
49	Alaska	927	0.2%
50	Wyoming	822	0.1%
	District of Columbia	3,042	0.5%

Source: American Medical Association (Chicago, Illinois)
    "Physician Characteristics and Distribution in the U.S." (1999 Edition)
*As of December 31, 1997. Comprised of federal and nonfederal physicians. Total does not include 8,811 male physicians in the U.S. territories and possessions, at APO's and FPO's and whose addresses are unknown.

Female Physicians in 1997

National Total = 163,734 Physicians*

ALPHA ORDER					RANK ORDER			
RANK	**STATE**	**PHYSICIANS**	**% of USA**		**RANK**	**STATE**	**PHYSICIANS**	**% of USA**
27	Alabama	1,576	1.0%		1	California	19,993	12.2%
46	Alaska	272	0.2%		2	New York	19,257	11.8%
24	Arizona	2,199	1.3%		3	Texas	8,876	5.4%
34	Arkansas	876	0.5%		4	Illinois	8,710	5.3%
1	California	19,993	12.2%		5	Pennsylvania	8,643	5.3%
21	Colorado	2,359	1.4%		6	Massachusetts	7,371	4.5%
17	Connecticut	2,890	1.8%		7	Florida	6,757	4.1%
44	Delaware	451	0.3%		8	Ohio	6,456	3.9%
7	Florida	6,757	4.1%		9	New Jersey	6,427	3.9%
14	Georgia	3,503	2.1%		10	Maryland	5,799	3.5%
36	Hawaii	790	0.5%		11	Michigan	5,514	3.4%
47	Idaho	266	0.2%		12	Virginia	4,171	2.5%
4	Illinois	8,710	5.3%		13	North Carolina	3,903	2.4%
22	Indiana	2,358	1.4%		14	Georgia	3,503	2.1%
32	Iowa	990	0.6%		15	Washington	3,357	2.1%
29	Kansas	1,237	0.8%		16	Minnesota	2,948	1.8%
26	Kentucky	1,700	1.0%		17	Connecticut	2,890	1.8%
23	Louisiana	2,213	1.4%		18	Missouri	2,780	1.7%
40	Maine	646	0.4%		19	Wisconsin	2,714	1.7%
10	Maryland	5,799	3.5%		20	Tennessee	2,626	1.6%
6	Massachusetts	7,371	4.5%		21	Colorado	2,359	1.4%
11	Michigan	5,514	3.4%		22	Indiana	2,358	1.4%
16	Minnesota	2,948	1.8%		23	Louisiana	2,213	1.4%
37	Mississippi	768	0.5%		24	Arizona	2,199	1.3%
18	Missouri	2,780	1.7%		25	Oregon	1,745	1.1%
45	Montana	285	0.2%		26	Kentucky	1,700	1.0%
38	Nebraska	732	0.4%		27	Alabama	1,576	1.0%
42	Nevada	506	0.3%		28	South Carolina	1,538	0.9%
41	New Hampshire	607	0.4%		29	Kansas	1,237	0.8%
9	New Jersey	6,427	3.9%		30	New Mexico	1,116	0.7%
30	New Mexico	1,116	0.7%		31	Oklahoma	1,095	0.7%
2	New York	19,257	11.8%		32	Iowa	990	0.6%
13	North Carolina	3,903	2.4%		33	Rhode Island	878	0.5%
49	North Dakota	233	0.1%		34	Arkansas	876	0.5%
8	Ohio	6,456	3.9%		35	West Virginia	817	0.5%
31	Oklahoma	1,095	0.7%		36	Hawaii	790	0.5%
25	Oregon	1,745	1.1%		37	Mississippi	768	0.5%
5	Pennsylvania	8,643	5.3%		38	Nebraska	732	0.4%
33	Rhode Island	878	0.5%		39	Utah	703	0.4%
28	South Carolina	1,538	0.9%		40	Maine	646	0.4%
48	South Dakota	237	0.1%		41	New Hampshire	607	0.4%
20	Tennessee	2,626	1.6%		42	Nevada	506	0.3%
3	Texas	8,876	5.4%		43	Vermont	473	0.3%
39	Utah	703	0.4%		44	Delaware	451	0.3%
43	Vermont	473	0.3%		45	Montana	285	0.2%
12	Virginia	4,171	2.5%		46	Alaska	272	0.2%
15	Washington	3,357	2.1%		47	Idaho	266	0.2%
35	West Virginia	817	0.5%		48	South Dakota	237	0.1%
19	Wisconsin	2,714	1.7%		49	North Dakota	233	0.1%
50	Wyoming	135	0.1%		50	Wyoming	135	0.1%
						District of Columbia	1,238	0.8%

Source: American Medical Association (Chicago, Illinois)
    "Physician Characteristics and Distribution in the U.S." (1999 Edition)
*As of December 31, 1997. Comprised of federal and nonfederal physicians. Total does not include 2,965 female physicians in the U.S. territories and possessions, at APO's and FPO's and whose addresses are unknown.

Percent of Physicians Who Are Female: 1997

National Percent = 22.0% of Physicians*

ALPHA ORDER				RANK ORDER		
RANK	STATE	PERCENT		RANK	STATE	PERCENT
40	Alabama	16.9		1	Massachusetts	27.4
13	Alaska	22.7		2	New Mexico	26.2
29	Arizona	19.8		3	Illinois	26.1
41	Arkansas	16.6		3	Maryland	26.1
18	California	21.9		3	New York	26.1
17	Colorado	22.4		6	New Jersey	25.4
11	Connecticut	23.1		7	Rhode Island	24.7
9	Delaware	23.5		8	Vermont	23.7
42	Florida	16.1		9	Delaware	23.5
28	Georgia	20.1		10	Michigan	23.3
20	Hawaii	21.2		11	Connecticut	23.1
50	Idaho	12.4		12	Pennsylvania	23.0
3	Illinois	26.1		13	Alaska	22.7
34	Indiana	18.8		14	Minnesota	22.6
38	Iowa	17.6		14	Virginia	22.6
27	Kansas	20.3		16	Ohio	22.5
32	Kentucky	19.2		17	Colorado	22.4
30	Louisiana	19.4		18	California	21.9
23	Maine	20.6		19	Washington	21.8
3	Maryland	26.1		20	Hawaii	21.2
1	Massachusetts	27.4		21	Missouri	20.8
10	Michigan	23.3		21	Wisconsin	20.8
14	Minnesota	22.6		23	Maine	20.6
43	Mississippi	15.5		23	Texas	20.6
21	Missouri	20.8		25	North Carolina	20.5
48	Montana	14.4		25	Oregon	20.5
35	Nebraska	18.5		27	Kansas	20.3
43	Nevada	15.5		28	Georgia	20.1
31	New Hampshire	19.3		29	Arizona	19.8
6	New Jersey	25.4		30	Louisiana	19.4
2	New Mexico	26.2		31	New Hampshire	19.3
3	New York	26.1		32	Kentucky	19.2
25	North Carolina	20.5		32	West Virginia	19.2
47	North Dakota	14.8		34	Indiana	18.8
16	Ohio	22.5		35	Nebraska	18.5
39	Oklahoma	17.5		36	Tennessee	18.3
25	Oregon	20.5		37	South Carolina	17.8
12	Pennsylvania	23.0		38	Iowa	17.6
7	Rhode Island	24.7		39	Oklahoma	17.5
37	South Carolina	17.8		40	Alabama	16.9
45	South Dakota	15.4		41	Arkansas	16.6
36	Tennessee	18.3		42	Florida	16.1
23	Texas	20.6		43	Mississippi	15.5
46	Utah	15.3		43	Nevada	15.5
8	Vermont	23.7		45	South Dakota	15.4
14	Virginia	22.6		46	Utah	15.3
19	Washington	21.8		47	North Dakota	14.8
32	West Virginia	19.2		48	Montana	14.4
21	Wisconsin	20.8		49	Wyoming	14.1
49	Wyoming	14.1		50	Idaho	12.4
					District of Columbia	28.9

Source: Morgan Quitno Press using data from American Medical Association (Chicago, Illinois)
       "Physician Characteristics and Distribution in the U.S." (1999 Edition)
*As of December 31, 1997. Comprised of federal and nonfederal physicians. National percent does not include physicians in the U.S. territories and possessions, at APO's and FPO's and whose addresses are unknown.

Physicians Under 35 Years Old in 1997

National Total = 132,101 Physicians*

ALPHA ORDER

RANK	STATE	PHYSICIANS	% of USA
24	Alabama	1,626	1.2%
48	Alaska	124	0.1%
26	Arizona	1,591	1.2%
33	Arkansas	839	0.6%
2	California	12,869	9.7%
25	Colorado	1,606	1.2%
20	Connecticut	2,126	1.6%
43	Delaware	317	0.2%
9	Florida	4,643	3.5%
14	Georgia	3,106	2.4%
39	Hawaii	518	0.4%
46	Idaho	219	0.2%
4	Illinois	7,527	5.7%
21	Indiana	2,053	1.6%
30	Iowa	1,033	0.8%
28	Kansas	1,067	0.8%
27	Kentucky	1,555	1.2%
18	Louisiana	2,447	1.9%
42	Maine	325	0.2%
10	Maryland	4,118	3.1%
7	Massachusetts	5,676	4.3%
8	Michigan	5,215	3.9%
17	Minnesota	2,513	1.9%
32	Mississippi	849	0.6%
15	Missouri	2,791	2.1%
50	Montana	109	0.1%
35	Nebraska	757	0.6%
41	Nevada	355	0.3%
40	New Hampshire	374	0.3%
11	New Jersey	3,869	2.9%
38	New Mexico	602	0.5%
1	New York	15,683	11.9%
12	North Carolina	3,782	2.9%
45	North Dakota	250	0.2%
6	Ohio	6,016	4.6%
31	Oklahoma	958	0.7%
29	Oregon	1,037	0.8%
5	Pennsylvania	7,395	5.6%
34	Rhode Island	786	0.6%
23	South Carolina	1,676	1.3%
47	South Dakota	186	0.1%
16	Tennessee	2,633	2.0%
3	Texas	8,511	6.4%
36	Utah	724	0.5%
44	Vermont	297	0.2%
13	Virginia	3,333	2.5%
22	Washington	2,045	1.5%
37	West Virginia	723	0.5%
19	Wisconsin	2,231	1.7%
48	Wyoming	124	0.1%

RANK ORDER

RANK	STATE	PHYSICIANS	% of USA
1	New York	15,683	11.9%
2	California	12,869	9.7%
3	Texas	8,511	6.4%
4	Illinois	7,527	5.7%
5	Pennsylvania	7,395	5.6%
6	Ohio	6,016	4.6%
7	Massachusetts	5,676	4.3%
8	Michigan	5,215	3.9%
9	Florida	4,643	3.5%
10	Maryland	4,118	3.1%
11	New Jersey	3,869	2.9%
12	North Carolina	3,782	2.9%
13	Virginia	3,333	2.5%
14	Georgia	3,106	2.4%
15	Missouri	2,791	2.1%
16	Tennessee	2,633	2.0%
17	Minnesota	2,513	1.9%
18	Louisiana	2,447	1.9%
19	Wisconsin	2,231	1.7%
20	Connecticut	2,126	1.6%
21	Indiana	2,053	1.6%
22	Washington	2,045	1.5%
23	South Carolina	1,676	1.3%
24	Alabama	1,626	1.2%
25	Colorado	1,606	1.2%
26	Arizona	1,591	1.2%
27	Kentucky	1,555	1.2%
28	Kansas	1,067	0.8%
29	Oregon	1,037	0.8%
30	Iowa	1,033	0.8%
31	Oklahoma	958	0.7%
32	Mississippi	849	0.6%
33	Arkansas	839	0.6%
34	Rhode Island	786	0.6%
35	Nebraska	757	0.6%
36	Utah	724	0.5%
37	West Virginia	723	0.5%
38	New Mexico	602	0.5%
39	Hawaii	518	0.4%
40	New Hampshire	374	0.3%
41	Nevada	355	0.3%
42	Maine	325	0.2%
43	Delaware	317	0.2%
44	Vermont	297	0.2%
45	North Dakota	250	0.2%
46	Idaho	219	0.2%
47	South Dakota	186	0.1%
48	Alaska	124	0.1%
48	Wyoming	124	0.1%
50	Montana	109	0.1%
	District of Columbia	892	0.7%

Source: American Medical Association (Chicago, Illinois)
    "Physician Characteristics and Distribution in the U.S." (1999 Edition)
*As of December 31, 1997. Comprised of federal and nonfederal physicians. Total does not include 1,739 physicians in the U.S. territories and possessions, at APO's and FPO's and whose addresses are unknown.

Percent of Physicians Under 35 Years Old in 1997

National Percent = 17.7% of Physicians*

ALPHA ORDER				RANK ORDER		
RANK	STATE	PERCENT		RANK	STATE	PERCENT
22	Alabama	17.4		1	Illinois	22.6
47	Alaska	10.3		2	Michigan	22.1
36	Arizona	14.3		2	Rhode Island	22.1
29	Arkansas	15.9		4	Louisiana	21.4
37	California	14.1		5	New York	21.2
32	Colorado	15.3		6	Massachusetts	21.1
25	Connecticut	17.0		7	Ohio	21.0
27	Delaware	16.5		8	Missouri	20.9
45	Florida	11.1		9	North Carolina	19.9
19	Georgia	17.8		10	Pennsylvania	19.7
39	Hawaii	13.9		10	Texas	19.7
49	Idaho	10.2		12	South Carolina	19.4
1	Illinois	22.6		13	Minnesota	19.2
28	Indiana	16.4		14	Nebraska	19.1
16	Iowa	18.3		15	Maryland	18.6
21	Kansas	17.5		16	Iowa	18.3
20	Kentucky	17.6		16	Tennessee	18.3
4	Louisiana	21.4		18	Virginia	18.1
47	Maine	10.3		19	Georgia	17.8
15	Maryland	18.6		20	Kentucky	17.6
6	Massachusetts	21.1		21	Kansas	17.5
2	Michigan	22.1		22	Alabama	17.4
13	Minnesota	19.2		23	Mississippi	17.2
23	Mississippi	17.2		24	Wisconsin	17.1
8	Missouri	20.9		25	Connecticut	17.0
50	Montana	5.5		25	West Virginia	17.0
14	Nebraska	19.1		27	Delaware	16.5
46	Nevada	10.9		28	Indiana	16.4
44	New Hampshire	11.9		29	Arkansas	15.9
32	New Jersey	15.3		29	North Dakota	15.9
37	New Mexico	14.1		31	Utah	15.8
5	New York	21.2		32	Colorado	15.3
9	North Carolina	19.9		32	New Jersey	15.3
29	North Dakota	15.9		32	Oklahoma	15.3
7	Ohio	21.0		35	Vermont	14.9
32	Oklahoma	15.3		36	Arizona	14.3
42	Oregon	12.2		37	California	14.1
10	Pennsylvania	19.7		37	New Mexico	14.1
2	Rhode Island	22.1		39	Hawaii	13.9
12	South Carolina	19.4		40	Washington	13.3
43	South Dakota	12.1		41	Wyoming	13.0
16	Tennessee	18.3		42	Oregon	12.2
10	Texas	19.7		43	South Dakota	12.1
31	Utah	15.8		44	New Hampshire	11.9
35	Vermont	14.9		45	Florida	11.1
18	Virginia	18.1		46	Nevada	10.9
40	Washington	13.3		47	Alaska	10.3
25	West Virginia	17.0		47	Maine	10.3
24	Wisconsin	17.1		49	Idaho	10.2
41	Wyoming	13.0		50	Montana	5.5

	District of Columbia	20.8

Source: Morgan Quitno Press using data from American Medical Association (Chicago, Illinois)
"Physician Characteristics and Distribution in the U.S." (1999 Edition)
*As of December 31, 1997. Comprised of federal and nonfederal physicians. National percent does not include physicians in the U.S. territories and possessions, at APO's and FPO's and whose addresses are unknown.

Physicians 35 to 44 Years Old in 1997

National Total = 209,906 Physicians*

ALPHA ORDER

RANK	STATE	PHYSICIANS	% of USA
25	Alabama	2,986	1.4%
49	Alaska	392	0.2%
23	Arizona	3,055	1.5%
32	Arkansas	1,629	0.8%
1	California	22,312	10.6%
24	Colorado	3,024	1.4%
21	Connecticut	3,563	1.7%
46	Delaware	535	0.3%
4	Florida	11,285	5.4%
13	Georgia	5,522	2.6%
38	Hawaii	1,056	0.5%
43	Idaho	641	0.3%
6	Illinois	9,196	4.4%
20	Indiana	3,813	1.8%
31	Iowa	1,637	0.8%
30	Kansas	1,725	0.8%
26	Kentucky	2,735	1.3%
22	Louisiana	3,129	1.5%
42	Maine	837	0.4%
10	Maryland	6,502	3.1%
8	Massachusetts	7,863	3.7%
11	Michigan	6,364	3.0%
19	Minnesota	3,952	1.9%
33	Mississippi	1,459	0.7%
18	Missouri	4,013	1.9%
44	Montana	577	0.3%
35	Nebraska	1,214	0.6%
39	Nevada	1,017	0.5%
41	New Hampshire	904	0.4%
9	New Jersey	7,239	3.4%
36	New Mexico	1,186	0.6%
2	New York	20,288	9.7%
12	North Carolina	5,951	2.8%
48	North Dakota	477	0.2%
7	Ohio	8,061	3.8%
29	Oklahoma	1,743	0.8%
28	Oregon	2,243	1.1%
5	Pennsylvania	10,814	5.2%
40	Rhode Island	1,004	0.5%
27	South Carolina	2,510	1.2%
47	South Dakota	492	0.2%
15	Tennessee	4,509	2.1%
3	Texas	12,507	6.0%
34	Utah	1,410	0.7%
45	Vermont	551	0.3%
14	Virginia	5,275	2.5%
16	Washington	4,334	2.1%
37	West Virginia	1,110	0.5%
17	Wisconsin	4,065	1.9%
50	Wyoming	245	0.1%

RANK ORDER

RANK	STATE	PHYSICIANS	% of USA
1	California	22,312	10.6%
2	New York	20,288	9.7%
3	Texas	12,507	6.0%
4	Florida	11,285	5.4%
5	Pennsylvania	10,814	5.2%
6	Illinois	9,196	4.4%
7	Ohio	8,061	3.8%
8	Massachusetts	7,863	3.7%
9	New Jersey	7,239	3.4%
10	Maryland	6,502	3.1%
11	Michigan	6,364	3.0%
12	North Carolina	5,951	2.8%
13	Georgia	5,522	2.6%
14	Virginia	5,275	2.5%
15	Tennessee	4,509	2.1%
16	Washington	4,334	2.1%
17	Wisconsin	4,065	1.9%
18	Missouri	4,013	1.9%
19	Minnesota	3,952	1.9%
20	Indiana	3,813	1.8%
21	Connecticut	3,563	1.7%
22	Louisiana	3,129	1.5%
23	Arizona	3,055	1.5%
24	Colorado	3,024	1.4%
25	Alabama	2,986	1.4%
26	Kentucky	2,735	1.3%
27	South Carolina	2,510	1.2%
28	Oregon	2,243	1.1%
29	Oklahoma	1,743	0.8%
30	Kansas	1,725	0.8%
31	Iowa	1,637	0.8%
32	Arkansas	1,629	0.8%
33	Mississippi	1,459	0.7%
34	Utah	1,410	0.7%
35	Nebraska	1,214	0.6%
36	New Mexico	1,186	0.6%
37	West Virginia	1,110	0.5%
38	Hawaii	1,056	0.5%
39	Nevada	1,017	0.5%
40	Rhode Island	1,004	0.5%
41	New Hampshire	904	0.4%
42	Maine	837	0.4%
43	Idaho	641	0.3%
44	Montana	577	0.3%
45	Vermont	551	0.3%
46	Delaware	535	0.3%
47	South Dakota	492	0.2%
48	North Dakota	477	0.2%
49	Alaska	392	0.2%
50	Wyoming	245	0.1%
	District of Columbia	955	0.5%

Source: American Medical Association (Chicago, Illinois)
 "Physician Characteristics and Distribution in the U.S." (1999 Edition)
*As of December 31, 1997. Comprised of federal and nonfederal physicians. Total does not include 3,496 physicians in the U.S. territories and possessions, at APO's and FPO's and whose addresses are unknown.

Physicians 45 to 54 Years Old in 1997

National Total = 173,024 Physicians*

ALPHA ORDER

RANK	STATE	PHYSICIANS	% of USA
26	Alabama	2,163	1.3%
49	Alaska	362	0.2%
24	Arizona	2,496	1.4%
32	Arkansas	1,257	0.7%
1	California	23,237	13.4%
22	Colorado	2,700	1.6%
21	Connecticut	2,879	1.7%
47	Delaware	421	0.2%
4	Florida	9,249	5.3%
15	Georgia	4,010	2.3%
37	Hawaii	933	0.5%
44	Idaho	535	0.3%
6	Illinois	7,395	4.3%
20	Indiana	2,910	1.7%
31	Iowa	1,308	0.8%
30	Kansas	1,380	0.8%
27	Kentucky	2,041	1.2%
23	Louisiana	2,623	1.5%
39	Maine	839	0.5%
10	Maryland	5,232	3.0%
9	Massachusetts	6,078	3.5%
11	Michigan	5,204	3.0%
17	Minnesota	3,066	1.8%
35	Mississippi	1,099	0.6%
19	Missouri	2,940	1.7%
43	Montana	556	0.3%
38	Nebraska	882	0.5%
40	Nevada	807	0.5%
41	New Hampshire	801	0.5%
7	New Jersey	6,244	3.6%
34	New Mexico	1,148	0.7%
2	New York	15,619	9.0%
14	North Carolina	4,129	2.4%
48	North Dakota	402	0.2%
8	Ohio	6,157	3.6%
29	Oklahoma	1,543	0.9%
25	Oregon	2,333	1.3%
5	Pennsylvania	8,347	4.8%
42	Rhode Island	675	0.4%
28	South Carolina	1,933	1.1%
46	South Dakota	423	0.2%
16	Tennessee	3,386	2.0%
3	Texas	9,916	5.7%
33	Utah	1,196	0.7%
45	Vermont	480	0.3%
12	Virginia	4,323	2.5%
13	Washington	4,154	2.4%
36	West Virginia	1,064	0.6%
18	Wisconsin	2,962	1.7%
50	Wyoming	248	0.1%

RANK ORDER

RANK	STATE	PHYSICIANS	% of USA
1	California	23,237	13.4%
2	New York	15,619	9.0%
3	Texas	9,916	5.7%
4	Florida	9,249	5.3%
5	Pennsylvania	8,347	4.8%
6	Illinois	7,395	4.3%
7	New Jersey	6,244	3.6%
8	Ohio	6,157	3.6%
9	Massachusetts	6,078	3.5%
10	Maryland	5,232	3.0%
11	Michigan	5,204	3.0%
12	Virginia	4,323	2.5%
13	Washington	4,154	2.4%
14	North Carolina	4,129	2.4%
15	Georgia	4,010	2.3%
16	Tennessee	3,386	2.0%
17	Minnesota	3,066	1.8%
18	Wisconsin	2,962	1.7%
19	Missouri	2,940	1.7%
20	Indiana	2,910	1.7%
21	Connecticut	2,879	1.7%
22	Colorado	2,700	1.6%
23	Louisiana	2,623	1.5%
24	Arizona	2,496	1.4%
25	Oregon	2,333	1.3%
26	Alabama	2,163	1.3%
27	Kentucky	2,041	1.2%
28	South Carolina	1,933	1.1%
29	Oklahoma	1,543	0.9%
30	Kansas	1,380	0.8%
31	Iowa	1,308	0.8%
32	Arkansas	1,257	0.7%
33	Utah	1,196	0.7%
34	New Mexico	1,148	0.7%
35	Mississippi	1,099	0.6%
36	West Virginia	1,064	0.6%
37	Hawaii	933	0.5%
38	Nebraska	882	0.5%
39	Maine	839	0.5%
40	Nevada	807	0.5%
41	New Hampshire	801	0.5%
42	Rhode Island	675	0.4%
43	Montana	556	0.3%
44	Idaho	535	0.3%
45	Vermont	480	0.3%
46	South Dakota	423	0.2%
47	Delaware	421	0.2%
48	North Dakota	402	0.2%
49	Alaska	362	0.2%
50	Wyoming	248	0.1%
	District of Columbia	939	0.5%

Source: American Medical Association (Chicago, Illinois)
    "Physician Characteristics and Distribution in the U.S." (1999 Edition)
As of December 31, 1997. Comprised of federal and nonfederal physicians. Total does not include 2,470 physicians in the U.S. territories and possessions, at APO's and FPO's and whose addresses are unknown.

Physicians 55 to 64 Years Old in 1997

National Total = 102,725 Physicians*

ALPHA ORDER

RANK	STATE	PHYSICIANS	% of USA
27	Alabama	1,175	1.1%
48	Alaska	205	0.2%
21	Arizona	1,588	1.5%
31	Arkansas	727	0.7%
1	California	14,102	13.7%
24	Colorado	1,443	1.4%
18	Connecticut	1,737	1.7%
45	Delaware	300	0.3%
3	Florida	6,088	5.9%
13	Georgia	2,398	2.3%
37	Hawaii	516	0.5%
43	Idaho	332	0.3%
6	Illinois	4,603	4.5%
20	Indiana	1,633	1.6%
34	Iowa	691	0.7%
30	Kansas	804	0.8%
26	Kentucky	1,220	1.2%
23	Louisiana	1,506	1.5%
41	Maine	449	0.4%
11	Maryland	3,105	3.0%
9	Massachusetts	3,339	3.3%
10	Michigan	3,205	3.1%
22	Minnesota	1,568	1.5%
32	Mississippi	721	0.7%
17	Missouri	1,744	1.7%
44	Montana	328	0.3%
39	Nebraska	480	0.5%
38	Nevada	490	0.5%
42	New Hampshire	423	0.4%
7	New Jersey	3,854	3.8%
35	New Mexico	619	0.6%
2	New York	9,987	9.7%
14	North Carolina	2,242	2.2%
47	North Dakota	221	0.2%
8	Ohio	3,799	3.7%
29	Oklahoma	959	0.9%
25	Oregon	1,287	1.3%
5	Pennsylvania	4,736	4.6%
40	Rhode Island	479	0.5%
28	South Carolina	1,092	1.1%
49	South Dakota	200	0.2%
16	Tennessee	1,768	1.7%
4	Texas	5,751	5.6%
36	Utah	570	0.6%
46	Vermont	258	0.3%
12	Virginia	2,530	2.5%
15	Washington	2,134	2.1%
33	West Virginia	701	0.7%
19	Wisconsin	1,680	1.6%
50	Wyoming	152	0.1%

RANK ORDER

RANK	STATE	PHYSICIANS	% of USA
1	California	14,102	13.7%
2	New York	9,987	9.7%
3	Florida	6,088	5.9%
4	Texas	5,751	5.6%
5	Pennsylvania	4,736	4.6%
6	Illinois	4,603	4.5%
7	New Jersey	3,854	3.8%
8	Ohio	3,799	3.7%
9	Massachusetts	3,339	3.3%
10	Michigan	3,205	3.1%
11	Maryland	3,105	3.0%
12	Virginia	2,530	2.5%
13	Georgia	2,398	2.3%
14	North Carolina	2,242	2.2%
15	Washington	2,134	2.1%
16	Tennessee	1,768	1.7%
17	Missouri	1,744	1.7%
18	Connecticut	1,737	1.7%
19	Wisconsin	1,680	1.6%
20	Indiana	1,633	1.6%
21	Arizona	1,588	1.5%
22	Minnesota	1,568	1.5%
23	Louisiana	1,506	1.5%
24	Colorado	1,443	1.4%
25	Oregon	1,287	1.3%
26	Kentucky	1,220	1.2%
27	Alabama	1,175	1.1%
28	South Carolina	1,092	1.1%
29	Oklahoma	959	0.9%
30	Kansas	804	0.8%
31	Arkansas	727	0.7%
32	Mississippi	721	0.7%
33	West Virginia	701	0.7%
34	Iowa	691	0.7%
35	New Mexico	619	0.6%
36	Utah	570	0.6%
37	Hawaii	516	0.5%
38	Nevada	490	0.5%
39	Nebraska	480	0.5%
40	Rhode Island	479	0.5%
41	Maine	449	0.4%
42	New Hampshire	423	0.4%
43	Idaho	332	0.3%
44	Montana	328	0.3%
45	Delaware	300	0.3%
46	Vermont	258	0.3%
47	North Dakota	221	0.2%
48	Alaska	205	0.2%
49	South Dakota	200	0.2%
50	Wyoming	152	0.1%
	District of Columbia	786	0.8%

Source: American Medical Association (Chicago, Illinois)
   "Physician Characteristics and Distribution in the U.S." (1999 Edition)
*As of December 31, 1997. Comprised of federal and nonfederal physicians. Total does not include 1,557
physicians in the U.S. territories and possessions, at APO's and FPO's and whose addresses are unknown.

Physicians 65 Years Old and Older in 1997

National Total = 127,178 Physicians*

ALPHA ORDER

RANK	STATE	PHYSICIANS	% of USA
27	Alabama	1,377	1.1%
50	Alaska	116	0.1%
16	Arizona	2,394	1.9%
32	Arkansas	835	0.7%
1	California	18,767	14.8%
23	Colorado	1,735	1.4%
17	Connecticut	2,226	1.8%
46	Delaware	343	0.3%
3	Florida	10,590	8.3%
15	Georgia	2,429	1.9%
36	Hawaii	695	0.5%
43	Idaho	420	0.3%
6	Illinois	4,638	3.6%
19	Indiana	2,101	1.7%
31	Iowa	967	0.8%
29	Kansas	1,127	0.9%
28	Kentucky	1,298	1.0%
24	Louisiana	1,712	1.3%
37	Maine	692	0.5%
11	Maryland	3,228	2.5%
9	Massachusetts	3,933	3.1%
10	Michigan	3,631	2.9%
21	Minnesota	1,974	1.6%
33	Mississippi	821	0.6%
22	Missouri	1,850	1.5%
45	Montana	411	0.3%
40	Nebraska	623	0.5%
42	Nevada	589	0.5%
39	New Hampshire	639	0.5%
8	New Jersey	4,123	3.2%
34	New Mexico	703	0.6%
2	New York	12,267	9.6%
13	North Carolina	2,911	2.3%
48	North Dakota	220	0.2%
7	Ohio	4,616	3.6%
30	Oklahoma	1,047	0.8%
25	Oregon	1,595	1.3%
5	Pennsylvania	6,236	4.9%
41	Rhode Island	608	0.5%
26	South Carolina	1,425	1.1%
47	South Dakota	241	0.2%
20	Tennessee	2,055	1.6%
4	Texas	6,445	5.1%
35	Utah	696	0.5%
44	Vermont	413	0.3%
12	Virginia	2,986	2.3%
14	Washington	2,756	2.2%
38	West Virginia	666	0.5%
18	Wisconsin	2,112	1.7%
49	Wyoming	188	0.1%

RANK ORDER

RANK	STATE	PHYSICIANS	% of USA
1	California	18,767	14.8%
2	New York	12,267	9.6%
3	Florida	10,590	8.3%
4	Texas	6,445	5.1%
5	Pennsylvania	6,236	4.9%
6	Illinois	4,638	3.6%
7	Ohio	4,616	3.6%
8	New Jersey	4,123	3.2%
9	Massachusetts	3,933	3.1%
10	Michigan	3,631	2.9%
11	Maryland	3,228	2.5%
12	Virginia	2,986	2.3%
13	North Carolina	2,911	2.3%
14	Washington	2,756	2.2%
15	Georgia	2,429	1.9%
16	Arizona	2,394	1.9%
17	Connecticut	2,226	1.8%
18	Wisconsin	2,112	1.7%
19	Indiana	2,101	1.7%
20	Tennessee	2,055	1.6%
21	Minnesota	1,974	1.6%
22	Missouri	1,850	1.5%
23	Colorado	1,735	1.4%
24	Louisiana	1,712	1.3%
25	Oregon	1,595	1.3%
26	South Carolina	1,425	1.1%
27	Alabama	1,377	1.1%
28	Kentucky	1,298	1.0%
29	Kansas	1,127	0.9%
30	Oklahoma	1,047	0.8%
31	Iowa	967	0.8%
32	Arkansas	835	0.7%
33	Mississippi	821	0.6%
34	New Mexico	703	0.6%
35	Utah	696	0.5%
36	Hawaii	695	0.5%
37	Maine	692	0.5%
38	West Virginia	666	0.5%
39	New Hampshire	639	0.5%
40	Nebraska	623	0.5%
41	Rhode Island	608	0.5%
42	Nevada	589	0.5%
43	Idaho	420	0.3%
44	Vermont	413	0.3%
45	Montana	411	0.3%
46	Delaware	343	0.3%
47	South Dakota	241	0.2%
48	North Dakota	220	0.2%
49	Wyoming	188	0.1%
50	Alaska	116	0.1%
	District of Columbia	708	0.6%

Source: American Medical Association (Chicago, Illinois)
    "Physician Characteristics and Distribution in the U.S." (1999 Edition)
*As of December 31, 1997. Comprised of federal and nonfederal physicians. Total does not include 2,514
physicians in the U.S. territories and possessions, at APO's and FPO's and whose addresses are unknown.

Percent of Physicians 65 Years Old and Older in 1997

National Percent = 17.1% of Physicians*

ALPHA ORDER

RANK ORDER

RANK	STATE	PERCENT		RANK	STATE	PERCENT
41	Alabama	14.8		1	Florida	25.3
50	Alaska	9.7		2	Maine	22.0
3	Arizona	21.5		3	Arizona	21.5
31	Arkansas	15.8		4	Montana	20.7
6	California	20.6		4	Vermont	20.7
24	Colorado	16.5		6	California	20.6
16	Connecticut	17.8		7	New Hampshire	20.3
14	Delaware	17.9		8	Idaho	19.6
1	Florida	25.3		8	Wyoming	19.6
47	Georgia	13.9		10	Oregon	18.8
11	Hawaii	18.7		11	Hawaii	18.7
8	Idaho	19.6		12	Kansas	18.5
47	Illinois	13.9		13	Nevada	18.1
19	Indiana	16.8		14	Delaware	17.9
17	Iowa	17.2		14	Washington	17.9
12	Kansas	18.5		16	Connecticut	17.8
42	Kentucky	14.7		17	Iowa	17.2
39	Louisiana	15.0		18	Rhode Island	17.1
2	Maine	22.0		19	Indiana	16.8
43	Maryland	14.6		19	Oklahoma	16.8
43	Massachusetts	14.6		21	Mississippi	16.6
35	Michigan	15.4		21	New York	16.6
37	Minnesota	15.1		21	Pennsylvania	16.6
21	Mississippi	16.6		24	Colorado	16.5
47	Missouri	13.9		24	New Mexico	16.5
4	Montana	20.7		24	South Carolina	16.5
32	Nebraska	15.7		27	New Jersey	16.3
13	Nevada	18.1		28	Virginia	16.2
7	New Hampshire	20.3		28	Wisconsin	16.2
27	New Jersey	16.3		30	Ohio	16.1
24	New Mexico	16.5		31	Arkansas	15.8
21	New York	16.6		32	Nebraska	15.7
36	North Carolina	15.3		33	South Dakota	15.6
46	North Dakota	14.0		33	West Virginia	15.6
30	Ohio	16.1		35	Michigan	15.4
19	Oklahoma	16.8		36	North Carolina	15.3
10	Oregon	18.8		37	Minnesota	15.1
21	Pennsylvania	16.6		37	Utah	15.1
18	Rhode Island	17.1		39	Louisiana	15.0
24	South Carolina	16.5		40	Texas	14.9
33	South Dakota	15.6		41	Alabama	14.8
45	Tennessee	14.3		42	Kentucky	14.7
40	Texas	14.9		43	Maryland	14.6
37	Utah	15.1		43	Massachusetts	14.6
4	Vermont	20.7		45	Tennessee	14.3
28	Virginia	16.2		46	North Dakota	14.0
14	Washington	17.9		47	Georgia	13.9
33	West Virginia	15.6		47	Illinois	13.9
28	Wisconsin	16.2		47	Missouri	13.9
8	Wyoming	19.6		50	Alaska	9.7
					District of Columbia	16.5

Source: Morgan Quitno Press using data from American Medical Association (Chicago, Illinois)
   "Physician Characteristics and Distribution in the U.S." (1999 Edition)
*As of December 31, 1997. Comprised of federal and nonfederal physicians. National percent does not include
physicians in the U.S. territories and possessions, at APO's and FPO's and whose addresses are unknown.

Federal Physicians in 1997

National Total = 18,286 Physicians*

<table>
<tr><td colspan="4">ALPHA ORDER</td><td colspan="4">RANK ORDER</td></tr>
<tr><td>RANK</td><td>STATE</td><td>PHYSICIANS</td><td>% of USA</td><td>RANK</td><td>STATE</td><td>PHYSICIANS</td><td>% of USA</td></tr>
<tr><td>24</td><td>Alabama</td><td>203</td><td>1.1%</td><td>1</td><td>California</td><td>2,134</td><td>11.7%</td></tr>
<tr><td>30</td><td>Alaska</td><td>160</td><td>0.9%</td><td>2</td><td>Maryland</td><td>2,031</td><td>11.1%</td></tr>
<tr><td>13</td><td>Arizona</td><td>353</td><td>1.9%</td><td>3</td><td>Texas</td><td>1,956</td><td>10.7%</td></tr>
<tr><td>34</td><td>Arkansas</td><td>118</td><td>0.6%</td><td>4</td><td>Virginia</td><td>1,040</td><td>5.7%</td></tr>
<tr><td>1</td><td>California</td><td>2,134</td><td>11.7%</td><td>5</td><td>Florida</td><td>957</td><td>5.2%</td></tr>
<tr><td>17</td><td>Colorado</td><td>269</td><td>1.5%</td><td>6</td><td>Georgia</td><td>813</td><td>4.4%</td></tr>
<tr><td>31</td><td>Connecticut</td><td>138</td><td>0.8%</td><td>7</td><td>New York</td><td>782</td><td>4.3%</td></tr>
<tr><td>46</td><td>Delaware</td><td>41</td><td>0.2%</td><td>8</td><td>Washington</td><td>664</td><td>3.6%</td></tr>
<tr><td>5</td><td>Florida</td><td>957</td><td>5.2%</td><td>9</td><td>North Carolina</td><td>516</td><td>2.8%</td></tr>
<tr><td>6</td><td>Georgia</td><td>813</td><td>4.4%</td><td>10</td><td>Illinois</td><td>510</td><td>2.8%</td></tr>
<tr><td>15</td><td>Hawaii</td><td>319</td><td>1.7%</td><td>11</td><td>Pennsylvania</td><td>450</td><td>2.5%</td></tr>
<tr><td>42</td><td>Idaho</td><td>55</td><td>0.3%</td><td>12</td><td>Ohio</td><td>445</td><td>2.4%</td></tr>
<tr><td>10</td><td>Illinois</td><td>510</td><td>2.8%</td><td>13</td><td>Arizona</td><td>353</td><td>1.9%</td></tr>
<tr><td>35</td><td>Indiana</td><td>103</td><td>0.6%</td><td>14</td><td>Massachusetts</td><td>343</td><td>1.9%</td></tr>
<tr><td>37</td><td>Iowa</td><td>80</td><td>0.4%</td><td>15</td><td>Hawaii</td><td>319</td><td>1.7%</td></tr>
<tr><td>28</td><td>Kansas</td><td>165</td><td>0.9%</td><td>16</td><td>Tennessee</td><td>294</td><td>1.6%</td></tr>
<tr><td>32</td><td>Kentucky</td><td>135</td><td>0.7%</td><td>17</td><td>Colorado</td><td>269</td><td>1.5%</td></tr>
<tr><td>19</td><td>Louisiana</td><td>236</td><td>1.3%</td><td>18</td><td>Mississippi</td><td>242</td><td>1.3%</td></tr>
<tr><td>47</td><td>Maine</td><td>40</td><td>0.2%</td><td>19</td><td>Louisiana</td><td>236</td><td>1.3%</td></tr>
<tr><td>2</td><td>Maryland</td><td>2,031</td><td>11.1%</td><td>20</td><td>Missouri</td><td>234</td><td>1.3%</td></tr>
<tr><td>14</td><td>Massachusetts</td><td>343</td><td>1.9%</td><td>21</td><td>Michigan</td><td>223</td><td>1.2%</td></tr>
<tr><td>21</td><td>Michigan</td><td>223</td><td>1.2%</td><td>22</td><td>New Jersey</td><td>219</td><td>1.2%</td></tr>
<tr><td>25</td><td>Minnesota</td><td>195</td><td>1.1%</td><td>22</td><td>South Carolina</td><td>219</td><td>1.2%</td></tr>
<tr><td>18</td><td>Mississippi</td><td>242</td><td>1.3%</td><td>24</td><td>Alabama</td><td>203</td><td>1.1%</td></tr>
<tr><td>20</td><td>Missouri</td><td>234</td><td>1.3%</td><td>25</td><td>Minnesota</td><td>195</td><td>1.1%</td></tr>
<tr><td>45</td><td>Montana</td><td>42</td><td>0.2%</td><td>26</td><td>Oklahoma</td><td>186</td><td>1.0%</td></tr>
<tr><td>43</td><td>Nebraska</td><td>54</td><td>0.3%</td><td>27</td><td>New Mexico</td><td>184</td><td>1.0%</td></tr>
<tr><td>40</td><td>Nevada</td><td>72</td><td>0.4%</td><td>28</td><td>Kansas</td><td>165</td><td>0.9%</td></tr>
<tr><td>44</td><td>New Hampshire</td><td>45</td><td>0.2%</td><td>29</td><td>Oregon</td><td>162</td><td>0.9%</td></tr>
<tr><td>22</td><td>New Jersey</td><td>219</td><td>1.2%</td><td>30</td><td>Alaska</td><td>160</td><td>0.9%</td></tr>
<tr><td>27</td><td>New Mexico</td><td>184</td><td>1.0%</td><td>31</td><td>Connecticut</td><td>138</td><td>0.8%</td></tr>
<tr><td>7</td><td>New York</td><td>782</td><td>4.3%</td><td>32</td><td>Kentucky</td><td>135</td><td>0.7%</td></tr>
<tr><td>9</td><td>North Carolina</td><td>516</td><td>2.8%</td><td>33</td><td>Wisconsin</td><td>131</td><td>0.7%</td></tr>
<tr><td>47</td><td>North Dakota</td><td>40</td><td>0.2%</td><td>34</td><td>Arkansas</td><td>118</td><td>0.6%</td></tr>
<tr><td>12</td><td>Ohio</td><td>445</td><td>2.4%</td><td>35</td><td>Indiana</td><td>103</td><td>0.6%</td></tr>
<tr><td>26</td><td>Oklahoma</td><td>186</td><td>1.0%</td><td>36</td><td>West Virginia</td><td>96</td><td>0.5%</td></tr>
<tr><td>29</td><td>Oregon</td><td>162</td><td>0.9%</td><td>37</td><td>Iowa</td><td>80</td><td>0.4%</td></tr>
<tr><td>11</td><td>Pennsylvania</td><td>450</td><td>2.5%</td><td>38</td><td>Utah</td><td>78</td><td>0.4%</td></tr>
<tr><td>41</td><td>Rhode Island</td><td>71</td><td>0.4%</td><td>39</td><td>South Dakota</td><td>74</td><td>0.4%</td></tr>
<tr><td>22</td><td>South Carolina</td><td>219</td><td>1.2%</td><td>40</td><td>Nevada</td><td>72</td><td>0.4%</td></tr>
<tr><td>39</td><td>South Dakota</td><td>74</td><td>0.4%</td><td>41</td><td>Rhode Island</td><td>71</td><td>0.4%</td></tr>
<tr><td>16</td><td>Tennessee</td><td>294</td><td>1.6%</td><td>42</td><td>Idaho</td><td>55</td><td>0.3%</td></tr>
<tr><td>3</td><td>Texas</td><td>1,956</td><td>10.7%</td><td>43</td><td>Nebraska</td><td>54</td><td>0.3%</td></tr>
<tr><td>38</td><td>Utah</td><td>78</td><td>0.4%</td><td>44</td><td>New Hampshire</td><td>45</td><td>0.2%</td></tr>
<tr><td>50</td><td>Vermont</td><td>33</td><td>0.2%</td><td>45</td><td>Montana</td><td>42</td><td>0.2%</td></tr>
<tr><td>4</td><td>Virginia</td><td>1,040</td><td>5.7%</td><td>46</td><td>Delaware</td><td>41</td><td>0.2%</td></tr>
<tr><td>8</td><td>Washington</td><td>664</td><td>3.6%</td><td>47</td><td>Maine</td><td>40</td><td>0.2%</td></tr>
<tr><td>36</td><td>West Virginia</td><td>96</td><td>0.5%</td><td>47</td><td>North Dakota</td><td>40</td><td>0.2%</td></tr>
<tr><td>33</td><td>Wisconsin</td><td>131</td><td>0.7%</td><td>49</td><td>Wyoming</td><td>36</td><td>0.2%</td></tr>
<tr><td>49</td><td>Wyoming</td><td>36</td><td>0.2%</td><td>50</td><td>Vermont</td><td>33</td><td>0.2%</td></tr>
<tr><td></td><td></td><td></td><td></td><td></td><td>District of Columbia</td><td>300</td><td>1.6%</td></tr>
</table>

Source: American Medical Association (Chicago, Illinois)
    "Physician Characteristics and Distribution in the U.S." (1999 Edition)
*As of December 31, 1997. Total does not include 1,161 physicians in U.S. territories and possessions.

Rate of Federal Physicians in 1997

National Rate = 6.8 Physicians per 100,000 Population*

ALPHA ORDER

RANK ORDER

RANK	STATE	RATE		RANK	STATE	RATE
30	Alabama	4.7		1	Maryland	39.9
3	Alaska	26.2		2	Hawaii	26.8
11	Arizona	7.8		3	Alaska	26.2
30	Arkansas	4.7		4	Virginia	15.4
16	California	6.6		5	Washington	11.8
14	Colorado	6.9		6	Georgia	10.9
37	Connecticut	4.2		7	New Mexico	10.7
21	Delaware	5.6		8	Texas	10.1
17	Florida	6.5		9	South Dakota	10.0
6	Georgia	10.9		10	Mississippi	8.9
2	Hawaii	26.8		11	Arizona	7.8
32	Idaho	4.5		12	Wyoming	7.5
33	Illinois	4.3		13	Rhode Island	7.2
50	Indiana	1.8		14	Colorado	6.9
46	Iowa	2.8		14	North Carolina	6.9
18	Kansas	6.3		16	California	6.6
43	Kentucky	3.5		17	Florida	6.5
26	Louisiana	5.4		18	Kansas	6.3
45	Maine	3.2		19	North Dakota	6.2
1	Maryland	39.9		20	South Carolina	5.8
21	Massachusetts	5.6		21	Delaware	5.6
49	Michigan	2.3		21	Massachusetts	5.6
37	Minnesota	4.2		21	Oklahoma	5.6
10	Mississippi	8.9		21	Vermont	5.6
33	Missouri	4.3		25	Tennessee	5.5
29	Montana	4.8		26	Louisiana	5.4
44	Nebraska	3.3		27	West Virginia	5.3
33	Nevada	4.3		28	Oregon	5.0
40	New Hampshire	3.8		29	Montana	4.8
47	New Jersey	2.7		30	Alabama	4.7
7	New Mexico	10.7		30	Arkansas	4.7
33	New York	4.3		32	Idaho	4.5
14	North Carolina	6.9		33	Illinois	4.3
19	North Dakota	6.2		33	Missouri	4.3
39	Ohio	4.0		33	Nevada	4.3
21	Oklahoma	5.6		33	New York	4.3
28	Oregon	5.0		37	Connecticut	4.2
42	Pennsylvania	3.7		37	Minnesota	4.2
13	Rhode Island	7.2		39	Ohio	4.0
20	South Carolina	5.8		40	New Hampshire	3.8
9	South Dakota	10.0		40	Utah	3.8
25	Tennessee	5.5		42	Pennsylvania	3.7
8	Texas	10.1		43	Kentucky	3.5
40	Utah	3.8		44	Nebraska	3.3
21	Vermont	5.6		45	Maine	3.2
4	Virginia	15.4		46	Iowa	2.8
5	Washington	11.8		47	New Jersey	2.7
27	West Virginia	5.3		48	Wisconsin	2.5
48	Wisconsin	2.5		49	Michigan	2.3
12	Wyoming	7.5		50	Indiana	1.8

District of Columbia 56.6

Source: Morgan Quitno Press using data from American Medical Association (Chicago, Illinois)
   "Physician Characteristics and Distribution in the U.S." (1999 Edition)
*As of December 31, 1997. National rate does not include physicians in U.S. territories and possessions.

Nonfederal Physicians in 1997

National Total = 726,648 Physicians*

RANK	STATE	PHYSICIANS	% of USA
25	Alabama	9,124	1.3%
49	Alaska	1,039	0.1%
23	Arizona	10,771	1.5%
32	Arkansas	5,169	0.7%
1	California	89,153	12.3%
24	Colorado	10,239	1.4%
21	Connecticut	12,393	1.7%
46	Delaware	1,875	0.3%
4	Florida	40,898	5.6%
14	Georgia	16,652	2.3%
39	Hawaii	3,399	0.5%
43	Idaho	2,092	0.3%
6	Illinois	32,849	4.5%
20	Indiana	12,407	1.7%
31	Iowa	5,556	0.8%
30	Kansas	5,938	0.8%
26	Kentucky	8,714	1.2%
22	Louisiana	11,181	1.5%
41	Maine	3,102	0.4%
11	Maryland	20,154	2.8%
8	Massachusetts	26,546	3.7%
10	Michigan	23,396	3.2%
19	Minnesota	12,878	1.8%
33	Mississippi	4,707	0.6%
17	Missouri	13,104	1.8%
45	Montana	1,939	0.3%
37	Nebraska	3,902	0.5%
40	Nevada	3,186	0.4%
42	New Hampshire	3,096	0.4%
9	New Jersey	25,110	3.5%
36	New Mexico	4,074	0.6%
2	New York	73,062	10.1%
12	North Carolina	18,499	2.5%
47	North Dakota	1,530	0.2%
7	Ohio	28,204	3.9%
29	Oklahoma	6,064	0.8%
28	Oregon	8,333	1.1%
5	Pennsylvania	37,078	5.1%
38	Rhode Island	3,481	0.5%
27	South Carolina	8,417	1.2%
48	South Dakota	1,468	0.2%
16	Tennessee	14,057	1.9%
3	Texas	41,174	5.7%
34	Utah	4,518	0.6%
44	Vermont	1,966	0.3%
13	Virginia	17,407	2.4%
15	Washington	14,759	2.0%
35	West Virginia	4,168	0.6%
18	Wisconsin	12,919	1.8%
50	Wyoming	921	0.1%

RANK	STATE	PHYSICIANS	% of USA
1	California	89,153	12.3%
2	New York	73,062	10.1%
3	Texas	41,174	5.7%
4	Florida	40,898	5.6%
5	Pennsylvania	37,078	5.1%
6	Illinois	32,849	4.5%
7	Ohio	28,204	3.9%
8	Massachusetts	26,546	3.7%
9	New Jersey	25,110	3.5%
10	Michigan	23,396	3.2%
11	Maryland	20,154	2.8%
12	North Carolina	18,499	2.5%
13	Virginia	17,407	2.4%
14	Georgia	16,652	2.3%
15	Washington	14,759	2.0%
16	Tennessee	14,057	1.9%
17	Missouri	13,104	1.8%
18	Wisconsin	12,919	1.8%
19	Minnesota	12,878	1.8%
20	Indiana	12,407	1.7%
21	Connecticut	12,393	1.7%
22	Louisiana	11,181	1.5%
23	Arizona	10,771	1.5%
24	Colorado	10,239	1.4%
25	Alabama	9,124	1.3%
26	Kentucky	8,714	1.2%
27	South Carolina	8,417	1.2%
28	Oregon	8,333	1.1%
29	Oklahoma	6,064	0.8%
30	Kansas	5,938	0.8%
31	Iowa	5,556	0.8%
32	Arkansas	5,169	0.7%
33	Mississippi	4,707	0.6%
34	Utah	4,518	0.6%
35	West Virginia	4,168	0.6%
36	New Mexico	4,074	0.6%
37	Nebraska	3,902	0.5%
38	Rhode Island	3,481	0.5%
39	Hawaii	3,399	0.5%
40	Nevada	3,186	0.4%
41	Maine	3,102	0.4%
42	New Hampshire	3,096	0.4%
43	Idaho	2,092	0.3%
44	Vermont	1,966	0.3%
45	Montana	1,939	0.3%
46	Delaware	1,875	0.3%
47	North Dakota	1,530	0.2%
48	South Dakota	1,468	0.2%
49	Alaska	1,039	0.1%
50	Wyoming	921	0.1%
	District of Columbia	3,980	0.5%

Source: American Medical Association (Chicago, Illinois)
    "Physician Characteristics and Distribution in the U.S." (1999 Edition)
*As of December 31, 1997. Total does not include 9,618 nonfederal physicians in U.S. territories and possessions.

Rate of Nonfederal Physicians in 1997

National Rate = 271 Physicians per 100,000 Population*

ALPHA ORDER

RANK	STATE	RATE		RANK	STATE	RATE
41	Alabama	211		1	Massachusetts	434
50	Alaska	170		2	New York	403
29	Arizona	237		3	Maryland	396
42	Arkansas	205		4	Connecticut	379
11	California	277		5	Rhode Island	353
15	Colorado	263		6	Vermont	334
4	Connecticut	379		7	New Jersey	312
21	Delaware	255		8	Pennsylvania	309
10	Florida	279		9	Hawaii	285
35	Georgia	222		10	Florida	279
9	Hawaii	285		11	California	277
48	Idaho	173		12	Minnesota	275
13	Illinois	274		13	Illinois	274
39	Indiana	212		14	New Hampshire	264
44	Iowa	195		15	Colorado	263
33	Kansas	228		15	Washington	263
34	Kentucky	223		17	Tennessee	262
19	Louisiana	257		18	Virginia	258
23	Maine	250		19	Louisiana	257
3	Maryland	396		19	Oregon	257
1	Massachusetts	434		21	Delaware	255
27	Michigan	239		22	Ohio	252
12	Minnesota	275		23	Maine	250
49	Mississippi	172		24	North Carolina	249
26	Missouri	242		25	Wisconsin	248
37	Montana	221		26	Missouri	242
31	Nebraska	235		27	Michigan	239
46	Nevada	190		27	North Dakota	239
14	New Hampshire	264		29	Arizona	237
7	New Jersey	312		30	New Mexico	236
30	New Mexico	236		31	Nebraska	235
2	New York	403		32	West Virginia	230
24	North Carolina	249		33	Kansas	228
27	North Dakota	239		34	Kentucky	223
22	Ohio	252		35	Georgia	222
47	Oklahoma	183		35	South Carolina	222
19	Oregon	257		37	Montana	221
8	Pennsylvania	309		38	Utah	219
5	Rhode Island	353		39	Indiana	212
35	South Carolina	222		39	Texas	212
43	South Dakota	199		41	Alabama	211
17	Tennessee	262		42	Arkansas	205
39	Texas	212		43	South Dakota	199
38	Utah	219		44	Iowa	195
6	Vermont	334		45	Wyoming	192
18	Virginia	258		46	Nevada	190
15	Washington	263		47	Oklahoma	183
32	West Virginia	230		48	Idaho	173
25	Wisconsin	248		49	Mississippi	172
45	Wyoming	192		50	Alaska	170
					District of Columbia	751

Source: Morgan Quitno Press using data from American Medical Association (Chicago, Illinois)
"Physician Characteristics and Distribution in the U.S." (1999 Edition)
*As of December 31, 1997.

Nonfederal Physicians in Patient Care in 1997

National Total = 595,618 Physicians*

ALPHA ORDER

RANK	STATE	PHYSICIANS	% of USA
25	Alabama	7,810	1.3%
49	Alaska	912	0.2%
23	Arizona	8,396	1.4%
32	Arkansas	4,398	0.7%
1	California	70,556	11.8%
24	Colorado	8,326	1.4%
21	Connecticut	9,979	1.7%
45	Delaware	1,555	0.3%
4	Florida	31,531	5.3%
14	Georgia	14,102	2.4%
39	Hawaii	2,753	0.5%
43	Idaho	1,739	0.3%
6	Illinois	27,733	4.7%
20	Indiana	10,441	1.8%
31	Iowa	4,457	0.7%
30	Kansas	4,878	0.8%
26	Kentucky	7,479	1.3%
22	Louisiana	9,594	1.6%
42	Maine	2,438	0.4%
11	Maryland	15,770	2.6%
8	Massachusetts	21,281	3.6%
10	Michigan	19,450	3.3%
19	Minnesota	10,561	1.8%
33	Mississippi	4,023	0.7%
17	Missouri	11,031	1.9%
44	Montana	1,563	0.3%
36	Nebraska	3,268	0.5%
40	Nevada	2,663	0.4%
41	New Hampshire	2,506	0.4%
9	New Jersey	20,925	3.5%
37	New Mexico	3,254	0.5%
2	New York	60,233	10.1%
12	North Carolina	15,220	2.6%
47	North Dakota	1,306	0.2%
7	Ohio	23,585	4.0%
29	Oklahoma	5,097	0.9%
28	Oregon	6,619	1.1%
5	Pennsylvania	30,611	5.1%
38	Rhode Island	2,891	0.5%
27	South Carolina	7,090	1.2%
48	South Dakota	1,247	0.2%
15	Tennessee	12,026	2.0%
3	Texas	34,929	5.9%
34	Utah	3,697	0.6%
46	Vermont	1,529	0.3%
13	Virginia	14,436	2.4%
16	Washington	11,698	2.0%
35	West Virginia	3,501	0.6%
18	Wisconsin	10,726	1.8%
50	Wyoming	741	0.1%

RANK ORDER

RANK	STATE	PHYSICIANS	% of USA
1	California	70,556	11.8%
2	New York	60,233	10.1%
3	Texas	34,929	5.9%
4	Florida	31,531	5.3%
5	Pennsylvania	30,611	5.1%
6	Illinois	27,733	4.7%
7	Ohio	23,585	4.0%
8	Massachusetts	21,281	3.6%
9	New Jersey	20,925	3.5%
10	Michigan	19,450	3.3%
11	Maryland	15,770	2.6%
12	North Carolina	15,220	2.6%
13	Virginia	14,436	2.4%
14	Georgia	14,102	2.4%
15	Tennessee	12,026	2.0%
16	Washington	11,698	2.0%
17	Missouri	11,031	1.9%
18	Wisconsin	10,726	1.8%
19	Minnesota	10,561	1.8%
20	Indiana	10,441	1.8%
21	Connecticut	9,979	1.7%
22	Louisiana	9,594	1.6%
23	Arizona	8,396	1.4%
24	Colorado	8,326	1.4%
25	Alabama	7,810	1.3%
26	Kentucky	7,479	1.3%
27	South Carolina	7,090	1.2%
28	Oregon	6,619	1.1%
29	Oklahoma	5,097	0.9%
30	Kansas	4,878	0.8%
31	Iowa	4,457	0.7%
32	Arkansas	4,398	0.7%
33	Mississippi	4,023	0.7%
34	Utah	3,697	0.6%
35	West Virginia	3,501	0.6%
36	Nebraska	3,268	0.5%
37	New Mexico	3,254	0.5%
38	Rhode Island	2,891	0.5%
39	Hawaii	2,753	0.5%
40	Nevada	2,663	0.4%
41	New Hampshire	2,506	0.4%
42	Maine	2,438	0.4%
43	Idaho	1,739	0.3%
44	Montana	1,563	0.3%
45	Delaware	1,555	0.3%
46	Vermont	1,529	0.3%
47	North Dakota	1,306	0.2%
48	South Dakota	1,247	0.2%
49	Alaska	912	0.2%
50	Wyoming	741	0.1%
	District of Columbia	3,064	0.5%

Source: American Medical Association (Chicago, Illinois)
    "Physician Characteristics and Distribution in the U.S." (1999 Edition)
*As of December 31, 1997. Total does not include 8,066 physicians in U.S. territories and possessions.

Rate of Nonfederal Physicians in Patient Care in 1997

National Rate = 222 Physicians per 100,000 Population*

ALPHA ORDER

RANK	STATE	RATE
37	Alabama	181
48	Alaska	150
36	Arizona	184
42	Arkansas	174
14	California	219
16	Colorado	214
4	Connecticut	305
19	Delaware	212
15	Florida	215
33	Georgia	188
9	Hawaii	231
50	Idaho	144
9	Illinois	231
40	Indiana	178
45	Iowa	156
33	Kansas	188
31	Kentucky	191
13	Louisiana	220
29	Maine	196
3	Maryland	310
1	Massachusetts	348
27	Michigan	199
11	Minnesota	225
49	Mississippi	147
24	Missouri	204
40	Montana	178
28	Nebraska	197
44	Nevada	159
16	New Hampshire	214
6	New Jersey	260
32	New Mexico	189
2	New York	332
23	North Carolina	205
24	North Dakota	204
20	Ohio	211
47	Oklahoma	153
24	Oregon	204
8	Pennsylvania	255
5	Rhode Island	293
35	South Carolina	187
43	South Dakota	169
12	Tennessee	224
38	Texas	180
39	Utah	179
6	Vermont	260
16	Virginia	214
21	Washington	208
30	West Virginia	193
22	Wisconsin	206
46	Wyoming	154

RANK ORDER

RANK	STATE	RATE
1	Massachusetts	348
2	New York	332
3	Maryland	310
4	Connecticut	305
5	Rhode Island	293
6	New Jersey	260
6	Vermont	260
8	Pennsylvania	255
9	Hawaii	231
9	Illinois	231
11	Minnesota	225
12	Tennessee	224
13	Louisiana	220
14	California	219
15	Florida	215
16	Colorado	214
16	New Hampshire	214
16	Virginia	214
19	Delaware	212
20	Ohio	211
21	Washington	208
22	Wisconsin	206
23	North Carolina	205
24	Missouri	204
24	North Dakota	204
24	Oregon	204
27	Michigan	199
28	Nebraska	197
29	Maine	196
30	West Virginia	193
31	Kentucky	191
32	New Mexico	189
33	Georgia	188
33	Kansas	188
35	South Carolina	187
36	Arizona	184
37	Alabama	181
38	Texas	180
39	Utah	179
40	Indiana	178
40	Montana	178
42	Arkansas	174
43	South Dakota	169
44	Nevada	159
45	Iowa	156
46	Wyoming	154
47	Oklahoma	153
48	Alaska	150
49	Mississippi	147
50	Idaho	144

District of Columbia	578

Source: Morgan Quitno Press using data from American Medical Association (Chicago, Illinois)
   "Physician Characteristics and Distribution in the U.S." (1999 Edition)
*As of December 31, 1997. National rate does not include physicians in U.S. territories and possessions.

Physicians in Primary Care in 1997

National Total = 256,968 Physicians*

ALPHA ORDER

RANK	STATE	PHYSICIANS	% of USA
25	Alabama	3,446	1.3%
49	Alaska	500	0.2%
24	Arizona	3,618	1.4%
31	Arkansas	1,991	0.8%
1	California	30,428	11.8%
23	Colorado	3,627	1.4%
21	Connecticut	4,162	1.6%
46	Delaware	638	0.2%
5	Florida	12,664	4.9%
14	Georgia	6,250	2.4%
38	Hawaii	1,351	0.5%
43	Idaho	784	0.3%
4	Illinois	12,770	5.0%
19	Indiana	4,530	1.8%
32	Iowa	1,965	0.8%
30	Kansas	2,218	0.9%
26	Kentucky	3,172	1.2%
22	Louisiana	3,889	1.5%
41	Maine	1,109	0.4%
11	Maryland	7,032	2.7%
9	Massachusetts	8,478	3.3%
10	Michigan	8,421	3.3%
17	Minnesota	4,858	1.9%
33	Mississippi	1,828	0.7%
20	Missouri	4,462	1.7%
45	Montana	667	0.3%
37	Nebraska	1,517	0.6%
40	Nevada	1,117	0.4%
42	New Hampshire	1,064	0.4%
8	New Jersey	9,109	3.5%
36	New Mexico	1,540	0.6%
2	New York	25,831	10.1%
12	North Carolina	6,623	2.6%
48	North Dakota	619	0.2%
7	Ohio	10,143	3.9%
29	Oklahoma	2,248	0.9%
28	Oregon	2,925	1.1%
6	Pennsylvania	12,328	4.8%
39	Rhode Island	1,263	0.5%
27	South Carolina	3,150	1.2%
47	South Dakota	625	0.2%
16	Tennessee	5,066	2.0%
3	Texas	14,787	5.8%
35	Utah	1,543	0.6%
44	Vermont	716	0.3%
13	Virginia	6,553	2.6%
15	Washington	5,296	2.1%
34	West Virginia	1,612	0.6%
18	Wisconsin	4,719	1.8%
50	Wyoming	396	0.2%

RANK ORDER

RANK	STATE	PHYSICIANS	% of USA
1	California	30,428	11.8%
2	New York	25,831	10.1%
3	Texas	14,787	5.8%
4	Illinois	12,770	5.0%
5	Florida	12,664	4.9%
6	Pennsylvania	12,328	4.8%
7	Ohio	10,143	3.9%
8	New Jersey	9,109	3.5%
9	Massachusetts	8,478	3.3%
10	Michigan	8,421	3.3%
11	Maryland	7,032	2.7%
12	North Carolina	6,623	2.6%
13	Virginia	6,553	2.6%
14	Georgia	6,250	2.4%
15	Washington	5,296	2.1%
16	Tennessee	5,066	2.0%
17	Minnesota	4,858	1.9%
18	Wisconsin	4,719	1.8%
19	Indiana	4,530	1.8%
20	Missouri	4,462	1.7%
21	Connecticut	4,162	1.6%
22	Louisiana	3,889	1.5%
23	Colorado	3,627	1.4%
24	Arizona	3,618	1.4%
25	Alabama	3,446	1.3%
26	Kentucky	3,172	1.2%
27	South Carolina	3,150	1.2%
28	Oregon	2,925	1.1%
29	Oklahoma	2,248	0.9%
30	Kansas	2,218	0.9%
31	Arkansas	1,991	0.8%
32	Iowa	1,965	0.8%
33	Mississippi	1,828	0.7%
34	West Virginia	1,612	0.6%
35	Utah	1,543	0.6%
36	New Mexico	1,540	0.6%
37	Nebraska	1,517	0.6%
38	Hawaii	1,351	0.5%
39	Rhode Island	1,263	0.5%
40	Nevada	1,117	0.4%
41	Maine	1,109	0.4%
42	New Hampshire	1,064	0.4%
43	Idaho	784	0.3%
44	Vermont	716	0.3%
45	Montana	667	0.3%
46	Delaware	638	0.2%
47	South Dakota	625	0.2%
48	North Dakota	619	0.2%
49	Alaska	500	0.2%
50	Wyoming	396	0.2%
	District of Columbia	1,320	0.5%

Source: American Medical Association (Chicago, Illinois)
      "Physician Characteristics and Distribution in the U.S." (1999 Edition)
Federal and nonfederal physicians as of December 31, 1997. National total does not include 4,819 physicians in U.S. territories and possessions. Primary Care Specialties include Family Practice, General Practice, Internal Medicine, Obstetrics/Gynecology and Pediatrics.

Rate of Physicians in Primary Care in 1997

National Rate = 96 Physicians per 100,000 Population*

ALPHA ORDER

RANK	STATE	RATE
39	Alabama	80
36	Alaska	82
40	Arizona	79
40	Arkansas	79
14	California	95
17	Colorado	93
5	Connecticut	127
28	Delaware	87
29	Florida	86
33	Georgia	83
7	Hawaii	113
50	Idaho	65
9	Illinois	107
42	Indiana	77
46	Iowa	69
31	Kansas	85
38	Kentucky	81
23	Louisiana	89
23	Maine	89
3	Maryland	138
2	Massachusetts	139
29	Michigan	86
10	Minnesota	104
48	Mississippi	67
33	Missouri	83
43	Montana	76
18	Nebraska	92
48	Nevada	67
19	New Hampshire	91
7	New Jersey	113
23	New Mexico	89
1	New York	142
23	North Carolina	89
12	North Dakota	97
19	Ohio	91
47	Oklahoma	68
22	Oregon	90
11	Pennsylvania	103
4	Rhode Island	128
33	South Carolina	83
31	South Dakota	85
15	Tennessee	94
43	Texas	76
45	Utah	75
6	Vermont	122
12	Virginia	97
15	Washington	94
23	West Virginia	89
19	Wisconsin	91
36	Wyoming	82

RANK ORDER

RANK	STATE	RATE
1	New York	142
2	Massachusetts	139
3	Maryland	138
4	Rhode Island	128
5	Connecticut	127
6	Vermont	122
7	Hawaii	113
7	New Jersey	113
9	Illinois	107
10	Minnesota	104
11	Pennsylvania	103
12	North Dakota	97
12	Virginia	97
14	California	95
15	Tennessee	94
15	Washington	94
17	Colorado	93
18	Nebraska	92
19	New Hampshire	91
19	Ohio	91
19	Wisconsin	91
22	Oregon	90
23	Louisiana	89
23	Maine	89
23	New Mexico	89
23	North Carolina	89
23	West Virginia	89
28	Delaware	87
29	Florida	86
29	Michigan	86
31	Kansas	85
31	South Dakota	85
33	Georgia	83
33	Missouri	83
33	South Carolina	83
36	Alaska	82
36	Wyoming	82
38	Kentucky	81
39	Alabama	80
40	Arizona	79
40	Arkansas	79
42	Indiana	77
43	Montana	76
43	Texas	76
45	Utah	75
46	Iowa	69
47	Oklahoma	68
48	Mississippi	67
48	Nevada	67
50	Idaho	65

	District of Columbia	249

Source: Morgan Quitno Press using data from American Medical Association (Chicago, Illinois)
    "Physician Characteristics and Distribution in the U.S." (1999 Edition)
*Federal and nonfederal physicians as of January 1, 1997. National rate does not include physicians in U.S.
territories and possessions. Primary Care Specialties include Family Practice, General Practice, Internal Medicine,
Obstetrics/Gynecology and Pediatrics.

Percent of Physicians in Primary Care in 1997

National Percent = 34.0% of Physicians*

ALPHA ORDER

RANK	STATE	PERCENT
10	Alabama	36.9
1	Alaska	41.7
47	Arizona	32.5
8	Arkansas	37.7
43	California	33.3
33	Colorado	34.5
45	Connecticut	33.2
43	Delaware	33.3
50	Florida	30.3
21	Georgia	35.8
14	Hawaii	36.3
12	Idaho	36.5
5	Illinois	38.3
16	Indiana	36.2
31	Iowa	34.9
14	Kansas	36.3
21	Kentucky	35.8
38	Louisiana	34.1
28	Maine	35.3
48	Maryland	31.7
49	Massachusetts	31.5
24	Michigan	35.7
9	Minnesota	37.2
10	Mississippi	36.9
42	Missouri	33.5
40	Montana	33.7
5	Nebraska	38.3
35	Nevada	34.3
39	New Hampshire	33.9
19	New Jersey	36.0
16	New Mexico	36.2
30	New York	35.0
32	North Carolina	34.8
4	North Dakota	39.4
27	Ohio	35.4
19	Oklahoma	36.0
34	Oregon	34.4
46	Pennsylvania	32.9
25	Rhode Island	35.6
12	South Carolina	36.5
3	South Dakota	40.5
28	Tennessee	35.3
35	Texas	34.3
41	Utah	33.6
21	Vermont	35.8
26	Virginia	35.5
35	Washington	34.3
7	West Virginia	37.8
16	Wisconsin	36.2
2	Wyoming	41.4

RANK ORDER

RANK	STATE	PERCENT
1	Alaska	41.7
2	Wyoming	41.4
3	South Dakota	40.5
4	North Dakota	39.4
5	Illinois	38.3
5	Nebraska	38.3
7	West Virginia	37.8
8	Arkansas	37.7
9	Minnesota	37.2
10	Alabama	36.9
10	Mississippi	36.9
12	Idaho	36.5
12	South Carolina	36.5
14	Hawaii	36.3
14	Kansas	36.3
16	Indiana	36.2
16	New Mexico	36.2
16	Wisconsin	36.2
19	New Jersey	36.0
19	Oklahoma	36.0
21	Georgia	35.8
21	Kentucky	35.8
21	Vermont	35.8
24	Michigan	35.7
25	Rhode Island	35.6
26	Virginia	35.5
27	Ohio	35.4
28	Maine	35.3
28	Tennessee	35.3
30	New York	35.0
31	Iowa	34.9
32	North Carolina	34.8
33	Colorado	34.5
34	Oregon	34.4
35	Nevada	34.3
35	Texas	34.3
35	Washington	34.3
38	Louisiana	34.1
39	New Hampshire	33.9
40	Montana	33.7
41	Utah	33.6
42	Missouri	33.5
43	California	33.3
43	Delaware	33.3
45	Connecticut	33.2
46	Pennsylvania	32.9
47	Arizona	32.5
48	Maryland	31.7
49	Massachusetts	31.5
50	Florida	30.3

District of Columbia	30.8

Source: American Medical Association (Chicago, Illinois)
   "Physician Characteristics and Distribution in the U.S." (1999 Edition)
Federal and nonfederal physicians as of January 1, 1997. National rate does not include physicians in U.S. territories and possessions. Primary Care Specialties include Family Practice, General Practice, Internal Medicine, Obstetrics/Gynecology and Pediatrics.

Percent of Population Lacking Access to Primary Care in 1998

National Percent = 9.6% of Population*

ALPHA ORDER				RANK ORDER		
RANK	STATE	PERCENT		RANK	STATE	PERCENT
6	Alabama	19.5		1	Louisiana	24.1
10	Alaska	14.6		2	Mississippi	22.1
30	Arizona	8.9		3	Utah	21.7
18	Arkansas	12.4		4	Idaho	21.0
40	California	6.7		5	South Dakota	20.1
34	Colorado	8.0		6	Alabama	19.5
41	Connecticut	6.5		7	Wyoming	18.7
47	Delaware	4.7		8	North Dakota	17.1
37	Florida	7.7		9	New Mexico	16.8
13	Georgia	13.6		10	Alaska	14.6
49	Hawaii	3.0		11	Missouri	13.8
4	Idaho	21.0		12	South Carolina	13.7
33	Illinois	8.2		13	Georgia	13.6
27	Indiana	9.6		14	Nevada	13.4
30	Iowa	8.9		15	Kentucky	13.2
27	Kansas	9.6		16	West Virginia	12.9
15	Kentucky	13.2		17	Michigan	12.6
1	Louisiana	24.1		18	Arkansas	12.4
35	Maine	7.9		19	Montana	12.3
50	Maryland	2.2		20	North Carolina	11.2
45	Massachusetts	5.4		21	Texas	11.1
17	Michigan	12.6		22	Wisconsin	10.3
48	Minnesota	4.2		23	Oregon	10.2
2	Mississippi	22.1		23	Tennessee	10.2
11	Missouri	13.8		25	Oklahoma	9.8
19	Montana	12.3		26	New York	9.7
35	Nebraska	7.9		27	Indiana	9.6
14	Nevada	13.4		27	Kansas	9.6
43	New Hampshire	5.9		27	Rhode Island	9.6
46	New Jersey	5.1		30	Arizona	8.9
9	New Mexico	16.8		30	Iowa	8.9
26	New York	9.7		32	Ohio	8.4
20	North Carolina	11.2		33	Illinois	8.2
8	North Dakota	17.1		34	Colorado	8.0
32	Ohio	8.4		35	Maine	7.9
25	Oklahoma	9.8		35	Nebraska	7.9
23	Oregon	10.2		37	Florida	7.7
44	Pennsylvania	5.7		38	Washington	7.5
27	Rhode Island	9.6		39	Vermont	7.4
12	South Carolina	13.7		40	California	6.7
5	South Dakota	20.1		41	Connecticut	6.5
23	Tennessee	10.2		42	Virginia	6.3
21	Texas	11.1		43	New Hampshire	5.9
3	Utah	21.7		44	Pennsylvania	5.7
39	Vermont	7.4		45	Massachusetts	5.4
42	Virginia	6.3		46	New Jersey	5.1
38	Washington	7.5		47	Delaware	4.7
16	West Virginia	12.9		48	Minnesota	4.2
22	Wisconsin	10.3		49	Hawaii	3.0
7	Wyoming	18.7		50	Maryland	2.2
					District of Columbia	21.4

Source: Morgan Quitno Press using data from U.S. Dept. of Health and Human Services, Div. of Shortage Designation
"Selected Statistics on Health Manpower Shortage Areas, As of September 30, 1998"
*Percent of population considered under-served by primary medical practitioners (Family & General Practice doctors, Internists, Ob/Gyns and Pediatricians). An under-served population does not have primary medical care within reasonable economic and geographic bounds.

Nonfederal Physicians in General/Family Practice in 1997

National Total = 77,624 Physicians*

RANK	STATE	PHYSICIANS	% of USA
22	Alabama	1,184	1.5%
47	Alaska	226	0.3%
20	Arizona	1,256	1.6%
28	Arkansas	1,033	1.3%
1	California	9,462	12.2%
18	Colorado	1,450	1.9%
36	Connecticut	573	0.7%
49	Delaware	210	0.3%
3	Florida	4,189	5.4%
15	Georgia	1,814	2.3%
45	Hawaii	293	0.4%
39	Idaho	463	0.6%
6	Illinois	3,446	4.4%
12	Indiana	2,167	2.8%
27	Iowa	1,065	1.4%
30	Kansas	1,013	1.3%
21	Kentucky	1,233	1.6%
25	Louisiana	1,141	1.5%
38	Maine	478	0.6%
23	Maryland	1,162	1.5%
26	Massachusetts	1,108	1.4%
8	Michigan	2,399	3.1%
10	Minnesota	2,293	3.0%
33	Mississippi	714	0.9%
24	Missouri	1,150	1.5%
44	Montana	330	0.4%
32	Nebraska	767	1.0%
40	Nevada	381	0.5%
41	New Hampshire	361	0.5%
17	New Jersey	1,500	1.9%
35	New Mexico	589	0.8%
5	New York	3,642	4.7%
11	North Carolina	2,209	2.8%
43	North Dakota	339	0.4%
7	Ohio	3,146	4.1%
31	Oklahoma	943	1.2%
29	Oregon	1,019	1.3%
4	Pennsylvania	3,781	4.9%
50	Rhode Island	207	0.3%
19	South Carolina	1,335	1.7%
42	South Dakota	344	0.4%
16	Tennessee	1,633	2.1%
2	Texas	5,166	6.7%
37	Utah	562	0.7%
46	Vermont	232	0.3%
13	Virginia	2,157	2.8%
9	Washington	2,373	3.1%
34	West Virginia	644	0.8%
14	Wisconsin	2,065	2.7%
48	Wyoming	217	0.3%

RANK	STATE	PHYSICIANS	% of USA
1	California	9,462	12.2%
2	Texas	5,166	6.7%
3	Florida	4,189	5.4%
4	Pennsylvania	3,781	4.9%
5	New York	3,642	4.7%
6	Illinois	3,446	4.4%
7	Ohio	3,146	4.1%
8	Michigan	2,399	3.1%
9	Washington	2,373	3.1%
10	Minnesota	2,293	3.0%
11	North Carolina	2,209	2.8%
12	Indiana	2,167	2.8%
13	Virginia	2,157	2.8%
14	Wisconsin	2,065	2.7%
15	Georgia	1,814	2.3%
16	Tennessee	1,633	2.1%
17	New Jersey	1,500	1.9%
18	Colorado	1,450	1.9%
19	South Carolina	1,335	1.7%
20	Arizona	1,256	1.6%
21	Kentucky	1,233	1.6%
22	Alabama	1,184	1.5%
23	Maryland	1,162	1.5%
24	Missouri	1,150	1.5%
25	Louisiana	1,141	1.5%
26	Massachusetts	1,108	1.4%
27	Iowa	1,065	1.4%
28	Arkansas	1,033	1.3%
29	Oregon	1,019	1.3%
30	Kansas	1,013	1.3%
31	Oklahoma	943	1.2%
32	Nebraska	767	1.0%
33	Mississippi	714	0.9%
34	West Virginia	644	0.8%
35	New Mexico	589	0.8%
36	Connecticut	573	0.7%
37	Utah	562	0.7%
38	Maine	478	0.6%
39	Idaho	463	0.6%
40	Nevada	381	0.5%
41	New Hampshire	361	0.5%
42	South Dakota	344	0.4%
43	North Dakota	339	0.4%
44	Montana	330	0.4%
45	Hawaii	293	0.4%
46	Vermont	232	0.3%
47	Alaska	226	0.3%
48	Wyoming	217	0.3%
49	Delaware	210	0.3%
50	Rhode Island	207	0.3%
	District of Columbia	160	0.2%

Source: American Medical Association (Chicago, Illinois)
    "Physician Characteristics and Distribution in the U.S." (1999 Edition)
*As of December 31, 1997. Total does not include 2,001 nonfederal physicians in U.S. territories and possessions.

Rate of Nonfederal Physicians in General/Family Practice in 1997

National Rate = 29 Physicians per 100,000 Population*

ALPHA ORDER

RANK	STATE	RATE
35	Alabama	27
14	Alaska	37
32	Arizona	28
7	Arkansas	41
28	California	29
14	Colorado	37
49	Connecticut	18
28	Delaware	29
28	Florida	29
42	Georgia	24
40	Hawaii	25
11	Idaho	38
28	Illinois	29
14	Indiana	37
14	Iowa	37
9	Kansas	39
21	Kentucky	32
38	Louisiana	26
11	Maine	38
43	Maryland	23
49	Massachusetts	18
40	Michigan	25
2	Minnesota	49
38	Mississippi	26
45	Missouri	21
11	Montana	38
4	Nebraska	46
43	Nevada	23
23	New Hampshire	31
48	New Jersey	19
20	New Mexico	34
47	New York	20
26	North Carolina	30
1	North Dakota	53
32	Ohio	28
32	Oklahoma	28
23	Oregon	31
23	Pennsylvania	31
45	Rhode Island	21
18	South Carolina	35
3	South Dakota	47
26	Tennessee	30
35	Texas	27
35	Utah	27
9	Vermont	39
21	Virginia	32
6	Washington	42
18	West Virginia	35
8	Wisconsin	40
5	Wyoming	45

RANK ORDER

RANK	STATE	RATE
1	North Dakota	53
2	Minnesota	49
3	South Dakota	47
4	Nebraska	46
5	Wyoming	45
6	Washington	42
7	Arkansas	41
8	Wisconsin	40
9	Kansas	39
9	Vermont	39
11	Idaho	38
11	Maine	38
11	Montana	38
14	Alaska	37
14	Colorado	37
14	Indiana	37
14	Iowa	37
18	South Carolina	35
18	West Virginia	35
20	New Mexico	34
21	Kentucky	32
21	Virginia	32
23	New Hampshire	31
23	Oregon	31
23	Pennsylvania	31
26	North Carolina	30
26	Tennessee	30
28	California	29
28	Delaware	29
28	Florida	29
28	Illinois	29
32	Arizona	28
32	Ohio	28
32	Oklahoma	28
35	Alabama	27
35	Texas	27
35	Utah	27
38	Louisiana	26
38	Mississippi	26
40	Hawaii	25
40	Michigan	25
42	Georgia	24
43	Maryland	23
43	Nevada	23
45	Missouri	21
45	Rhode Island	21
47	New York	20
48	New Jersey	19
49	Connecticut	18
49	Massachusetts	18

| | District of Columbia | 30 |

Source: Morgan Quitno Press using data from American Medical Association (Chicago, Illinois)
    "Physician Characteristics and Distribution in the U.S." (1999 Edition)
*As of December 31, 1997. National rate does not include physicians in U.S. territories and possessions.

Percent of Family Physicians Who Practice Pediatrics in 1998

National Percent = 87.9% of Family Physicians*

RANK	STATE	PERCENT
37	Alabama	86.7
33	Alaska	87.5
38	Arizona	86.4
33	Arkansas	87.5
42	California	85.8
5	Colorado	93.1
36	Connecticut	87.1
22	Delaware	89.7
50	Florida	76.5
38	Georgia	86.4
21	Hawaii	89.8
11	Idaho	91.9
32	Illinois	87.6
12	Indiana	91.8
13	Iowa	91.6
15	Kansas	91.3
26	Kentucky	89.0
41	Louisiana	86.0
16	Maine	90.7
49	Maryland	82.1
9	Massachusetts	92.1
26	Michigan	89.0
8	Minnesota	92.2
35	Mississippi	87.3
30	Missouri	87.8
9	Montana	92.1
2	Nebraska	95.2
28	Nevada	88.8
4	New Hampshire	93.5
43	New Jersey	85.6
18	New Mexico	90.1
45	New York	83.5
29	North Carolina	87.9
30	North Dakota	87.8
25	Ohio	89.1
19	Oklahoma	90.0
20	Oregon	89.9
23	Pennsylvania	89.4
16	Rhode Island	90.7
43	South Carolina	85.6
1	South Dakota	97.1
38	Tennessee	86.4
47	Texas	82.5
5	Utah	93.1
14	Vermont	91.4
24	Virginia	89.3
7	Washington	92.8
46	West Virginia	82.6
3	Wisconsin	93.8
47	Wyoming	82.5

RANK	STATE	PERCENT
1	South Dakota	97.1
2	Nebraska	95.2
3	Wisconsin	93.8
4	New Hampshire	93.5
5	Colorado	93.1
5	Utah	93.1
7	Washington	92.8
8	Minnesota	92.2
9	Massachusetts	92.1
9	Montana	92.1
11	Idaho	91.9
12	Indiana	91.8
13	Iowa	91.6
14	Vermont	91.4
15	Kansas	91.3
16	Maine	90.7
16	Rhode Island	90.7
18	New Mexico	90.1
19	Oklahoma	90.0
20	Oregon	89.9
21	Hawaii	89.8
22	Delaware	89.7
23	Pennsylvania	89.4
24	Virginia	89.3
25	Ohio	89.1
26	Kentucky	89.0
26	Michigan	89.0
28	Nevada	88.8
29	North Carolina	87.9
30	Missouri	87.8
30	North Dakota	87.8
32	Illinois	87.6
33	Alaska	87.5
33	Arkansas	87.5
35	Mississippi	87.3
36	Connecticut	87.1
37	Alabama	86.7
38	Arizona	86.4
38	Georgia	86.4
38	Tennessee	86.4
41	Louisiana	86.0
42	California	85.8
43	New Jersey	85.6
43	South Carolina	85.6
45	New York	83.5
46	West Virginia	82.6
47	Texas	82.5
47	Wyoming	82.5
49	Maryland	82.1
50	Florida	76.5

	District of Columbia	80.0

Source: The American Academy of Family Physicians
    "Facts About Family Practice 1998"
As of January 1, 1998. Includes members of the Academy who are in direct patient care and who practice pediatrics "in some fashion".

Percent of Family Physicians Who Practice Obstetrics in 1998

National Percent = 30.4% of Family Physicians*

ALPHA ORDER

RANK ORDER

RANK	STATE	PERCENT		RANK	STATE	PERCENT
44	Alabama	12.9		1	South Dakota	71.4
3	Alaska	59.7		2	North Dakota	63.3
26	Arizona	26.0		3	Alaska	59.7
30	Arkansas	23.0		4	Nebraska	59.4
30	California	23.0		5	Minnesota	58.8
14	Colorado	45.5		6	Wisconsin	58.4
42	Connecticut	14.7		7	Idaho	53.7
40	Delaware	15.5		8	Montana	52.5
50	Florida	6.3		9	Kansas	51.9
36	Georgia	17.3		10	Washington	51.6
29	Hawaii	25.4		11	Iowa	49.6
7	Idaho	53.7		12	Wyoming	49.2
23	Illinois	31.1		13	Utah	45.8
15	Indiana	44.0		14	Colorado	45.5
11	Iowa	49.6		15	Indiana	44.0
9	Kansas	51.9		16	Oklahoma	42.5
47	Kentucky	12.6		17	Oregon	42.0
38	Louisiana	16.3		18	Maine	39.8
18	Maine	39.8		19	Michigan	38.7
46	Maryland	12.7		20	Vermont	37.0
25	Massachusetts	28.1		21	New Hampshire	34.1
19	Michigan	38.7		22	New Mexico	33.8
5	Minnesota	58.8		23	Illinois	31.1
49	Mississippi	11.3		24	Rhode Island	30.2
28	Missouri	25.7		25	Massachusetts	28.1
8	Montana	52.5		26	Arizona	26.0
4	Nebraska	59.4		26	New York	26.0
48	Nevada	12.5		28	Missouri	25.7
21	New Hampshire	34.1		29	Hawaii	25.4
41	New Jersey	14.8		30	Arkansas	23.0
22	New Mexico	33.8		30	California	23.0
26	New York	26.0		32	Tennessee	21.7
34	North Carolina	20.2		33	Texas	20.3
2	North Dakota	63.3		34	North Carolina	20.2
35	Ohio	18.1		35	Ohio	18.1
16	Oklahoma	42.5		36	Georgia	17.3
17	Oregon	42.0		37	South Carolina	16.7
39	Pennsylvania	16.1		38	Louisiana	16.3
24	Rhode Island	30.2		39	Pennsylvania	16.1
37	South Carolina	16.7		40	Delaware	15.5
1	South Dakota	71.4		41	New Jersey	14.8
32	Tennessee	21.7		42	Connecticut	14.7
33	Texas	20.3		43	West Virginia	13.9
13	Utah	45.8		44	Alabama	12.9
20	Vermont	37.0		44	Virginia	12.9
44	Virginia	12.9		46	Maryland	12.7
10	Washington	51.6		47	Kentucky	12.6
43	West Virginia	13.9		48	Nevada	12.5
6	Wisconsin	58.4		49	Mississippi	11.3
12	Wyoming	49.2		50	Florida	6.3
					District of Columbia	20.0

Source: The American Academy of Family Physicians
     "Facts About Family Practice 1998"
*As of January 1, 1998. Includes members of the Academy who are in direct patient care and who practice obstetrics "in some fashion".

Percent of Nonfederal Physicians Who Are Specialists in 1997

National Percent = 76.9% of Physicians*

ALPHA ORDER

RANK	STATE	PERCENT
17	Alabama	77.2
38	Alaska	70.2
36	Arizona	70.8
41	Arkansas	68.9
24	California	74.0
29	Colorado	72.9
4	Connecticut	83.4
18	Delaware	77.0
36	Florida	70.8
10	Georgia	79.0
14	Hawaii	77.5
49	Idaho	62.8
9	Illinois	79.4
34	Indiana	71.3
46	Iowa	66.9
40	Kansas	69.6
20	Kentucky	75.9
8	Louisiana	80.3
44	Maine	67.8
6	Maryland	82.9
1	Massachusetts	84.6
13	Michigan	78.3
39	Minnesota	69.7
26	Mississippi	73.4
7	Missouri	81.3
47	Montana	66.4
41	Nebraska	68.9
23	Nevada	75.3
25	New Hampshire	73.9
5	New Jersey	83.0
35	New Mexico	71.2
2	New York	84.1
19	North Carolina	76.3
45	North Dakota	67.1
15	Ohio	77.4
28	Oklahoma	73.1
33	Oregon	71.5
11	Pennsylvania	78.8
3	Rhode Island	83.5
29	South Carolina	72.9
48	South Dakota	64.2
11	Tennessee	78.8
16	Texas	77.3
22	Utah	75.4
31	Vermont	72.4
21	Virginia	75.6
43	Washington	68.8
27	West Virginia	73.3
32	Wisconsin	72.1
50	Wyoming	61.6

RANK ORDER

RANK	STATE	PERCENT
1	Massachusetts	84.6
2	New York	84.1
3	Rhode Island	83.5
4	Connecticut	83.4
5	New Jersey	83.0
6	Maryland	82.9
7	Missouri	81.3
8	Louisiana	80.3
9	Illinois	79.4
10	Georgia	79.0
11	Pennsylvania	78.8
11	Tennessee	78.8
13	Michigan	78.3
14	Hawaii	77.5
15	Ohio	77.4
16	Texas	77.3
17	Alabama	77.2
18	Delaware	77.0
19	North Carolina	76.3
20	Kentucky	75.9
21	Virginia	75.6
22	Utah	75.4
23	Nevada	75.3
24	California	74.0
25	New Hampshire	73.9
26	Mississippi	73.4
27	West Virginia	73.3
28	Oklahoma	73.1
29	Colorado	72.9
29	South Carolina	72.9
31	Vermont	72.4
32	Wisconsin	72.1
33	Oregon	71.5
34	Indiana	71.3
35	New Mexico	71.2
36	Arizona	70.8
36	Florida	70.8
38	Alaska	70.2
39	Minnesota	69.7
40	Kansas	69.6
41	Arkansas	68.9
41	Nebraska	68.9
43	Washington	68.8
44	Maine	67.8
45	North Dakota	67.1
46	Iowa	66.9
47	Montana	66.4
48	South Dakota	64.2
49	Idaho	62.8
50	Wyoming	61.6
	District of Columbia	86.2

Source: Morgan Quitno Press using data from American Medical Association (Chicago, Illinois) "Physician Characteristics and Distribution in the U.S." (1999 Edition)

**As of December 31, 1997. National rate does not include physicians in U.S. territories and possessions. Includes physicians in medical, surgical and other specialties.*

Nonfederal Physicians in Medical Specialties in 1997

National Total = 224,596 Physicians*

ALPHA ORDER

RANK	STATE	PHYSICIANS	% of USA
24	Alabama	2,808	1.3%
49	Alaska	224	0.1%
23	Arizona	2,881	1.3%
32	Arkansas	1,281	0.6%
2	California	25,981	11.6%
25	Colorado	2,736	1.2%
15	Connecticut	4,518	2.0%
44	Delaware	545	0.2%
4	Florida	11,708	5.2%
14	Georgia	4,892	2.2%
38	Hawaii	1,053	0.5%
46	Idaho	381	0.2%
6	Illinois	11,130	5.0%
22	Indiana	3,206	1.4%
33	Iowa	1,273	0.6%
30	Kansas	1,448	0.6%
26	Kentucky	2,464	1.1%
21	Louisiana	3,374	1.5%
42	Maine	770	0.3%
11	Maryland	7,107	3.2%
7	Massachusetts	10,072	4.5%
10	Michigan	7,374	3.3%
19	Minnesota	3,591	1.6%
34	Mississippi	1,229	0.5%
16	Missouri	4,394	2.0%
45	Montana	407	0.2%
39	Nebraska	975	0.4%
40	Nevada	894	0.4%
41	New Hampshire	826	0.4%
8	New Jersey	9,651	4.3%
37	New Mexico	1,066	0.5%
1	New York	27,912	12.4%
12	North Carolina	5,451	2.4%
47	North Dakota	349	0.2%
9	Ohio	8,720	3.9%
29	Oklahoma	1,608	0.7%
27	Oregon	2,221	1.0%
5	Pennsylvania	11,537	5.1%
31	Rhode Island	1,319	0.6%
28	South Carolina	2,108	0.9%
48	South Dakota	337	0.2%
17	Tennessee	4,330	1.9%
3	Texas	11,761	5.2%
35	Utah	1,227	0.5%
43	Vermont	554	0.2%
13	Virginia	5,113	2.3%
18	Washington	3,634	1.6%
36	West Virginia	1,136	0.5%
20	Wisconsin	3,450	1.5%
50	Wyoming	162	0.1%

RANK ORDER

RANK	STATE	PHYSICIANS	% of USA
1	New York	27,912	12.4%
2	California	25,981	11.6%
3	Texas	11,761	5.2%
4	Florida	11,708	5.2%
5	Pennsylvania	11,537	5.1%
6	Illinois	11,130	5.0%
7	Massachusetts	10,072	4.5%
8	New Jersey	9,651	4.3%
9	Ohio	8,720	3.9%
10	Michigan	7,374	3.3%
11	Maryland	7,107	3.2%
12	North Carolina	5,451	2.4%
13	Virginia	5,113	2.3%
14	Georgia	4,892	2.2%
15	Connecticut	4,518	2.0%
16	Missouri	4,394	2.0%
17	Tennessee	4,330	1.9%
18	Washington	3,634	1.6%
19	Minnesota	3,591	1.6%
20	Wisconsin	3,450	1.5%
21	Louisiana	3,374	1.5%
22	Indiana	3,206	1.4%
23	Arizona	2,881	1.3%
24	Alabama	2,808	1.3%
25	Colorado	2,736	1.2%
26	Kentucky	2,464	1.1%
27	Oregon	2,221	1.0%
28	South Carolina	2,108	0.9%
29	Oklahoma	1,608	0.7%
30	Kansas	1,448	0.6%
31	Rhode Island	1,319	0.6%
32	Arkansas	1,281	0.6%
33	Iowa	1,273	0.6%
34	Mississippi	1,229	0.5%
35	Utah	1,227	0.5%
36	West Virginia	1,136	0.5%
37	New Mexico	1,066	0.5%
38	Hawaii	1,053	0.5%
39	Nebraska	975	0.4%
40	Nevada	894	0.4%
41	New Hampshire	826	0.4%
42	Maine	770	0.3%
43	Vermont	554	0.2%
44	Delaware	545	0.2%
45	Montana	407	0.2%
46	Idaho	381	0.2%
47	North Dakota	349	0.2%
48	South Dakota	337	0.2%
49	Alaska	224	0.1%
50	Wyoming	162	0.1%
	District of Columbia	1,408	0.6%

Source: American Medical Association (Chicago, Illinois)
    "Physician Characteristics and Distribution in the U.S." (1999 Edition)
*As of December 31, 1997. Total does not include 2,657 physicians in U.S. territories and possessions. Medical Specialties are Allergy/Immunology, Cardiovascular Diseases, Dermatology, Gastroenterology, Internal Medicine, Pediatrics, Pediatric Cardiology and Pulmonary Diseases.

Rate of Nonfederal Physicians in Medical Specialties in 1997

National Rate = 84 Physicians per 100,000 Population*

ALPHA ORDER

RANK	STATE	RATE
26	Alabama	65
48	Alaska	37
29	Arizona	63
42	Arkansas	51
11	California	81
22	Colorado	70
4	Connecticut	138
20	Delaware	74
14	Florida	80
26	Georgia	65
10	Hawaii	88
50	Idaho	32
9	Illinois	93
39	Indiana	55
46	Iowa	45
37	Kansas	56
29	Kentucky	63
16	Louisiana	77
32	Maine	62
3	Maryland	139
1	Massachusetts	165
19	Michigan	75
16	Minnesota	77
46	Mississippi	45
11	Missouri	81
44	Montana	46
35	Nebraska	59
41	Nevada	53
22	New Hampshire	70
6	New Jersey	120
32	New Mexico	62
2	New York	154
21	North Carolina	73
40	North Dakota	54
15	Ohio	78
43	Oklahoma	48
24	Oregon	68
7	Pennsylvania	96
5	Rhode Island	134
37	South Carolina	56
44	South Dakota	46
11	Tennessee	81
34	Texas	61
35	Utah	59
8	Vermont	94
18	Virginia	76
26	Washington	65
29	West Virginia	63
25	Wisconsin	66
49	Wyoming	34

RANK ORDER

RANK	STATE	RATE
1	Massachusetts	165
2	New York	154
3	Maryland	139
4	Connecticut	138
5	Rhode Island	134
6	New Jersey	120
7	Pennsylvania	96
8	Vermont	94
9	Illinois	93
10	Hawaii	88
11	California	81
11	Missouri	81
11	Tennessee	81
14	Florida	80
15	Ohio	78
16	Louisiana	77
16	Minnesota	77
18	Virginia	76
19	Michigan	75
20	Delaware	74
21	North Carolina	73
22	Colorado	70
22	New Hampshire	70
24	Oregon	68
25	Wisconsin	66
26	Alabama	65
26	Georgia	65
26	Washington	65
29	Arizona	63
29	Kentucky	63
29	West Virginia	63
32	Maine	62
32	New Mexico	62
34	Texas	61
35	Nebraska	59
35	Utah	59
37	Kansas	56
37	South Carolina	56
39	Indiana	55
40	North Dakota	54
41	Nevada	53
42	Arkansas	51
43	Oklahoma	48
44	Montana	46
44	South Dakota	46
46	Iowa	45
46	Mississippi	45
48	Alaska	37
49	Wyoming	34
50	Idaho	32

District of Columbia — 266

Source: Morgan Quitno Press using data from American Medical Association (Chicago, Illinois)
    "Physician Characteristics and Distribution in the U.S." (1999 Edition)

*As of December 31, 1997. National rate does not include physicians in U.S. territories and possessions. Medical Specialties are Allergy/Immunology, Cardiovascular Diseases, Dermatology, Gastroenterology, Internal Medicine, Pediatrics, Pediatric Cardiology and Pulmonary Diseases.

Nonfederal Physicians in Internal Medicine in 1997

National Total = 122,793 Physicians*

ALPHA ORDER

RANK	STATE	PHYSICIANS	% of USA
23	Alabama	1,533	1.2%
49	Alaska	112	0.1%
24	Arizona	1,431	1.2%
36	Arkansas	585	0.5%
2	California	13,653	11.1%
25	Colorado	1,417	1.2%
14	Connecticut	2,668	2.2%
44	Delaware	267	0.2%
7	Florida	5,748	4.7%
15	Georgia	2,568	2.1%
35	Hawaii	597	0.5%
47	Idaho	187	0.2%
3	Illinois	6,568	5.3%
22	Indiana	1,624	1.3%
34	Iowa	629	0.5%
30	Kansas	808	0.7%
27	Kentucky	1,265	1.0%
21	Louisiana	1,749	1.4%
42	Maine	431	0.4%
11	Maryland	4,030	3.3%
5	Massachusetts	6,108	5.0%
10	Michigan	4,243	3.5%
18	Minnesota	2,027	1.7%
32	Mississippi	638	0.5%
16	Missouri	2,424	2.0%
45	Montana	210	0.2%
39	Nebraska	503	0.4%
40	Nevada	491	0.4%
41	New Hampshire	441	0.4%
8	New Jersey	5,236	4.3%
37	New Mexico	563	0.5%
1	New York	16,587	13.5%
12	North Carolina	2,831	2.3%
46	North Dakota	208	0.2%
9	Ohio	4,655	3.8%
29	Oklahoma	834	0.7%
26	Oregon	1,332	1.1%
4	Pennsylvania	6,497	5.3%
31	Rhode Island	767	0.6%
28	South Carolina	1,042	0.8%
48	South Dakota	184	0.1%
17	Tennessee	2,298	1.9%
6	Texas	5,848	4.8%
38	Utah	558	0.5%
43	Vermont	324	0.3%
13	Virginia	2,685	2.2%
19	Washington	1,982	1.6%
33	West Virginia	636	0.5%
20	Wisconsin	1,901	1.5%
50	Wyoming	84	0.1%

RANK ORDER

RANK	STATE	PHYSICIANS	% of USA
1	New York	16,587	13.5%
2	California	13,653	11.1%
3	Illinois	6,568	5.3%
4	Pennsylvania	6,497	5.3%
5	Massachusetts	6,108	5.0%
6	Texas	5,848	4.8%
7	Florida	5,748	4.7%
8	New Jersey	5,236	4.3%
9	Ohio	4,655	3.8%
10	Michigan	4,243	3.5%
11	Maryland	4,030	3.3%
12	North Carolina	2,831	2.3%
13	Virginia	2,685	2.2%
14	Connecticut	2,668	2.2%
15	Georgia	2,568	2.1%
16	Missouri	2,424	2.0%
17	Tennessee	2,298	1.9%
18	Minnesota	2,027	1.7%
19	Washington	1,982	1.6%
20	Wisconsin	1,901	1.5%
21	Louisiana	1,749	1.4%
22	Indiana	1,624	1.3%
23	Alabama	1,533	1.2%
24	Arizona	1,431	1.2%
25	Colorado	1,417	1.2%
26	Oregon	1,332	1.1%
27	Kentucky	1,265	1.0%
28	South Carolina	1,042	0.8%
29	Oklahoma	834	0.7%
30	Kansas	808	0.7%
31	Rhode Island	767	0.6%
32	Mississippi	638	0.5%
33	West Virginia	636	0.5%
34	Iowa	629	0.5%
35	Hawaii	597	0.5%
36	Arkansas	585	0.5%
37	New Mexico	563	0.5%
38	Utah	558	0.5%
39	Nebraska	503	0.4%
40	Nevada	491	0.4%
41	New Hampshire	441	0.4%
42	Maine	431	0.4%
43	Vermont	324	0.3%
44	Delaware	267	0.2%
45	Montana	210	0.2%
46	North Dakota	208	0.2%
47	Idaho	187	0.2%
48	South Dakota	184	0.1%
49	Alaska	112	0.1%
50	Wyoming	84	0.1%
	District of Columbia	786	0.6%

Source: American Medical Association (Chicago, Illinois)
"Physician Characteristics and Distribution in the U.S." (1999 Edition)
As of December 31, 1997. Total does not include 1,230 physicians in U.S. territories and possessions. Internal Medicine includes Diabetes, Endocrinology, Geriatrics, Hematology, Infectious Diseases, Nephrology, Nutrition, Medical Oncology and Rheumatology.

Rate of Nonfederal Physicians in Internal Medicine in 1997

National Rate = 46 Physicians per 100,000 Population*

RANK	STATE	RATE
26	Alabama	35
48	Alaska	18
34	Arizona	31
45	Arkansas	23
15	California	42
24	Colorado	36
3	Connecticut	82
24	Delaware	36
20	Florida	39
30	Georgia	34
10	Hawaii	50
50	Idaho	15
7	Illinois	55
39	Indiana	28
47	Iowa	22
34	Kansas	31
32	Kentucky	32
18	Louisiana	40
26	Maine	35
4	Maryland	79
1	Massachusetts	100
12	Michigan	43
12	Minnesota	43
45	Mississippi	23
11	Missouri	45
44	Montana	24
36	Nebraska	30
38	Nevada	29
21	New Hampshire	38
6	New Jersey	65
31	New Mexico	33
2	New York	91
21	North Carolina	38
32	North Dakota	32
15	Ohio	42
42	Oklahoma	25
17	Oregon	41
9	Pennsylvania	54
5	Rhode Island	78
39	South Carolina	28
42	South Dakota	25
12	Tennessee	43
36	Texas	30
41	Utah	27
7	Vermont	55
18	Virginia	40
26	Washington	35
26	West Virginia	35
23	Wisconsin	37
49	Wyoming	17

RANK	STATE	RATE
1	Massachusetts	100
2	New York	91
3	Connecticut	82
4	Maryland	79
5	Rhode Island	78
6	New Jersey	65
7	Illinois	55
7	Vermont	55
9	Pennsylvania	54
10	Hawaii	50
11	Missouri	45
12	Michigan	43
12	Minnesota	43
12	Tennessee	43
15	California	42
15	Ohio	42
17	Oregon	41
18	Louisiana	40
18	Virginia	40
20	Florida	39
21	New Hampshire	38
21	North Carolina	38
23	Wisconsin	37
24	Colorado	36
24	Delaware	36
26	Alabama	35
26	Maine	35
26	Washington	35
26	West Virginia	35
30	Georgia	34
31	New Mexico	33
32	Kentucky	32
32	North Dakota	32
34	Arizona	31
34	Kansas	31
36	Nebraska	30
36	Texas	30
38	Nevada	29
39	Indiana	28
39	South Carolina	28
41	Utah	27
42	Oklahoma	25
42	South Dakota	25
44	Montana	24
45	Arkansas	23
45	Mississippi	23
47	Iowa	22
48	Alaska	18
49	Wyoming	17
50	Idaho	15

District of Columbia	148

Source: Morgan Quitno Press using data from American Medical Association (Chicago, Illinois)
    "Physician Characteristics and Distribution in the U.S." (1999 Edition)
*As of December 31, 1997. National rate does not include physicians in U.S. territories and possessions. Internal Medicine includes Diabetes, Endocrinology, Geriatrics, Hematology, Infectious Diseases, Nephrology, Nutrition, Medical Oncology and Rheumatology.

Nonfederal Physicians in Pediatrics in 1997

National Total = 53,609 Physicians*

ALPHA ORDER

RANK	STATE	PHYSICIANS	% of USA
25	Alabama	646	1.2%
47	Alaska	70	0.1%
23	Arizona	723	1.3%
30	Arkansas	371	0.7%
1	California	6,587	12.3%
24	Colorado	696	1.3%
17	Connecticut	956	1.8%
42	Delaware	168	0.3%
4	Florida	2,691	5.0%
14	Georgia	1,265	2.4%
37	Hawaii	279	0.5%
46	Idaho	80	0.1%
5	Illinois	2,495	4.7%
22	Indiana	763	1.4%
35	Iowa	297	0.6%
32	Kansas	333	0.6%
26	Kentucky	625	1.2%
19	Louisiana	860	1.6%
41	Maine	178	0.3%
11	Maryland	1,708	3.2%
9	Massachusetts	2,055	3.8%
10	Michigan	1,710	3.2%
21	Minnesota	770	1.4%
33	Mississippi	323	0.6%
16	Missouri	984	1.8%
45	Montana	81	0.2%
39	Nebraska	236	0.4%
43	Nevada	164	0.3%
40	New Hampshire	206	0.4%
6	New Jersey	2,378	4.4%
36	New Mexico	282	0.5%
2	New York	6,341	11.8%
12	North Carolina	1,379	2.6%
49	North Dakota	65	0.1%
8	Ohio	2,252	4.2%
29	Oklahoma	374	0.7%
28	Oregon	444	0.8%
7	Pennsylvania	2,360	4.4%
34	Rhode Island	302	0.6%
27	South Carolina	555	1.0%
48	South Dakota	67	0.1%
15	Tennessee	1,099	2.1%
3	Texas	3,185	5.9%
31	Utah	360	0.7%
44	Vermont	150	0.3%
13	Virginia	1,329	2.5%
18	Washington	871	1.6%
38	West Virginia	269	0.5%
20	Wisconsin	803	1.5%
50	Wyoming	44	0.1%

RANK ORDER

RANK	STATE	PHYSICIANS	% of USA
1	California	6,587	12.3%
2	New York	6,341	11.8%
3	Texas	3,185	5.9%
4	Florida	2,691	5.0%
5	Illinois	2,495	4.7%
6	New Jersey	2,378	4.4%
7	Pennsylvania	2,360	4.4%
8	Ohio	2,252	4.2%
9	Massachusetts	2,055	3.8%
10	Michigan	1,710	3.2%
11	Maryland	1,708	3.2%
12	North Carolina	1,379	2.6%
13	Virginia	1,329	2.5%
14	Georgia	1,265	2.4%
15	Tennessee	1,099	2.1%
16	Missouri	984	1.8%
17	Connecticut	956	1.8%
18	Washington	871	1.6%
19	Louisiana	860	1.6%
20	Wisconsin	803	1.5%
21	Minnesota	770	1.4%
22	Indiana	763	1.4%
23	Arizona	723	1.3%
24	Colorado	696	1.3%
25	Alabama	646	1.2%
26	Kentucky	625	1.2%
27	South Carolina	555	1.0%
28	Oregon	444	0.8%
29	Oklahoma	374	0.7%
30	Arkansas	371	0.7%
31	Utah	360	0.7%
32	Kansas	333	0.6%
33	Mississippi	323	0.6%
34	Rhode Island	302	0.6%
35	Iowa	297	0.6%
36	New Mexico	282	0.5%
37	Hawaii	279	0.5%
38	West Virginia	269	0.5%
39	Nebraska	236	0.4%
40	New Hampshire	206	0.4%
41	Maine	178	0.3%
42	Delaware	168	0.3%
43	Nevada	164	0.3%
44	Vermont	150	0.3%
45	Montana	81	0.2%
46	Idaho	80	0.1%
47	Alaska	70	0.1%
48	South Dakota	67	0.1%
49	North Dakota	65	0.1%
50	Wyoming	44	0.1%
	District of Columbia	380	0.7%

Source: American Medical Association (Chicago, Illinois)
"Physician Characteristics and Distribution in the U.S." (1999 Edition)
*As of December 31, 1997. Total does not include 961 physicians in U.S. territories and possessions. Pediatrics includes Adolescent Medicine, Neonatal-Perinatal, Pediatric Allergy, Pediatric Endocrinology, Pediatric Pulmonology, Pediatric Hematology-Oncology and Pediatric Nephrology.

Rate of Nonfederal Physicians in Pediatrics in 1997

National Rate = 77 Physicians per 100,000 Population 17 Years and Younger*

RANK	STATE	RATE
27	Alabama	60
45	Alaska	37
32	Arizona	57
34	Arkansas	56
16	California	74
21	Colorado	69
5	Connecticut	121
8	Delaware	95
15	Florida	78
25	Georgia	64
9	Hawaii	92
50	Idaho	23
13	Illinois	79
39	Indiana	51
43	Iowa	41
40	Kansas	48
23	Kentucky	65
18	Louisiana	72
27	Maine	60
3	Maryland	135
1	Massachusetts	142
22	Michigan	68
26	Minnesota	62
41	Mississippi	43
19	Missouri	70
47	Montana	35
37	Nebraska	53
45	Nevada	37
19	New Hampshire	70
6	New Jersey	120
34	New Mexico	56
2	New York	139
16	North Carolina	74
44	North Dakota	39
13	Ohio	79
41	Oklahoma	43
36	Oregon	55
11	Pennsylvania	82
4	Rhode Island	129
31	South Carolina	58
48	South Dakota	34
10	Tennessee	83
32	Texas	57
38	Utah	52
7	Vermont	103
12	Virginia	81
27	Washington	60
23	West Virginia	65
27	Wisconsin	60
49	Wyoming	33

RANK	STATE	RATE
1	Massachusetts	142
2	New York	139
3	Maryland	135
4	Rhode Island	129
5	Connecticut	121
6	New Jersey	120
7	Vermont	103
8	Delaware	95
9	Hawaii	92
10	Tennessee	83
11	Pennsylvania	82
12	Virginia	81
13	Illinois	79
13	Ohio	79
15	Florida	78
16	California	74
16	North Carolina	74
18	Louisiana	72
19	Missouri	70
19	New Hampshire	70
21	Colorado	69
22	Michigan	68
23	Kentucky	65
23	West Virginia	65
25	Georgia	64
26	Minnesota	62
27	Alabama	60
27	Maine	60
27	Washington	60
27	Wisconsin	60
31	South Carolina	58
32	Arizona	57
32	Texas	57
34	Arkansas	56
34	New Mexico	56
36	Oregon	55
37	Nebraska	53
38	Utah	52
39	Indiana	51
40	Kansas	48
41	Mississippi	43
41	Oklahoma	43
43	Iowa	41
44	North Dakota	39
45	Alaska	37
45	Nevada	37
47	Montana	35
48	South Dakota	34
49	Wyoming	33
50	Idaho	23

District of Columbia   354

Source: Morgan Quitno Press using data from American Medical Association (Chicago, Illinois)
     "Physician Characteristics and Distribution in the U.S." (1999 Edition)
*As of December 31, 1997. National rate does not include physicians in U.S. territories and possessions. Pediatrics includes Adolescent Medicine, Neonatal-Perinatal, Pediatric Allergy, Pediatric Endocrinology, Pediatric Pulmonology, Pediatric Hematology-Oncology and Pediatric Nephrology.

Nonfederal Physicians in Surgical Specialties in 1997

National Total = 147,422 Physicians*

ALPHA ORDER

RANK ORDER

RANK	STATE	PHYSICIANS	% of USA
23	Alabama	2,165	1.5%
49	Alaska	221	0.1%
24	Arizona	2,083	1.4%
33	Arkansas	1,065	0.7%
1	California	17,088	11.6%
25	Colorado	2,048	1.4%
21	Connecticut	2,458	1.7%
45	Delaware	385	0.3%
4	Florida	8,173	5.5%
12	Georgia	3,931	2.7%
40	Hawaii	694	0.5%
43	Idaho	487	0.3%
6	Illinois	6,423	4.4%
20	Indiana	2,471	1.7%
31	Iowa	1,154	0.8%
30	Kansas	1,161	0.8%
26	Kentucky	1,918	1.3%
17	Louisiana	2,779	1.9%
42	Maine	580	0.4%
13	Maryland	3,873	2.6%
10	Massachusetts	4,479	3.0%
9	Michigan	4,825	3.3%
22	Minnesota	2,316	1.6%
32	Mississippi	1,150	0.8%
16	Missouri	2,938	2.0%
44	Montana	424	0.3%
36	Nebraska	812	0.6%
39	Nevada	702	0.5%
41	New Hampshire	638	0.4%
8	New Jersey	5,109	3.5%
37	New Mexico	759	0.5%
2	New York	13,941	9.5%
11	North Carolina	4,019	2.7%
48	North Dakota	304	0.2%
7	Ohio	5,971	4.1%
29	Oklahoma	1,296	0.9%
28	Oregon	1,643	1.1%
5	Pennsylvania	7,500	5.1%
38	Rhode Island	706	0.5%
27	South Carolina	1,907	1.3%
47	South Dakota	309	0.2%
15	Tennessee	3,226	2.2%
3	Texas	9,160	6.2%
34	Utah	1,003	0.7%
46	Vermont	343	0.2%
14	Virginia	3,669	2.5%
18	Washington	2,698	1.8%
35	West Virginia	916	0.6%
19	Wisconsin	2,497	1.7%
50	Wyoming	191	0.1%

RANK	STATE	PHYSICIANS	% of USA
1	California	17,088	11.6%
2	New York	13,941	9.5%
3	Texas	9,160	6.2%
4	Florida	8,173	5.5%
5	Pennsylvania	7,500	5.1%
6	Illinois	6,423	4.4%
7	Ohio	5,971	4.1%
8	New Jersey	5,109	3.5%
9	Michigan	4,825	3.3%
10	Massachusetts	4,479	3.0%
11	North Carolina	4,019	2.7%
12	Georgia	3,931	2.7%
13	Maryland	3,873	2.6%
14	Virginia	3,669	2.5%
15	Tennessee	3,226	2.2%
16	Missouri	2,938	2.0%
17	Louisiana	2,779	1.9%
18	Washington	2,698	1.8%
19	Wisconsin	2,497	1.7%
20	Indiana	2,471	1.7%
21	Connecticut	2,458	1.7%
22	Minnesota	2,316	1.6%
23	Alabama	2,165	1.5%
24	Arizona	2,083	1.4%
25	Colorado	2,048	1.4%
26	Kentucky	1,918	1.3%
27	South Carolina	1,907	1.3%
28	Oregon	1,643	1.1%
29	Oklahoma	1,296	0.9%
30	Kansas	1,161	0.8%
31	Iowa	1,154	0.8%
32	Mississippi	1,150	0.8%
33	Arkansas	1,065	0.7%
34	Utah	1,003	0.7%
35	West Virginia	916	0.6%
36	Nebraska	812	0.6%
37	New Mexico	759	0.5%
38	Rhode Island	706	0.5%
39	Nevada	702	0.5%
40	Hawaii	694	0.5%
41	New Hampshire	638	0.4%
42	Maine	580	0.4%
43	Idaho	487	0.3%
44	Montana	424	0.3%
45	Delaware	385	0.3%
46	Vermont	343	0.2%
47	South Dakota	309	0.2%
48	North Dakota	304	0.2%
49	Alaska	221	0.1%
50	Wyoming	191	0.1%
	District of Columbia	814	0.6%

Source: American Medical Association (Chicago, Illinois)
"Physician Characteristics and Distribution in the U.S." (1999 Edition)
*As of December 31, 1997. Total does not include 1,513 physicians in U.S. territories and possessions. Surgical Specialties include Colon and Rectal, General, Neurological, Obstetrics & Gynecology, Ophthalmology, Orthopedic, Otolaryngology, Plastic, Thoracic and Urological Surgeries.

Rate of Nonfederal Physicians in Surgical Specialties in 1997

National Rate = 55 Physicians per 100,000 Population*

ALPHA ORDER

RANK ORDER

RANK	STATE	RATE
24	Alabama	50
50	Alaska	36
38	Arizona	46
41	Arkansas	42
18	California	53
18	Colorado	53
3	Connecticut	75
21	Delaware	52
12	Florida	56
21	Georgia	52
10	Hawaii	58
46	Idaho	40
13	Illinois	54
41	Indiana	42
46	Iowa	40
39	Kansas	45
27	Kentucky	49
6	Louisiana	64
35	Maine	47
2	Maryland	76
4	Massachusetts	73
27	Michigan	49
27	Minnesota	49
41	Mississippi	42
13	Missouri	54
32	Montana	48
27	Nebraska	49
41	Nevada	42
13	New Hampshire	54
7	New Jersey	63
40	New Mexico	44
1	New York	77
13	North Carolina	54
35	North Dakota	47
18	Ohio	53
49	Oklahoma	39
23	Oregon	51
8	Pennsylvania	62
5	Rhode Island	72
24	South Carolina	50
41	South Dakota	42
9	Tennessee	60
35	Texas	47
27	Utah	49
10	Vermont	58
13	Virginia	54
32	Washington	48
24	West Virginia	50
32	Wisconsin	48
46	Wyoming	40

RANK	STATE	RATE
1	New York	77
2	Maryland	76
3	Connecticut	75
4	Massachusetts	73
5	Rhode Island	72
6	Louisiana	64
7	New Jersey	63
8	Pennsylvania	62
9	Tennessee	60
10	Hawaii	58
10	Vermont	58
12	Florida	56
13	Illinois	54
13	Missouri	54
13	New Hampshire	54
13	North Carolina	54
13	Virginia	54
18	California	53
18	Colorado	53
18	Ohio	53
21	Delaware	52
21	Georgia	52
23	Oregon	51
24	Alabama	50
24	South Carolina	50
24	West Virginia	50
27	Kentucky	49
27	Michigan	49
27	Minnesota	49
27	Nebraska	49
27	Utah	49
32	Montana	48
32	Washington	48
32	Wisconsin	48
35	Maine	47
35	North Dakota	47
35	Texas	47
38	Arizona	46
39	Kansas	45
40	New Mexico	44
41	Arkansas	42
41	Indiana	42
41	Mississippi	42
41	Nevada	42
41	South Dakota	42
46	Idaho	40
46	Iowa	40
46	Wyoming	40
49	Oklahoma	39
50	Alaska	36

District of Columbia   154

Source: Morgan Quitno Press using data from American Medical Association (Chicago, Illinois)
   "Physician Characteristics and Distribution in the U.S." (1999 Edition)
*As of December 31, 1997. National rate does not include physicians in U.S. territories and possessions. Surgical
Specialties include Colon and Rectal, General, Neurological, Obstetrics & Gynecology, Ophthalmology,
Orthopedic, Otolaryngology, Plastic, Thoracic and Urological Surgeries.

Nonfederal Physicians in General Surgery in 1997

National Total = 39,241 Physicians*

ALPHA ORDER

RANK	STATE	PHYSICIANS	% of USA
22	Alabama	612	1.6%
49	Alaska	51	0.1%
25	Arizona	512	1.3%
34	Arkansas	286	0.7%
2	California	4,032	10.3%
27	Colorado	505	1.3%
21	Connecticut	627	1.6%
44	Delaware	111	0.3%
5	Florida	1,936	4.9%
11	Georgia	1,033	2.6%
41	Hawaii	171	0.4%
43	Idaho	112	0.3%
6	Illinois	1,731	4.4%
19	Indiana	636	1.6%
30	Iowa	343	0.9%
29	Kansas	345	0.9%
24	Kentucky	584	1.5%
17	Louisiana	751	1.9%
41	Maine	171	0.4%
13	Maryland	1,001	2.6%
10	Massachusetts	1,324	3.4%
8	Michigan	1,392	3.5%
23	Minnesota	590	1.5%
32	Mississippi	310	0.8%
16	Missouri	806	2.1%
45	Montana	104	0.3%
35	Nebraska	242	0.6%
39	Nevada	183	0.5%
40	New Hampshire	180	0.5%
9	New Jersey	1,377	3.5%
38	New Mexico	198	0.5%
1	New York	4,054	10.3%
12	North Carolina	1,016	2.6%
47	North Dakota	92	0.2%
7	Ohio	1,714	4.4%
31	Oklahoma	317	0.8%
28	Oregon	396	1.0%
4	Pennsylvania	2,248	5.7%
37	Rhode Island	201	0.5%
25	South Carolina	512	1.3%
48	South Dakota	89	0.2%
15	Tennessee	908	2.3%
3	Texas	2,338	6.0%
36	Utah	211	0.5%
45	Vermont	104	0.3%
14	Virginia	924	2.4%
20	Washington	630	1.6%
33	West Virginia	297	0.8%
18	Wisconsin	643	1.6%
50	Wyoming	45	0.1%

RANK ORDER

RANK	STATE	PHYSICIANS	% of USA
1	New York	4,054	10.3%
2	California	4,032	10.3%
3	Texas	2,338	6.0%
4	Pennsylvania	2,248	5.7%
5	Florida	1,936	4.9%
6	Illinois	1,731	4.4%
7	Ohio	1,714	4.4%
8	Michigan	1,392	3.5%
9	New Jersey	1,377	3.5%
10	Massachusetts	1,324	3.4%
11	Georgia	1,033	2.6%
12	North Carolina	1,016	2.6%
13	Maryland	1,001	2.6%
14	Virginia	924	2.4%
15	Tennessee	908	2.3%
16	Missouri	806	2.1%
17	Louisiana	751	1.9%
18	Wisconsin	643	1.6%
19	Indiana	636	1.6%
20	Washington	630	1.6%
21	Connecticut	627	1.6%
22	Alabama	612	1.6%
23	Minnesota	590	1.5%
24	Kentucky	584	1.5%
25	Arizona	512	1.3%
25	South Carolina	512	1.3%
27	Colorado	505	1.3%
28	Oregon	396	1.0%
29	Kansas	345	0.9%
30	Iowa	343	0.9%
31	Oklahoma	317	0.8%
32	Mississippi	310	0.8%
33	West Virginia	297	0.8%
34	Arkansas	286	0.7%
35	Nebraska	242	0.6%
36	Utah	211	0.5%
37	Rhode Island	201	0.5%
38	New Mexico	198	0.5%
39	Nevada	183	0.5%
40	New Hampshire	180	0.5%
41	Hawaii	171	0.4%
41	Maine	171	0.4%
43	Idaho	112	0.3%
44	Delaware	111	0.3%
45	Montana	104	0.3%
45	Vermont	104	0.3%
47	North Dakota	92	0.2%
48	South Dakota	89	0.2%
49	Alaska	51	0.1%
50	Wyoming	45	0.1%
	District of Columbia	246	0.6%

Source: American Medical Association (Chicago, Illinois)
   "Physician Characteristics and Distribution in the U.S." (1999 Edition)
*As of December 31, 1997. Total does not include 416 physicians in U.S. territories and possessions. General Surgery includes Abdominal, Cardiovascular, Hand, Head and Neck, Pediatric, Traumatic and Vascular Surgeries.

Rate of Nonfederal Physicians in General Surgery in 1997

National Rate = 14.7 Physicians per 100,000 Population*

ALPHA ORDER

RANK	STATE	RATE
21	Alabama	14.2
50	Alaska	8.4
42	Arizona	11.2
40	Arkansas	11.3
32	California	12.5
30	Colorado	13.0
5	Connecticut	19.2
14	Delaware	15.1
29	Florida	13.2
23	Georgia	13.8
20	Hawaii	14.3
49	Idaho	9.3
18	Illinois	14.4
45	Indiana	10.8
37	Iowa	12.0
28	Kansas	13.3
15	Kentucky	14.9
8	Louisiana	17.2
23	Maine	13.8
4	Maryland	19.6
2	Massachusetts	21.7
21	Michigan	14.2
31	Minnesota	12.6
40	Mississippi	11.3
15	Missouri	14.9
38	Montana	11.8
17	Nebraska	14.6
44	Nevada	10.9
12	New Hampshire	15.4
9	New Jersey	17.1
39	New Mexico	11.5
1	New York	22.3
25	North Carolina	13.7
18	North Dakota	14.4
13	Ohio	15.3
47	Oklahoma	9.5
34	Oregon	12.2
6	Pennsylvania	18.7
3	Rhode Island	20.4
27	South Carolina	13.5
35	South Dakota	12.1
10	Tennessee	16.9
35	Texas	12.1
46	Utah	10.2
7	Vermont	17.7
25	Virginia	13.7
42	Washington	11.2
11	West Virginia	16.4
33	Wisconsin	12.4
48	Wyoming	9.4

RANK ORDER

RANK	STATE	RATE
1	New York	22.3
2	Massachusetts	21.7
3	Rhode Island	20.4
4	Maryland	19.6
5	Connecticut	19.2
6	Pennsylvania	18.7
7	Vermont	17.7
8	Louisiana	17.2
9	New Jersey	17.1
10	Tennessee	16.9
11	West Virginia	16.4
12	New Hampshire	15.4
13	Ohio	15.3
14	Delaware	15.1
15	Kentucky	14.9
15	Missouri	14.9
17	Nebraska	14.6
18	Illinois	14.4
18	North Dakota	14.4
20	Hawaii	14.3
21	Alabama	14.2
21	Michigan	14.2
23	Georgia	13.8
23	Maine	13.8
25	North Carolina	13.7
25	Virginia	13.7
27	South Carolina	13.5
28	Kansas	13.3
29	Florida	13.2
30	Colorado	13.0
31	Minnesota	12.6
32	California	12.5
33	Wisconsin	12.4
34	Oregon	12.2
35	South Dakota	12.1
35	Texas	12.1
37	Iowa	12.0
38	Montana	11.8
39	New Mexico	11.5
40	Arkansas	11.3
40	Mississippi	11.3
42	Arizona	11.2
42	Washington	11.2
44	Nevada	10.9
45	Indiana	10.8
46	Utah	10.2
47	Oklahoma	9.5
48	Wyoming	9.4
49	Idaho	9.3
50	Alaska	8.4

District of Columbia 46.4

Source: Morgan Quitno Press using data from American Medical Association (Chicago, Illinois)
"Physician Characteristics and Distribution in the U.S." (1999 Edition)
*As of December 31, 1997. National rate does not include physicians in U.S. territories and possessions. General Surgery includes Abdominal, Cardiovascular, Hand, Head and Neck, Pediatric, Traumatic and Vascular Surgeries.

Nonfederal Physicians in Obstetrics and Gynecology in 1997

National Total = 38,142 Physicians*

ALPHA ORDER

RANK	STATE	PHYSICIANS	% of USA
23	Alabama	529	1.4%
49	Alaska	52	0.1%
21	Arizona	568	1.5%
33	Arkansas	227	0.6%
1	California	4,499	11.8%
23	Colorado	529	1.4%
18	Connecticut	698	1.8%
44	Delaware	94	0.2%
4	Florida	1,966	5.2%
10	Georgia	1,150	3.0%
34	Hawaii	221	0.6%
43	Idaho	101	0.3%
5	Illinois	1,848	4.8%
20	Indiana	601	1.6%
36	Iowa	211	0.6%
31	Kansas	263	0.7%
27	Kentucky	440	1.2%
17	Louisiana	700	1.8%
42	Maine	132	0.3%
11	Maryland	1,106	2.9%
13	Massachusetts	1,101	2.9%
9	Michigan	1,345	3.5%
26	Minnesota	487	1.3%
30	Mississippi	293	0.8%
16	Missouri	719	1.9%
45	Montana	87	0.2%
40	Nebraska	168	0.4%
37	Nevada	208	0.5%
41	New Hampshire	160	0.4%
8	New Jersey	1,462	3.8%
38	New Mexico	202	0.5%
2	New York	3,676	9.6%
12	North Carolina	1,102	2.9%
48	North Dakota	55	0.1%
7	Ohio	1,521	4.0%
29	Oklahoma	313	0.8%
28	Oregon	402	1.1%
6	Pennsylvania	1,770	4.6%
39	Rhode Island	187	0.5%
25	South Carolina	515	1.4%
47	South Dakota	63	0.2%
15	Tennessee	830	2.2%
3	Texas	2,491	6.5%
32	Utah	253	0.7%
46	Vermont	79	0.2%
14	Virginia	1,022	2.7%
19	Washington	648	1.7%
35	West Virginia	218	0.6%
22	Wisconsin	544	1.4%
50	Wyoming	49	0.1%

RANK ORDER

RANK	STATE	PHYSICIANS	% of USA
1	California	4,499	11.8%
2	New York	3,676	9.6%
3	Texas	2,491	6.5%
4	Florida	1,966	5.2%
5	Illinois	1,848	4.8%
6	Pennsylvania	1,770	4.6%
7	Ohio	1,521	4.0%
8	New Jersey	1,462	3.8%
9	Michigan	1,345	3.5%
10	Georgia	1,150	3.0%
11	Maryland	1,106	2.9%
12	North Carolina	1,102	2.9%
13	Massachusetts	1,101	2.9%
14	Virginia	1,022	2.7%
15	Tennessee	830	2.2%
16	Missouri	719	1.9%
17	Louisiana	700	1.8%
18	Connecticut	698	1.8%
19	Washington	648	1.7%
20	Indiana	601	1.6%
21	Arizona	568	1.5%
22	Wisconsin	544	1.4%
23	Alabama	529	1.4%
23	Colorado	529	1.4%
25	South Carolina	515	1.4%
26	Minnesota	487	1.3%
27	Kentucky	440	1.2%
28	Oregon	402	1.1%
29	Oklahoma	313	0.8%
30	Mississippi	293	0.8%
31	Kansas	263	0.7%
32	Utah	253	0.7%
33	Arkansas	227	0.6%
34	Hawaii	221	0.6%
35	West Virginia	218	0.6%
36	Iowa	211	0.6%
37	Nevada	208	0.5%
38	New Mexico	202	0.5%
39	Rhode Island	187	0.5%
40	Nebraska	168	0.4%
41	New Hampshire	160	0.4%
42	Maine	132	0.3%
43	Idaho	101	0.3%
44	Delaware	94	0.2%
45	Montana	87	0.2%
46	Vermont	79	0.2%
47	South Dakota	63	0.2%
48	North Dakota	55	0.1%
49	Alaska	52	0.1%
50	Wyoming	49	0.1%
	District of Columbia	237	0.6%

Source: American Medical Association (Chicago, Illinois)
"Physician Characteristics and Distribution in the U.S." (1999 Edition)
*As of December 31, 1997. Total does not include 536 physicians in U.S. territories and possessions. Obstetrics and Gynecology includes Gynecology and Oncology, Maternal and Fetal Medicine and Reproductive Endocrinology.

Rate of Nonfederal Physicians in Obstetrics and Gynecology in 1997

National Rate = 28 Physicians per 100,000 Female Population*

ALPHA ORDER

RANK ORDER

RANK	STATE	RATE		RANK	STATE	RATE
29	Alabama	24		1	Connecticut	42
44	Alaska	18		1	Maryland	42
24	Arizona	25		3	New York	39
46	Arkansas	17		4	Hawaii	37
14	California	28		4	Rhode Island	37
16	Colorado	27		6	Massachusetts	35
1	Connecticut	42		6	New Jersey	35
24	Delaware	25		8	Louisiana	31
20	Florida	26		9	Georgia	30
9	Georgia	30		9	Illinois	30
4	Hawaii	37		9	Tennessee	30
46	Idaho	17		9	Virginia	30
9	Illinois	30		13	North Carolina	29
40	Indiana	20		14	California	28
50	Iowa	14		14	Pennsylvania	28
40	Kansas	20		16	Colorado	27
34	Kentucky	22		16	Michigan	27
8	Louisiana	31		16	New Hampshire	27
35	Maine	21		16	South Carolina	27
1	Maryland	42		20	Florida	26
6	Massachusetts	35		20	Missouri	26
16	Michigan	27		20	Ohio	26
35	Minnesota	21		20	Vermont	26
35	Mississippi	21		24	Arizona	25
20	Missouri	26		24	Delaware	25
40	Montana	20		24	Nevada	25
40	Nebraska	20		24	Oregon	25
24	Nevada	25		24	Texas	25
16	New Hampshire	27		29	Alabama	24
6	New Jersey	35		29	Utah	24
31	New Mexico	23		31	New Mexico	23
3	New York	39		31	Washington	23
13	North Carolina	29		31	West Virginia	23
46	North Dakota	17		34	Kentucky	22
20	Ohio	26		35	Maine	21
44	Oklahoma	18		35	Minnesota	21
24	Oregon	25		35	Mississippi	21
14	Pennsylvania	28		35	Wisconsin	21
4	Rhode Island	37		35	Wyoming	21
16	South Carolina	27		40	Indiana	20
46	South Dakota	17		40	Kansas	20
9	Tennessee	30		40	Montana	20
24	Texas	25		40	Nebraska	20
29	Utah	24		44	Alaska	18
20	Vermont	26		44	Oklahoma	18
9	Virginia	30		46	Arkansas	17
31	Washington	23		46	Idaho	17
31	West Virginia	23		46	North Dakota	17
35	Wisconsin	21		46	South Dakota	17
35	Wyoming	21		50	Iowa	14
					District of Columbia	84

Source: Morgan Quitno Press using data from American Medical Association (Chicago, Illinois)
      "Physician Characteristics and Distribution in the U.S." (1999 Edition)
*As of December 31, 1997. National rate does not include physicians in U.S. territories and possessions. Obstetrics and Gynecology includes Gynecology and Oncology, Maternal and Fetal Medicine and Reproductive Endocrinology.

Nonfederal Physicians in Ophthalmology in 1997

National Total = 17,354 Physicians*

ALPHA ORDER

RANK	STATE	PHYSICIANS	% of USA
26	Alabama	205	1.2%
49	Alaska	27	0.2%
23	Arizona	257	1.5%
32	Arkansas	139	0.8%
1	California	2,102	12.1%
24	Colorado	248	1.4%
20	Connecticut	298	1.7%
45	Delaware	43	0.2%
3	Florida	1,087	6.3%
14	Georgia	385	2.2%
37	Hawaii	86	0.5%
43	Idaho	61	0.4%
6	Illinois	712	4.1%
22	Indiana	282	1.6%
29	Iowa	162	0.9%
30	Kansas	154	0.9%
28	Kentucky	197	1.1%
15	Louisiana	340	2.0%
40	Maine	68	0.4%
11	Maryland	492	2.8%
10	Massachusetts	540	3.1%
9	Michigan	554	3.2%
21	Minnesota	297	1.7%
33	Mississippi	133	0.8%
15	Missouri	340	2.0%
44	Montana	50	0.3%
36	Nebraska	92	0.5%
39	Nevada	73	0.4%
42	New Hampshire	66	0.4%
8	New Jersey	619	3.6%
38	New Mexico	77	0.4%
2	New York	1,770	10.2%
12	North Carolina	407	2.3%
47	North Dakota	38	0.2%
7	Ohio	642	3.7%
31	Oklahoma	147	0.8%
27	Oregon	199	1.1%
5	Pennsylvania	898	5.2%
41	Rhode Island	67	0.4%
25	South Carolina	223	1.3%
48	South Dakota	34	0.2%
18	Tennessee	333	1.9%
4	Texas	1,001	5.8%
34	Utah	115	0.7%
46	Vermont	42	0.2%
13	Virginia	404	2.3%
19	Washington	303	1.7%
35	West Virginia	99	0.6%
15	Wisconsin	340	2.0%
50	Wyoming	17	0.1%

RANK ORDER

RANK	STATE	PHYSICIANS	% of USA
1	California	2,102	12.1%
2	New York	1,770	10.2%
3	Florida	1,087	6.3%
4	Texas	1,001	5.8%
5	Pennsylvania	898	5.2%
6	Illinois	712	4.1%
7	Ohio	642	3.7%
8	New Jersey	619	3.6%
9	Michigan	554	3.2%
10	Massachusetts	540	3.1%
11	Maryland	492	2.8%
12	North Carolina	407	2.3%
13	Virginia	404	2.3%
14	Georgia	385	2.2%
15	Louisiana	340	2.0%
15	Missouri	340	2.0%
15	Wisconsin	340	2.0%
18	Tennessee	333	1.9%
19	Washington	303	1.7%
20	Connecticut	298	1.7%
21	Minnesota	297	1.7%
22	Indiana	282	1.6%
23	Arizona	257	1.5%
24	Colorado	248	1.4%
25	South Carolina	223	1.3%
26	Alabama	205	1.2%
27	Oregon	199	1.1%
28	Kentucky	197	1.1%
29	Iowa	162	0.9%
30	Kansas	154	0.9%
31	Oklahoma	147	0.8%
32	Arkansas	139	0.8%
33	Mississippi	133	0.8%
34	Utah	115	0.7%
35	West Virginia	99	0.6%
36	Nebraska	92	0.5%
37	Hawaii	86	0.5%
38	New Mexico	77	0.4%
39	Nevada	73	0.4%
40	Maine	68	0.4%
41	Rhode Island	67	0.4%
42	New Hampshire	66	0.4%
43	Idaho	61	0.4%
44	Montana	50	0.3%
45	Delaware	43	0.2%
46	Vermont	42	0.2%
47	North Dakota	38	0.2%
48	South Dakota	34	0.2%
49	Alaska	27	0.2%
50	Wyoming	17	0.1%
	District of Columbia	89	0.5%

Source: American Medical Association (Chicago, Illinois)
    "Physician Characteristics and Distribution in the U.S." (1999 Edition)
*As of December 31, 1997. Total does not include 181 physicians in U.S. territories and possessions.
Ophthalmology is the branch of medicine dealing with the anatomy, functions and diseases of the eye.

Rate of Nonfederal Physicians in Ophthalmology in 1997

National Rate = 6.5 Physicians per 100,000 Population*

ALPHA ORDER

RANK	STATE	RATE
44	Alabama	4.7
47	Alaska	4.4
29	Arizona	5.6
33	Arkansas	5.5
12	California	6.5
14	Colorado	6.4
3	Connecticut	9.1
24	Delaware	5.8
8	Florida	7.4
39	Georgia	5.1
9	Hawaii	7.2
40	Idaho	5.0
20	Illinois	5.9
43	Indiana	4.8
25	Iowa	5.7
20	Kansas	5.9
40	Kentucky	5.0
5	Louisiana	7.8
33	Maine	5.5
2	Maryland	9.7
4	Massachusetts	8.8
25	Michigan	5.7
15	Minnesota	6.3
42	Mississippi	4.9
15	Missouri	6.3
25	Montana	5.7
29	Nebraska	5.6
49	Nevada	4.3
29	New Hampshire	5.6
6	New Jersey	7.7
46	New Mexico	4.5
1	New York	9.8
33	North Carolina	5.5
20	North Dakota	5.9
25	Ohio	5.7
47	Oklahoma	4.4
18	Oregon	6.1
7	Pennsylvania	7.5
11	Rhode Island	6.8
20	South Carolina	5.9
45	South Dakota	4.6
17	Tennessee	6.2
38	Texas	5.2
29	Utah	5.6
10	Vermont	7.1
19	Virginia	6.0
37	Washington	5.4
33	West Virginia	5.5
12	Wisconsin	6.5
50	Wyoming	3.5

RANK ORDER

RANK	STATE	RATE
1	New York	9.8
2	Maryland	9.7
3	Connecticut	9.1
4	Massachusetts	8.8
5	Louisiana	7.8
6	New Jersey	7.7
7	Pennsylvania	7.5
8	Florida	7.4
9	Hawaii	7.2
10	Vermont	7.1
11	Rhode Island	6.8
12	California	6.5
12	Wisconsin	6.5
14	Colorado	6.4
15	Minnesota	6.3
15	Missouri	6.3
17	Tennessee	6.2
18	Oregon	6.1
19	Virginia	6.0
20	Illinois	5.9
20	Kansas	5.9
20	North Dakota	5.9
20	South Carolina	5.9
24	Delaware	5.8
25	Iowa	5.7
25	Michigan	5.7
25	Montana	5.7
25	Ohio	5.7
29	Arizona	5.6
29	Nebraska	5.6
29	New Hampshire	5.6
29	Utah	5.6
33	Arkansas	5.5
33	Maine	5.5
33	North Carolina	5.5
33	West Virginia	5.5
37	Washington	5.4
38	Texas	5.2
39	Georgia	5.1
40	Idaho	5.0
40	Kentucky	5.0
42	Mississippi	4.9
43	Indiana	4.8
44	Alabama	4.7
45	South Dakota	4.6
46	New Mexico	4.5
47	Alaska	4.4
47	Oklahoma	4.4
49	Nevada	4.3
50	Wyoming	3.5

District of Columbia   16.8

Source: Morgan Quitno Press using data from American Medical Association (Chicago, Illinois)
    "Physician Characteristics and Distribution in the U.S." (1999 Edition)
*As of December 31, 1997. National rate does not include physicians in U.S. territories and possessions.
Ophthalmology is the branch of medicine dealing with the anatomy, functions and diseases of the eye.

Nonfederal Physicians in Orthopedic Surgery in 1997

National Total = 22,281 Physicians*

ALPHA ORDER

RANK	STATE	PHYSICIANS	% of USA
25	Alabama	328	1.5%
49	Alaska	47	0.2%
24	Arizona	332	1.5%
33	Arkansas	178	0.8%
1	California	2,809	12.6%
23	Colorado	367	1.6%
22	Connecticut	368	1.7%
46	Delaware	55	0.2%
4	Florida	1,255	5.6%
12	Georgia	573	2.6%
43	Hawaii	94	0.4%
41	Idaho	105	0.5%
7	Illinois	895	4.0%
20	Indiana	413	1.9%
31	Iowa	184	0.8%
32	Kansas	179	0.8%
27	Kentucky	283	1.3%
21	Louisiana	397	1.8%
40	Maine	109	0.5%
14	Maryland	521	2.3%
9	Massachusetts	675	3.0%
10	Michigan	635	2.8%
18	Minnesota	436	2.0%
34	Mississippi	159	0.7%
19	Missouri	430	1.9%
44	Montana	87	0.4%
36	Nebraska	136	0.6%
42	Nevada	97	0.4%
37	New Hampshire	116	0.5%
8	New Jersey	715	3.2%
35	New Mexico	147	0.7%
2	New York	1,769	7.9%
11	North Carolina	616	2.8%
48	North Dakota	48	0.2%
6	Ohio	905	4.1%
29	Oklahoma	213	1.0%
28	Oregon	282	1.3%
5	Pennsylvania	1,081	4.9%
37	Rhode Island	116	0.5%
26	South Carolina	295	1.3%
46	South Dakota	55	0.2%
16	Tennessee	466	2.1%
3	Texas	1,344	6.0%
30	Utah	185	0.8%
45	Vermont	61	0.3%
13	Virginia	540	2.4%
15	Washington	498	2.2%
37	West Virginia	116	0.5%
17	Wisconsin	442	2.0%
50	Wyoming	45	0.2%

RANK ORDER

RANK	STATE	PHYSICIANS	% of USA
1	California	2,809	12.6%
2	New York	1,769	7.9%
3	Texas	1,344	6.0%
4	Florida	1,255	5.6%
5	Pennsylvania	1,081	4.9%
6	Ohio	905	4.1%
7	Illinois	895	4.0%
8	New Jersey	715	3.2%
9	Massachusetts	675	3.0%
10	Michigan	635	2.8%
11	North Carolina	616	2.8%
12	Georgia	573	2.6%
13	Virginia	540	2.4%
14	Maryland	521	2.3%
15	Washington	498	2.2%
16	Tennessee	466	2.1%
17	Wisconsin	442	2.0%
18	Minnesota	436	2.0%
19	Missouri	430	1.9%
20	Indiana	413	1.9%
21	Louisiana	397	1.8%
22	Connecticut	368	1.7%
23	Colorado	367	1.6%
24	Arizona	332	1.5%
25	Alabama	328	1.5%
26	South Carolina	295	1.3%
27	Kentucky	283	1.3%
28	Oregon	282	1.3%
29	Oklahoma	213	1.0%
30	Utah	185	0.8%
31	Iowa	184	0.8%
32	Kansas	179	0.8%
33	Arkansas	178	0.8%
34	Mississippi	159	0.7%
35	New Mexico	147	0.7%
36	Nebraska	136	0.6%
37	New Hampshire	116	0.5%
37	Rhode Island	116	0.5%
37	West Virginia	116	0.5%
40	Maine	109	0.5%
41	Idaho	105	0.5%
42	Nevada	97	0.4%
43	Hawaii	94	0.4%
44	Montana	87	0.4%
45	Vermont	61	0.3%
46	Delaware	55	0.2%
46	South Dakota	55	0.2%
48	North Dakota	48	0.2%
49	Alaska	47	0.2%
50	Wyoming	45	0.2%
	District of Columbia	79	0.4%

Source: American Medical Association (Chicago, Illinois)
"Physician Characteristics and Distribution in the U.S." (1999 Edition)
*As of December 31, 1997. Total does not include 115 physicians in U.S. territories and possessions.
Orthopedics is the branch of medicine dealing with the skeletal system.

Rate of Nonfederal Physicians in Orthopedic Surgery in 1997

National Rate = 8.3 Physicians per 100,000 Population*

ALPHA ORDER

RANK	STATE	RATE
34	Alabama	7.6
32	Alaska	7.7
39	Arizona	7.3
41	Arkansas	7.1
18	California	8.7
9	Colorado	9.4
2	Connecticut	11.3
35	Delaware	7.5
22	Florida	8.6
32	Georgia	7.7
30	Hawaii	7.9
18	Idaho	8.7
35	Illinois	7.5
42	Indiana	7.0
46	Iowa	6.4
43	Kansas	6.9
40	Kentucky	7.2
12	Louisiana	9.1
17	Maine	8.8
5	Maryland	10.2
3	Massachusetts	11.0
45	Michigan	6.5
11	Minnesota	9.3
49	Mississippi	5.8
28	Missouri	8.0
6	Montana	9.9
26	Nebraska	8.2
49	Nevada	5.8
6	New Hampshire	9.9
15	New Jersey	8.9
23	New Mexico	8.5
8	New York	9.7
25	North Carolina	8.3
35	North Dakota	7.5
27	Ohio	8.1
46	Oklahoma	6.4
18	Oregon	8.7
13	Pennsylvania	9.0
1	Rhode Island	11.7
31	South Carolina	7.8
35	South Dakota	7.5
18	Tennessee	8.7
43	Texas	6.9
13	Utah	9.0
4	Vermont	10.4
28	Virginia	8.0
15	Washington	8.9
46	West Virginia	6.4
23	Wisconsin	8.5
9	Wyoming	9.4

RANK ORDER

RANK	STATE	RATE
1	Rhode Island	11.7
2	Connecticut	11.3
3	Massachusetts	11.0
4	Vermont	10.4
5	Maryland	10.2
6	Montana	9.9
6	New Hampshire	9.9
8	New York	9.7
9	Colorado	9.4
9	Wyoming	9.4
11	Minnesota	9.3
12	Louisiana	9.1
13	Pennsylvania	9.0
13	Utah	9.0
15	New Jersey	8.9
15	Washington	8.9
17	Maine	8.8
18	California	8.7
18	Idaho	8.7
18	Oregon	8.7
18	Tennessee	8.7
22	Florida	8.6
23	New Mexico	8.5
23	Wisconsin	8.5
25	North Carolina	8.3
26	Nebraska	8.2
27	Ohio	8.1
28	Missouri	8.0
28	Virginia	8.0
30	Hawaii	7.9
31	South Carolina	7.8
32	Alaska	7.7
32	Georgia	7.7
34	Alabama	7.6
35	Delaware	7.5
35	Illinois	7.5
35	North Dakota	7.5
35	South Dakota	7.5
39	Arizona	7.3
40	Kentucky	7.2
41	Arkansas	7.1
42	Indiana	7.0
43	Kansas	6.9
43	Texas	6.9
45	Michigan	6.5
46	Iowa	6.4
46	Oklahoma	6.4
46	West Virginia	6.4
49	Mississippi	5.8
49	Nevada	5.8

	District of Columbia	14.9

Source: Morgan Quitno Press using data from American Medical Association (Chicago, Illinois)
   "Physician Characteristics and Distribution in the U.S." (1999 Edition)
As of December 31, 1997. National rate does not include physicians in U.S. territories and possessions.
Orthopedics is the branch of medicine dealing with the skeletal system.

Nonfederal Physicians in Plastic Surgery in 1997

National Total = 5,892 Physicians*

ALPHA ORDER

RANK	STATE	PHYSICIANS	% of USA
21	Alabama	81	1.4%
47	Alaska	8	0.1%
17	Arizona	118	2.0%
33	Arkansas	32	0.5%
1	California	903	15.3%
19	Colorado	89	1.5%
21	Connecticut	81	1.4%
44	Delaware	17	0.3%
3	Florida	440	7.5%
14	Georgia	136	2.3%
34	Hawaii	31	0.5%
42	Idaho	20	0.3%
6	Illinois	209	3.5%
23	Indiana	80	1.4%
37	Iowa	25	0.4%
30	Kansas	47	0.8%
25	Kentucky	79	1.3%
20	Louisiana	88	1.5%
45	Maine	14	0.2%
11	Maryland	145	2.5%
10	Massachusetts	162	2.7%
9	Michigan	175	3.0%
23	Minnesota	80	1.4%
34	Mississippi	31	0.5%
15	Missouri	135	2.3%
43	Montana	18	0.3%
36	Nebraska	28	0.5%
32	Nevada	36	0.6%
39	New Hampshire	23	0.4%
8	New Jersey	181	3.1%
38	New Mexico	24	0.4%
2	New York	561	9.5%
12	North Carolina	142	2.4%
46	North Dakota	10	0.2%
7	Ohio	203	3.4%
31	Oklahoma	46	0.8%
28	Oregon	58	1.0%
5	Pennsylvania	245	4.2%
39	Rhode Island	23	0.4%
29	South Carolina	57	1.0%
49	South Dakota	6	0.1%
16	Tennessee	133	2.3%
4	Texas	419	7.1%
27	Utah	64	1.1%
48	Vermont	7	0.1%
12	Virginia	142	2.4%
18	Washington	109	1.8%
39	West Virginia	23	0.4%
26	Wisconsin	78	1.3%
50	Wyoming	3	0.1%

RANK ORDER

RANK	STATE	PHYSICIANS	% of USA
1	California	903	15.3%
2	New York	561	9.5%
3	Florida	440	7.5%
4	Texas	419	7.1%
5	Pennsylvania	245	4.2%
6	Illinois	209	3.5%
7	Ohio	203	3.4%
8	New Jersey	181	3.1%
9	Michigan	175	3.0%
10	Massachusetts	162	2.7%
11	Maryland	145	2.5%
12	North Carolina	142	2.4%
12	Virginia	142	2.4%
14	Georgia	136	2.3%
15	Missouri	135	2.3%
16	Tennessee	133	2.3%
17	Arizona	118	2.0%
18	Washington	109	1.8%
19	Colorado	89	1.5%
20	Louisiana	88	1.5%
21	Alabama	81	1.4%
21	Connecticut	81	1.4%
23	Indiana	80	1.4%
23	Minnesota	80	1.4%
25	Kentucky	79	1.3%
26	Wisconsin	78	1.3%
27	Utah	64	1.1%
28	Oregon	58	1.0%
29	South Carolina	57	1.0%
30	Kansas	47	0.8%
31	Oklahoma	46	0.8%
32	Nevada	36	0.6%
33	Arkansas	32	0.5%
34	Hawaii	31	0.5%
34	Mississippi	31	0.5%
36	Nebraska	28	0.5%
37	Iowa	25	0.4%
38	New Mexico	24	0.4%
39	New Hampshire	23	0.4%
39	Rhode Island	23	0.4%
39	West Virginia	23	0.4%
42	Idaho	20	0.3%
43	Montana	18	0.3%
44	Delaware	17	0.3%
45	Maine	14	0.2%
46	North Dakota	10	0.2%
47	Alaska	8	0.1%
48	Vermont	7	0.1%
49	South Dakota	6	0.1%
50	Wyoming	3	0.1%
	District of Columbia	27	0.5%

Source: American Medical Association (Chicago, Illinois)
"Physician Characteristics and Distribution in the U.S." (1999 Edition)
*As of December 31, 1997. Total does not include 31 physicians in U.S. territories and possessions.

Rate of Nonfederal Physicians in Plastic Surgery in 1997

National Rate = 2.2 Physicians per 100,000 Population*

ALPHA ORDER				RANK ORDER		
RANK	STATE	RATE		RANK	STATE	RATE
24	Alabama	1.9		1	New York	3.1
42	Alaska	1.3		1	Utah	3.1
6	Arizona	2.6		3	Florida	3.0
42	Arkansas	1.3		4	California	2.8
4	California	2.8		4	Maryland	2.8
12	Colorado	2.3		6	Arizona	2.6
9	Connecticut	2.5		6	Hawaii	2.6
12	Delaware	2.3		6	Massachusetts	2.6
3	Florida	3.0		9	Connecticut	2.5
27	Georgia	1.8		9	Missouri	2.5
6	Hawaii	2.6		9	Tennessee	2.5
32	Idaho	1.7		12	Colorado	2.3
32	Illinois	1.7		12	Delaware	2.3
39	Indiana	1.4		12	Rhode Island	2.3
48	Iowa	0.9		15	New Jersey	2.2
27	Kansas	1.8		15	Texas	2.2
19	Kentucky	2.0		17	Nevada	2.1
19	Louisiana	2.0		17	Virginia	2.1
46	Maine	1.1		19	Kentucky	2.0
4	Maryland	2.8		19	Louisiana	2.0
6	Massachusetts	2.6		19	Montana	2.0
27	Michigan	1.8		19	New Hampshire	2.0
32	Minnesota	1.7		19	Pennsylvania	2.0
46	Mississippi	1.1		24	Alabama	1.9
9	Missouri	2.5		24	North Carolina	1.9
19	Montana	2.0		24	Washington	1.9
32	Nebraska	1.7		27	Georgia	1.8
17	Nevada	2.1		27	Kansas	1.8
19	New Hampshire	2.0		27	Michigan	1.8
15	New Jersey	2.2		27	Ohio	1.8
39	New Mexico	1.4		27	Oregon	1.8
1	New York	3.1		32	Idaho	1.7
24	North Carolina	1.9		32	Illinois	1.7
36	North Dakota	1.6		32	Minnesota	1.7
27	Ohio	1.8		32	Nebraska	1.7
39	Oklahoma	1.4		36	North Dakota	1.6
27	Oregon	1.8		37	South Carolina	1.5
19	Pennsylvania	2.0		37	Wisconsin	1.5
12	Rhode Island	2.3		39	Indiana	1.4
37	South Carolina	1.5		39	New Mexico	1.4
49	South Dakota	0.8		39	Oklahoma	1.4
9	Tennessee	2.5		42	Alaska	1.3
15	Texas	2.2		42	Arkansas	1.3
1	Utah	3.1		42	West Virginia	1.3
45	Vermont	1.2		45	Vermont	1.2
17	Virginia	2.1		46	Maine	1.1
24	Washington	1.9		46	Mississippi	1.1
42	West Virginia	1.3		48	Iowa	0.9
37	Wisconsin	1.5		49	South Dakota	0.8
50	Wyoming	0.6		50	Wyoming	0.6
					District of Columbia	5.1

Source: Morgan Quitno Press using data from American Medical Association (Chicago, Illinois)
"Physician Characteristics and Distribution in the U.S." (1999 Edition)
*As of December 31, 1997. National rate does not include physicians in U.S. territories and possessions.

462

Nonfederal Physicians in Other Specialties in 1997

National Total = 187,070 Physicians*

<table>
<thead>
<tr><th colspan="4">ALPHA ORDER</th><th colspan="4">RANK ORDER</th></tr>
<tr><th>RANK</th><th>STATE</th><th>PHYSICIANS</th><th>% of USA</th><th>RANK</th><th>STATE</th><th>PHYSICIANS</th><th>% of USA</th></tr>
</thead>
<tbody>
<tr><td>28</td><td>Alabama</td><td>2,069</td><td>1.1%</td><td>1</td><td>California</td><td>22,920</td><td>12.3%</td></tr>
<tr><td>49</td><td>Alaska</td><td>284</td><td>0.2%</td><td>2</td><td>New York</td><td>19,608</td><td>10.5%</td></tr>
<tr><td>24</td><td>Arizona</td><td>2,663</td><td>1.4%</td><td>3</td><td>Texas</td><td>10,894</td><td>5.8%</td></tr>
<tr><td>32</td><td>Arkansas</td><td>1,215</td><td>0.6%</td><td>4</td><td>Pennsylvania</td><td>10,176</td><td>5.4%</td></tr>
<tr><td>1</td><td>California</td><td>22,920</td><td>12.3%</td><td>5</td><td>Florida</td><td>9,068</td><td>4.8%</td></tr>
<tr><td>23</td><td>Colorado</td><td>2,680</td><td>1.4%</td><td>6</td><td>Illinois</td><td>8,524</td><td>4.6%</td></tr>
<tr><td>18</td><td>Connecticut</td><td>3,362</td><td>1.8%</td><td>7</td><td>Massachusetts</td><td>7,917</td><td>4.2%</td></tr>
<tr><td>44</td><td>Delaware</td><td>514</td><td>0.3%</td><td>8</td><td>Ohio</td><td>7,149</td><td>3.8%</td></tr>
<tr><td>5</td><td>Florida</td><td>9,068</td><td>4.8%</td><td>9</td><td>Michigan</td><td>6,116</td><td>3.3%</td></tr>
<tr><td>14</td><td>Georgia</td><td>4,324</td><td>2.3%</td><td>10</td><td>New Jersey</td><td>6,078</td><td>3.2%</td></tr>
<tr><td>38</td><td>Hawaii</td><td>887</td><td>0.5%</td><td>11</td><td>Maryland</td><td>5,724</td><td>3.1%</td></tr>
<tr><td>46</td><td>Idaho</td><td>446</td><td>0.2%</td><td>12</td><td>North Carolina</td><td>4,636</td><td>2.5%</td></tr>
<tr><td>6</td><td>Illinois</td><td>8,524</td><td>4.6%</td><td>13</td><td>Virginia</td><td>4,374</td><td>2.3%</td></tr>
<tr><td>20</td><td>Indiana</td><td>3,167</td><td>1.7%</td><td>14</td><td>Georgia</td><td>4,324</td><td>2.3%</td></tr>
<tr><td>31</td><td>Iowa</td><td>1,289</td><td>0.7%</td><td>15</td><td>Washington</td><td>3,821</td><td>2.0%</td></tr>
<tr><td>30</td><td>Kansas</td><td>1,522</td><td>0.8%</td><td>16</td><td>Tennessee</td><td>3,519</td><td>1.9%</td></tr>
<tr><td>25</td><td>Kentucky</td><td>2,228</td><td>1.2%</td><td>17</td><td>Wisconsin</td><td>3,363</td><td>1.8%</td></tr>
<tr><td>22</td><td>Louisiana</td><td>2,822</td><td>1.5%</td><td>18</td><td>Connecticut</td><td>3,362</td><td>1.8%</td></tr>
<tr><td>42</td><td>Maine</td><td>754</td><td>0.4%</td><td>19</td><td>Missouri</td><td>3,328</td><td>1.8%</td></tr>
<tr><td>11</td><td>Maryland</td><td>5,724</td><td>3.1%</td><td>20</td><td>Indiana</td><td>3,167</td><td>1.7%</td></tr>
<tr><td>7</td><td>Massachusetts</td><td>7,917</td><td>4.2%</td><td>21</td><td>Minnesota</td><td>3,073</td><td>1.6%</td></tr>
<tr><td>9</td><td>Michigan</td><td>6,116</td><td>3.3%</td><td>22</td><td>Louisiana</td><td>2,822</td><td>1.5%</td></tr>
<tr><td>21</td><td>Minnesota</td><td>3,073</td><td>1.6%</td><td>23</td><td>Colorado</td><td>2,680</td><td>1.4%</td></tr>
<tr><td>35</td><td>Mississippi</td><td>1,075</td><td>0.6%</td><td>24</td><td>Arizona</td><td>2,663</td><td>1.4%</td></tr>
<tr><td>19</td><td>Missouri</td><td>3,328</td><td>1.8%</td><td>25</td><td>Kentucky</td><td>2,228</td><td>1.2%</td></tr>
<tr><td>45</td><td>Montana</td><td>457</td><td>0.2%</td><td>26</td><td>South Carolina</td><td>2,119</td><td>1.1%</td></tr>
<tr><td>37</td><td>Nebraska</td><td>902</td><td>0.5%</td><td>27</td><td>Oregon</td><td>2,092</td><td>1.1%</td></tr>
<tr><td>41</td><td>Nevada</td><td>803</td><td>0.4%</td><td>28</td><td>Alabama</td><td>2,069</td><td>1.1%</td></tr>
<tr><td>40</td><td>New Hampshire</td><td>823</td><td>0.4%</td><td>29</td><td>Oklahoma</td><td>1,529</td><td>0.8%</td></tr>
<tr><td>10</td><td>New Jersey</td><td>6,078</td><td>3.2%</td><td>30</td><td>Kansas</td><td>1,522</td><td>0.8%</td></tr>
<tr><td>34</td><td>New Mexico</td><td>1,077</td><td>0.6%</td><td>31</td><td>Iowa</td><td>1,289</td><td>0.7%</td></tr>
<tr><td>2</td><td>New York</td><td>19,608</td><td>10.5%</td><td>32</td><td>Arkansas</td><td>1,215</td><td>0.6%</td></tr>
<tr><td>12</td><td>North Carolina</td><td>4,636</td><td>2.5%</td><td>33</td><td>Utah</td><td>1,176</td><td>0.6%</td></tr>
<tr><td>47</td><td>North Dakota</td><td>374</td><td>0.2%</td><td>34</td><td>New Mexico</td><td>1,077</td><td>0.6%</td></tr>
<tr><td>8</td><td>Ohio</td><td>7,149</td><td>3.8%</td><td>35</td><td>Mississippi</td><td>1,075</td><td>0.6%</td></tr>
<tr><td>29</td><td>Oklahoma</td><td>1,529</td><td>0.8%</td><td>36</td><td>West Virginia</td><td>1,003</td><td>0.5%</td></tr>
<tr><td>27</td><td>Oregon</td><td>2,092</td><td>1.1%</td><td>37</td><td>Nebraska</td><td>902</td><td>0.5%</td></tr>
<tr><td>4</td><td>Pennsylvania</td><td>10,176</td><td>5.4%</td><td>38</td><td>Hawaii</td><td>887</td><td>0.5%</td></tr>
<tr><td>39</td><td>Rhode Island</td><td>881</td><td>0.5%</td><td>39</td><td>Rhode Island</td><td>881</td><td>0.5%</td></tr>
<tr><td>26</td><td>South Carolina</td><td>2,119</td><td>1.1%</td><td>40</td><td>New Hampshire</td><td>823</td><td>0.4%</td></tr>
<tr><td>48</td><td>South Dakota</td><td>296</td><td>0.2%</td><td>41</td><td>Nevada</td><td>803</td><td>0.4%</td></tr>
<tr><td>16</td><td>Tennessee</td><td>3,519</td><td>1.9%</td><td>42</td><td>Maine</td><td>754</td><td>0.4%</td></tr>
<tr><td>3</td><td>Texas</td><td>10,894</td><td>5.8%</td><td>43</td><td>Vermont</td><td>527</td><td>0.3%</td></tr>
<tr><td>33</td><td>Utah</td><td>1,176</td><td>0.6%</td><td>44</td><td>Delaware</td><td>514</td><td>0.3%</td></tr>
<tr><td>43</td><td>Vermont</td><td>527</td><td>0.3%</td><td>45</td><td>Montana</td><td>457</td><td>0.2%</td></tr>
<tr><td>13</td><td>Virginia</td><td>4,374</td><td>2.3%</td><td>46</td><td>Idaho</td><td>446</td><td>0.2%</td></tr>
<tr><td>15</td><td>Washington</td><td>3,821</td><td>2.0%</td><td>47</td><td>North Dakota</td><td>374</td><td>0.2%</td></tr>
<tr><td>36</td><td>West Virginia</td><td>1,003</td><td>0.5%</td><td>48</td><td>South Dakota</td><td>296</td><td>0.2%</td></tr>
<tr><td>17</td><td>Wisconsin</td><td>3,363</td><td>1.8%</td><td>49</td><td>Alaska</td><td>284</td><td>0.2%</td></tr>
<tr><td>50</td><td>Wyoming</td><td>214</td><td>0.1%</td><td>50</td><td>Wyoming</td><td>214</td><td>0.1%</td></tr>
<tr><td></td><td></td><td></td><td></td><td></td><td>District of Columbia</td><td>1,208</td><td>0.6%</td></tr>
</tbody>
</table>

Source: American Medical Association (Chicago, Illinois)
"Physician Characteristics and Distribution in the U.S." (1999 Edition)
*As of December 31, 1997. Total does not include 2,320 physicians in U.S. territories and possessions. Other Specialties include Aerospace Medicine, Anesthesiology, Child Psychiatry, Diagnostic Radiology, Emergency Medicine, Forensic Pathology, Nuclear Medicine, Occupational Medicine, Neurology, Psychiatry, Public Health, Anatomic/Clinical Pathology, Radiology, Radiation Oncology and other specialties.

Rate of Nonfederal Physicians in Other Specialties in 1997

National Rate = 70 Physicians per 100,000 Population*

ALPHA ORDER

RANK	STATE	RATE
41	Alabama	48
44	Alaska	47
30	Arizona	58
41	Arkansas	48
10	California	71
14	Colorado	69
4	Connecticut	103
12	Delaware	70
24	Florida	62
30	Georgia	58
9	Hawaii	74
50	Idaho	37
10	Illinois	71
38	Indiana	54
46	Iowa	45
29	Kansas	59
33	Kentucky	57
18	Louisiana	65
28	Maine	61
2	Maryland	112
1	Massachusetts	129
23	Michigan	63
16	Minnesota	66
49	Mississippi	39
24	Missouri	62
40	Montana	52
38	Nebraska	54
41	Nevada	48
12	New Hampshire	70
8	New Jersey	75
24	New Mexico	62
3	New York	108
24	North Carolina	62
30	North Dakota	58
22	Ohio	64
45	Oklahoma	46
18	Oregon	65
7	Pennsylvania	85
6	Rhode Island	89
35	South Carolina	56
48	South Dakota	40
16	Tennessee	66
35	Texas	56
33	Utah	57
5	Vermont	90
18	Virginia	65
15	Washington	68
37	West Virginia	55
18	Wisconsin	65
46	Wyoming	45

RANK ORDER

RANK	STATE	RATE
1	Massachusetts	129
2	Maryland	112
3	New York	108
4	Connecticut	103
5	Vermont	90
6	Rhode Island	89
7	Pennsylvania	85
8	New Jersey	75
9	Hawaii	74
10	California	71
10	Illinois	71
12	Delaware	70
12	New Hampshire	70
14	Colorado	69
15	Washington	68
16	Minnesota	66
16	Tennessee	66
18	Louisiana	65
18	Oregon	65
18	Virginia	65
18	Wisconsin	65
22	Ohio	64
23	Michigan	63
24	Florida	62
24	Missouri	62
24	New Mexico	62
24	North Carolina	62
28	Maine	61
29	Kansas	59
30	Arizona	58
30	Georgia	58
30	North Dakota	58
33	Kentucky	57
33	Utah	57
35	South Carolina	56
35	Texas	56
37	West Virginia	55
38	Indiana	54
38	Nebraska	54
40	Montana	52
41	Alabama	48
41	Arkansas	48
41	Nevada	48
44	Alaska	47
45	Oklahoma	46
46	Iowa	45
46	Wyoming	45
48	South Dakota	40
49	Mississippi	39
50	Idaho	37

	District of Columbia	228

Source: Morgan Quitno Press using data from American Medical Association (Chicago, Illinois)
    "Physician Characteristics and Distribution in the U.S." (1999 Edition)
*As of December 31, 1997. National rate does not include physicians in U.S. territories and possessions. Other Specialties include Aerospace Medicine, Anesthesiology, Child Psychiatry, Diagnostic Radiology, Emergency Medicine, Forensic Pathology, Nuclear Medicine, Occupational Medicine, Neurology, Psychiatry, Public Health, Anatomic/Clinical Pathology, Radiology, Radiation Oncology and other specialties.

Nonfederal Physicians in Anesthesiology in 1997

National Total = 32,840 Physicians*

ALPHA ORDER

RANK ORDER

RANK	STATE	PHYSICIANS	% of USA	RANK	STATE	PHYSICIANS	% of USA
26	Alabama	404	1.2%	1	California	4,043	12.3%
47	Alaska	52	0.2%	2	New York	3,041	9.3%
19	Arizona	590	1.8%	3	Texas	2,401	7.3%
33	Arkansas	230	0.7%	4	Florida	1,916	5.8%
1	California	4,043	12.3%	5	Illinois	1,579	4.8%
22	Colorado	476	1.4%	6	Pennsylvania	1,561	4.8%
21	Connecticut	482	1.5%	7	Ohio	1,289	3.9%
46	Delaware	62	0.2%	8	New Jersey	1,208	3.7%
4	Florida	1,916	5.8%	9	Massachusetts	1,199	3.7%
13	Georgia	763	2.3%	10	Maryland	879	2.7%
40	Hawaii	129	0.4%	11	Washington	807	2.5%
44	Idaho	76	0.2%	12	Michigan	796	2.4%
5	Illinois	1,579	4.8%	13	Georgia	763	2.3%
16	Indiana	711	2.2%	14	North Carolina	731	2.2%
31	Iowa	251	0.8%	15	Virginia	715	2.2%
32	Kansas	236	0.7%	16	Indiana	711	2.2%
23	Kentucky	462	1.4%	17	Tennessee	661	2.0%
25	Louisiana	442	1.3%	18	Wisconsin	647	2.0%
39	Maine	131	0.4%	19	Arizona	590	1.8%
10	Maryland	879	2.7%	20	Missouri	564	1.7%
9	Massachusetts	1,199	3.7%	21	Connecticut	482	1.5%
12	Michigan	796	2.4%	22	Colorado	476	1.4%
24	Minnesota	453	1.4%	23	Kentucky	462	1.4%
34	Mississippi	223	0.7%	24	Minnesota	453	1.4%
20	Missouri	564	1.7%	25	Louisiana	442	1.3%
42	Montana	102	0.3%	26	Alabama	404	1.2%
37	Nebraska	162	0.5%	27	Oregon	402	1.2%
35	Nevada	200	0.6%	28	South Carolina	350	1.1%
41	New Hampshire	128	0.4%	29	Oklahoma	302	0.9%
8	New Jersey	1,208	3.7%	30	Utah	265	0.8%
36	New Mexico	172	0.5%	31	Iowa	251	0.8%
2	New York	3,041	9.3%	32	Kansas	236	0.7%
14	North Carolina	731	2.2%	33	Arkansas	230	0.7%
48	North Dakota	51	0.2%	34	Mississippi	223	0.7%
7	Ohio	1,289	3.9%	35	Nevada	200	0.6%
29	Oklahoma	302	0.9%	36	New Mexico	172	0.5%
27	Oregon	402	1.2%	37	Nebraska	162	0.5%
6	Pennsylvania	1,561	4.8%	38	West Virginia	146	0.4%
43	Rhode Island	91	0.3%	39	Maine	131	0.4%
28	South Carolina	350	1.1%	40	Hawaii	129	0.4%
49	South Dakota	42	0.1%	41	New Hampshire	128	0.4%
17	Tennessee	661	2.0%	42	Montana	102	0.3%
3	Texas	2,401	7.3%	43	Rhode Island	91	0.3%
30	Utah	265	0.8%	44	Idaho	76	0.2%
45	Vermont	67	0.2%	45	Vermont	67	0.2%
15	Virginia	715	2.2%	46	Delaware	62	0.2%
11	Washington	807	2.5%	47	Alaska	52	0.2%
38	West Virginia	146	0.4%	48	North Dakota	51	0.2%
18	Wisconsin	647	2.0%	49	South Dakota	42	0.1%
49	Wyoming	42	0.1%	49	Wyoming	42	0.1%
					District of Columbia	108	0.3%

Source: American Medical Association (Chicago, Illinois)
"Physician Characteristics and Distribution in the U.S." (1999 Edition)
As of December 31, 1997. Total does not include 203 physicians in U.S. territories and possessions.

Rate of Nonfederal Physicians in Anesthesiology in 1997

National Rate = 12.3 Physicians per 100,000 Population*

ALPHA ORDER

RANK ORDER

RANK	STATE	RATE
35	Alabama	9.3
43	Alaska	8.5
9	Arizona	13.0
38	Arkansas	9.1
12	California	12.6
17	Colorado	12.2
5	Connecticut	14.8
44	Delaware	8.4
8	Florida	13.1
29	Georgia	10.2
25	Hawaii	10.8
49	Idaho	6.3
7	Illinois	13.2
18	Indiana	12.1
41	Iowa	8.8
38	Kansas	9.1
20	Kentucky	11.8
29	Louisiana	10.2
27	Maine	10.5
2	Maryland	17.3
1	Massachusetts	19.6
46	Michigan	8.1
34	Minnesota	9.7
45	Mississippi	8.2
28	Missouri	10.4
21	Montana	11.6
32	Nebraska	9.8
19	Nevada	11.9
24	New Hampshire	10.9
4	New Jersey	15.0
31	New Mexico	10.0
3	New York	16.8
32	North Carolina	9.8
47	North Dakota	8.0
22	Ohio	11.5
38	Oklahoma	9.1
13	Oregon	12.4
9	Pennsylvania	13.0
36	Rhode Island	9.2
36	South Carolina	9.2
50	South Dakota	5.7
16	Tennessee	12.3
13	Texas	12.4
11	Utah	12.8
23	Vermont	11.4
26	Virginia	10.6
6	Washington	14.4
47	West Virginia	8.0
13	Wisconsin	12.4
42	Wyoming	8.7

RANK	STATE	RATE
1	Massachusetts	19.6
2	Maryland	17.3
3	New York	16.8
4	New Jersey	15.0
5	Connecticut	14.8
6	Washington	14.4
7	Illinois	13.2
8	Florida	13.1
9	Arizona	13.0
9	Pennsylvania	13.0
11	Utah	12.8
12	California	12.6
13	Oregon	12.4
13	Texas	12.4
13	Wisconsin	12.4
16	Tennessee	12.3
17	Colorado	12.2
18	Indiana	12.1
19	Nevada	11.9
20	Kentucky	11.8
21	Montana	11.6
22	Ohio	11.5
23	Vermont	11.4
24	New Hampshire	10.9
25	Hawaii	10.8
26	Virginia	10.6
27	Maine	10.5
28	Missouri	10.4
29	Georgia	10.2
29	Louisiana	10.2
31	New Mexico	10.0
32	Nebraska	9.8
32	North Carolina	9.8
34	Minnesota	9.7
35	Alabama	9.3
36	Rhode Island	9.2
36	South Carolina	9.2
38	Arkansas	9.1
38	Kansas	9.1
38	Oklahoma	9.1
41	Iowa	8.8
42	Wyoming	8.7
43	Alaska	8.5
44	Delaware	8.4
45	Mississippi	8.2
46	Michigan	8.1
47	North Dakota	8.0
47	West Virginia	8.0
49	Idaho	6.3
50	South Dakota	5.7

District of Columbia	20.4

Source: Morgan Quitno Press using data from American Medical Association (Chicago, Illinois)
   "Physician Characteristics and Distribution in the U.S." (1999 Edition)
*As of December 31, 1997. National rate does not include physicians in U.S. territories and possessions.

Nonfederal Physicians in Psychiatry in 1997

National Total = 36,970 Physicians*

ALPHA ORDER					RANK ORDER			
RANK	STATE	PHYSICIANS	% of USA		RANK	STATE	PHYSICIANS	% of USA
29	Alabama	275	0.7%		1	New York	5,528	15.0%
48	Alaska	55	0.1%		2	California	4,988	13.5%
23	Arizona	448	1.2%		3	Massachusetts	1,960	5.3%
34	Arkansas	187	0.5%		4	Pennsylvania	1,913	5.2%
2	California	4,988	13.5%		5	Texas	1,685	4.6%
17	Colorado	550	1.5%		6	Florida	1,540	4.2%
12	Connecticut	910	2.5%		7	Illinois	1,479	4.0%
44	Delaware	99	0.3%		8	New Jersey	1,306	3.5%
6	Florida	1,540	4.2%		9	Maryland	1,279	3.5%
15	Georgia	768	2.1%		10	Ohio	1,098	3.0%
35	Hawaii	186	0.5%		11	Michigan	1,062	2.9%
47	Idaho	61	0.2%		12	Connecticut	910	2.5%
7	Illinois	1,479	4.0%		13	North Carolina	878	2.4%
24	Indiana	445	1.2%		14	Virginia	836	2.3%
35	Iowa	186	0.5%		15	Georgia	768	2.1%
28	Kansas	349	0.9%		16	Washington	680	1.8%
27	Kentucky	374	1.0%		17	Colorado	550	1.5%
21	Louisiana	496	1.3%		18	Wisconsin	548	1.5%
37	Maine	173	0.5%		19	Missouri	531	1.4%
9	Maryland	1,279	3.5%		20	Tennessee	515	1.4%
3	Massachusetts	1,960	5.3%		21	Louisiana	496	1.3%
11	Michigan	1,062	2.9%		22	Minnesota	460	1.2%
22	Minnesota	460	1.2%		23	Arizona	448	1.2%
41	Mississippi	148	0.4%		24	Indiana	445	1.2%
19	Missouri	531	1.4%		25	South Carolina	420	1.1%
46	Montana	64	0.2%		26	Oregon	387	1.0%
40	Nebraska	154	0.4%		27	Kentucky	374	1.0%
43	Nevada	111	0.3%		28	Kansas	349	0.9%
33	New Hampshire	198	0.5%		29	Alabama	275	0.7%
8	New Jersey	1,306	3.5%		30	Oklahoma	242	0.7%
31	New Mexico	231	0.6%		31	New Mexico	231	0.6%
1	New York	5,528	15.0%		32	Rhode Island	206	0.6%
13	North Carolina	878	2.4%		33	New Hampshire	198	0.5%
45	North Dakota	75	0.2%		34	Arkansas	187	0.5%
10	Ohio	1,098	3.0%		35	Hawaii	186	0.5%
30	Oklahoma	242	0.7%		35	Iowa	186	0.5%
26	Oregon	387	1.0%		37	Maine	173	0.5%
4	Pennsylvania	1,913	5.2%		38	West Virginia	161	0.4%
32	Rhode Island	206	0.6%		39	Utah	155	0.4%
25	South Carolina	420	1.1%		40	Nebraska	154	0.4%
49	South Dakota	53	0.1%		41	Mississippi	148	0.4%
20	Tennessee	515	1.4%		42	Vermont	143	0.4%
5	Texas	1,685	4.6%		43	Nevada	111	0.3%
39	Utah	155	0.4%		44	Delaware	99	0.3%
42	Vermont	143	0.4%		45	North Dakota	75	0.2%
14	Virginia	836	2.3%		46	Montana	64	0.2%
16	Washington	680	1.8%		47	Idaho	61	0.2%
38	West Virginia	161	0.4%		48	Alaska	55	0.1%
18	Wisconsin	548	1.5%		49	South Dakota	53	0.1%
50	Wyoming	33	0.1%		50	Wyoming	33	0.1%
					District of Columbia		341	0.9%

Source: American Medical Association (Chicago, Illinois)
    "Physician Characteristics and Distribution in the U.S." (1999 Edition)
*As of December 31, 1997. Total does not include 353 physicians in U.S. territories and possessions. Psychiatry includes psychoanalysis.

Rate of Nonfederal Physicians in Psychiatry in 1997

National Rate = 13.8 Physicians per 100,000 Population*

ALPHA ORDER				RANK ORDER		
RANK	STATE	RATE		RANK	STATE	RATE
48	Alabama	6.4		1	Massachusetts	32.1
36	Alaska	9.0		2	New York	30.5
29	Arizona	9.8		3	Connecticut	27.9
41	Arkansas	7.4		4	Maryland	25.1
11	California	15.5		5	Vermont	24.3
12	Colorado	14.1		6	Rhode Island	20.9
3	Connecticut	27.9		7	New Hampshire	16.9
14	Delaware	13.5		8	New Jersey	16.2
26	Florida	10.5		9	Pennsylvania	15.9
28	Georgia	10.3		10	Hawaii	15.6
10	Hawaii	15.6		11	California	15.5
50	Idaho	5.0		12	Colorado	14.1
18	Illinois	12.3		13	Maine	13.9
39	Indiana	7.6		14	Delaware	13.5
47	Iowa	6.5		15	Kansas	13.4
15	Kansas	13.4		15	New Mexico	13.4
33	Kentucky	9.6		17	Virginia	12.4
23	Louisiana	11.4		18	Illinois	12.3
13	Maine	13.9		19	Washington	12.1
4	Maryland	25.1		20	Oregon	11.9
1	Massachusetts	32.1		21	North Carolina	11.8
25	Michigan	10.9		22	North Dakota	11.7
29	Minnesota	9.8		23	Louisiana	11.4
49	Mississippi	5.4		24	South Carolina	11.1
29	Missouri	9.8		25	Michigan	10.9
42	Montana	7.3		26	Florida	10.5
35	Nebraska	9.3		26	Wisconsin	10.5
46	Nevada	6.6		28	Georgia	10.3
7	New Hampshire	16.9		29	Arizona	9.8
8	New Jersey	16.2		29	Minnesota	9.8
15	New Mexico	13.4		29	Missouri	9.8
2	New York	30.5		29	Ohio	9.8
21	North Carolina	11.8		33	Kentucky	9.6
22	North Dakota	11.7		33	Tennessee	9.6
29	Ohio	9.8		35	Nebraska	9.3
42	Oklahoma	7.3		36	Alaska	9.0
20	Oregon	11.9		37	West Virginia	8.9
9	Pennsylvania	15.9		38	Texas	8.7
6	Rhode Island	20.9		39	Indiana	7.6
24	South Carolina	11.1		40	Utah	7.5
44	South Dakota	7.2		41	Arkansas	7.4
33	Tennessee	9.6		42	Montana	7.3
38	Texas	8.7		42	Oklahoma	7.3
40	Utah	7.5		44	South Dakota	7.2
5	Vermont	24.3		45	Wyoming	6.9
17	Virginia	12.4		46	Nevada	6.6
19	Washington	12.1		47	Iowa	6.5
37	West Virginia	8.9		48	Alabama	6.4
26	Wisconsin	10.5		49	Mississippi	5.4
45	Wyoming	6.9		50	Idaho	5.0

District of Columbia 64.4

Source: Morgan Quitno Press using data from American Medical Association (Chicago, Illinois)
   "Physician Characteristics and Distribution in the U.S." (1999 Edition)
*As of December 31, 1997. National rate does not include physicians in U.S. territories and possessions.
Psychiatry includes psychoanalysis.

Percent of Population Lacking Access to Mental Health Care in 1998

National Percent = 11.7% of Population*

ALPHA ORDER

RANK	STATE	PERCENT
2	Alabama	53.6
44	Alaska	1.5
18	Arizona	19.9
3	Arkansas	44.2
45	California	1.2
34	Colorado	5.3
47	Connecticut	0.5
7	Delaware	30.9
42	Florida	2.6
22	Georgia	17.5
41	Hawaii	2.8
5	Idaho	38.9
36	Illinois	4.8
37	Indiana	4.1
14	Iowa	22.4
10	Kansas	27.6
19	Kentucky	18.9
20	Louisiana	18.2
23	Maine	16.3
40	Maryland	3.3
46	Massachusetts	0.8
21	Michigan	17.6
28	Minnesota	10.7
12	Mississippi	23.6
9	Missouri	27.8
6	Montana	34.4
11	Nebraska	26.3
38	Nevada	3.4
32	New Hampshire	6.6
43	New Jersey	2.4
4	New Mexico	39.4
33	New York	5.8
30	North Carolina	8.2
27	North Dakota	11.8
38	Ohio	3.4
17	Oklahoma	20.2
25	Oregon	13.2
31	Pennsylvania	7.6
49	Rhode Island	0.0
8	South Carolina	30.6
48	South Dakota	0.3
24	Tennessee	13.9
15	Texas	20.9
35	Utah	5.1
49	Vermont	0.0
28	Virginia	10.7
26	Washington	12.2
15	West Virginia	20.9
13	Wisconsin	22.8
1	Wyoming	85.9

RANK ORDER

RANK	STATE	PERCENT
1	Wyoming	85.9
2	Alabama	53.6
3	Arkansas	44.2
4	New Mexico	39.4
5	Idaho	38.9
6	Montana	34.4
7	Delaware	30.9
8	South Carolina	30.6
9	Missouri	27.8
10	Kansas	27.6
11	Nebraska	26.3
12	Mississippi	23.6
13	Wisconsin	22.8
14	Iowa	22.4
15	Texas	20.9
15	West Virginia	20.9
17	Oklahoma	20.2
18	Arizona	19.9
19	Kentucky	18.9
20	Louisiana	18.2
21	Michigan	17.6
22	Georgia	17.5
23	Maine	16.3
24	Tennessee	13.9
25	Oregon	13.2
26	Washington	12.2
27	North Dakota	11.8
28	Minnesota	10.7
28	Virginia	10.7
30	North Carolina	8.2
31	Pennsylvania	7.6
32	New Hampshire	6.6
33	New York	5.8
34	Colorado	5.3
35	Utah	5.1
36	Illinois	4.8
37	Indiana	4.1
38	Nevada	3.4
38	Ohio	3.4
40	Maryland	3.3
41	Hawaii	2.8
42	Florida	2.6
43	New Jersey	2.4
44	Alaska	1.5
45	California	1.2
46	Massachusetts	0.8
47	Connecticut	0.5
48	South Dakota	0.3
49	Rhode Island	0.0
49	Vermont	0.0

District of Columbia 12.8

Source: Morgan Quitno Press using data from U.S. Dept. of Health and Human Services, Div. of Shortage Designation
"Selected Statistics on Health Manpower Shortage Areas, As of September 30, 1998"
*Percent of population considered under-served by mental health practitioners. An under-served population does
not have primary medical care within reasonable economic and geographic bounds.

International Medical School Graduates Practicing in the U.S. in 1997

National Total = 167,873 Nonfederal Physicians*

ALPHA ORDER

RANK	STATE	PHYSICIANS	% of USA
26	Alabama	1,115	0.7%
48	Alaska	65	0.0%
20	Arizona	1,658	1.0%
36	Arkansas	491	0.3%
2	California	18,618	11.1%
33	Colorado	572	0.3%
13	Connecticut	3,169	1.9%
38	Delaware	484	0.3%
3	Florida	13,596	8.1%
15	Georgia	2,557	1.5%
35	Hawaii	524	0.3%
49	Idaho	61	0.0%
4	Illinois	11,205	6.7%
16	Indiana	2,107	1.3%
30	Iowa	812	0.5%
27	Kansas	954	0.6%
21	Kentucky	1,554	0.9%
22	Louisiana	1,516	0.9%
42	Maine	350	0.2%
10	Maryland	5,584	3.3%
11	Massachusetts	5,104	3.0%
9	Michigan	7,034	4.2%
23	Minnesota	1,466	0.9%
39	Mississippi	449	0.3%
14	Missouri	2,566	1.5%
47	Montana	75	0.0%
41	Nebraska	364	0.2%
32	Nevada	621	0.4%
40	New Hampshire	372	0.2%
5	New Jersey	11,091	6.6%
37	New Mexico	488	0.3%
1	New York	30,587	18.2%
18	North Carolina	1,860	1.1%
43	North Dakota	294	0.2%
8	Ohio	7,254	4.3%
29	Oklahoma	909	0.5%
34	Oregon	530	0.3%
7	Pennsylvania	8,154	4.9%
28	Rhode Island	916	0.5%
31	South Carolina	763	0.5%
45	South Dakota	150	0.1%
19	Tennessee	1,810	1.1%
6	Texas	8,798	5.2%
44	Utah	239	0.1%
46	Vermont	147	0.1%
12	Virginia	3,371	2.0%
25	Washington	1,313	0.8%
24	West Virginia	1,413	0.8%
17	Wisconsin	1,940	1.2%
50	Wyoming	48	0.0%

RANK ORDER

RANK	STATE	PHYSICIANS	% of USA
1	New York	30,587	18.2%
2	California	18,618	11.1%
3	Florida	13,596	8.1%
4	Illinois	11,205	6.7%
5	New Jersey	11,091	6.6%
6	Texas	8,798	5.2%
7	Pennsylvania	8,154	4.9%
8	Ohio	7,254	4.3%
9	Michigan	7,034	4.2%
10	Maryland	5,584	3.3%
11	Massachusetts	5,104	3.0%
12	Virginia	3,371	2.0%
13	Connecticut	3,169	1.9%
14	Missouri	2,566	1.5%
15	Georgia	2,557	1.5%
16	Indiana	2,107	1.3%
17	Wisconsin	1,940	1.2%
18	North Carolina	1,860	1.1%
19	Tennessee	1,810	1.1%
20	Arizona	1,658	1.0%
21	Kentucky	1,554	0.9%
22	Louisiana	1,516	0.9%
23	Minnesota	1,466	0.9%
24	West Virginia	1,413	0.8%
25	Washington	1,313	0.8%
26	Alabama	1,115	0.7%
27	Kansas	954	0.6%
28	Rhode Island	916	0.5%
29	Oklahoma	909	0.5%
30	Iowa	812	0.5%
31	South Carolina	763	0.5%
32	Nevada	621	0.4%
33	Colorado	572	0.3%
34	Oregon	530	0.3%
35	Hawaii	524	0.3%
36	Arkansas	491	0.3%
37	New Mexico	488	0.3%
38	Delaware	484	0.3%
39	Mississippi	449	0.3%
40	New Hampshire	372	0.2%
41	Nebraska	364	0.2%
42	Maine	350	0.2%
43	North Dakota	294	0.2%
44	Utah	239	0.1%
45	South Dakota	150	0.1%
46	Vermont	147	0.1%
47	Montana	75	0.0%
48	Alaska	65	0.0%
49	Idaho	61	0.0%
50	Wyoming	48	0.0%
	District of Columbia	755	0.4%

Source: American Medical Association (Chicago, Illinois)
    "Physician Characteristics and Distribution in the U.S." (1999 Edition)
*As of December 31, 1997. Total does not include 5,133 physicians in U.S. territories and possessions.

Rate of International Medical School Graduates Practicing in the U.S. in 1997

National Rate = 63 Nonfederal Physicians per 100,000 Population*

ALPHA ORDER			RANK ORDER		
RANK	STATE	RATE	RANK	STATE	RATE
35	Alabama	26	1	New York	169
47	Alaska	11	2	New Jersey	138
24	Arizona	36	3	Maryland	110
42	Arkansas	19	4	Connecticut	97
14	California	58	5	Florida	93
45	Colorado	15	5	Illinois	93
4	Connecticut	97	5	Rhode Island	93
12	Delaware	66	8	Massachusetts	83
5	Florida	93	9	West Virginia	78
27	Georgia	34	10	Michigan	72
19	Hawaii	44	11	Pennsylvania	68
50	Idaho	5	12	Delaware	66
5	Illinois	93	13	Ohio	65
24	Indiana	36	14	California	58
31	Iowa	28	15	Virginia	50
21	Kansas	37	16	Missouri	47
20	Kentucky	40	17	North Dakota	46
26	Louisiana	35	18	Texas	45
31	Maine	28	19	Hawaii	44
3	Maryland	110	20	Kentucky	40
8	Massachusetts	83	21	Kansas	37
10	Michigan	72	21	Nevada	37
30	Minnesota	31	21	Wisconsin	37
43	Mississippi	16	24	Arizona	36
16	Missouri	47	24	Indiana	36
49	Montana	9	26	Louisiana	35
39	Nebraska	22	27	Georgia	34
21	Nevada	37	27	Tennessee	34
29	New Hampshire	32	29	New Hampshire	32
2	New Jersey	138	30	Minnesota	31
31	New Mexico	28	31	Iowa	28
1	New York	169	31	Maine	28
36	North Carolina	25	31	New Mexico	28
17	North Dakota	46	34	Oklahoma	27
13	Ohio	65	35	Alabama	26
34	Oklahoma	27	36	North Carolina	25
43	Oregon	16	36	Vermont	25
11	Pennsylvania	68	38	Washington	23
5	Rhode Island	93	39	Nebraska	22
40	South Carolina	20	40	South Carolina	20
40	South Dakota	20	40	South Dakota	20
27	Tennessee	34	42	Arkansas	19
18	Texas	45	43	Mississippi	16
46	Utah	12	43	Oregon	16
36	Vermont	25	45	Colorado	15
15	Virginia	50	46	Utah	12
38	Washington	23	47	Alaska	11
9	West Virginia	78	48	Wyoming	10
21	Wisconsin	37	49	Montana	9
48	Wyoming	10	50	Idaho	5
				District of Columbia	142

Source: Morgan Quitno Press using data from American Medical Association (Chicago, Illinois)
  "Physician Characteristics and Distribution in the U.S." (1999 Edition)
*As of December 31, 1997. National rate does not include physicians in U.S. territories and possessions.

International Medical School Graduates
As a Percent of Nonfederal Physicians in 1997
National Percent = 23.1% of Nonfederal Physicians*

ALPHA ORDER

RANK	STATE	PERCENT
31	Alabama	12.2
45	Alaska	6.3
23	Arizona	15.4
38	Arkansas	9.5
14	California	20.9
46	Colorado	5.6
11	Connecticut	25.6
9	Delaware	25.8
5	Florida	33.2
23	Georgia	15.4
23	Hawaii	15.4
50	Idaho	2.9
3	Illinois	34.1
21	Indiana	17.0
28	Iowa	14.6
22	Kansas	16.1
20	Kentucky	17.8
29	Louisiana	13.6
35	Maine	11.3
7	Maryland	27.7
18	Massachusetts	19.2
6	Michigan	30.1
34	Minnesota	11.4
38	Mississippi	9.5
15	Missouri	19.6
49	Montana	3.9
40	Nebraska	9.3
16	Nevada	19.5
32	New Hampshire	12.0
1	New Jersey	44.2
32	New Mexico	12.0
2	New York	41.9
37	North Carolina	10.1
18	North Dakota	19.2
10	Ohio	25.7
26	Oklahoma	15.0
44	Oregon	6.4
12	Pennsylvania	22.0
8	Rhode Island	26.3
41	South Carolina	9.1
36	South Dakota	10.2
30	Tennessee	12.9
13	Texas	21.4
47	Utah	5.3
43	Vermont	7.5
17	Virginia	19.4
42	Washington	8.9
4	West Virginia	33.9
26	Wisconsin	15.0
48	Wyoming	5.2

RANK ORDER

RANK	STATE	PERCENT
1	New Jersey	44.2
2	New York	41.9
3	Illinois	34.1
4	West Virginia	33.9
5	Florida	33.2
6	Michigan	30.1
7	Maryland	27.7
8	Rhode Island	26.3
9	Delaware	25.8
10	Ohio	25.7
11	Connecticut	25.6
12	Pennsylvania	22.0
13	Texas	21.4
14	California	20.9
15	Missouri	19.6
16	Nevada	19.5
17	Virginia	19.4
18	Massachusetts	19.2
18	North Dakota	19.2
20	Kentucky	17.8
21	Indiana	17.0
22	Kansas	16.1
23	Arizona	15.4
23	Georgia	15.4
23	Hawaii	15.4
26	Oklahoma	15.0
26	Wisconsin	15.0
28	Iowa	14.6
29	Louisiana	13.6
30	Tennessee	12.9
31	Alabama	12.2
32	New Hampshire	12.0
32	New Mexico	12.0
34	Minnesota	11.4
35	Maine	11.3
36	South Dakota	10.2
37	North Carolina	10.1
38	Arkansas	9.5
38	Mississippi	9.5
40	Nebraska	9.3
41	South Carolina	9.1
42	Washington	8.9
43	Vermont	7.5
44	Oregon	6.4
45	Alaska	6.3
46	Colorado	5.6
47	Utah	5.3
48	Wyoming	5.2
49	Montana	3.9
50	Idaho	2.9
	District of Columbia	19.0

Source: Morgan Quitno Press using data from American Medical Association (Chicago, Illinois)
    "Physician Characteristics and Distribution in the U.S." (1999 Edition)
*As of December 31, 1997. National rate does not include physicians in U.S. territories and possessions.

Osteopathic Physicians in 1998

National Total = 40,288 Osteopathic Physicians*

ALPHA ORDER

RANK	STATE	OSTEOPATHS	% of USA
28	Alabama	251	0.6%
45	Alaska	65	0.2%
12	Arizona	1,120	2.8%
38	Arkansas	167	0.4%
8	California	1,828	4.5%
14	Colorado	669	1.7%
31	Connecticut	188	0.5%
36	Delaware	171	0.4%
4	Florida	2,842	7.1%
18	Georgia	484	1.2%
43	Hawaii	87	0.2%
39	Idaho	99	0.2%
10	Illinois	1,610	4.0%
15	Indiana	591	1.5%
13	Iowa	925	2.3%
16	Kansas	542	1.3%
32	Kentucky	184	0.5%
42	Louisiana	91	0.2%
21	Maine	418	1.0%
26	Maryland	274	0.7%
23	Massachusetts	389	1.0%
1	Michigan	4,876	12.1%
30	Minnesota	208	0.5%
34	Mississippi	175	0.4%
9	Missouri	1,750	4.3%
44	Montana	71	0.2%
46	Nebraska	63	0.2%
27	Nevada	257	0.6%
40	New Hampshire	97	0.2%
6	New Jersey	2,393	5.9%
32	New Mexico	184	0.5%
7	New York	2,236	5.6%
29	North Carolina	232	0.6%
48	North Dakota	51	0.1%
3	Ohio	3,269	8.1%
11	Oklahoma	1,147	2.8%
22	Oregon	402	1.0%
2	Pennsylvania	4,815	12.0%
35	Rhode Island	174	0.4%
36	South Carolina	171	0.4%
47	South Dakota	58	0.1%
25	Tennessee	312	0.8%
5	Texas	2,438	6.1%
41	Utah	93	0.2%
49	Vermont	50	0.1%
24	Virginia	329	0.8%
17	Washington	491	1.2%
19	West Virginia	455	1.1%
20	Wisconsin	432	1.1%
50	Wyoming	34	0.1%

RANK ORDER

RANK	STATE	OSTEOPATHS	% of USA
1	Michigan	4,876	12.1%
2	Pennsylvania	4,815	12.0%
3	Ohio	3,269	8.1%
4	Florida	2,842	7.1%
5	Texas	2,438	6.1%
6	New Jersey	2,393	5.9%
7	New York	2,236	5.6%
8	California	1,828	4.5%
9	Missouri	1,750	4.3%
10	Illinois	1,610	4.0%
11	Oklahoma	1,147	2.8%
12	Arizona	1,120	2.8%
13	Iowa	925	2.3%
14	Colorado	669	1.7%
15	Indiana	591	1.5%
16	Kansas	542	1.3%
17	Washington	491	1.2%
18	Georgia	484	1.2%
19	West Virginia	455	1.1%
20	Wisconsin	432	1.1%
21	Maine	418	1.0%
22	Oregon	402	1.0%
23	Massachusetts	389	1.0%
24	Virginia	329	0.8%
25	Tennessee	312	0.8%
26	Maryland	274	0.7%
27	Nevada	257	0.6%
28	Alabama	251	0.6%
29	North Carolina	232	0.6%
30	Minnesota	208	0.5%
31	Connecticut	188	0.5%
32	Kentucky	184	0.5%
32	New Mexico	184	0.5%
34	Mississippi	175	0.4%
35	Rhode Island	174	0.4%
36	Delaware	171	0.4%
36	South Carolina	171	0.4%
38	Arkansas	167	0.4%
39	Idaho	99	0.2%
40	New Hampshire	97	0.2%
41	Utah	93	0.2%
42	Louisiana	91	0.2%
43	Hawaii	87	0.2%
44	Montana	71	0.2%
45	Alaska	65	0.2%
46	Nebraska	63	0.2%
47	South Dakota	58	0.1%
48	North Dakota	51	0.1%
49	Vermont	50	0.1%
50	Wyoming	34	0.1%
	District of Columbia	30	0.1%

Source: American Osteopathic Association
"AOA Yearbook and Directory of Osteopathic Physicians 1999"
Excludes retired, disabled, foreign and federal osteopaths. Osteopaths practice a system of medicine based on the theory that disturbances in the musculoskeletal system affect other body parts, causing many disorders that can be corrected by various manipulative techniques in conjunction with conventional medical, surgical, pharmacological, and other therapeutic procedures.

Rate of Osteopathic Physicians in 1998

National Rate = 14.9 Osteopaths per 100,000 Population*

ALPHA ORDER

RANK	STATE	RATE
38	Alabama	5.8
21	Alaska	10.6
10	Arizona	24.0
34	Arkansas	6.6
41	California	5.6
15	Colorado	16.8
39	Connecticut	5.7
11	Delaware	23.0
13	Florida	19.1
36	Georgia	6.3
32	Hawaii	7.3
28	Idaho	8.1
17	Illinois	13.4
23	Indiana	10.0
5	Iowa	32.3
12	Kansas	20.6
44	Kentucky	4.7
50	Louisiana	2.1
4	Maine	33.6
42	Maryland	5.3
36	Massachusetts	6.3
1	Michigan	49.7
46	Minnesota	4.4
35	Mississippi	6.4
6	Missouri	32.2
28	Montana	8.1
48	Nebraska	3.8
16	Nevada	14.7
27	New Hampshire	8.2
7	New Jersey	29.5
21	New Mexico	10.6
18	New York	12.3
49	North Carolina	3.1
30	North Dakota	8.0
8	Ohio	29.2
3	Oklahoma	34.3
20	Oregon	12.2
2	Pennsylvania	40.1
14	Rhode Island	17.6
45	South Carolina	4.5
31	South Dakota	7.9
39	Tennessee	5.7
18	Texas	12.3
46	Utah	4.4
25	Vermont	8.5
43	Virginia	4.8
24	Washington	8.6
9	West Virginia	25.1
26	Wisconsin	8.3
33	Wyoming	7.1

RANK ORDER

RANK	STATE	RATE
1	Michigan	49.7
2	Pennsylvania	40.1
3	Oklahoma	34.3
4	Maine	33.6
5	Iowa	32.3
6	Missouri	32.2
7	New Jersey	29.5
8	Ohio	29.2
9	West Virginia	25.1
10	Arizona	24.0
11	Delaware	23.0
12	Kansas	20.6
13	Florida	19.1
14	Rhode Island	17.6
15	Colorado	16.8
16	Nevada	14.7
17	Illinois	13.4
18	New York	12.3
18	Texas	12.3
20	Oregon	12.2
21	Alaska	10.6
21	New Mexico	10.6
23	Indiana	10.0
24	Washington	8.6
25	Vermont	8.5
26	Wisconsin	8.3
27	New Hampshire	8.2
28	Idaho	8.1
28	Montana	8.1
30	North Dakota	8.0
31	South Dakota	7.9
32	Hawaii	7.3
33	Wyoming	7.1
34	Arkansas	6.6
35	Mississippi	6.4
36	Georgia	6.3
36	Massachusetts	6.3
38	Alabama	5.8
39	Connecticut	5.7
39	Tennessee	5.7
41	California	5.6
42	Maryland	5.3
43	Virginia	4.8
44	Kentucky	4.7
45	South Carolina	4.5
46	Minnesota	4.4
46	Utah	4.4
48	Nebraska	3.8
49	North Carolina	3.1
50	Louisiana	2.1

| | District of Columbia | 5.7 |

Source: Morgan Quitno Press using data from American Osteopathic Association
"AOA Yearbook and Directory of Osteopathic Physicians 1999"
*Excludes retired, disabled, foreign and federal osteopaths. Osteopaths practice a system of medicine based on the theory that disturbances in the musculoskeletal system affect other body parts, causing many disorders that can be corrected by various manipulative techniques in conjunction with conventional medical, surgical, pharmacological, and other therapeutic procedures.

Osteopathic Physicians in Primary Care in 1996

National Total = 21,638 Osteopathic Physicians*

ALPHA ORDER

RANK ORDER

RANK	STATE	OSTEOPATHS	% of USA	RANK	STATE	OSTEOPATHS	% of USA
28	Alabama	132	0.61%	1	Pennsylvania	2,751	12.71%
40	Alaska	52	0.24%	2	Michigan	2,363	10.92%
12	Arizona	546	2.52%	3	Ohio	1,625	7.51%
33	Arkansas	97	0.45%	4	Florida	1,425	6.59%
8	California	1,041	4.81%	5	Texas	1,396	6.45%
14	Colorado	428	1.98%	6	New Jersey	1,288	5.95%
36	Connecticut	87	0.40%	7	New York	1,213	5.61%
29	Delaware	111	0.51%	8	California	1,041	4.81%
4	Florida	1,425	6.59%	9	Missouri	943	4.36%
18	Georgia	286	1.32%	10	Illinois	778	3.60%
39	Hawaii	63	0.29%	11	Oklahoma	677	3.13%
42	Idaho	50	0.23%	12	Arizona	546	2.52%
10	Illinois	778	3.60%	13	Iowa	527	2.44%
17	Indiana	304	1.40%	14	Colorado	428	1.98%
13	Iowa	527	2.44%	15	Washington	324	1.50%
16	Kansas	310	1.43%	16	Kansas	310	1.43%
37	Kentucky	84	0.39%	17	Indiana	304	1.40%
44	Louisiana	44	0.20%	18	Georgia	286	1.32%
21	Maine	253	1.17%	19	West Virginia	273	1.26%
26	Maryland	139	0.64%	20	Wisconsin	256	1.18%
23	Massachusetts	203	0.94%	21	Maine	253	1.17%
2	Michigan	2,363	10.92%	22	Oregon	228	1.05%
31	Minnesota	110	0.51%	23	Massachusetts	203	0.94%
34	Mississippi	93	0.43%	24	Virginia	196	0.91%
9	Missouri	943	4.36%	25	Tennessee	160	0.74%
46	Montana	32	0.15%	26	Maryland	139	0.64%
45	Nebraska	36	0.17%	27	Nevada	135	0.62%
27	Nevada	135	0.62%	28	Alabama	132	0.61%
40	New Hampshire	52	0.24%	29	Delaware	111	0.51%
6	New Jersey	1,288	5.95%	29	New Mexico	111	0.51%
29	New Mexico	111	0.51%	31	Minnesota	110	0.51%
7	New York	1,213	5.61%	32	Rhode Island	98	0.45%
35	North Carolina	92	0.43%	33	Arkansas	97	0.45%
50	North Dakota	12	0.06%	34	Mississippi	93	0.43%
3	Ohio	1,625	7.51%	35	North Carolina	92	0.43%
11	Oklahoma	677	3.13%	36	Connecticut	87	0.40%
22	Oregon	228	1.05%	37	Kentucky	84	0.39%
1	Pennsylvania	2,751	12.71%	38	South Carolina	81	0.37%
32	Rhode Island	98	0.45%	39	Hawaii	63	0.29%
38	South Carolina	81	0.37%	40	Alaska	52	0.24%
47	South Dakota	28	0.13%	40	New Hampshire	52	0.24%
25	Tennessee	160	0.74%	42	Idaho	50	0.23%
5	Texas	1,396	6.45%	43	Utah	47	0.22%
43	Utah	47	0.22%	44	Louisiana	44	0.20%
48	Vermont	25	0.12%	45	Nebraska	36	0.17%
24	Virginia	196	0.91%	46	Montana	32	0.15%
15	Washington	324	1.50%	47	South Dakota	28	0.13%
19	West Virginia	273	1.26%	48	Vermont	25	0.12%
20	Wisconsin	256	1.18%	49	Wyoming	19	0.09%
49	Wyoming	19	0.09%	50	North Dakota	12	0.06%
					District of Columbia	14	0.06%

Source: Morgan Quitno Press using data from American Osteopathic Association "AOA Biographical Records" (February 1997)

As of June 1, 1996. Excludes retired, disabled, foreign and federal osteopaths. Osteopaths practice a system of medicine based on the theory that disturbances in the musculoskeletal system affect other body parts, causing many disorders that can be corrected by various manipulative techniques in conjunction with conventional medical, surgical, pharmacological, and other therapeutic procedures.

Podiatric Physicians in 1995

National Total = 11,628 Podiatric Physicians*

<table>
<thead>
<tr><th colspan="4">ALPHA ORDER</th><th colspan="4">RANK ORDER</th></tr>
<tr><th>RANK</th><th>STATE</th><th>PODIATRISTS</th><th>% of USA</th><th>RANK</th><th>STATE</th><th>PODIATRISTS</th><th>% of USA</th></tr>
</thead>
<tbody>
<tr><td>31</td><td>Alabama</td><td>61</td><td>0.52%</td><td>1</td><td>California</td><td>1,415</td><td>12.17%</td></tr>
<tr><td>49</td><td>Alaska</td><td>15</td><td>0.13%</td><td>2</td><td>New York</td><td>1,154</td><td>9.92%</td></tr>
<tr><td>17</td><td>Arizona</td><td>199</td><td>1.71%</td><td>3</td><td>Pennsylvania</td><td>994</td><td>8.55%</td></tr>
<tr><td>39</td><td>Arkansas</td><td>39</td><td>0.34%</td><td>4</td><td>Florida</td><td>877</td><td>7.54%</td></tr>
<tr><td>1</td><td>California</td><td>1,415</td><td>12.17%</td><td>5</td><td>New Jersey</td><td>747</td><td>6.42%</td></tr>
<tr><td>24</td><td>Colorado</td><td>115</td><td>0.99%</td><td>6</td><td>Illinois</td><td>670</td><td>5.76%</td></tr>
<tr><td>12</td><td>Connecticut</td><td>282</td><td>2.43%</td><td>7</td><td>Ohio</td><td>490</td><td>4.21%</td></tr>
<tr><td>43</td><td>Delaware</td><td>37</td><td>0.32%</td><td>8</td><td>Michigan</td><td>457</td><td>3.93%</td></tr>
<tr><td>4</td><td>Florida</td><td>877</td><td>7.54%</td><td>9</td><td>Massachusetts</td><td>429</td><td>3.69%</td></tr>
<tr><td>13</td><td>Georgia</td><td>248</td><td>2.13%</td><td>10</td><td>Texas</td><td>422</td><td>3.63%</td></tr>
<tr><td>46</td><td>Hawaii</td><td>20</td><td>0.17%</td><td>11</td><td>Maryland</td><td>330</td><td>2.84%</td></tr>
<tr><td>37</td><td>Idaho</td><td>44</td><td>0.38%</td><td>12</td><td>Connecticut</td><td>282</td><td>2.43%</td></tr>
<tr><td>6</td><td>Illinois</td><td>670</td><td>5.76%</td><td>13</td><td>Georgia</td><td>248</td><td>2.13%</td></tr>
<tr><td>14</td><td>Indiana</td><td>227</td><td>1.95%</td><td>14</td><td>Indiana</td><td>227</td><td>1.95%</td></tr>
<tr><td>19</td><td>Iowa</td><td>148</td><td>1.27%</td><td>15</td><td>Virginia</td><td>209</td><td>1.80%</td></tr>
<tr><td>27</td><td>Kansas</td><td>86</td><td>0.74%</td><td>16</td><td>North Carolina</td><td>206</td><td>1.77%</td></tr>
<tr><td>28</td><td>Kentucky</td><td>82</td><td>0.71%</td><td>17</td><td>Arizona</td><td>199</td><td>1.71%</td></tr>
<tr><td>30</td><td>Louisiana</td><td>72</td><td>0.62%</td><td>18</td><td>Wisconsin</td><td>180</td><td>1.55%</td></tr>
<tr><td>34</td><td>Maine</td><td>54</td><td>0.46%</td><td>19</td><td>Iowa</td><td>148</td><td>1.27%</td></tr>
<tr><td>11</td><td>Maryland</td><td>330</td><td>2.84%</td><td>19</td><td>Washington</td><td>148</td><td>1.27%</td></tr>
<tr><td>9</td><td>Massachusetts</td><td>429</td><td>3.69%</td><td>21</td><td>Minnesota</td><td>130</td><td>1.12%</td></tr>
<tr><td>8</td><td>Michigan</td><td>457</td><td>3.93%</td><td>22</td><td>Tennessee</td><td>129</td><td>1.11%</td></tr>
<tr><td>21</td><td>Minnesota</td><td>130</td><td>1.12%</td><td>23</td><td>Missouri</td><td>128</td><td>1.10%</td></tr>
<tr><td>44</td><td>Mississippi</td><td>28</td><td>0.24%</td><td>24</td><td>Colorado</td><td>115</td><td>0.99%</td></tr>
<tr><td>23</td><td>Missouri</td><td>128</td><td>1.10%</td><td>25</td><td>Utah</td><td>99</td><td>0.85%</td></tr>
<tr><td>38</td><td>Montana</td><td>40</td><td>0.34%</td><td>26</td><td>Oregon</td><td>98</td><td>0.84%</td></tr>
<tr><td>32</td><td>Nebraska</td><td>56</td><td>0.48%</td><td>27</td><td>Kansas</td><td>86</td><td>0.74%</td></tr>
<tr><td>35</td><td>Nevada</td><td>53</td><td>0.46%</td><td>28</td><td>Kentucky</td><td>82</td><td>0.71%</td></tr>
<tr><td>33</td><td>New Hampshire</td><td>55</td><td>0.47%</td><td>29</td><td>Oklahoma</td><td>74</td><td>0.64%</td></tr>
<tr><td>5</td><td>New Jersey</td><td>747</td><td>6.42%</td><td>30</td><td>Louisiana</td><td>72</td><td>0.62%</td></tr>
<tr><td>41</td><td>New Mexico</td><td>38</td><td>0.33%</td><td>31</td><td>Alabama</td><td>61</td><td>0.52%</td></tr>
<tr><td>2</td><td>New York</td><td>1,154</td><td>9.92%</td><td>32</td><td>Nebraska</td><td>56</td><td>0.48%</td></tr>
<tr><td>16</td><td>North Carolina</td><td>206</td><td>1.77%</td><td>33</td><td>New Hampshire</td><td>55</td><td>0.47%</td></tr>
<tr><td>48</td><td>North Dakota</td><td>16</td><td>0.14%</td><td>34</td><td>Maine</td><td>54</td><td>0.46%</td></tr>
<tr><td>7</td><td>Ohio</td><td>490</td><td>4.21%</td><td>35</td><td>Nevada</td><td>53</td><td>0.46%</td></tr>
<tr><td>29</td><td>Oklahoma</td><td>74</td><td>0.64%</td><td>35</td><td>West Virginia</td><td>53</td><td>0.46%</td></tr>
<tr><td>26</td><td>Oregon</td><td>98</td><td>0.84%</td><td>37</td><td>Idaho</td><td>44</td><td>0.38%</td></tr>
<tr><td>3</td><td>Pennsylvania</td><td>994</td><td>8.55%</td><td>38</td><td>Montana</td><td>40</td><td>0.34%</td></tr>
<tr><td>39</td><td>Rhode Island</td><td>39</td><td>0.34%</td><td>39</td><td>Arkansas</td><td>39</td><td>0.34%</td></tr>
<tr><td>41</td><td>South Carolina</td><td>38</td><td>0.33%</td><td>39</td><td>Rhode Island</td><td>39</td><td>0.34%</td></tr>
<tr><td>45</td><td>South Dakota</td><td>24</td><td>0.21%</td><td>41</td><td>New Mexico</td><td>38</td><td>0.33%</td></tr>
<tr><td>22</td><td>Tennessee</td><td>129</td><td>1.11%</td><td>41</td><td>South Carolina</td><td>38</td><td>0.33%</td></tr>
<tr><td>10</td><td>Texas</td><td>422</td><td>3.63%</td><td>43</td><td>Delaware</td><td>37</td><td>0.32%</td></tr>
<tr><td>25</td><td>Utah</td><td>99</td><td>0.85%</td><td>44</td><td>Mississippi</td><td>28</td><td>0.24%</td></tr>
<tr><td>46</td><td>Vermont</td><td>20</td><td>0.17%</td><td>45</td><td>South Dakota</td><td>24</td><td>0.21%</td></tr>
<tr><td>15</td><td>Virginia</td><td>209</td><td>1.80%</td><td>46</td><td>Hawaii</td><td>20</td><td>0.17%</td></tr>
<tr><td>19</td><td>Washington</td><td>148</td><td>1.27%</td><td>46</td><td>Vermont</td><td>20</td><td>0.17%</td></tr>
<tr><td>35</td><td>West Virginia</td><td>53</td><td>0.46%</td><td>48</td><td>North Dakota</td><td>16</td><td>0.14%</td></tr>
<tr><td>18</td><td>Wisconsin</td><td>180</td><td>1.55%</td><td>49</td><td>Alaska</td><td>15</td><td>0.13%</td></tr>
<tr><td>50</td><td>Wyoming</td><td>10</td><td>0.09%</td><td>50</td><td>Wyoming</td><td>10</td><td>0.09%</td></tr>
<tr><td></td><td></td><td></td><td></td><td></td><td>District of Columbia</td><td>43</td><td>0.37%</td></tr>
</tbody>
</table>

Source: American Podiatric Medical Association, Inc.
   "Podiatric Physicians in Active Practice"
*As of December 1995. Includes only Podiatric physicians considered in "active practice." Podiatry deals with the diagnosis, treatment, and prevention of diseases of the human foot. National total does not include eight podiatrists in Puerto Rico.

Rate of Podiatric Physicians in 1995

National Rate = 4.4 Podiatrists per 100,000 Population*

ALPHA ORDER

RANK ORDER

RANK	STATE	RATE		RANK	STATE	RATE
48	Alabama	1.4		1	New Jersey	9.4
36	Alaska	2.5		2	Connecticut	8.6
14	Arizona	4.6		3	Pennsylvania	8.2
47	Arkansas	1.6		4	Massachusetts	7.1
16	California	4.5		5	Maryland	6.5
30	Colorado	3.1		6	New York	6.3
2	Connecticut	8.6		7	Florida	6.2
9	Delaware	5.2		8	Illinois	5.7
7	Florida	6.2		9	Delaware	5.2
24	Georgia	3.4		9	Iowa	5.2
45	Hawaii	1.7		11	Utah	5.1
21	Idaho	3.8		12	Michigan	4.8
8	Illinois	5.7		12	New Hampshire	4.8
19	Indiana	3.9		14	Arizona	4.6
9	Iowa	5.2		14	Montana	4.6
24	Kansas	3.4		16	California	4.5
43	Kentucky	2.1		17	Maine	4.4
45	Louisiana	1.7		17	Ohio	4.4
17	Maine	4.4		19	Indiana	3.9
5	Maryland	6.5		19	Rhode Island	3.9
4	Massachusetts	7.1		21	Idaho	3.8
12	Michigan	4.8		22	Nevada	3.5
34	Minnesota	2.8		22	Wisconsin	3.5
49	Mississippi	1.0		24	Georgia	3.4
39	Missouri	2.4		24	Kansas	3.4
14	Montana	4.6		24	Nebraska	3.4
24	Nebraska	3.4		24	Vermont	3.4
22	Nevada	3.5		28	South Dakota	3.3
12	New Hampshire	4.8		29	Virginia	3.2
1	New Jersey	9.4		30	Colorado	3.1
41	New Mexico	2.2		30	Oregon	3.1
6	New York	6.3		32	North Carolina	2.9
32	North Carolina	2.9		32	West Virginia	2.9
36	North Dakota	2.5		34	Minnesota	2.8
17	Ohio	4.4		35	Washington	2.7
40	Oklahoma	2.3		36	Alaska	2.5
30	Oregon	3.1		36	North Dakota	2.5
3	Pennsylvania	8.2		36	Tennessee	2.5
19	Rhode Island	3.9		39	Missouri	2.4
49	South Carolina	1.0		40	Oklahoma	2.3
28	South Dakota	3.3		41	New Mexico	2.2
36	Tennessee	2.5		41	Texas	2.2
41	Texas	2.2		43	Kentucky	2.1
11	Utah	5.1		43	Wyoming	2.1
24	Vermont	3.4		45	Hawaii	1.7
29	Virginia	3.2		45	Louisiana	1.7
35	Washington	2.7		47	Arkansas	1.6
32	West Virginia	2.9		48	Alabama	1.4
22	Wisconsin	3.5		49	Mississippi	1.0
43	Wyoming	2.1		49	South Carolina	1.0
					District of Columbia	7.7

*Source: Morgan Quitno Press using data from American Podiatric Medical Association, Inc.
"Podiatric Physicians in Active Practice"*
*Includes only Podiatric physicians considered in "active practice." Podiatry deals with the diagnosis, treatment, and prevention of diseases of the human foot. National rate does not include podiatrists in Puerto Rico.

Doctors of Chiropractic in 1997

National Total = 75,282 Chiropractors*

ALPHA ORDER

RANK	STATE	CHIROPRACTORS	% of USA
28	Alabama	749	0.99%
49	Alaska	179	0.24%
9	Arizona	2,490	3.31%
33	Arkansas	532	0.71%
1	California	11,332	15.05%
11	Colorado	1,970	2.62%
26	Connecticut	869	1.15%
46	Delaware	212	0.28%
3	Florida	4,224	5.61%
10	Georgia	2,474	3.29%
35	Hawaii	502	0.67%
40	Idaho	328	0.44%
7	Illinois	2,835	3.77%
25	Indiana	905	1.20%
21	Iowa	1,363	1.81%
29	Kansas	623	0.83%
23	Kentucky	1,037	1.38%
32	Louisiana	559	0.74%
37	Maine	367	0.49%
34	Maryland	518	0.69%
16	Massachusetts	1,663	2.21%
8	Michigan	2,527	3.36%
17	Minnesota	1,622	2.15%
39	Mississippi	335	0.44%
13	Missouri	1,827	2.43%
44	Montana	256	0.34%
42	Nebraska	296	0.39%
38	Nevada	356	0.47%
36	New Hampshire	497	0.66%
6	New Jersey	3,160	4.20%
30	New Mexico	590	0.78%
2	New York	5,909	7.85%
19	North Carolina	1,399	1.86%
47	North Dakota	201	0.27%
12	Ohio	1,944	2.58%
24	Oklahoma	1,013	1.35%
20	Oregon	1,370	1.82%
5	Pennsylvania	3,490	4.64%
50	Rhode Island	171	0.23%
22	South Carolina	1,139	1.51%
41	South Dakota	324	0.43%
27	Tennessee	778	1.03%
4	Texas	3,960	5.26%
31	Utah	575	0.76%
45	Vermont	246	0.33%
18	Virginia	1,462	1.94%
15	Washington	1,803	2.39%
43	West Virginia	273	0.36%
14	Wisconsin	1,804	2.40%
48	Wyoming	182	0.24%

RANK ORDER

RANK	STATE	CHIROPRACTORS	% of USA
1	California	11,332	15.05%
2	New York	5,909	7.85%
3	Florida	4,224	5.61%
4	Texas	3,960	5.26%
5	Pennsylvania	3,490	4.64%
6	New Jersey	3,160	4.20%
7	Illinois	2,835	3.77%
8	Michigan	2,527	3.36%
9	Arizona	2,490	3.31%
10	Georgia	2,474	3.29%
11	Colorado	1,970	2.62%
12	Ohio	1,944	2.58%
13	Missouri	1,827	2.43%
14	Wisconsin	1,804	2.40%
15	Washington	1,803	2.39%
16	Massachusetts	1,663	2.21%
17	Minnesota	1,622	2.15%
18	Virginia	1,462	1.94%
19	North Carolina	1,399	1.86%
20	Oregon	1,370	1.82%
21	Iowa	1,363	1.81%
22	South Carolina	1,139	1.51%
23	Kentucky	1,037	1.38%
24	Oklahoma	1,013	1.35%
25	Indiana	905	1.20%
26	Connecticut	869	1.15%
27	Tennessee	778	1.03%
28	Alabama	749	0.99%
29	Kansas	623	0.83%
30	New Mexico	590	0.78%
31	Utah	575	0.76%
32	Louisiana	559	0.74%
33	Arkansas	532	0.71%
34	Maryland	518	0.69%
35	Hawaii	502	0.67%
36	New Hampshire	497	0.66%
37	Maine	367	0.49%
38	Nevada	356	0.47%
39	Mississippi	335	0.44%
40	Idaho	328	0.44%
41	South Dakota	324	0.43%
42	Nebraska	296	0.39%
43	West Virginia	273	0.36%
44	Montana	256	0.34%
45	Vermont	246	0.33%
46	Delaware	212	0.28%
47	North Dakota	201	0.27%
48	Wyoming	182	0.24%
49	Alaska	179	0.24%
50	Rhode Island	171	0.23%
	District of Columbia	42	0.06%

Source: Federation of Chiropractic Licensing Boards
"1998-99 Official Directory"

As of December 1997. Licensed active doctors. There is some duplication as some doctors are licensed in more than one state.

Rate of Doctors of Chiropractic in 1997

National Rate = 28 Chiropractors per 100,000 Population*

ALPHA ORDER

RANK	STATE	RATE
42	Alabama	17
23	Alaska	29
1	Arizona	55
37	Arkansas	21
11	California	35
2	Colorado	51
29	Connecticut	27
23	Delaware	29
23	Florida	29
16	Georgia	33
5	Hawaii	42
29	Idaho	27
34	Illinois	24
45	Indiana	15
3	Iowa	48
34	Kansas	24
29	Kentucky	27
48	Louisiana	13
21	Maine	30
50	Maryland	10
29	Massachusetts	27
33	Michigan	26
11	Minnesota	35
49	Mississippi	12
14	Missouri	34
23	Montana	29
41	Nebraska	18
37	Nevada	21
5	New Hampshire	42
9	New Jersey	39
14	New Mexico	34
16	New York	33
40	North Carolina	19
19	North Dakota	31
42	Ohio	17
19	Oklahoma	31
5	Oregon	42
23	Pennsylvania	29
42	Rhode Island	17
21	South Carolina	30
4	South Dakota	44
47	Tennessee	14
39	Texas	20
28	Utah	28
5	Vermont	42
36	Virginia	22
18	Washington	32
45	West Virginia	15
11	Wisconsin	35
10	Wyoming	38

RANK ORDER

RANK	STATE	RATE
1	Arizona	55
2	Colorado	51
3	Iowa	48
4	South Dakota	44
5	Hawaii	42
5	New Hampshire	42
5	Oregon	42
5	Vermont	42
9	New Jersey	39
10	Wyoming	38
11	California	35
11	Minnesota	35
11	Wisconsin	35
14	Missouri	34
14	New Mexico	34
16	Georgia	33
16	New York	33
18	Washington	32
19	North Dakota	31
19	Oklahoma	31
21	Maine	30
21	South Carolina	30
23	Alaska	29
23	Delaware	29
23	Florida	29
23	Montana	29
23	Pennsylvania	29
28	Utah	28
29	Connecticut	27
29	Idaho	27
29	Kentucky	27
29	Massachusetts	27
33	Michigan	26
34	Illinois	24
34	Kansas	24
36	Virginia	22
37	Arkansas	21
37	Nevada	21
39	Texas	20
40	North Carolina	19
41	Nebraska	18
42	Alabama	17
42	Ohio	17
42	Rhode Island	17
45	Indiana	15
45	West Virginia	15
47	Tennessee	14
48	Louisiana	13
49	Mississippi	12
50	Maryland	10

District of Columbia   8

Source: Morgan Quitno Press using data from Federation of Chiropractic Licensing Boards
    "1998-99 Official Directory"

*As of December 1997. Licensed active doctors. There is some duplication as some doctors are licensed in more than one state.

Physician Assistants in Clinical Practice in 1999

National Total = 34,192 Physician Assistants*

RANK	STATE (ALPHA ORDER)	PA's	% of USA		RANK	STATE (RANK ORDER)	PA's	% of USA
38	Alabama	211	0.6%		1	New York	4,211	12.3%
33	Alaska	265	0.8%		2	California	3,561	10.4%
17	Arizona	583	1.7%		3	Texas	2,151	6.3%
50	Arkansas	5	0.0%		4	North Carolina	1,866	5.5%
2	California	3,561	10.4%		5	Florida	1,839	5.4%
12	Colorado	790	2.3%		6	Pennsylvania	1,812	5.3%
14	Connecticut	660	1.9%		7	Michigan	1,281	3.7%
48	Delaware	68	0.2%		8	Georgia	1,194	3.5%
5	Florida	1,839	5.4%		9	Washington	1,086	3.2%
8	Georgia	1,194	3.5%		10	Ohio	1,016	3.0%
46	Hawaii	89	0.3%		11	Maryland	1,013	3.0%
40	Idaho	174	0.5%		12	Colorado	790	2.3%
16	Illinois	637	1.9%		13	Massachusetts	746	2.2%
36	Indiana	225	0.7%		14	Connecticut	660	1.9%
21	Iowa	451	1.3%		15	Wisconsin	652	1.9%
24	Kansas	405	1.2%		16	Illinois	637	1.9%
26	Kentucky	369	1.1%		17	Arizona	583	1.7%
35	Louisiana	233	0.7%		18	Oklahoma	513	1.5%
27	Maine	351	1.0%		19	Virginia	497	1.5%
11	Maryland	1,013	3.0%		20	Minnesota	453	1.3%
13	Massachusetts	746	2.2%		21	Iowa	451	1.3%
7	Michigan	1,281	3.7%		22	Tennessee	414	1.2%
20	Minnesota	453	1.3%		23	West Virginia	408	1.2%
49	Mississippi	34	0.1%		24	Kansas	405	1.2%
32	Missouri	271	0.8%		25	Nebraska	397	1.2%
43	Montana	136	0.4%		26	Kentucky	369	1.1%
25	Nebraska	397	1.2%		27	Maine	351	1.0%
39	Nevada	190	0.6%		28	New Jersey	346	1.0%
42	New Hampshire	167	0.5%		29	New Mexico	331	1.0%
28	New Jersey	346	1.0%		30	Oregon	322	0.9%
29	New Mexico	331	1.0%		31	Utah	311	0.9%
1	New York	4,211	12.3%		32	Missouri	271	0.8%
4	North Carolina	1,866	5.5%		33	Alaska	265	0.8%
40	North Dakota	174	0.5%		34	South Carolina	261	0.8%
10	Ohio	1,016	3.0%		35	Louisiana	233	0.7%
18	Oklahoma	513	1.5%		36	Indiana	225	0.7%
30	Oregon	322	0.9%		37	South Dakota	222	0.6%
6	Pennsylvania	1,812	5.3%		38	Alabama	211	0.6%
44	Rhode Island	127	0.4%		39	Nevada	190	0.6%
34	South Carolina	261	0.8%		40	Idaho	174	0.5%
37	South Dakota	222	0.6%		40	North Dakota	174	0.5%
22	Tennessee	414	1.2%		42	New Hampshire	167	0.5%
3	Texas	2,151	6.3%		43	Montana	136	0.4%
31	Utah	311	0.9%		44	Rhode Island	127	0.4%
45	Vermont	101	0.3%		45	Vermont	101	0.3%
19	Virginia	497	1.5%		46	Hawaii	89	0.3%
9	Washington	1,086	3.2%		46	Wyoming	89	0.3%
23	West Virginia	408	1.2%		48	Delaware	68	0.2%
15	Wisconsin	652	1.9%		49	Mississippi	34	0.1%
46	Wyoming	89	0.3%		50	Arkansas	5	0.0%
						District of Columbia	199	0.6%

Source: The American Academy of Physician Assistants
   "Projected Number of PAs in Clinical Practice as of January 1, 1999" (Information Update, October 20, 1998)
*Projected.

Rate of Physician Assistants in Clinical Practice in 1999

National Rate = 12.6 PA's per 100,000 Population*

ALPHA ORDER

RANK	STATE	RATE
46	Alabama	4.8
1	Alaska	43.2
27	Arizona	12.5
50	Arkansas	0.2
31	California	10.9
10	Colorado	19.9
9	Connecticut	20.2
37	Delaware	9.1
29	Florida	12.3
17	Georgia	15.6
40	Hawaii	7.5
23	Idaho	14.2
43	Illinois	5.3
48	Indiana	3.8
16	Iowa	15.8
18	Kansas	15.4
36	Kentucky	9.4
43	Louisiana	5.3
3	Maine	28.2
11	Maryland	19.7
30	Massachusetts	12.1
25	Michigan	13.0
35	Minnesota	9.6
49	Mississippi	1.2
45	Missouri	5.0
18	Montana	15.4
6	Nebraska	23.9
31	Nevada	10.9
24	New Hampshire	14.1
47	New Jersey	4.3
12	New Mexico	19.1
7	New York	23.2
5	North Carolina	24.7
4	North Dakota	27.3
37	Ohio	9.1
20	Oklahoma	15.3
34	Oregon	9.8
21	Pennsylvania	15.1
26	Rhode Island	12.8
42	South Carolina	6.8
2	South Dakota	30.1
39	Tennessee	7.6
31	Texas	10.9
22	Utah	14.8
15	Vermont	17.1
41	Virginia	7.3
12	Washington	19.1
8	West Virginia	22.5
27	Wisconsin	12.5
14	Wyoming	18.5

RANK ORDER

RANK	STATE	RATE
1	Alaska	43.2
2	South Dakota	30.1
3	Maine	28.2
4	North Dakota	27.3
5	North Carolina	24.7
6	Nebraska	23.9
7	New York	23.2
8	West Virginia	22.5
9	Connecticut	20.2
10	Colorado	19.9
11	Maryland	19.7
12	New Mexico	19.1
12	Washington	19.1
14	Wyoming	18.5
15	Vermont	17.1
16	Iowa	15.8
17	Georgia	15.6
18	Kansas	15.4
18	Montana	15.4
20	Oklahoma	15.3
21	Pennsylvania	15.1
22	Utah	14.8
23	Idaho	14.2
24	New Hampshire	14.1
25	Michigan	13.0
26	Rhode Island	12.8
27	Arizona	12.5
27	Wisconsin	12.5
29	Florida	12.3
30	Massachusetts	12.1
31	California	10.9
31	Nevada	10.9
31	Texas	10.9
34	Oregon	9.8
35	Minnesota	9.6
36	Kentucky	9.4
37	Delaware	9.1
37	Ohio	9.1
39	Tennessee	7.6
40	Hawaii	7.5
41	Virginia	7.3
42	South Carolina	6.8
43	Illinois	5.3
43	Louisiana	5.3
45	Missouri	5.0
46	Alabama	4.8
47	New Jersey	4.3
48	Indiana	3.8
49	Mississippi	1.2
50	Arkansas	0.2

| | District of Columbia | 38.0 |

Source: Morgan Quitno Press using data from The American Academy of Physician Assistants
"Projected Number of PAs in Clinical Practice as of January 1, 1999" (Information Update, October 20, 1998)
*Projected. Rates calculated using 1998 Census population estimates.

Registered Nurses in 1996

National Total = 2,161,700 Registered Nurses*

<u>ALPHA ORDER</u>

RANK	STATE	NURSES	% of USA
23	Alabama	32,800	1.5%
48	Alaska	6,300	0.3%
22	Arizona	33,200	1.5%
33	Arkansas	17,900	0.8%
1	California	179,700	8.3%
25	Colorado	30,900	1.4%
21	Connecticut	33,400	1.5%
43	Delaware	7,700	0.4%
5	Florida	119,300	5.5%
13	Georgia	53,600	2.5%
42	Hawaii	8,900	0.4%
45	Idaho	7,100	0.3%
6	Illinois	104,700	4.8%
15	Indiana	46,900	2.2%
27	Iowa	29,100	1.3%
30	Kansas	21,600	1.0%
26	Kentucky	30,400	1.4%
24	Louisiana	32,400	1.5%
36	Maine	13,300	0.6%
20	Maryland	43,000	2.0%
9	Massachusetts	73,300	3.4%
8	Michigan	79,600	3.7%
17	Minnesota	46,200	2.1%
31	Mississippi	19,900	0.9%
14	Missouri	51,200	2.4%
45	Montana	7,100	0.3%
34	Nebraska	15,200	0.7%
41	Nevada	9,900	0.5%
40	New Hampshire	11,200	0.5%
10	New Jersey	67,100	3.1%
38	New Mexico	11,700	0.5%
2	New York	167,600	7.8%
11	North Carolina	62,000	2.9%
47	North Dakota	7,000	0.3%
7	Ohio	101,200	4.7%
32	Oklahoma	19,600	0.9%
29	Oregon	26,500	1.2%
3	Pennsylvania	126,300	5.8%
39	Rhode Island	11,400	0.5%
28	South Carolina	27,400	1.3%
43	South Dakota	7,700	0.4%
16	Tennessee	46,400	2.1%
4	Texas	124,200	5.7%
37	Utah	13,000	0.6%
49	Vermont	5,300	0.2%
12	Virginia	54,400	2.5%
19	Washington	43,500	2.0%
35	West Virginia	15,000	0.7%
18	Wisconsin	45,600	2.1%
50	Wyoming	4,200	0.2%

<u>RANK ORDER</u>

RANK	STATE	NURSES	% of USA
1	California	179,700	8.3%
2	New York	167,600	7.8%
3	Pennsylvania	126,300	5.8%
4	Texas	124,200	5.7%
5	Florida	119,300	5.5%
6	Illinois	104,700	4.8%
7	Ohio	101,200	4.7%
8	Michigan	79,600	3.7%
9	Massachusetts	73,300	3.4%
10	New Jersey	67,100	3.1%
11	North Carolina	62,000	2.9%
12	Virginia	54,400	2.5%
13	Georgia	53,600	2.5%
14	Missouri	51,200	2.4%
15	Indiana	46,900	2.2%
16	Tennessee	46,400	2.1%
17	Minnesota	46,200	2.1%
18	Wisconsin	45,600	2.1%
19	Washington	43,500	2.0%
20	Maryland	43,000	2.0%
21	Connecticut	33,400	1.5%
22	Arizona	33,200	1.5%
23	Alabama	32,800	1.5%
24	Louisiana	32,400	1.5%
25	Colorado	30,900	1.4%
26	Kentucky	30,400	1.4%
27	Iowa	29,100	1.3%
28	South Carolina	27,400	1.3%
29	Oregon	26,500	1.2%
30	Kansas	21,600	1.0%
31	Mississippi	19,900	0.9%
32	Oklahoma	19,600	0.9%
33	Arkansas	17,900	0.8%
34	Nebraska	15,200	0.7%
35	West Virginia	15,000	0.7%
36	Maine	13,300	0.6%
37	Utah	13,000	0.6%
38	New Mexico	11,700	0.5%
39	Rhode Island	11,400	0.5%
40	New Hampshire	11,200	0.5%
41	Nevada	9,900	0.5%
42	Hawaii	8,900	0.4%
43	Delaware	7,700	0.4%
43	South Dakota	7,700	0.4%
45	Idaho	7,100	0.3%
45	Montana	7,100	0.3%
47	North Dakota	7,000	0.3%
48	Alaska	6,300	0.3%
49	Vermont	5,300	0.2%
50	Wyoming	4,200	0.2%
	District of Columbia	8,900	0.4%

*Source: U.S. Department of Health and Human Services, Health Resources and Services Administration
    unpublished data*
As of December 1996.

Rate of Registered Nurses in 1996

National Rate = 815 Nurses per 100,000 Population*

ALPHA ORDER

RANK ORDER

RANK	STATE	RATE		RANK	STATE	RATE
36	Alabama	764		1	Massachusetts	1,205
8	Alaska	1,041		2	Rhode Island	1,154
38	Arizona	749		3	North Dakota	1,089
43	Arkansas	715		4	Maine	1,074
50	California	566		5	Delaware	1,059
31	Colorado	810		6	Pennsylvania	1,050
9	Connecticut	1,023		7	South Dakota	1,044
5	Delaware	1,059		8	Alaska	1,041
27	Florida	827		9	Connecticut	1,023
42	Georgia	731		10	Iowa	1,022
37	Hawaii	750		11	Minnesota	994
48	Idaho	599		12	New Hampshire	966
19	Illinois	877		13	Missouri	954
33	Indiana	805		14	New York	924
10	Iowa	1,022		15	Nebraska	922
25	Kansas	836		16	Ohio	906
35	Kentucky	783		17	Vermont	904
39	Louisiana	747		18	Wisconsin	881
4	Maine	1,074		19	Illinois	877
22	Maryland	850		20	Wyoming	875
1	Massachusetts	1,205		21	Tennessee	874
29	Michigan	818		22	Maryland	850
11	Minnesota	994		23	North Carolina	848
40	Mississippi	734		24	New Jersey	838
13	Missouri	954		25	Kansas	836
31	Montana	810		26	Oregon	829
15	Nebraska	922		27	Florida	827
47	Nevada	619		28	West Virginia	824
12	New Hampshire	966		29	Michigan	818
24	New Jersey	838		30	Virginia	816
44	New Mexico	685		31	Colorado	810
14	New York	924		31	Montana	810
23	North Carolina	848		33	Indiana	805
3	North Dakota	1,089		34	Washington	788
16	Ohio	906		35	Kentucky	783
49	Oklahoma	595		36	Alabama	764
26	Oregon	829		37	Hawaii	750
6	Pennsylvania	1,050		38	Arizona	749
2	Rhode Island	1,154		39	Louisiana	747
41	South Carolina	733		40	Mississippi	734
7	South Dakota	1,044		41	South Carolina	733
21	Tennessee	874		42	Georgia	731
45	Texas	653		43	Arkansas	715
46	Utah	643		44	New Mexico	685
17	Vermont	904		45	Texas	653
30	Virginia	816		46	Utah	643
34	Washington	788		47	Nevada	619
28	West Virginia	824		48	Idaho	599
18	Wisconsin	881		49	Oklahoma	595
20	Wyoming	875		50	California	566

District of Columbia   1,649

Source: Morgan Quitno Press using data from U.S. Dept. of Health & Human Services, Health Resources/Services Admn. unpublished data

*As of December 1996. Calculated with updated Census population estimates for July 1, 1996.

Dentists in 1997

National Total = 160,529 Dentists*

ALPHA ORDER

RANK	STATE	DENTISTS	% of USA		RANK	STATE	DENTISTS	% of USA
27	Alabama	1,697	1.06%		1	California	20,676	12.88%
45	Alaska	338	0.21%		2	New York	12,864	8.01%
26	Arizona	1,878	1.17%		3	Texas	8,078	5.03%
34	Arkansas	995	0.62%		4	Illinois	7,559	4.71%
1	California	20,676	12.88%		5	Pennsylvania	7,259	4.52%
19	Colorado	2,501	1.56%		6	Florida	6,740	4.20%
22	Connecticut	2,378	1.48%		7	New Jersey	5,826	3.63%
48	Delaware	301	0.19%		8	Michigan	5,736	3.57%
6	Florida	6,740	4.20%		9	Ohio	5,662	3.53%
14	Georgia	3,024	1.88%		10	Massachusetts	4,462	2.78%
36	Hawaii	902	0.56%		11	Virginia	3,380	2.07%
40	Idaho	612	0.38%		12	Washington	3,263	2.03%
4	Illinois	7,559	4.71%		13	Maryland	3,136	1.95%
18	Indiana	2,683	1.67%		14	Georgia	3,024	1.88%
30	Iowa	1,424	0.89%		15	Wisconsin	2,889	1.80%
32	Kansas	1,204	0.75%		16	North Carolina	2,815	1.75%
25	Kentucky	1,912	1.19%		17	Minnesota	2,787	1.74%
24	Louisiana	1,920	1.20%		18	Indiana	2,683	1.67%
41	Maine	586	0.37%		19	Colorado	2,501	1.56%
13	Maryland	3,136	1.95%		20	Tennessee	2,492	1.55%
10	Massachusetts	4,462	2.78%		21	Missouri	2,461	1.53%
8	Michigan	5,736	3.57%		22	Connecticut	2,378	1.48%
17	Minnesota	2,787	1.74%		23	Oregon	2,049	1.28%
35	Mississippi	986	0.61%		24	Louisiana	1,920	1.20%
21	Missouri	2,461	1.53%		25	Kentucky	1,912	1.19%
44	Montana	449	0.28%		26	Arizona	1,878	1.17%
33	Nebraska	997	0.62%		27	Alabama	1,697	1.06%
41	Nevada	586	0.37%		28	Oklahoma	1,483	0.92%
38	New Hampshire	664	0.41%		29	South Carolina	1,459	0.91%
7	New Jersey	5,826	3.63%		30	Iowa	1,424	0.89%
39	New Mexico	645	0.40%		31	Utah	1,237	0.77%
2	New York	12,864	8.01%		32	Kansas	1,204	0.75%
16	North Carolina	2,815	1.75%		33	Nebraska	997	0.62%
49	North Dakota	285	0.18%		34	Arkansas	995	0.62%
9	Ohio	5,662	3.53%		35	Mississippi	986	0.61%
28	Oklahoma	1,483	0.92%		36	Hawaii	902	0.56%
23	Oregon	2,049	1.28%		37	West Virginia	765	0.48%
5	Pennsylvania	7,259	4.52%		38	New Hampshire	664	0.41%
43	Rhode Island	544	0.34%		39	New Mexico	645	0.40%
29	South Carolina	1,459	0.91%		40	Idaho	612	0.38%
47	South Dakota	310	0.19%		41	Maine	586	0.37%
20	Tennessee	2,492	1.55%		41	Nevada	586	0.37%
3	Texas	8,078	5.03%		43	Rhode Island	544	0.34%
31	Utah	1,237	0.77%		44	Montana	449	0.28%
46	Vermont	328	0.20%		45	Alaska	338	0.21%
11	Virginia	3,330	2.07%		46	Vermont	328	0.20%
12	Washington	3,263	2.03%		47	South Dakota	310	0.19%
37	West Virginia	765	0.48%		48	Delaware	301	0.19%
15	Wisconsin	2,889	1.80%		49	North Dakota	285	0.18%
50	Wyoming	235	0.15%		50	Wyoming	235	0.15%
						District of Columbia	583	0.36%

Source: American Dental Association
   "1997 ADA Dentist Masterfile"
*National total includes 14,534 dentists working for the military, Public Health Service or whose address is unknown. These are not distributed among the states. Does not include 4,411 dental graduate students.

Rate of Dentists in 1997

National Rate = 60 Dentists per 100,000 Population*

ALPHA ORDER			RANK ORDER		
RANK	STATE	RATE	RANK	STATE	RATE
44	Alabama	39	1	Hawaii	76
20	Alaska	55	2	Connecticut	73
41	Arizona	41	2	Massachusetts	73
44	Arkansas	39	4	New Jersey	72
6	California	64	5	New York	71
6	Colorado	64	6	California	64
2	Connecticut	73	6	Colorado	64
41	Delaware	41	6	Illinois	64
30	Florida	46	9	Oregon	63
43	Georgia	40	10	Maryland	62
1	Hawaii	76	11	Nebraska	60
22	Idaho	51	11	Pennsylvania	60
6	Illinois	64	11	Utah	60
30	Indiana	46	14	Michigan	59
25	Iowa	50	14	Minnesota	59
30	Kansas	46	16	Washington	58
26	Kentucky	49	17	New Hampshire	57
36	Louisiana	44	18	Vermont	56
29	Maine	47	18	Wisconsin	56
10	Maryland	62	20	Alaska	55
2	Massachusetts	73	20	Rhode Island	55
14	Michigan	59	22	Idaho	51
14	Minnesota	59	22	Montana	51
49	Mississippi	36	22	Ohio	51
30	Missouri	46	25	Iowa	50
22	Montana	51	26	Kentucky	49
11	Nebraska	60	26	Virginia	49
50	Nevada	35	26	Wyoming	49
17	New Hampshire	57	29	Maine	47
4	New Jersey	72	30	Florida	46
48	New Mexico	37	30	Indiana	46
5	New York	71	30	Kansas	46
47	North Carolina	38	30	Missouri	46
36	North Dakota	44	30	Tennessee	46
22	Ohio	51	35	Oklahoma	45
35	Oklahoma	45	36	Louisiana	44
9	Oregon	63	36	North Dakota	44
11	Pennsylvania	60	38	South Dakota	42
20	Rhode Island	55	38	Texas	42
44	South Carolina	39	38	West Virginia	42
38	South Dakota	42	41	Arizona	41
30	Tennessee	46	41	Delaware	41
38	Texas	42	43	Georgia	40
11	Utah	60	44	Alabama	39
18	Vermont	56	44	Arkansas	39
26	Virginia	49	44	South Carolina	39
16	Washington	58	47	North Carolina	38
38	West Virginia	42	48	New Mexico	37
18	Wisconsin	56	49	Mississippi	36
26	Wyoming	49	50	Nevada	35
				District of Columbia	110

Source: Morgan Quitno Press using data from American Dental Association
"1997 ADA Dentist Masterfile"
*National total includes dentists working for the military, Public Health Service or whose address is unknown.
These are not distributed among the states. Does not include dental graduate students.

485

Percent of Population Lacking Access to Dental Care in 1998

National Percent = 5.1% of Population*

ALPHA ORDER

RANK	STATE	PERCENT
11	Alabama	8.5
48	Alaska	0.0
27	Arizona	4.0
25	Arkansas	4.3
28	California	3.7
24	Colorado	4.4
21	Connecticut	4.6
14	Delaware	7.9
23	Florida	4.5
21	Georgia	4.6
30	Hawaii	3.3
5	Idaho	14.3
41	Illinois	1.8
33	Indiana	2.6
43	Iowa	1.3
29	Kansas	3.4
26	Kentucky	4.2
17	Louisiana	6.2
13	Maine	8.3
40	Maryland	1.9
42	Massachusetts	1.6
7	Michigan	12.3
47	Minnesota	0.2
6	Mississippi	12.6
35	Missouri	2.3
48	Montana	0.0
32	Nebraska	2.7
4	Nevada	14.6
48	New Hampshire	0.0
43	New Jersey	1.3
1	New Mexico	17.8
18	New York	6.0
36	North Carolina	2.2
19	North Dakota	5.4
39	Ohio	2.0
20	Oklahoma	4.9
3	Oregon	15.8
30	Pennsylvania	3.3
11	Rhode Island	8.5
8	South Carolina	9.4
16	South Dakota	6.5
2	Tennessee	17.2
9	Texas	8.7
15	Utah	7.5
43	Vermont	1.3
36	Virginia	2.2
9	Washington	8.7
34	West Virginia	2.4
36	Wisconsin	2.2
46	Wyoming	0.5

RANK ORDER

RANK	STATE	PERCENT
1	New Mexico	17.8
2	Tennessee	17.2
3	Oregon	15.8
4	Nevada	14.6
5	Idaho	14.3
6	Mississippi	12.6
7	Michigan	12.3
8	South Carolina	9.4
9	Texas	8.7
9	Washington	8.7
11	Alabama	8.5
11	Rhode Island	8.5
13	Maine	8.3
14	Delaware	7.9
15	Utah	7.5
16	South Dakota	6.5
17	Louisiana	6.2
18	New York	6.0
19	North Dakota	5.4
20	Oklahoma	4.9
21	Connecticut	4.6
21	Georgia	4.6
23	Florida	4.5
24	Colorado	4.4
25	Arkansas	4.3
26	Kentucky	4.2
27	Arizona	4.0
28	California	3.7
29	Kansas	3.4
30	Hawaii	3.3
30	Pennsylvania	3.3
32	Nebraska	2.7
33	Indiana	2.6
34	West Virginia	2.4
35	Missouri	2.3
36	North Carolina	2.2
36	Virginia	2.2
36	Wisconsin	2.2
39	Ohio	2.0
40	Maryland	1.9
41	Illinois	1.8
42	Massachusetts	1.6
43	Iowa	1.3
43	New Jersey	1.3
43	Vermont	1.3
46	Wyoming	0.5
47	Minnesota	0.2
48	Alaska	0.0
48	Montana	0.0
48	New Hampshire	0.0

District of Columbia   1.2

Source: Morgan Quitno Press using data from U.S. Dept. of Health and Human Services, Div. of Shortage Designation
"Selected Statistics on Health Manpower Shortage Areas, As of September 30, 1998"
*Percent of population considered under-served by dental practitioners. An under-served population does not have primary medical care within reasonable economic and geographic bounds.

Employment in Health Services Industries in 1996

National Total = 10,990,227 Employees*

ALPHA ORDER

RANK	STATE	EMPLOYEES	% of USA		RANK	STATE	EMPLOYEES	% of USA
22	Alabama	177,626	1.6%		1	California	1,017,633	9.3%
49	Alaska	18,385	0.2%		2	New York	925,424	8.4%
25	Arizona	143,116	1.3%		3	Texas	728,886	6.6%
32	Arkansas	101,222	0.9%		4	Florida	615,332	5.6%
1	California	1,017,633	9.3%		5	Pennsylvania	583,827	5.3%
26	Colorado	139,845	1.3%		6	Ohio	515,760	4.7%
23	Connecticut	171,166	1.6%		7	Illinois	482,723	4.4%
47	Delaware	31,179	0.3%		8	Michigan	392,117	3.6%
4	Florida	615,332	5.6%		9	Massachusetts	360,073	3.3%
12	Georgia	278,939	2.5%		10	New Jersey	338,822	3.1%
43	Hawaii	37,791	0.3%		11	North Carolina	280,037	2.5%
42	Idaho	38,857	0.4%		12	Georgia	278,939	2.5%
7	Illinois	482,723	4.4%		13	Indiana	252,306	2.3%
13	Indiana	252,306	2.3%		14	Missouri	252,233	2.3%
28	Iowa	136,694	1.2%		15	Minnesota	235,553	2.1%
29	Kansas	124,149	1.1%		16	Tennessee	234,431	2.1%
24	Kentucky	162,358	1.5%		17	Wisconsin	229,839	2.1%
19	Louisiana	208,862	1.9%		18	Virginia	225,766	2.1%
37	Maine	59,259	0.5%		19	Louisiana	208,862	1.9%
20	Maryland	205,887	1.9%		20	Maryland	205,887	1.9%
9	Massachusetts	360,073	3.3%		21	Washington	201,237	1.8%
8	Michigan	392,117	3.6%		22	Alabama	177,626	1.6%
15	Minnesota	235,553	2.1%		23	Connecticut	171,166	1.6%
33	Mississippi	100,696	0.9%		24	Kentucky	162,358	1.5%
14	Missouri	252,233	2.3%		25	Arizona	143,116	1.3%
46	Montana	33,586	0.3%		26	Colorado	139,845	1.3%
35	Nebraska	73,201	0.7%		27	Oklahoma	138,056	1.3%
41	Nevada	45,771	0.4%		28	Iowa	136,694	1.2%
40	New Hampshire	48,928	0.4%		29	Kansas	124,149	1.1%
10	New Jersey	338,822	3.1%		30	South Carolina	123,250	1.1%
38	New Mexico	58,370	0.5%		31	Oregon	109,363	1.0%
2	New York	925,424	8.4%		32	Arkansas	101,222	0.9%
11	North Carolina	280,037	2.5%		33	Mississippi	100,696	0.9%
45	North Dakota	34,995	0.3%		34	West Virginia	76,059	0.7%
6	Ohio	515,760	4.7%		35	Nebraska	73,201	0.7%
27	Oklahoma	138,056	1.3%		36	Utah	67,638	0.6%
31	Oregon	109,363	1.0%		37	Maine	59,259	0.5%
5	Pennsylvania	583,827	5.3%		38	New Mexico	58,370	0.5%
39	Rhode Island	51,706	0.5%		39	Rhode Island	51,706	0.5%
30	South Carolina	123,250	1.1%		40	New Hampshire	48,928	0.4%
44	South Dakota	37,582	0.3%		41	Nevada	45,771	0.4%
16	Tennessee	234,431	2.1%		42	Idaho	38,857	0.4%
3	Texas	728,886	6.6%		43	Hawaii	37,791	0.3%
36	Utah	67,638	0.6%		44	South Dakota	37,582	0.3%
48	Vermont	21,564	0.2%		45	North Dakota	34,995	0.3%
18	Virginia	225,766	2.1%		46	Montana	33,586	0.3%
21	Washington	201,237	1.8%		47	Delaware	31,179	0.3%
34	West Virginia	76,059	0.7%		48	Vermont	21,564	0.2%
17	Wisconsin	229,839	2.1%		49	Alaska	18,385	0.2%
50	Wyoming	16,732	0.2%		50	Wyoming	16,732	0.2%
						District of Columbia	45,396	0.4%

Source: U.S. Bureau of the Census
"1996 County Business Patterns"
Total of employment in 1996 at establishments classified in Standard Industrial Classification (S.I.C.) code 8000.
An establishment is a single physical location at which business is conducted or where services or industrial operations are performed. It is not necessarily identical with a company or enterprise, which may consist of one establishment or more.

VII. PHYSICAL FITNESS

Users of Exercise Equipment in 1997

National Total = 47,868,000 Users

ALPHA ORDER

RANK	STATE	USERS	% of USA
26	Alabama	633,000	1.3%
NA	Alaska*	NA	NA
20	Arizona	836,000	1.7%
33	Arkansas	424,000	0.9%
1	California	6,208,000	13.0%
21	Colorado	788,000	1.6%
32	Connecticut	480,000	1.0%
46	Delaware	84,000	0.2%
4	Florida	2,478,000	5.2%
11	Georgia	1,344,000	2.8%
NA	Hawaii*	NA	NA
38	Idaho	265,000	0.6%
5	Illinois	2,397,000	5.0%
12	Indiana	1,161,000	2.4%
25	Iowa	657,000	1.4%
35	Kansas	310,000	0.6%
19	Kentucky	882,000	1.8%
23	Louisiana	678,000	1.4%
36	Maine	282,000	0.6%
16	Maryland	996,000	2.1%
17	Massachusetts	968,000	2.0%
6	Michigan	2,247,000	4.7%
27	Minnesota	600,000	1.3%
37	Mississippi	276,000	0.6%
15	Missouri	1,010,000	2.1%
47	Montana	81,000	0.2%
39	Nebraska	255,000	0.5%
34	Nevada	372,000	0.8%
43	New Hampshire	122,000	0.3%
9	New Jersey	1,381,000	2.9%
40	New Mexico	182,000	0.4%
2	New York	3,484,000	7.3%
14	North Carolina	1,150,000	2.4%
41	North Dakota	161,000	0.3%
7	Ohio	1,983,000	4.1%
29	Oklahoma	548,000	1.1%
24	Oregon	658,000	1.4%
8	Pennsylvania	1,962,000	4.1%
48	Rhode Island	44,000	0.1%
31	South Carolina	504,000	1.1%
42	South Dakota	129,000	0.3%
22	Tennessee	691,000	1.4%
3	Texas	3,297,000	6.9%
28	Utah	567,000	1.2%
45	Vermont	108,000	0.2%
10	Virginia	1,345,000	2.8%
13	Washington	1,160,000	2.4%
30	West Virginia	534,000	1.1%
18	Wisconsin	919,000	1.9%
44	Wyoming	113,000	0.2%

RANK ORDER

RANK	STATE	USERS	% of USA
1	California	6,208,000	13.0%
2	New York	3,484,000	7.3%
3	Texas	3,297,000	6.9%
4	Florida	2,478,000	5.2%
5	Illinois	2,397,000	5.0%
6	Michigan	2,247,000	4.7%
7	Ohio	1,983,000	4.1%
8	Pennsylvania	1,962,000	4.1%
9	New Jersey	1,381,000	2.9%
10	Virginia	1,345,000	2.8%
11	Georgia	1,344,000	2.8%
12	Indiana	1,161,000	2.4%
13	Washington	1,160,000	2.4%
14	North Carolina	1,150,000	2.4%
15	Missouri	1,010,000	2.1%
16	Maryland	996,000	2.1%
17	Massachusetts	968,000	2.0%
18	Wisconsin	919,000	1.9%
19	Kentucky	882,000	1.8%
20	Arizona	836,000	1.7%
21	Colorado	788,000	1.6%
22	Tennessee	691,000	1.4%
23	Louisiana	678,000	1.4%
24	Oregon	658,000	1.4%
25	Iowa	657,000	1.4%
26	Alabama	633,000	1.3%
27	Minnesota	600,000	1.3%
28	Utah	567,000	1.2%
29	Oklahoma	548,000	1.1%
30	West Virginia	534,000	1.1%
31	South Carolina	504,000	1.1%
32	Connecticut	480,000	1.0%
33	Arkansas	424,000	0.9%
34	Nevada	372,000	0.8%
35	Kansas	310,000	0.6%
36	Maine	282,000	0.6%
37	Mississippi	276,000	0.6%
38	Idaho	265,000	0.6%
39	Nebraska	255,000	0.5%
40	New Mexico	182,000	0.4%
41	North Dakota	161,000	0.3%
42	South Dakota	129,000	0.3%
43	New Hampshire	122,000	0.3%
44	Wyoming	113,000	0.2%
45	Vermont	108,000	0.2%
46	Delaware	84,000	0.2%
47	Montana	81,000	0.2%
48	Rhode Island	44,000	0.1%
NA	Alaska*	NA	NA
NA	Hawaii*	NA	NA
	District of Columbia*	NA	NA

Source: The National Sporting Goods Association
"NSGA Sports Participation Survey, January-December 1997 (Copyright 1998, reprinted with permission)
Not available.

Participants in Golf

National Total = 26,216,000 Golfers

ALPHA ORDER				RANK ORDER			
RANK	STATE	GOLFERS	% of USA	RANK	STATE	GOLFERS	% of USA
24	Alabama	368,000	1.4%	1	California	2,937,000	11.2%
NA	Alaska*	NA	NA	2	New York	1,953,000	7.4%
20	Arizona	470,000	1.8%	3	Illinois	1,555,000	5.9%
35	Arkansas	172,000	0.7%	4	Ohio	1,471,000	5.6%
1	California	2,937,000	11.2%	5	Texas	1,380,000	5.3%
22	Colorado	402,000	1.5%	6	Pennsylvania	1,350,000	5.1%
23	Connecticut	390,000	1.5%	7	Michigan	1,225,000	4.7%
46	Delaware	69,000	0.3%	8	Florida	1,196,000	4.6%
8	Florida	1,196,000	4.6%	9	Wisconsin	739,000	2.8%
13	Georgia	658,000	2.5%	10	Massachusetts	727,000	2.8%
NA	Hawaii*	NA	NA	11	North Carolina	690,000	2.6%
34	Idaho	174,000	0.7%	12	Washington	687,000	2.6%
3	Illinois	1,555,000	5.9%	13	Georgia	658,000	2.5%
15	Indiana	601,000	2.3%	14	Missouri	616,000	2.3%
25	Iowa	361,000	1.4%	15	Indiana	601,000	2.3%
37	Kansas	144,000	0.5%	16	Maryland	586,000	2.2%
28	Kentucky	304,000	1.2%	17	New Jersey	584,000	2.2%
32	Louisiana	196,000	0.7%	18	Virginia	518,000	2.0%
39	Maine	137,000	0.5%	19	Minnesota	472,000	1.8%
16	Maryland	586,000	2.2%	20	Arizona	470,000	1.8%
10	Massachusetts	727,000	2.8%	21	South Carolina	438,000	1.7%
7	Michigan	1,225,000	4.7%	22	Colorado	402,000	1.5%
19	Minnesota	472,000	1.8%	23	Connecticut	390,000	1.5%
29	Mississippi	271,000	1.0%	24	Alabama	368,000	1.4%
14	Missouri	616,000	2.3%	25	Iowa	361,000	1.4%
41	Montana	118,000	0.5%	26	Utah	338,000	1.3%
27	Nebraska	336,000	1.3%	27	Nebraska	336,000	1.3%
38	Nevada	142,000	0.5%	28	Kentucky	304,000	1.2%
48	New Hampshire	43,000	0.2%	29	Mississippi	271,000	1.0%
17	New Jersey	584,000	2.2%	30	Oregon	245,000	0.9%
42	New Mexico	114,000	0.4%	31	Tennessee	237,000	0.9%
2	New York	1,953,000	7.4%	32	Louisiana	196,000	0.7%
11	North Carolina	690,000	2.6%	33	North Dakota	176,000	0.7%
33	North Dakota	176,000	0.7%	34	Idaho	174,000	0.7%
4	Ohio	1,471,000	5.6%	35	Arkansas	172,000	0.7%
36	Oklahoma	162,000	0.6%	36	Oklahoma	162,000	0.6%
30	Oregon	245,000	0.9%	37	Kansas	144,000	0.5%
6	Pennsylvania	1,350,000	5.1%	38	Nevada	142,000	0.5%
45	Rhode Island	80,000	0.3%	39	Maine	137,000	0.5%
21	South Carolina	438,000	1.7%	40	West Virginia	136,000	0.5%
44	South Dakota	81,000	0.3%	41	Montana	118,000	0.5%
31	Tennessee	237,000	0.9%	42	New Mexico	114,000	0.4%
5	Texas	1,380,000	5.3%	43	Wyoming	95,000	0.4%
26	Utah	338,000	1.3%	44	South Dakota	81,000	0.3%
47	Vermont	48,000	0.2%	45	Rhode Island	80,000	0.3%
18	Virginia	518,000	2.0%	46	Delaware	69,000	0.3%
12	Washington	687,000	2.6%	47	Vermont	48,000	0.2%
40	West Virginia	136,000	0.5%	48	New Hampshire	43,000	0.2%
9	Wisconsin	739,000	2.8%	NA	Alaska*	NA	NA
43	Wyoming	95,000	0.4%	NA	Hawaii*	NA	NA
					District of Columbia*	NA	NA

Source: The National Sporting Goods Association
"NSGA Sports Participation Survey, January-December 1997 (Copyright 1998, reprinted with permission)
*Not available.

Participants in Running/Jogging in 1997

National Total = 21,688,000 Runners/Joggers

ALPHA ORDER				RANK ORDER			
RANK	STATE	RUNNERS	% of USA	RANK	STATE	RUNNERS	% of USA
21	Alabama	338,000	1.6%	1	California	3,268,000	15.1%
NA	Alaska*	NA	NA	2	New York	1,736,000	8.0%
14	Arizona	474,000	2.2%	3	Texas	1,572,000	7.2%
34	Arkansas	203,000	0.9%	4	Illinois	979,000	4.5%
1	California	3,268,000	15.1%	5	Florida	905,000	4.2%
17	Colorado	402,000	1.9%	6	Pennsylvania	849,000	3.9%
31	Connecticut	232,000	1.1%	7	Virginia	796,000	3.7%
47	Delaware	30,000	0.1%	8	Ohio	768,000	3.5%
5	Florida	905,000	4.2%	9	Georgia	669,000	3.1%
9	Georgia	669,000	3.1%	10	Michigan	619,000	2.9%
NA	Hawaii*	NA	NA	11	New Jersey	575,000	2.7%
36	Idaho	152,000	0.7%	12	North Carolina	557,000	2.6%
4	Illinois	979,000	4.5%	13	Washington	476,000	2.2%
16	Indiana	432,000	2.0%	14	Arizona	474,000	2.2%
25	Iowa	285,000	1.3%	15	Louisiana	455,000	2.1%
37	Kansas	119,000	0.5%	16	Indiana	432,000	2.0%
20	Kentucky	345,000	1.6%	17	Colorado	402,000	1.9%
15	Louisiana	455,000	2.1%	18	Massachusetts	392,000	1.8%
41	Maine	85,000	0.4%	19	Missouri	364,000	1.7%
21	Maryland	338,000	1.6%	20	Kentucky	345,000	1.6%
18	Massachusetts	392,000	1.8%	21	Alabama	338,000	1.6%
10	Michigan	619,000	2.9%	21	Maryland	338,000	1.6%
24	Minnesota	331,000	1.5%	23	South Carolina	336,000	1.5%
42	Mississippi	70,000	0.3%	24	Minnesota	331,000	1.5%
19	Missouri	364,000	1.7%	25	Iowa	285,000	1.3%
44	Montana	64,000	0.3%	26	Utah	274,000	1.3%
33	Nebraska	208,000	1.0%	27	Oklahoma	273,000	1.3%
38	Nevada	112,000	0.5%	27	Tennessee	273,000	1.3%
46	New Hampshire	53,000	0.2%	29	Oregon	241,000	1.1%
11	New Jersey	575,000	2.7%	30	Wisconsin	240,000	1.1%
35	New Mexico	167,000	0.8%	31	Connecticut	232,000	1.1%
2	New York	1,736,000	8.0%	32	West Virginia	221,000	1.0%
12	North Carolina	557,000	2.6%	33	Nebraska	208,000	1.0%
44	North Dakota	64,000	0.3%	34	Arkansas	203,000	0.9%
8	Ohio	768,000	3.5%	35	New Mexico	167,000	0.8%
27	Oklahoma	273,000	1.3%	36	Idaho	152,000	0.7%
29	Oregon	241,000	1.1%	37	Kansas	119,000	0.5%
6	Pennsylvania	849,000	3.9%	38	Nevada	112,000	0.5%
43	Rhode Island	68,000	0.3%	39	Wyoming	109,000	0.5%
23	South Carolina	336,000	1.5%	40	South Dakota	106,000	0.5%
40	South Dakota	106,000	0.5%	41	Maine	85,000	0.4%
27	Tennessee	273,000	1.3%	42	Mississippi	70,000	0.3%
3	Texas	1,572,000	7.2%	43	Rhode Island	68,000	0.3%
26	Utah	274,000	1.3%	44	Montana	64,000	0.3%
48	Vermont	18,000	0.1%	44	North Dakota	64,000	0.3%
7	Virginia	796,000	3.7%	46	New Hampshire	53,000	0.2%
13	Washington	476,000	2.2%	47	Delaware	30,000	0.1%
32	West Virginia	221,000	1.0%	48	Vermont	18,000	0.1%
30	Wisconsin	240,000	1.1%	NA	Alaska*	NA	NA
39	Wyoming	109,000	0.5%	NA	Hawaii*	NA	NA
					District of Columbia*	NA	NA

Source: The National Sporting Goods Association
"NSGA Sports Participation Survey, January-December 1997 (Copyright 1998, reprinted with permission)
Not available.

Participants in Soccer in 1997

National Total = 13,651,000 Soccer Players

RANK	STATE	PARTICIPANTS	% of USA
22	Alabama	195,000	1.4%
NA	Alaska*	NA	NA
25	Arizona	173,000	1.3%
35	Arkansas	84,000	0.6%
1	California	2,020,000	14.8%
20	Colorado	219,000	1.6%
27	Connecticut	152,000	1.1%
NA	Delaware*	NA	NA
6	Florida	575,000	4.2%
18	Georgia	225,000	1.6%
NA	Hawaii*	NA	NA
32	Idaho	112,000	0.8%
5	Illinois	648,000	4.7%
14	Indiana	294,000	2.2%
30	Iowa	136,000	1.0%
38	Kansas	58,000	0.4%
31	Kentucky	119,000	0.9%
28	Louisiana	150,000	1.1%
36	Maine	71,000	0.5%
10	Maryland	427,000	3.1%
15	Massachusetts	291,000	2.1%
9	Michigan	436,000	3.2%
24	Minnesota	175,000	1.3%
33	Mississippi	109,000	0.8%
13	Missouri	332,000	2.4%
NA	Montana*	NA	NA
26	Nebraska	171,000	1.3%
43	Nevada	35,000	0.3%
42	New Hampshire	36,000	0.3%
7	New Jersey	509,000	3.7%
45	New Mexico	23,000	0.2%
2	New York	1,273,000	9.3%
19	North Carolina	221,000	1.6%
46	North Dakota	20,000	0.1%
12	Ohio	360,000	2.6%
23	Oklahoma	181,000	1.3%
29	Oregon	139,000	1.0%
4	Pennsylvania	653,000	4.8%
40	Rhode Island	43,000	0.3%
17	South Carolina	262,000	1.9%
41	South Dakota	40,000	0.3%
37	Tennessee	65,000	0.5%
3	Texas	1,011,000	7.4%
16	Utah	272,000	2.0%
39	Vermont	44,000	0.3%
8	Virginia	501,000	3.7%
11	Washington	383,000	2.8%
33	West Virginia	109,000	0.8%
21	Wisconsin	213,000	1.6%
44	Wyoming	28,000	0.2%

RANK	STATE	PARTICIPANTS	% of USA
1	California	2,020,000	14.8%
2	New York	1,273,000	9.3%
3	Texas	1,011,000	7.4%
4	Pennsylvania	653,000	4.8%
5	Illinois	648,000	4.7%
6	Florida	575,000	4.2%
7	New Jersey	509,000	3.7%
8	Virginia	501,000	3.7%
9	Michigan	436,000	3.2%
10	Maryland	427,000	3.1%
11	Washington	383,000	2.8%
12	Ohio	360,000	2.6%
13	Missouri	332,000	2.4%
14	Indiana	294,000	2.2%
15	Massachusetts	291,000	2.1%
16	Utah	272,000	2.0%
17	South Carolina	262,000	1.9%
18	Georgia	225,000	1.6%
19	North Carolina	221,000	1.6%
20	Colorado	219,000	1.6%
21	Wisconsin	213,000	1.6%
22	Alabama	195,000	1.4%
23	Oklahoma	181,000	1.3%
24	Minnesota	175,000	1.3%
25	Arizona	173,000	1.3%
26	Nebraska	171,000	1.3%
27	Connecticut	152,000	1.1%
28	Louisiana	150,000	1.1%
29	Oregon	139,000	1.0%
30	Iowa	136,000	1.0%
31	Kentucky	119,000	0.9%
32	Idaho	112,000	0.8%
33	Mississippi	109,000	0.8%
33	West Virginia	109,000	0.8%
35	Arkansas	84,000	0.6%
36	Maine	71,000	0.5%
37	Tennessee	65,000	0.5%
38	Kansas	58,000	0.4%
39	Vermont	44,000	0.3%
40	Rhode Island	43,000	0.3%
41	South Dakota	40,000	0.3%
42	New Hampshire	36,000	0.3%
43	Nevada	35,000	0.3%
44	Wyoming	28,000	0.2%
45	New Mexico	23,000	0.2%
46	North Dakota	20,000	0.1%
NA	Alaska*	NA	NA
NA	Delaware*	NA	NA
NA	Hawaii*	NA	NA
NA	Montana*	NA	NA
	District of Columbia*	NA	NA

Source: The National Sporting Goods Association
"NSGA Sports Participation Survey, January-December 1997 (Copyright 1998, reprinted with permission)
*Not available.

Participants in Swimming in 1997

National Total = 59,547,000 Swimmers

ALPHA ORDER

RANK	STATE	SWIMMERS	% of USA
25	Alabama	833,000	1.4%
NA	Alaska*	NA	NA
18	Arizona	1,116,000	1.9%
35	Arkansas	433,000	0.7%
1	California	7,642,000	12.8%
30	Colorado	724,000	1.2%
23	Connecticut	872,000	1.5%
39	Delaware	234,000	0.4%
4	Florida	3,472,000	5.8%
10	Georgia	1,704,000	2.9%
NA	Hawaii*	NA	NA
36	Idaho	403,000	0.7%
6	Illinois	2,514,000	4.2%
14	Indiana	1,371,000	2.3%
31	Iowa	575,000	1.0%
37	Kansas	320,000	0.5%
22	Kentucky	925,000	1.6%
26	Louisiana	822,000	1.4%
40	Maine	228,000	0.4%
17	Maryland	1,173,000	2.0%
15	Massachusetts	1,287,000	2.2%
8	Michigan	2,000,000	3.4%
19	Minnesota	971,000	1.6%
34	Mississippi	465,000	0.8%
13	Missouri	1,397,000	2.3%
48	Montana	84,000	0.1%
33	Nebraska	516,000	0.9%
38	Nevada	317,000	0.5%
44	New Hampshire	130,000	0.2%
9	New Jersey	1,803,000	3.0%
42	New Mexico	183,000	0.3%
2	New York	4,404,000	7.4%
12	North Carolina	1,412,000	2.4%
43	North Dakota	156,000	0.3%
7	Ohio	2,420,000	4.1%
28	Oklahoma	762,000	1.3%
27	Oregon	812,000	1.4%
5	Pennsylvania	3,117,000	5.2%
46	Rhode Island	115,000	0.2%
24	South Carolina	862,000	1.4%
47	South Dakota	110,000	0.2%
16	Tennessee	1,269,000	2.1%
3	Texas	4,351,000	7.3%
29	Utah	742,000	1.2%
45	Vermont	119,000	0.2%
11	Virginia	1,639,000	2.8%
21	Washington	930,000	1.6%
32	West Virginia	569,000	1.0%
20	Wisconsin	935,000	1.6%
41	Wyoming	213,000	0.4%

RANK ORDER

RANK	STATE	SWIMMERS	% of USA
1	California	7,642,000	12.8%
2	New York	4,404,000	7.4%
3	Texas	4,351,000	7.3%
4	Florida	3,472,000	5.8%
5	Pennsylvania	3,117,000	5.2%
6	Illinois	2,514,000	4.2%
7	Ohio	2,420,000	4.1%
8	Michigan	2,000,000	3.4%
9	New Jersey	1,803,000	3.0%
10	Georgia	1,704,000	2.9%
11	Virginia	1,639,000	2.8%
12	North Carolina	1,412,000	2.4%
13	Missouri	1,397,000	2.3%
14	Indiana	1,371,000	2.3%
15	Massachusetts	1,287,000	2.2%
16	Tennessee	1,269,000	2.1%
17	Maryland	1,173,000	2.0%
18	Arizona	1,116,000	1.9%
19	Minnesota	971,000	1.6%
20	Wisconsin	935,000	1.6%
21	Washington	930,000	1.6%
22	Kentucky	925,000	1.6%
23	Connecticut	872,000	1.5%
24	South Carolina	862,000	1.4%
25	Alabama	833,000	1.4%
26	Louisiana	822,000	1.4%
27	Oregon	812,000	1.4%
28	Oklahoma	762,000	1.3%
29	Utah	742,000	1.2%
30	Colorado	724,000	1.2%
31	Iowa	575,000	1.0%
32	West Virginia	569,000	1.0%
33	Nebraska	516,000	0.9%
34	Mississippi	465,000	0.8%
35	Arkansas	433,000	0.7%
36	Idaho	403,000	0.7%
37	Kansas	320,000	0.5%
38	Nevada	317,000	0.5%
39	Delaware	234,000	0.4%
40	Maine	228,000	0.4%
41	Wyoming	213,000	0.4%
42	New Mexico	183,000	0.3%
43	North Dakota	156,000	0.3%
44	New Hampshire	130,000	0.2%
45	Vermont	119,000	0.2%
46	Rhode Island	115,000	0.2%
47	South Dakota	110,000	0.2%
48	Montana	84,000	0.1%
NA	Alaska*	NA	NA
NA	Hawaii*	NA	NA
	District of Columbia*	NA	NA

Source: The National Sporting Goods Association
   "NSGA Sports Participation Survey, January-December 1997 (Copyright 1998, reprinted with permission)
Not available.

Participants in Tennis in 1997

National Total = 11,106,000 Tennis Players

ALPHA ORDER

RANK	STATE	PLAYERS	% of USA
21	Alabama	173,000	1.6%
NA	Alaska*	NA	NA
30	Arizona	102,000	0.9%
33	Arkansas	65,000	0.6%
1	California	1,527,000	13.7%
25	Colorado	138,000	1.2%
26	Connecticut	125,000	1.1%
39	Delaware	27,000	0.2%
4	Florida	620,000	5.6%
10	Georgia	327,000	2.9%
NA	Hawaii*	NA	NA
18	Idaho	218,000	2.0%
7	Illinois	514,000	4.6%
19	Indiana	217,000	2.0%
24	Iowa	141,000	1.3%
36	Kansas	44,000	0.4%
17	Kentucky	224,000	2.0%
29	Louisiana	104,000	0.9%
44	Maine	13,000	0.1%
11	Maryland	310,000	2.8%
14	Massachusetts	258,000	2.3%
13	Michigan	290,000	2.6%
16	Minnesota	236,000	2.1%
31	Mississippi	72,000	0.6%
9	Missouri	352,000	3.2%
45	Montana	12,000	0.1%
40	Nebraska	26,000	0.2%
41	Nevada	23,000	0.2%
42	New Hampshire	21,000	0.2%
15	New Jersey	251,000	2.3%
NA	New Mexico*	NA	NA
2	New York	923,000	8.3%
12	North Carolina	304,000	2.7%
32	North Dakota	66,000	0.6%
6	Ohio	573,000	5.2%
35	Oklahoma	46,000	0.4%
27	Oregon	120,000	1.1%
8	Pennsylvania	501,000	4.5%
NA	Rhode Island*	NA	NA
23	South Carolina	159,000	1.4%
37	South Dakota	40,000	0.4%
22	Tennessee	164,000	1.5%
3	Texas	750,000	6.8%
38	Utah	30,000	0.3%
NA	Vermont*	NA	NA
5	Virginia	602,000	5.4%
28	Washington	113,000	1.0%
34	West Virginia	63,000	0.6%
20	Wisconsin	188,000	1.7%
43	Wyoming	18,000	0.2%

RANK ORDER

RANK	STATE	PLAYERS	% of USA
1	California	1,527,000	13.7%
2	New York	923,000	8.3%
3	Texas	750,000	6.8%
4	Florida	620,000	5.6%
5	Virginia	602,000	5.4%
6	Ohio	573,000	5.2%
7	Illinois	514,000	4.6%
8	Pennsylvania	501,000	4.5%
9	Missouri	352,000	3.2%
10	Georgia	327,000	2.9%
11	Maryland	310,000	2.8%
12	North Carolina	304,000	2.7%
13	Michigan	290,000	2.6%
14	Massachusetts	258,000	2.3%
15	New Jersey	251,000	2.3%
16	Minnesota	236,000	2.1%
17	Kentucky	224,000	2.0%
18	Idaho	218,000	2.0%
19	Indiana	217,000	2.0%
20	Wisconsin	188,000	1.7%
21	Alabama	173,000	1.6%
22	Tennessee	164,000	1.5%
23	South Carolina	159,000	1.4%
24	Iowa	141,000	1.3%
25	Colorado	138,000	1.2%
26	Connecticut	125,000	1.1%
27	Oregon	120,000	1.1%
28	Washington	113,000	1.0%
29	Louisiana	104,000	0.9%
30	Arizona	102,000	0.9%
31	Mississippi	72,000	0.6%
32	North Dakota	66,000	0.6%
33	Arkansas	65,000	0.6%
34	West Virginia	63,000	0.6%
35	Oklahoma	46,000	0.4%
36	Kansas	44,000	0.4%
37	South Dakota	40,000	0.4%
38	Utah	30,000	0.3%
39	Delaware	27,000	0.2%
40	Nebraska	26,000	0.2%
41	Nevada	23,000	0.2%
42	New Hampshire	21,000	0.2%
43	Wyoming	18,000	0.2%
44	Maine	13,000	0.1%
45	Montana	12,000	0.1%
NA	Alaska*	NA	NA
NA	Hawaii*	NA	NA
NA	New Mexico*	NA	NA
NA	Rhode Island*	NA	NA
NA	Vermont*	NA	NA
	District of Columbia*	NA	NA

Source: The National Sporting Goods Association
    "NSGA Sports Participation Survey, January-December 1997 (Copyright 1998, reprinted with permission)
*Not available.

Apparent Alcohol Consumption in 1996

National Total = 450,251,000 Gallons*

ALPHA ORDER					RANK ORDER			
RANK	**STATE**	**GALLONS**	**% of USA**		**RANK**	**STATE**	**GALLONS**	**% of USA**
25	Alabama	6,275,000	1.39%		1	California	53,266,000	11.83%
48	Alaska	1,179,000	0.26%		2	Texas	33,277,000	7.39%
16	Arizona	9,072,000	2.01%		3	Florida	29,796,000	6.62%
34	Arkansas	3,531,000	0.78%		4	New York	27,313,000	6.07%
1	California	53,266,000	11.83%		5	Illinois	21,349,000	4.74%
23	Colorado	7,832,000	1.74%		6	Pennsylvania	18,065,000	4.01%
27	Connecticut	5,534,000	1.23%		7	Ohio	17,075,000	3.79%
45	Delaware	1,556,000	0.35%		8	Michigan	15,788,000	3.51%
3	Florida	29,796,000	6.62%		9	New Jersey	13,865,000	3.08%
10	Georgia	12,530,000	2.78%		10	Georgia	12,530,000	2.78%
39	Hawaii	2,196,000	0.49%		11	Massachusetts	11,519,000	2.56%
42	Idaho	1,802,000	0.40%		12	North Carolina	11,260,000	2.50%
5	Illinois	21,349,000	4.74%		13	Wisconsin	10,724,000	2.38%
18	Indiana	8,768,000	1.95%		14	Virginia	10,129,000	2.25%
32	Iowa	4,257,000	0.95%		15	Washington	9,241,000	2.05%
35	Kansas	3,439,000	0.76%		16	Arizona	9,072,000	2.01%
28	Kentucky	5,331,000	1.18%		17	Missouri	8,900,000	1.98%
20	Louisiana	8,258,000	1.83%		18	Indiana	8,768,000	1.95%
40	Maine	2,178,000	0.48%		19	Minnesota	8,547,000	1.90%
21	Maryland	8,206,000	1.82%		20	Louisiana	8,258,000	1.83%
11	Massachusetts	11,519,000	2.56%		21	Maryland	8,206,000	1.82%
8	Michigan	15,788,000	3.51%		22	Tennessee	7,943,000	1.76%
19	Minnesota	8,547,000	1.90%		23	Colorado	7,832,000	1.74%
31	Mississippi	4,437,000	0.99%		24	South Carolina	6,868,000	1.53%
17	Missouri	8,900,000	1.98%		25	Alabama	6,275,000	1.39%
44	Montana	1,660,000	0.37%		26	Oregon	5,732,000	1.27%
37	Nebraska	2,765,000	0.61%		27	Connecticut	5,534,000	1.23%
29	Nevada	5,161,000	1.15%		28	Kentucky	5,331,000	1.18%
33	New Hampshire	3,752,000	0.83%		29	Nevada	5,161,000	1.15%
9	New Jersey	13,865,000	3.08%		30	Oklahoma	4,560,000	1.01%
36	New Mexico	3,131,000	0.70%		31	Mississippi	4,437,000	0.99%
4	New York	27,313,000	6.07%		32	Iowa	4,257,000	0.95%
12	North Carolina	11,260,000	2.50%		33	New Hampshire	3,752,000	0.83%
47	North Dakota	1,217,000	0.27%		34	Arkansas	3,531,000	0.78%
7	Ohio	17,075,000	3.79%		35	Kansas	3,439,000	0.76%
30	Oklahoma	4,560,000	1.01%		36	New Mexico	3,131,000	0.70%
26	Oregon	5,732,000	1.27%		37	Nebraska	2,765,000	0.61%
6	Pennsylvania	18,065,000	4.01%		38	West Virginia	2,392,000	0.53%
43	Rhode Island	1,796,000	0.40%		39	Hawaii	2,196,000	0.49%
24	South Carolina	6,868,000	1.53%		40	Maine	2,178,000	0.48%
46	South Dakota	1,256,000	0.28%		41	Utah	1,881,000	0.42%
22	Tennessee	7,943,000	1.76%		42	Idaho	1,802,000	0.40%
2	Texas	33,277,000	7.39%		43	Rhode Island	1,796,000	0.40%
41	Utah	1,881,000	0.42%		44	Montana	1,660,000	0.37%
49	Vermont	1,097,000	0.24%		45	Delaware	1,556,000	0.35%
14	Virginia	10,129,000	2.25%		46	South Dakota	1,256,000	0.28%
15	Washington	9,241,000	2.05%		47	North Dakota	1,217,000	0.27%
38	West Virginia	2,392,000	0.53%		48	Alaska	1,179,000	0.26%
13	Wisconsin	10,724,000	2.38%		49	Vermont	1,097,000	0.24%
50	Wyoming	890,000	0.20%		50	Wyoming	890,000	0.20%
						District of Columbia	1,653,000	0.37%

*Source: Distilled Spirits Council of the United States, Inc., Steve L. Barsby Assoc.'s & Beer Institute
"1996 Statistical Information for the Distilled Spirits Industry" (August 1997)*
*This is apparent consumption of actual alcohol, not entire volume of an alcoholic beverage (e.g. wine is roughly
11% absolute alcohol content). Apparent consumption is based on several sources which together approximate
sales but do not actually measure consumption. Reported state volumes reflect only in-state purchases.
Accordingly, figures for some states may be skewed by purchases by nonresidents.*

Adult Per Capita Apparent Alcohol Consumption in 1996

National Per Capita = 2.43 Gallons Consumed per Adult Age 21 Years & Older*

ALPHA ORDER

RANK	STATE	PER CAPITA
43	Alabama	2.09
3	Alaska	3.00
6	Arizona	2.94
45	Arkansas	2.03
25	California	2.45
6	Colorado	2.94
33	Connecticut	2.34
4	Delaware	2.99
8	Florida	2.84
24	Georgia	2.46
14	Hawaii	2.66
34	Idaho	2.31
18	Illinois	2.60
38	Indiana	2.14
39	Iowa	2.12
48	Kansas	1.94
47	Kentucky	1.95
8	Louisiana	2.84
26	Maine	2.44
35	Maryland	2.28
20	Massachusetts	2.58
32	Michigan	2.37
15	Minnesota	2.65
27	Mississippi	2.43
31	Missouri	2.38
12	Montana	2.74
27	Nebraska	2.43
1	Nevada	4.57
2	New Hampshire	4.55
27	New Jersey	2.43
10	New Mexico	2.76
41	New York	2.11
36	North Carolina	2.17
12	North Dakota	2.74
36	Ohio	2.17
46	Oklahoma	2.01
22	Oregon	2.53
44	Pennsylvania	2.08
23	Rhode Island	2.50
16	South Carolina	2.64
21	South Dakota	2.54
42	Tennessee	2.10
18	Texas	2.60
50	Utah	1.57
17	Vermont	2.62
39	Virginia	2.12
30	Washington	2.39
49	West Virginia	1.81
5	Wisconsin	2.98
11	Wyoming	2.75

RANK ORDER

RANK	STATE	PER CAPITA
1	Nevada	4.57
2	New Hampshire	4.55
3	Alaska	3.00
4	Delaware	2.99
5	Wisconsin	2.98
6	Arizona	2.94
6	Colorado	2.94
8	Florida	2.84
8	Louisiana	2.84
10	New Mexico	2.76
11	Wyoming	2.75
12	Montana	2.74
12	North Dakota	2.74
14	Hawaii	2.66
15	Minnesota	2.65
16	South Carolina	2.64
17	Vermont	2.62
18	Illinois	2.60
18	Texas	2.60
20	Massachusetts	2.58
21	South Dakota	2.54
22	Oregon	2.53
23	Rhode Island	2.50
24	Georgia	2.46
25	California	2.45
26	Maine	2.44
27	Mississippi	2.43
27	Nebraska	2.43
27	New Jersey	2.43
30	Washington	2.39
31	Missouri	2.38
32	Michigan	2.37
33	Connecticut	2.34
34	Idaho	2.31
35	Maryland	2.28
36	North Carolina	2.17
36	Ohio	2.17
38	Indiana	2.14
39	Iowa	2.12
39	Virginia	2.12
41	New York	2.11
42	Tennessee	2.10
43	Alabama	2.09
44	Pennsylvania	2.08
45	Arkansas	2.03
46	Oklahoma	2.01
47	Kentucky	1.95
48	Kansas	1.94
49	West Virginia	1.81
50	Utah	1.57

| | District of Columbia | 3.97 |

Source: MQ Press using data from Steve L. Barsby & Assoc. & Beer Institute as published by the Distilled Spirits
Council of the United States, Inc. "1996 Statistical Information for the Distilled Spirits Industry" (August 1997) and Census
*This is apparent consumption of actual alcohol, not the liquid volume of an alcoholic beverage (e.g. wine is roughly
11% absolute alcohol content). Apparent consumption is based on several sources which together approximate
sales but do not actually measure consumption. Reported state volumes reflect only in-state purchases.
Accordingly, figures for some states may be skewed by purchases by nonresidents.

Apparent Beer Consumption in 1996

National Total = 5,851,579,000 Gallons of Beer Consumed*

ALPHA ORDER					RANK ORDER			
RANK	STATE	GALLONS	% of USA		RANK	STATE	GALLONS	% of USA
25	Alabama	89,534,000	1.53%		1	California	609,522,000	10.42%
49	Alaska	13,612,000	0.23%		2	Texas	519,248,000	8.87%
16	Arizona	121,932,000	2.08%		3	Florida	364,567,000	6.23%
33	Arkansas	50,321,000	0.86%		4	New York	320,410,000	5.48%
1	California	609,522,000	10.42%		5	Illinois	271,621,000	4.64%
23	Colorado	94,622,000	1.62%		6	Pennsylvania	269,542,000	4.61%
32	Connecticut	56,369,000	0.96%		7	Ohio	260,599,000	4.45%
45	Delaware	17,838,000	0.30%		8	Michigan	206,990,000	3.54%
3	Florida	364,567,000	6.23%		9	Georgia	161,436,000	2.76%
9	Georgia	161,436,000	2.76%		10	North Carolina	154,430,000	2.64%
39	Hawaii	30,042,000	0.51%		11	New Jersey	145,996,000	2.49%
42	Idaho	24,477,000	0.42%		12	Wisconsin	142,468,000	2.43%
5	Illinois	271,621,000	4.64%		13	Virginia	137,318,000	2.35%
17	Indiana	118,596,000	2.03%		14	Massachusetts	127,075,000	2.17%
29	Iowa	65,868,000	1.13%		15	Missouri	126,254,000	2.16%
34	Kansas	48,698,000	0.83%		16	Arizona	121,932,000	2.08%
26	Kentucky	74,050,000	1.27%		17	Indiana	118,596,000	2.03%
18	Louisiana	115,389,000	1.97%		18	Louisiana	115,389,000	1.97%
41	Maine	26,432,000	0.45%		19	Tennessee	114,468,000	1.96%
22	Maryland	94,627,000	1.62%		20	Washington	111,326,000	1.90%
14	Massachusetts	127,075,000	2.17%		21	Minnesota	104,404,000	1.78%
8	Michigan	206,990,000	3.54%		22	Maryland	94,627,000	1.62%
21	Minnesota	104,404,000	1.78%		23	Colorado	94,622,000	1.62%
28	Mississippi	66,057,000	1.13%		24	South Carolina	93,873,000	1.60%
15	Missouri	126,254,000	2.16%		25	Alabama	89,534,000	1.53%
43	Montana	23,491,000	0.40%		26	Kentucky	74,050,000	1.27%
36	Nebraska	40,254,000	0.69%		27	Oregon	71,380,000	1.22%
31	Nevada	56,460,000	0.96%		28	Mississippi	66,057,000	1.13%
38	New Hampshire	36,123,000	0.62%		29	Iowa	65,868,000	1.13%
11	New Jersey	145,996,000	2.49%		30	Oklahoma	65,669,000	1.12%
35	New Mexico	46,564,000	0.80%		31	Nevada	56,460,000	0.96%
4	New York	320,410,000	5.48%		32	Connecticut	56,369,000	0.96%
10	North Carolina	154,430,000	2.64%		33	Arkansas	50,321,000	0.86%
47	North Dakota	17,112,000	0.29%		34	Kansas	48,698,000	0.83%
7	Ohio	260,599,000	4.45%		35	New Mexico	46,564,000	0.80%
30	Oklahoma	65,669,000	1.12%		36	Nebraska	40,254,000	0.69%
27	Oregon	71,380,000	1.22%		37	West Virginia	38,272,000	0.65%
6	Pennsylvania	269,542,000	4.61%		38	New Hampshire	36,123,000	0.62%
44	Rhode Island	21,448,000	0.37%		39	Hawaii	30,042,000	0.51%
24	South Carolina	93,873,000	1.60%		40	Utah	26,452,000	0.45%
46	South Dakota	17,789,000	0.30%		41	Maine	26,432,000	0.45%
19	Tennessee	114,468,000	1.96%		42	Idaho	24,477,000	0.42%
2	Texas	519,248,000	8.87%		43	Montana	23,491,000	0.40%
40	Utah	26,452,000	0.45%		44	Rhode Island	21,448,000	0.37%
48	Vermont	13,708,000	0.23%		45	Delaware	17,838,000	0.30%
13	Virginia	137,318,000	2.35%		46	South Dakota	17,789,000	0.30%
20	Washington	111,326,000	1.90%		47	North Dakota	17,112,000	0.29%
37	West Virginia	38,272,000	0.65%		48	Vermont	13,708,000	0.23%
12	Wisconsin	142,468,000	2.43%		49	Alaska	13,612,000	0.23%
50	Wyoming	11,832,000	0.20%		50	Wyoming	11,832,000	0.20%
						District of Columbia	15,013,000	0.26%

Source: Beer Institute as published by the Distilled Spirits Council of the United States, Inc.
  "1996 Statistical Information for the Distilled Spirits Industry" (August 1997)
*Apparent consumption is based on several sources which together approximate sales but do not actually measure consumption. Reported state volumes reflect only in-state purchases. Accordingly, figures for some states may be skewed by purchases by nonresidents.

Adult Per Capita Apparent Beer Consumption in 1996

National Per Capita = 31.57 Gallons Consumed per Adult 21 Years and Older*

ALPHA ORDER

RANK	STATE	PER CAPITA
33	Alabama	29.78
18	Alaska	34.69
7	Arizona	39.46
38	Arkansas	28.93
43	California	28.04
15	Colorado	35.49
49	Connecticut	23.85
19	Delaware	34.25
17	Florida	34.79
26	Georgia	31.73
11	Hawaii	36.36
28	Idaho	31.44
22	Illinois	33.08
36	Indiana	29.01
23	Iowa	32.82
44	Kansas	27.48
45	Kentucky	27.05
5	Louisiana	39.70
35	Maine	29.56
46	Maryland	26.27
42	Massachusetts	28.51
29	Michigan	31.09
25	Minnesota	32.43
12	Mississippi	36.18
20	Missouri	33.73
8	Montana	38.77
16	Nebraska	35.44
1	Nevada	50.01
2	New Hampshire	43.76
47	New Jersey	25.56
3	New Mexico	41.07
48	New York	24.74
34	North Carolina	29.75
9	North Dakota	38.50
21	Ohio	33.15
39	Oklahoma	28.89
27	Oregon	31.54
30	Pennsylvania	30.97
32	Rhode Island	29.83
13	South Carolina	36.14
14	South Dakota	36.04
31	Tennessee	30.31
4	Texas	40.53
50	Utah	22.09
24	Vermont	32.72
40	Virginia	28.79
41	Washington	28.78
37	West Virginia	29.00
6	Wisconsin	39.61
10	Wyoming	36.53

RANK ORDER

RANK	STATE	PER CAPITA
1	Nevada	50.01
2	New Hampshire	43.76
3	New Mexico	41.07
4	Texas	40.53
5	Louisiana	39.70
6	Wisconsin	39.61
7	Arizona	39.46
8	Montana	38.77
9	North Dakota	38.50
10	Wyoming	36.53
11	Hawaii	36.36
12	Mississippi	36.18
13	South Carolina	36.14
14	South Dakota	36.04
15	Colorado	35.49
16	Nebraska	35.44
17	Florida	34.79
18	Alaska	34.69
19	Delaware	34.25
20	Missouri	33.73
21	Ohio	33.15
22	Illinois	33.08
23	Iowa	32.82
24	Vermont	32.72
25	Minnesota	32.43
26	Georgia	31.73
27	Oregon	31.54
28	Idaho	31.44
29	Michigan	31.09
30	Pennsylvania	30.97
31	Tennessee	30.31
32	Rhode Island	29.83
33	Alabama	29.78
34	North Carolina	29.75
35	Maine	29.56
36	Indiana	29.01
37	West Virginia	29.00
38	Arkansas	28.93
39	Oklahoma	28.89
40	Virginia	28.79
41	Washington	28.78
42	Massachusetts	28.51
43	California	28.04
44	Kansas	27.48
45	Kentucky	27.05
46	Maryland	26.27
47	New Jersey	25.56
48	New York	24.74
49	Connecticut	23.85
50	Utah	22.09
	District of Columbia	36.01

Source: Beer Institute as published by the Distilled Spirits Council of the United States, Inc.
"1996 Statistical Information for the Distilled Spirits Industry" (August 1997)
*Apparent consumption is based on several sources which together approximate sales but do not actually measure consumption. Reported state volumes reflect only in-state purchases. Accordingly, figures for some states may be skewed by purchases by nonresidents.

Apparent Wine Consumption in 1996

National Total = 497,931,000 Gallons of Wine Consumed*

ALPHA ORDER				RANK ORDER			
RANK	STATE	GALLONS	% of USA	RANK	STATE	GALLONS	% of USA
28	Alabama	4,074,000	0.82%	1	California	94,301,000	18.94%
45	Alaska	1,224,000	0.25%	2	New York	41,862,000	8.41%
16	Arizona	9,379,000	1.88%	3	Florida	34,558,000	6.94%
41	Arkansas	1,907,000	0.38%	4	Texas	25,041,000	5.03%
1	California	94,301,000	18.94%	5	Illinois	24,960,000	5.01%
17	Colorado	9,259,000	1.86%	6	New Jersey	22,219,000	4.46%
15	Connecticut	9,653,000	1.94%	7	Massachusetts	18,559,000	3.73%
39	Delaware	1,993,000	0.40%	8	Pennsylvania	14,612,000	2.93%
3	Florida	34,558,000	6.94%	9	Washington	13,813,000	2.77%
14	Georgia	10,915,000	2.19%	10	Michigan	13,047,000	2.62%
32	Hawaii	2,765,000	0.56%	11	Virginia	12,510,000	2.51%
38	Idaho	2,160,000	0.43%	12	Ohio	12,398,000	2.49%
5	Illinois	24,960,000	5.01%	13	North Carolina	11,105,000	2.23%
23	Indiana	7,105,000	1.43%	14	Georgia	10,915,000	2.19%
37	Iowa	2,262,000	0.45%	15	Connecticut	9,653,000	1.94%
36	Kansas	2,284,000	0.46%	16	Arizona	9,379,000	1.88%
30	Kentucky	3,108,000	0.62%	17	Colorado	9,259,000	1.86%
25	Louisiana	5,883,000	1.18%	18	Maryland	9,174,000	1.84%
34	Maine	2,575,000	0.52%	19	Oregon	8,865,000	1.78%
18	Maryland	9,174,000	1.84%	20	Wisconsin	7,871,000	1.58%
7	Massachusetts	18,559,000	3.73%	21	Minnesota	7,524,000	1.51%
10	Michigan	13,047,000	2.62%	22	Missouri	7,273,000	1.46%
21	Minnesota	7,524,000	1.51%	23	Indiana	7,105,000	1.43%
43	Mississippi	1,477,000	0.30%	24	Nevada	6,013,000	1.21%
22	Missouri	7,273,000	1.46%	25	Louisiana	5,883,000	1.18%
44	Montana	1,476,000	0.30%	26	Tennessee	5,461,000	1.10%
40	Nebraska	1,930,000	0.39%	27	South Carolina	5,047,000	1.01%
24	Nevada	6,013,000	1.21%	28	Alabama	4,074,000	0.82%
29	New Hampshire	3,973,000	0.80%	29	New Hampshire	3,973,000	0.80%
6	New Jersey	22,219,000	4.46%	30	Kentucky	3,108,000	0.62%
35	New Mexico	2,369,000	0.48%	31	Oklahoma	2,847,000	0.57%
2	New York	41,862,000	8.41%	32	Hawaii	2,765,000	0.56%
13	North Carolina	11,105,000	2.23%	33	Rhode Island	2,733,000	0.55%
49	North Dakota	523,000	0.11%	34	Maine	2,575,000	0.52%
12	Ohio	12,398,000	2.49%	35	New Mexico	2,369,000	0.48%
31	Oklahoma	2,847,000	0.57%	36	Kansas	2,284,000	0.46%
19	Oregon	8,865,000	1.78%	37	Iowa	2,262,000	0.45%
8	Pennsylvania	14,612,000	2.93%	38	Idaho	2,160,000	0.43%
33	Rhode Island	2,733,000	0.55%	39	Delaware	1,993,000	0.40%
27	South Carolina	5,047,000	1.01%	40	Nebraska	1,930,000	0.39%
48	South Dakota	604,000	0.12%	41	Arkansas	1,907,000	0.38%
26	Tennessee	5,461,000	1.10%	42	Vermont	1,683,000	0.34%
4	Texas	25,041,000	5.03%	43	Mississippi	1,477,000	0.30%
46	Utah	1,168,000	0.23%	44	Montana	1,476,000	0.30%
42	Vermont	1,683,000	0.34%	45	Alaska	1,224,000	0.25%
11	Virginia	12,510,000	2.51%	46	Utah	1,168,000	0.23%
9	Washington	13,813,000	2.77%	47	West Virginia	1,121,000	0.23%
47	West Virginia	1,121,000	0.23%	48	South Dakota	604,000	0.12%
20	Wisconsin	7,871,000	1.58%	49	North Dakota	523,000	0.11%
50	Wyoming	492,000	0.10%	50	Wyoming	492,000	0.10%
					District of Columbia	2,716,000	0.55%

Source: Steve L. Barsby and Associates, Inc. as published by the Distilled Spirits Council of the United States, Inc. "1996 Statistical Information for the Distilled Spirits Industry" (August 1997)

*Apparent consumption is based on several sources which together approximate sales but do not actually measure consumption. Reported state volumes reflect only in-state purchases. Accordingly, figures for some states may be skewed by purchases by nonresidents.

Adult Per Capita Apparent Wine Consumption in 1996

National Per Capita = 2.69 Gallons Consumed per Adult Age 21 Years and Older*

ALPHA ORDER			RANK ORDER		
RANK	STATE	PER CAPITA	RANK	STATE	PER CAPITA
40	Alabama	1.36	1	Nevada	5.33
16	Alaska	3.12	2	New Hampshire	4.81
17	Arizona	3.04	3	California	4.34
47	Arkansas	1.10	4	Massachusetts	4.16
3	California	4.34	5	Connecticut	4.08
12	Colorado	3.47	6	Vermont	4.02
5	Connecticut	4.08	7	Oregon	3.92
9	Delaware	3.83	8	New Jersey	3.89
14	Florida	3.30	9	Delaware	3.83
26	Georgia	2.15	10	Rhode Island	3.80
13	Hawaii	3.35	11	Washington	3.57
20	Idaho	2.77	12	Colorado	3.47
17	Illinois	3.04	13	Hawaii	3.35
34	Indiana	1.75	14	Florida	3.30
46	Iowa	1.13	15	New York	3.23
41	Kansas	1.29	16	Alaska	3.12
45	Kentucky	1.14	17	Arizona	3.04
29	Louisiana	2.02	17	Illinois	3.04
19	Maine	2.88	19	Maine	2.88
22	Maryland	2.55	20	Idaho	2.77
4	Massachusetts	4.16	21	Virginia	2.62
30	Michigan	1.96	22	Maryland	2.55
24	Minnesota	2.34	23	Montana	2.44
50	Mississippi	0.81	24	Minnesota	2.34
32	Missouri	1.94	25	Wisconsin	2.19
23	Montana	2.44	26	Georgia	2.15
35	Nebraska	1.70	27	North Carolina	2.14
1	Nevada	5.33	28	New Mexico	2.09
2	New Hampshire	4.81	29	Louisiana	2.02
8	New Jersey	3.89	30	Michigan	1.96
28	New Mexico	2.09	31	Texas	1.95
15	New York	3.23	32	Missouri	1.94
27	North Carolina	2.14	32	South Carolina	1.94
44	North Dakota	1.18	34	Indiana	1.75
37	Ohio	1.58	35	Nebraska	1.70
42	Oklahoma	1.25	36	Pennsylvania	1.68
7	Oregon	3.92	37	Ohio	1.58
36	Pennsylvania	1.68	38	Wyoming	1.52
10	Rhode Island	3.80	39	Tennessee	1.45
32	South Carolina	1.94	40	Alabama	1.36
43	South Dakota	1.22	41	Kansas	1.29
39	Tennessee	1.45	42	Oklahoma	1.25
31	Texas	1.95	43	South Dakota	1.22
48	Utah	0.98	44	North Dakota	1.18
6	Vermont	4.02	45	Kentucky	1.14
21	Virginia	2.62	46	Iowa	1.13
11	Washington	3.57	47	Arkansas	1.10
49	West Virginia	0.85	48	Utah	0.98
25	Wisconsin	2.19	49	West Virginia	0.85
38	Wyoming	1.52	50	Mississippi	0.81
				District of Columbia	6.52

Source: Steve L. Barsby and Associates, Inc. as published by the Distilled Spirits Council of the United States, Inc.
"1996 Statistical Information for the Distilled Spirits Industry" (August 1997)
*Apparent consumption is based on several sources which together approximate sales but do not actually measure consumption. Reported state volumes reflect only in-state purchases. Accordingly, figures for some states may be skewed by purchases by nonresidents.

Apparent Distilled Spirits Consumption in 1996

National Total = 330,393,000 Gallons of Distilled Spirits Consumed*

ALPHA ORDER

RANK	STATE	GALLONS	% of USA
27	Alabama	4,493,000	1.36%
46	Alaska	1,080,000	0.33%
20	Arizona	6,383,000	1.93%
33	Arkansas	2,643,000	0.80%
1	California	38,662,000	11.70%
19	Colorado	6,390,000	1.93%
26	Connecticut	4,838,000	1.46%
42	Delaware	1,336,000	0.40%
2	Florida	23,973,000	7.26%
9	Georgia	10,161,000	3.08%
41	Hawaii	1,349,000	0.41%
44	Idaho	1,157,000	0.35%
5	Illinois	15,951,000	4.83%
17	Indiana	6,608,000	2.00%
34	Iowa	2,610,000	0.79%
35	Kansas	2,491,000	0.75%
29	Kentucky	4,143,000	1.25%
21	Louisiana	6,047,000	1.83%
38	Maine	1,762,000	0.53%
15	Maryland	7,346,000	2.22%
11	Massachusetts	9,397,000	2.84%
6	Michigan	12,595,000	3.81%
14	Minnesota	7,553,000	2.29%
31	Mississippi	3,254,000	0.98%
21	Missouri	6,047,000	1.83%
45	Montana	1,102,000	0.33%
37	Nebraska	1,852,000	0.56%
25	Nevada	4,897,000	1.48%
28	New Hampshire	4,224,000	1.28%
7	New Jersey	12,128,000	3.67%
36	New Mexico	1,938,000	0.59%
3	New York	20,725,000	6.27%
13	North Carolina	7,724,000	2.34%
47	North Dakota	973,000	0.29%
10	Ohio	9,960,000	3.01%
32	Oklahoma	3,230,000	0.98%
30	Oregon	3,862,000	1.17%
8	Pennsylvania	10,820,000	3.27%
43	Rhode Island	1,325,000	0.40%
24	South Carolina	5,221,000	1.58%
48	South Dakota	972,000	0.29%
23	Tennessee	5,479,000	1.66%
4	Texas	17,892,000	5.42%
39	Utah	1,405,000	0.43%
50	Vermont	738,000	0.22%
18	Virginia	6,435,000	1.95%
16	Washington	6,780,000	2.05%
40	West Virginia	1,367,000	0.41%
12	Wisconsin	8,618,000	2.61%
49	Wyoming	759,000	0.23%

RANK ORDER

RANK	STATE	GALLONS	% of USA
1	California	38,662,000	11.70%
2	Florida	23,973,000	7.26%
3	New York	20,725,000	6.27%
4	Texas	17,892,000	5.42%
5	Illinois	15,951,000	4.83%
6	Michigan	12,595,000	3.81%
7	New Jersey	12,128,000	3.67%
8	Pennsylvania	10,820,000	3.27%
9	Georgia	10,161,000	3.08%
10	Ohio	9,960,000	3.01%
11	Massachusetts	9,397,000	2.84%
12	Wisconsin	8,618,000	2.61%
13	North Carolina	7,724,000	2.34%
14	Minnesota	7,553,000	2.29%
15	Maryland	7,346,000	2.22%
16	Washington	6,780,000	2.05%
17	Indiana	6,608,000	2.00%
18	Virginia	6,435,000	1.95%
19	Colorado	6,390,000	1.93%
20	Arizona	6,383,000	1.93%
21	Louisiana	6,047,000	1.83%
21	Missouri	6,047,000	1.83%
23	Tennessee	5,479,000	1.66%
24	South Carolina	5,221,000	1.58%
25	Nevada	4,897,000	1.48%
26	Connecticut	4,838,000	1.46%
27	Alabama	4,493,000	1.36%
28	New Hampshire	4,224,000	1.28%
29	Kentucky	4,143,000	1.25%
30	Oregon	3,862,000	1.17%
31	Mississippi	3,254,000	0.98%
32	Oklahoma	3,230,000	0.98%
33	Arkansas	2,643,000	0.80%
34	Iowa	2,610,000	0.79%
35	Kansas	2,491,000	0.75%
36	New Mexico	1,938,000	0.59%
37	Nebraska	1,852,000	0.56%
38	Maine	1,762,000	0.53%
39	Utah	1,405,000	0.43%
40	West Virginia	1,367,000	0.41%
41	Hawaii	1,349,000	0.41%
42	Delaware	1,336,000	0.40%
43	Rhode Island	1,325,000	0.40%
44	Idaho	1,157,000	0.35%
45	Montana	1,102,000	0.33%
46	Alaska	1,080,000	0.33%
47	North Dakota	973,000	0.29%
48	South Dakota	972,000	0.29%
49	Wyoming	759,000	0.23%
50	Vermont	738,000	0.22%
	District of Columbia	1,695,000	0.51%

Source: Distilled Spirits Council of the United States, Inc.
    "1996 Statistical Information for the Distilled Spirits Industry" (August 1997)
*Apparent consumption is based on several sources which together approximate sales but do not actually measure consumption. Reported state volumes reflect only in-state purchases. Accordingly, figures for some states may be skewed by purchases by nonresidents.

Adult Per Capita Apparent Distilled Spirits Consumption in 1996

National Per Capita = 1.78 Gallons Consumed per Adult Age 21 and Older*

<u>ALPHA ORDER</u>

RANK	STATE	PER CAPITA
38	Alabama	1.49
3	Alaska	2.75
14	Arizona	2.07
36	Arkansas	1.52
25	California	1.78
5	Colorado	2.40
15	Connecticut	2.05
4	Delaware	2.57
9	Florida	2.29
18	Georgia	2.00
31	Hawaii	1.63
38	Idaho	1.49
21	Illinois	1.94
33	Indiana	1.62
46	Iowa	1.30
43	Kansas	1.41
37	Kentucky	1.51
13	Louisiana	2.08
19	Maine	1.97
16	Maryland	2.04
12	Massachusetts	2.11
22	Michigan	1.89
7	Minnesota	2.35
25	Mississippi	1.78
33	Missouri	1.62
24	Montana	1.82
31	Nebraska	1.63
2	Nevada	4.34
1	New Hampshire	5.12
11	New Jersey	2.12
29	New Mexico	1.71
35	New York	1.60
38	North Carolina	1.49
10	North Dakota	2.19
47	Ohio	1.27
42	Oklahoma	1.42
29	Oregon	1.71
48	Pennsylvania	1.24
23	Rhode Island	1.84
17	South Carolina	2.01
19	South Dakota	1.97
41	Tennessee	1.45
44	Texas	1.40
49	Utah	1.17
27	Vermont	1.76
45	Virginia	1.35
28	Washington	1.75
50	West Virginia	1.04
5	Wisconsin	2.40
8	Wyoming	2.34

<u>RANK ORDER</u>

RANK	STATE	PER CAPITA
1	New Hampshire	5.12
2	Nevada	4.34
3	Alaska	2.75
4	Delaware	2.57
5	Colorado	2.40
5	Wisconsin	2.40
7	Minnesota	2.35
8	Wyoming	2.34
9	Florida	2.29
10	North Dakota	2.19
11	New Jersey	2.12
12	Massachusetts	2.11
13	Louisiana	2.08
14	Arizona	2.07
15	Connecticut	2.05
16	Maryland	2.04
17	South Carolina	2.01
18	Georgia	2.00
19	Maine	1.97
19	South Dakota	1.97
21	Illinois	1.94
22	Michigan	1.89
23	Rhode Island	1.84
24	Montana	1.82
25	California	1.78
25	Mississippi	1.78
27	Vermont	1.76
28	Washington	1.75
29	New Mexico	1.71
29	Oregon	1.71
31	Hawaii	1.63
31	Nebraska	1.63
33	Indiana	1.62
33	Missouri	1.62
35	New York	1.60
36	Arkansas	1.52
37	Kentucky	1.51
38	Alabama	1.49
38	Idaho	1.49
38	North Carolina	1.49
41	Tennessee	1.45
42	Oklahoma	1.42
43	Kansas	1.41
44	Texas	1.40
45	Virginia	1.35
46	Iowa	1.30
47	Ohio	1.27
48	Pennsylvania	1.24
49	Utah	1.17
50	West Virginia	1.04
	District of Columbia	4.07

Source: Distilled Spirits Council of the United States, Inc.
  "1996 Statistical Information for the Distilled Spirits Industry" (August 1997)
*Apparent consumption is based on several sources which together approximate sales but do not actually measure consumption. Reported state volumes reflect only in-state purchases. Accordingly, figures for some states may be skewed by purchases by nonresidents.

Percent of Adults Who Are Binge Drinkers: 1997

National Median = 14.5% of Adults*

<table>
<tr><td colspan="3">ALPHA ORDER</td><td colspan="3">RANK ORDER</td></tr>
<tr><td>RANK</td><td>STATE</td><td>PERCENT</td><td>RANK</td><td>STATE</td><td>PERCENT</td></tr>
<tr><td>36</td><td>Alabama</td><td>11.4</td><td>1</td><td>Wisconsin</td><td>23.3</td></tr>
<tr><td>10</td><td>Alaska</td><td>16.5</td><td>2</td><td>South Dakota</td><td>20.9</td></tr>
<tr><td>44</td><td>Arizona</td><td>8.8</td><td>3</td><td>Nevada</td><td>19.2</td></tr>
<tr><td>41</td><td>Arkansas</td><td>9.2</td><td>4</td><td>Michigan</td><td>18.9</td></tr>
<tr><td>19</td><td>California</td><td>15.2</td><td>5</td><td>North Dakota</td><td>18.4</td></tr>
<tr><td>18</td><td>Colorado</td><td>15.3</td><td>6</td><td>Iowa</td><td>17.9</td></tr>
<tr><td>15</td><td>Connecticut</td><td>15.6</td><td>6</td><td>Massachusetts</td><td>17.9</td></tr>
<tr><td>35</td><td>Delaware</td><td>11.9</td><td>8</td><td>Texas</td><td>17.4</td></tr>
<tr><td>32</td><td>Florida</td><td>13.1</td><td>9</td><td>Hawaii</td><td>17.1</td></tr>
<tr><td>39</td><td>Georgia</td><td>9.4</td><td>10</td><td>Alaska</td><td>16.5</td></tr>
<tr><td>9</td><td>Hawaii</td><td>17.1</td><td>11</td><td>Illinois</td><td>16.3</td></tr>
<tr><td>22</td><td>Idaho</td><td>14.9</td><td>11</td><td>Nebraska</td><td>16.3</td></tr>
<tr><td>11</td><td>Illinois</td><td>16.3</td><td>13</td><td>New Hampshire</td><td>16.1</td></tr>
<tr><td>34</td><td>Indiana</td><td>12.6</td><td>13</td><td>Vermont</td><td>16.1</td></tr>
<tr><td>6</td><td>Iowa</td><td>17.9</td><td>15</td><td>Connecticut</td><td>15.6</td></tr>
<tr><td>31</td><td>Kansas</td><td>13.3</td><td>15</td><td>Minnesota</td><td>15.6</td></tr>
<tr><td>39</td><td>Kentucky</td><td>9.4</td><td>17</td><td>Wyoming</td><td>15.4</td></tr>
<tr><td>19</td><td>Louisiana</td><td>15.2</td><td>18</td><td>Colorado</td><td>15.3</td></tr>
<tr><td>30</td><td>Maine</td><td>13.8</td><td>19</td><td>California</td><td>15.2</td></tr>
<tr><td>50</td><td>Maryland</td><td>6.3</td><td>19</td><td>Louisiana</td><td>15.2</td></tr>
<tr><td>6</td><td>Massachusetts</td><td>17.9</td><td>21</td><td>Missouri</td><td>15.1</td></tr>
<tr><td>4</td><td>Michigan</td><td>18.9</td><td>22</td><td>Idaho</td><td>14.9</td></tr>
<tr><td>15</td><td>Minnesota</td><td>15.6</td><td>22</td><td>Rhode Island</td><td>14.9</td></tr>
<tr><td>38</td><td>Mississippi</td><td>9.5</td><td>24</td><td>New Mexico</td><td>14.6</td></tr>
<tr><td>21</td><td>Missouri</td><td>15.1</td><td>24</td><td>Pennsylvania</td><td>14.6</td></tr>
<tr><td>29</td><td>Montana</td><td>14.0</td><td>26</td><td>Virginia</td><td>14.5</td></tr>
<tr><td>11</td><td>Nebraska</td><td>16.3</td><td>26</td><td>Washington</td><td>14.5</td></tr>
<tr><td>3</td><td>Nevada</td><td>19.2</td><td>28</td><td>Oregon</td><td>14.3</td></tr>
<tr><td>13</td><td>New Hampshire</td><td>16.1</td><td>29</td><td>Montana</td><td>14.0</td></tr>
<tr><td>32</td><td>New Jersey</td><td>13.1</td><td>30</td><td>Maine</td><td>13.8</td></tr>
<tr><td>24</td><td>New Mexico</td><td>14.6</td><td>31</td><td>Kansas</td><td>13.3</td></tr>
<tr><td>41</td><td>New York</td><td>9.2</td><td>32</td><td>Florida</td><td>13.1</td></tr>
<tr><td>43</td><td>North Carolina</td><td>9.0</td><td>32</td><td>New Jersey</td><td>13.1</td></tr>
<tr><td>5</td><td>North Dakota</td><td>18.4</td><td>34</td><td>Indiana</td><td>12.6</td></tr>
<tr><td>46</td><td>Ohio</td><td>8.7</td><td>35</td><td>Delaware</td><td>11.9</td></tr>
<tr><td>44</td><td>Oklahoma</td><td>8.8</td><td>36</td><td>Alabama</td><td>11.4</td></tr>
<tr><td>28</td><td>Oregon</td><td>14.3</td><td>37</td><td>South Carolina</td><td>9.7</td></tr>
<tr><td>24</td><td>Pennsylvania</td><td>14.6</td><td>38</td><td>Mississippi</td><td>9.5</td></tr>
<tr><td>22</td><td>Rhode Island</td><td>14.9</td><td>39</td><td>Georgia</td><td>9.4</td></tr>
<tr><td>37</td><td>South Carolina</td><td>9.7</td><td>39</td><td>Kentucky</td><td>9.4</td></tr>
<tr><td>2</td><td>South Dakota</td><td>20.9</td><td>41</td><td>Arkansas</td><td>9.2</td></tr>
<tr><td>49</td><td>Tennessee</td><td>7.2</td><td>41</td><td>New York</td><td>9.2</td></tr>
<tr><td>8</td><td>Texas</td><td>17.4</td><td>43</td><td>North Carolina</td><td>9.0</td></tr>
<tr><td>48</td><td>Utah</td><td>7.7</td><td>44</td><td>Arizona</td><td>8.8</td></tr>
<tr><td>13</td><td>Vermont</td><td>16.1</td><td>44</td><td>Oklahoma</td><td>8.8</td></tr>
<tr><td>26</td><td>Virginia</td><td>14.5</td><td>46</td><td>Ohio</td><td>8.7</td></tr>
<tr><td>26</td><td>Washington</td><td>14.5</td><td>47</td><td>West Virginia</td><td>8.4</td></tr>
<tr><td>47</td><td>West Virginia</td><td>8.4</td><td>48</td><td>Utah</td><td>7.7</td></tr>
<tr><td>1</td><td>Wisconsin</td><td>23.3</td><td>49</td><td>Tennessee</td><td>7.2</td></tr>
<tr><td>17</td><td>Wyoming</td><td>15.4</td><td>50</td><td>Maryland</td><td>6.3</td></tr>
<tr><td></td><td></td><td></td><td colspan="2">District of Columbia</td><td>12.1</td></tr>
</table>

Source: U.S. Department of Health and Human Services, Centers for Disease Control and Prevention
   "1997 Behavioral Risk Factor Surveillance Summary Prevalence Report" (August 17, 1998)
*Persons 18 and older reporting consumption of five or more alcoholic drinks on one or more occasions during the previous month.

Percent of Adults Who Smoke: 1997

National Median = 23.2% of Adults*

<table>
<tr><td colspan="3">ALPHA ORDER</td><td colspan="3">RANK ORDER</td></tr>
<tr><td>RANK</td><td>STATE</td><td>PERCENT</td><td>RANK</td><td>STATE</td><td>PERCENT</td></tr>
<tr><td>13</td><td>Alabama</td><td>24.7</td><td>1</td><td>Kentucky</td><td>30.7</td></tr>
<tr><td>8</td><td>Alaska</td><td>26.5</td><td>2</td><td>Missouri</td><td>28.6</td></tr>
<tr><td>42</td><td>Arizona</td><td>21.1</td><td>3</td><td>Arkansas</td><td>28.4</td></tr>
<tr><td>3</td><td>Arkansas</td><td>28.4</td><td>4</td><td>Nevada</td><td>28.0</td></tr>
<tr><td>49</td><td>California</td><td>18.4</td><td>5</td><td>West Virginia</td><td>27.4</td></tr>
<tr><td>32</td><td>Colorado</td><td>22.6</td><td>6</td><td>Tennessee</td><td>26.9</td></tr>
<tr><td>40</td><td>Connecticut</td><td>21.6</td><td>7</td><td>Delaware</td><td>26.6</td></tr>
<tr><td>7</td><td>Delaware</td><td>26.6</td><td>8</td><td>Alaska</td><td>26.5</td></tr>
<tr><td>23</td><td>Florida</td><td>23.6</td><td>9</td><td>Indiana</td><td>26.4</td></tr>
<tr><td>35</td><td>Georgia</td><td>22.4</td><td>10</td><td>Michigan</td><td>26.0</td></tr>
<tr><td>48</td><td>Hawaii</td><td>18.7</td><td>11</td><td>North Carolina</td><td>25.9</td></tr>
<tr><td>47</td><td>Idaho</td><td>19.9</td><td>12</td><td>Ohio</td><td>25.1</td></tr>
<tr><td>26</td><td>Illinois</td><td>23.2</td><td>13</td><td>Alabama</td><td>24.7</td></tr>
<tr><td>9</td><td>Indiana</td><td>26.4</td><td>13</td><td>New Hampshire</td><td>24.7</td></tr>
<tr><td>28</td><td>Iowa</td><td>23.1</td><td>15</td><td>Oklahoma</td><td>24.6</td></tr>
<tr><td>32</td><td>Kansas</td><td>22.6</td><td>16</td><td>Louisiana</td><td>24.5</td></tr>
<tr><td>1</td><td>Kentucky</td><td>30.7</td><td>17</td><td>Virginia</td><td>24.4</td></tr>
<tr><td>16</td><td>Louisiana</td><td>24.5</td><td>18</td><td>Rhode Island</td><td>24.3</td></tr>
<tr><td>31</td><td>Maine</td><td>22.7</td><td>18</td><td>South Dakota</td><td>24.3</td></tr>
<tr><td>46</td><td>Maryland</td><td>20.4</td><td>20</td><td>Pennsylvania</td><td>24.2</td></tr>
<tr><td>44</td><td>Massachusetts</td><td>20.5</td><td>21</td><td>Wyoming</td><td>24.0</td></tr>
<tr><td>10</td><td>Michigan</td><td>26.0</td><td>22</td><td>Washington</td><td>23.8</td></tr>
<tr><td>39</td><td>Minnesota</td><td>21.9</td><td>23</td><td>Florida</td><td>23.6</td></tr>
<tr><td>28</td><td>Mississippi</td><td>23.1</td><td>24</td><td>South Carolina</td><td>23.4</td></tr>
<tr><td>2</td><td>Missouri</td><td>28.6</td><td>25</td><td>Vermont</td><td>23.3</td></tr>
<tr><td>44</td><td>Montana</td><td>20.5</td><td>26</td><td>Illinois</td><td>23.2</td></tr>
<tr><td>37</td><td>Nebraska</td><td>22.1</td><td>26</td><td>Wisconsin</td><td>23.2</td></tr>
<tr><td>4</td><td>Nevada</td><td>28.0</td><td>28</td><td>Iowa</td><td>23.1</td></tr>
<tr><td>13</td><td>New Hampshire</td><td>24.7</td><td>28</td><td>Mississippi</td><td>23.1</td></tr>
<tr><td>41</td><td>New Jersey</td><td>21.4</td><td>28</td><td>New York</td><td>23.1</td></tr>
<tr><td>37</td><td>New Mexico</td><td>22.1</td><td>31</td><td>Maine</td><td>22.7</td></tr>
<tr><td>28</td><td>New York</td><td>23.1</td><td>32</td><td>Colorado</td><td>22.6</td></tr>
<tr><td>11</td><td>North Carolina</td><td>25.9</td><td>32</td><td>Kansas</td><td>22.6</td></tr>
<tr><td>36</td><td>North Dakota</td><td>22.3</td><td>32</td><td>Texas</td><td>22.6</td></tr>
<tr><td>12</td><td>Ohio</td><td>25.1</td><td>35</td><td>Georgia</td><td>22.4</td></tr>
<tr><td>15</td><td>Oklahoma</td><td>24.6</td><td>36</td><td>North Dakota</td><td>22.3</td></tr>
<tr><td>43</td><td>Oregon</td><td>20.7</td><td>37</td><td>Nebraska</td><td>22.1</td></tr>
<tr><td>20</td><td>Pennsylvania</td><td>24.2</td><td>37</td><td>New Mexico</td><td>22.1</td></tr>
<tr><td>18</td><td>Rhode Island</td><td>24.3</td><td>39</td><td>Minnesota</td><td>21.9</td></tr>
<tr><td>24</td><td>South Carolina</td><td>23.4</td><td>40</td><td>Connecticut</td><td>21.6</td></tr>
<tr><td>18</td><td>South Dakota</td><td>24.3</td><td>41</td><td>New Jersey</td><td>21.4</td></tr>
<tr><td>6</td><td>Tennessee</td><td>26.9</td><td>42</td><td>Arizona</td><td>21.1</td></tr>
<tr><td>32</td><td>Texas</td><td>22.6</td><td>43</td><td>Oregon</td><td>20.7</td></tr>
<tr><td>50</td><td>Utah</td><td>13.8</td><td>44</td><td>Massachusetts</td><td>20.5</td></tr>
<tr><td>25</td><td>Vermont</td><td>23.3</td><td>44</td><td>Montana</td><td>20.5</td></tr>
<tr><td>17</td><td>Virginia</td><td>24.4</td><td>46</td><td>Maryland</td><td>20.4</td></tr>
<tr><td>22</td><td>Washington</td><td>23.8</td><td>47</td><td>Idaho</td><td>19.9</td></tr>
<tr><td>5</td><td>West Virginia</td><td>27.4</td><td>48</td><td>Hawaii</td><td>18.7</td></tr>
<tr><td>26</td><td>Wisconsin</td><td>23.2</td><td>49</td><td>California</td><td>18.4</td></tr>
<tr><td>21</td><td>Wyoming</td><td>24.0</td><td>50</td><td>Utah</td><td>13.8</td></tr>
<tr><td></td><td></td><td></td><td></td><td>District of Columbia</td><td>18.8</td></tr>
</table>

Source: U.S. Department of Health and Human Services, Centers for Disease Control and Prevention
"1997 Behavioral Risk Factor Surveillance Summary Prevalence Report" (August 17, 1998)
*Persons 18 and older who have ever smoked 100 cigarettes and currently smoke.

Percent of Men Who Smoke: 1997

National Median = 25.3% of Men*

ALPHA ORDER				RANK ORDER		
RANK	STATE	PERCENT		RANK	STATE	PERCENT
10	Alabama	28.6		1	Kentucky	33.0
16	Alaska	27.2		2	Arkansas	32.0
42	Arizona	22.0		3	Missouri	31.6
2	Arkansas	32.0		4	North Carolina	29.7
40	California	22.4		5	Michigan	29.6
37	Colorado	24.0		6	South Carolina	29.5
48	Connecticut	21.3		7	Delaware	29.2
7	Delaware	29.2		7	Indiana	29.2
20	Florida	26.0		7	Louisiana	29.2
27	Georgia	25.2		10	Alabama	28.6
47	Hawaii	21.5		11	Mississippi	28.3
43	Idaho	21.8		12	South Dakota	28.0
31	Illinois	25.0		12	Texas	28.0
7	Indiana	29.2		14	Tennessee	27.9
25	Iowa	25.5		15	West Virginia	27.3
17	Kansas	26.7		16	Alaska	27.2
1	Kentucky	33.0		17	Kansas	26.7
7	Louisiana	29.2		18	Ohio	26.3
27	Maine	25.2		19	Pennsylvania	26.2
45	Maryland	21.7		20	Florida	26.0
43	Massachusetts	21.8		20	Virginia	26.0
5	Michigan	29.6		22	New Hampshire	25.9
36	Minnesota	24.1		23	Nevada	25.6
11	Mississippi	28.3		23	Wisconsin	25.6
3	Missouri	31.6		25	Iowa	25.5
49	Montana	20.8		25	Rhode Island	25.5
34	Nebraska	24.3		27	Georgia	25.2
23	Nevada	25.6		27	Maine	25.2
22	New Hampshire	25.9		27	Oklahoma	25.2
39	New Jersey	23.4		27	Vermont	25.2
46	New Mexico	21.6		31	Illinois	25.0
33	New York	24.9		31	Washington	25.0
4	North Carolina	29.7		33	New York	24.9
34	North Dakota	24.3		34	Nebraska	24.3
18	Ohio	26.3		34	North Dakota	24.3
27	Oklahoma	25.2		36	Minnesota	24.1
41	Oregon	22.1		37	Colorado	24.0
19	Pennsylvania	26.2		38	Wyoming	23.9
25	Rhode Island	25.5		39	New Jersey	23.4
6	South Carolina	29.5		40	California	22.4
12	South Dakota	28.0		41	Oregon	22.1
14	Tennessee	27.9		42	Arizona	22.0
12	Texas	28.0		43	Idaho	21.8
50	Utah	16.1		43	Massachusetts	21.8
27	Vermont	25.2		45	Maryland	21.7
20	Virginia	26.0		46	New Mexico	21.6
31	Washington	25.0		47	Hawaii	21.5
15	West Virginia	27.3		48	Connecticut	21.3
23	Wisconsin	25.6		49	Montana	20.8
38	Wyoming	23.9		50	Utah	16.1
					District of Columbia	22.7

Source: U.S. Department of Health and Human Services, Centers for Disease Control and Prevention
"1997 Behavioral Risk Factor Surveillance Summary Prevalence Report" (August 17, 1998)
*Persons 18 and older who have ever smoked 100 cigarettes and currently smoke.

Percent of Women Who Smoke: 1997

National Percent = 21.1% of Women*

RANK	STATE	PERCENT
26	Alabama	21.2
6	Alaska	25.8
34	Arizona	20.2
7	Arkansas	25.2
49	California	14.5
27	Colorado	21.1
21	Connecticut	21.9
8	Delaware	24.2
25	Florida	21.4
37	Georgia	19.8
48	Hawaii	15.8
45	Idaho	18.1
22	Illinois	21.6
12	Indiana	23.8
28	Iowa	21.0
43	Kansas	18.8
2	Kentucky	28.7
32	Louisiana	20.3
31	Maine	20.4
40	Maryland	19.3
40	Massachusetts	19.3
16	Michigan	22.8
37	Minnesota	19.8
44	Mississippi	18.5
4	Missouri	26.0
34	Montana	20.2
36	Nebraska	20.1
1	Nevada	30.5
13	New Hampshire	23.6
39	New Jersey	19.5
18	New Mexico	22.5
23	New York	21.5
19	North Carolina	22.4
32	North Dakota	20.3
9	Ohio	24.0
9	Oklahoma	24.0
40	Oregon	19.3
19	Pennsylvania	22.4
14	Rhode Island	23.2
46	South Carolina	18.0
30	South Dakota	20.8
4	Tennessee	26.0
47	Texas	17.4
50	Utah	11.5
23	Vermont	21.5
15	Virginia	22.9
17	Washington	22.7
3	West Virginia	27.6
29	Wisconsin	20.9
9	Wyoming	24.0

RANK	STATE	PERCENT
1	Nevada	30.5
2	Kentucky	28.7
3	West Virginia	27.6
4	Missouri	26.0
4	Tennessee	26.0
6	Alaska	25.8
7	Arkansas	25.2
8	Delaware	24.2
9	Ohio	24.0
9	Oklahoma	24.0
9	Wyoming	24.0
12	Indiana	23.8
13	New Hampshire	23.6
14	Rhode Island	23.2
15	Virginia	22.9
16	Michigan	22.8
17	Washington	22.7
18	New Mexico	22.5
19	North Carolina	22.4
19	Pennsylvania	22.4
21	Connecticut	21.9
22	Illinois	21.6
23	New York	21.5
23	Vermont	21.5
25	Florida	21.4
26	Alabama	21.2
27	Colorado	21.1
28	Iowa	21.0
29	Wisconsin	20.9
30	South Dakota	20.8
31	Maine	20.4
32	Louisiana	20.3
32	North Dakota	20.3
34	Arizona	20.2
34	Montana	20.2
36	Nebraska	20.1
37	Georgia	19.8
37	Minnesota	19.8
39	New Jersey	19.5
40	Maryland	19.3
40	Massachusetts	19.3
40	Oregon	19.3
43	Kansas	18.8
44	Mississippi	18.5
45	Idaho	18.1
46	South Carolina	18.0
47	Texas	17.4
48	Hawaii	15.8
49	California	14.5
50	Utah	11.5
	District of Columbia	15.4

Source: U.S. Department of Health and Human Services, Centers for Disease Control and Prevention
"1997 Behavioral Risk Factor Surveillance Summary Prevalence Report" (August 17, 1998)
*Persons 18 and older who have ever smoked 100 cigarettes and currently smoke.

Percent of Adults Overweight: 1997

National Median = 31.1% of Adults*

ALPHA ORDER				RANK ORDER		
RANK	STATE	PERCENT		RANK	STATE	PERCENT
12	Alabama	32.7		1	West Virginia	36.3
6	Alaska	34.1		2	Kentucky	35.6
49	Arizona	25.4		3	Mississippi	35.1
18	Arkansas	32.1		4	Michigan	34.9
35	California	29.1		5	Indiana	34.6
50	Colorado	25.1		6	Alaska	34.1
35	Connecticut	29.1		7	Louisiana	33.5
14	Delaware	32.5		8	Iowa	33.3
28	Florida	30.4		9	North Dakota	32.9
27	Georgia	30.8		10	Texas	32.8
46	Hawaii	26.6		10	Wisconsin	32.8
34	Idaho	29.6		12	Alabama	32.7
19	Illinois	32.0		13	Ohio	32.6
5	Indiana	34.6		14	Delaware	32.5
8	Iowa	33.3		15	North Carolina	32.4
23	Kansas	31.5		15	Oregon	32.4
2	Kentucky	35.6		17	Pennsylvania	32.2
7	Louisiana	33.5		18	Arkansas	32.1
29	Maine	30.2		19	Illinois	32.0
24	Maryland	31.2		20	South Carolina	31.8
48	Massachusetts	25.5		21	Missouri	31.6
4	Michigan	34.9		21	Tennessee	31.6
33	Minnesota	29.7		23	Kansas	31.5
3	Mississippi	35.1		24	Maryland	31.2
21	Missouri	31.6		25	Nebraska	31.1
42	Montana	27.9		25	South Dakota	31.1
25	Nebraska	31.1		27	Georgia	30.8
47	Nevada	26.2		28	Florida	30.4
44	New Hampshire	27.5		29	Maine	30.2
40	New Jersey	28.2		30	Virginia	30.0
32	New Mexico	29.8		31	Vermont	29.9
38	New York	28.4		32	New Mexico	29.8
15	North Carolina	32.4		33	Minnesota	29.7
9	North Dakota	32.9		34	Idaho	29.6
13	Ohio	32.6		35	California	29.1
38	Oklahoma	28.4		35	Connecticut	29.1
15	Oregon	32.4		35	Washington	29.1
17	Pennsylvania	32.2		38	New York	28.4
41	Rhode Island	28.1		38	Oklahoma	28.4
20	South Carolina	31.8		40	New Jersey	28.2
25	South Dakota	31.1		41	Rhode Island	28.1
21	Tennessee	31.6		42	Montana	27.9
10	Texas	32.8		42	Wyoming	27.9
45	Utah	27.0		44	New Hampshire	27.5
31	Vermont	29.9		45	Utah	27.0
30	Virginia	30.0		46	Hawaii	26.6
35	Washington	29.1		47	Nevada	26.2
1	West Virginia	36.3		48	Massachusetts	25.5
10	Wisconsin	32.8		49	Arizona	25.4
42	Wyoming	27.9		50	Colorado	25.1
					District of Columbia	28.0

Source: U.S. Department of Health and Human Services, Centers for Disease Control and Prevention
  "1997 Behavioral Risk Factor Surveillance Summary Prevalence Report" (August 17, 1998)
*Persons 18 and older. Overweight is defined as men with a Body Mass Index (BMI) of 27.8 or greater and women with an index of 27.3 or greater.   BMI is a ratio of height to weight. As an example, a person 5' 8" and weighing 185 pounds has a BMI of 28. See http://www.mealformation.com/bmassidx.htm.

Number of Days in the Past Month When Physical Health was "Not Good": 1997

National Median = 3.1 Days*

ALPHA ORDER

RANK	STATE	DAYS
2	Alabama	3.8
32	Alaska	2.9
50	Arizona	1.1
9	Arkansas	3.4
22	California	3.1
38	Colorado	2.8
22	Connecticut	3.1
3	Delaware	3.7
5	Florida	3.5
48	Georgia	2.2
28	Hawaii	3.0
9	Idaho	3.4
14	Illinois	3.3
9	Indiana	3.4
32	Iowa	2.9
49	Kansas	2.1
1	Kentucky	4.1
17	Louisiana	3.2
5	Maine	3.5
45	Maryland	2.4
14	Massachusetts	3.3
14	Michigan	3.3
28	Minnesota	3.0
22	Mississippi	3.1
5	Missouri	3.5
40	Montana	2.7
32	Nebraska	2.9
5	Nevada	3.5
22	New Hampshire	3.1
28	New Jersey	3.0
17	New Mexico	3.2
22	New York	3.1
32	North Carolina	2.9
32	North Dakota	2.9
42	Ohio	2.6
47	Oklahoma	2.3
17	Oregon	3.2
17	Pennsylvania	3.2
28	Rhode Island	3.0
32	South Carolina	2.9
42	South Dakota	2.6
9	Tennessee	3.4
17	Texas	3.2
4	Utah	3.6
40	Vermont	2.7
45	Virginia	2.4
22	Washington	3.1
9	West Virginia	3.4
38	Wisconsin	2.8
42	Wyoming	2.6

RANK ORDER

RANK	STATE	DAYS
1	Kentucky	4.1
2	Alabama	3.8
3	Delaware	3.7
4	Utah	3.6
5	Florida	3.5
5	Maine	3.5
5	Missouri	3.5
5	Nevada	3.5
9	Arkansas	3.4
9	Idaho	3.4
9	Indiana	3.4
9	Tennessee	3.4
9	West Virginia	3.4
14	Illinois	3.3
14	Massachusetts	3.3
14	Michigan	3.3
17	Louisiana	3.2
17	New Mexico	3.2
17	Oregon	3.2
17	Pennsylvania	3.2
17	Texas	3.2
22	California	3.1
22	Connecticut	3.1
22	Mississippi	3.1
22	New Hampshire	3.1
22	New York	3.1
22	Washington	3.1
28	Hawaii	3.0
28	Minnesota	3.0
28	New Jersey	3.0
28	Rhode Island	3.0
32	Alaska	2.9
32	Iowa	2.9
32	Nebraska	2.9
32	North Carolina	2.9
32	North Dakota	2.9
32	South Carolina	2.9
38	Colorado	2.8
38	Wisconsin	2.8
40	Montana	2.7
40	Vermont	2.7
42	Ohio	2.6
42	South Dakota	2.6
42	Wyoming	2.6
45	Maryland	2.4
45	Virginia	2.4
47	Oklahoma	2.3
48	Georgia	2.2
49	Kansas	2.1
50	Arizona	1.1
	District of Columbia	1.5

Source: U.S. Department of Health and Human Services, Centers for Disease Control and Prevention
"1997 Behavioral Risk Factor Surveillance Summary Prevalence Report" (August 17, 1998)
*Persons 18 and older.

Average Number of Days in the Past Month When Mental Health was "Not Good": 1997
National Median = 2.9 Days*

ALPHA ORDER

RANK	STATE	DAYS
9	Alabama	3.3
13	Alaska	3.2
50	Arizona	1.5
22	Arkansas	3.0
7	California	3.4
13	Colorado	3.2
31	Connecticut	2.8
13	Delaware	3.2
7	Florida	3.4
31	Georgia	2.8
38	Hawaii	2.6
18	Idaho	3.1
18	Illinois	3.1
3	Indiana	3.6
26	Iowa	2.9
49	Kansas	1.7
1	Kentucky	4.9
4	Louisiana	3.5
26	Maine	2.9
46	Maryland	1.8
18	Massachusetts	3.1
9	Michigan	3.3
22	Minnesota	3.0
39	Mississippi	2.5
13	Missouri	3.2
39	Montana	2.5
39	Nebraska	2.5
2	Nevada	3.7
9	New Hampshire	3.3
26	New Jersey	2.9
9	New Mexico	3.3
22	New York	3.0
39	North Carolina	2.5
22	North Dakota	3.0
45	Ohio	2.2
46	Oklahoma	1.8
13	Oregon	3.2
26	Pennsylvania	2.9
33	Rhode Island	2.7
46	South Carolina	1.8
33	South Dakota	2.7
4	Tennessee	3.5
26	Texas	2.9
4	Utah	3.5
33	Vermont	2.7
33	Virginia	2.7
18	Washington	3.1
44	West Virginia	2.3
39	Wisconsin	2.5
33	Wyoming	2.7

RANK ORDER

RANK	STATE	DAYS
1	Kentucky	4.9
2	Nevada	3.7
3	Indiana	3.6
4	Louisiana	3.5
4	Tennessee	3.5
4	Utah	3.5
7	California	3.4
7	Florida	3.4
9	Alabama	3.3
9	Michigan	3.3
9	New Hampshire	3.3
9	New Mexico	3.3
13	Alaska	3.2
13	Colorado	3.2
13	Delaware	3.2
13	Missouri	3.2
13	Oregon	3.2
18	Idaho	3.1
18	Illinois	3.1
18	Massachusetts	3.1
18	Washington	3.1
22	Arkansas	3.0
22	Minnesota	3.0
22	New York	3.0
22	North Dakota	3.0
26	Iowa	2.9
26	Maine	2.9
26	New Jersey	2.9
26	Pennsylvania	2.9
26	Texas	2.9
31	Connecticut	2.8
31	Georgia	2.8
33	Rhode Island	2.7
33	South Dakota	2.7
33	Vermont	2.7
33	Virginia	2.7
33	Wyoming	2.7
38	Hawaii	2.6
39	Mississippi	2.5
39	Montana	2.5
39	Nebraska	2.5
39	North Carolina	2.5
39	Wisconsin	2.5
44	West Virginia	2.3
45	Ohio	2.2
46	Maryland	1.8
46	Oklahoma	1.8
46	South Carolina	1.8
49	Kansas	1.7
50	Arizona	1.5

District of Columbia	2.1

Source: U.S. Department of Health and Human Services, Centers for Disease Control and Prevention
"1997 Behavioral Risk Factor Surveillance Summary Prevalence Report" (August 17, 1998)
*Persons 18 and older.

Percent of Adults Who Have Ever Been Tested for AIDS: 1997

National Median = 42.3% of Adults*

ALPHA ORDER

RANK	STATE	PERCENT
9	Alabama	49.5
4	Alaska	54.1
47	Arizona	31.7
27	Arkansas	41.7
NA	California**	NA
14	Colorado	47.1
24	Connecticut	43.0
6	Delaware	52.1
3	Florida	55.8
28	Georgia	41.2
16	Hawaii	45.5
21	Idaho	44.1
25	Illinois	42.3
35	Indiana	38.2
46	Iowa	31.9
49	Kansas	24.4
37	Kentucky	37.8
8	Louisiana	50.1
40	Maine	36.3
5	Maryland	52.6
19	Massachusetts	44.9
20	Michigan	44.5
45	Minnesota	32.0
10	Mississippi	49.2
29	Missouri	41.1
35	Montana	38.2
42	Nebraska	34.8
1	Nevada	60.5
39	New Hampshire	37.4
11	New Jersey	48.5
16	New Mexico	45.5
23	New York	43.3
30	North Carolina	40.5
48	North Dakota	31.0
43	Ohio	33.7
40	Oklahoma	36.3
22	Oregon	43.4
26	Pennsylvania	42.0
15	Rhode Island	46.0
13	South Carolina	47.9
38	South Dakota	37.6
16	Tennessee	45.5
7	Texas	51.2
32	Utah	38.8
33	Vermont	38.7
2	Virginia	57.1
12	Washington	48.3
44	West Virginia	33.1
31	Wisconsin	40.3
33	Wyoming	38.7

RANK ORDER

RANK	STATE	PERCENT
1	Nevada	60.5
2	Virginia	57.1
3	Florida	55.8
4	Alaska	54.1
5	Maryland	52.6
6	Delaware	52.1
7	Texas	51.2
8	Louisiana	50.1
9	Alabama	49.5
10	Mississippi	49.2
11	New Jersey	48.5
12	Washington	48.3
13	South Carolina	47.9
14	Colorado	47.1
15	Rhode Island	46.0
16	Hawaii	45.5
16	New Mexico	45.5
16	Tennessee	45.5
19	Massachusetts	44.9
20	Michigan	44.5
21	Idaho	44.1
22	Oregon	43.4
23	New York	43.3
24	Connecticut	43.0
25	Illinois	42.3
26	Pennsylvania	42.0
27	Arkansas	41.7
28	Georgia	41.2
29	Missouri	41.1
30	North Carolina	40.5
31	Wisconsin	40.3
32	Utah	38.8
33	Vermont	38.7
33	Wyoming	38.7
35	Indiana	38.2
35	Montana	38.2
37	Kentucky	37.8
38	South Dakota	37.6
39	New Hampshire	37.4
40	Maine	36.3
40	Oklahoma	36.3
42	Nebraska	34.8
43	Ohio	33.7
44	West Virginia	33.1
45	Minnesota	32.0
46	Iowa	31.9
47	Arizona	31.7
48	North Dakota	31.0
49	Kansas	24.4
NA	California**	NA

District of Columbia   60.2

Source: U.S. Department of Health and Human Services, Centers for Disease Control and Prevention
"1997 Behavioral Risk Factor Surveillance Summary Prevalence Report" (August 17, 1998)
*Persons 18 to 64 years old.
**Not available.

Percent of Adults Who Believe They Have a Chance of Getting AIDS: 1997

National Median = 6.1% of Adults*

ALPHA ORDER			RANK ORDER		
RANK	STATE	PERCENT	RANK	STATE	PERCENT
27	Alabama	5.8	1	Texas	12.1
29	Alaska	5.7	2	West Virginia	9.1
49	Arizona	3.3	3	South Dakota	8.9
13	Arkansas	7.2	4	Kansas	8.7
NA	California**	NA	5	Nebraska	8.3
45	Colorado	4.6	6	Missouri	8.0
24	Connecticut	6.1	7	Florida	7.9
14	Delaware	7.0	7	New Mexico	7.9
7	Florida	7.9	7	Wyoming	7.9
40	Georgia	4.9	10	Illinois	7.6
14	Hawaii	7.0	11	New York	7.3
36	Idaho	5.2	11	Rhode Island	7.3
10	Illinois	7.6	13	Arkansas	7.2
24	Indiana	6.1	14	Delaware	7.0
32	Iowa	5.5	14	Hawaii	7.0
4	Kansas	8.7	14	Tennessee	7.0
27	Kentucky	5.8	17	Mississippi	6.8
40	Louisiana	4.9	17	Pennsylvania	6.8
40	Maine	4.9	19	North Carolina	6.7
38	Maryland	5.0	20	Vermont	6.6
24	Massachusetts	6.1	21	New Jersey	6.4
35	Michigan	5.4	22	Nevada	6.3
29	Minnesota	5.7	23	Ohio	6.2
17	Mississippi	6.8	24	Connecticut	6.1
6	Missouri	8.0	24	Indiana	6.1
47	Montana	4.3	24	Massachusetts	6.1
5	Nebraska	8.3	27	Alabama	5.8
22	Nevada	6.3	27	Kentucky	5.8
48	New Hampshire	4.2	29	Alaska	5.7
21	New Jersey	6.4	29	Minnesota	5.7
7	New Mexico	7.9	31	Wisconsin	5.6
11	New York	7.3	32	Iowa	5.5
19	North Carolina	6.7	32	Oregon	5.5
40	North Dakota	4.9	32	South Carolina	5.5
23	Ohio	6.2	35	Michigan	5.4
40	Oklahoma	4.9	36	Idaho	5.2
32	Oregon	5.5	36	Utah	5.2
17	Pennsylvania	6.8	38	Maryland	5.0
11	Rhode Island	7.3	38	Virginia	5.0
32	South Carolina	5.5	40	Georgia	4.9
3	South Dakota	8.9	40	Louisiana	4.9
14	Tennessee	7.0	40	Maine	4.9
1	Texas	12.1	40	North Dakota	4.9
36	Utah	5.2	40	Oklahoma	4.9
20	Vermont	6.6	45	Colorado	4.6
38	Virginia	5.0	46	Washington	4.5
46	Washington	4.5	47	Montana	4.3
2	West Virginia	9.1	48	New Hampshire	4.2
31	Wisconsin	5.6	49	Arizona	3.3
7	Wyoming	7.9	NA	California**	NA
				District of Columbia	7.2

Source: U.S. Department of Health and Human Services, Centers for Disease Control and Prevention
"1997 Behavioral Risk Factor Surveillance Summary Prevalence Report" (August 17, 1998)
*For persons 18 to 64 years old who believe their chances of getting the AIDS virus are "medium" or "high."
**Not available.

Safety Belt Usage Rate in 1998

National Rate = 65% Use Safety Belts*

ALPHA ORDER

RANK ORDER

RANK	STATE	PERCENT		RANK	STATE	PERCENT
46	Alabama	52		1	California	88
16	Alaska	69		2	New Mexico	87
25	Arizona	63		3	Oregon	85
48	Arkansas	48		4	North Carolina	83
1	California	88		5	Washington	82
38	Colorado	59		6	Hawaii	80
23	Connecticut	64		7	Iowa	75
35	Delaware	60		7	Texas	75
35	Florida	60		7	Wyoming	75
17	Georgia	68		10	New York	74
6	Hawaii	80		11	Montana	73
43	Idaho	54		12	Maryland	71
23	Illinois	64		12	Vermont	71
25	Indiana	63		14	Michigan	70
7	Iowa	75		14	Nevada	70
42	Kansas	56		16	Alaska	69
43	Kentucky	54		17	Georgia	68
18	Louisiana	67		18	Louisiana	67
32	Maine	61		18	Virginia	67
12	Maryland	71		20	Minnesota	65
45	Massachusetts	53		20	Ohio	65
14	Michigan	70		20	Pennsylvania	65
20	Minnesota	65		23	Connecticut	64
48	Mississippi	48		23	Illinois	64
29	Missouri	62		25	Arizona	63
11	Montana	73		25	Indiana	63
25	Nebraska	63		25	Nebraska	63
14	Nevada	70		25	Utah	63
NA	New Hampshire**	NA		29	Missouri	62
29	New Jersey	62		29	New Jersey	62
2	New Mexico	87		29	Wisconsin	62
10	New York	74		32	Maine	61
4	North Carolina	83		32	South Carolina	61
47	North Dakota	49		32	Tennessee	61
20	Ohio	65		35	Delaware	60
35	Oklahoma	60		35	Florida	60
3	Oregon	85		35	Oklahoma	60
20	Pennsylvania	65		38	Colorado	59
40	Rhode Island	58		38	South Dakota	59
32	South Carolina	61		40	Rhode Island	58
38	South Dakota	59		40	West Virginia	58
32	Tennessee	61		42	Kansas	56
7	Texas	75		43	Idaho	54
25	Utah	63		43	Kentucky	54
12	Vermont	71		45	Massachusetts	53
18	Virginia	67		46	Alabama	52
5	Washington	82		47	North Dakota	49
40	West Virginia	58		48	Arkansas	48
29	Wisconsin	62		48	Mississippi	48
7	Wyoming	75		NA	New Hampshire**	NA
					District of Columbia	66

Source: U.S. Department of Transportation, National Highway Safety Traffic Safety Administration
  "Key Provisions of Safety Belt Use" (October 1998)
*As of January 1998. National average is a simple average of reporting states' rates.
**Not reported.

Percent of Adults Whose Children Use a Car Safety Seat: 1997

National Median = 94.4% of Adults*

ALPHA ORDER

RANK	STATE	PERCENT
28	Alabama	93.9
38	Alaska	92.8
12	Arizona	96.7
49	Arkansas	85.9
35	California	93.3
21	Colorado	94.9
13	Connecticut	96.3
5	Delaware	97.7
15	Florida	96.2
2	Georgia	99.3
45	Hawaii	90.6
47	Idaho	88.8
19	Illinois	95.7
42	Indiana	91.2
40	Iowa	91.9
20	Kansas	95.2
4	Kentucky	98.1
30	Louisiana	93.8
1	Maine	99.6
10	Maryland	97.1
23	Massachusetts	94.7
45	Michigan	90.6
28	Minnesota	93.9
30	Mississippi	93.8
5	Missouri	97.7
39	Montana	92.0
26	Nebraska	94.4
23	Nevada	94.7
7	New Hampshire	97.6
17	New Jersey	96.0
30	New Mexico	93.8
25	New York	94.6
34	North Carolina	93.5
11	North Dakota	96.8
27	Ohio	94.3
35	Oklahoma	93.3
37	Oregon	93.0
21	Pennsylvania	94.9
18	Rhode Island	95.8
9	South Carolina	97.4
43	South Dakota	91.0
8	Tennessee	97.5
49	Texas	85.9
44	Utah	90.7
3	Vermont	98.3
16	Virginia	96.1
48	Washington	87.3
13	West Virginia	96.3
33	Wisconsin	93.6
41	Wyoming	91.5

RANK ORDER

RANK	STATE	PERCENT
1	Maine	99.6
2	Georgia	99.3
3	Vermont	98.3
4	Kentucky	98.1
5	Delaware	97.7
5	Missouri	97.7
7	New Hampshire	97.6
8	Tennessee	97.5
9	South Carolina	97.4
10	Maryland	97.1
11	North Dakota	96.8
12	Arizona	96.7
13	Connecticut	96.3
13	West Virginia	96.3
15	Florida	96.2
16	Virginia	96.1
17	New Jersey	96.0
18	Rhode Island	95.8
19	Illinois	95.7
20	Kansas	95.2
21	Colorado	94.9
21	Pennsylvania	94.9
23	Massachusetts	94.7
23	Nevada	94.7
25	New York	94.6
26	Nebraska	94.4
27	Ohio	94.3
28	Alabama	93.9
28	Minnesota	93.9
30	Louisiana	93.8
30	Mississippi	93.8
30	New Mexico	93.8
33	Wisconsin	93.6
34	North Carolina	93.5
35	California	93.3
35	Oklahoma	93.3
37	Oregon	93.0
38	Alaska	92.8
39	Montana	92.0
40	Iowa	91.9
41	Wyoming	91.5
42	Indiana	91.2
43	South Dakota	91.0
44	Utah	90.7
45	Hawaii	90.6
45	Michigan	90.6
47	Idaho	88.8
48	Washington	87.3
49	Arkansas	85.9
49	Texas	85.9
	District of Columbia	85.0

Source: U.S. Department of Health and Human Services, Centers for Disease Control and Prevention
"1997 Behavioral Risk Factor Surveillance Summary Prevalence Report" (August 17, 1998)
Persons whose children under 5 years old "always or nearly always use a safety seat".

VIII. APPENDIX

Population Charts

Population in 1998

National Total = 270,298,524*

ALPHA ORDER

RANK	STATE	POPULATION	% of USA
23	Alabama	4,351,999	1.6%
48	Alaska	614,010	0.2%
21	Arizona	4,668,631	1.7%
33	Arkansas	2,538,303	0.9%
1	California	32,666,550	12.1%
24	Colorado	3,970,971	1.5%
29	Connecticut	3,274,069	1.2%
45	Delaware	743,603	0.3%
4	Florida	14,915,980	5.5%
10	Georgia	7,642,207	2.8%
41	Hawaii	1,193,001	0.4%
40	Idaho	1,228,684	0.5%
5	Illinois	12,045,326	4.5%
14	Indiana	5,899,195	2.2%
30	Iowa	2,862,447	1.1%
32	Kansas	2,629,067	1.0%
25	Kentucky	3,936,499	1.5%
22	Louisiana	4,368,967	1.6%
39	Maine	1,244,250	0.5%
19	Maryland	5,134,808	1.9%
13	Massachusetts	6,147,132	2.3%
8	Michigan	9,817,242	3.6%
20	Minnesota	4,725,419	1.7%
31	Mississippi	2,752,092	1.0%
16	Missouri	5,438,559	2.0%
44	Montana	880,453	0.3%
38	Nebraska	1,662,719	0.6%
36	Nevada	1,746,898	0.6%
42	New Hampshire	1,185,048	0.4%
9	New Jersey	8,115,011	3.0%
37	New Mexico	1,736,931	0.6%
3	New York	18,175,301	6.7%
11	North Carolina	7,546,493	2.8%
47	North Dakota	638,244	0.2%
7	Ohio	11,209,493	4.1%
27	Oklahoma	3,346,713	1.2%
28	Oregon	3,281,974	1.2%
6	Pennsylvania	12,001,451	4.4%
43	Rhode Island	988,480	0.4%
26	South Carolina	3,835,962	1.4%
46	South Dakota	738,171	0.3%
17	Tennessee	5,430,621	2.0%
2	Texas	19,759,614	7.3%
34	Utah	2,099,758	0.8%
49	Vermont	590,883	0.2%
12	Virginia	6,791,345	2.5%
15	Washington	5,689,263	2.1%
35	West Virginia	1,811,156	0.7%
18	Wisconsin	5,223,500	1.9%
50	Wyoming	480,907	0.2%

RANK ORDER

RANK	STATE	POPULATION	% of USA
1	California	32,666,550	12.1%
2	Texas	19,759,614	7.3%
3	New York	18,175,301	6.7%
4	Florida	14,915,980	5.5%
5	Illinois	12,045,326	4.5%
6	Pennsylvania	12,001,451	4.4%
7	Ohio	11,209,493	4.1%
8	Michigan	9,817,242	3.6%
9	New Jersey	8,115,011	3.0%
10	Georgia	7,642,207	2.8%
11	North Carolina	7,546,493	2.8%
12	Virginia	6,791,345	2.5%
13	Massachusetts	6,147,132	2.3%
14	Indiana	5,899,195	2.2%
15	Washington	5,689,263	2.1%
16	Missouri	5,438,559	2.0%
17	Tennessee	5,430,621	2.0%
18	Wisconsin	5,223,500	1.9%
19	Maryland	5,134,808	1.9%
20	Minnesota	4,725,419	1.7%
21	Arizona	4,668,631	1.7%
22	Louisiana	4,368,967	1.6%
23	Alabama	4,351,999	1.6%
24	Colorado	3,970,971	1.5%
25	Kentucky	3,936,499	1.5%
26	South Carolina	3,835,962	1.4%
27	Oklahoma	3,346,713	1.2%
28	Oregon	3,281,974	1.2%
29	Connecticut	3,274,069	1.2%
30	Iowa	2,862,447	1.1%
31	Mississippi	2,752,092	1.0%
32	Kansas	2,629,067	1.0%
33	Arkansas	2,538,303	0.9%
34	Utah	2,099,758	0.8%
35	West Virginia	1,811,156	0.7%
36	Nevada	1,746,898	0.6%
37	New Mexico	1,736,931	0.6%
38	Nebraska	1,662,719	0.6%
39	Maine	1,244,250	0.5%
40	Idaho	1,228,684	0.5%
41	Hawaii	1,193,001	0.4%
42	New Hampshire	1,185,048	0.4%
43	Rhode Island	988,480	0.4%
44	Montana	880,453	0.3%
45	Delaware	743,603	0.3%
46	South Dakota	738,171	0.3%
47	North Dakota	638,244	0.2%
48	Alaska	614,010	0.2%
49	Vermont	590,883	0.2%
50	Wyoming	480,907	0.2%
	District of Columbia	523,124	0.2%

Source: U.S. Bureau of the Census
Press Release (CB98-242, December 31, 1998)
Includes armed forces residing in each state.

Population in 1997

National Total = 267,743,595*

ALPHA ORDER				RANK ORDER			
RANK	STATE	POPULATION	% of USA	RANK	STATE	POPULATION	% of USA
23	Alabama	4,322,113	1.6%	1	California	32,182,118	12.0%
48	Alaska	609,655	0.2%	2	Texas	19,385,699	7.2%
21	Arizona	4,553,249	1.7%	3	New York	18,146,200	6.8%
33	Arkansas	2,523,186	0.9%	4	Florida	14,677,181	5.5%
1	California	32,182,118	12.0%	5	Pennsylvania	12,011,278	4.5%
25	Colorado	3,892,029	1.5%	6	Illinois	11,989,352	4.5%
28	Connecticut	3,267,240	1.2%	7	Ohio	11,192,932	4.2%
46	Delaware	735,143	0.3%	8	Michigan	9,779,984	3.7%
4	Florida	14,677,181	5.5%	9	New Jersey	8,058,384	3.0%
10	Georgia	7,489,982	2.8%	10	Georgia	7,489,982	2.8%
41	Hawaii	1,192,057	0.4%	11	North Carolina	7,430,675	2.8%
40	Idaho	1,208,865	0.5%	12	Virginia	6,737,489	2.5%
6	Illinois	11,989,352	4.5%	13	Massachusetts	6,114,440	2.3%
14	Indiana	5,864,847	2.2%	14	Indiana	5,864,847	2.2%
30	Iowa	2,854,330	1.1%	15	Washington	5,614,151	2.1%
32	Kansas	2,601,437	1.0%	16	Missouri	5,408,455	2.0%
24	Kentucky	3,910,366	1.5%	17	Tennessee	5,371,693	2.0%
22	Louisiana	4,353,646	1.6%	18	Wisconsin	5,201,226	1.9%
39	Maine	1,241,895	0.5%	19	Maryland	5,094,924	1.9%
19	Maryland	5,094,924	1.9%	20	Minnesota	4,687,408	1.8%
13	Massachusetts	6,114,440	2.3%	21	Arizona	4,553,249	1.7%
8	Michigan	9,779,984	3.7%	22	Louisiana	4,353,646	1.6%
20	Minnesota	4,687,408	1.8%	23	Alabama	4,322,113	1.6%
31	Mississippi	2,731,644	1.0%	24	Kentucky	3,910,366	1.5%
16	Missouri	5,408,455	2.0%	25	Colorado	3,892,029	1.5%
44	Montana	878,730	0.3%	26	South Carolina	3,788,119	1.4%
38	Nebraska	1,657,009	0.6%	27	Oklahoma	3,321,611	1.2%
37	Nevada	1,678,691	0.6%	28	Connecticut	3,267,240	1.2%
42	New Hampshire	1,172,140	0.4%	29	Oregon	3,243,272	1.2%
9	New Jersey	8,058,384	3.0%	30	Iowa	2,854,330	1.1%
36	New Mexico	1,723,965	0.6%	31	Mississippi	2,731,644	1.0%
3	New York	18,146,200	6.8%	32	Kansas	2,601,437	1.0%
11	North Carolina	7,430,675	2.8%	33	Arkansas	2,523,186	0.9%
47	North Dakota	640,965	0.2%	34	Utah	2,065,001	0.8%
7	Ohio	11,192,932	4.2%	35	West Virginia	1,815,231	0.7%
27	Oklahoma	3,321,611	1.2%	36	New Mexico	1,723,965	0.6%
29	Oregon	3,243,272	1.2%	37	Nevada	1,678,691	0.6%
5	Pennsylvania	12,011,278	4.5%	38	Nebraska	1,657,009	0.6%
43	Rhode Island	987,263	0.4%	39	Maine	1,241,895	0.5%
26	South Carolina	3,788,119	1.4%	40	Idaho	1,208,865	0.5%
45	South Dakota	737,755	0.3%	41	Hawaii	1,192,057	0.4%
17	Tennessee	5,371,693	2.0%	42	New Hampshire	1,172,140	0.4%
2	Texas	19,385,699	7.2%	43	Rhode Island	987,263	0.4%
34	Utah	2,065,001	0.8%	44	Montana	878,730	0.3%
49	Vermont	588,632	0.2%	45	South Dakota	737,755	0.3%
12	Virginia	6,737,489	2.5%	46	Delaware	735,143	0.3%
15	Washington	5,614,151	2.1%	47	North Dakota	640,965	0.2%
35	West Virginia	1,815,231	0.7%	48	Alaska	609,655	0.2%
18	Wisconsin	5,201,226	1.9%	49	Vermont	588,632	0.2%
50	Wyoming	480,043	0.2%	50	Wyoming	480,043	0.2%
					District of Columbia	529,895	0.2%

Source: U.S. Bureau of the Census
   Press Release (CB98-242, December 31, 1998)
*Includes armed forces residing in each state. This updates earlier 1997 population estimates.

Male Population in 1997

National Total = 131,017,669 Males

<table>
<tr><td colspan="4">ALPHA ORDER</td><td colspan="4">RANK ORDER</td></tr>
<tr><th>RANK</th><th>STATE</th><th>MALES</th><th>% of USA</th><th>RANK</th><th>STATE</th><th>MALES</th><th>% of USA</th></tr>
<tr><td>23</td><td>Alabama</td><td>2,076,894</td><td>1.6%</td><td>1</td><td>California</td><td>16,162,155</td><td>12.3%</td></tr>
<tr><td>47</td><td>Alaska</td><td>320,238</td><td>0.2%</td><td>2</td><td>Texas</td><td>9,611,078</td><td>7.3%</td></tr>
<tr><td>21</td><td>Arizona</td><td>2,258,329</td><td>1.7%</td><td>3</td><td>New York</td><td>8,742,751</td><td>6.7%</td></tr>
<tr><td>33</td><td>Arkansas</td><td>1,221,537</td><td>0.9%</td><td>4</td><td>Florida</td><td>7,123,245</td><td>5.4%</td></tr>
<tr><td>1</td><td>California</td><td>16,162,155</td><td>12.3%</td><td>5</td><td>Illinois</td><td>5,811,208</td><td>4.4%</td></tr>
<tr><td>24</td><td>Colorado</td><td>1,931,218</td><td>1.5%</td><td>6</td><td>Pennsylvania</td><td>5,788,677</td><td>4.4%</td></tr>
<tr><td>29</td><td>Connecticut</td><td>1,589,630</td><td>1.2%</td><td>7</td><td>Ohio</td><td>5,418,599</td><td>4.1%</td></tr>
<tr><td>46</td><td>Delaware</td><td>356,526</td><td>0.3%</td><td>8</td><td>Michigan</td><td>4,764,800</td><td>3.6%</td></tr>
<tr><td>4</td><td>Florida</td><td>7,123,245</td><td>5.4%</td><td>9</td><td>New Jersey</td><td>3,907,778</td><td>3.0%</td></tr>
<tr><td>10</td><td>Georgia</td><td>3,650,375</td><td>2.8%</td><td>10</td><td>Georgia</td><td>3,650,375</td><td>2.8%</td></tr>
<tr><td>41</td><td>Hawaii</td><td>596,755</td><td>0.5%</td><td>11</td><td>North Carolina</td><td>3,610,888</td><td>2.8%</td></tr>
<tr><td>40</td><td>Idaho</td><td>605,252</td><td>0.5%</td><td>12</td><td>Virginia</td><td>3,298,271</td><td>2.5%</td></tr>
<tr><td>5</td><td>Illinois</td><td>5,811,208</td><td>4.4%</td><td>13</td><td>Massachusetts</td><td>2,954,329</td><td>2.3%</td></tr>
<tr><td>14</td><td>Indiana</td><td>2,859,316</td><td>2.2%</td><td>14</td><td>Indiana</td><td>2,859,316</td><td>2.2%</td></tr>
<tr><td>30</td><td>Iowa</td><td>1,391,648</td><td>1.1%</td><td>15</td><td>Washington</td><td>2,796,136</td><td>2.1%</td></tr>
<tr><td>32</td><td>Kansas</td><td>1,277,681</td><td>1.0%</td><td>16</td><td>Missouri</td><td>2,621,192</td><td>2.0%</td></tr>
<tr><td>25</td><td>Kentucky</td><td>1,899,716</td><td>1.4%</td><td>17</td><td>Tennessee</td><td>2,595,576</td><td>2.0%</td></tr>
<tr><td>22</td><td>Louisiana</td><td>2,097,289</td><td>1.6%</td><td>18</td><td>Wisconsin</td><td>2,544,836</td><td>1.9%</td></tr>
<tr><td>39</td><td>Maine</td><td>606,937</td><td>0.5%</td><td>19</td><td>Maryland</td><td>2,480,619</td><td>1.9%</td></tr>
<tr><td>19</td><td>Maryland</td><td>2,480,619</td><td>1.9%</td><td>20</td><td>Minnesota</td><td>2,312,594</td><td>1.8%</td></tr>
<tr><td>13</td><td>Massachusetts</td><td>2,954,329</td><td>2.3%</td><td>21</td><td>Arizona</td><td>2,258,329</td><td>1.7%</td></tr>
<tr><td>8</td><td>Michigan</td><td>4,764,800</td><td>3.6%</td><td>22</td><td>Louisiana</td><td>2,097,289</td><td>1.6%</td></tr>
<tr><td>20</td><td>Minnesota</td><td>2,312,594</td><td>1.8%</td><td>23</td><td>Alabama</td><td>2,076,894</td><td>1.6%</td></tr>
<tr><td>31</td><td>Mississippi</td><td>1,311,959</td><td>1.0%</td><td>24</td><td>Colorado</td><td>1,931,218</td><td>1.5%</td></tr>
<tr><td>16</td><td>Missouri</td><td>2,621,192</td><td>2.0%</td><td>25</td><td>Kentucky</td><td>1,899,716</td><td>1.4%</td></tr>
<tr><td>44</td><td>Montana</td><td>438,030</td><td>0.3%</td><td>26</td><td>South Carolina</td><td>1,816,821</td><td>1.4%</td></tr>
<tr><td>38</td><td>Nebraska</td><td>812,173</td><td>0.6%</td><td>27</td><td>Oklahoma</td><td>1,623,255</td><td>1.2%</td></tr>
<tr><td>36</td><td>Nevada</td><td>855,083</td><td>0.7%</td><td>28</td><td>Oregon</td><td>1,604,344</td><td>1.2%</td></tr>
<tr><td>42</td><td>New Hampshire</td><td>577,841</td><td>0.4%</td><td>29</td><td>Connecticut</td><td>1,589,630</td><td>1.2%</td></tr>
<tr><td>9</td><td>New Jersey</td><td>3,907,778</td><td>3.0%</td><td>30</td><td>Iowa</td><td>1,391,648</td><td>1.1%</td></tr>
<tr><td>37</td><td>New Mexico</td><td>852,920</td><td>0.7%</td><td>31</td><td>Mississippi</td><td>1,311,959</td><td>1.0%</td></tr>
<tr><td>3</td><td>New York</td><td>8,742,751</td><td>6.7%</td><td>32</td><td>Kansas</td><td>1,277,681</td><td>1.0%</td></tr>
<tr><td>11</td><td>North Carolina</td><td>3,610,888</td><td>2.8%</td><td>33</td><td>Arkansas</td><td>1,221,537</td><td>0.9%</td></tr>
<tr><td>48</td><td>North Dakota</td><td>319,678</td><td>0.2%</td><td>34</td><td>Utah</td><td>1,025,615</td><td>0.8%</td></tr>
<tr><td>7</td><td>Ohio</td><td>5,418,599</td><td>4.1%</td><td>35</td><td>West Virginia</td><td>876,665</td><td>0.7%</td></tr>
<tr><td>27</td><td>Oklahoma</td><td>1,623,255</td><td>1.2%</td><td>36</td><td>Nevada</td><td>855,083</td><td>0.7%</td></tr>
<tr><td>28</td><td>Oregon</td><td>1,604,344</td><td>1.2%</td><td>37</td><td>New Mexico</td><td>852,920</td><td>0.7%</td></tr>
<tr><td>6</td><td>Pennsylvania</td><td>5,788,677</td><td>4.4%</td><td>38</td><td>Nebraska</td><td>812,173</td><td>0.6%</td></tr>
<tr><td>43</td><td>Rhode Island</td><td>475,424</td><td>0.4%</td><td>39</td><td>Maine</td><td>606,937</td><td>0.5%</td></tr>
<tr><td>26</td><td>South Carolina</td><td>1,816,821</td><td>1.4%</td><td>40</td><td>Idaho</td><td>605,252</td><td>0.5%</td></tr>
<tr><td>45</td><td>South Dakota</td><td>363,783</td><td>0.3%</td><td>41</td><td>Hawaii</td><td>596,755</td><td>0.5%</td></tr>
<tr><td>17</td><td>Tennessee</td><td>2,595,576</td><td>2.0%</td><td>42</td><td>New Hampshire</td><td>577,841</td><td>0.4%</td></tr>
<tr><td>2</td><td>Texas</td><td>9,611,078</td><td>7.3%</td><td>43</td><td>Rhode Island</td><td>475,424</td><td>0.4%</td></tr>
<tr><td>34</td><td>Utah</td><td>1,025,615</td><td>0.8%</td><td>44</td><td>Montana</td><td>438,030</td><td>0.3%</td></tr>
<tr><td>49</td><td>Vermont</td><td>290,209</td><td>0.2%</td><td>45</td><td>South Dakota</td><td>363,783</td><td>0.3%</td></tr>
<tr><td>12</td><td>Virginia</td><td>3,298,271</td><td>2.5%</td><td>46</td><td>Delaware</td><td>356,526</td><td>0.3%</td></tr>
<tr><td>15</td><td>Washington</td><td>2,796,136</td><td>2.1%</td><td>47</td><td>Alaska</td><td>320,238</td><td>0.2%</td></tr>
<tr><td>35</td><td>West Virginia</td><td>876,665</td><td>0.7%</td><td>48</td><td>North Dakota</td><td>319,678</td><td>0.2%</td></tr>
<tr><td>18</td><td>Wisconsin</td><td>2,544,836</td><td>1.9%</td><td>49</td><td>Vermont</td><td>290,209</td><td>0.2%</td></tr>
<tr><td>50</td><td>Wyoming</td><td>241,601</td><td>0.2%</td><td>50</td><td>Wyoming</td><td>241,601</td><td>0.2%</td></tr>
<tr><td></td><td></td><td></td><td></td><td></td><td>District of Columbia</td><td>248,195</td><td>0.2%</td></tr>
</table>

Source: U.S. Bureau of the Census
"Estimates of the Population of the States by Selected Age Groups and Sex" (ST-97-5, July 1, 1998)
(http://www.census.gov/population/estimates/state/97agesex.txt)

Female Population in 1997

National Total = 136,618,392 Females

RANK	STATE	FEMALES	% of USA
23	Alabama	2,242,260	1.6%
49	Alaska	289,073	0.2%
21	Arizona	2,296,637	1.7%
33	Arkansas	1,301,282	1.0%
1	California	16,106,146	11.8%
25	Colorado	1,961,426	1.4%
28	Connecticut	1,680,228	1.2%
45	Delaware	375,055	0.3%
4	Florida	7,530,700	5.5%
10	Georgia	3,835,867	2.8%
42	Hawaii	589,847	0.4%
40	Idaho	604,980	0.4%
6	Illinois	6,084,641	4.5%
14	Indiana	3,004,792	2.2%
30	Iowa	1,460,775	1.1%
32	Kansas	1,317,159	1.0%
24	Kentucky	2,008,408	1.5%
22	Louisiana	2,254,480	1.7%
39	Maine	635,114	0.5%
19	Maryland	2,613,670	1.9%
13	Massachusetts	3,163,191	2.3%
8	Michigan	5,009,092	3.7%
20	Minnesota	2,372,955	1.7%
31	Mississippi	1,418,542	1.0%
16	Missouri	2,780,866	2.0%
44	Montana	440,780	0.3%
37	Nebraska	844,697	0.6%
38	Nevada	821,726	0.6%
41	New Hampshire	594,868	0.4%
9	New Jersey	4,145,071	3.0%
36	New Mexico	876,831	0.6%
3	New York	9,394,475	6.9%
11	North Carolina	3,814,295	2.8%
47	North Dakota	321,205	0.2%
7	Ohio	5,767,732	4.2%
27	Oklahoma	1,693,836	1.2%
29	Oregon	1,639,143	1.2%
5	Pennsylvania	6,230,984	4.6%
43	Rhode Island	512,005	0.4%
26	South Carolina	1,943,360	1.4%
46	South Dakota	374,190	0.3%
17	Tennessee	2,772,622	2.0%
2	Texas	9,828,259	7.2%
34	Utah	1,033,533	0.8%
48	Vermont	298,769	0.2%
12	Virginia	3,435,725	2.5%
15	Washington	2,814,226	2.1%
35	West Virginia	939,122	0.7%
18	Wisconsin	2,624,841	1.9%
50	Wyoming	238,142	0.2%

RANK	STATE	FEMALES	% of USA
1	California	16,106,146	11.8%
2	Texas	9,828,259	7.2%
3	New York	9,394,475	6.9%
4	Florida	7,530,700	5.5%
5	Pennsylvania	6,230,984	4.6%
6	Illinois	6,084,641	4.5%
7	Ohio	5,767,732	4.2%
8	Michigan	5,009,092	3.7%
9	New Jersey	4,145,071	3.0%
10	Georgia	3,835,867	2.8%
11	North Carolina	3,814,295	2.8%
12	Virginia	3,435,725	2.5%
13	Massachusetts	3,163,191	2.3%
14	Indiana	3,004,792	2.2%
15	Washington	2,814,226	2.1%
16	Missouri	2,780,866	2.0%
17	Tennessee	2,772,622	2.0%
18	Wisconsin	2,624,841	1.9%
19	Maryland	2,613,670	1.9%
20	Minnesota	2,372,955	1.7%
21	Arizona	2,296,637	1.7%
22	Louisiana	2,254,480	1.7%
23	Alabama	2,242,260	1.6%
24	Kentucky	2,008,408	1.5%
25	Colorado	1,961,426	1.4%
26	South Carolina	1,943,360	1.4%
27	Oklahoma	1,693,836	1.2%
28	Connecticut	1,680,228	1.2%
29	Oregon	1,639,143	1.2%
30	Iowa	1,460,775	1.1%
31	Mississippi	1,418,542	1.0%
32	Kansas	1,317,159	1.0%
33	Arkansas	1,301,282	1.0%
34	Utah	1,033,533	0.8%
35	West Virginia	939,122	0.7%
36	New Mexico	876,831	0.6%
37	Nebraska	844,697	0.6%
38	Nevada	821,726	0.6%
39	Maine	635,114	0.5%
40	Idaho	604,980	0.4%
41	New Hampshire	594,868	0.4%
42	Hawaii	589,847	0.4%
43	Rhode Island	512,005	0.4%
44	Montana	440,780	0.3%
45	Delaware	375,055	0.3%
46	South Dakota	374,190	0.3%
47	North Dakota	321,205	0.2%
48	Vermont	298,769	0.2%
49	Alaska	289,073	0.2%
50	Wyoming	238,142	0.2%
	District of Columbia	280,769	0.2%

Source: U.S. Bureau of the Census
"Estimates of the Population of the States by Selected Age Groups and Sex" (ST-97-5, July 1, 1998)
(http://www.census.gov/population/estimates/state/97agesex.txt)

Population in 1993

National Total = 257,746,103*

ALPHA ORDER				RANK ORDER			
RANK	STATE	POPULATION	% of USA	RANK	STATE	POPULATION	% of USA
22	Alabama	4,191,879	1.6%	1	California	31,124,200	12.1%
48	Alaska	596,906	0.2%	2	New York	18,139,051	7.0%
23	Arizona	3,993,563	1.5%	3	Texas	18,009,031	7.0%
33	Arkansas	2,423,980	0.9%	4	Florida	13,712,052	5.3%
1	California	31,124,200	12.1%	5	Pennsylvania	12,022,460	4.7%
26	Colorado	3,562,064	1.4%	6	Illinois	11,718,133	4.5%
27	Connecticut	3,269,944	1.3%	7	Ohio	11,063,366	4.3%
46	Delaware	700,112	0.3%	8	Michigan	9,523,247	3.7%
4	Florida	13,712,052	5.3%	9	New Jersey	7,873,468	3.1%
11	Georgia	6,895,071	2.7%	10	North Carolina	6,948,740	2.7%
40	Hawaii	1,163,835	0.5%	11	Georgia	6,895,071	2.7%
42	Idaho	1,100,328	0.4%	12	Virginia	6,466,977	2.5%
6	Illinois	11,718,133	4.5%	13	Massachusetts	6,008,044	2.3%
14	Indiana	5,700,920	2.2%	14	Indiana	5,700,920	2.2%
30	Iowa	2,820,625	1.1%	15	Washington	5,248,735	2.0%
32	Kansas	2,538,069	1.0%	16	Missouri	5,237,813	2.0%
24	Kentucky	3,793,694	1.5%	17	Tennessee	5,082,456	2.0%
21	Louisiana	4,285,622	1.7%	18	Wisconsin	5,055,710	2.0%
39	Maine	1,236,178	0.5%	19	Maryland	4,943,092	1.9%
19	Maryland	4,943,092	1.9%	20	Minnesota	4,523,560	1.8%
13	Massachusetts	6,008,044	2.3%	21	Louisiana	4,285,622	1.7%
8	Michigan	9,523,247	3.7%	22	Alabama	4,191,879	1.6%
20	Minnesota	4,523,560	1.8%	23	Arizona	3,993,563	1.5%
31	Mississippi	2,635,647	1.0%	24	Kentucky	3,793,694	1.5%
16	Missouri	5,237,813	2.0%	25	South Carolina	3,634,842	1.4%
44	Montana	840,052	0.3%	26	Colorado	3,562,064	1.4%
37	Nebraska	1,612,336	0.6%	27	Connecticut	3,269,944	1.3%
38	Nevada	1,382,223	0.5%	28	Oklahoma	3,229,393	1.3%
41	New Hampshire	1,122,141	0.4%	29	Oregon	3,034,869	1.2%
9	New Jersey	7,873,468	3.1%	30	Iowa	2,820,625	1.1%
36	New Mexico	1,615,385	0.6%	31	Mississippi	2,635,647	1.0%
2	New York	18,139,051	7.0%	32	Kansas	2,538,069	1.0%
10	North Carolina	6,948,740	2.7%	33	Arkansas	2,423,980	0.9%
47	North Dakota	637,315	0.2%	34	Utah	1,872,018	0.7%
7	Ohio	11,063,366	4.3%	35	West Virginia	1,816,508	0.7%
28	Oklahoma	3,229,393	1.3%	36	New Mexico	1,615,385	0.6%
29	Oregon	3,034,869	1.2%	37	Nebraska	1,612,336	0.6%
5	Pennsylvania	12,022,460	4.7%	38	Nevada	1,382,223	0.5%
43	Rhode Island	997,817	0.4%	39	Maine	1,236,178	0.5%
25	South Carolina	3,634,842	1.4%	40	Hawaii	1,163,835	0.5%
45	South Dakota	722,550	0.3%	41	New Hampshire	1,122,141	0.4%
17	Tennessee	5,082,456	2.0%	42	Idaho	1,100,328	0.4%
3	Texas	18,009,031	7.0%	43	Rhode Island	997,817	0.4%
34	Utah	1,872,018	0.7%	44	Montana	840,052	0.3%
49	Vermont	573,837	0.2%	45	South Dakota	722,550	0.3%
12	Virginia	6,466,977	2.5%	46	Delaware	700,112	0.3%
15	Washington	5,248,735	2.0%	47	North Dakota	637,315	0.2%
35	West Virginia	1,816,508	0.7%	48	Alaska	596,906	0.2%
18	Wisconsin	5,055,710	2.0%	49	Vermont	573,837	0.2%
50	Wyoming	469,065	0.2%	50	Wyoming	469,065	0.2%
					District of Columbia	577,180	0.2%

Source: U.S. Bureau of the Census
Press Release (CB98-242, December 31, 1998)
*Includes armed forces residing in each state. This updates earlier 1993 population estimates.

IX. SOURCES

American Academy of Family Physicians
8880 Ward Parkway
Kansas City, MO   64114-2797
816-333-9700
Internet: www.aafp.org

American Academy of Physicians Assistants
950 North Washington Street
Alexandria, VA 22314-1552
703-836-2272
Internet: www.aapa.org

American Association of Health Plans
1129 20th Street, NW., Suite 600
Washington, DC   20036-3421
202-778-3200
Internet: www.aahp.org

American Cancer Society, Inc.
1599 Clifton Road, NE.
Atlanta, GA   30329-4251
800-227-2345
Internet: http://www.cancer.org

American Dental Association
211 E. Chicago Ave.
Chicago, IL   60611
312-440-2500
Internet: www.ada.org

American Hospital Association
One North Franklin
Chicago, IL   60606-3401
312-422-3000
Internet: www.aha.org

American Medical Association
515 North State Street
Chicago, IL   60610
312-464-5000
Internet: http://www.ama-assn.org

American Osteopathic Association
142 East Ontario Street
Chicago, IL   60611
312-202-8000
Internet: www.am-osteo-assn.org

American Podiatric Medical Association
9312 Old Georgetown Road
Bethesda, MD   20814-1698
301-571-9200
Internet: www.apma.org

Census Bureau
3 Silver Hill and Suitland Roads
Suitland, MD   20746
301-457-2794
Internet: http://www.census.gov

Centers for Disease Control and Prevention
1600 Clifton Road, NE.
Atlanta, GA   30333
404-639-3535 (Public Affairs)
800-458-5231 (AIDS Clearinghouse)
Internet: http://www.cdc.gov

Distilled Spirits Council of the U.S., Inc.
1250 Eye Street, NW., Ste. 900
Washington, DC   20005
202-628-3544
Internet: http://www.discus.health.org

Federation of Chiropractic Licensing Boards
901 54th Ave., Ste. 101
Greeley, CO   80634
970-356-3500
Internet: www.sni.net/fclb/

Health Care Financing Administration
U.S. Department of Health and Human Services
7500 Security Boulevard
Baltimore, MD   21244
410-786-3000
Internet: http://www.hcfa.gov

Health Insurance Association of America
555 13th Street, NW., Suite 600 East
Washington, DC   20004
202-824-1600
Internet: www.hiaa.org

National Center for Health Statistics
U.S. Department of Health and Human Services
6525 Belcrest Road
Hyattsville, MD   20782-2003
301-436-8951 (vital statistics division)
Internet: http://www.cdc.gov/nchswww/

National Sporting Goods Association
1699 Wall Street, Suite 700
Mt. Prospect, IL   60056-5780
847-439-4000
Internet: www.nsga.org

Smoking and Health Office
Centers for Disease Control and Prevention
4770 Buford Hwy, NE., Mail Stop K-50
Atlanta, GA   30341-3724
770-488-5705
www.cdc.gov/nccdphp/osh/oshresfa.htm

X. INDEX

X. INDEX (continued)

X. INDEX (continued)

Births and Reproductive Health

Deaths

Facilities

Finance

Incidence of Disease

Providers

Physical Fitness

CHAPTER INDEX

6928264

3 1378 00692 8264

LIBRARY USE ONLY

HOW TO USE THIS INDEX

Place left thumb on the outer edge of this page. To locate the desired entry, fold back the remaining page edges and align the index edge mark with the appropriate page edge mark.

Other books by Morgan Quitno Press:

- *State Statistical Trends (monthly journal)*
- *State Rankings 1999 ($49.95)*
- *Crime State Rankings 1999 ($49.95)*
- *City Crime Rankings, 5th Edition ($37.95)*

Call toll free: 1-800-457-0742 or
visit us at www.morganquitno.com